# *Essentials of*
# Plastic Surgery

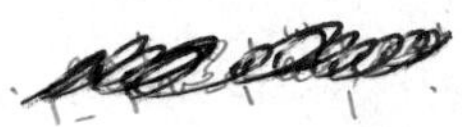

# *Essentials of*
# Plastic Surgery

*Second Edition*

Edited by

**Jeffrey E. Janis, MD, FACS**

Professor and Executive Vice Chairman,
Department of Plastic Surgery, Ohio State University;
Chief of Plastic Surgery, University Hospital,
Columbus, Ohio

With Illustrations by
**Amanda L. Good, MA and Sarah J. Taylor, MS, BA**

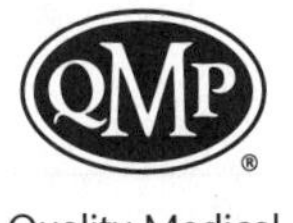


Quality Medical
Publishing, Inc.

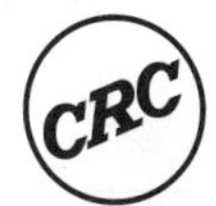


CRC Press
Taylor & Francis Group

2014

CRC Press
Taylor & Francis Group
6000 Broken Sound Parkway NW, Suite 300
Boca Raton, FL 33487-2742



Printed on acid-free paper
Version Date: 20150603

International Standard Book Number-13: 978-1-57626-385-3 (Pack - Book and Ebook)



**Library of Congress Cataloging-in-Publication Data**

Essentials of plastic surgery / edited by Jeffrey E. Janis. -- Second edition.
p. ; cm.
Includes bibliographical references and index.
ISBN 978-1-57626-385-3 (paperback : alk. paper)
I. Janis, Jeffrey E., editor of compilation.
[DNLM: 1. Reconstructive Surgical Procedures--outlines. Wo 18.2]

RD118
617.9'5--dc23
2013047997

**Visit the Taylor & Francis Web site at**
**http://www.taylorandfrancis.com**

**and the CRC Press Web site at**
**http://www.crcpress.com**

*To my wife, Emily, our children, Jackson and Brinkley,
and to my mother and father—all of whom have
shaped, molded, and influenced my life and career beyond measure—
and to all of plastic surgery, to whom this book belongs*

# Contributors

**Samer Abouzeid, MD**
Fellow, Craniofacial and Pediatric Plastic Surgery, Department of Plastic Surgery, University of Texas Southwestern Medical Center, Dallas, Texas

**Lee W.T. Alkureishi, MBChB, MRCS**
Doctor, Department of Surgery, Section of Plastic and Reconstructive Surgery, University of Chicago, Pritzker School of Medicine, Chicago, Illinois

**Jonathan Bank, MD**
Resident, Department of Surgery, Section of Plastic and Reconstructive Surgery, University of Chicago, Pritzker School of Medicine, Chicago, Illinois

**Zach J. Barnes, MD**
Clinical Assistant Professor of Plastic Surgery, Department of Plastic Surgery, Ohio State University, Columbus, Ohio

**Deniz Basci, MD**
Resident, Department of Plastic and Reconstructive Surgery, University of Texas Southwestern Medical Center, Dallas, Texas

**Daniel O. Beck, MD**
Aesthetic Fellow, Department of Plastic Surgery, University of Texas Southwestern Medical Center, Dallas, Texas

**Amanda Y. Behr, MA, CMI, FAMI**
Assistant Professor, Department of Medical Illustration, Georgia Regents University, Augusta, Georgia

**Prosper Benhaim, MD**
Associate Professor and Chief of Hand Surgery, Department of Orthopaedic Surgery and Division of Plastic and Reconstructive Surgery, University of California, Los Angeles, Los Angeles, California

**Brian P. Bradow, MD**
Assistant Clinical Professor, Department of Surgery, University of Illinois College of Medicine, Peoria, Illinois

**John L. Burns, Jr., MD**
Clinic Instructor, Department of Plastic Surgery, University of Texas Southwestern Medical Center; Dallas Plastic Surgery Institute, Dallas, Texas

**Daniel R. Butz, MD**
Resident, Department of Surgery, Section of Plastic and Reconstructive Surgery, University of Chicago, Pritzker School of Medicine, Chicago, Illinois

**Carey Faber Campbell, MD**
Resident, Department of Plastic Surgery, University of Texas Southwestern Medical Center, Dallas, Texas

**David S. Chang, MD**
Assistant Clinical Professor, Department of Surgery, University of California, San Francisco, San Francisco, California

**Tae Chong, MD**
Assistant Professor, Department of Plastic Surgery, University of Texas Southwestern Medical Center, Dallas, Texas

**James B. Collins, MD**
Resident, Department of Plastic Surgery, Scott and White Healthcare and Texas A&M Health Sciences Center College of Medicine, Temple, Texas

**Fadi C. Constantine, MD**
Aesthetic Surgery Fellow, Department of Plastic Surgery, Manhattan Eye, Ear, and Throat Hospital, New York, New York

**Kristin K. Constantine, MD**
Fellow, Otolaryngology-Head & Neck Surgery, New York Head & Neck Institute, New York, New York

**Melissa A. Crosby, MD, FACS**
Associate Professor, Department of Plastic Surgery, University of Texas MD Anderson Cancer Center, Houston, Texas

**Marcin Czerwinski, MD, FRCSC, FACS**
Assistant Professor of Surgery, Division of Plastic Surgery, Department of Surgery, Scott and White Healthcare and Texas A&M Health Sciences Center College of Medicine, Temple, Texas

**Phillip B. Dauwe, MD**
Resident, Department of Plastic Surgery, University of Texas Southwestern Medical Center, Dallas, Texas

**Michael E. Decherd, MD, FACS**
Clinical Assistant Professor, Department of Surgery, University of Texas Health Science Center at San Antonio, San Antonio, Texas

**Chantelle M. DeCroff, MD**
Resident, Department of Plastic Surgery, Scott and White Healthcare and Texas A&M Health Sciences Center College of Medicine, Temple, Texas

**Christopher A. Derderian, MD**
Assistant Professor, Department of Plastic Surgery, University of Texas Southwestern Medical Center, Children's Medical Center, Dallas, Texas

**Michael S. Dolan, MD, FACS**
Hand Surgeon, Department of Orthopedic Surgery, Jackson-Madison County General Hospital, Jackson, Tennessee

**Jordan P. Farkas, MD**
Chief Resident, Department of Plastic Surgery, University of Texas Southwestern Medical Center, Dallas, Texas; Private Practice, Department of Plastic Surgery, Paramus, New Jersey

**Douglas S. Fornfeist, MD**
Assistant Professor, Department of Orthopedic Surgery, Scott and White Healthcare and Texas A&M Health Sciences Center College of Medicine, Temple, Texas

**Sam Fuller, MD**
Resident, Department of Surgery, Section of Plastic and Reconstructive Surgery, University of Chicago, Pritzker School of Medicine, Chicago, Illinois

**C. Alejandra Garcia de Mitchell, MD**
Adjunct Assistant Professor, Department of Surgery, Division of Plastic and Reconstructive Surgery, University of Texas Health Science Center San Antonio, San Antonio, Texas

**Patrick B. Garvey, MD, FACS**
Associate Professor, Department of Plastic Surgery, University of Texas MD Anderson Cancer Center, Houston, Texas

**Ashkan Ghavami, MD**
Assistant Clinical Professor, Department of Plastic Surgery, David Geffen UCLA School of Medicine, Los Angeles, California; Private Practice, Ghavami Plastic Surgery, Beverly Hills, California

**Amanda A. Gosman, MD**
Associate Clinical Professor, Residency Training Program Director, Division of Plastic and Reconstructive Surgery, University of California, San Diego, San Diego, California

**Matthew R. Greives, MD**
Craniofacial Fellow, Children's Hospital of Pittsburgh, University of Pittsburgh Department of Plastic Surgery, Pittsburgh, Pennsylvania

**Adam H. Hamawy, MD, FACS**
Private Practice, The Juventus Clinic, New York, New York

**Bridget Harrison, MD**
Resident, Department of Plastic Surgery, University of Texas Southwestern Medical Center, Dallas, Texas

**Bishr Hijazi, MD**
Private Practice, Nevada Surgical Institute, Las Vegas, Nevada

**John E. Hoopman, CMLSO**
Certified Medical Laser Specialist, Department of Plastic Surgery, University of Texas Southwestern Medical Center, Dallas, Texas

**Tarik M. Husain, MD**
Attending Orthopaedic/Sports Medicine Surgeon and Hand Surgeon, OrthoNOW, Doral, Florida; Attending Plastic and Hand Surgeon, MOSA Medspa, Miami Beach, Florida

**Jeffrey E. Janis, MD, FACS**
Professor and Executive Vice Chairman, Department of Plastic Surgery, Ohio State University; Chief of Plastic Surgery, University Hospital, Columbus, Ohio

**Charles F. Kallina IV, MD, MS**
Assistant Professor, Department of Surgery; Hand Surgeon, Department of Orthopedic Surgery, Scott and White Healthcare and Texas A&M Health Sciences Center College of Medicine, Temple, Texas

**Phillip D. Khan, MD**
Aesthetic Surgery Fellow, The Hunstad-Kortesis Center for Cosmetic Plastic Surgery & Medspa, Charlotte, North Carolina

**Rohit K. Khosla, MD**
Assistant Professor, Division of Plastic and Reconstructive Surgery, Stanford University Medical Center, Palo Alto, California

**Grant M. Kleiber, MD**
Resident, Department of Surgery, Section of Plastic and Reconstructive Surgery, University of Chicago, Pritzker School of Medicine, Chicago, Illinois

**Reza Kordestani, MD**
Resident, Department of Plastic Surgery, University of Texas Southwestern Medical Center, Dallas, Texas

**Essie Kueberuwa, MD, BSc (Hons)**
Resident, Department of Surgery, Section of Plastic and Reconstructive Surgery, University of Chicago, Pritzker School of Medicine, Chicago, Illinois

**Huay-Zong Law, MD**
Resident, Department of Plastic Surgery, University of Texas Southwestern Medical Center, Dallas, Texas

**Danielle M. LeBlanc, MD, FACS**
Private Practice, Department of Plastic and Reconstructive Surgery, Forth Worth Plastic Surgery Institute, Fort Worth, Texas

**Michael R. Lee, MD**
Plastic Surgeon, The Wall Center for Plastic Surgery, Shreveport, Louisiana

**Jason E. Leedy, MD**
Private Practice, Mayfield Heights, Ohio

**Benjamin T. Lemelman, MD**
Resident, Department of Surgery, Section of Plastic and Reconstructive Surgery, University of Chicago, Pritzker School of Medicine, Chicago, Illinois

**Joshua A. Lemmon, MD**
Plastic and Hand Surgeon, Regional Plastic Surgery Associates, Richardson, Texas

**Raman C. Mahabir, MD, MSc, FRCSC, FACS**
Vice Chair, Associate Professor, Chief of Microsurgery, Department of Surgery, Scott and White Healthcare and Texas A&M Health Sciences Center College of Medicine, Temple, Texas

**Janae L. Maher, MD**
Resident, Division of Plastic Surgery, Scott and White Healthcare and Texas A&M Health Sciences Center College of Medicine, Temple, Texas

**Menyoli Malafa, MD**
Resident, Department of Plastic Surgery, University of Texas Southwestern Medical Center, Dallas, Texas

**David W. Mathes, MD**
Associate Professor of Surgery, Division of Plastic and Reconstructive Surgery, University of Washington, Seattle, Washington

**Ricardo A. Meade, MD**
Plastic Surgeon, Department of Plastic Surgery, University of Texas Southwestern Medical Center; Private Practice, Dallas Plastic Surgery Institute, Dallas, Texas

**Blake A. Morrison, MD**
Medical Director, The Advanced Wound Center, Clear Lake Regional Medical Center, Webster, Texas

**Scott W. Mosser, MD**
Private Practice, San Francisco, California

**Purushottam A. Nagarkar, MD**
Resident, Department of Plastic Surgery, University of Texas Southwestern Medical Center, Dallas, Texas

**Karthik Naidu, DMD, MD**
Attending Surgeon, Division of Oral and Maxillofacial Surgery, Scott and White Healthcare and Texas A&M Health Sciences Center College of Medicine, Temple, Texas

**Kailash Narasimhan, MD**
Chief Resident, Department of Plastic Surgery, University of Texas Southwestern Medical Center, Dallas, Texas

**Trang Q. Nguyen, MD**
Fellow, Plastic and Reconstructive Surgical Service, Memorial Sloan-Kettering Cancer Center, New York, New York

**Sacha I. Obaid, MD**
Medical Director, North Texas Plastic Surgery, Southlake, Texas

**Babatunde Ogunnaike, MD**
Vice Chairman and Chief of Anesthesia Services, Parkland Hospital, Department of Anesthesiology and Pain Management, University of Texas Southwestern Medical Center, Dallas, Texas

**Eamon B. O'Reilly, MD, LCDR MC US Navy**
Staff Surgeon, Department of Plastic Surgery, Naval Medical Center San Diego, San Diego, California

**Thornwell Hay Parker III, MD, FACMS**
Volunteer Faculty, Department of Plastic Surgery, University of Texas Southwestern Medical Center; Staff, Department of Plastic Surgery, Texas Health Presbyterian Hospital of Dallas, Dallas, Texas

**Wendy L. Parker, MD, PhD, FRCSC, FACS**
Associate Professor, Division of Plastic Surgery, Department of Surgery, Scott and White Healthcare and Texas A&M Health Sciences Center College of Medicine, Temple, Texas

**Jason K. Potter, MD**
Clinical Assistant Professor, Department of Plastic Surgery, University of Texas Southwestern Medical Center, Dallas, Texas

**Benson J. Pulikkottil, MD**
Plastic Surgeon, Department of Plastic Surgery, University of Texas Southwestern Medical Center, Dallas, Texas

**Smita R. Ramanadham, MD**
Senior Resident, Department of Plastic Surgery, University of Texas Southwestern Medical Center, Dallas, Texas

**Rey N. Ramirez, MD**
Pediatric Hand Surgeon, Shriners Hospital of Erie, Erie, Pennsylvania

**Timmothy R. Randell, MD**
Orthopedic Surgery Resident, Department of Orthopedic Surgery, Scott and White Healthcare and Texas A&M Health Sciences Center College of Medicine, Temple, Texas

**Lance A. Read, DDS**
Assistant Professor of Surgery; Director, Division of Oral and Maxillofacial Surgery, Department of Surgery, Scott and White Healthcare and Texas A&M Health Sciences Center College of Medicine, Temple, Texas

**Gangadasu Reddy, MD, MS**
Fellow in Hand and Microsurgery, Department of Plastic Surgery, University of Texas Southwestern Medical Center, Dallas, Texas

**Edward M. Reece, MD, MS**
Attending Surgeon, St. Joseph's Medical and Trauma Center, Phoenix, Arizona

**José L. Rios, MD**
Private Practice, Joliet, Illinois

**Luis M. Rios, Jr., MD**
Adjunct Clinical Professor, Department of Surgery, University of Texas Health Science Center–RAHC, San Antonio, Texas

**Kendall R. Roehl, MD**
Assistant Professor, Division of Plastic Surgery, Scott and White Healthcare and Texas A&M Health Sciences Center College of Medicine, Temple, Texas

**Jason Roostaeian, MD**
Clinical Instructor, Division of Plastic and Reconstructive Surgery, David Geffen School of Medicine at University of California Los Angeles, Los Angeles, California

**Michel Saint-Cyr, MD, FRCSC**
Professor of Plastic Surgery, Practice Chair, Department of Plastic Surgery, Mayo Clinic, Rochester, Minnesota

**Douglas M. Sammer, MD**
Assistant Professor, Program Director, Hand Surgery Fellowship, Department of Plastic Surgery, University of Texas Southwestern Medical Center, Dallas, Texas

**Christopher M. Shale, MD**
Private Practice, Department of Plastic and Reconstructive Surgery, McKay-Dee Dermatology and Plastic Surgery, Ogden, Utah

**Deana S. Shenaq, MD**
Resident, Department of Surgery, Section of Plastic and Reconstructive Surgery, University of Chicago, Pritzker School of Medicine, Chicago, Illinois

**Alison M. Shore, MD**
Zaccone Family Fellow in Reconstructive Microsurgery, Department of Surgery, Section of Plastic and Reconstructive Surgery, University of Chicago, Pritzker School of Medicine, Chicago, Illinois

**Kevin Shultz, MD**
Plastic Surgeon, Department of Plastic Surgery, Scott and White Healthcare and Texas A&M Health Services Center College of Medicine, Temple, Texas

**Amanda K. Silva, MD**
Resident, Department of Surgery, Section of Plastic and Reconstructive Surgery, University of Chicago, Pritzker School of Medicine, Chicago, Illinois

**Holly P. Smith, BFA**
Owner and Creative Director, HP Smith Design, Dallas, Texas

**Georges N. Tabbal, MD**
Resident, Department of Plastic Surgery, University of Texas Southwestern Medical Center, Dallas, Texas

**Sumeet S. Teotia, MD**
Assistant Professor of Plastic Surgery, Department of Plastic Surgery, University of Texas Southwestern Medical Center, Dallas, Texas; Charter Plastic Surgeon, Alliance of Smiles, San Francisco, California

**Chad M. Teven, MD**
Resident, Department of Surgery, Section of Plastic and Reconstructive Surgery, University of Chicago, Pritzker School of Medicine, Chicago, Illinois

**Jacob G. Unger, MD**
Chief Resident, Department of Plastic Surgery, University of Texas Southwestern Medical Center, Dallas, Texas

**Dinah Wan, MD**
Medical Doctor, Department of Plastic Surgery, University of Texas Southwestern Medical Center, Dallas, Texas

**Russell A. Ward, MD**
Assistant Professor, Department of Surgery; Director, Musculoskeletal Oncology, Department of Orthopedic Surgery, Scott and White Healthcare and Texas A&M Health Sciences Center College of Medicine, Temple, Texas

**Robert A. Weber, MD**
Professor and Vice Chair of Education, Department of Surgery; Chief, Section of Hand Surgery, Division of Plastic Surgery, Scott and White Healthcare and Texas A&M Health Sciences Center College of Medicine, Temple, Texas

**Adam Bryce Weinfeld, MD**
Faculty, Department of Pediatric Plastic Surgery, University of Texas Southwestern Medical Center Residency Programs at Seton Healthcare Family; Attending Plastic Surgeon, Institute for Reconstructive Plastic Surgery of Central Texas & Dell Children's Medical Center of Central Texas, Austin, Texas

**Dawn D. Wells, PA-C, MPAS**
Physician Assistant, Advanced Dermasurgery Associates, Highland Village, Texas

**Daniel S. Wu, MD**
Medical Doctor, Department of Plastic Surgery, Scott and White Healthcare and Texas A&M Health Sciences Center College of Medicine, Temple, Texas

# Foreword

When the first edition of *Essentials of Plastic Surgery* by Dr. Jeffrey Janis was published in 2007, it immediately achieved spectacular success worldwide, fulfilling its defined role (according to the Oxford English Dictionary) as an "indispensible, absolutely necessary" publication. This compact yet comprehensive paperback handbook quickly became the "go-to" resource for plastic surgery residents and faculty alike. As a testament to its popularity, it could be seen stuffed into lab coat pockets of residents throughout the world, its cover worn with use.

*Essentials,* which is filled with valuable information on topics across the entire spectrum of our broad-based specialty, provides an excellent, portable resource for day-to-day education and the practice of plastic surgery. Its easy-to-use outline format is enhanced by numerous illustrations, tips, tables, algorithms, references, and key points. Now, seven years later, the dynamic nature of plastic surgery has mandated another edition of this beloved manual. This edition is even better than the previous one.

The architect of *Essentials* is Dr. Jeffrey Janis, a young, talented surgeon who I have had the pleasure to know and to help mentor when he was a medical student at Case Western Reserve. Even at that early stage of his training, he expressed a strong interest in plastic surgery. Jeff impressed everyone with his intellect, work ethic, and organizational skills. His early promise has borne fruit during his time at the University of Texas Southwestern Medical Center at Dallas and now in his new position at Ohio State University Medical Center. He has become a recognized leader in academic plastic surgery and a respected educator and author.

This second edition of *Essentials of Plastic Surgery* continues its emphasis on core content in plastic surgery, as encapsulated by Dr. Janis and a superb group of contributors. The substantial advances in our specialty have been fully incorporated, with 13 new chapters and dozens of new illustrations. New chapters on topics such as fat grafting, perforator flaps, lymphedema, surgical treatment of migraine headaches, and vascularized composite allografts and transplant immunology attest to the new information and extensive updating that is evident in this edition. While remaining compact, the book has grown to 102 chapters and more than 1000 pages, expanding the book's coverage while making it both current and timely. Updated content is included in every chapter This comprehensive yet concise edition will ensure that *Essentials of Plastic Surgery* will retain its role as an indispensible element in the fabric of graduate and continuing medical education in plastic surgery.

**Edward Luce, MD**
Professor, Department of Plastic Surgery,
The University of Tennessee Health Science Center,
Memphis, Tennessee

# Preface

It's hard to believe that it's been 10 years since I sat at the kitchen table of one of my best friends, José Rios, in Dallas, Texas, where the idea for *Essentials of Plastic Surgery* was born. At the time, we wanted to create a "quick and dirty one-stop shopping" utility book for medical students, residents, and fellows to provide high-impact information across the spectrum and variety of plastic surgery to better prepare them for their training programs. *Essentials* was intentionally designed to be a portable reference book, whether for an emergency department consult, an operating room case, a clinic patient, or for teaching conferences.

Neither of us had any idea that the book would turn into an item that is used by so many people in the United States and around the world. A testament to its success has been not only the number of copies sold, but the number of requests for a second edition. In the 6 years that have passed since the first edition was released, there have been many significant changes in the field of plastic surgery, so it was high time to produce an updated book.

In this second edition, we have expanded the number of chapters from 88 to 102. This reflects the increasing knowledge and understanding of plastic surgery that has occurred since 2007. New chapters such as Fundamentals of Perforator Flaps, Vascularized Composite Allografts and Transplant Immunology, Negative Pressure Wound Therapy, Surgical Treatment of Migraine Headaches, Face Transplantation, Augmentation-Mastopexy, Nipple-Areolar Reconstruction, Foot Ulcers, Lymphedema, Distal Radius Fractures, Hand Transplantation, Facial Analysis, and Fat Grafting join updated chapters across the entire table of contents. The book retains its familiarity, though, in that it is still divided into seven parts: Fundamentals and Basics; Skin and Soft Tissue; Head and Neck; Breast; Trunk and Lower Extremity; Hand, Wrist, and Upper Extremity; and Aesthetic Surgery. Also retained are the familiar bullet point style, format, and pocket size of the first edition that made it both useful and successful. References have been updated and expanded to guide the reader to classic and definitive articles and chapters.

Since this book belongs to all of plastic surgery, authors from around the country were solicited to update, and in many cases completely rewrite, chapters to make the information current, accurate, and contemporary. There have been significant additions of graphics, specifically tables, charts, diagrams, and illustrations, all of which have been created by in-house Quality Medical Publishing illustrators so that the consistency and quality are uniform. This richly augmented graphical content should make the text even more clear to the reader.

Ultimately, this book reflects the tremendous effort of a great number of authors and contributors, taking all of the most useful aspects of the first edition and building on that foundation with improvements in content, graphics, and utility. To that end, an electronic format of this book will be released to serve as a useful adjunct to readers as they journey through residency training, fellowship training, or preparation for maintenance of certification.The true test of the book's utility will lie with you, the reader, as you decide what book to keep in your pocket or on your shelf. My hope is that this one is the book with a cracked and worn spine, creased pages, and absolutely no dust.

**Jeffrey E. Janis**

# Acknowledgments

This book truly is a labor of love that simply could not have come to life without the tremendous time and effort invested in it by so many people.

First credit must go to the authors across the country who have taken a significant amount of time to pour through the literature to carefully craft these chapters, and who endured a rigorous editing process where every word and illustration were carefully scrutinized. As they will clearly attest, meticulous attention to detail and emphasis on quality and accuracy demanded much energy and determination. To them, I am sincerely grateful for their time and for the fruits of their efforts.

Distinct recognition must also go to Karen Berger, Amy Debrecht, Suzanne Wakefield, Carolyn Reich, Carol Hollett, Makalah Boyer, Hilary Rice, and all of the amazing, hard-working staff at Quality Medical Publishing, who poured their heart and soul into this book and have created a book that could not be done by anyone else. Special gratitude goes to Amanda Good and Sarah Taylor, the illustrators, who deserve an incredible amount of credit for all of the illustrations that make this book pop alive with color, clarity, and flavor.

Most of all, with tremendous sincerity, I want to thank my wife, Emily, and our children, Jackson and Brinkley, for their understanding and patience, and above all else, their unconditional love and support. Without them, this book would not be possible, and what is most important, my life would not be complete.

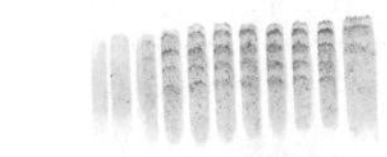

# Contents

## Part I ◆ Fundamentals and Basics

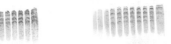

## Part II ◆ Skin and Soft Tissue



## Part III ◆ Head and Neck

## Part IV ◆ Breast



## Part V ◆ Trunk and Lower Extremity

## Part VI ◆ Hand, Wrist, and Upper Extremity

# *Essentials of* Plastic Surgery

# PART I

## Fundamentals and Basics

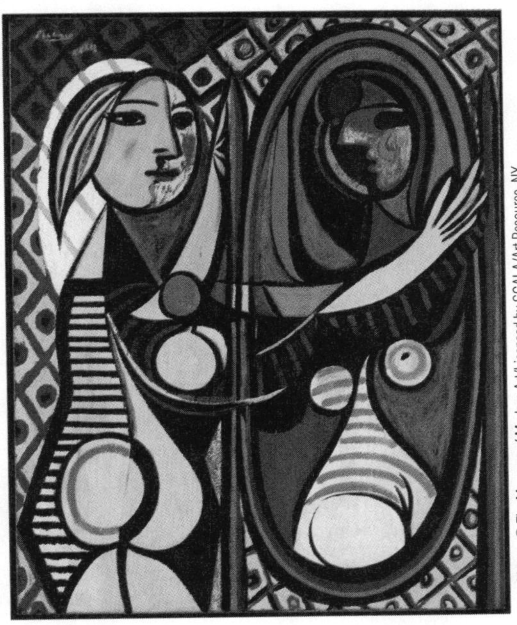

Part I opening art: Picasso, Pablo (1881-1973) © Artist Rights Society (ARS), NY. Girl Before a Mirror. 1932. Oil on canvas, 64″ × 51¼″. Gift of Mrs. Simon Guggenheim. (2.1938). The Museum of Modern Art, New York, NY, USA. Digital Image © The Museum of Modern Art/Licensed by SCALA/Art Resource, NY. © 2006 Estate of Pablo Picasso/ARS, New York.

# 1. Wound Healing

**Thornwell Hay Parker III, Bridget Harrison**

## THREE PHASES OF WOUND HEALING[1-4]

1. Inflammatory phase (days 1 to 6)
2. Fibroproliferative phase (day 4 to week 3)
3. Maturation/remodeling phase (week 3 to 1 year)

### INFLAMMATORY PHASE (DAYS 1 TO 6)

- **Vasoconstriction:** Constriction of injured vessels for 5-10 minutes after injury
- **Coagulation:** Clot formed by platelets and fibrin, contains growth factors to signal wound repair
- **Vasodilation and increased permeability:** Mediated by histamine, serotonin (from platelets), and nitrous oxide (from endothelial cells)
- **Chemotaxis:** Signaled by platelet products (from alpha granules), coagulation cascade, complement activation (C5a), tissue products, and bacterial products
- **Cell migration**
  - Margination: Increased adhesion to vessel walls
  - Diapedesis: Movement through vessel wall
  - Fibrin: Creates initial matrix for cell migration
- **Cellular response**
  - Neutrophils (24-48 hours): Produce inflammatory products and phagocytosis, **not critical to wound healing**
  - Macrophages (48-96 hours): Become dominant cell population (until fibroblast proliferation), **most critical to wound healing;** orchestrate growth factors
  - Lymphocytes (5-7 days): Role poorly defined, possible regulation of collagenase and extracellular matrix (ECM) remodeling

### FIBROPROLIFERATIVE PHASE (DAY 4 TO WEEK 3)

- **Matrix formation**
  - Fibroblasts: Move into wound days 2-3, dominant cell at 7 days, high rate of collagen synthesis from day 5 to week 3
  - Glycosaminoglycan (GAG) production
    - Hyaluronic acid first
    - Then chondroitin-4 sulfate, dermatan sulfate, and heparin sulfate
    - Followed by collagen production (see later)
  - Tensile strength begins to increase at days 4-5
- **Angiogenesis:** Increased vascularity from parent vessels; vascular endothelial growth factor (VEGF)/nitrous oxide
- **Epithelialization** (see later)

> **TIP:** Angiogenesis is the formation of new blood vessels from existing ones. Vasculogenesis is the process of blood vessel formation de novo.

## Maturation/Remodeling Phase (Week 3 to 1 Year)

- After 3-5 weeks, equilibrium reached between collagen breakdown and synthesis
- Subsequently no net change in quantity
- Increased collagen organization and stronger cross-links
- Type I collagen replacement of type III collagen, restoring normal 4:1 ratio
- Decrease in GAGs, water content, vascularity, and cellular population
- **Peak tensile strength at approximately 60 days—80% preinjury strength**

## COLLAGEN PRODUCTION

- Collagen composed of three polypeptides wound together into a helix
- High concentration of hydroxyproline and hydroxylysine amino acids
- More than 20 types of collagen based on amino acid sequences
- **Type I:** Most abundant (90% of body collagen); dominant in skin, tendon, and bone
- **Type II:** Cornea and hyaline cartilage
- **Type III:** Vessel and bowel walls, uterus, and skin
- **Type IV:** Basement membrane only

## GROWTH FACTORS (Table 1-1)

**Table 1-1** *Growth Factors*

| Growth Factor | Function |
|---|---|
| FGF | Fibroblast and keratinocyte proliferation; Fibroblast chemotaxis |
| VEGF | Endothelial cell proliferation |
| TGF-beta | Fibroblast migration and proliferation |
| PDGF | Proliferation of fibroblasts, endothelial and smooth muscle cells |
| EGF | Keratinocyte and fibroblasts division and migration |

## EPITHELIALIZATION

- **Mobilization:** Loss of contact inhibition—cells at edge of wound or in appendages (in partial thickness wounds) flatten and break contact (integrins) with neighboring cells.
- **Migration:** Cells move across wound until meeting cells from other side, then contact inhibition is reestablished.
- **Mitosis:** As cells at edge are migrating, basal cells further back from the wound edge proliferate to support cell numbers needed to bridge wound.
- **Differentiation:** Reestablishment of epithelial layers are from basal layer to stratum corneum after migration ceases.

epidermis

## CONTRACTION

- **Myofibroblast:** Specialized fibroblast with contractile cytoplasmic microfilaments and distinct cellular adhesion structures (desmosomes and maculae adherens)
- Dispersed throughout granulating wound, act in concert to contract entire wound bed
- Appear day 3; maximal at days 10-21; disappear as contraction is complete
- **Less contraction when more dermis is present in wound**, just as full-thickness skin grafts have less secondary contraction than split-thickness grafts

1° contraction: More dermis = more contraction
2° contraction: More dermis = less contraction

## TYPES OF WOUND HEALING

- **Primary:** Closed within hours of creation by reapproximating edges of wound
- **Secondary:** Wound allowed to heal on its own by contraction and epithelialization
- **Delayed primary:** Subacute or chronic wound converted to acute wound by sharp debridement, then closed primarily; healing comparable to primary closure

## FACTORS AFFECTING WOUND HEALING

### GENETIC

- Predisposition to hypertrophic or keloid scarring
- Hereditary conditions (Table 1-2)
- Skin type: Pigmentation (Fitzpatrick type), elasticity, thickness, sebaceous quality, and location (e.g., shoulder, sternum, earlobe)
- Age: Affects healing rate

**Table 1-2** *Diseases and Conditions*

| | Defect | Characteristics | Surgical Intervention |
|---|---|---|---|
| Ehlers-Danlos syndrome | Abnormal collagen structure, production of processing | Hyperflexible joints<br>Stretchy, fragile skin<br>Easy bruising<br>Vascular aneurysms | Not recommended |
| Progeria | Mutation in *LMNA* gene | Limited growth<br>Full body alopecia<br>Wrinkled skin<br>Atherosclerosis<br>Large head, narrow face, beaked nose | Not recommended |
| Werner syndrome | Mutation in *WRN* gene | Graying of hair<br>Hoarse voice<br>Thickened skin<br>Diabetes mellitus<br>Atherosclerosis<br>Cataracts | Not recommended, but reported for temporary improvements |
| Pseudoxanthoma elasticum | Fragmentation and mineralization of elastic fibers | Cutaneous laxity<br>Yellow skin papules<br>Vision loss | Redundant skin folds can be treated with surgical excision |
| Cutis laxa | Mutation in elastic fibers | Loose, wrinkled skin<br>Hypermobile joints | Surgical excision of redundant skin produces temporary benefit but patients do **not** have wound healing problems |

### SYSTEMIC HEALTH

- Comorbidities
  - Diabetes
  - Atherosclerotic disease
  - Renal failure
  - Immunodeficiency
  - Nutritional deficiencies

## Vitamins

> **TIP:** Supplements typically only help when deficiencies exist.

- **Vitamin A:** Reverses delayed wound healing from steroids; does not affect immunosuppression.
  - 25,000 IU by mouth once per day increases tensile strength, or 200,000 IU topical every 8 hours increases epithelialization.
- **Vitamin C:** Vital for hydroxylation reactions in collagen synthesis.
  - Deficiency leads to scurvy: Immature fibroblasts, deficient collagen synthesis, capillary hemorrhage, decreased tensile strength.
- **Vitamin E:** Antioxidant; stabilizes membranes.
  - Large doses inhibit healing, but unproven to reduce scarring and may cause dermatitis.
- **Zinc:** Cofactor for many enzymes.
  - Deficiency causes impaired epithelial and fibroblast proliferation.

## Drugs

- **Smoking:** Cigarette smoke contains more than 4000 constituents
  - Nicotine: Constricts blood vessels, increases platelet adhesiveness
  - Carbon monoxide: Binds to hemoglobin and reduces oxygen delivery
  - Hydrogen cyanide: Inhibits oxygen transport
- **Steroids**
  - Decrease inflammation
  - Inhibit epithelialization
  - Decrease collagen production
- **Antineoplastic agents**
  - Early evidence suggested diminished wound healing, but clinical reports have not substantiated this[5]
  - Few or no adverse effects if administration delayed for 10-14 days after wound closure
- **Anti-inflammatories:** May decrease collagen synthesis
- **Lathyrogens:** Prevent cross-linking of collagen, decreasing tensile strength
  - Beta-aminopropionitrile (BAPN): Product of ground peas and d-penicillamine
  - Possible therapeutic use for decreasing scar tissue

## Local Wound Factors

- **Oxygen delivery**

> **TIP:** The most common cause of failure to heal and wound infection is poor oxygen delivery associated with various disease states and local conditions (microvascular disease).

  - Atherosclerosis, Raynaud's disease, scleroderma
  - Adequate cardiac output, distal perfusion, oxygen delivery (hematocrit, oxygen dissociation curve)
  - Hyperbaric oxygen: Increases angiogenesis and new fibroblasts
- **Infection**
  - Clinical infection: Decreases oxygen tension, lowers pH, increases collagenase activity, retards epithelialization and angiogenesis, prolongs inflammation and edema
- **Chronic wound**
  - Metalloproteases abundant, promote extracellular matrix turnover, slow wound healing
  - Debridement of chronic wound: Removes excess granulation tissue and metalloproteases, transforms it to an acute wound state, and expedites healing

- **Radiation therapy**
  - Causes stasis/occlusion of small vessels, damages fibroblasts, chronic damage to nuclei
- **Moisture**
  - Speeds epithelialization
- **Warmth**
  - Increased tensile strength (better perfusion)
- **Free radicals**
  - Reactive oxygen species increased by ischemia, reperfusion, inflammation, radiation, vitamin deficiencies, and chemical agents

## SCARRING

- **Hypertrophic scars (HTS)** (Fig.1-1)
  - Primarily type III collagen oriented parallel to epidermal surface with abundant myofibroblasts and extracellular collagen
  - Scar elevated but **within borders of original scar;** more common than keloids (5%-15% of wounds)
    - Predisposition to areas of tension, flexor surfaces
    - Less recurrence following excision and adjuvant therapy

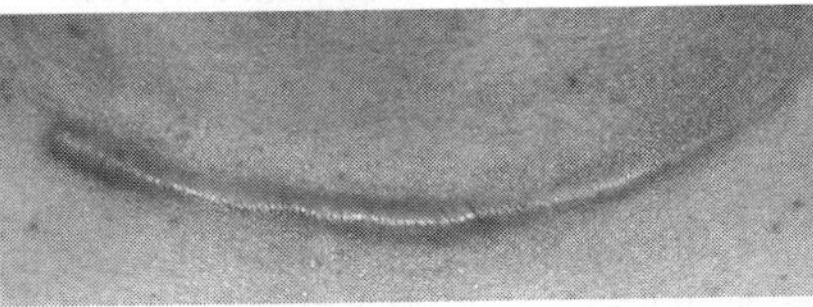

**Fig. 1-1** Hypertrophic scar.

- **Keloid scars** (Fig. 1-2)
  - Derived from Greek *chele*, or crab's claw
  - **Grow outside original wound borders**
  - Disorganized type I and III collagen, hypocellular collagen bundles
  - Only seen in humans; rare in newborns or elderly
  - May occur with deep injuries (less common than HTS)
    - Genetic and endocrine influences (increased growth in puberty and pregnancy)
    - Rarely regress and more resistant to excision and therapy
  - Because of high recurrence rates, **multimodality therapy recommended**[6,7] (Table 1-3)

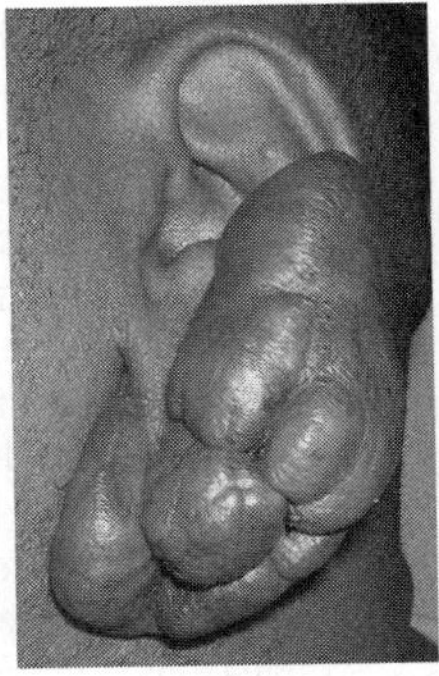

**Fig. 1-2** Keloid scar.

**Table 1-3** *Keloid Treatments*

| Treatment | Mechanism | Recurrence Rates |
|---|---|---|
| Silicone sheeting | Hydration, increased temperature | Most effective as preventive method |
| Corticosteroids | Reduce collagen synthesis and inflammatory mediators | 9%-50% |
| Interferon | Reduce fibroblast production of glycosaminoglycans, increase collagenase | 54% |
| 5-Fluorouracil | Inhibits fibroblast proliferation | 19% |
| Cryotherapy | Modifies collagen synthesis and fibroblast differentiation | 50%-80% obtain volume reduction |
| Excision | Removal of abnormal tissue | 50%-100% |
| Radiation | Inhibition of angiogenesis and fibroblasts | 2%-33% |

- **Widened scars** (Fig. 1-3)
  - Wide and depressed from wound tension perpendicular to wound and mobility during maturation phase
- **Fetal healing**
  - Potentially scarless healing in first two trimesters
  - Higher concentrations of type III collagen and hyaluronic acid, no inflammation, no angiogenesis, relative hypoxia

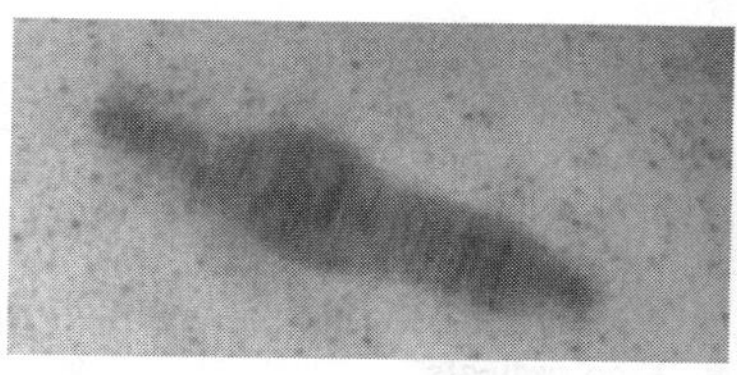

**Fig. 1-3** Widened scar.

- **Scar management**[8]
  - Silicone sheeting recommended as soon as epithelialization is complete and should be continued for at least one month
    - **Mechanism of action not known, but suggested mechanisms include increases in temperature and collagenase activity, increased hydration, and polarization of the scar tissue**
  - If silicone sheeting unsuccessful, corticosteroid injections may be used
    - Potential risks include subcutaneous atrophy, telangiectasia, and pigment changes
  - Pressure therapy and massage have been recommended and may reduce scar thickness, but support is weak[9]
  - Improvement with topical vitamin E not supported—may cause contact dermatitis[10]
  - Topical onion extract (Mederma, Merz Pharmaceuticals, Greensboro, NC) has not shown improvement in scar erythema, hypertrophy, or overall cosmetic appearance.[11]

## Key Points

- ✓ The three stages of wound healing are inflammatory phase (macrophage most important), fibroproliferative phase, and maturation phase.
- ✓ Peak tensile strength occurs at 42-60 days (80% of original strength).
- ✓ Epithelialization is initiated by loss of contact inhibition.
- ✓ The amount of dermis present is inversely proportional to the amount of secondary contraction (i.e., more dermis equates to less secondary contraction).
- ✓ Vitamin A is used to reverse detrimental effects of steroids on wound healing.
- ✓ Hypertrophic scars and keloids are distinguished clinically; both have high recurrence rates unless combined modalities are used.

## References

1. Broughton G, Rohrich RJ. Wounds and scars. Sel Read Plast Surg 10:5-7, 2005.
2. Glat P, Longaker M. Wound healing. In Aston SJ, Beasley RW, Thorne CH, et al, eds. Grabb and Smith's Plastic Surgery, 5th ed. Philadelphia: Lippincott-Raven, 1997.
3. Janis JE, Kwon RK, Lalonde DH. A practical guide to wound healing. Plast Reconstr Surg 125:230e-244e, 2010.
4. Janis JE, Morrison B. Wound healing. Part I: Basic science (accepted by Plast Reconstr Surg 2013).
5. Falcone RE, Nappi JF. Chemotherapy and wound healing. Surg Clin North Am 64:779-794, 1984.
6. Sidle DM, Kim H. Keloids: prevention and management. Facial Plast Surg Clin North Am 19:505-515, 2011.
7. Chike-Obi CJ, Cole PD, Brissett AE. Keloids: pathogenesis, clinical features, and management. Semin Plast Surg 23:178-184, 2009.

8. Mustoe TA, Cooter RD, Gold MH, et al. International clinical recommendations on scar management. Plast Reconstr Surg 110: 560-571, 2002.
9. Shin TM, Bordeaux JS. The role of massage in scar management: a literature review. Dermatol Surg 38:414-423, 2012.
10. Khoo TL, Halim AS, Zakaria Z, et al. A prospective, randomized, double-blinded trial to study the efficacy of topical tocotrienol in the prevention of hypertrophic scars. J Plast Reconstr Aesthet Surg 64:e137-e145, 2011.
11. Chung VQ, Kelley L, Marra D, et al. Onion extract gel versus petrolatum emollient on new surgical scars: prospective double-blinded study. Dermatol Surg 32:193-219, 2006.

# 2. General Management of Complex Wounds

**Jeffrey E. Janis, Bridget Harrison**

## GENERAL POINTS[1]

### ALGORITHMIC APPROACH

- Thorough and comprehensive patient evaluation
- Examination and evaluation of the wound
- Lab tests and imaging
- Assessment, plan, and execution

### HISTORY

- Age
- General health
- Presence of comorbidities
- Prewound functional and ambulatory capacity
- Associated factors that influence wound healing
  - Diabetes mellitus
  - End-stage renal disease
  - Cardiac disease
  - Peripheral vascular disease
  - Tobacco use
  - Vasculitis
  - Malnutrition
  - Steroid therapy
  - Radiation
  - Hemophilia
    - **80%** of normal factor VIII levels are recommended in perioperative period

### PHYSICAL EXAMINATION

- Assessment of vascular system
  - Palpable pulses
  - Temperature
  - Hair growth
  - Skin changes
- Assessment of **neurosensory** system
  - Reflexes
  - Two-point discrimination/vibratory testing (128 Hz)

## WOUND EVALUATION

- **Wound history**
  - Circumstances surrounding injury
  - History of wound healing problems
  - Chronicity
  - Previous diagnostics
  - Previous treatments
- **Components of wound evaluation**
  - Location (helps determine underlying causes)
  - Size
    - Length, width, depth
    - Area
  - Extent of defect
    - Skin; subcutaneous tissue; muscle, tendon, nerve; bone
- **Condition of surrounding tissue and wound margins**
  - Color
  - Pigmentation
  - Inflammation/induration
  - Satellite lesions
  - Edema
- **Condition of wound bed**
  - Odor
  - Necrosis
  - Granulation tissue
  - Exposed structures
  - Fibrin, exudate, eschar
  - Foreign bodies
  - Inflammation/infection
  - Tunneling/sinuses

## LABORATORY STUDIES

- Complete blood count (CBC)
  - Elevated white-cell count? Left shift?
- Blood urine nitrogen (BUN)/creatinine
  - Assessment of renal function and hydration status
- Glucose/hemoglobin $A_1C$
  - Assessment of hyperglycemia and its trend
    - Questions remain regarding appropriate insulin therapy and glucose levels in surgical patients.[2]
    - Tight blood glucose control with intensive insulin therapy and normoglycemia (<110 mg/dl) has shown absolute reduction in risk of hospital death by 3%-4% in some trials.[3]
    - When intensive glucose control leads to hypoglycemia (<70 mg/dl), there is an increased risk of death in critically ill patients.[4]
    - In patients with or without diabetes, perioperative hyperglycemia (>180 mg/dl) carries a significantly increased risk of infection.[5]
  - **Normal $A_1C$: 6.0**
    - Represents average glucose over previous **120 days.**
    - Although postoperative hyperglycemia and undiagnosed diabetes increase the risk of surgical site infections, elevated hemoglobin $A_1C$ values do not correlate.[6,7]

- Albumin and prealbumin
  - **Albumin ($t_{1/2}$ ~ 20 days)**
    - Mild malnutrition: 2.8-3.5 g/dl
    - Moderate malnutrition: 2.1-2.7 g/dl
    - Severe malnutrition: Less than 2.1 g/dl
    - Of 34 preoperative risk factors evaluated in a national VA surgical risk study, preoperative serum albumin level was the most important predictor of 30-day mortality.[8]
  - **Prealbumin ($t_{1/2}$ ~ 3 days)**
    - Rule of fives
      - Normal: Greater than 15 mg/dl
      - Mild deficiency: Less than 15 mg/dl
      - Moderate deficiency: Less than 10 mg/dl
      - Severe deficiency: Less than 5 mg/dl
- Unreliable in infections, inflammation, or recent trauma
- Erythrocyte sedimentation rate/C-reactive protein (ESR/CRP)
  - Nonspecific inflammatory markers
  - Obtain baseline
  - Subsequent measurements to help follow potential recurrence of osteomyelitis

## Imaging

- **Plain films**
  - Fractures
  - Foreign bodies
  - Osteomyelitis (14%-54% sensitivity; 70% specificity)
- **CT scan**
  - Abscess
  - Extent of wound
  - Tracking/tunneling
- **MRI/MRA**
  - Osteomyelitis (80%-90% sensitivity; 60%-90% specificity)
  - Assessment of vascular status
- **Angiography**
  - Assessment of vascular status
    - Contrast-enhanced MRA has overall better diagnostic accuracy for peripheral arterial disease than CTA or ultrasound and is preferred by patients over contrast angiography.[9]
    - Recommendations for preoperative imaging of lower extremities before free flap reconstruction vary. Some authors advocate angiography,[10] and others recommend preoperative and intraoperative clinical assessment.[11,12]
    - Normal imaging does not guarantee finding vessels suitable for anastomosis.

## Diagnostic Tests

- **Handheld Doppler**
- **Ankle-brachial index**
  - Greater than 1.2: Noncompressible (calcified)
  - 0.9-1.2: Normal
  - 0.5-0.9: Mixed arterial/venous disease
  - Less than 0.5: Critical stenosis
  - Less than 0.2: Ischemic gangrene likely

- **Transcutaneous oxygen tension ($TcPO_2$)**
  - Evaluation of response to oxygen administration as a surrogate marker for reversible hypoxia
  - Greater than 40 mm Hg: Normal
  - Less than 30 mm Hg: Abnormal
- **Cultures**
  - Identification of specific microorganisms and sensitivities
- **Biopsy**
  - Vasculitis
  - Marjolin's ulcer/malignancy
    - Time to malignant transformation averages 30-year latency period
  - Pyogenic granuloma

## Assessment

- Working diagnosis
- Set treatment goals
- Define monitoring parameters

## Plan (Reconstructive Ladder)

- Mathes and Nahai[13] suggested the **reconstructive triangle,** including tissue expansion, local flaps and microsurgery.
- Gottlieb and Krieger[14] introduced the **reconstructive elevator** to emphasize the freedom to rise directly to a more complex level when appropriate.
- Janis et al[15] modified the traditional reconstructive ladder to include **dermal matrices** and negative pressure wound therapy (Fig. 2-1).
  - Dermal matrices generally consist of collagen and are vascularized from the native wound bed.
    - Bilaminate neodermis contains outer layer of silicone and inner matrix of collagen and glycosaminoglycans.
  - Can be used to cover exposed critical structures, improve cosmesis from skin grafting, and simplify scalp reconstruction.[16]
  - May prevent need for free flap reconstruction, but require attention to potential complications such as seromas, hematomas, and infection.

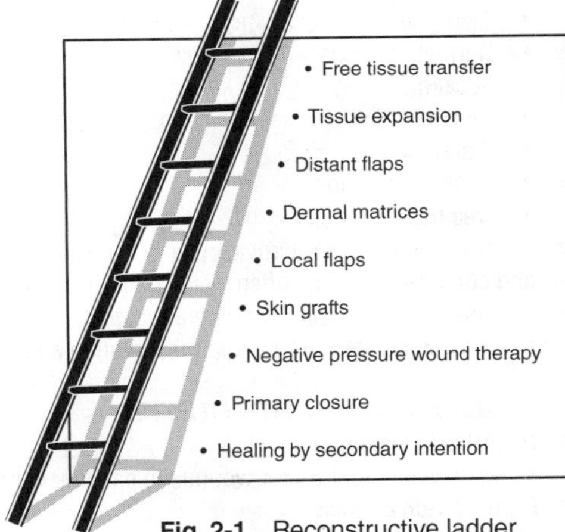

• Free tissue transfer
• Tissue expansion
• Distant flaps
• Dermal matrices
• Local flaps
• Skin grafts
• Negative pressure wound therapy
• Primary closure
• Healing by secondary intention


**Fig. 2-1** Reconstructive ladder.

- Erba et al[17] proposed a reconstructive matrix with three axes representing technologic sophistication, surgical complexity, and patient-surgical risk.
  - Within the infinite number of possibilities in this 3D grid exists a reconstructive matrix of the optimal solutions for a given patient and surgeon (Fig. 2-2).

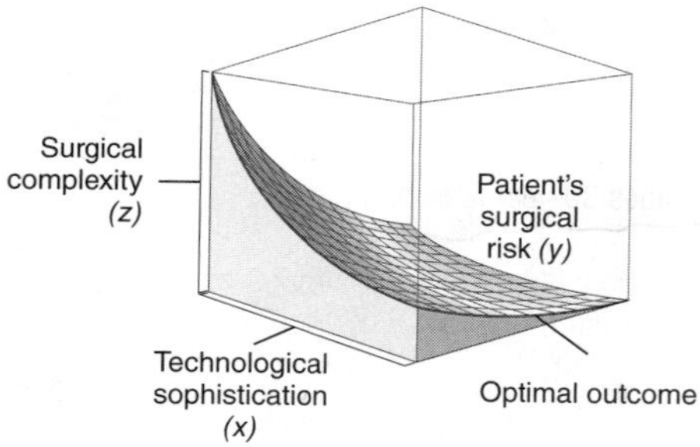


**Fig. 2-2** Hyperbolic representation of the optimal solutions for a given patient and surgeon.

- Modified reconstructive ladder
  - Useful: Organizes reconstructive solutions in order of complexity
  - Systematic consideration of the most simple to the most complex solution
  - Primary closure
  - Healing by secondary intention
  - Negative pressure wound therapy
  - Skin graft
  - Dermal matrices
  - Local flap
  - Regional flap
  - Distant flap
  - Tissue expansion
  - Free tissue transfer
- In the current era of microvascular proficiency, free tissue transfer is no longer a last resort, and complex solutions often yield superior results to simpler options.
- The use of tissue expansion, prefabrication, and composite flaps enables surgeons to optimize the balance between donor site preservation and restoration of defect form and function.

## Wound Healing Adjuncts

- **Hyberbaric oxygen**
  - May be helpful for foot wounds in patients with diabetes and for osteoradionecrosis
- **Platelet-rich plasma**
  - Contains high concentration of growth factors in small amount of plasma
  - Lacks high-level evidence for its use; production methods vary
- **Stem cells**
  - Potential for regeneration of skin, bone, and cartilage
  - Adult stem cells may be derived from bone marrow, blood, or adipose tissue
  - Lack high-level evidence
- **Honey**
  - Used by ancient Greeks and Egyptians
  - Antibacterial action against *Staphylococcus aureus, Escherichia coli, Haemophilus influenzae,* and *Pseudomonas* spp.[18]

- **Biologic dressings** (Table 2-1)
- **Vacuum-assisted closure** (VAC)
  - First reported by Argenta and Morykwas in 1997[19]
  - Increases local blood flow and granulation tissue
  - Functions by inducing cellular deformation that increases mitotic activity, removing fluid exudate, and potentially damaging cytokines.
  - Not recommended if there are exposed blood vessels, malignancy, untreated osteomyelitis, unexplored fistulas, or grossly infected tissues.

**Table 2-1** *Biologic Dressings*

| Product | Composition |
|---|---|
| AlloDerm (LifeCell, Branchburg, NJ) | Cadaveric human acellular dermis |
| SurgiMend (TEI Biosciences, Boston, MA) | Bovine-derived acellular dermal matrix |
| Integra Meshed Bilayer Wound Matrix (Integra LifeSciences, Plainsboro, NJ) | Bilayer of outer silicone and inner bovine collagen and glycosaminoglycan matrix |
| Transcyte (Smith & Nephew, London) | Cultured neonatal dermal fibroblasts on silicone/collagen matrix |
| Dermagraft (Advanced Tissue Sciences, La Jolla, CA) | Human fibroblast–derived dermal substitute |
| Apligraf (Organogenesis, Canton, MA) | Bilayer of bovine collagen and human fibroblast matrix under human keratinocytes |
| Biobrane (Smith & Nephew, London) | Nylon fibers embedded in silicone with chemically bound collagen |

## Considerations

- Functional impact
- Durability
- Individualize treatment to the patient (socioeconomic impact)
  - Does the patient need to minimize hospital stay, decrease the need for staged procedures, or get back to work quickly?
- Appearance
- Make sure solution not more complicated than problem

### Key Points

- ✓ Successful treatment of any wound first requires comprehensive clinical evaluation of the wound and patient comorbidities.
- ✓ Blood glucose and nutritional parameters must be optimized preoperatively and postoperatively to prevent surgical site complications.
- ✓ Preoperative serum albumin is a predictor of postoperative mortality.
- ✓ New algorithms for reconstruction expand on the reconstructive ladder to allow plans tailored to the defect, donor site morbidity, patient, and surgeon preference.

## References


1. Janis JE, Morrison B. Wound healing. Part II: Clinical applications (accepted by Plast Reconstr Surg 2013).
2. Devos P, Preiser JC. Current controversies around tight glucose control in critically ill patients. Curr Opi Clin Nutr Metab Care 10:206-209, 2007.
3. Vanhorebeek I, Langouche L, Van den Berghe G. Tight blood glucose control: what is the evidence? Crit Care Med 35(9 Suppl):S496-S502, 2007.
4. Finfer S, Liu B, Chittock DR, et al. Hypoglycemia and risk of death in critically ill patients. New Engl J Med 367:1108-1118, 2012.
5. Kwon S, Thompson R, Dellinger P, et al. Importance of perioperative glycemic control in general surgery: a report from the Surgical Care and Outcomes Assessment Program. Ann Surg 257:8-14, 2013.
6. King JT Jr, Goulet JL, Perkal MF, et al. Glycemic control and infections in patients with diabetes undergoing noncardiac surgery. Ann Surg 253:158-165, 2011.
7. Latham R, Lancaster AD, Covington JF, et al. The association of diabetes and glucose control with surgical-site infections among cardiothoracic surgery patients. Infect Control Hosp Epidemiol 22:607-612, 2001.
8. Gibbs J, Cull W, Henderson W, et al. Preoperative serum albumin level as a predictor of operative mortality and morbidity: results from the National VA Surgical Risk Study. Arch Surg 134:36-42, 1999.
9. Collins R, Cranny G, Burch J, et al. A systematic review of duplex ultrasound, magnetic resonance angiography and computed tomography angiography for the diagnosis and assessment of symptomatic, lower limb peripheral arterial disease. Health Technol Assess 11:iii-iv, xi-xiii, 1-184, 2007.
10. Haddock NT, Weichman KE, Reformat DD, et al. Lower extremity arterial injury patterns and reconstructive outcomes in patients with severe lower extremity trauma: a 26-year review. J Am Coll Surg 210:66-72, 2010.
11. Isenberg JS, Sherman R. The limited value of preoperative angiography in microsurgical reconstruction of the lower limb. J Reconstr Microsurg 12:303-305, 1996.
12. Lutz BS, Ng SH, Cabailo R, et al. Value of routine angiography before traumatic lower-limb reconstruction with microvascular free tissue transplantation. J Trauma 44:682-686, 1998.
13. Mathes SJ, Nahai F. Reconstructive Surgery: Principles, Anatomy, & Technique. St Louis: Quality Medical Publishing, 1997.
14. Gottlieb LJ, Krieger LM. From the reconstructive ladder to the reconstructive elevator. Plast Reconstr Surg 93:1503-1504, 1994.
15. Janis JE, Kwon RK, Attinger CE. The new reconstructive ladder: modifications to the traditional model. Plast Reconstr Surg 127(Suppl 1):S205-S212, 2011.
16. Komorowska-Timek E, Gabriel A, Bennett DC, et al. Artificial dermis as an alternative for coverage of complex scalp defects following excision of malignant tumors. Plast Reconstr Surg 115:1010-1017, 2005.
17. Erba P, Ogawa R, Vyas R, et al. The reconstructive matrix: a new paradigm in reconstructive plastic surgery. Plast Reconstr Surg 126:492-498, 2010.
18. Song JJ, Salcido R. Use of honey in wound care: an update. Adv Skin Wound Care 24:40-44, 2011.
19. Argenta LC, Morykwas MJ. Vacuum-assisted closure: a new method for wound control and treatment: clinical experience. Ann Plast Surg 38:563-576, 1997.

# 3. Sutures and Needles

**Huay-Zong Law, Scott W. Mosser**

## QUALITIES OF SUTURE MATERIALS: ESSENTIAL VOCABULARY[1]

### PERMANENCE: ABSORBABLE VERSUS NONABSORBABLE

- **Absorbable**
  - Lose at least 50% of their strength in 4 weeks
  - Eventually completely absorbed
  - Degradation process
    - **Hydrolytic**
      - Process for **synthetic sutures**
      - Minimal inflammation
    - **Proteolytic**
      - Enzyme-mediated
      - Process for **natural sutures** (e.g., gut, from beef or sheep intestine)
      - More inflammation leads to more scarring around the suture site.
- **Nonabsorbable**
  - Induce a cell-mediated reaction until the suture becomes encapsulated

### CONFIGURATION

- **Monofilament** versus **multifilament** (twisted or braided)
  - Monofilament sutures slide through tissue with less friction and are less likely to harbor infective organisms.
  - Multifilament sutures are stronger, more pliable, and less sensitive to crimping and crushing, which may create a weak spot.

**TIP:** Gut sutures do not fit into either category but behave more like monofilament sutures.

- **Barbed** versus **nonbarbed** (twisted or braided)[2-5]
  - Addition of one-way barbs to maintain tension in knotless closure
  - Similar strength and postoperative complication profile to nonbarbed suture
  - Faster deployment than nonbarbed suture, but unable to backtrack and may trap fibers from laparotomy sponges and surgical drapes
  - Range of absorbable and nonabsorbable barbed sutures available from multiple vendors

### KNOT SECURITY

*The force necessary to cause a knot to slip*

- Knot security is proportional to the coefficient of friction and the ability of the suture to stretch.
- More knot security means fewer throws are necessary to tie a reliable knot.
- Braided sutures (e.g., silk, Vicryl) generally have better knot security than monofilament sutures (e.g., Prolene, nylon).

### Elasticity

*The tendency of a suture to return to its original length after stretching*

- Elastic sutures stretch in edematous wounds, then return to their original size while maintaining tension.
- Inelastic sutures (e.g., steel) cut through edematous tissues instead of forgiving the added tension.

### Memory

*The tendency of a suture material to return to its original shape (similar to stiffness)*

- Sutures with more memory are less pliable and more difficult to handle.
- More memory leads to less knot security.

### Fluid Absorption and Capillarity

*Fluid absorption is the amount of fluid retained by a suture.*
*Capillarity is the tendency of fluid to travel along the suture.*

- Capillarity correlates with increased adhesion of bacteria and infection.[6,7]

### Cost

- Cost includes both the suture material and the needle.
- Sutures attached to precision needles (which are sharper and made of high-grade alloys) are more expensive than sutures with standard needles.

### Visibility

- Dyeing aids in visibility during placement and removal, but buried sutures may be undesirably visible.
- Braided sutures are usually visible even if undyed, because they become saturated with blood intraoperatively.

> **TIP:** The United States Pharmacopoeia (USP) rating system is often used.[8]
>
> Diameters are given in #-0 values based on USP breaking strength rating, not the width of the suture.
>
> Two different sutures with the same number can have different diameters (e.g., a 3-0 stainless steel suture is thinner than a 3-0 silk suture but has the same breaking strength).

## NEEDLE CONFIGURATIONS[9]

### Point Configuration (Fig. 3-1)

- **Cutting needles**
  - Have sharp edges along the length of the needle tip; better at penetrating tough tissues
  - Skin and dermis are sutured with cutting needles.
  - **Conventional cutting versus reverse cutting needles**
    - *Conventional cutting* needles: Sharp edge on the interior of the curve that creates a weak point on the tract where suture can cut through skin
    - *Reverse cutting* needles: Sharp edge on the exterior of the curve; preferable for skin closure
- **Taper needles**
  - Taper needles have a sharp tip but no sharp edge.
  - Tissue spreads around the needle instead of being cut by it.
  - Suture material is less likely to cut through tissue if the tract is made with a taper needle.
  - Taper needles are typically used for tendon and deep tissue closure (fascia).

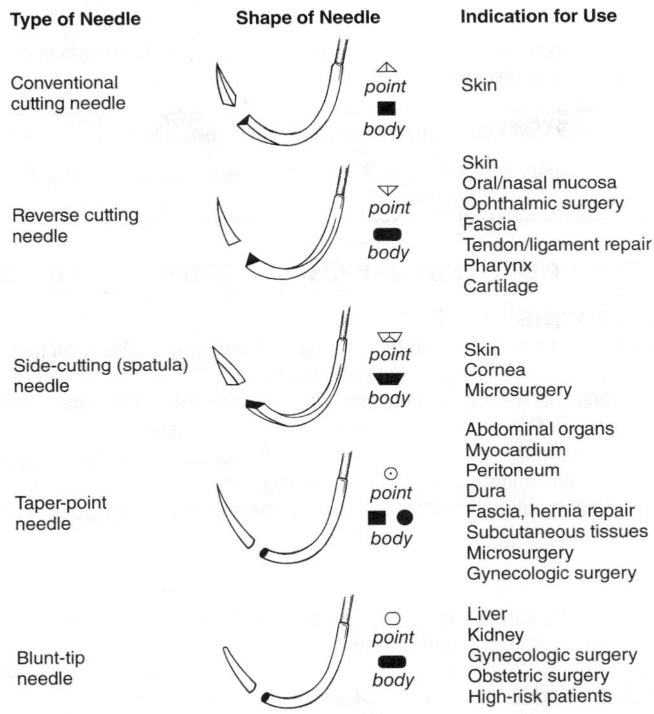

Type of Needle
Shape of Needle
Indication for Use
Conventional cutting needle
point
body
Skin
Reverse cutting needle
point
body
Skin
Oral/nasal mucosa
Ophthalmic surgery
Fascia
Tendon/ligament repair
Pharynx
Cartilage
Side-cutting (spatula) needle
point
body
Skin
Cornea
Microsurgery
Taper-point needle
point
body
Abdominal organs
Myocardium
Peritoneum
Dura
Fascia, hernia repair
Subcutaneous tissues
Microsurgery
Gynecologic surgery
Blunt-tip needle
point
body
Liver
Kidney
Gynecologic surgery
Obstetric surgery
High-risk patients


**Fig. 3-1** Types of commonly used needles.

## SIZE (Figs. 3-2 and 3-3)

- **Curvature**
  - Most needles used in plastic surgery have a three-eighths circle curvature.
  - A one-fourth curve may be better for microsurgical applications.
  - Some wound geometries require a one-half or five-eighths curve to facilitate tissue handling.
- **Length**
  - *Needle length:* Circumferential distance along the curve
  - *Chord length:* Straight-line distance between the point and the eye (nearly always swaged)

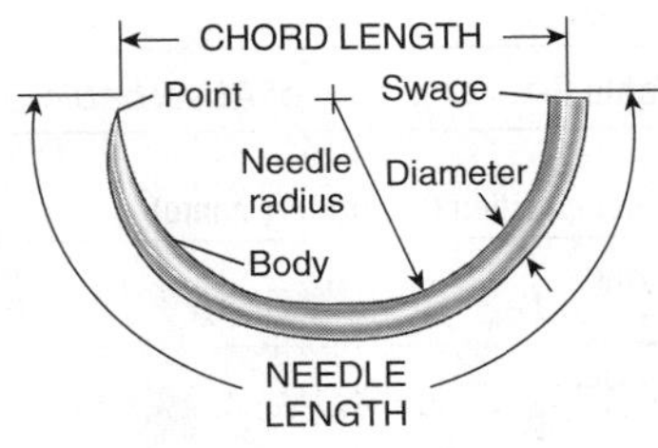


**Fig. 3-2** Anatomy of a needle.

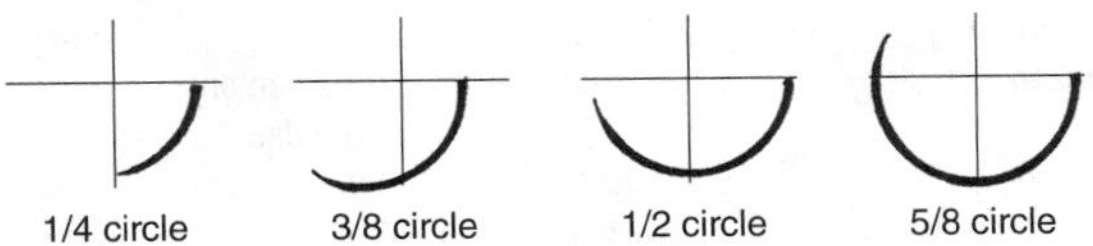


**Fig. 3-3** Curvature of a needle.

- **Diameter**
  - Determined by the balance between providing sufficient material strength and the smallest diameter possible for the required suture size

**TIP:** Vendors use needle codes for specific needle configurations.

Common plastic surgery codes include *BV* (blood vessel), *CT* (circle taper), *P/PS* (plastic surgery), *RB* (renal bypass), *SH* (small half [circle]).

## FACTORS THAT GUIDE SUTURE CHOICE (Tables 3-1 and 3-2)[9-12]

### ABSORBABLE VERSUS NONABSORABLE

- Rapidly absorbing suture can be used for layers closed under minimal tension (e.g., gut suture to close mucosa or skin after deep sutures are placed).
- Absorbable sutures that maintain strength for 4-6 weeks are used for closures under short-term tension (e.g., Vicryl or PDS to close fascia and subcutaneous tissue).
- Considerable long-term tension requires permanent sutures (e.g., nylon, polypropylene, or polyester for bone anchoring, ligament, and tendon repair).
- Choose an absorbable suture that loses strength comparable to the timing of wound strength recovery[12] (Fig. 3-4).

### CALIBER

- Caliber is largely dictated by the strength of suture needed.
- Choose the smallest-caliber suture that provides sufficient strength.

### TYPE OF TISSUE AND NEEDLE CHOICE

- Generally, use permanent sutures on taper needles for fascia, tendon, or cartilage under tension.
- Use absorbable sutures on cutting needles for subcutaneous, dermis, and skin closures.

**Table 3-1** *Qualities of Absorbable Sutures*

| Composition (proprietary name) | Time to 50% Strength | Configuration | Reactivity | Memory |
|---|---|---|---|---|
| Gut | Unpredictable | | | |
| Fast | 5-7 days | Monofilament | High | Low |
| Plain | 7-10 days | Monofilament | High | Low |
| Chromic | 10-14 days | Monofilament | High | Low |
| Polyglytone 6211 (Caprosyn*) | 5-7 days | Monofilament | Low | Medium |
| Poliglecaprone 25 (Monocryl†) | 7-10 days | Monofilament | Low | Medium |
| Glycomer 631 (Biosyn†) | 2-3 weeks | Monofilament | Low | Medium |
| Glycolide/lactide copolymer | 5 days | Braided | Low | Low |
| Low molecular weight (Vicryl Rapide*) | | | | |
| Regular (Polysorb†, Vicryl*) | 2-3 weeks | Braided | Low | Low |
| Polyglycolic acid (Dexon S†) | 2-3 weeks | Monofilament or braided | Low | Low |
| Polyglyconate (Maxon†) | 4 weeks | Monofilament | Low | High |
| Polydioxanone (PDS II*) | 4 weeks | Monofilament | Low | High |

*Ethicon.
†U.S. Surgical Corporation.

**Table 3-2** *Qualities of Nonabsorbable Sutures*

| Composition (proprietary name) | Tensile Strength | Configuration | Reactivity | Memory/ Handling |
|---|---|---|---|---|
| Silk | Lost in 1 year | Braided | High | − −/Good |
| Nylon | 81% at 1 year, | | | |
| Monofilament (Ethilon*, Monosof-Dermalon†) | 72% at 2 years, | Monofilament | Low | +/Fair |
| Braided (Nurolon*, Surgilon†) | 66% at 11 years | Braided | Low | − −/Good |
| Polypropylene (Prolene*, Surgipro†) | Indefinite | Monofilament | Low | + +/Poor |
| Polybutester | | | | |
| Uncoated (Novafil†) | Indefinite | Monofilament | Low | +/Fair |
| Coated (Vascufil†) | Indefinite | Monofilament | Low | −/Good |
| Polyester | | | | |
| Uncoated (Mersilene*) | Indefinite | Braided | Moderate | − −/Good |
| Coated (Ethibond*, Surgidac†, Ticron†) | Indefinite | Braided | Moderate | − −/Good |
| Surgical steel | Indefinite | Monofilament or braided | Low | + +/Poor |

*Ethicon.
†U.S. Surgical Corporation.

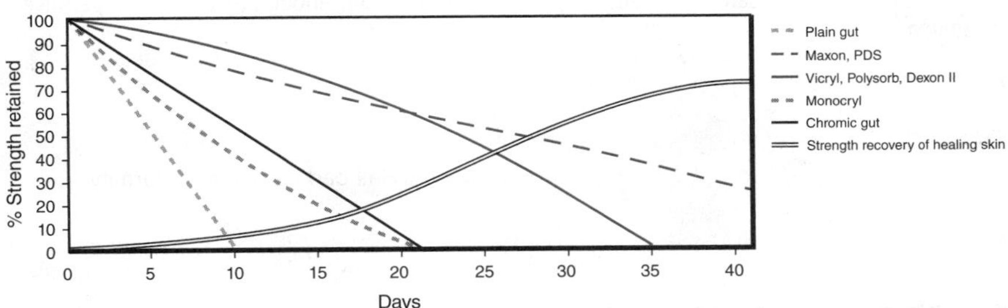


**Fig. 3-4** Suture absorption and wound strength recovery. After a procedure, skin strength can be expected to regain 5% of its original strength within a week, nearly 50% within 4 weeks, and 80% within 6 weeks of skin closure. Even after collagen maturation is complete (6 months to 1 year postoperatively), a wound will only regain 80% of its original strength.

## Wound Contamination and Inflammation

**TIP:** Monofilament sutures should be used for contaminated and infected wounds to prevent harboring bacteria in the suture material.

- Wound infection accelerates the process of suture absorption.

## Patient Factors

- Patient reliability, age, and overall wound-healing capability affect how long the sutures must maintain closure tension.

**TIP:** In thin patients, buried knot configurations with braided, absorbable suture will prevent palpability of sutures after surgery.

## Microsutures and Needles (see Chapter 8)

- Suture choice depends on vessel or structure size.
  - 8-0 is used for large (4 mm) vessels (e.g., radial and ulnar arteries).
  - 9-0 is used for 3-4 mm vessels (e.g., internal mammary, dorsalis pedis, and posterior tibial arteries).
  - 10-0 is used for 1-2 mm structures (e.g., digital arteries and nerves).
  - 11-0 is used for very small (<1 mm) vessels, such as those in children and infants.
- Microsutures behave similarly in tying and memory characteristics at these diameters.
- Sutures are nearly always *monofilament synthetic* (e.g., nylon or polypropylene).

# SUTURE REMOVAL

## Potential Complication: Railroad Track Scar (Fig. 3-5)

*A "railroad track" scar is the formation of punctate scars and parallel rows of scar beneath them.*

- The *punctate component* of the scars results from delayed suture removal.
  - Epithelial cells that abut a skin suture form a cylindrical cuff and grow downward along the suture.
  - The cells continue to develop after suture removal and keratinize the length of the suture tract, resulting in inflammation and punctate scar formation.
- *Parallel rows* result from pressure necrosis of the skin and subcutaneous tissue beneath the external suture. This can be prevented by tying sutures loosely enough to allow postoperative edema.

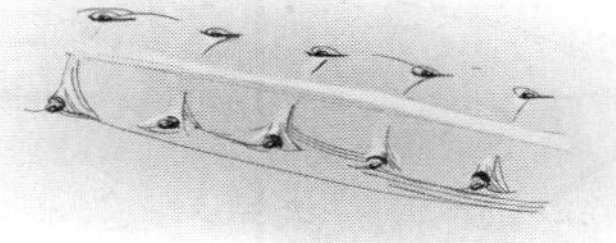

**Fig. 3-5** Railroad track scar deformity.

# OTHER CLOSURE MATERIALS

## Stainless Steel Staples[13]

- Nonreactive, but inelastic and offer imprecise epidermal approximation
- Least ischemic method of closure
- Faster than sutures without clinically significant difference in cosmetic result, infection, or ease of removal

## Cyanoacrylate

- Rapid and effective for well-aligned wounds under no tension, but imprecise edge approximation
- Does not support significant skin edge tension during healing
- Decreased rates of postoperative surgical site infections in some studies[14,15]
- Use in combination with polyester mesh (e.g., Prineo) compared with intradermal sutures resulted in faster closure (1.5 versus 6.7 minutes for 22 cm incision on average) with no statistical difference in cosmetic outcome[16]
  - No difference in infection rate was seen.
  - Blistering occurred in 2.4% (2 of 83 patients) of polyester/cyanoacrylate closure sites compared with 0% of the intradermal suture sites.

## Key Points

- ✓ In a contaminated wound, monofilament suture should be used.
- ✓ Tissue under significant long-term tension should be closed with permanent suture only.
- ✓ Choose an absorbable suture that loses strength comparable to the timing of wound strength recovery.[12]
- ✓ Of the absorbable sutures available for skin closure, only fast-absorbing plain gut and Vicryl Rapide are absorbed in time to prevent punctate scar formation.
- ✓ To avoid *railroad track scars,* sutures in the skin layer should be removed promptly. Therefore the final skin layer should not be closed under tension, and a gaping skin wound should be approximated first with deep sutures.

## References


1. Friedman J, Mosser SW. Closure material. In Evans G, ed. Operative Plastic Surgery. New York: McGraw-Hill, 2000.
2. Oni G, Brown SA, Kenkel JM. A comparison between barbed and nonbarbed absorbable suture for fascial closure in a porcine model. Plast Reconstr Surg 130:536e-541e, 2012.
3. Rosen A, Hartman T. Repair of the midline fascial defect in abdominoplasty with long-acting barbed and smooth absorbable sutures. Aesthet Surg J 31:668-673, 2011.
4. Covidien, 2012. Available at *www.covidien.com.*
5. Angiotech, 2012. Available at *www.angioedupro.com.*
6. Osterberg B, Blomstedt B. Effect of suture materials on bacterial survival in infected wounds. An experimental study. Acta Chir Scand 145:431-434, 1979.
7. Katz S, Izhar M, Mirelman D. Bacterial adherence to surgical sutures: a possible factor in suture induced infection. Ann Surg 94:35-41, 1981.
8. United States Pharmacopoeia, vol 29. Rockville, MD: United States Pharmacopeia, 2006.
9. Ethicon. Wound Closure Manual. Somerville, NJ: Ethicon, 2005.
10. Weinzwig J, Weinzwig N. Plastic surgery techniques. In Guyuron B, Eriksson E, Persing JA, eds. Plastic Surgery: Indications and Practice. Philadelphia: Saunders Elsevier, 2009.
11. Mirastschjiski U, Jokuszies A, Vogt PM. Skin wound healing: repair biology, wound, and scar treatment. In Neligan PC, ed. Plastic Surgery, 3rd ed. London: Saunders Elsevier, 2013.
12. Levenson SM, Geever EF, Crowley LV, et al. The healing of rat skin wounds. Ann Surg 161:293-308, 1965.
13. Shuster M. Comparing skin staples to sutures. Can Fam Phys 35:505-509, 1989.
14. Chambers A, Scarci M. Is skin closure with cyanoacrylate glue effective for the prevention of sternal wound infections? Interact Cardiovasc Thorac Surg 10:793-796, 2010.
15. Eymann R, Kiefer M. Glue instead of stitches: a minor change of the operative technique with a serious impact on the shunt infection rate. Acta Neurochir Suppl 106:87-89, 2010.
16. Richter D, Stoff A, Ramakrishnan V, et al. A comparison of a new skin closure device and intradermal sutures in the closure of full-thickness surgical incisions. Plast Reconstr Surg 130:843-850, 2012.

# 4. Basics of Flaps

Deniz Basci, Amanda A. Gosman

## DEFINITION

A flap is a unit of tissue that maintains its own blood supply while being transferred from a donor site to a recipient site.

## CLASSIFICATION

Most flaps can be classified according to **three principles**

1. Vascularity
2. Tissue composition
3. Method of movement

> **TIP:** The intrinsic vascularity of a flap is the most critical determinant of successful transfer and is therefore the most clinically valid method of classification.

### VASCULARITY

- **Vascular anatomy of the skin**[1] (Fig. 4-1)
  - Microvascular plexuses run parallel to the skin with numerous collaterals supplied by septocutaneous and myocutaneous arteries.
  - **Septocutaneous perforators** are found in the fascial septa between muscles and are most abundant in thin long muscles of the extremities.
  - **Myocutaneous perforators** pass perpendicularly through muscles and are found most commonly in broad flat muscles of the torso.
  - The epidermis, with its higher metabolic activity, receives nutrients via diffusion from the dermal vascular plexus.

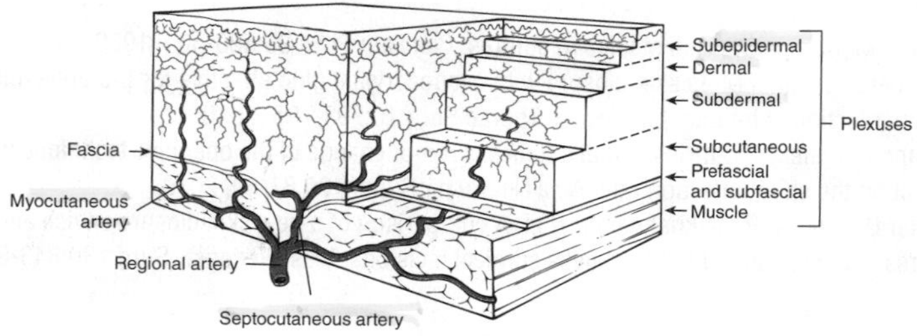


**Fig. 4-1** Cutaneous circulation.

## ■ Two theories of blood supply to the skin

1. **Angiosome:** A composite unit of skin and its underlying deep tissue supplied by a single source artery and its branches
   - In 1987, Taylor and Palmer[2] proposed **40 angiosomes** (Fig. 4-2) linked to one other by either *true* anastomotic arteries of similar caliber or reduced-caliber *choke* anastomotic vessels.[3]
   - Choke vessels serve to regulate blood flow between neighboring angiosomes and can potentially dilate to the caliber of a true anastomotic vessel after surgical delay or with a decrease in sympathetic tone.
   - A single source vessel may supply multiple angiosomes.

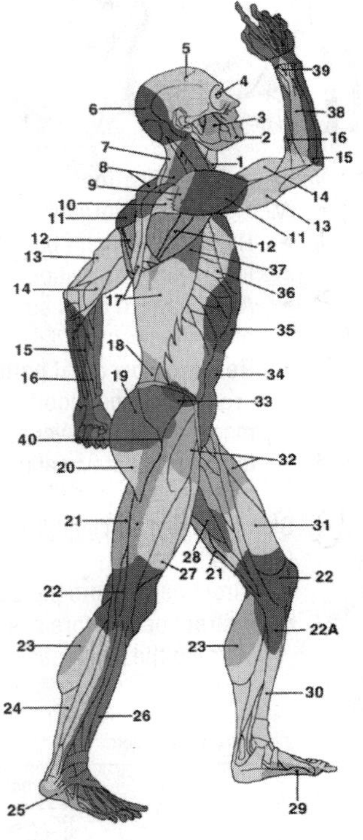


**Fig. 4-2** The angiosomes of the source arteries of the body. *1,* Thyroid; *2,* facial; *3,* buccal internal maxillary; *4,* ophthalmic; *5,* superficial temporal; *6,* occipital; *7,* deep cervical; *8,* transverse cervical; *9,* acromiothoracic; *10,* suprascapular; *11,* posterior circumflex humeral; *12,* circumflex scapular; *13,* profunda brachii; *14,* brachial; *15,* ulnar; *16,* radial; *17,* posterior intercostals; *18,* lumbar; *19,* superior gluteal; *20,* inferior gluteal; *21,* profunda femoris; *22,* popliteal; *22A,* decending geniculate saphenous; *23,* sural; *24,* peroneal; *25,* lateral plantar; *26,* anterior tibial; *27,* lateral femoral circumflex; *28,* adductor profunda; *29,* medial plantar; *30,* posterior tibial; *31,* superficial femoral; *32,* common femoral; *33,* deep circumflex iliac; *34,* deep inferior epigastric; *35,* internal thoracic; *36,* lateral thoracic; *37,* thoracodorsal; *38,* posterior interosseous; *39,* anterior interosseous; 40, internal pudendal.

> **TIP:** Knowledge of angiosome boundaries and locations of source vessels can guide flap designs to improve flap viability.

2. **Fasciocutaneous plexus:** A communicating network of the subfascial intrafascial, suprafascial, subcutaneous, and subdermal vascular plexuses fed by different configurations of inflow vessels
   - This network extends throughout the body as a continuous system encompassing the dermal, subdermal, superficial, and deep adipofascial layers.
   - All skin flaps are based on the fasciocutaneous plexus, which is supplied from perforating vessels that penetrate the deep fascia either directly or indirectly.
   - Nakajima et al[4] identified six vessel types that perforate the deep fascia to supply the fasciocutaneous plexus (Fig. 4-3).
   - Two systems for venous drainage of skin[5] are tied together via anastomotic connections that permit flow reversal in distally based flaps.
     1. Valvular superficial and deep cutaneous veins parallel the course of adjacent arteries.
     2. Avalvular oscillating veins permit bidirectional flow between adjacent venous territories.

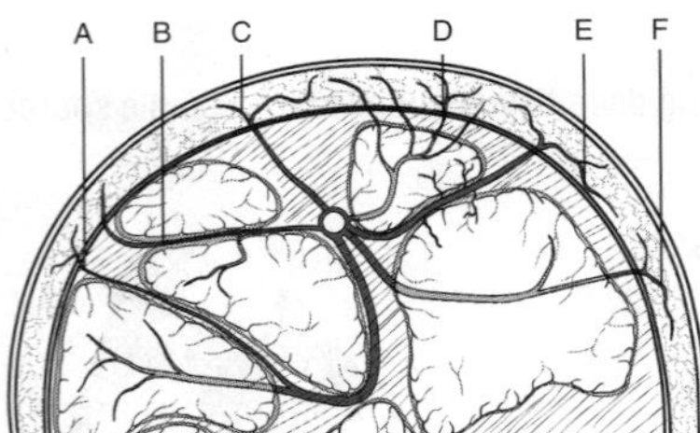


**Fig. 4-3** The six distinctive deep fascia perforators. A separate type of fasciocutaneous flap may be named for each different perforator. *A,* Direct cutaneous branch of a muscular vessel; *B,* septocutaneous perforator; *C,* direct cutaneous; *D,* myocutaneous perforator; *E,* direct septocutaneous; *F,* perforating cutaneous branch of a muscular vessel.

- **Vascular Classification**
  - McGregor and Morgan[6] categorized cutaneous flaps as follows.
    - **Random flaps** are based off the subdermal plexus and are traditionally limited to 3:1 length-to-width ratios.
    - **Axial pattern flaps** contain a single direct cutaneous artery within the longitudinal axis of the flap.
    - **Reverse-flow axial pattern flaps** are axial flaps in which the source vessel is divided proximally, and blood flows in a retrograde fashion through the distal vessel. This is made possible by venae comitantes, bypass vessels, and valvular incompetence.
    - **Island flaps** are axial pattern flaps raised on a pedicle devoid of skin to facilitate distant transfer.
  - Skin flaps can be classified simply and accurately as a **direct** or an **indirect** perforator flaps[7] (Fig. 4-4).
    - **Direct** perforators pierce the deep fascia without traversing any deeper structures.
    - **Indirect** perforators pass through deeper tissues, usually muscle or septum, before entering the deep fascia.

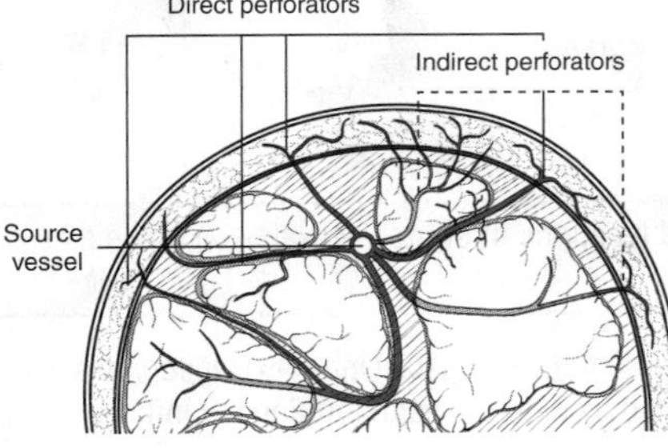


**Fig. 4-4** The distinct deep fascial perforators of Nakajima can be considered more simply to be either *direct* or *indirect* perforators. These perforators all arise from the same source vessel, but only indirect perforators *(dotted lines)* first course through some other intermediary tissue (here depicted as muscle), before piercing the deep fascia.

- **Perforator flaps**[8-14] (Box 4-1)
  - Consist of skin or subcutaneous fat supplied by isolated perforator vessel (or vessels).
  - May pass from their source vessel origin either through or between the deep tissues.
  - Classified into three categories based on the three different kinds of perforator vessels[15] (Fig. 4-5).
    - **Indirect muscle perforator:** Myocutaneous perforator flap
    - **Indirect septal perforator:** Septocutaneous perforator flap
    - **Direct cutaneous perforator:** Direct cutaneous perforator flap

- Perforator flaps are named for their nutrient vessel (e.g., deep inferior epigastric perforator [DIEP] flap), except in areas where multiple perforator flaps can be raised from a single vessel; then the flap is named for its anatomic region or muscle (e.g., anterolateral thigh [ALT] flap).

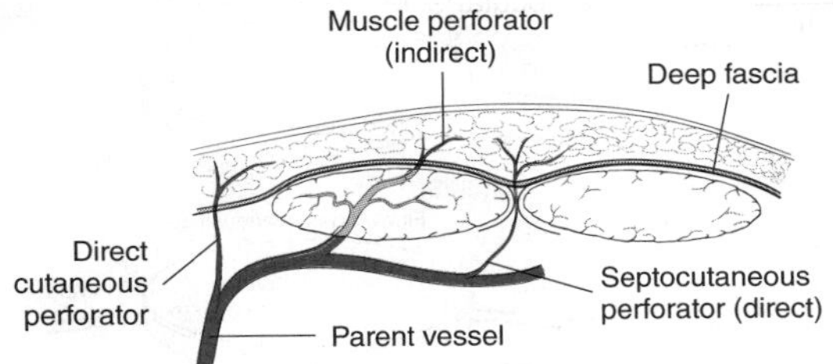


**Fig. 4-5** Different types of direct and indirect perforator vessels with regard to their surgical importance: Direct perforator perforating the deep fascia only, indirect muscle perforator traveling through muscle before piercing the deep fascia, and indirect septal perforator traveling through the intermuscular septum before piercing the deep fascia.

**Box 4-1** *ADVANTAGES AND DISADVANTAGES OF PERFORATOR FLAPS*

| Advantages | Disadvantages |
|---|---|
| Numerous potential donor sites | Tedious pedicle dissection |
| Often able to incorporate muscle, fat, and bone into flap design | Variation in perforator anatomy and size |
| Preserve muscle function | Increased risk of fat necrosis compared with myocutaneous flaps |
| Minimal donor site morbidity | |
| Reduced postoperative recovery time and pain medication requirements | |
| Versatility of size and thickness | |

- **Neurocutaneous and venocutaneous flaps** (e.g., sural nerve and saphenous vein flaps)

*Skin flaps based off the perforating arteries accompanying cutaneous nerves and veins*[16]
  - Run in the deep adipofascial layer of the skin[17]
  - Sensate (neurocutaneous flaps)
  - Commonly used as pedicled flaps for coverage of local or regional extremity defects
- **Venous flaps**[18-22] (Box 4-2)

*Skin flaps supplied through a venous pedicle*

**Box 4-2** *ADVANTAGES AND DISADVANTAGES OF VENOUS FLAPS*

| Advantages | Disadvantages |
|---|---|
| Minimal donor site morbidity requiring only the sacrifice of a vein and no artery | Poorly understood physiology |
| Long and very thin | Unpredictable survival, making application controversial |
| Anatomically constant pedicle (e.g., saphenous vein) | |
| Fast and expedient flap elevation | |

- Thatte and Thatte[23] classify venous flaps into three groups (Fig. 4-6).[21]
  - **Type I** is an unipedicled venous flap, or a pure venous flap with a single cephalad vein as the only vascular conduit.
  - **Type II** venous flaps are bipedicled "flow-through" flaps with afferent and efferent veins exhibiting flow from caudal to cephalad.
  - **Type III** venous flaps are arterialized through a proximal arteriovenous anastomosis and drained by a distal vein.
- The mechanism of venous flap perfusion is still not completely understood and has been attributed to a number of factors, including[19]:
  - Plasmatic imbibition
  - Perfusion pressure
  - Sites of arteriovenous anastomosis
  - Perivenous arterial networks
  - Vein-to-vein interconnections
  - Circumvention of venous valves

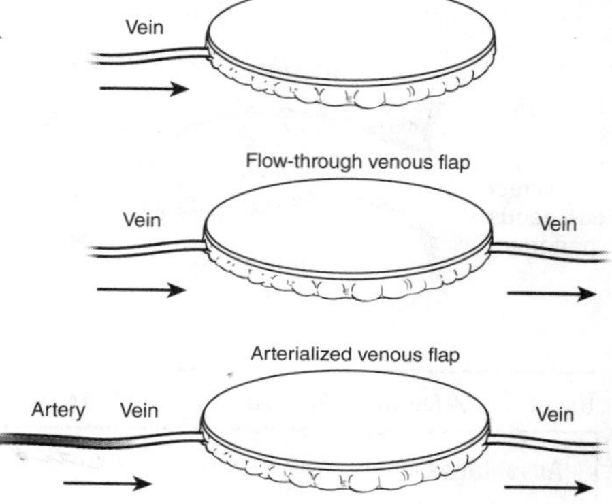


**Fig. 4-6** Three types of venous flaps.

## TISSUE COMPOSITION

■ Fascial and fasciocutaneous flap

*Fasciocutaneous flaps are created by elevating skin with its underlying deep fascia.*

- **Fasciocutaneous flaps:** Supplied by the fasciocutaneous plexus

> **TIP:** Including the deep fascia is not necessary for flap survival, although some authors advocate its preservation to protect the suprafascial portion of the fasciocutaneous plexus.

- **Fascial and adipofascial flaps:** Created by elevating the deep fascia with or without subcutaneous adipose tissue **without** the overlying skin component (Box 4-3)
- Mathes[24] classified fasciocutaneous flaps as those supplied by:
  - Direct cutaneous pedicle
  - Septocutaneous pedicle
  - Myocutaneous pedicle
- Can be used as pedicled flaps for coverage of local, regional, and distant defects, or as free tissue transfer flaps

**Box 4-3** *ADVANTAGES AND DISADVANTAGES OF FASCIAL AND FASCIOCUTANEOUS FLAPS*

| Advantages | Disadvantages |
|---|---|
| Preservation of muscle | Donor site morbidity (may require skin graft) |
| Thin and pliable | Less resistant to infection than muscle flaps |
| Amenable to tissue expansion | |
| Can incorporate sensory nerves | |

- **Muscle and myocutaneous flaps**
  - Muscle flaps can be transferred as pedicled flaps or as a free tissue transfer based on their dominant vascular pedicle.
  - Myocutaneous flaps are composites of skin and underlying muscle supplied by a dominant vascular pedicle.
  - Myocutaneous flaps are primarily used for breast, head and neck, and pressure sore reconstruction.
  - Muscle flaps are indicated for coverage of infected, radiated, or traumatic wounds.
  - Myocutaneous versus fasciocutaneous flaps (Box 4-4):
    - Myocutaneous and fasciocutaneous flaps demonstrate a marked increase in blood flow to all levels of tissue after elevation.[25]
    - The decrease in bacterial concentration is significantly greater in wounds covered with myocutaneous flaps than in those covered with fasciocutaneous flaps ($10^4$ versus $10^2$).[25]
    - Myocutaneous flaps exhibit more collagen deposition than fasciocutaneous flaps.[26]
  - **Mathes and Nahai**[27] developed a classification of muscles based on circulatory patterns (Fig. 4-7).
    - Type I, III, and V muscle flaps have the most reliable vascularity.
    - Type II and IV muscle flaps are less reliable because the vascular pedicle to distal muscle must be divided to achieve adequate arc of rotation.

**Box 4-4** *ADVANTAGES AND DISADVANTAGES OF MUSCLE AND MYOCUTANEOUS FLAPS*

| Advantages | Disadvantages |
|---|---|
| Potential to obliterate dead space with vascularized tissue | Donor site morbidity (functional deficit) |
| Increased resistance to infection | Flap bulk |

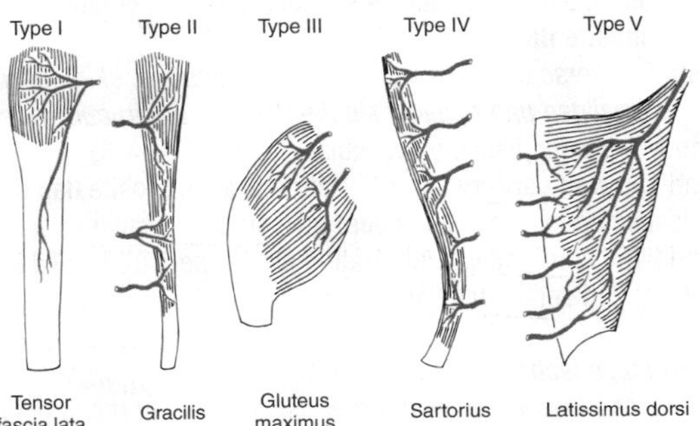


**Fig. 4-7** Patterns of vascular anatomy. *Type I,* one vascular pedicle; *type II,* dominant pedicle(s) and minor pedicle(s); *type III,* two dominant pedicles; *type IV,* segmental vascular pedicles; *type V,* one dominant pedicle and secondary segmental pedicles.

- **Vascularized bone flaps** (Box 4-5)
  - Vascularized bone flaps can be transferred in a pedicled or free fashion based on their nutrient vessels.
  - Most commonly transferred vascularized bone flaps:
    - Fibula (peroneal artery)
    - Iliac crest (deep circumflex iliac artery)
    - Scapula (transverse branch of circumflex scapular artery)
    - Radius (radial artery)

**Box 4-5** *ADVANTAGES AND DISADVANTAGES OF VASCULARIZED BONE FLAPS*

| Advantages | Disadvantages |
|---|---|
| Can reconstruct large bony defects | Donor site morbidity |
| Undergo primary bony healing | |
| Withstand radiation and implantation | |
| Can be transferred as a composite with other tissue types (e.g., scapular flap and free toe transfers) | |

- **Visceral flaps**
  - The omentum, colon, and jejunum can be transferred as visceral flaps based on their dominant pedicles or vascular arcades.
  - Intestinal flaps are primarily useful in pharyngoesophageal reconstruction.
  - The omentum is a versatile flap that can be tailored to many different defects.
- **Innervated flaps**

*Functional muscle flaps and sensory flaps can be created by inclusion of the appropriate motor or sensory nerve for coaptation at the recipient site after flap transfer.*

  - **To restore muscle function after transfer, the original tension and length/width ratio of the fibers need to be recreated during inset.**
  - The gracilis, latissimus dorsi, and serratus muscles are often used for functional muscle transfers.
  - Many flaps can be modified to include a sensory nerve for creating a sensory flap.
- **Compound and composite flaps**

*Compound flaps contain diverse tissue components such as bone, skin, fascia, and muscle that are incorporated into an interrelated unit to allow single-stage reconstruction of complex defects.*

  - Classified into two groups based on vascularization[28] (Fig. 4-8)
    1. Compound flap with **solitary** vascularization is a composite flap that incorporates multiple tissue components dependent on a single vascular supply.
    2. Compound flaps of **mixed** vascularization are further subdivided into Siamese flaps, conjoint flaps, and sequential flaps.
- **Prefabricated flaps**

*Prefabrication is a two-stage technique in which a flap is surgically altered by partial elevation, structural manipulation, and incorporation of other tissue layers at the first stage to create a specialized composite flap.*

  - The altered flap is allowed to heal, and transfer is delayed for the second stage.
  - Prefabrication is useful for nasal reconstruction where skin grafts and cartilage can be used to reconstruct lining and framework in a forehead or free radial forearm flap.

- Prefabrication can also be used to create vascular pedicle for a flap subsequent to transfer by transposing an adjacent artery and vein into the area of flap design. This technique is named *prelamination* and is unreliable.

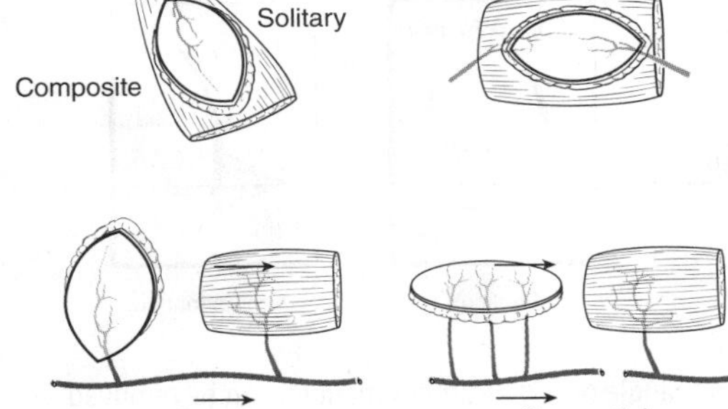


**Fig. 4-8** Compound flaps can be classified based on solitary or combined vascularity.

## Method of Movement

- **Local flaps:** Adjacent tissue used to close defects that are large and require significant tension to close
  - **Advancement flaps:** Unidirectional tissue advancement into a defect by stretching the skin, without rotation or lateral movement (Fig. 4-9)
    - Single-pedicle advancement
    - Double-pedicle advancement (always design and elevate the first flap completely to verify necessity of second flap before incising)
    - V-Y advancement (Fig. 4-10)

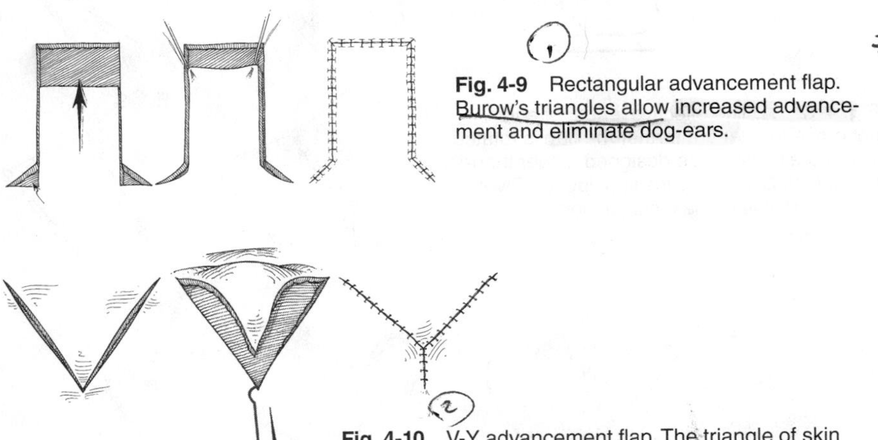

**Fig. 4-9** Rectangular advancement flap. Burow's triangles allow increased advancement and eliminate dog-ears.

**Fig. 4-10** V-Y advancement flap. The triangle of skin should have a length 2-3 times the diameter of the primary defect and a width equal to the greatest width of the primary defect.

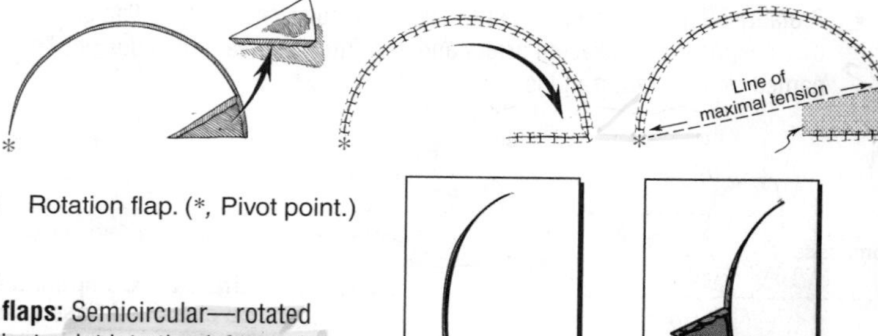


Fig. 4-11 Rotation flap. (*, Pivot point.)

- **Rotation flaps:** Semicircular—rotated about a pivot point into the defect to be closed (Fig. 4-11)
  - Donor site can be closed primarily or with a skin graft.
  - To facilitate rotation, the base can be back-cut at the pivot point, or a triangle of skin (Burow's triangle) can be removed **external** to the pivot point.
- **Transposition flaps:** Rotated laterally about a pivot point into an immediately adjacent defect
  - **Effective length of the flap becomes shorter the farther the flap is rotated;** therefore the flap must be designed longer than the defect to be covered, otherwise a back-cut may be necessary (Fig. 4-12).
  - Donor site can be closed by skin graft, direct suture, or secondary flap (e.g., bilobed flap) (Fig. 4-13).

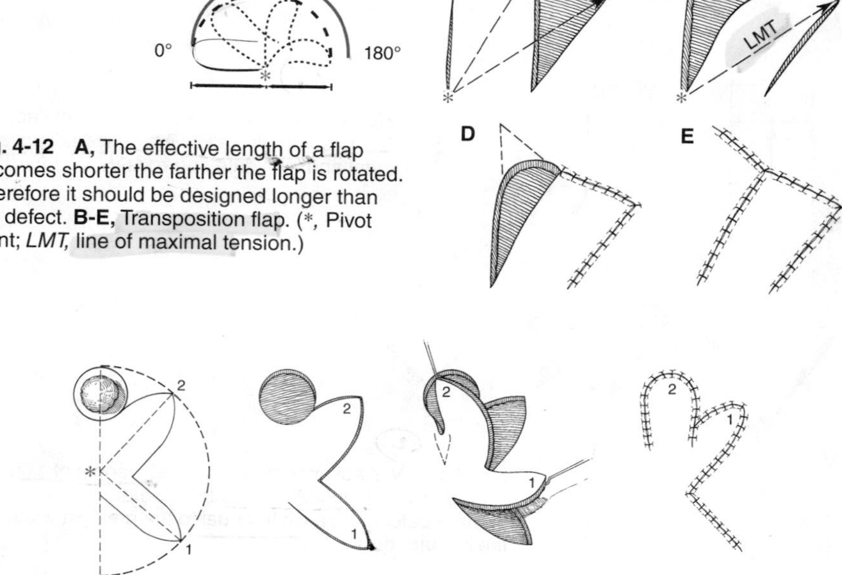


**Fig. 4-12 A,** The effective length of a flap becomes shorter the farther the flap is rotated. Therefore it should be designed longer than the defect. **B-E,** Transposition flap. (*, Pivot point; *LMT,* line of maximal tension.)

**Fig. 4-13** Bilobed flap. (*, Pivot point.)

- Z-plasty is a variation of the transposition flap in which two adjacent triangular flaps are reversed.
  - **The three limbs of the Z must be of equal length, and the two lateral-limb to central-limb angles should be equivalent.**
  - Gain in length is related to the angles between the central and lateral limbs[29] (Table 4-1).

> **TIP:** The 60-degree Z-plasty is most effective, because it lengthens the central limb without placing too much tension laterally (Fig. 4-14).

**Table 4-1** *Theoretical Gain in Length of the Central Limb With Various Angles in Z-Plasty*

| Angle of Each Lateral Limb of Z-Plasty (Degrees) | Theoretical Gain in Length of Central Limb (%) |
|---|---|
| 30 | 25 |
| 45 | 50 |
| 60 | 75 |
| 75 | 100 |
| 90 | 120 |

- Gain in central limb length is estimated to be 55%-84% of predicted and varies with local skin tension.[30]
- Multiple Z-plasties can be designed in series, but the geometry of one large Z-plasty is more effective for achieving skin lengthening.[31]
- Curvilinear modification of the Z-plasty using double opposing semicircular flaps can close circular defects[32] (Fig. 4-15).

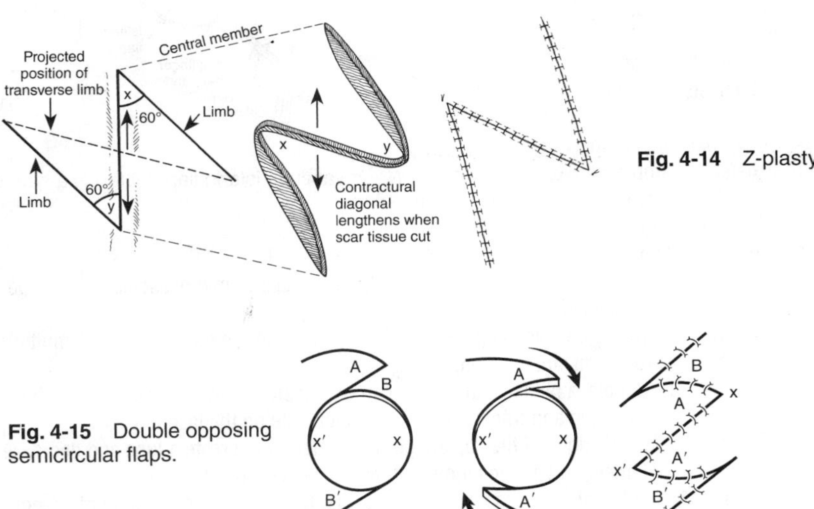


**Fig. 4-14** Z-plasty.

**Fig. 4-15** Double opposing semicircular flaps.

- **Rhomboid (Limberg) flap** is a variation of the transposition flap in which the longitudinal axis of the rhomboid excision parallels the line of minimal skin tension.
  - Rhomboid defect must have **60-degree** and **120-degree** angles (Fig. 4-16).
  - Technique can be expanded to create a double or triple rhomboid flap.
- **Dufourmentel flap** is similar to the rhomboid flap but can be drawn with angles up to 90 degrees.

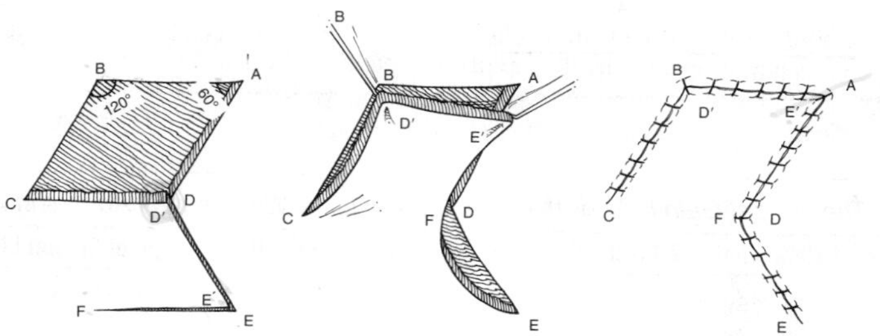


**Fig. 4-16** Rhomboid (Limberg) flap.

- **Interpolation flaps:** Rotate on a pivot point into a defect that is near but not adjacent to the donor site—flap pedicle must pass over or under intervening tissue. Examples:
  - Deltopectoral (Bakamjian) flap
  - Island flaps such as the Littler neurovascular digital pulp flap[1] (Fig. 4-17)
- **Distant flaps:** Donor and recipient sites not close to one another
  - Direct flaps can be used when the donor site can be approximated to the defect. Examples:
    - Thenar flap
    - Cross-leg flap
    - Groin flap

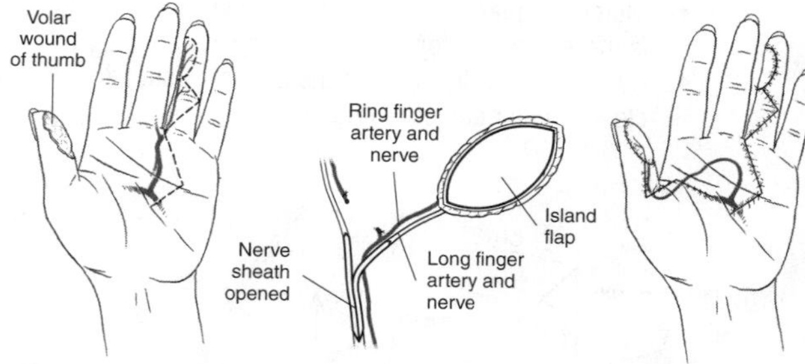


**Fig. 4-17** Neurovascular island flap (Littler) is a type of interpolation flap.

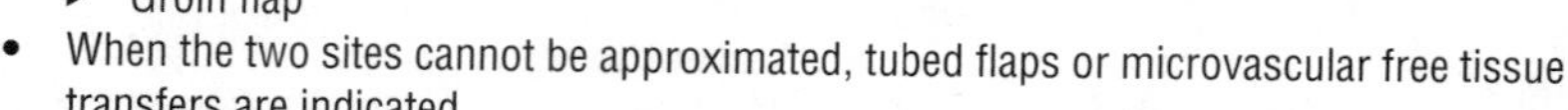

  - When the two sites cannot be approximated, tubed flaps or microvascular free tissue transfers are indicated.
    - Tubed flaps are pedicled flaps that can be "walked" to the recipient site, in multiple stages, from a distant location.
      - For example, a pedicled groin flap can be transferred to the forearm, and then later it can be divided and transferred to a recipient site on the face.
      - The lateral edges of the flap are sutured together to create a tube and decrease the risk of infection and the amount of raw surface exposed.
    - Free tissue transfer moves a unit of tissue that has a pedicle consisting of a feeding artery and a draining vein. The pedicle is anastomosed to an artery and vein at the recipient site to reestablish blood flow to the unit of tissue.

# FLAP PHYSIOLOGY

## Regulation of Blood Flow to Skin

- Systemic and local factors regulate cutaneous blood flow at the level of microcirculation.[33]
- **Systemic control**
  - **Neural regulation:** Occurs primarily through sympathetic adrenergic fibers.
    - Alpha-adrenergic receptors: Vasoconstriction
      Beta-adrenergic receptors: Vasodilation.
    - Sympathetic adrenergic fibers: Maintain basal tone of vascular smooth muscle at the arteriovenous anastomoses, arterioles, and arteries.
    - Cholinergic fibers: Bradykinin release → vasodilation.
  - Humoral regulation
    - **Mediators of vasoconstriction**
      - Epinephrine
      - Norepinephrine
      - Serotonin
      - Thromboxane $A_2$
      - Prostaglandin $F_{2\alpha}$
    - **Mediators of vasodilation**
      - Bradykinin
      - Histamine
      - Prostaglandin-$E_1$
- **Local control (autoregulation)**
  - **Metabolic factors** (act primarily as vasodilators)
    - Hypercapnia
    - Hypoxia
    - Acidosis
    - Hyperkalemia
  - Physical factors
    - Myogenic reflex triggers vasoconstriction in response to distention of isolated cutaneous vessels and maintains capillary flow at a constant level, independent of arterial pressure.
    - Local hypothermia (which acts directly on the smooth muscle in vessel walls) decreases flow.
    - Increased blood viscosity (hematocrit >45%) decreases flow.
- **Differences in blood flow regulation for skin and muscle** (Table 4-2).

**Table 4-2** *Differences in Blood Flow Regulation for Skin and Muscle*

| | Skin | Muscle |
|---|---|---|
| **Neuronal Control** | | |
| Sympathetic vasoconstriction | Most important | Less important |
| **Humoral Control** | | |
| Epinephrine | Vasoconstriction | Vasodilation |
| **Metabolic Factors** | | |
| Autoregulation | Important | Most important |
| **Physical Factors** | | |
| Temperature | Important | Not important |
| Myogenic tone | Less important | More important |

### Flap Transfer

- **Elevating a skin flap disrupts the equilibrium of homeostasis through:**
  - Loss of sympathetic innervation
  - Ischemia
  - Change from aerobic to anaerobic metabolism
  - Increased lactate production
  - Increased levels of superoxide radicals
  - Changes in blood viscosity and clotting
- **Ischemia-induced reperfusion injury (IIRI):** Direct cytotoxic injury results from accumulation of oxygen-derived free radicals during flap ischemia. After reperfusion, the free radicals are attacked by free radical scavengers, causing further injury to the cells.
  - The transition from normal reperfusion to reperfusion injury differs according to tissue type.
  - Skin and bone can usually tolerate ischemia for up to 3 hours, but muscle and intestinal mucosa are much less tolerant.[34]

## FLAP DELAY

*The surgical interruption of a portion of the blood supply to a flap at a preliminary stage before transfer*

- **Purpose:** To increase the surviving length of a flap or to improve the circulation of a flap and diminish the insult of transfer.
- **Two theories**
  1. The delay conditions tissue to ischemia, allowing it to survive on less nutrient blood flow than normally needed.
  2. The delay improves or increases vascularity through the dilation of choke vessels connecting adjacent vascular territories.
- Contribution to flap survival is likely a combination of both mechanisms acting to a greater or lesser extent at various times during surgical delay.
- **Five mechanisms of delay**
  1. Sympathectomy
  2. Vascular reorganization
  3. Reactive hyperemia
  4. Acclimatization to hypoxia
  5. Nonspecific inflammatory reaction
- **Timing of delay**
  - Flaps can be divided as early as the third day after delay in animal models; however, the clinical delay period should be lengthened to suit specific anatomy, expected flap viability, and characteristics of the recipient site.
- Most flaps can be divided safely at **10 days to 3 weeks.**
- *Tissue expansion is a form of delay that has histologic features similar to incisional delay.*

## FLAP CHOICE[35,36] (Box 4-6)

- The goals of surgical reconstruction are preservation and restoration of form and function while minimizing morbidity.
- An optimal reconstructive solution can be designed through a systematic analysis of the following:
  - Wound defect
  - Medical and functional status of the patient
  - Available reconstructive options

**Box 4-6** *CONSIDERATIONS IN FLAP SELECTION*

| Patient Factors | Local Factors | Flap Factors |
|---|---|---|
| Medical comorbidities<br>Concurrent adjuvant therapy<br>Ability to undergo surgery<br>Willingness to accept scars<br>Desired recovery time<br>Patient reliability | Location on the body<br>Previous surgery<br>Previous or anticipated radiation therapy<br>Tissue quality<br>Local tissue availability | Surface area and volume<br>Color and texture match<br>Component parts (muscle, skin, fascia, bone)<br>Pedicle length<br>Arc of rotation<br>Need for sensibility<br>Need for function (functional muscle, toe transfer)<br>Special characteristics (hair, mucosa) |

## Defect Analysis

- Location
- Size and surface area of wound after adequate debridement
- Tissue components missing or exposed in defect (e.g., skin, hair, mucosa, subcutaneous tissue, muscle, vessels, nerves, cartilage, bone)
  - Which components need to be replaced?
  - Which components can feasibly be replaced?
- Vascular status of wound
  - Presence of vascular disease
  - Evaluation of zone of injury (trauma)
  - Adequate microcirculation to support grafts or local flaps
  - Suitable recipient vessels available for free tissue transfer
  - Previous radiation
  - Previous surgery or trauma
- Infection and bacteriology of wound
- Future management concerns (e.g., need for postoperative radiation, future surgical needs)

## Patient Factors

- Reconstructing wounds that are not life threatening is secondary to treating any vital organ system dysfunction.
- Conditions that influence the safety and success of reconstructive options:
  - Diabetes
  - Peripheral vascular disease
  - Hypertension
  - Obesity
  - Hematologic disorders
  - Immunosuppression
  - Pulmonary dysfunction
  - Tobacco use
- Functional status, lifestyle, and rehabilitative capacity of the patient also require consideration.
- Complex reconstruction may be questionable in a patient with a limited life expectancy or with central nervous system dysfunction.
- The sacrifice of specific muscles for flap coverage affects individuals differently, depending on other disabilities present (e.g., paraplegia) or their occupation and lifestyle (e.g., professional athlete versus accountant).

## Reconstructive Options

- Reconstructive ladder (Fig. 4-18)
  - A useful paradigm that organizes reconstructive solutions by complexity[37]
  - Systematic consideration of the most simple to the most complex solution
  - Primary closure
  - Healing by secondary intention
  - Negative pressure wound therapy
  - Skin graft
  - Dermal matrices
  - Local flap
  - Regional flap
  - Distant flap
  - Tissue expansion
  - Free tissue transfer

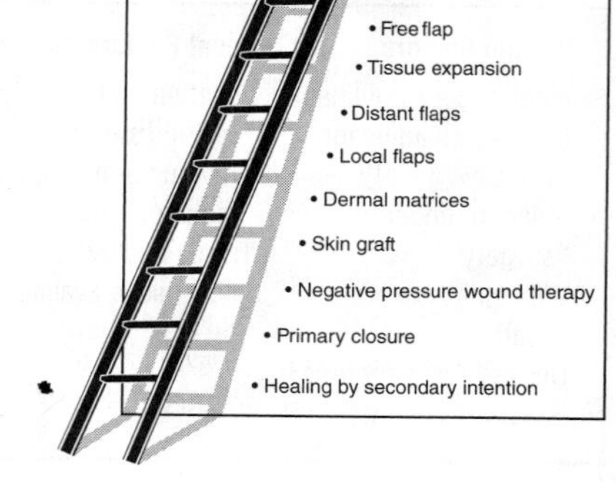


**Fig. 4-18** A new reconstruction ladder.

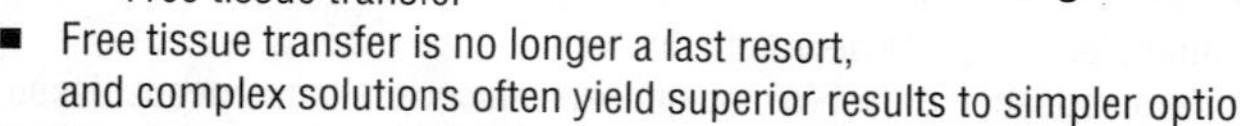

- Free tissue transfer is no longer a last resort, and complex solutions often yield superior results to simpler options.
- Tissue expansion, prefabrication, and composite flaps enable surgeons to optimize the balance between donor site preservation and restoration of defect form and function.

# FLAP SURVIVAL

## Physical Factors

- Physical factors that have experimentally demonstrated a survival advantage include[38-40]:
  - Maintenance of a moist environment along flap edges
  - Avoidance of local hypothermia

## Pharmacologic Factors

- **Anticoagulants**
  - **Dextran**
    - Originally designed as a volume expander
    - Effects:
      - Decreased platelet adhesiveness and procoagulant activity
      - Inhibition of platelet aggregation
      - Increased bleeding time
      - Decreased blood viscosity
    - Has been shown to improve short-term microcirculatory patency[41-43]
    - Associated with significant systemic morbidity, including:
      - Anaphylaxis
      - Pulmonary edema
      - Cardiac complications
      - Adult respiratory distress syndrome
      - Renal failure
    - Routine use in free tissue transfer is discouraged[44,45]
  - **Heparin**
    - Anticoagulant
    - Acts in conjunction with antithrombin III to inhibit thrombosis by inactivation of factor X
    - More effective at preventing venous thrombosis than arterial thrombosis

        - Both unfractionated and low-molecular-weight heparin (LMWH) improve microcirculatory perfusion, but only LMWH has been shown to improve anastomotic patency while minimizing hemorrhage.[46]
    - **Thrombolytic agents**
        - Stimulates the conversion of plasminogen to plasmin, which acts to cleave fibrin within a thrombus
        - First generation agents
            - Streptokinase
            - Urokinase
        - Second generation agents
            - Tissue plasminogen activator (t-PA)
            - Acylated plasminogen-streptokinase activator complex (APSAC)
        - Have been effective in salvaging flaps after microvascular thrombosis[47,48]
    - **Medicinal leeches** *(Hirudo medicinalis)*
        - Exert their effect by injecting **hirudin** at the site of bite.
            - *Hirudin:* A naturally occurring anticoagulant that inhibits the conversion of fibrin to fibrinogen, but, unlike heparin, does not require antithrombin III for activation
        - Also secrete[49]:
            - Hyaluronidase: Facilitates spread of the anticoagulant within the tissues.
            - A vasodilator: Contributes to prolonged bleeding (up to 48 hours).
        - Mechanical effect of creating physical channels through which venous drainage can occur
        - Risks:
            - Bacterial infection from the gram-negative rod *Aeromonas hydrophila*
            - Anaphylaxis
            - Persistent bleeding
            - Excessive scarring
        - Use of antibiotic prophylaxis against *Aeromonas hydrophila* recommended
            - Fluoroquinolones
            - Resistance to amoxicillin/clavulanate and all generations of cephalosporins reported
- **Vasodilators**
    - **Calcium-channel blockers**
        - Act on the vascular smooth muscles
        - Increased flap survival in experimental models after topical and intravenous administration
        - No clinical evidence to support use
    - **Topical nitroglycerin**
        - Potent vasodilator with a greater effect on venous circulation than arterial
        - Improved survival of axial flaps reported from treatment with transdermal nitroglycerin[50]
    - **Topical lidocaine and pentobarbital**
        - Inhibit endothelium-dependent relaxation on the vascular smooth muscle[51]
        - Have demonstrated effective resolution of mechanically induced vasospasm
- **Anti-inflammatory agents**
    - Steroids
        - Increased flap survival in some experimental models, but no evidence to support clinical use of corticosteroids to enhance flap viability
    - **Aspirin (ASA)**
        - Aspirin acetylates the enzyme cyclooxygenase, thereby decreasing the synthesis of thromboxane $A_2$ ($TxA_2$), a potent vasoconstrictor in platelets, and prostacyclin ($PGI_2$), a potent vasodilator in vessel walls.

- At low doses the effect of aspirin is selective, and only the cyclooxygenase system in platelets is inhibited, blocking the formation of thromboxane.
- Experimentally, preoperative aspirin decreases thrombus formation at venous anastomoses and improves capillary perfusion in the microcirculation.[52]
- Studies demonstrate increased early anastomotic patency, but there is no difference from controls after 24 hours to 1 week.[34]
- There is no empiric evidence in the literature for using aspirin postoperatively.[34]

**CAUTION: Acute exposure of human skin vasculature to nicotine is associated with amplification of norepinephrine-induced skin vasoconstriction and impaired of endothelium-dependent skin vasorelaxation.[53]**

## Flap Monitoring

- Strict evaluation of flap perfusion is essential to prevent, recognize, and treat complications.
- **Venous insufficiency is the most common cause of flap failure.**
- The failure rate of free tissue transfer is reported to be less than 5%. However, the incidence of pedicle thrombosis is higher than the failure rate reflects, because the salvage rate after pedicle thrombosis ranges from 36% to 70%.[48]
- Because of more successful salvage within the first 24 hours after initial surgery, hourly monitoring is recommended for the first 24 hours and then every 4 hours for 48 hours.[54]

## Subjective and Physical Criteria

- **Clinical observation remains the most effective method of flap monitoring.**
  - Subjective evaluation of flap viability by color, capillary blanching, and warmth can be unreliable.[1]
  - Bleeding from a stab wound is the most accurate clinical test.
  - Clinical signs can be used to differentiate venous from arterial insufficiency in flaps[55] (Table 4-3).
- **Temperature monitoring can be accomplished by measuring surface temperature and differential thermometry.**
  - Surface temperature is clinically useful for monitoring extrinsic complications but is an inadequate indicator of intrinsic flap failure.
  - Differential thermometry is useful for monitoring vascular patency in buried free tissue transfers for which a temperature gradient exceeding **3° C** is considered significant.[1]

**Table 4-3** *Signs of Arterial Occlusion and Venous Congestion*

| | Arterial Occlusion | Venous Congestion |
|---|---|---|
| **Skin color** | Pale, mottled, bluish, or white | Cyanotic, bluish, or dusky |
| **Capillary refill** | Sluggish | Brisker than normal |
| **Tissue turgor** | Prunelike; turgor decreased | Tense, swollen; turgor increased |
| **Dermal bleeding** | Scant amount of dark blood or serum | Rapid bleeding of dark blood |
| **Temperature** | Cool | Cool |

## Vital Dye Measurements

- Fluorescein is reported to be more than 70% accurate as an indicator of circulatory status of a flap.[56]
  - Fluorescein is usually given as a bolus injection of 500 to 1000 mg (15 mg/kg).
  - After waiting 20-30 minutes, the extent of dye staining in tissues that are adequately perfused can be seen with a Wood's lamp.
  - **Indocyanine green** (Spy Elite, LifeCell, Branchburg, NJ)
    - Helps identify zones of perfusion before commiting to flap design.

## Photoelectric Assessment[57]

- **Two types of Doppler instruments currently in clinical use**
  1. **Ultrasound Doppler** uses reflected sound to pick up pulsatile vessels.
  2. **Laser Doppler** measures the frequency shift of light and therefore has limited penetration (1.5 mm).
- **Advantages of Doppler probing**
  - High reliability (approaching 100% at 24 hours after flap transfer)
  - Continuous monitoring by a noninvasive technique
- **Disadvantages of Doppler probing**
  - Not quantitative
  - Obtains information from a single site
  - Sensitive to movement of the subject
  - Limited accuracy below the critical threshold at which tissue necrosis is guaranteed

## Metabolic

- *Transcutaneous oxygen tension* measures the partial-pressure of oxygen and has been shown to be an accurate predictor of the effectiveness of delay procedures.[58]
- *Photoplethysmography* measures fluid volume by detecting variations in infrared light absorption by the skin.
  - A *pulse oximeter* displays photoplethysmographic waveforms and measures light absorption to derive oxygen saturation of arterial hemoglobin.
  - This method has been inaccurate and disappointing in clinical settings.[1]

## Key Points

✓ Vascularity is the most valid method of flap classification, because it is the most critical determinant of successful flap transfer.

✓ The fasciocutaneous plexus is an intercommunicating network between the deep fascia and the dermis fed by different configurations of deep fascial perforators.

✓ All skin and fascial flaps are supplied by the fasciocutaneous plexus. Inclusion of the deep fascia is not required for the survival of cutaneous or fasciocutaneous flaps.

✓ Anastomotic connections between valvular veins (venae comitantes) and avalvular oscillating veins permit reversal of flow in distally based flaps.

✓ Myocutaneous flaps exhibit more collagen deposition and are more resistant to infection than fasciocutaneous flaps.

✓ Muscle flaps with a segmental vascular pattern (type IV) have the most limited arc of rotation and are the least reliable for transfer (e.g., the sartorius muscle).

✓ The sympathetic nervous system is the most important factor for regulating blood flow to the skin.

✓ Metabolic autoregulation plays a more important role for regulating blood flow to muscle because muscle has a higher metabolic demand than skin.

✓ Venous insufficiency is the most common cause of flap failure.

✓ Clinical observation is the most effective method of flap monitoring.

## REFERENCES


1. Daniel RK, Kerrigan CL. Principles and physiology of skin flap surgery. In McCarthy JG, ed. Plastic Surgery, vol 1. Philadelphia: Saunders, 1990.
2. Taylor GI, Palmer JH. The vascular territories (angiosomes) of the body: experimental study and clinical applications. Br J Plast Surg 40:113, 1987.
3. Taylor G. The blood supply to the skin. In Aston SJ, Beasley RW, Thorne CH, et al, eds. Grabb and Smith's Plastic Surgery, 5th ed. Philadelphia: Lippincott-Raven, 1997.
4. Nakajima H, Fujino T, Adachi S. A new concept of vascular supply to the skin and classification of skin flaps according to their vascularization. Ann Plast Surg 16:1, 1986.
5. Taylor GI, Caddy CM, Watterson PA, et al. The venous territories (venosomes) of the human body: experimental study and clinical implications. Plast Reconstr Surg 86:185, 1990.
6. McGregor IA, Morgan G. Axial and random pattern flaps. Br J Plast Surg 26:202, 1973.
7. Hallock G. Direct and indirect perforator flaps: the history and the controversy. Plast Reconstr Surg 111:855, 2003.
8. Geddes CR, Morris SF, Neligan PC. Perforator flaps: evolution, classification, and applications. Ann Plast Surg 50:90, 2003.
9. Nahabedian MY, Momen B, Galdino G, et al. Breast reconstruction with the free TRAM or DIEP flap: patient selection, choice of flap, and outcome. Plast Reconstr Surg 110:466, 2002.
10. Celik N, Wei FC, Lin CH, et al. Technique and strategy in anterolateral thigh perforator flap surgery, based on an analysis of 15 complete and partial failures in 439 cases. Plast Reconstr Surg 109:2211, 2002.
11. Chen HC, Tang YB. Anterolateral thigh flap: an ideal soft tissue flap. Clin Plast Surg 30:383, 2003.
12. Kimata Y, Uchiyama K, Ebihara S, et al. Anatomic variations and technical problems of the anterolateral thigh flap: a report of 74 cases. Plast Reconstr Surg 102:1517, 1998.
13. Craigie JE, Allen RJ, DellaCroce FJ, et al. Autogenous breast reconstruction with the deep inferior epigastric perforator flap. Clin Plast Surg 30:359, 2003.
14. Kroll SS. Fat necrosis in free transverse rectus abdominis myocutaneous and deep inferior epigastric perforator flaps. Plast Reconstr Surg 106:576, 2000.
15. Blondeel PN, Van Landuyt K, Hamdi M, et al. Perforator flap terminology: update 2002. Clin Plast Surg 30:343, 2003.
16. Masquelet AC, Romana MC, Wolf G. Skin island flaps supplied by the vascular axis of the sensitive superficial nerves: anatomic study and clinical experience in the leg. Plast Reconstr Surg 89:1115, 1992.
17. Nakajima H, Imanishi N, Fukuzumi S, et al. Accompanying arteries of the cutaneous veins and cutaneous nerves in the extremities: anatomical study and a concept of the venoadipofascial and/or neuroadipofascial pedicled fasciocutaneous flap. Plast Reconstr Surg 102:779, 1998.
18. Thornton JT, Gosman AA. Skin grafts and skin substitutes and principles of flaps. Sel Read Plast Surg 10(1), 2004.
19. De Lorenzi F, van der Hulst R, den Dunnen WFA, et al. Arterialized venous free flaps for soft-tissue reconstruction of digits: a 40-case series. J Reconstr Microsurg 18:569, 2002.
20. Koshima I, Soeda S, Nakayama Y, et al. An arterialised venous flap using the long saphenous vein. Br J Plast Surg 44:23, 1991.
21. Inoue G, Suzuki K. Arterialized venous flap for treating multiple skin defects of the hand. Plast Reconstr Surg 91:299, 1993.
22. Lee W. Discussion of "Arterialized venous flap for treating multiple skin defects of the hand," by G. Inoue and K. Suzuki. Plast Reconstr Surg 91:303, 1993.
23. Thatte MR, Thatte RL. Venous flaps. Plast Reconstr Surg 91:747, 1993.
24. Mathes SJ. Clinical Applications for Muscle and Myocutaneous Flaps. St Louis: Mosby, 1981.

25. Gosain A, Chang N, Mathes S, et al. A study of the relationship between blood flow and bacterial inoculation in musculocutaneous and fasciocutaneous flaps. Plast Reconstr Surg 86:1152, 1990.
26. Calderon W, Chang N, Mathes SJ. Comparison of the effect of bacterial inoculation in musculocutaneous and fasciocutaneous flaps. Plast Reconstr Surg 77:785, 1986.
27. Mathes SJ, Nahai F. Classification of the vascular anatomy of muscles: experimental and clinical correlation. Plast Reconstr Surg 67:177, 1981.
28. Hallock G. Simplified nomenclature for compound flaps. Plast Reconstr Surg 105:1465, 2000.
29. Rohrich RJ, Zbar PI. A simplified algorithm for the use of Z-plasty. Plast Reconstr Surg 103:1513, 1999.
30. Furnas DW, Fischer GW. The Z-plasty: biomechanics and mathematics. Br J Plast Surg 24:144, 1971.
31. Seyhan A. A V-shaped ruler to detect the largest transposable Z-plasty. Plast Reconstr Surg 101:870, 1994.
32. Keser A, Sensoz O, Mengi AS. Double opposing semicircular flap: a modification of opposing Z-plasty for closing circular defects. Plast Reconstr Surg 102:1001, 1998.
33. Daniel RK, Kerrigan CL. Skin flaps: an anatomical and hemodynamic approach. Clin Plast Surg 6:181, 1979.
34. Carroll WR, Esclamado RM. Ischemia/reperfusion injury in microvascular surgery. Head Neck 22:700, 2000.
35. Hoopes JE. Pedicle flaps: an overview. In Hoopes JE, Krizek TJ, eds. Symposium on Basic Science in Plastic Surgery. St Louis: Mosby, 1976.
36. Zenn MR, Jones G. Reconstructive Surgery: Anatomy, Technique, & Clinical Application. St Louis: Quality Medical Publishing, 2012.
37. Janis JE, Kwon RK, Attinger CE. The new reconstructive ladder: modifications to the traditional model. Plast Reconstr Surg 127(Suppl 1):205S, 2011.
38. Sasaki A, Fukuda O, Soeda S. Attempts to increase the surviving length in skin flaps by a moist environment. Plast Reconstr Surg 64:526, 1979.
39. McGrath M. How topical dressings salvage "questionable" flaps: experimental study. Plast Reconstr Surg 67:653, 1981.
40. Awwad AM, White RJ, Webster MH, et al. The effect of temperature on blood flow in island and free skin flaps: an experimental study. Br J Plast Surg 36:373, 1983.
41. Rothkopf DM, Chu B, Bern S, et al. The effect of dextran on microvascular thrombosis in an experimental rabbit model. Plast Reconstr Surg 92:511, 1993.
42. Zhang B, Wieslander JB. Improvement of patency in small veins following dextran and/or low-molecular-weight heparin treatment. Plast Reconstr Surg 94:352, 1994.
43. Salemark L, Knudsen F, Dougan P. The effect of dextran 40 on patency following severe trauma in small arteries and veins. Br J Plast Surg 48:121, 1995.
44. Hein KD, Wechsler M, Schwartzstein RM, et al. The adult respiratory distress syndrome after dextran infusion as an antithrombotic agent in free TRAM flap breast reconstruction. Plast Reconstr Surg 103:1706, 1999.
45. Brooks D, Okeefe P, Buncke HJ. Dextran-induced acute renal failure after microvascular muscle transplantation. Plast Reconstr Surg 108:2057, 2001.
46. Ritter EF, Cronan JC, Rudner AM, et al. Improved microsurgical anastomotic patency with low molecular weight heparin. J Reconstr Microsurg 14:331, 1998.
47. Serletti JM, Moran SL, Orlando GS, et al. Urokinase protocol for free-flap salvage following prolonged venous thrombosis. Plast Reconstr Surg 102:1947, 1998.
48. Yii NW, Evans GR, Miller MJ, et al. Thrombolytic therapy: what is its role in free flap salvage? Ann Plast Surg 46:601, 2001.
49. Soucacos PN, Beris AE, Malizos KN, et al. The use of medicinal leeches, *Hirudo medicinalis,* to restore venous circulation in trauma and reconstructive surgery. Int Angiol 13:251, 1994.

50. Rohrich RJ, Cherry GW, Spira M. Enhancement of skin-flap survival using nitroglycerin ointment. Plast Reconstr Surg 73:943, 1984.
51. Wadstrom J, Gerdin B. Modulatory effects of topically administered lidocaine and pentobarbital on traumatic vasospasm in the rabbit ear artery. Br J Plast Surg 44:341, 1991.
52. Peter FW, Franken RJ, Wang WZ, et al. Effect of low dose aspirin on thrombus formation at arterial and venous microanastomoses and on the tissue microcirculation. Plast Reconstr Surg 99:1112, 1997.
53. Black CE, Huang N, Neligan PC, et al. Effect of nicotine on vasoconstrictor and vasodilator responses in human skin vasculature. Am J Physiol Regul Integr Comp Physiol 281:R1097, 2001.
54. Brown JS, Devine JC, Magennis P, et al. Factors that influence the outcome of salvage in free tissue transfer. Br J Oral Maxillofac Surg 41:16, 2003.
55. Adams JF, Lassen LF. Leech therapy for venous congestion following myocutaneous pectoralis flap reconstruction. ORL Head Neck Nurs 13:12, 1995.
56. Lange K, Boyd LJ. The use of fluorescein to determine the adequacy of the circulation. Med Clin North Am 26:943, 1942.
57. Hallock GG, Altobelli JA. Assessment of TRAM flap perfusion using laser Doppler flowmetry: an adjunct to microvascular augmentation. Ann Plast Surg 29:122, 1992.
58. Tsur H, Orenstein A, Mazkereth R. The use of transcutaneous oxygen pressure measurement in flap surgery. Ann Plast Surg 8:510, 1982.

# 5. Fundamentals of Perforator Flaps

**Brian P. Bradow**

*"Just what constitutes a perforator flap can be an enigma, but most of us know it when we see it."*

**G.G. Hallock**

## DEFINITIONS

A **perforator flap** is a vascularized area of skin and/or subcutaneous tissue that receives its blood supply from one or more blood vessels or *perforators* originating from a named source vessel below the deep fascia (Fig. 5-1) (Table 5-1).[1,2] These vessels course, directly or indirectly, to the deep fascia, which they cross en route to the subdermal plexus and respective superficial target tissue (the *perforasome*).

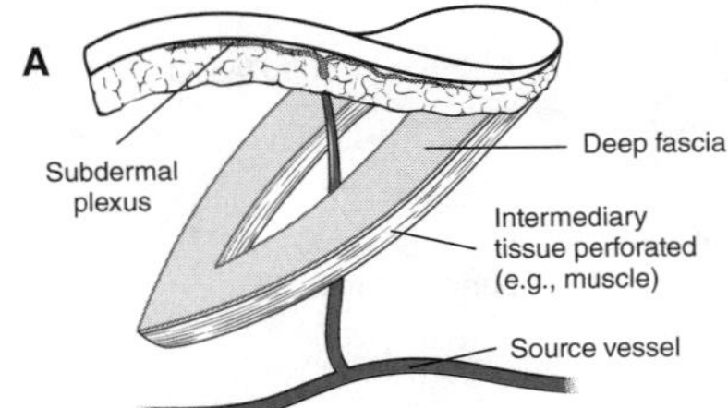


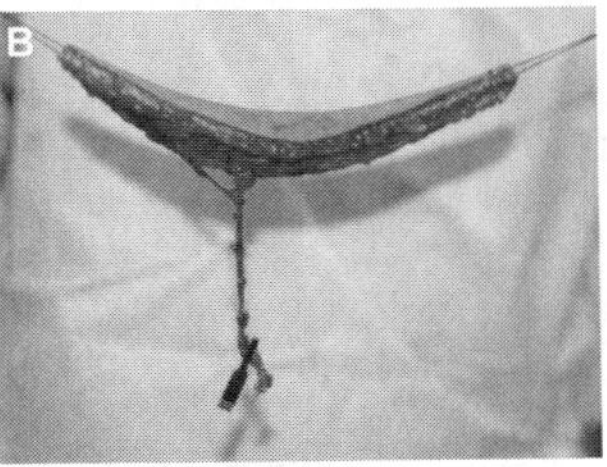


**Fig. 5-1 A,** Common perforator flap (myocutaneous type). **B,** Harvested perforator flap. Notice that the perforating vessel has been released from the source vessel and intermediary tissue (e.g., muscle).

**Table 5-1** *Pros and Cons of Perforator and Muscle Flaps*

| | Perforator Flaps | Muscle Flaps |
|---|---|---|
| Accessibility | + | − |
| Anatomic anomalies | − | + |
| Availability | + | − |
| Composite flaps | ± | + |
| Use in infected or irradiated wound | ± | + |
| Donor site morbidity | − | + |
| Dynamic transfer | − | + |
| Expendable | + | − |
| Malleability | − | + |

+, Asset; −, detriment; =, no significant difference; ±, variable.

*Continued*

**Table 5-1** *Pros and Cons of Perforator and Muscle Flaps—cont'd*

| | Perforator Flaps | Muscle Flaps |
|---|---|---|
| Microsurgical tissue transfer | = | = |
| Reliability | = | = |
| Sensate | + | − |
| Size | + | ± |
| Thinness | ± | + |
| Recovery time | + | − |
| Fat necrosis | − | ± |

+, Asset; −, detriment; =, no significant difference; ±, variable.

## Direct Perforator (Figs. 5-2 and 5-3)

A **direct perforator** originates from the source artery and pierces the deep fascia without traversing any deeper structures.

- ***Direct cutaneous:*** Branches from the source artery directly to the skin
- ***Septocutaneous:*** Traverses the septa between muscles en route to the skin

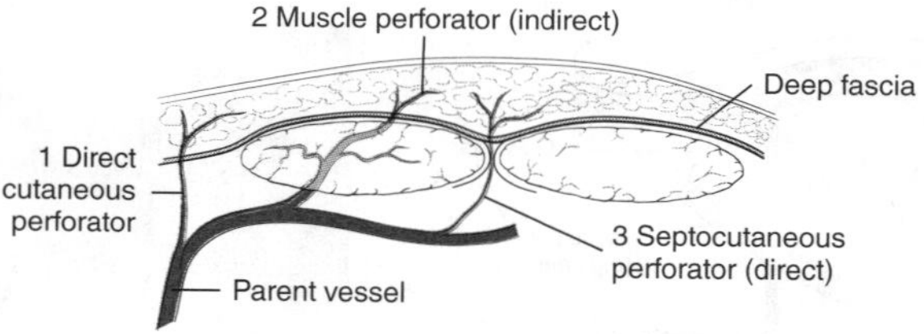


**Fig. 5-2** Basic types of direct and indirect perforator vessels. *1, Direct perforator* perforating the deep fascia only. *2, Indirect muscle perforator* passing through muscle before piercing the deep fascia. *3, Direct septal perforator* traveling between the intermuscular septum before piercing the deep fascia.

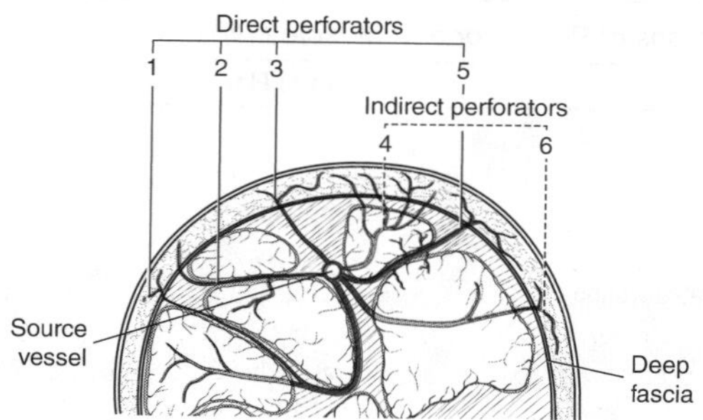


**Fig. 5-3** The classic six distinct types of deep fascia perforators originally described by Nakajima.[4]

## Indirect Perforator (see Figs. 5-2 and 5-3)

An **indirect perforator** passes through an intermediary structure before crossing the deep fascia en route to the skin.

- **Musculocutaneous/myocutaneous type:** Travels through muscle
  - Most common
- **Other intermediate tissues**[3-5]
  - Nerve
  - Vein
  - Bone/periosteum
  - Tendon
  - Gland
- **Flap dissection**
  - Goal is to free perforating vessel(s) from intermediate tissue
    - This may not always be possible, or even desired
      - Danger of injuring the vessel(s)
      - Tenuous blood supply to flap
      - Risk of defunctionalizing the intermediate tissue
      - Scarring (such as from previous radiation)
      - Need for a bulkier flap
- **Controversy**
  - Some have argued that indirect perforators are the only true perforators because they actually perforate defined tissue (usually muscle).[6]
  - Direct perforator vessel patterns are still included in most perforator classification systems.

## Perforator and Fasciocutaneous Flaps

- **Clarification**
  - Fasciocutaneous flaps traditionally have included the deep fascia and its associated vascular plexus when elevated.[7]
    - Retention of the fascia theoretically improves vascular reliability and connections to the subcutaneous tissue and skin.
    - The need to include the fascia has been challenged.[8]
  - Both flap types rely on the same supplying vessels (i.e., perforators) that arise from below the deep fascia (see Figs. 5-1 and 5-2), as indicated by the Mathes-Nahai definition of fasciocutaneous flaps[9]:
    - *Type A:* Direct cutaneous
    - *Type B:* Septocutaneous (direct)
    - *Type C:* Myocutaneous (indirect)
  - Harvest
    - Including or excluding the fascia can alter the type of flap raised (e.g., radial forearm)[10]
      - *Fasciocutaneous flap:* Includes deep forearm fascia
      - *Perforator flap:* Same perforators, excludes fascia
    - The deep fascia and adipocutaneous tissue layers are not usually separated in fasciocutaneous flaps as they are in perforator flap dissection (see Fig. 5-1, *A,* where the deep fascia would instead be on the undersurface of the adipocutaneous layer)
      - Quantity, caliber, and location of perforators may not be clear
      - Fasciocutaneous flap dimensions can be more trial and error

**TIP:** The *myocutaneous flap* (or musculocutaneous flap) and its sister, the *myocutaneous perforator flap,* share many, if not all, supplying vessels. They differ only in that the latter involves dissection of the intramuscular perforating vessels from the muscle en route to the skin to preserve muscle function. That is why a deep inferior epigastric artery perforator (DIEP) flap can be converted to a full, or muscle-sparing, free transverse rectus abdominis myocutaneous (TRAM) flap when necessary.

## Angiosomes and Perforasomes

- **Angiosome** (Fig. 5-4)
  - Three-dimensional block of composite tissue, including skin and its underlying tissue, supplied by *all* the perforators of a source artery
  - Approximately 40 described by Taylor in 1987[11,12]
  - Concept now augmented by *perforasome theory*
- **Perforasome**[13] (Fig. 5-5)
  - More than 300 individual perforators have been identified, arising from varying source vessels.
    - Each supplies its own three-dimensional vascular territory (perforasome).
    - A custom flap, free or pedicled, can be elevated on each perforator.

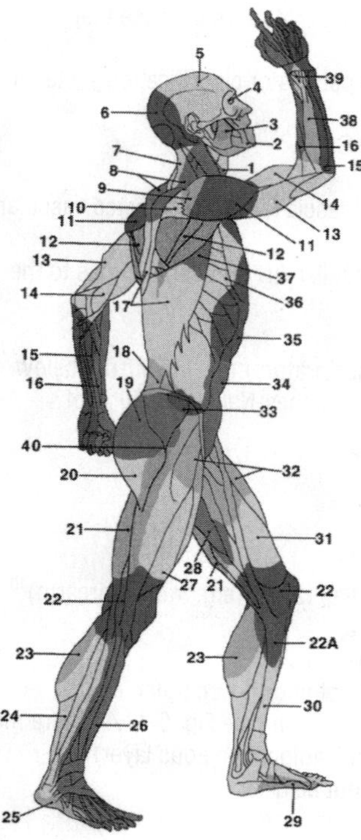


**Fig. 5-4** The angiosomes of the source arteries of the body. *1,* Thyroid; *2,* facial; *3,* buccal internal maxillary; *4,* ophthalmic; *5,* superficial temporal; *6,* occipital; *7,* deep cervical; *8,* transverse cervical; *9,* acromiothoracic; *10,* suprascapular; *11,* posterior circumflex humeral; *12,* circumflex scapular; *13,* profunda brachii; *14,* brachial; *15,* ulnar; *16,* radial; *17,* posterior intercostals; *18,* lumbar; *19,* superior gluteal; *20,* inferior gluteal; *21,* profunda femoris; *22,* popliteal; *22A,* descending geniculate saphenous; *23,* sural; *24,* peroneal; *25,* lateral plantar; *26,* anterior tibial; *27,* lateral femoral circumflex; *28,* adductor profunda; *29,* medial plantar; *30,* posterior tibial; *31,* superficial femoral; *32,* common femoral; *33,* deep circumflex iliac; *34,* deep inferior epigastric; *35,* internal thoracic; *36,* lateral thoracic; *37,* thoracodorsal; *38,* posterior interosseous; *39,* anterior interosseous; 40, internal pudendal.

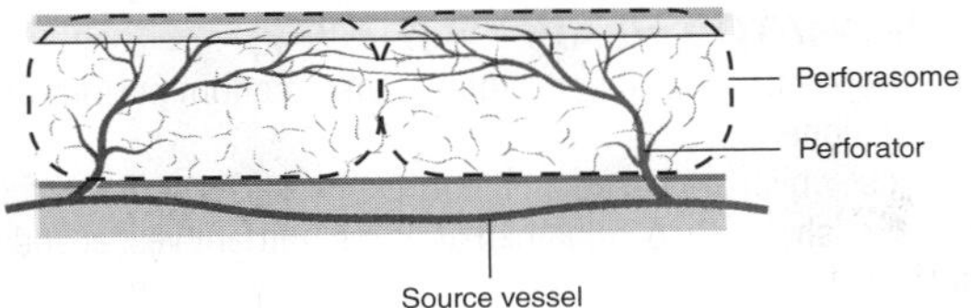


**Fig. 5-5** Perforasome concept. Each perforator originating from the source vessel supplies its own vascular territory *(ellipses).*

- Each perforasome is connected to adjacent ones by linking vessels that are analogous to choke vessels, described by Taylor.[11]
- In essence, multiple perforasomes compose the angiosome of a source vessel.

## CLASSIFICATION

- No universal nomenclature system exists.
- The Gent consensus and Canadian systems are most widely used.
- American, Korean, and other systems also have been proposed.

### Gent Consensus[14]

- Flap named after the nutrient source vessel (e.g., deep inferior epigastric perforator [DIEP] flap)
- When a source vessel can supply more than one flap, the name is based on either:
  - Associated muscle (e.g., tensor fascia lata perforator [TFLP])
  - Anatomic region (e.g., anterior lateral thigh perforator [ALTP])

### Canadian System[1,15] (Fig. 5-6)

- Flap also named after the associated source vessel but with addition of "artery" (e.g., deep inferior epigastric *artery* perforator [DIEAP] flap).
- When the source vessel supplies more than one flap, additional abbreviations are added.
  - *-muscle abbreviation* suffix added (e.g., lateral circumflex femoral artery perforator flap involving the tensor fascia lata [LCFAP-*tfl*])
  - *-s* suffix added if septocutaneous type (e.g., superficial femoral artery perforator [SFAP-*s*])

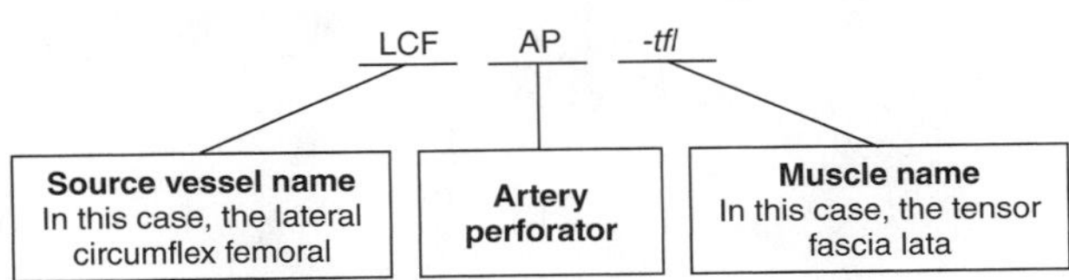


**Fig. 5-6** An example of standardized muscle perforator nomenclature per the Canadian system using the tensor fascia lata.

## Freestyle Perforator Flap[16-19] (Fig. 5-7)

A locoregional adipocutaneous flap raised and centered on a random perforator identified preoperatively by Doppler signal

- Includes propeller flaps, which are based on an off-center perforator (see Fig. 5-7)
- Per the Gent consensus, should also be named after the nutrient vessel and not after the underlying muscle[14]
- Availability and usefulness depends on location and quality of perforator(s) in relationship to defect

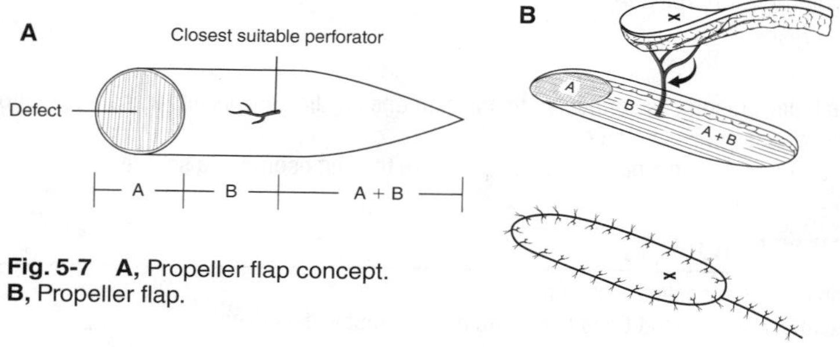


**Fig. 5-7 A,** Propeller flap concept. **B,** Propeller flap.

# COMMON PERFORATOR FLAPS

## Background

- Perforator flaps have become mainstream.[18]
- In addition to free tissue transfer, they are now commonly used as local flaps.
- Of the most popular donor sites, the deep inferior epigastric artery and anterolateral thigh flaps are the most frequently used (Fig. 5-8).[18]

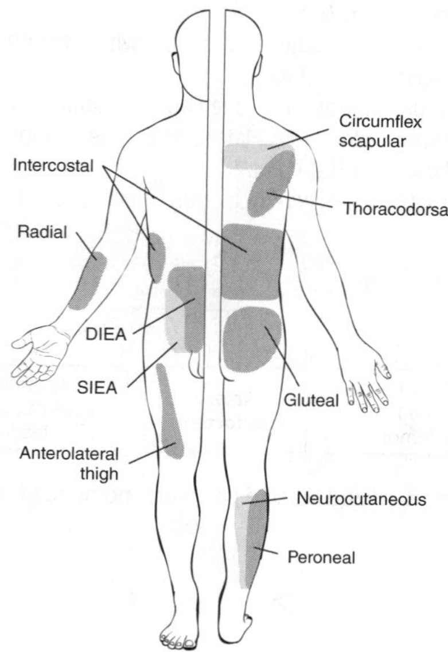


**Fig. 5-8** Ten currently most-used perforator flap donor site regions by source vessel territory.

## ANTERIOR LATERAL THIGH[19-21]

- **Source vessel**
  - Lateral circumflex femoral artery
    - *Descending branch* (dominant): Myocutaneous and/or septocutaneous perforator(s)
    - *Transverse branch* (minor): Myocutaneous perforator(s)
- **Classification**
  - *Gent consensus:* Anterior lateral thigh perforator (ALTP)
  - *Canadian system:* Lateral circumflex femoral artery perforator (LCFAP)
    - *LCFAP-vl:* When the vastus lateralis is perforated (myocutaneous)
    - *LCFAP-s:* When purely septocutaneous type
  - *Mathes & Nahai:* Fasciocutaneous Types A and B
- **Advantages**
  - Favorable donor site (when closed primarily)
  - Relative ease of dissection
  - Long pedicle
  - Small, large (up to 25 × 35 cm), sensate, flow-through, or chimeric flaps possible
  - For additional bulk when needed, vastus lateralis can be included
- **Disadvantages**
  - Unsightly donor site (when not closed primarily)
  - Obese patients
    - Flap thickness variable
    - Intramuscular dissection more difficult
- **Common uses**
  - Locoregional (pedicled) reconstruction
    - Ipsilateral and contralateral groin
    - Posterior trunk, ischium
    - Lower abdomen
    - Scrotum, perineum
    - Pelvic exenteration
    - Lower thigh and knee (reverse flap)
  - Free tissue transfer
    - All areas of the body

## DEEP INFERIOR EPIGASTRIC ARTERY[1]

- **Source vessel**
  - Deep inferior epigastric artery: Myocutaneous perforators
- **Classification**
  - *Gent consensus:* Deep inferior epigastric perforator (DIEP) flap
  - *Canadian system:* Deep inferior epigastric artery perforator (DIEAP) flap
- **Advantages**
  - Favorable donor site
  - Rectus muscle and fascia preserved to maintain abdominal wall integrity
  - Long pedicle
  - Contralateral flap can be lifeboat if only hemiflap elevated
  - Conversion to traditional myocutaneous flap possible when necessary
  - Can supercharge if ipsilateral or contralateral superficial inferior epigastric vessels harvested (i.e., SIEA and SIEV)

- **Disadvantages**
  - Significant anatomic variation from patient to patient and side to side
  - Difficult dissection
    - Large perforators commonly pass through inscriptions of rectus abdominis and/or run intramuscular for some variable length.
    - Wrong choice of perforator(s) can result in partial or full flap loss.
  - Inadequate native connections between the deep and superficial inferior epigastric venous systems may result in vascular compromise (such as venous congestion).
- **Common uses**
  - Locoregional (pedicled) reconstruction
    - Abdomen
    - Genitals
    - Proximal thighs, groin
    - Buttock
  - Free tissue transfer
    - Breast reconstruction most common
    - All areas of the body (but often bulky)

# IMAGING, VASCULAR MAPPING, AND MONITORING

## Preoperative Imaging

- **Doppler** (handheld)
  - Transcutaneous signal(s) of the underlying perforator(s) can often be located easily
  - Useful in flap design (such as in freestyle type)
- **CT angiography**
  - Best method for donor sites of perforator flaps with variable anatomy (e.g., ALT and DIEP)
  - Able to evaluate multiple potential donor sites simultaneously (e.g., DIEP, SGAP)
  - Not essential, especially when handheld Doppler suffices
- **Duplex ultrasonography**
- **MRA**

## Intraoperative Imaging

- **Doppler** (handheld)
- **Indocyanine green** (SPY *Elite,* LifeCell, Branchburg, NJ)
  - Helps identify zones of adequate perfusion before committing to flap design

## Postoperative Monitoring[22]

- **Noninvasive monitoring**
  - Conventional methods (e.g., clinical examination, handheld Doppler)
    - Hands-on flap evaluation is the baseline standard and also serves as the follow-up to any flap concerns arising from other monitoring techniques.
    - Reliability can depend on clinician and frequency.
  - *Laser Doppler flowmetry*
    - Measures blood velocity within tissue
    - High positive and negative predictive values
    - Can be used in combination with tissue spectrometry and temperature sensors
    - Sensitive to vibration and motion of the tissue/probe
    - Limited tissue penetration
    - Moderately expensive

- *Tissue oximetry* (e.g., the T.Ox Tissue Oximeter, ViOptix, Fremont, CA)
    - Utilizes near-infrared spectroscopy
    - Early detection of flow failure
    - Higher tissue penetration than laser Doppler
    - High positive and negative predictive values
    - Smart phone monitoring via Wi-Fi
    - Expensive
    - Requires adequate skin paddle

- **Invasive monitoring**
    - *Implantable Doppler*
        - Easy to use and interpret (all-or-none phenomenon)
        - Informative during flap inset
        - Applicable to all flap types especially buried
        - Probe and/or wire can dislodge
        - Lower positive predictive value

## TECHNICAL PEARLS

### PERFORATOR SELECTION

- **General principles**
    - Obtain wide surgical exposure.
    - Maintaining a bloodless operative field is imperative.
    - Be aware of scarring and other causes of aberrant anatomy.
    - Limit vessel manipulation (such as twisting, stretching, and grasping).
    - Dissect close to perforator(s) in loose areolar plane.
    - Quantify and qualify all possible perforators before committing to perforator choice and flap design.
    - Vessel spasms may be alleviated with antispasmodics (such as lidocaine or papaverine) or adventitial stripping.
- **Quantity**
    - Flap type and design may dictate how many perforators are needed.
    - For DIEP flap, using fewer than five perforators is linked to increased risk of fat necrosis.[23]
    - Some argue that perforator quality, not quantity, determines flap viability.[24]
- **Quality**
    - *Size:* Minimum external diameter of 0.5 mm recommended
    - *Pulse:* A visible or palpable pulse is strong indicator of a good perforator

### FLAP DESIGN

- **Size limit**
    - Largely remains clinical trial and error because of perforator variability
    - Indocyanine green angiography is only available objective intraoperative method
    - Common flaps (e.g., DIEP, ALT, radial forearm)
        - Relatively more defined because upper limits known
        - Remains dependent on proper identification and selection of perforator(s), especially with smaller flaps
    - Freestyle flaps
        - Depend on the location and caliber of perforator(s) related to defect
    - In theory, distance from one perforator to the next adjacent should survive

## Complications and Salvage

- Similar to that of traditional free flaps (see Chapter 8)
- Inflow problems
  - Inadequate quality or quantity of perforator(s)
  - Vessel spasm
  - Twisting, tension, pressure, or compression of perforator(s) or source vessel
  - Injury to perforator(s) or source artery at time of dissection
  - Conversion to full muscle flap may salvage flap if problem noted early in dissection
- Outflow problems
  - Twisting, tension, pressure, or compression of vein(s)
  - Inadequate connections between the superficial and deep venous systems
  - Course of perforator vein(s) within subcutaneous tissue often anomalous and venae comitantes of source vessel may be smaller caliber
  - Other large perforators or superficial veins (e.g., SIEV in DIEP flap) should be identified in case the need to supercharge outflow arises

## NEW INNOVATIONS

- Supermicrosurgery (vessel diameter <0.5 mm)[25-27]
- Superthin flaps[1,28,29]
- Combined DIEP and vascularized lymph node transfer for postmastectomy lymphedema[30,31]
- Abdominal wall soft tissue coverage[32]
- Intraoperative navigation-assisted identification of DIEA perforators[33]

## Key Points

- ✓ Perforator flap are now a mainstream option for the treatment of distant, locoregional, and local defects.
- ✓ Nomenclature and the appropriate classification system are controversial.
- ✓ Understanding this controversy and the history of perforator flaps is essential to understanding the anatomy and the need for a classification system.
- ✓ The most common perforator flaps are those supplied by indirect perforating vessels (musculocutaneous/myocutaneous type).
- ✓ Perforator flaps are generally more sleek and pliable than their traditional myocutaneous flap counterparts, because the muscle is both excluded and preserved.
- ✓ Flap success is largely dependent on appropriate perforator selection (quality, quantity, and/or location).

## References

1. Blondeel PN, Morris SF, Hallock GG, Neligan PC, eds. Perforator Flaps: Anatomy, Technique, & Clinical Application, 2nd ed. St Louis: Quality Medical Publishing, 2013.
2. Weinzweig J. Plastic Surgery Secrets Plus. Philadelphia: Elsevier, 2010.
3. Niranjan NS, Price RD, Govilkar P. Fascial feeder and perforator-based V-Y advancement flaps in the reconstruction of lower limb defects. Br J Plast Surg 53:679-689, 2000.
4. Nakajima H, Fujino T, Adachi S. A new concept of vascular supply to the skin and classification of skin flaps according to their vascularization. Ann Plast Surg 16:1-19, 1986.

5. Masquelet AC, Romana MC, Wolf G. Skin island flaps supplied by the vascular axis of the sensitive superficial nerves: anatomical study and clinical experience in the leg. Plast Reconstr Surg 89:1115-1121, 1992.
6. Wei FC, Jain V, Suominen S, et al. Confusion among perforator flaps: what is a true perforator flap? Plast Reconstr Surg 107:874–876, 2001.
7. Nahai F. Surgical indications for fasciocutaneous flaps. Ann Plast Surg 13:495-503, 1984.
8. Hallock GG. Principles of fascia and fasciocutaneous flaps. In Weinzweig J. Plastic Surgery Secrets Plus. Philadelphia: Elsevier, 2010.
9. Mathes SJ, Nahai F. Reconstructive Surgery: Principles, Anatomy, & Technique. St Louis: Quality Medical Publishing, 1997.
10. Kim JT. New nomenclature concept of perforator flap. Br J Plast Surg 58:431-440, 2005.
11. Taylor GI, Palmer JH. The vascular territories (angiosomes) of the body: experimental study and clinical applications. Br J Plast Surg 40:113-141, 1987.
12. Taylor GI. The angiosomes of the body and their supply to perforator flaps. Clin Plast Surg 30:331-342, 2003.
13. Saint-Cyr M, Wong C, Schaverien M, et al. The perforasome theory: vascular anatomy and clinical implications. Plast Reconstr Surg 124:1529-1544, 2009.
14. Blondeel PN, Van Landuyt KH, Monstrey SJ, et al. The "Gent" consensus on perforator flap terminology: preliminary definitions. Plast Reconstr Surg 112:1378-1382, 2003.
15. Geddes CR, Morris SF, Neligan PC. Perforator flaps: evolution, classification, and applications. Ann Plast Surg 50:90-99, 2003.
16. Wei FC, Mardini S. Free-style free flaps. Plast Reconstr Surg 114:910-916, 2004.
17. Pignatti M, Ogawa R, Hallock GG, et al. The "Tokyo" consensus on propeller flaps. Plast Reconstr Surg 127:716-722, 2011.
18. Hallock GG. If based on citation volume, perforator flaps have landed mainstream. Plast Reconstr Surg 130:769e-771e, 2012.
19. Zenn M, Jones G. Reconstructive Surgery: Anatomy, Technique, & Clinical Applications. St Louis: Quality Medical Publishing, 2012.
20. Wei FC, Jain V, Celik N, Chen HC, et al. Have we found an ideal soft-tissue flap? An experience with 672 anterolateral thigh flaps. Plast Reconstr Surg 109:2219-2226, 2002.
21. Hallock GG. Skin grafts and local flaps. Plast Reconstr Surg 27:5e-22e, 2011.
22. Smit JM, Zeebregts CJ, Acosta R, et al. Advancements in free flap monitoring in the last decade: a critical review. Plast Reconstr Surg 125:177-185, 2010.
23. Baumann DP, Lin HY, Chevray PM. Perforator number predicts fat necrosis in a prospective analysis of breast reconstruction with free TRAM, DIEP, and SIEA flaps. Plast Reconstr Surg 125:1335-1341, 2010.
24. Lindsey JT. Perforator number does not predict fat necrosis. Plast Reconstr Surg 127:1391-1392, 2011.
25. Koshima I, Yamamoto T, Narushima M, et al. Perforator flaps and supermicrosurgery. Clin Plast Surg 37:683-689, 2010.
26. Hong JP. The use of supermicrosurgery in lower extremity reconstruction: the next step in evolution. Plast Reconstr Surg 123:230-235, 2009.
27. Mihara M, Hayashi Y, Iida T, et al. Instruments for supermicrosurgery in Japan. Plast Reconstr Surg 129:404e-406e, 2012.
28. Kimura N, Satoh K, Hosaka Y. Microdissected thin perforator flaps: 46 cases. Plast Reconstr Surg 112:1875-1885, 2003.
29. Ogawa R, Hyakusoku H. Flap thinning technique: the effect of primary flap defatting. Plast Reconstr Surg 122:987-988, 2008.

30. Becker C, Assouad J, Riquet M, et al. Postmastectomy lymphedema: long-term results following microsurgical lymph node transplantation. Ann Surg 243:313-315, 2006.
31. Saaristo AM, Niemi TS, Viitanen TP, et al. Microvascular breast reconstruction and lymph node transfer for postmastectomy lymphedema patients. Ann Plast Surg 255:468-473, 2012.
32. Hallock GG. A paradigm shift for soft-tissue coverage of the zones of the abdominal wall using perforator flaps. Plast Reconstr Surg 130:590-599, 2012.
33. Durden F, Carruthers KH, Haran O, et al. Intraoperative navigation-assisted identification of deep inferior epigastric artery perforators. Plast Reconstr Surg 129:880e-882e, 2012.

# 6. Tissue Expansion

Janae L. Maher, Raman C. Mahabir, Joshua A. Lemmon

## GOALS

To obtain additional tissue of a specific quantity and quality (color, texture, hair-bearing, sensate, minimal donor defect).

## PHYSIOLOGY

### STRUCTURE OF SKIN

For more detailed review, see Chapter 14.

- **Epidermis**
  - Stratum corneum, stratum lucidem, stratum granulosum, stratum spinosum, and stratum basale
- **Dermis**
  - Two layers: Papillary and reticular
  - Structural components: Collagen, elastin, ground substance

### VISCOELASTIC PROPERTIES OF SKIN (Fig. 6-1)[1]

- **Creep**

*Mechanical and biologic creep occur when a constant mechanical stress is applied to skin over time.*

- **Mechanical creep:** Occurs when tissue is *acutely* stretched.
  - Collagen fibers straighten and realign parallel to one another and with the vector of force.
  - Elastic fibers microfragment.
  - Water is displaced from the ground substance.
  - Adjacent tissue is recruited into the expanded field.

**TIP:** Mechanical creep is the basis of intraoperative tissue expansion for acute wound closure.

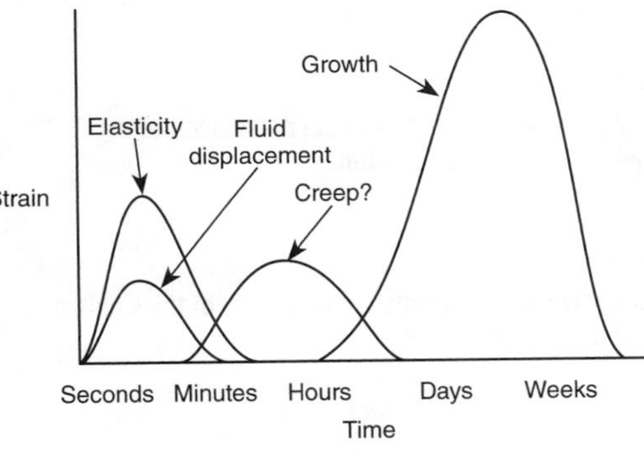


**Fig. 6-1** Viscoelastic properties of skin as a function of time.

- **Biologic creep:** Occurs when tissue is *chronically* stretched.
  - Cellular growth and tissue regeneration is initiated.
  - Stretch-induced signal transduction pathways lead to increased production of collagen, angiogenesis, fibroblast mitosis, and epidermal proliferation (flattened cells divide more frequently than round cells).
  - Multiple molecular cascades involving growth factors and protein kinases have been discovered that are initiated by mechanical force.[2]

■ **Stress relaxation**

*The force required to maintain tissue elongation decreases over time.*

- Corollary of creep, not a separate process

## HISTOLOGY[3-5]

Predictable changes occur to the layers of the skin and soft tissue in response to tissue expansion.

### Epidermis

- Mitotic activity increases.
- Thickens through hyperkeratosis.
- Intercellular spaces narrow.
- Normalizes after 6 months.[6]

### Dermis

- Thins 30% to 50%
- Increased fibroblasts and myofibroblasts
- Increased collagen deposition and realignment of collagen fibers along the lines of tension
- Fragmentation of elastin fibers
- Flattening of dermal papillae
- Dermal appendages (sweat glands and hair follicles) farther apart
- Thickness returns to normal 2 years after expansion

### Muscle

- Decreased thickness and mass
- Myofibril and myofilament arrangement disorganized
- Increased size and number of mitochondria
- Function unchanged

### Fat

- Extremely sensitive to mechanical force.
- Subcutaneous fat layer thins and some permanent loss of total fat mass occurs.
- Fat necrosis and fibrosis may occur with aggressive expansion.

### Capsule

- Forms around the expander within days
- Composed of elongated fibroblasts and few myofibroblasts within a layer of thick collagen bundles oriented parallel to the surface of the expander
  - **Inner layer:** Synovial-like lining
  - **Central layer:** Elongated fibroblasts and myofibroblasts
  - **Transitional layer:** Loose collagen
  - **Outer layer:** Vasculature and collagen

### Vascularity

- Angiogenesis occurs rapidly in expanded soft tissue with increased number and size of capillaries.
- Highest density of vessels is found at junction of capsule and host tissue.
- Tissue expansion is regarded as a form of delay phenomenon because of the similarity between expanded and delayed flaps in vessel caliber.[7]

**TIP:** Flaps raised on expanded skin have improved survival compared with flaps raised on nonexpanded skin because of the increased vascularity.[8-10]

## TYPES OF INTERNAL EXPANDERS

### Basic Design

- Most of the literature about tissue expansion refers to internal tissue expanders. There is a section at the end of this chapter on external tissue expansion.
- Inflatable silicone elastomer reservoir
- Variables: Style of injection port, base style, +/− differential expansion, surface texture, shape/dimensions (length, width, projection, volume)

### Injection Ports

- **Remote port**
  - Connected to the reservoir with tubing
  - Placed in the subcutaneous tissue (palpable) and accessed percutaneously or placed externally to obviate the need for skin puncture
  - **Pros:** Removes danger of prosthesis perforation during port access
  - **Cons:** Internal remote ports have potential complications of port flipping (the port turns over and you can no longer access it), tube obstruction, and migration
- **Integrated port**
  - Incorporated into the reservoir itself
  - Located by palpation or magnetic finder and accessed with 23-gauge needle
  - **Pros:** Subcutaneous tunneling and separate port site not necessary
  - **Cons:** Risk of expander puncture with port access

### Base

- Stable base (most common): Rigid back, permits unidirectional expansion
- Soft base: Allows expansion in all directions

### Surface

- Smooth
- Textured: Allows ingrowth of capsule into device, which decreases migration and capsular contracture

### Differential Expansion

- Differential thickness of expander envelope allows greater expansion in selected dimensions (e.g., breast reconstruction tissue expander that creates natural ptosis contour)

### Shape

- Available in many shapes and can be custom designed
- Amount of tissue expanded in vivo only a fraction of that expected by mathematical calculation
- Expander geometry influences the amount of surface area gained[11]
  - **Round expander:** 25% of calculated tissue expansion
  - **Crescent expander:** 32% of calculated tissue expansion
  - **Rectangular expander:** 38% of calculated tissue expansion

### Permanent Expanders[12]

- Used for breast reconstruction
- Two compartments
  - *Outer compartment:* Filled with silicone gel
  - *Inner compartment:* Saline-filled reservoir connected to a remote port
- Port intended to be removed when expansion complete
- Designed to remain in position permanently

### Self-Inflating Expanders

- Contain hypertonic sodium chloride crystals and fill by osmosis
- Rarely used and largely experimental

## CONTRAINDICATIONS

- Relative
  - Previous or anticipated radiation therapy
  - Psychiatric patient
  - Near an open wound
- Absolute
  - Near malignancy
  - Under skin graft
  - Open infection
  - Already tight tissue

## ADVANTAGES OF TISSUE EXPANSION

- Larger defects can be closed than by using local flaps alone.
  - Expansion usually used for simple advancement flaps, but some prefer transposition flaps[13]
  - May also be used in preparation for expanded axial, myocutaneous, or fasciocutaneous flaps
- Donor tissue is adjacent tissue and shares similar color, texture, thickness, sensation, and hair-bearing characteristics.
- Primary closure is often an option, thus limiting donor site morbidity.
- Scar location can be manipulated.
- Expanded tissue can be expanded repeatedly.
- Methods are reliable.

## DISADVANTAGES OF TISSUE EXPANSION

- Multiple operations (at least two) are required.
- Reconstruction is delayed until expansion is complete.

- Multiple outpatient visits are required.
- A temporary dramatic aesthetic deformity exists during expansion process.
- Risks and complications (e.g., pain during expansion, exposure, or infection).

## TECHNIQUE

### CHOICE OF EXPANDER

- **Size**
  - Base diameter of expander should be 2 to 2.5 times the diameter of the defect to be covered.[11,14]

> **TIP:** Volume is a minor issue because most expanders can be overfilled many times their listed volume.

- **Shape**
  - Mostly depends on location
  - Rectangular expanders well suited to long, narrow extremities
  - Circular shapes excellent for the breast
  - Crescent shapes often used in the scalp
- **Number**
  - May use multiple expanders for a single defect
  - Depends on availability of adjacent tissue

### INCISION

- Made perpendicular to the direction of expansion (long axis of the expander) to avoid tension across the incision.
- May also be made in existing incisional scars, through the lesion to be excised, or at the edge of the defect to be excised so that the scar can be removed at the time of reconstruction (Fig. 6-2).

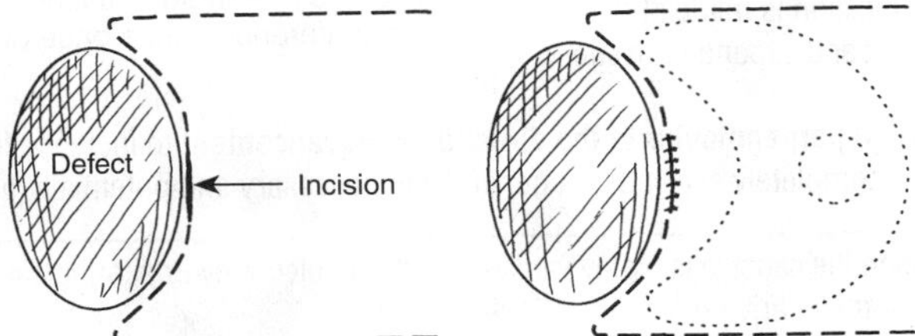


**Fig. 6-2** The access incision may be placed at the margin of the defect. (Although this is not the "preferable" incision, it is probably the one most often used.)

### POCKET

- Subcutaneous, suprafascial, submuscular, or subgaleal, depending on location
- Must be large enough for expander to lie flat without creases, but not so large that it allows migration or excessive movement of the expander
- Hemostasis and meticulous dissection essential for preserving overlying vascularity
- Closed suction drains to control dead space from undermining
- Layered closure

- Partial saline inflation (10% to 20%) to fill dead space and properly position expander without surface folds

### Expansion Process

- Expansion usually started within 1-3 weeks of expander placement and takes 6-12 weeks to complete
- 23-gauge (or smaller) needle or Huber needle used to access the filling port
- Expander filled until patient senses discomfort or the overlying skin blanches
- Frequency
  - Expansion can be repeated after 3-4 days, but is usually done weekly to facilitate scheduled clinic visits.
  - Rapid expansion can be associated with higher extrusion rates.
- Completion
  - Expansion is complete when enough soft tissue is available to cover the defect.
  - Determining when expansion is complete can be a difficult clinical decision.

> **TIP:** The amount of tissue available for advancement is equal to the circumference minus the base width of the expander.[5,11]

### Reconstruction

- Undertaken when expander inflated to desired volume
  - **Expanded circumference (dome length) minus the base diameter of the expander estimates the amount of tissue available for a simple advancement flap (Fig. 6-3).**
- When placed before excising a defect (scar, nevi, etc.), the incision is made at the junction of defect and expanded tissue.
- Capsule
  - May be scored **perpendicular to the direction of advancement** to increase flap mobilization
  - May also be completely excised, but generally unnecessary and potentially harmful

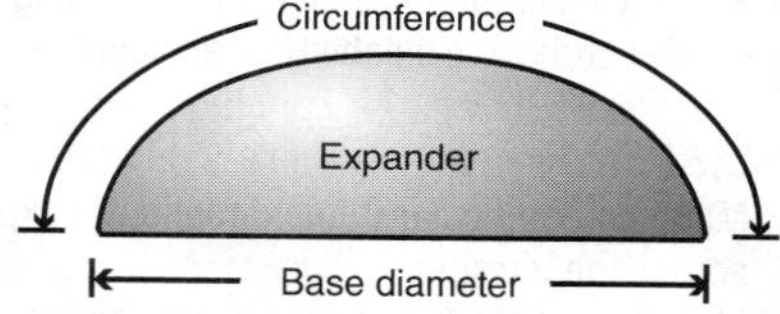


**Fig. 6-3** Amount of tissue available equals circumference minus base diameter.

> **TIP:** Remember, the capsule is highly vascular, and capsulectomy or scoring can compromise the vascularity of the overlying skin.[15]

## CLINICAL APPLICATIONS

### Scalp

- Defects involving up to **50%** of the scalp can be reconstructed with tissue expansion without significant thinning of the remaining hair.[16]
- Expanders with remote filling ports are placed in the subgaleal plane.
- Multiple expansions and combinations of rotation and advancement flaps are used.
- Applications
  - Male pattern baldness
  - Traumatic defects

- Burn alopecia
- Congenital nevi
- Skin malignancy reconstruction

## Face and Neck

For optimal aesthetic result, adhere to the subunit principle and create expander placement and flap incisions so that final scars are hidden in the natural creases.

- **Ear**
  - Postauricular skin can be expanded before reconstruction of congenital and acquired auricular deformities.[17,18]
  - Thin, non-hair-bearing skin may be draped over the reconstructed cartilage framework.
- **Nose**
  - Forehead tissue expanders can be placed before using forehead flaps for nasal reconstruction.
    - Flap dimensions are increased, which allows for primary closure of the donor site.
    - Authors argue that expanded forehead flaps are not ideal and that the donor site is best left to heal by secondary intention.[19]

## Trunk

- **Breast**

For a more detailed review, see Chapter 50.

  - Tissue expanders are commonly used for immediate and delayed breast reconstruction.
  - An expander with an integrated port is most often used.
  - Generally placed beneath the pectoral muscle, and either acellular dermal matrix or portions of the rectus abdominus and/or serratus anterior muscle can be recruited for total implant coverage.
- **Giant congenital melanocytic nevi**
  - Tissue expansion is indicated for large lesions involving the back, abdomen, and chest that cannot be serially excised in three stages or fewer.[20]
  - Allows for excision of nevus and resurfacing with normal skin of appropriate color and texture.
- **Abdominal wall reconstruction**
  - Skin grafting is often performed in the management of complex abdominal wounds following trauma, infection, and dehiscence of midline incisions.
  - Tissue expansion allows for excision of the grafted skin and coverage with vascularized and innervated local tissue.
  - For reconstructing large myofascial defects, expanders can be placed between the external and internal oblique muscles.
    - After expansion, component separation allows primary closure of defects that involve more than 50% of the abdominal surface area.[21,22]
  - Can also be placed subcutaneously to generate additional soft tissue coverage.

## Extremities

- Expanders are placed suprafascial.
- Primary application is to excise nevi or resurface areas of unstable soft tissue, burn contractures, or unsightly scar or contour deformities.[23]
- Extremity tissue expansion has been associated with higher levels of complications.[24-27]
- Remote incisions lead to lower infection, extrusion, and flap failure rates.

**TIP:** Keep in mind other expansion options to reconstruct extremity defects: expanded transposition flaps from the back or shoulder for proximal upper extremity coverage; expansion of the flank, creating a pedicled flap for distal upper extremity coverage followed by pedicle division; expanded full-thickness skin graft from abdomen or groin for the digits, webs, and hand; and expanded free flaps (TRAM, scapular) for large circumferential upper extremity or large lower extremity defects.

## COMPLICATIONS

### Minor Complications

- Pain
- Scar widening
- Dog-ears at the donor site
- Transient neuropraxia
- Temporary body contour distortion
- Seroma

### Major Complications

- Exposure
- Infection
- Hematoma
- Expander deflation
- Skin ischemia and necrosis

**TIP:** An exposed expander can be salvaged and expansion resumed in some cases.[27]

### Risk Factors Associated With Higher Complication Rates

- Children, especially under age 7
- Use in extremities: Lower extremities associated with more complications than upper extremities (particularly below the knee)
- Burn reconstruction
- Irradiated field

## EXTERNAL TISSUE EXPANSION

### Mechanical

- Recent proliferation of multiple devices: Abra (Canica Design, Almonte, Ontario, Canada), ClozeX (Closex Medical, Wellesley, MA), DermaClose (Wound Care Technologies, Chanhassen, MN), Dynaclose (Canica Design)
- Creates continuous tension across an open wound to gradually reapproximate the edges and achieve delayed primary closure through both mechanical and biologic creep.
- Recent literature demonstrates successful delayed primary closure with low associated morbidity and may reduce the need for more complex reconstruction.[28-31]
- More evidence will help to define indications, contraindications, safety, and outcomes.

## Negative Pressure

- Brava is a negative pressure therapy device that when used appropriately may enlarge the breast without surgery.[32]
- Concerns with compliance, longevity of results, and lack of information on biologic mechanism and safety have limited its wide acceptance.[33]
- Recent efforts combining Brava followed by fat grafting have more promising results[34] (see Chapter 89).

## Key Points

- ✓ Tissue expansion takes advantage of the viscoelastic properties of the skin, specifically creep and stress relaxation.
- ✓ The epidermis is the only layer that thickens in response to tissue expansion. The other layers become thinner.
- ✓ Rectangular expanders give the most skin expansion (relative to what is mathematically expected) of all shapes of expanders.
- ✓ The base diameter of the expander should be 2.5 times the diameter of the defect to be covered.
- ✓ Wait 1-3 weeks after placement of the expander to begin expansion, which can then be carried out every week.
- ✓ The amount of tissue available for advancement equals the circumference minus the base width of the expander.
- ✓ The breast is the most frequently expanded region, followed by the scalp.
- ✓ Up to 50% of the scalp can be reconstructed using tissue expansion without causing significant alopecia.
- ✓ Tissue expansion in the extremity is associated with the highest levels of complications.
- ✓ External tissue expansion is a developing field. New devices are available and being evaluated.

## References


1. Siegert R, Weerda H, Hoffmann S, et al. Clinical and experimental evaluation of intermittent intra-operative short-term expansion. Plast Reconstr Surg 92:248-254, 1993.
2. Takei T, Mills I, Arai K, et al. Molecular basis for tissue expansion: clinical implications for the surgeon. Plast Reconstr Surg 102:247-258, 1998.
3. Austad ED, Pasyk KA, McClatchey KD, et al. Histomorphologic evaluation of guinea pig skin and soft tissue after controlled tissue expansion. Plast Reconstr Surg 70:704-710, 1982.
4. Johnson TM, Lowe L, Brown MD, et al. Histology and physiology of tissue expansion. J Dermatol Surg Oncol 19:1074-1078, 1993.
5. Malata CM, Williams NW, Sharpe DT. Tissue expansion: an overview. J Wound Care 4:37-44, 1995.
6. Olenius M, Johansson O. Variations in epidermal thickness in expanded human breast skin. Scand J Plast Reconstr Hand Surg 29:15-20, 1995.
7. Bauer B. Tissue expansion. In Grabb & Smith's Plastic Surgery, 6th ed. Philadelphia: Lippincott-Raven, 2007.
8. Cherry GW, Austad E, Pasyk K, et al. Increased survival and vascularity of random-pattern skin flaps elevated in controlled, expanded skin. Plast Reconstr Surg 72:680-687, 1983.
9. Sasaki GH, Pang CY. Pathophysiology of skin flaps raised on expanded pig skin. Plast Reconstr Surg 74:59-67, 1984.

10. Saxby PJ. Survival of island flaps after tissue expansion: a pig model. Plast Reconstr Surg 81:30-34, 1988.
11. van Rappard JH, Molenaar J, van Doorn K, et al. Surface-area increase in tissue expansion. Plast Reconstr Surg 82:833-837, 1988.
12. Becker H. Breast reconstruction using an inflatable breast implant with detachable reservoir. Plast Reconstr Surg 73:678-683, 1984.
13. Joss GS, Zoltie N, Chapman P. Tissue expansion technique and the transposition flap. Brit J Plast Surg 43:328-333, 1990.
14. Wilhelmi BJ, Blackwell SJ, Mancoll JS, et al. Creep vs. stretch: a review of the viscoelastic properties of skin. Ann Plast Surg 41:215-219, 1998.
15. Manders EK, Schenden MJ, Furrey JA, et al. Soft-tissue expansion: concepts and complications. Plast Reconstr Surg 74:493-507, 1984.
16. MacLennan SE, Corcoran JF, Neale HW. Tissue expansion in head and neck burn reconstruction. Clin Plast Surg 27:121-132, 2000.
17. Hata Y, Hosokawa K, Yano K, et al. Correction of congenital microtia using the tissue expander. Plast Reconstr Surg 84:741-751, 1989.
18. Sasaki GH. Tissue expansion in reconstruction of acquired auricular defects. Clin Plast Surg 17:327-338, 1990.
19. Burget GC. Axial paramedian forehead flap. In Strauch B, ed. Grabb's Encyclopedia of Flaps. Philadelphia: Lippincott, 1998.
20. Ameja JS, Gosain AK. Giant congenital melanocytic nevi of the trunk and an algorithm for treatment. J Craniofac Surg 16:886-893, 2005.
21. Byrd HS, Hobar PC. Abdominal wall expansion in congenital defects. Plast Reconstr Surg 84:347-352, 1989.
22. Jacobsen WM, Petty PM, Bite U, et al. Massive abdominal-wall hernia reconstruction with expanded external/internal oblique and transversalis musculofascia. Plast Reconstr Surg 100:326-335, 1997.
23. Radovan C: Tissue expansion in soft-tissue reconstruction. Plast Reconstr Surg 74:482, 1984.
24. Antonyshyn O, Gruss JS, Mackinnon SE, et al. Complications of soft tissue expansion. Brit J Plast Surg 41:239-250, 1988.
25. Casanova D, Bali D, Bardot J, et al. Tissue expansion of the lower limb: complications in a cohort of 103 cases. Br J Plast Surg 54:310-316, 2001.
26. Manders EK, Oaks TE, Au VK, et al. Soft-tissue expansion in the lower extremities. Plast Reconstr Surg 81:208, 1988.
27. Pandya AN, Vadodaria S, Coleman DJ. Tissue expansion in the limbs: a comparative analysis of limb and non-limb sites. Brit J Plast Surg 55:302-306, 2002.
28. Santiago GF, Bograd B, Basile PL, et al. Soft tissue injury management with a continuous external tissue expander. Ann Plast Surg 69:418-421, 2012.
29. O'Reilly AG, Schmitt WR, Roenigk RK, et al. Closure of scalp and forehead defects using external tissue expander. Arch Facial Plast Surg 14:419-422, 2012.
30. Laurence VG, Martin JB, Wirth GA. External tissue expanders as adjunct therapy in closing difficult wounds. J Plast Reconstr Aesthet Surg 65:e297-e299, 2012.
31. Formby P, Flint J, Gordon WT, et al. Use of a continuous external tissue expander in the conversion of a type IIIB fracture to a type IIIA fracture. Orthopedics 36:e249-e251, 2013.
32. Schlenz I, Kaider A. The Brava external tissue expander: is breast enlargement without surgery a reality? Plast Reconstr Surg 120:1680-1689, 2007.
33. Slavin SA. Discussion of Schlenz I, Kaider A. The Brava external tissue expander: is breast enlargement without surgery a reality? Plast Reconstr Surg 120:1690-1691, 2007.
34. Khouri RK, Eisenmann-Klein M, Cardoso E, et al. Brava and autologous fat transfer is a safe and effective breast augmentation alternative: results of a 6-year, 81-patient, prospective multicenter study. Plast Reconstr Surg 129:1173-1187, 2012.

# 7. Vascularized Composite Allografts and Transplant Immunology

**Menyoli Malafa, Tae Chong**

## DEFINITIONS[1]

- Graft: Tissue that requires growth of new vessels from recipient tissue
- Autograft: Transplanted tissue from self
- Allograft: Transplanted tissue from an unrelated same-species individual
- Isograft: Transplanted tissue from genetically identical individual (e.g., monozygotic twin)
- Xenograft: Transplanted tissue from another species
- Vascularized graft: Tissue that becomes revascularized via anastomoses to recipient vessels
- Composite graft: Transplant consisting of multiple tissue types

## MAJOR HISTOCOMPATIBILITY COMPLEX (MHC) ANTIGENS[1-3]

- Regulates cell-mediated adaptive immune response
  - In humans, it is referred to as *human leukocyte antigen* (HLA) *molecules.*
    - Immunologic fingerprint
    - Differences between individuals can be directly responsible for allograft rejection.
  - **Class I molecules**
    - HLA-A, HLA-B, HLA-C
    - Present on surface of all nucleated cells
    - Display peptides generated **within the cell** (e.g., peptides from normal cellular processes or from intracellular pathogens such as viruses)
  - **Class II molecules**
    - HLA-DP, HLA-DQ, HLA-DR
    - Present on surface of antigen-presenting cells (e.g., monocytes, macrophages, dendritic cells, B-cells)
    - Display peptides sampled from **outside cell** via phagocytosis (newly acquired antigen)

## ADAPTIVE (ACQUIRED) IMMUNE SYSTEM[1-4]

- Plays a primary role in rejection of transplanted tissue
  - **Lymphocytes (B-cells and T-cells) with antigen-specific surface receptors are the primary mediators.**
  - Activation results in antigen-targeted immune response.
    - Capable of memory
    - Enhanced secondary response that is more vigorous and with a faster onset of immune response
- T-cell activation: Requires three signals
  - **Foreign antigen (Ag) recognition:** T-cell receptor (TCR) recognizes donor-derived peptide–self-MHC complexes.
    - CD8 (present on cytotoxic T-cells) stabilizes TCR interaction with MHC class I.
    - CD4 (present on helper T-cells) stabilizes TCR interaction with MHC class II.

- **Costimulatory signal**
- **Cytokine release:** Cytokine release (e.g., IL-2) leads to proliferation, differentiation, and activation of T-cell effector functions.
  - Cytotoxic (CD8+) cells carry out destruction of abnormal cells.
  - Helper (CD4+) T-cells release many cytokines and play a central role in regulating the overall immune response.
    - Activate monocytes, macrophages, neutrophils, eosinophils, mast cells
    - Activate B-cells and promote humoral response
    - Promote cell-mediated cytotoxicity (CD8+/natural killer [NK] cells)

## DONOR ORGAN RECOGNITION PATHWAYS[2-3]

There are two mechanisms by which the immune system recognizes the donor organ.

- **Direct pathway**
  - Antigen-presenting cells from the donor migrate to the recipient's lymphoid tissue and directly stimulate a T-cell response.
    - This is seen predominantly during **early, acute rejection.**
- **Indirect pathway**
  - Donor antigens are processed by recipient antigen-presenting cells and presented to T-cells.
    - Predominant mechanism in **chronic rejection**

## TYPES OF ALLOGRAFT REJECTION[1-3,5]

- **Hyperacute rejection**
  - **Occurs within minutes to hours**
  - Mediated by donor-specific antibodies (DSAs), which are circulating in the body before transplantation
    - DSAs are acquired by prior exposure to alloantigen.
      - Pregnancy
      - Blood transfusions
      - Prior transplants
  - Antibodies bind the antigen on donor endothelial cells and elicit endothelial damage and vessel thrombosis via the complement and coagulation cascades.
  - Preventable with detection of alloreactive antibodies in recipient before transplantation
    - ABO blood-group matching
    - Crossmatch assay
      - Donor cells are mixed with recipient serum, and complement is added.
      - Lysis indicates presence of antidonor antibodies (positive crossmatch).
    - Panel-reactive antibody (PRA) assay
      - Recipient serum is screened against panel of random donor cells that are representative of regional donor pool.
      - Results are expressed as percentage of donor cell set that lyses. (A high score indicates highly sensitized individual.)
- **Accelerated rejection**
  - **Occurs within first days**
  - Secondary immune response mediated by sensitized (memory) T-cells
  - **Treatment**
    - Pulse steroids
    - Lymphocyte-depleting agents

- **Acute rejection**
  - **Occurs within weeks to months**
  - Immune response results in inflammatory damage to the tissue components, which may impair function and increase risk of chronic rejection.
  - Acute cellular (cell-mediated) rejection
    - T-cell mediated immune response
    - **Treatment**
      - Pulse steroids
      - Optimize drug levels of maintenance immunosuppression
      - Lymphocyte-depleting agents
  - Acute humoral (antibody-mediated) rejection
    - B cells stimulated to produce DSAs
    - **Treatment:** Plasmapheresis, IVIg, rituximab
  - **The only type of acute rejection reported in vascularized composite allograft (VCA) is cell-mediated.**[2]
- **Chronic rejection**
  - Occurs over months to years
  - Development of chronic vasculopathy leads to graft fibrosis.
    - Endothelial injury → inflammation → vascular smooth muscle cell proliferation → blockage of vessel lumen → fibrosis → graft dysfunction
  - **No good treatment exists.**
  - **Immunologic factors**
    - Prior acute rejection episodes
    - Recipient sensitization
    - Inadequate immunosuppression
  - **Nonimmunologic factors**
    - Prolonged total ischemia time
    - Donor brain death
    - Recipient medical history: Hypertension, hyperlipidemia, smoking
  - These immunologic and nonimmunologic factors have been linked to increased risk of chronic graft rejection in solid organ grafts. To date, chronic rejection has not been confirmed in VCAs.
- **Current data suggest that VCAs are relatively resistant to chronic rejection.**

## INNATE IMMUNE SYSTEM

- Less well-defined role in transplant rejection
- Can be activated through the adaptive immune system response
- Components
  - Epithelial barriers: Block entry of microbes
  - Neutrophils, macrophages: Phagocytosis, inflammation
  - Dendritic cells: Most potent antigen-presenting cells
  - Natural killer (NK) cells: Cell-mediated cytotoxicity
  - Plasma proteins: Complement proteins, opsonins
  - Pattern recognition receptors (PRRs): Bind pathogen-associated molecular patterns (PAMPs) leading to immune response
- Toll-like receptors (TLRs)
  - A type of pattern-recognition receptor (PRR)
  - Expressed on both parenchymal and hematopoietic cells
  - Activation triggers inflammatory response

- Recognized/activated by:
  - PAMPs such as lipopolysaccharide (LPS), bacterial DNA, viral RNA, fungi glucans
  - **Endogenous ligands such as factors released from necrotic cells and during ischemia-reperfusion injury**

> **TIP:** Although the endogenous immune system is primarily responsible for initiating targeted response against transplanted tissue, the innate immune system is recruited to exert its effects via signals from the adaptive immune system (e.g., antibodies, cytokines) and by recognizing damaged tissue (e.g., ischemic graft tissue).

## TRANSPLANT IMMUNOLOGY (Fig. 7-1)

### VCA TRANSPLANTATION[1-3,6]

- VCA also referred to as *composite tissue allograft* (CTA)
- Transfer of multiple tissue types within one graft:
  - Skin
  - Fat
  - Muscle
  - Tendon
  - Bone
  - Cartilage
  - Nerves
  - Vessels
- Direct visual inspection of skin can facilitate early recognition and treatment of acute rejection.
  - **Skin is the most antigenic tissue and main target of immune response in acute rejection.**
  - Acute rejection manifests as erythematous macules, diffuse redness, or asymptomatic papules.
  - **Banff 2007 grading scheme for acute rejection**[7]
    - **Grade 0 (no rejection)**
      - No or rare inflammatory infiltrates
    - **Grade I (mild rejection)**
      - Mild perivascular infiltration
      - No involvement of overlying epidermis
    - **Grade II (moderate rejection)**
      - Moderate to severe perivascular inflammation with or without mild epidermal and/or adnexal involvement (limited to spongiosis and exocytosis)
      - No epidermal dyskeratosis or apoptosis
    - **Grade III (severe rejection)**
      - Dense inflammation and epidermal involvement, with epithelial apoptosis, dyskeratosis and/or keratinolysis
    - **Grade IV (necrotizing acute rejection)**
      - Frank necrosis of epidermis or other skin structures

> **TIP:** In face allografts, oral mucosa may have similar changes that are more pronounced, compared with the skin on the graft.

- Chronic rejection has not been clearly identified in VCAs.

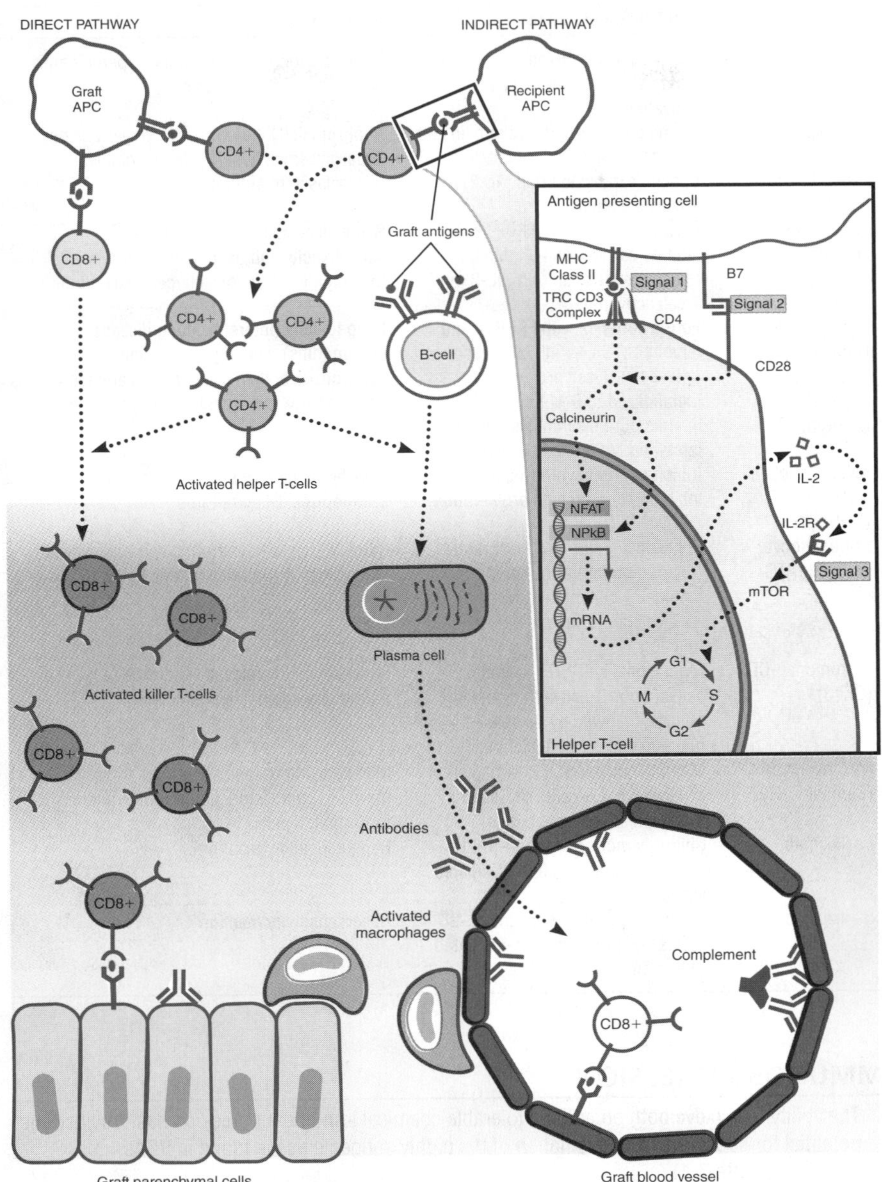


**Fig. 7-1** Transplant immunology.

**Table 7-1** *Immunosuppression Drugs*

| Drug | Mechanism of Action | Side Effects |
|---|---|---|
| Prednisone | Inhibits NF-kB, thereby inhibiting gene expression and T-cell activation | Hypertension, hyperglycemia, hyperlipidemia, weight gain, osteoporosis |
| Cyclosporine | Forms complex with cyclophilin and inhibits calcineurin → inhibition of gene expression (e.g., IL-2) and T-cell activation | Nephrotoxicity, neurotoxicity, hypertension, hyperglycemia, hyperlipidemia, gingival hyperplasia, hirsutism |
| Tacrolimus (Prograf) | Forms complex with FKBP12 and inhibits calcineurin → inhibition of gene expression (e.g., IL-2) and T-cell activation | Same as cyclosporine but increased neurotoxicity and decreased hypertension, hyperlipidemia, gingival hyperplasia, hirsutism |
| Sirolimus (rapamycin) | Forms complex with FKBP12 and inhibits mTOR → inhibits response to IL-2 and T-cell proliferation | Lung toxicity (interstitial lung disease, pneumonitis), hyperlipidemia, less nephrotoxicity than cyclosporine and tacrolimus |
| Azathioprine (Imuran) | Metabolized to 6-MP by liver → inhibits purine synthesis, thereby inhibiting lymphocyte proliferation | Bone marrow suppression, GI symptoms |
| Mycophenolate mofetil (CellCept) | Inhibits purine synthesis, thereby inhibiting lymphocyte proliferation | Less bone marrow suppression than azathioprine, GI symptoms |
| Antithymocyte globulin (ATG) | Polyclonal antibodies from rabbit (thymoglobulin) or horse (Atgam) → block T-cell membrane proteins → T-cell depletion and altered function | Cytokine release syndrome, serum sickness, leukopenia, thrombocytopenia |
| Muromonab-CD3 (OKT3) | Monoclonal anti-CD3 → initial activation of T-cell with cytokine release, followed by decreased function and T-cell depletion | Severe cytokine release syndrome (e.g., pulmonary edema, hypotension) |
| Alemtuzumab (Campath-1H) | Monoclonal anti-CD52 → depletion of T-cells and B-cells, NKCs, and monocytes/macrophages | Mild cytokine release syndrome, bone marrow suppression, autoimmune anemia/thrombocytopenia |
| Basiliximab | Chimeric monoclonal anti-IL-2R (CD25) → prevents IL-2–mediated activation | Hypersensitivity reaction |
| Daclizumab | Humanized monoclonal anti-IL-2R (CD25) → prevents IL-2–mediated activation | Hypersensitivity reaction |

## IMMUNOSUPPRESSION

- The ability to achieve both potent and tolerable chemical immunosuppression has provided the potential for successful transplantation of the highly antigenic tissue found in VCAs.
- **Drugs**[3,8,9] **(Table 7-1)**
- **Regimens**[3-5,9,10]
  - Induction therapy
    - Goal: Modulate the immune system at time of transplantation to prevent and/or decrease severity of acute rejection

  - Benefits: Decrease incidence/severity/frequency of acute rejection, minimize steroid requirement in the maintenance phase
  - Drawbacks: The profound degree of immunosuppression can increase the risk of opportunistic infection and posttransplant lymphoproliferative disease (PTLD).
  - Typical agents used
    - Polyclonal ATGs
    - Monoclonal anti-IL-2 receptor antibodies (daclizumab, basiliximab)
    - Monoclonal anti-CD3 antibodies (OKT3)
- Maintenance therapy
  - Goal: Abrogate the immune response to the allograft while ensuring that normal immune surveillance occurs for infection and malignancy
  - Lifelong therapy required so regimen adjusted to minimize toxicity
  - Typical regimen: Calcineurin inhibitor (tacrolimus), antimetabolite (mycophenolate mofetil), and corticosteroid (prednisone)
- **Rescue therapy**
  - Goal: Treatment of acute rejection episodes
  - First line: Corticosteroids, ensure that calcineurin inhibitors are at therapeutic levels, and topical immunosuppressants (clobetasol and Protopic)
  - Second-line agents
    - Induction therapy agents
    - Sirolimus
    - High-dose tacrolimus

- **Risks**[1-3,9]
  - Drug side effects (metabolic, hematologic, organ toxicity, etc.)
  - Infection (bacterial, viral, fungal)
  - Malignancy
    - Skin cancer
      - **Most common malignancy after transplant**
      - **Squamous cell carcinoma is most common.**
    - PTLD
      - Epstein-Barr virus–related
      - Treatment: Discontinue immunosuppression, chemotherapy/radiotherapy

## TOLERANCE[1,3,10]

- **Self-tolerance:** Immune system's ability to distinguish between self and non-self
  - **Central tolerance**
    - Occurs in thymus
    - Self-reactive T-cells undergo deletion (negative selection)
  - **Peripheral tolerance**
    - Occurs outside thymus by various mechanisms
    - Extrathymic deletion of self-reactive T-cells
    - Induction of T-cell anergy (no co-stimulatory signal provided by APC → T-cell remains inactive/unable to respond to antigen)
    - Active suppression of response by regulatory T-cells
  - Loss of self-tolerance leads to autoimmune disease.
- **Donor-specific (transplantation) tolerance:** Immune system does not respond to graft in the absence of immunosuppression, but it maintains ability to respond to other antigens.
  - Represents the ultimate goal of transplant immunology research
    - Long-term graft survival

    - Eliminates risks associated with immunosuppression drug therapy
- Proposed strategies
    - Early T-cell depletion
    - Immunotherapy with regulatory T-cells
    - Co-stimulation blockade
    - Bone marrow transplant to induce mixed chimerism

## Key Points

✓ Transplant rejection is primarily an adaptive immune system response against non-self tissue differentiated by unique cell-surface receptors, the human leukocyte antigens.
✓ The innate immune system plays a secondary and less well-defined role in mediating transplant tissue damage.
✓ There are two mechanisms by which the immune system recognizes non-self. The direct pathway is the predominant mechanism in acute rejection, whereas the indirect pathway is more closely associated with chronic rejection.
✓ The important mechanism in VCA rejection is acute cell-mediated rejection.
✓ Skin is the most antigenic tissue and the main target of acute rejection in VCA. The Banff grading scheme for acute VCA rejection is based on histologic features of the skin.
✓ Immunosuppressive therapy targets specific arms of the adaptive immune system, thereby promoting nonspecific tolerance to transplanted tissue at the expense of systemic side effects.
✓ The ultimate goal of transplant immunology research is to develop a method to induce complete, stable, donor-specific tolerance in which the immune system does not respond to the transplant in the absence of immunosuppression therapy, while maintaining its ability to respond to other foreign antigens.

## References

1. Thorne CH, Bartlett SP, Beasley RW, et al, eds. Grabb and Smith's Plastic Surgery, 6th ed. Philadelphia: Lippincott Williams & Wilkins, 2007.
2. Siemionow M, Klimczak A. Basics of immune responses in transplantation in preparation for application of composite tissue allografts in plastic and reconstructive surgery. Part I. Plast Reconstr Surg 121:4e-12e, 2008.
3. Townsend CM Jr, Beauchamp RD, Evers BM, et al, eds. Sabiston Textbook of Surgery: The Biological Basis of Modern Surgical Practice, 19th ed. Philadelphia: Saunders Elsevier, 2012.
4. Ravindra K, Haeberle M, Levin LS, et al. Immunology of vascularized composite allotransplantation: a primer for hand surgeons. J Hand Surg 37:842-850, 2012.
5. Swearingen B, Ravindra K, Xu H, et al. Science of composite tissue allotransplantation. Transplantation 86:627-635, 2008.
6. Morelon E, Kanitakis J, Petruzzo P. Immunological issues in clinical composite tissue transplantation: Where do we stand today? Transplantation 93:855-859, 2012.
7. Cendales LC, Kanitakis J, Schneeberger S, et al. The Banff 2007 working classification of skin-containing composite tissue allograft pathology. Am J Transplant 8:1396-1400, 2008.
8. Taylor AL, Watson CJE, Bradley JA. Immunosuppressive agents in solid organ transplantation: mechanisms of action and therapeutic efficacy. Crit Rev Oncol Hematol 56:23-46, 2005.
9. Whitaker IS, Duggan EM, Alloway RR, et al. Composite tissue allotransplantation: a review of relevant immunological issues for plastic surgeons. J Plast Reconstr Aesthetic Surg 61:481-492, 2008.
10. Siemionow M, Klimczak A. Tolerance and future directions for composite tissue allograft transplants. Part II. Plast Reconstr Surg 123:7e-17e, 2009.

# 8. Basics of Microsurgery

David S. Chang, Jeffrey E. Janis, Patrick B. Garvey

## INDICATIONS FOR MICROSURGICAL RECONSTRUCTION

Microsurgical reconstruction traditionally has been considered the highest level on the *reconstructive ladder;* however, many now describe the *reconstructive elevator* on which free tissue transfer represents the first choice for reconstruction of certain defects, particularly complex, composite defects.[1]

- Consider for reconstruction of composite wounds (e.g., reconstruction of mandible after cancer extirpation, covering open fractures) when simpler or local options for wound coverage are either unavailable or inadequate to restore function and form
- Possible to transplant composite tissue (e.g., bone, skin, subcutaneous tissue, fascia, muscle) to reconstruct distant sites

### OTHER INDICATIONS

- Hand and digit replantation or reconstruction
- Functional muscle transfer
- Vascularized bone and nerve grafts

## POTENTIAL CONTRAINDICATIONS

In general, there are no *absolute* contraindications to microsurgical reconstruction.

- **Age:** Extremes of age alone are not a contraindication.
- **Systemic disease:** There are no absolute contraindications to microsurgical reconstruction. However, the patient must be able to tolerate prolonged general anesthesia. Hypercoagulable disorders represent a relative contraindication to free tissue transfer.
  - Associated conditions that should raise suspicion for hypercoagulable disorders include a history of miscarriages or thromboembolic events such as deep venous thrombosis or pulmonary emboli.
- **Smoking:** Free flaps do not have greater flap loss, so smoking is not an absolute contraindication; however, smokers have approximately 50% greater chance of wound healing complications.[2] Most microsurgeons avoid elective free tissue transfer in active smokers when possible.

**CAUTION: Smoking after digital replantation has been associated with 80%-90% failure rate.[3] Patients must be counseled before replantation.**

- **Preoperative radiation:** Not a contraindication. Free flaps have similar failure rates in irradiated and nonirradiated tissue.[4] Free tissue transfer is often the best choice for reconstruction in the setting of prior radiation, because it brings nonirradiated tissue into the wound to facilitate wound healing.

**TIP:** Exercise great care when working with irradiated vessels. Limit dissection, use the finest-caliber suture and needle, and pass the needle from inside out when possible to avoid separation of vessel layers.

## EQUIPMENT AND INSTRUMENTS[5]

- **Magnification**
  - Ocular loupes at least 2.5× for flap dissection. Although most microsurgeons prefer to perform microvascular anastomoses under the microscope, some feel comfortable creating anastomoses with 4.5× loupes.
  - Microscope: 200-250 mm focal length, typically up to 25× magnification, although most set scope to 10×-12.5× magnification
  - Double-headed system for two surgeons
  - Video output to monitor so that surgical scrub technician can follow the procedure and anticipate the next instruments needed by the microsurgeon; video monitor useful for teaching purposes
  - Some scopes now equipped with laser fluorescent angiography technology to assess vessel patency after completion of the anastomoses
- **Forceps**
  - No. 2 through No. 5 jeweler's forceps
  - Round or flat handles
  - 4-6 inches long
- **Microscissors**
  - Fine-tipped, spring-handled
  - Curved microscissors used for dissecting and trimming vessels
  - Straight microscissors used for cutting suture
- **Vessel dilator**
  - Smooth, fine-tipped
  - Can be used to gently dilate vessel to relieve spasm or correct size mismatch
- **Needle holder:** Curved or straight, nonlocking; some prefer to use jeweler's forceps
- Microvascular clamps
  - Single clamps of various sizes temporarily occlude vessels during microvascular anastomosis.
  - Closing pressure $<30$ g/mm$^2$ prevents trauma to endothelium.
  - Adjustable double clamps can be used for tension-free approximation of vessel ends.
- **Background**
  - MicroMat (PMT Corp, Chanhassen, MN) or other thin sheet of plastic in a color that maximizes contrast of suture and tissue (e.g., light blue or green)
- **Irrigation**
  - 3 ml syringe with 27-gauge angiocath or blunt-tip needle
  - Heparinized saline (100 U/ml)[6]
  - Topical papaverine: Calcium channel blocker, used to stop vasospasm
- **Other equipment**
  - Cellulose sponges (Weck-Cel spears [Medtronic, Jacksonville, FL] or half-inch cottonoids) to blot blood from field
  - Microscopic hemoclips: For any vessel branches
  - "Bird bath": Specimen cup filled with heparinized saline and gauze to clean instruments
  - Merocel (Medtronic) (moistened with saline) used to clear debris from instruments

## SUTURE AND NEEDLES

- Suture is typically monofilament nylon or polypropylene in sizes 8-0 to 11-0 depending on vessel size. 9-0 and 10-0 are most commonly used sutures for microvascular surgery (Table 8-1).

### MICRONEEDLE (Fig. 8-1)

- **Chord length:** Straight-line distance from swage to point
- **Diameter:** 75 to 135 μm
- **Length:** Circumference of needle (distance from swage to point along the curve of the needle)
- **Radius:** Distance from center of circle to needle
- **Shape:** Three-eighths circle or one-half circle
- **Size** of needle diameter determines size of suture hole.
- **Swage:** Where needle is attached to suture

BV 130-4

SHAPE
BV—3/8 circle
BVH—1/2 circle
ST—Straight

DIAMETER
in microns

CHORD LENGTH
in millimeters

**Fig. 8-1** Nomenclature of a microsuture needle.

### MICROVASCULAR VENOUS COUPLER[6a,7] (GEM COUPLER SYSTEM; SYNOVIS, BIRMINGHAM, AL) (Fig. 8-2)

- Coupled, rigid rings create sutureless venous anastomosis
- Decreases ischemic time
- Rigid rings stent vascular anastomosis open
- Sizes 1.5 to 4.0 mm
- Can be used to create end-to-end or end-to-side venous anastomoses
- Associated with <1% venous thrombosis rate and a minimal learning curve[7]

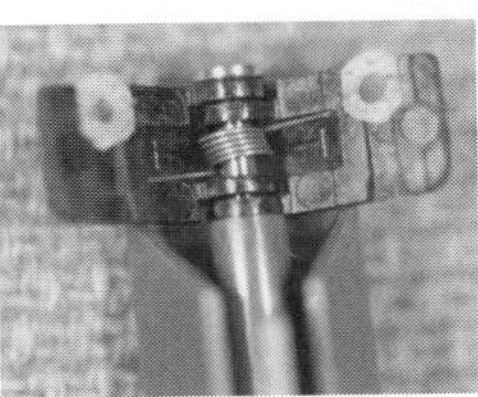

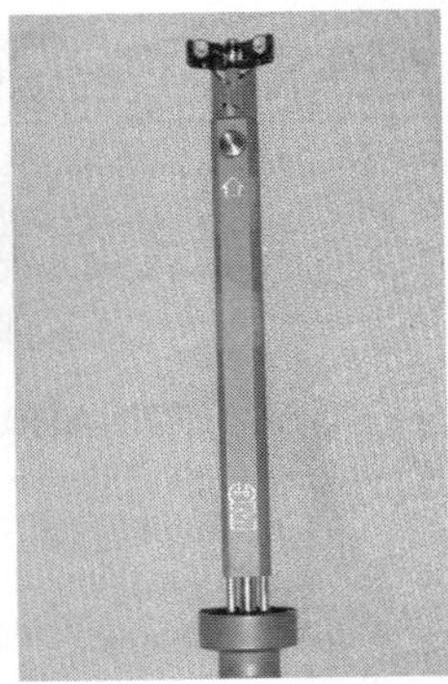

**Fig. 8-2** Microvascular coupler.

**Table 8-1** *Commonly Used Sutures and Needles*

| Suture | Needle | Typical Vessels |
|---|---|---|
| 8-0 | BV130-5 | Radial, ulnar, anterior tibial, peroneal |
| 9-0 | BV100-4 | Dorsalis pedis, posterior tibial |
| 10-0 | BV75-3 | Digital vessels |
| 11-0 | BV50-3 | Children |

## PLANNING

- Discuss plan with anesthesiologist; avoid placing IVs, arterial lines, or blood pressure cuffs in flap harvest sites (e.g., free radial forearm flaps). A "No IV Sticks" medical alert bracelet can be placed on the arm or leg from which the flap is to be harvested during the patient's initial consultation or preoperative clinic visit.
- Prepare widely: Anticipate need for skin graft and include donor site in preparations.
- Surgeon posture and position are essential to prevent fatigue, tremor, and cervical disc disease.
  - Feet flat on floor; hips, knees, and elbows at right angles; back and neck straight
  - Support hands and forearms with stacks of towels if necessary to minimize intention tremor.
- Caffeine: Routine consumption should not have adverse effects; therefore drink your normal amount.[8,9]
- Exposure is critical: Use self-retaining retractors, keep operative field dry, position patient and microscope to optimize visualization.

> **TIP:** Elastic Stay Hooks (Lone Star Medical, Stafford, TX) clamped to drapes work well as retractors.

> **TIP:** It is useful to longitudinally mark donor vessels with a marking pen (i.e., "racing stripe") before dividing the pedicle to prevent twisting of the pedicle. Twisting that occurs after completion of the anastomosis and microvascular clamp release necessitates repeating the anastomosis to prevent flap thrombosis.

## TECHNICAL CONSIDERATIONS[10,11]

- Keep vessels moist.
- Prevent traumatizing vessels by grasping only adventitia.
- Tension-free anastomosis is critical for patency; mobilize donor pedicle and recipient vessels from their surrounding connective tissue.

### VESSEL PREPARATION (Fig. 8-3)

- Cut back to healthy vessel if ends are traumatized.
- If wounds are traumatic, choose vessels outside zone of injury.
- Prepare vessels by dissecting 2-5 mm of adventitia from vessel end.
- Watch for signs of microvascular trauma (Fig. 8-4).

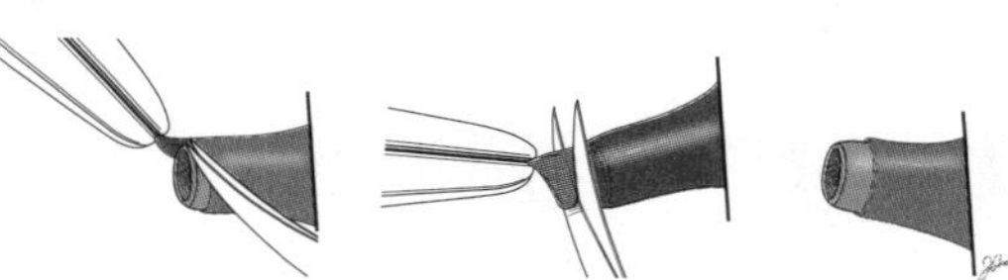

**Fig. 8-3** Proper vessel preparation.

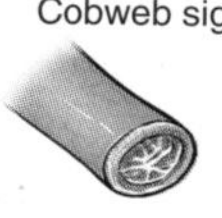

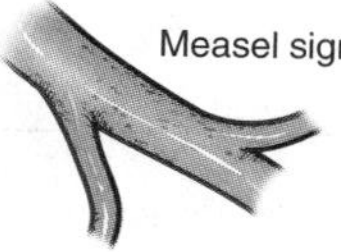

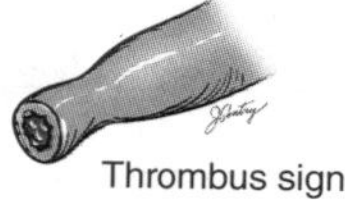

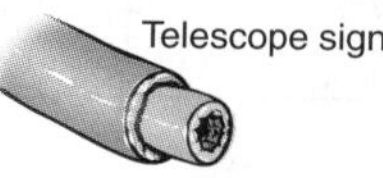


**Fig. 8-4** Signs of microvascular trauma.

- Flush artery and vein with heparinized saline.
- Always release arterial clamp to test inflow before anastomosis ("spurt test") (Fig 8-5).

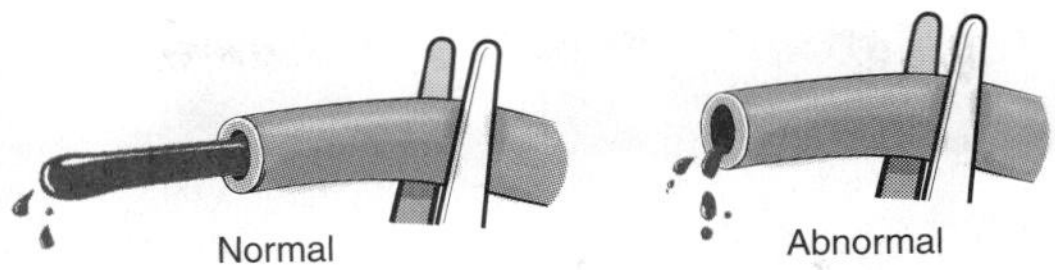


**Fig. 8-5** Spurt test.

## Establishing Anastomosis

- Needles should enter vessel at 90 degrees, full thickness, and follow curve of needle.
- Tie all knots square (usually three throws) and place precisely without excessive tension.
- Sutures should coapt vessel edges; exposure of vascular endothelium to adventitia can promote platelet aggregation and thrombus.

> **TIP:** Cut one limb of suture long to use as a handle.

- Directly visualize the needle tip as it passes across the two vessel ends and check the lumen of the vessel after each suture placement to confirm that no "back walling" has occurred.
- Number of stitches:
  - Size of vessel determines number of stitches.
  - Use just enough sutures necessary to approximate vessel. However, leaking anastomoses can promote platelet plugging that might promote vessel thrombosis. Leakage after clamp removal should be repaired with "rescue stitches."

## Completion of Anastomosis

- Release the microvascular clamp from the vein first, then release the artery. The opposite sequence can cause damage to flap vessels (e.g., mural thrombus) from high resistance to arterial flow before the vein is released.
- **Strip test:** Gently grasp the vessel distal to the anastomosis with two forceps; gently milk blood distally so the vessel is collapsed between the two forceps; release the proximal forceps; blood should fill the collapsed vessel if the anastomosis is patent (Fig. 8-6).
- Clip or suture-ligate any bleeding side branches.

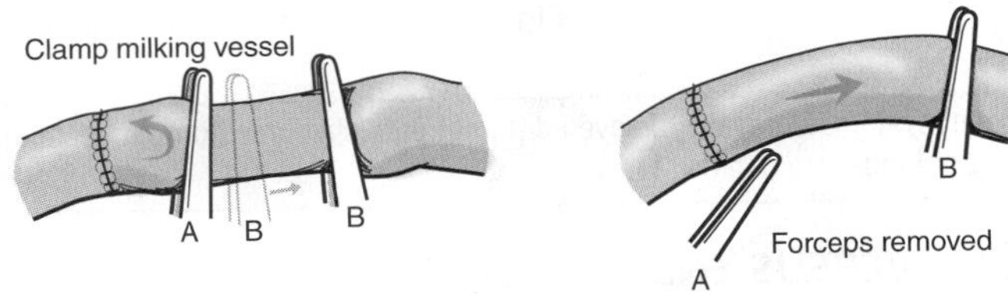


**Fig. 8-6** Strip test to check vessel.

## SEVEN MAIN ANASTOMOTIC TECHNIQUES[12,13] (Fig. 8-7)

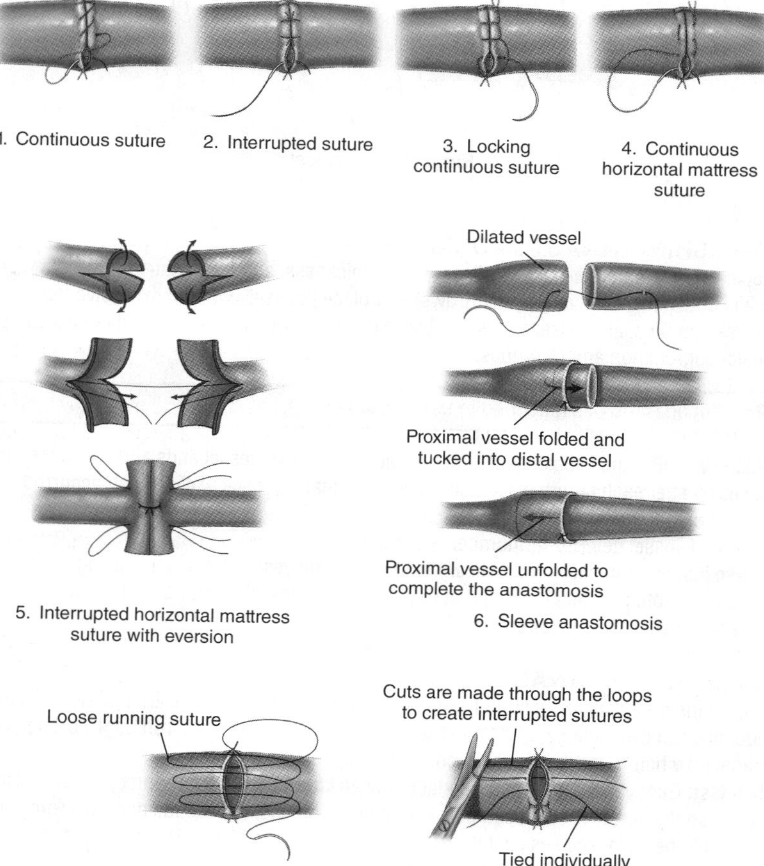


**Fig. 8-7**

> **TIP:** A recent systematic review of seven different published anastomotic techniques found no short- and/or long-term patency rates.

## END-TO-END VERSUS END-TO-SIDE[12]

### END-TO-END

- **Halving technique** (Fig. 8-8)
  - First two sutures are placed 180 degrees apart, beginning with the midpoint of the back wall.

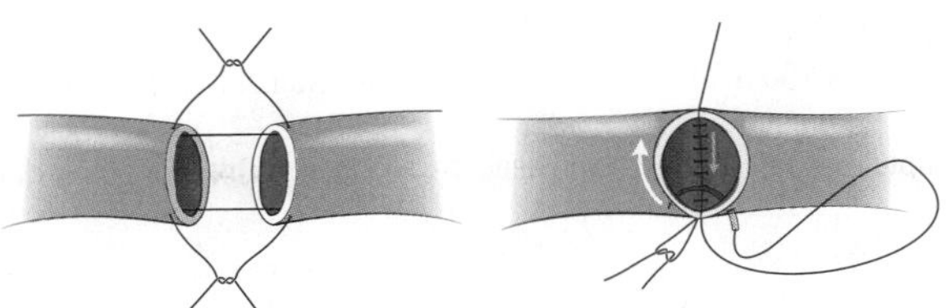

**Fig. 8-8** End-to-end anastomosis (halving technique).

- Vessel is then rotated 90 degrees in either direction to place sutures between the first two sutures by halving the distance between.
- Two additional sutures are placed between each of the four sutures spaced 90 degrees from each other (total of 12 sutures).
- Technique is particularly useful for minor vessel size mismatch.

■ **Back wall up technique**
- Interrupted sutures placed, beginning at the midpoint of the back wall, up one side then the other
- Facilitates visualization of the lumen until the final suture is placed
- Particularly useful when the vessel cannot safely be rotated 180 degrees to expose the back wall (e.g., in friable, irradiated vessels)

■ **Triangulation technique**
- Three sutures placed 120 degrees apart
- Vessel rotated to place sutures between the first three sutures, spacing appropriately
- Least commonly used technique today

## End-to-Side

■ Useful for significant vessel size discrepancy or to preserve in-line flow and distal perfusion

■ Patency is equivalent to end-to-end technique.[12]

■ Ideal angle of entry is between 30 and 75 degrees.

■ Ideal anastomosis/vessel diameter is 2:1 (Fig. 8-9).

■ Arteriotomy is key step (three suggested techniques) (Fig. 8-10).
- Use No. 11 blade or eye knife to make initial arteriotomy, then cut out ellipse with scissors.
- Place single microsuture full-thickness, tent up vessel, and cut out ellipse with curved serrated microscissors to create arteriotomy.
- Use 2.5 mm vascular punch.

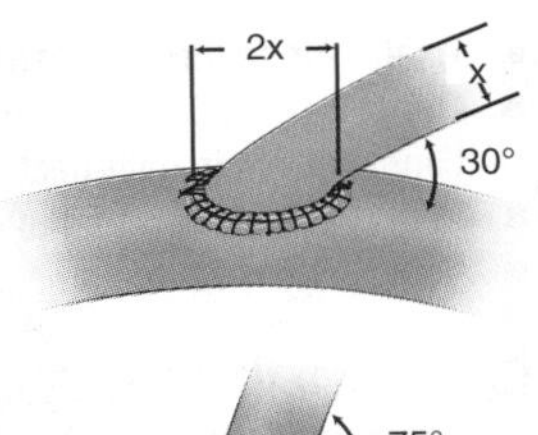


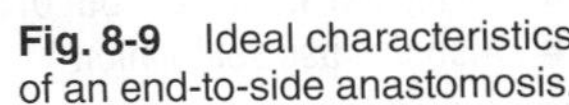


**Fig. 8-9** Ideal characteristics of an end-to-side anastomosis.

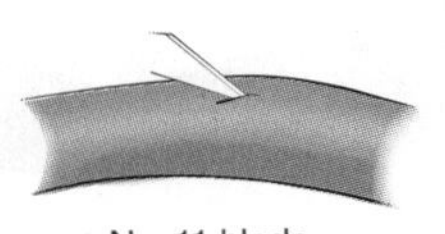

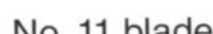

No. 11 blade

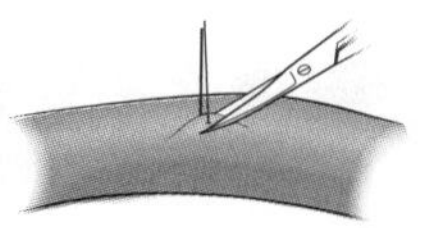

Tenting technique

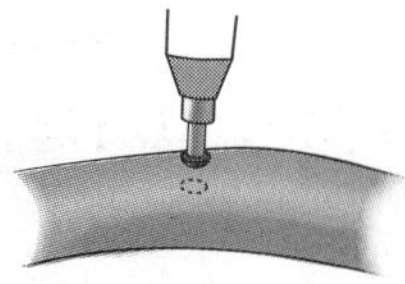

Vascular punch

**Fig. 8-10** Methods of performing an arteriotomy.

- Interrupted sutures
  - Place first sutures 180 degrees apart, then the front wall and back wall.
- Running sutures
  - Place interrupted sutures at the toe and heel, leave long, and run in opposite directions (Fig. 8-11).

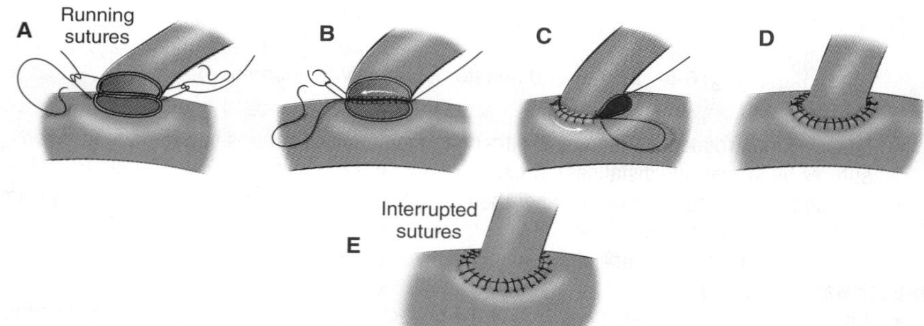


**Fig. 8-11** End-to-side anastomosis. **A-D,** Running suture technique. **E,** Interrupted sutures.

## Vein Grafts

> **TIP:** Excessive tension can compromise anastomosis; consider a vein graft any time there is tension.

- Useful for spanning a gap in either arterial or venous anastomosis.
- Donor sites: Volar wrist or forearm, dorsum of foot, greater or lesser saphenous veins of legs, cephalic vein in deltopectoral groove
- Vein longitudinally marked before completing harvest to prevent twisting
- Vein grafts reversed so that valves do not occlude flow

## Overcoming Size Discrepancy (Fig. 8-12)

- Interposition vein graft
- End-to-side anastomosis
- Sleeving technique
  - Similar patency if proximal vessel is telescoped into distal vessel
- Triangular wedge cut out of larger vessel to cone down and anastomose to smaller vessel
- Also can use spatulation

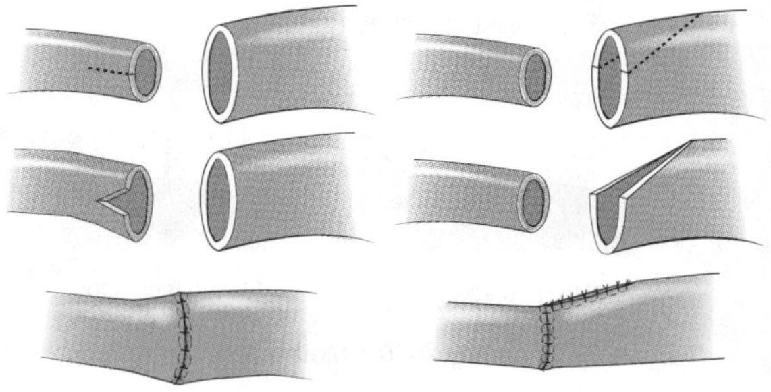

**Fig. 8-12** Size discrepancies can be corrected by spatulation or longitudinal wedge resection.

## POSTOPERATIVE CARE[14] (see Chapters 4 and 5)

### MONITORING ANASTOMOSIS

- **Clinical examination**
  - Assess color, capillary refill, bleeding from cut edges, temperature, and handheld Doppler signals.
  - Flap or digit should be warm and pink with capillary refill time of ~2 seconds.
  - Venous congestion: Flap appears blue and swollen. Skin demonstrates petechiae with rapid capillary refill.
  - Arterial insufficiency: Flap appears pale and flaccid and feels cool; slow or no capillary refill.
  - If unsure, scratch skin with 18-gauge needle and assess bleeding; bright red blood should gradually appear. No bleeding suggests arterial insufficiency. Briskly flowing dark red blood suggests venous outflow obstruction.
  - Arterial Doppler signals sound rhythmic; venous Doppler signals are continuous.
  - When in doubt return to the OR.
- **Venous Doppler**
  - Implantable Doppler probe placed directly on vein and/or artery distal to venous and/or arterial anastomoses before insetting of flap to detect problem before clinical signs
  - Although 100% salvage rate reported using implantable Doppler, many avoid routine use because of high false-negative rate (i.e., signal lost when flap is otherwise fine) and potential for kinking vessels
  - Particularly useful for flaps without a cutaneous skin island for external monitoring ("buried flaps")
- **Transcutanous tissue oximetry**
  - Noninvasive way of continuously measuring perfusion quality of flap postoperatively
  - Oximetry probe measures tissue oxygen saturation ($StO_2$)
  - Probe placed intraoperatively on cutaneous skin island to determine baseline $StO_2$ for the flap
  - Detects vascular compromise of the flap earlier than the development of clinical signs, facilitating earlier intervention
  - May lead to higher flap salvage rates

## FLAP FAILURE

- Success rates are greater than 98% in experienced hands.
- **Flap salvage:** Time to restoration of perfusion is critical.
  - Prompt return to OR increases the chances of flap salvage.
- No-reflow phenomenon
  - Potential source of flap failure despite patent anastomosis
  - Thought to be caused by endothelial swelling, platelet aggregation, and leaky capillaries, resulting in poor tissue perfusion
  - Reversible at 4-8 hours, irreversible after 12 hours

## USE OF ANTICOAGULANTS IN MICROSURGERY

- The best way to prevent flap thrombosis is to harvest a well-designed flap with optimal perfusion, select recipient vessels with robust inflow and outflow, and execute a technically perfect anastomosis. There have been no randomized controlled trials showing improved patency for microsurgery with any of these medications; nevertheless, some microsurgeons routinely prescribe postoperative anticoagulants as a strategy to prevent thrombotic complications.

### Aspirin

- Aspirin inhibits platelet aggregation through inhibition of cyclooxygenase.
- Lower doses (81 and 325 mg) inhibit thromboxane, but not prostacyclin.[15]
- Dose per rectum may be given preoperatively or immediately postoperatively, then continued daily for 2-4 weeks.

### Heparin

- Binds antithrombin III, inducing conformational change and accelerating inhibition of thrombin and factor Xa
- No evidence that systemic heparinization increases anastomotic patency, but does increase risk for postoperative bleeding and hematoma[16,17]
- Systemic anticoagulation with heparin only advocated if intraoperative clot appears at anastomosis or anastomosis is revised suggesting hypercoagulable disorder[18]
  - Partial thromboplastin time maintained at 1.5 to 2 times control
  - Continue 5-7 days postoperatively

### 10% Dextran 40[19]

- Low-molecular-weight polysaccharide
- Exact mechanism unknown, but has the following effects:
  - Volume expansion
  - Inactivates von Willebrand's factor
  - Imparts negative charge on platelets
  - Fibrinolytic effects
- Use is controversial: Evidence that routine use increases complications without increasing microvascular patency rates[20]
- Potential adverse effects of dextran include anaphylaxis, pulmonary edema, and nephrotoxicity.[21]

## MICRONEURAL REPAIR

### General Principles of Repair

- Assess preoperative function.
- Coapt nerves without tension.
- Use interposition graft if there is tension.
- None of the repair types is superior to the others.

### Types of Repair

- **Epineurial**
  - Standard for small nerves
  - 10-0 or 11-0 suture
  - Fascicles lined up and trimmed to prevent buckling of fibers
  - Suture passes through epineurium only (two to three sutures)
  - 180-degree technique
- **Perineurial (fascicular)**
  - Technically more difficult
  - Individual fascicles lined up and sutured
  - Theoretically improves coaptation of fascicles, but no superior results
- **Grouped fascicular**
  - Distinct fascicular groups sutured together at inner epineurial level
  - Can be used for larger nerves at level where specific branches can be identified

## Nerve Grafts and Conduits[22]

- Used if gap or excessive tension is present
- Common donor nerves: Sural nerve, lateral or medial antebrachial cutaneous nerve
- Vein grafts and polyglycolic acid (PGA) nerve tubes can be used for sensory nerve defects of up to 3 cm with results comparable to nerve grafts.[23-26]
- Processed human allograft conduits (AxoGen, Alachua, FL) provide scaffolds (microtubes) through which axons regenerate in a more organized fashion than through simple PGA macrotubes. Allografts may support nerve regeneration better than PGA nerve tubes.[27,28]

### Key Points

- ✓ There are no absolute contraindications to microsurgical reconstruction.
- ✓ Surgeon comfort and exposure of the working field are essential for successful microsurgery.
- ✓ Tension-free anastomoses of vessels and coaptation of nerves are critical.
- ✓ Monitoring devices are helpful postoperatively, but should not supplant a good clinical examination.
- ✓ If you are concerned about the patency of an anastomosis, do not hesitate to take the patient back to the OR—timely reexploration can save a flap.

## References

1. Gottlieb LJ, Krieger LM. From the reconstructive ladder to the reconstructive elevator. Plast Reconstr Surg 93:1503-1504, 1994.
2. Reus WF, Colen LB, Straker DJ. Tobacco smoking and complications in elective microsurgery. Plast Reconstr Surg 89:490-494, 1992.
3. Chang LD, Buncke G, Slezak S, et al. Cigarette smoking, plastic surgery, and microsurgery. J Reconstr Microsurg 12:467-474, 1996.
4. Bengtson BP, Schusterman MA, Baldwin BJ, et al. Influence of prior radiotherapy on the development of postoperative complications and success of free tissue transfers in head and neck cancer reconstruction. Am J of Surg 166:326-330, 1993.
5. Acland RD. Instrumentation for microsurgery. Orthop Clin North Am 8:281-294, 1973.
6. Cox GW, Runnels S, Hsu HS, et al. A comparison of heparinised saline irrigation solutions in a model of microvascular thrombosis. Br J Plast Surg 45:345-348, 1992.

6a. Gilbert RW, Ragnarsson R, Berggren A, et al. Strength of microvascular anastomosis: comparison between the unilink anastomotic system and sutures. Microsurgery 10:40-46, 1989.

7. Jandali S, Wu LC, Vega SJ, et al. 1000 consecutive venous anastomoses using the microvascular anastomotic coupler in breast reconstruction. Plast Reconstr Surg 125:792-799, 2010.
8. Arnold RW, Springer DT, Engel WK, et al. The effect of wrist rest, caffeine, and oral timolol on the hand steadiness of ophthalmologists. Ann Ophthalmol 25:250-253, 1993.
9. Pederson WC. Principles of microsurgery. In Green DP, Hotchkiss RN, Pederson WC, Wolfe SW, eds. Green's Operative Hand Surgery, 5th ed. Philadelphia: Elsevier Churchill Livingstone, 2005.
10. Weiss DD, Pribaz JJ. Microsurgery. In Achauer BM, ed. Plastic Surgery, Indications, Operations, and Outcomes. St Louis: Mosby–Year Book, 2000.
11. Yap, LH, Butler CE. Principles of microsurgery. In Thorne CH, ed. Grabb and Smith's Plastic Surgery. Philadelphia: Lippincott Williams & Wilkins, 2007.
12. Alghoul MS, Gordon CR, Yetman R, et al. From simple interrupted to complex spiral: a systematic review of various suture techniques for microvascular anastomosis. Microsurgery 31:72-80, 2011.

13. Turan T, Ozcelik D, Kuran I, et al. Eversion with four sutures: an easy, fast, and reliable technique for microvascular anastomosis. Plast Reconstr Surg 107:463-470, 2001.
14. Roehl KR, Mahabir RC. A practical guide to free tissue transfer. Plast Reconstr Surg 132:147e-159e, 2013.
15. Weksler BB, Pett SB, Alonso D, et al. Differential inhibition by aspirin of vascular and platelet prostaglandin synthesis in atherosclerotic patients. N Engl J Med 308:800-805, 1983.
16. Pugh CM, Dennis RH II, Massac EA. Evaluation of intraoperative anticoagulants in microvascular free-flap surgery. J Natl Med Assoc 88:655-657, 1996.
17. Kroll SS, Miller MJ, Reece GP, et al. Anticoagulants and hematomas in free flap surgery. Plast Reconstr Surg 96:643-647, 1995.
18. Conrad MH, Adams WP Jr. Pharmacologic optimization of microsurgery in the new millennium. Plast Reconstr Surg 108:2088-2096, 2001.
19. Jallali N. Dextrans in microsurgery. Microsurgery 23:78-80, 2003.
20. Disa JJ, Polvora VP, Pusic AL, et al. Dextran-related complications in head and neck microsurgery: Do the benefits outweigh the risks? A prospective randomized analysis. Plast Reconstr Surg 112:1534-1539, 2003.
21. Riva FM, Chen YC, Tan NC, et al. The outcome of prostaglandin-E1 and dextran-40 compared to no antithrombotic therapy in head and neck free tissue transfer: analysis of 1,351 cases in a single center. Microsurgery 32:339-343, 2012.
22. Walton RL, Brown RE, Matory WE Jr, et al. Autogenous vein graft repair of digital nerve defects in the finger: a retrospective clinical study. Plast Reconstr Surg 84:944-949, 1989.
23. Wang H, Lineaweaver WC. Nerve conduits for nerve reconstruction. Oper Tech Plast Reconstr Surg 9:59-66, 2003.
24. Chiu DT, Strauch B. A prospective clinical evaluation of autogenous vein grafts used as a nerve conduit for distal sensory nerve defects of 3 cm or less. Plast Reconstr Surg 86:928-934, 1990.
25. Mackinnon SE, Dellon AL. Clinical nerve reconstruction with a bioabsorbable polyglycolic acid tube. Plast Reconstr Surg 85:419-424, 1990.
26. Weber RA, Breidenbach WC, Brown RE, et al. A randomized prospective study of polyglycolic acid conduits for digital nerve reconstruction in humans. Plast Reconstr Surg 106:1036-1045, 2000.
27. Karabekmez FE, Dymaz Z, Moran SL. Early clinical outcomes with the use of decellularized nerve allograft for repair of sensory defects within the hand. Hand 4:245-249, 2009.
28. Whitlock EL, Tuffaha SH, Luciano JP, et al. Processed allografts and type I collagen conduits for the repair of peripheral nerve gaps. Muscle Nerve 39:787-799, 2009.

# 9. Biomaterials

**Dinah Wan, Jason K. Potter**

## DEFINITION

*Biomaterials are synthetic and naturally occurring materials used to replace, reconstruct, or augment tissues in the human body.*

## CHOOSING A BIOMATERIAL

- *Permanence* is long-term biocompatibility between the host and implant (Box 9-1).
- Permanence is the most important clinical aspect of an implanted material

**Box 9-1** *IDEAL PROPERTIES FOR BIOMATERIALS*

Biocompatible
Chemically inert
Nonallergenic
Noncarcinogenic
Sterilizable
Cost effective
Easy handling

- The interaction between host and implant commonly is not ideal, and various biologic reactions may be observed (Box 9-2).

**Box 9-2** *BIOLOGIC REACTIONS TO A FOREIGN BODY*

Rejection
Fibrous encapsulation
Resorption
Incorporation

## CLASSIFICATION OF BIOMATERIALS (Table 9-1)

**Table 9-1** *Characteristics of Biomaterials*

| | Incorporation | Resistance to Infection | Antigenicity | Host Tissue Inflammatory Reaction | Infectious Disease Transmission | Availability |
|---|---|---|---|---|---|---|
| **Autograft** | ++++ | +++ | − | + | − | + |
| **Allograft** | +++ | ++ | + | ++ | + | ++ |
| **Xenograft** | ++ | ++ | ++ | ++ | + | ++ |
| **Alloplast** | + | − | − | +++ | − | +++ |

**Autograft:** Living tissue derived from the host

**TIP:** Autografts are the benchmark against which all biomaterials are compared because of their high tolerance and incorporation in the host. Their main disadvantage is the requirement of a donor site.

**Allograft:** Nonliving or living tissue derived from a donor of the same species (e.g., cadaveric, neonatal). Also called *homograft.*
**Xenograft:** Nonliving tissue derived from different species donor (e.g., bovine, porcine)
**Alloplast** Implant derived from synthetic material

**TIP:** Alloplasts have the lowest degree of incorporation into host tissue and are the least tolerant of infection. They almost always require removal if infection occurs.

## SKIN SUBSTITUTES

### SKIN AUTOGRAFTS

- Skin of various thicknesses harvested from the host
- Ideal permanent skin substitute, limited only by availability
- **Split-thickness skin graft (STSG)** (Box 9-3)

**Box 9-3** *STAGES OF STSG TAKE*

*Imbibition* (24-48 hours): Graft obtains nutrients via capillary action
*Inosculation* (48-72 hours): Recipient and donor end capillaries align
*Revascularization* (4-6 days): Full ingrowth of host capillaries into graft

- Includes all of epidermis and part of dermis
  - Thin: 5/1000-12/1000 inch
  - Medium: 12/1000-16/1000 inch
  - Thick: 16/1000-30/1000 inch
- Donor site reepithelializes in 7-14 days
- **Donor sites**
  - Thigh
  - Buttock
  - Back

    - Scalp
    - Arm
  - **Advantages**
    - High chance of graft survival
    - Fast revascularization (4-6 days)
    - Can reharvest from the same donor site
    - Donor site can regenerate hair, because hair follicles left intact in dermis
  - **Disadvantages**
    - High degree of secondary contracture (thinner graft yields more contracture)
    - Poor color and texture match
- **Full-thickness skin graft (FTSG)**
  - Includes all of epidermis and dermis
  - Dermis never regenerates at donor site
  - **Donor sites**
    - Preauricular and postauricular
    - Supraclavicular
    - Groin
    - Axillary
  - **Advantages**
    - Less secondary contracture
    - Better color and texture match
    - Improved sensory return
  - **Disadvantages**
    - Lower chance of graft survival
    - Slower revascularization
    - Must be able to close donor site primarily
- **Cultured epidermal autografts (CEA)**
  - Living keratinocytes cultured from a biopsy specimen of autologous skin and allowed to proliferate
  - **Advantage**
    - Useful in difficult clinical scenarios with limited autologous skin
  - **Disadvantages**
    - Expensive
    - Time-intensive (3 weeks for 10,000-fold keratinocyte expansion)
    - Grown with murine fibroblasts and fetal calf serum, thus potentiating possible immunogenic reaction and rejection of the CEA
    - Extremely fragile
  - ***Epicel*** (Genzyme, Cambridge, MA)
    - Indicated for deep partial and full-thickness burns with total body surface area (TBSA) >30%

## Skin Allografts and Xenografts

- Allografts are derived from cadaveric (nonliving) or neonatal (living) donors.
- Xenografts are derived from bovine or porcine donors.
- Grafts can be *dermal* (includes only dermal elements) or *bilayered* (includes two layers, simulating the dermal and epidermal layers of native skin).
- Grafts can be *acellular* or *cellular*, depending on whether living cells are retained (Box 9-4).

**Box 9-4** *ACELLULAR VERSUS CELLULAR GRAFTS*

***Acellular:*** No living cells remain in graft
- Immunologically inert
- Acellular allografts are derived from decellularized cadaveric source
- Xenografts must be acellular to prevent strong immunogenic host response

***Cellular:*** Living cells (e.g., fibroblasts, keratinocytes) retained in graft
- Can only be from a human source
- Cellular allografts are often cultured from neonatal foreskin
- May cause some degree of immunogenic host response

## ACELLULAR DERMAL MATRIX (ADM)

- Nonliving dermal components from an allogenic or a xenogenic donor
- Composed of collagen, elastin, laminin, and glycosaminoglycans
- Incorporate well into host tissue, with revascularization initiated 1 to 2 weeks after implantation[1]
- More for reinforcing soft tissue repairs and facilitating wound healing rather than actual skin substitutes
- **Clinical applications**
  - **Breast reconstruction**
    - Provides support and additional tissue coverage in implant or expander-based breast reconstructions
    - Shown to help increase intraoperative tissue expansion volume and decrease capsular contracture rate[1-4]
    - Associated with increased seroma rate, although evidence is inconsistent [1-3,5]

**TIP:** Use of ADM with implants or tissue expanders may cause breast erythema mimicking breast cellulitis, also called *red breast syndrome.*[6]

  - **Abdominal wall reconstruction**
    - Provides additional strength in hernia repairs
    - Helps bridge large abdominal wall defects
    - Generally favored over synthetic materials in contaminated wounds

**TIP:** Biologic materials such as ADMs are favored over synthetic materials in contaminated fields, because biologics are better incorporated and more resistant to infection.[7]

  - **Chest wall reconstruction**
  - **Wound healing**
    - Serves as a regenerative tissue matrix for chronic wounds
    - Has been shown to be an effective bridge to definitive STSG coverage in wounds with exposed nerve, vessel, tendon, bone, or cartilage[8]
  - **Head and neck reconstruction**[9]
    - Covers intraoral mucosal defects (e.g., floor of mouth, tongue)
    - Has been shown to reduce fistula rate in cleft palate repairs[10]

- Corrects contour deformities of the nose
- Eyelid reconstruction
- Covers dural defects

- **Allogenic ADMs (Table 9-2)**[11,12]
  - Derived from minimally processed, decellularized, human cadaveric dermis
  - Classified by the FDA as banked human tissue and regulated as human cell and tissue-based products (HCT/P) as of 2001
  - Relatively tolerant to hostile environments, such as irradiated or infected tissues[2]
  - ***AlloDerm*** (LifeCell, Branchburg, NJ)
    - Requires 10-40 minutes of rehydration before application[13]
    - Orientation
      - Dermal side (smooth, shiny): Absorbs blood, usually placed against most vascular tissue or wound bed
      - Basement membrane (rough, dull): Repels blood, usually placed against viscera or expander/implant
    - Used extensively in breast reconstruction
    - Was among the first human ADMs to be used in abdominal wall reconstruction, but soon fell out of favor because of high rates of postoperative bulge and hernia compared with xenogenic ADMs[14,15]
  - ***AlloDerm Ready To Use*** (LifeCell)
    - Similar to AlloDerm, except sterile and requires only 2 minutes for rehydration

**TIP:** AlloDerm is the most extensively used ADM in breast surgery and has the largest body of published evidence supporting this indication.[5]

  - ***DermaMatrix*** (MTF, Edison, NJ)
    - Used in breast, abdominal wall, facial, and intraoral reconstructions
  - ***FlexHD*** (MTF)
    - Used in breast and abdominal wall reconstruction
  - ***GraftJacket*** (Wright Medical Technology, Arlington, TN)
    - Used in diabetic/venous/pressure ulcers and tendon/ligament reconstruction[16]
  - ***DermACELL*** (Arthrex, Naples, FL)
    - Indicated for diabetic foot ulcers and chronic nonhealing wounds
  - ***Repriza*** (Specialty Surgical Products, Victor, MT)
    - Indicated in breast and abdominal wall reconstruction and augmentation of soft tissue irregularities
  - ***DermaSpan*** (Biomet, Warsaw, IN)
    - Used for wound or tendon coverage
  - ***AlloMax*** (CR Bard, Warwick, RI)
    - Used in abdominal wall reconstruction and hiatal hernia repairs

- **Xenogenic ADMs (see Table 9-2)**
  - Derived from porcine or bovine source
  - Classified by FDA as a medical device, which requires 510(k) clearance before marketing
  - Requires more extensive processing than allografts to reduce immunogenicity
  - Processing may involve *cross-linking*, which inhibits collagen degradation by collagenase

**Table 9-2** *Summary of Current Acellular Dermal Matrices (ADMs)*

| ADM | Source | FDA Regulation | Processor | Preparation Time | Preparation | Cross-linked |
|---|---|---|---|---|---|---|
| **Allografts*** | | | | | | |
| AlloDerm | Cadaveric dermis | Regulated as HCT/P | LifeCell | 10-40 min | Room-temp or warm NS/LR | No |
| AlloDerm Ready to Use | Cadaveric dermis | Regulated as HCT/P | LifeCell | 2 min | Room-temp NS/LR | No |
| DermaMatrix | Cadaveric dermis | Regulated as HCT/P | MTF | <3 min | Room-temp NS/LR | No |
| FlexHD | Cadaveric dermis | Regulated as HCT/P | MTF | None | None | No |
| GraftJacket | Cadaveric dermis | Regulated as HCT/P | Wright Medical | 10 min | Room-temp or warm NS/LR | No |
| DermACELL | Cadaveric dermis | Regulated as HCT/P | Arthrex | None | None | No |
| Repriza | Cadaveric dermis | Regulated as HCT/P | SSP | None | None | No |
| DermaSpan | Cadaveric dermis | Regulated as HCT/P | Biomet | 15-45 min | Room-temp NS | No |
| AlloMax | Cadaveric dermis | Regulated as HCT/P | CR Bard | 3 min | Room-temp NS | No |
| **Xenografts‡** | | | | | | |
| Surgisis Biodesign | Porcine submucosa | 510(k) clearance in 1998 | Cook Surgical | 3-10 min | Room-temp NS | No |
| Oasis | Porcine submucosa | 510(k) clearance in 2000 | Cook Biotech | None | None | No |
| Tutopatch | Bovine pericardium | 510(k) clearance in 2000 | RTI Biologics | Several min | Room-temp NS | No |
| Permacol | Porcine dermis | 510(k) clearance in 2000 | Covidien | None | None | Yes |
| Veritas | Bovine pericardium | 510(k) clearance in 2000 | Synovis Surgical | None | None | No |

*All allograft materials are considered banked human tissue and are regulated by the FDA as Human Cell and Tissue-based Products (HCT/P) as of 2001. Manufacturers of allogenic ADMs are required to register *annually* with the FDA to be considered an accredited tissue bank of the American Association of Tissue Banks (AATB).

†Provided in a nonsterile pouch.

‡Xenografts are considered medical devices and require FDA 510(k) clearance prior to marketing.

| Sterile | Type of Sterilization | Refrigeration | Hydration | Orientation | Additional Features | Shelf Life |
|---|---|---|---|---|---|---|
| | | | | | | |
| No | Aseptically processed† | Yes | Dehydrated | Yes | Freeze-dried | 2 yr |
| Yes | eBeam radiation | No | Hydrated | Yes | Terminally sterilized | 2 yr |
| No | Aseptically processed; passes USP <71> for sterility | No | Dehydrated | Yes | Freeze-dried<br>High tensile strength | 3 yr |
| No | Aseptically processed; passes USP <71> for sterility | No | Hydrated | Yes | Resistance to stretching | 3 yr |
| No | Aseptically processed† | Yes | Dehydrated | Yes | Freeze-dried<br>High tensile strength<br>Pre-meshed | 2 yr |
| Yes | Terminally sterilized (10-6 SAL) | No | Hydrated | Yes | >97% DNA removed | 2 yr |
| Yes | Undefined | No | Hydrated | No | Custom sizing available | 2 yr |
| Yes | Gamma radiation | No | Dehydrated | Yes | Freeze-dried<br>High tensile strength | Not specified |
| Yes | Gamma radiation | No | Dehydrated | No | Not freeze-dried | 5 yr |
| | | | | | | |
| Yes | Ethylene oxide | No | Dehydrated | No | Multilaminate | 18 mo |
| Yes | Ethylene oxide | No | Dehydrated | No | Rehydrate with NS *after* application | 2 yr |
| Yes | Gamma radiation | No | Dehydrated | Yes | Flexible | 5 yr |
| Yes | Gamma radiation | No | Hydrated | No | Durable | 3 yr |
| Yes | Irradiated | No | Hydrated | No | Less DNA in end-product | 3 yr |

*Continued*

**Table 9-2** *Summary of Current Acellular Dermal Matrices (ADMs)—cont'd*

| ADM | Source | FDA Regulation | Processor | Preparation Time | Preparation | Cross-linked |
|---|---|---|---|---|---|---|
| CollaMend | Porcine dermis | 510(k) clearance in 2006 | CR Bard | 3 min | Room-temp NS | Yes |
| SurgiMend | Fetal bovine dermis | 510(k) clearance in 2007 | TEI BioSciences | 60 sec | Room-temp NS | No |
| Strattice | Porcine dermis | 510(k) clearance in 2007 | LifeCell | 2 min | Room-temp NS/LR | No |
| XenMatrix | Porcine dermis | 510(k) clearance in 2008 | CR Bard | None | None | No |

**TIP:** Cross-linking strengthens the material, prolongs its lifespan, and decreases its antigenicity. However, it also delays incorporation, prolongs inflammation, promotes bowel adhesions, and increases infection rate. Generally speaking, cross-linking causes a biologic material to behave more like a synthetic material.[14,15,17-20]

- ***Surgisis Biodesign*** (Cook Surgical, Bloomington, IN)
  - Non-cross-linked porcine small intestine submucosal collagen matrix
  - Non-dermis-based matrix contains only trace amounts of elastin, thus limiting stretch
  - One of the first biologic grafts used for hernia repair (FDA clearance in 1998)
  - Indicated for ventral/hiatal/inguinal hernia repair, fistula repair, and pelvic floor reconstruction
- ***Oasis*** (Cook Biotech, Lafayette, IN)
  - Non-cross-linked porcine small intestine submucosal collagen matrix
  - Primarily used as a regenerative wound matrix
  - Indicated for diabetic and venous stasis ulcers, surgical wounds, draining wounds, burns, and trauma wounds
- ***Tutopatch*** (RTI Biologics, Alachua, FL)
  - Non-cross-linked bovine pericardium
  - Used in ventral and hiatal hernia repairs, ligament and tendon reconstructions, orbital floor and maxillary wall reconstructions
  - Can also implant subdermally to smooth facial wrinkles and fill subcutaneous defects
- ***Permacol*** (Covidien, Mansfield, MA)
  - Cross-linked porcine dermal matrix
  - Used in abdominal wall reconstruction
- ***Veritas*** (Synovis Surgical Innovations, St. Paul, MN)
  - Non-cross-linked bovine pericardium
  - Used in abdominal wall reconstruction
- ***CollaMend*** (CR Bard)
  - Cross-linked porcine dermal matrix
  - Relatively high infection and low incorporation rate because of heavy cross-linking[18]
  - Indicated in abdominal and chest wall reconstruction

| Sterile | Type of Sterilization | Refrigeration | Hydration | Orientation | Additional Features | Shelf Life |
|---|---|---|---|---|---|---|
| Yes | Ethylene oxide | No | Dehydrated | No | Fenestrated. Heavily cross-linked | 9.5 mo |
| Yes | Ethylene oxide | No | Dehydrated | No | Type III collagen | 3 yr |
| Yes | eBeam radiation | No | Hydrated | No | Nonsided | 18 mo |
| Yes | eBeam radiation | No | Hydrated | No | Open collagen structure | Not specified |

- ***SurgiMend*** (TEI Biosciences, Boston, MA)
  - Non-cross-linked bovine dermal matrix
  - Used in abdominal wall reconstruction and inguinal hernia repairs
- ***Strattice*** (LifeCell)
  - Non-cross-linked porcine dermal matrix
  - Used in breast and abdominal wall reconstruction
- ***XenMatrix*** (CR Bard)
  - Non-cross-linked porcine dermal matrix
  - Used in abdominal wall reconstruction
  - Certain lots recalled in 2011 for high endotoxin levels

■ **Acellular Bilayered Matrix**

- The "dermal" layer serves as an acellular scaffold for fibrovascular ingrowth
- The "epidermal" layer is often a synthetic substitute and serves as a semipermeable barrier to microbes and moisture loss
- Primarily used as a tissue regeneration matrix or temporary biologic dressing for wounds
- ***Integra Dermal Regeneration Template*** (Integra LifeSciences, Plainsboro, NJ)
  - Bilayered matrix composed of bovine collagen cross-linked with shark glycosaminoglycans, with a semipermeable silicone outer layer
  - Neovascularization of the dermal component complete at 3 weeks
  - Top silicone layer removed at 2 to 4 weeks for application of autologous skin graft
  - **Advantages**
    - Allows for thinner STSG (4/1000-6/1000 inch) to be placed over the vascularized dermal matrix
    - Provides a vascularized bed over exposed bone, tendon, or joint
  - **Disadvantages**
    - Expensive
    - Requires two procedures

- **Clinical applications**[16]
  - FDA approved in 1996 for postexcisional treatment of full or deep partial-thickness burns where sufficient autograft is not available
  - FDA approved in 2002 for reconstruction of scar contractures where other therapies have failed
- ***Integra Meshed Bilayer Wound Matrix*** (Integra LifeSciences)
  - Bilayered matrix with meshed silicone layer to allow drainage of wound exudate
  - Designed for use with negative-pressure therapy
  - Indicated for diabetic/pressure/venous ulcers, surgical wounds, trauma wounds, draining wounds, and burns
- ***Integra Matrix Wound Dressing*** (Integra LifeSciences)
- ***Integra Dermal Regeneration Template–Single Layer*** (Integra LifeSciences)
  - Consists of dermal collagen matrix without silicone outer layer
  - Can be used as an extra layer under the bilayered Integra matrix to add thickness in deep or tunneled wounds
  - Thin (1.3 mm) dermal matrix revascularizes quickly, allowing placement of autologous STSG over the dermal matrix in the same-stage procedure
  - Animal and clinical studies have shown successful STSG take when placed in the same procedure over a single-layered Integra dermal matrix[21,22]
- ***Biobrane*** (Smith & Nephew, Largo, FL)
  - Porcine collagen embedded in nylon mesh, with a semipermeable silicone outer layer
  - Must be removed 7 to 14 days after application prior to permanent skin grafting
  - Indicated for temporary coverage of freshly excised superficial burn wounds

- **Cellular Dermal Matrix**
  - ***Dermagraft*** (Advanced Tissue Sciences, La Jolla, CA)
    - Neonatal foreskin fibroblasts prepared on a biodegradable polyglactin mesh
    - Indicated for noninfected, full-thickness, diabetic foot ulcers that do not involve tendon, muscle, joint, or bone
- **Cellular Bilayered Matrix**
  - Includes neonatal fibroblasts in the dermal layer and keratinocytes in the epidermal layer
  - Most closely mimics the biologic activity of autologous skin
  - ***Apligraf*** (Organogenesis, Canton, MA)
    - Neonatal fibroblasts and keratinocytes cultured onto a bovine collagen matrix
    - 10-day shelf life
    - Indicated for noninfected venous and diabetic ulcers that do not involve tendon, muscle, joint, or bone
  - ***OrCel*** (Ortec International, New York, NY)
    - Neonatal fibroblasts and keratinocytes cultured onto a bovine collagen matrix
    - Cryopreserved, thus longer shelf-life
    - Indicated in diabetic and venous ulcers and burn wounds
  - ***TransCyte*** (Advanced BioHealing, La Jolla, CA)
    - Neonatal fibroblasts seeded in Biobrane (porcine collagen matrix with silicone outer layer)
    - Indicated for temporary coverage of surgically excised deep partial and full-thickness burn wounds prior to permanent skin grafting

## BONE SUBSTITUTES (Table 9-3)[23]

**Table 9-3** *Comparison of Bone Grafts and Their Biologic Properties*

| | Strength | Osteoconduction | Osteoinduction | Osteogenesis |
|---|---|---|---|---|
| ***Autograft*** | | | | |
| Cancellous | No | +++ | +++ | +++ |
| Cortical | +++ | ++ | ++ | ++ |
| ***Allograft*** | | | | |
| Cancellous | | | | |
| *Fresh-frozen* | No | ++ | + | No |
| *Freeze-dried* | No | ++ | + | No |
| Cortical | | | | |
| *Fresh-frozen* | +++ | + | No | No |
| *Freeze-dried* | + | + | No | No |
| ***Alloplast*** | +++ | + | No | No |

- Most clinically relevant bone grafts are autologous, allogenic, or synthetic, with xenografts playing a limited role.
- The stages of bone graft incorporation are similar to the stages of bone healing (Box 9-5).

**Box 9-5** *STAGES OF BONE GRAFT INCORPORATION*

Hematoma formation
Inflammation
Vascular ingrowth
Focal osteoclastic resorption of graft
New bone formation on graft surfaces

- Incorporation of the bone graft depends on its biologic properties (Box 9-6).

**Box 9-6** *BIOLOGIC PROPERTIES OF BONE GRAFTS*

*Osteogenesis:* Osteoblasts within the graft directly produce bone.
*Osteoinduction:* Growth factors (principally BMP) within the graft stimulate osteogenesis in host tissue.
*Osteoconduction:* The graft serves as a nonviable scaffold for bony ingrowth.

## BONE AUTOGRAFTS

- Cancellous or cortical bone derived from the host
- Retains all biologic properties (osteogenesis, osteoinduction, osteoconduction)
- Highest rate of incorporation, but requires a donor site
- **Cancellous bone**
  - Includes high concentrations of osteoblasts and growth factors
  - Heals primarily by osteogenesis

- Donor sites
  - Iliac crest
  - Metaphyseal bone (femur, tibia, distal radius)
- **Advantage**
  - Rapid revascularization: Incorporates within 2 weeks of grafting
- **Disadvantage**
  - Minimal to no immediate structural support
- **Clinical applications**
  - Nonunions or small bone gaps (<6 cm) where immediate structural rigidity is not needed

■ **Cortical bone**
- Less biologically active than cancellous bone
- Heals primarily by osteoconduction
- Common donor sites
  - Fibula
  - Radius
  - Iliac crest
  - Calvarium
  - Rib

**TIP:** Remove cartilaginous cap to prevent bony overgrowth.

- **Advantages**
  - Immediate structural support
  - Maintains significantly more volume than cancellous grafts over time[24]
- **Disadvantage**
  - Slow revascularization: Takes up to 2 months to fully incorporate
- **Clinical applications**
  - Segmental bony defects larger than 5 cm where structural support is immediately needed

## Bone Allografts

- Cortical or cancellous bone derived from cadaveric donors
- Cadaveric grafts are processed to remove osteoblasts and growth factors, thus limiting osteogenic and osteoinductive properties
- Principally osteoconductive
- Slow union time (1-2 years)
- Fresh-frozen allografts
  - Sterilized, washed, then frozen at −70° C
  - Relatively immunogenic
  - Retains more strength than freeze-dried grafts
- Freeze-dried (lyophilized) allografts
  - Sterilized, washed, frozen, then vacuum-desiccated
  - Can be stored at room temperature
  - Lower risk of infectious disease transmission and less immunogenic than fresh-frozen grafts

## Synthetic Bone Substitutes (Alloplasts)

- Principally osteoconductive, with little to no osteogenic or osteoinductive properties
- Varied resorption rates
- **Calcium sulfate *(Plaster of Paris)***
  - One of the earliest materials used as a bone void filler
  - Undergoes rapid and complete resorption at 5-8 weeks[25,26]

- **Advantages**
  - Safe and well tolerated
  - Rapid resorption permits use if there is infection
- **Disadvantages**
  - Relatively low compressive strength with little structural support[26]
  - Requires a dry environment
- **Clinical applications**
  - Augments autologous bone grafts in fractures or nonunions
  - Bony void filler if there is osteomyelitis
- ***Osteoset*** (Wright Medical Technology): Antibiotic-impregnated calcium sulfate

- **Calcium phosphates**
  - Good compressive strength, but poor tensile strength (brittle)[25]
  - Highly inert with relatively limited resorption[27]
  - Favorable infection rate ($<$3% in craniofacial reconstruction)[28]
  - Clinical applications[26]
    - Void filler for metaphyseal defects (fractures, nonunions)
    - Reconstruction of craniofacial defects
    - Soft tissue filler (e.g., facial augmentation)
  - **Hydroxyapatite (HA)**
    - HA = $Ca_{10}(PO_4)_6(OH)_2$, the principle mineral component of human bone
    - *Ceramic HA:* Synthetic HA crystals sintered at high heat to form a highly crystalline and dense structure
      - Considered clinically permanent with resorption rate of $<$5% per year[25,27,29]
      - ***Calcitite*** (Calcitek, San Diego, CA)
    - *Coralline HA:* naturally derived from marine coral exoskeletons, yielding a porous structure similar to cancellous bone
      - Porous structure allows for more fibro-osseous ingrowth
      - ***ProOsteon*** (Interpore Cross, Irvine, CA)
    - *Cementable HA:* forms dense paste when mixed with water which can be molded to shape intraoperatively
      - Sets isothermally
      - Used to resurface bony contour irregularities
      - ***BoneSource*** (Stryker, Portage, MI)
      - ***NorianSRS*** (Norian, Westchester, PA)
  - **Beta tricalcium phosphate (βTCP)**
    - Unpredictable resorption rate (6-18 months)[25]
    - Porous structure is similar to cancellous bone
    - ***Vitoss*** (Orthovita, Malvern, PA)
    - ***Orthograft*** (DePuy, Warsaw, IN)

- **Methylmethacrylate (MMA)**
  - A nonresorbable, high-density, porous polymer
  - Used as a bone cement
  - **Advantages**
    - Inexpensive
    - Easily molded
    - Inert, biocompatible
    - High compression strength
    - Can be impregnated with antibiotic for use in infected fractures

- **Disadvantages**
  - Exothermic reaction when mixed, requiring continual cooling
  - Dense structure inhibits bony incorporation
  - Becomes encapsulated rather than incorporated
- **Clinical applications**
  - Cranial reconstruction
  - Forehead augmentation
  - Fixation of joint replacements
  - Void filler in bony gaps and fractures

## CARTILAGE SUBSTITUTES

### CARTILAGE AUTOGRAFTS

- **Biologic properties**
  - Avascular, dense extracellular matrix supported by chondroblasts
  - Low metabolic rate (1/100 to 1/500 the rate of other human tissues)
- **Donor sites**
  - Cartilaginous nasal septum
  - Conchal cartilage
  - Rib
- **Advantages**
  - Low resorption rate: Retains bulk and shape[30]
  - Can be sculpted to precise form
  - Rarely becomes infected
- **Disadvantages**
  - Dense matrix impedes cellular ingrowth and graft incorporation
  - Warping: Cartilage carved on one side curves toward the intact, taut opposite side
- **Clinical applications**
  - Facial reconstruction (e.g., nose, ear, eyelid)
  - Nipple augmentation

### CARTILAGE ALLOGRAFTS

- Cadaveric source
- Has been shown to undergo ossification and calcification with time[31]
- Higher resorption and infection rate than autologous cartilage[32]

## MISCELLANEOUS ALLOPLASTIC MATERIALS

### METALS

- High tensile and compressive strength
- Frequently used in reconstructive plates and screws for craniofacial and bony surgery
- **Stainless steel**
  - Alloy of iron, nickel, and molybdenum, with a surface layer of chromium oxide
  - **Advantage**
    - High tensile and compressive strength
  - **Disadvantages**
    - Undergoes corrosion after several years
    - Risk of allergic reaction due to high nickel content
    - High scatter on CT/MRI

- **Clinical applications**
  - Reconstructive plates and screws

- **Vitallium**
  - Alloy of cobalt and chromium
  - **Advantages**
    - Relatively resistant to corrosion
    - Similar or higher strength than stainless steel
    - Produces less radiographic scatter than stainless steel
  - **Disadvantage**
    - Difficult to bend and shape
  - **Clinical applications**
    - Reconstructive plates and screws
- **Titanium**
  - Pure metal, not an alloy[24]
  - **Advantages**
    - 10× strength of bone
    - Resistant to corrosion
    - High degree of fibro-osseous ingrowth
    - Little radiologic scatter
    - Easily contoured
  - **Clinical applications**
    - Used as mesh or plates for large and complex orbital wall defects
    - Reconstructive plates and screws (often alloyed with other metals)

> **TIP:** Titanium has largely replaced stainless steel and vitallium in reconstructive surgery because of its many advantages.

- **Gold**
  - **Advantage**
    - Highly resistant to corrosion
  - **Disadvantages**
    - Expensive
    - Soft, lacks strength (not indicated in craniofacial fixation)
  - **Clinical applications**
    - Main utility is in weighting the upper eyelid in facial paralysis

## POLYMERS

- Synthetic chemical compounds consisting of repeating structural units
- Can be synthesized with varied degrees of porosity[33] (Box 9-7)
- Often used as surgical mesh or implants

**Box 9-7** *POROSITY OF POLYMERS*

*Macroporous* (pores >75 μm): Enables the highest degree of cellular ingrowth and graft incorporation (e.g., Prolene, Marlex).

*Microporous* (pores <10 μm): Allows some degree of cellular ingrowth and incorporation without excessive inflammation and host tissue adhesion (e.g., Gore-Tex).

*Nonporous:* Dense and smooth surface does not allow for any cellular ingrowth. These implants become encapsulated without incorporation.

## Nonresorbable Polymers

- Highly biocompatible, inert, and stable
- High tensile strength
- ***Medpor*** (Porex Surgical, Newnan, GA)
  - *High-density polyethylene* (HDPE)
  - Large pore size (100-200 mm) allows significant fibrovascular ingrowth, but also makes difficult to remove[34]
  - Available as mesh and implants of various shapes and sizes
  - **Clinical applications**
    - Implants for facial augmentation (chin, nasal, malar, temporal, etc.)
    - Mesh for simple orbital floor defects
    - Auricular reconstruction
- ***Gore-Tex*** (WL Gore, Flagstaff, AZ)
  - Microporous *expanded polytetrafluoroethylene* (ePTFE)
  - Available as mesh, tubes, and blocks
  - **Clinical applications**
    - Implants for facial augmentation (e.g., lip, chin, nasal, malar, forehead)
    - Mesh for chest and abdominal wall reconstruction
    - Tubes for vascular grafts
    - Muscle slings for facial palsy
- ***Gore DualMesh*** (WL Gore)
  - Dual-surfaced ePTFE mesh designed for abdominal hernia repair
  - Smooth microporous surface placed against viscera to limit bowel adhesions
  - Rough corduroy surface with larger pores placed against abdominal wall to encourage host tissue incorporation
- ***Marlex*** (CR Bard), ***Prolene*** (Ethicon, Somerville, NJ)
  - Macroporous heavyweight *polypropylene* (PE) mesh
  - Used in chest and abdominal wall reconstruction
- ***Mersilene*** (Ethicon)
  - Macroporous *polyethylene terephthalate* (PET) mesh with microporous components
  - Used in abdominal hernia repair

> **TIP:** Macroporous mesh such as Marlex and Prolene has been shown to cause significantly denser bowel adhesions than microporous mesh such as Gore-Tex.[14]

## Resorbable Polymers

- Variable absorption rates
- May cause some inflammation during the absorption process
- ***Dexon*** (Covidien), ***Vicryl*** (Ethicon)
  - Absorbable mesh composed of polyglycolic acid (Dexon) or polyglactin 910 (Vicryl)
  - Used in abdominal wall reconstruction
  - Maintains integrity for 4-6 weeks, providing support while granulation tissue forms[35]
  - Favored over synthetic materials in infected fields
  - Also used as absorbable suture material
- ***TIGR*** (Novus Scientific, San Diego, CA)
  - 100% synthetic, long-term, dual-stage, resorbable mesh
  - Two fiber types:
    - **Fast-resorbing fiber** (copolymer of lactide, glycolide, and trimethylene carbonate): Maintains strength for 1-2 weeks, completely resorbed in 4 months

        - **Slow-resorbing fiber** (copolymer of lactide and trimethylene carbonate): Maintains strength for 6-9 months, completely resorbed in 3 years
    - Overall mesh maintains strength for 6 months, completely resorbed within 3 years
    - Dual-staged: Mechanics designed for gradually increasing compliance
    - Indicated for reinforcement of soft tissue where weakness exists

**TIP:** Although resorbable meshes, such as Vicryl or Dexon, are suitable temporary solutions in the setting of infection, they inevitably lead to hernia recurrence after the graft is completely absorbed.[14]

- ***LactoSorb*** (Walter Lorenz Surgical, Jacksonville, FL)
    - A resorbable plating system for pediatric craniomaxillofacial fixation
    - Made of 82% polylactide and 18% polygycolic acid
    - Retains 70% of its strength at 8 weeks, allowing for complete osseous union
    - Complete degradation within 9-15 months prevents growth interference or late complications[36]

## Composite Mesh

- Surgical mesh composed of two or more materials with different chemical and physical properties
- Mostly used in ventral hernia repairs
- **Tissue-separating mesh**
    - Includes a nonresorbable polymer on one surface with a biologic or resorbable material on the other surface.
    - The porous, synthetic surface is placed against the abdominal wall to encourage host tissue incorporation, whereas the bioresorbable surface is placed against the viscera to limit bowel adhesions.
    - Proper orientation is integral to success of repair.
    - ***Proceed*** (Ethicon)
        - Two-sided mesh with polypropylene on one side and oxidized regenerated cellulose (a plant-based biologic material) on the other side
        - Two sides bonded by an intervening layer of polydiaxanone (PDS), a resorbable polymer
    - ***SepraMesh*** (CR Bard)
        - Two-sided mesh with polypropylene on one side and absorbable polyglycolic acid (PGA) coated with bioresorbable hydrogel (hyaluronate and carboxymethylcellulose) on the other side.
        - PGA fibers maintain 50% of strength at 4 weeks.
        - Hydrogel protects viscera until completely resorbed (within 4 weeks).
    - ***Parietex*** (Covidien)
        - Macroporous polyester mesh coated with resorbable collagen film on one side
- **Coated Mesh**
    - Synthetic mesh coated on both sides with a low-inflammatory material
    - ***C-Qur*** (Atrium, Hudson, NH)
        - Lightweight polypropylene mesh coated with omega-3 fatty acid (O3FA)
        - O3FA allows more natural healing with less visceral adhesions and inflammation
        - O3FA coating is ~70% absorbed in 120 days
    - ***TiMesh*** (Atrium)
        - Lightweight polypropylene mesh with covalent-bonded titanized surface
        - Highly biocompatible titanium surface limits inflammatory response

## SILICONE

- A nonresorbable polymer based on the element silicon
- Can take the form of liquid, gel, or solid, depending on the length of chains and degree of cross-linking (solid form consists of the longest chains and the most cross-linking)
- Injectable silicone (liquid or gel) is *not* FDA-approved because of the risk of granulomas and siliconomas
- **Advantages**
  - Inert and resistant to degradation
  - Sterilizable
  - Concerns for systemic disease associated with silicone implants have been refuted[37]
- **Disadvantages**
  - Nonporous, thus no tissue ingrowth
  - Becomes encapsulated, not incorporated
- **Clinical applications**
  - Breast implant fillers (FDA-reapproved in 2006) and outer shells
  - Implants for soft tissue augmentation (malar, chin, nasal, chest, calf), joint replacement, and tendon reconstruction

## KEY POINTS

✓ Autografts are the benchmark against which all biomaterials are compared because of their high tolerance and incorporation in the host.

✓ Split-thickness skin grafts revascularize quicker and have higher rates of graft survival, whereas full-thickness skin grafts offer improved cosmesis with less secondary contracture.

✓ Acellular dermal matrices are frequently used to provide additional support and coverage in breast and abdominal wall reconstructions.

✓ *AlloDerm* is the most extensively used acellular dermal matrix in breast surgery and has the largest body of evidence supporting this indication.

✓ Cross-linking strengthens the dermal collagen matrix and prolongs its lifespan, but also increases inflammation, delays incorporation, and increases infection rate.

✓ Bilayered skin matrices are often used as temporary wound dressings and provide a vascularized bed over exposed bone, tendon, or joint for autologous skin grafting.

✓ Cortical bone grafts provide greater initial strength and maintain more volume with time, whereas cancellous grafts incorporate quicker and retain more biologic properties.

✓ Cartilage autografts are highly inert and stable, retaining bulk and shape with low incidences of cellular ingrowth, inflammation, and infection.

✓ Titanium has largely replaced stainless steel and vitallium for craniofacial reconstruction because of its many advantages.

✓ Macroporous polymers enable a high degree of cellular infiltration and host tissue adhesions, making them difficult to remove.

✓ Biologic and resorbable meshes are favored if there is infection, but they offer less strength than synthetic meshes.

✓ Composite mesh offers the dual advantage of strength and tissue incorporation on the synthetic surface while limiting visceral adhesions on the bioresorbable surface.

✓ Resorbable alloplasts are useful in pediatric patients.

## REFERENCES


1. Nahabedian MY. Acellular dermal matrices in primary breast reconstruction: principles, concepts, and indications. Plast Reconstr Surg 130(5 Suppl 2):S44-S53, 2012.
2. Clemens MW, Kronowitz SJ. Acellular dermal matrix in irradiated tissue expander/implant-based breast reconstruction: evidence-based review. Plast Reconstr Surg 130(5 Suppl 2):S27-S34, 2012.
3. Basu CB, Jeffers L. The role of acellular dermal matrices in capsular contracture: a review of the evidence. Plast Reconstr Surg 130(5 Suppl 2):S118-S124, 2012.
4. Bengtson B. Acellular dermal matrices in secondary aesthetic breast surgery: indications, techniques, and outcomes. Plast Reconstr Surg 130(5 Suppl 2):S142-S156, 2012.
5. Israeli R. Complications of acellular dermal matrices in breast surgery. Plast Reconstr Surg 130 (5 Suppl 2):S159-S172, 2012.
6. Kim JY, Connor CM. Focus on technique: two-stage implant-based breast reconstruction. Plast Reconstr Surg 130(5 Suppl 2):S104-S115, 2012.
7. Janis JE, O'Neill AC, Ahmad J, et al. Acellular dermal matrices in abdominal wall reconstruction: a systematic review of the current evidence. Plast Reconstr Surg 130(5 Suppl 2):S183-S193, 2012.
8. Ellis CV, Kulber DA. Acellular dermal matrices in hand reconstruction. Plast Reconstr Surg 130 (5 Suppl 2):S256-S269, 2012.
9. Shridharani SM, Tufaro AP. A systematic review of acelluar dermal matrices in head and neck reconstruction. Plast Reconstr Surg 130(5 Suppl 2):S35-S43, 2012.
10. Aldekhayel SA, Sinno H, Gilardino MS. Acellular dermal matrix in cleft palate repair: an evidence-based review. Plast Reconstr Surg 130:177-182, 2012.
11. Moyer HR, Losken A. The science behind tissue biologics. Plastic Surgery Pulse News 3(4):43-49, 2011.
12. Cheng A, Saint-Cyr M. Comparison of different ADM materials in breast surgery. Clin Plastic Surg 39:167-175, 2012.
13. Becker S, Saint-Cyr M, Wong C, et al. AlloDerm versus DermaMatrix in immediate expander-based breast reconstruction: a preliminary comparison of complication profiles and material compliance. Plast Reconstr Surg 123:1-6, 2009.
14. Turza KC, Butler CE. Adhesions and meshes: synthetic versus bioprosthetic. Plast Reconstr Surg 130(5 Suppl 2):S206-S213, 2012.
15. Patel KM, Bhanot P. Complications of acellular dermal matrices in abdominal wall reconstruction. Plast Reconstr Surg 130(5 Suppl 2):S216-S224, 2012.
16. Iorio ML, Shuck J, Attinger CE. Wound healing in the upper and lower extremities: a systematic review on the use of acellular dermal matrices. Plast Reconstr Surg 130(5 Suppl 2):S232-S241, 2012.
17. Dunn RM. Cross-linking in biomaterials: a primer for clinicians. Plast Reconstr Surg 130(5 Suppl 2): S18-S26, 2012.
18. Novitsky YW, Rosen MJ. The biology of biologics: basic science and clinical concepts. Plast Reconstr Surg 130(5 Suppl 2):S9-S17, 2012.
19. Bengtson B. Discussion: use of dermal matrix to prevent capsular contracture in aesthetic breast surgery. Plast Reconstr Surg 130(5 Suppl 2):S137-S141, 2012.
20. Butler CE, Burns NK, Campbell KT, et al. Comparison of cross-linked and non-cross-linked porcine acellular dermal matrices for ventral hernia repair. J Am Coll Surg 211:368-376, 2010.
21. Bottcher-Haberzeth S, Biedermann T, Schiestl C, et al. Matriderm 1 mm versus Integra Single Layer 1.3 mm for one-step closure of full thickness skin defects: a comparative experimental study in rats. Pediatr Surg Int 28:171-177, 2012.
22. Koenen W, Felcht M, Vockenroth K, et al. One-stage reconstruction of deep facial defects with a single layer dermal regeneration template. J Eur Acad Dermatol Venereol 25:788-793, 2011.
23. Parikh SN. Bone graft substitutes: past, present, future. J Postgrad Med 48:142-148, 2002.

24. Ozaki W, Buchman SR. Volume maintenance of onlay bone grafts in the craniofacial skeleton: micro-architecture versus embryologic origin. Plast Reconstr Surg 102:291-299, 1998.
25. Moore WR, Graves SE, Bain GI. Synthetic bone graft substitutes. ANZ J Surg 71:354-361, 2001.
26. Kakar S, Tsiridia E, Einhorn T. Bone grafting and enhancement of fracture repair. In: Bucholz R, Heckman J, Court-Brown C, eds. Rockwood & Green's Fractures in Adults, vol 1, 6th ed. Philadelphia: Lippincott Williams & Wilkins, 2006.
27. Holmes RE, Hagler HK. Porous hydroxyapatite as a bone graft substitute in cranial reconstruction: a histometric study. Plast Reconstr Surg 81:662-671, 1988.
28. Rubin JP, Yaremchuk MJ. Complications and toxicities of implantable biomaterials used in facial reconstructive and aesthetic surgery: a comprehensive review of the literature. Plast Reconstr Surg 100:1336-1353, 1997.
29. Jamali A, Hilpert A, Debes J, et al. Hydroxyapatite/calcium carbonate (HA/CC) vs. plaster of Paris: a histomorphometric and radiographic study in a rabbit tibial defect model. Calcif Tissue Int 71:172-178, 2002.
30. Peer LA. The neglected septal cartilage graft, with experimental observations on the growth of human cartilage grafts. Arch Otolaryngol 42:384-396, 1945.
31. Chen JM, Zingg M, Laedrach K, et al. Early surgical intervention for orbital floor fractures: a clinical evaluation of lyophilized dura and cartilage reconstruction. J Oral Maxillofac Surg 50:935-941, 1992.
32. Vuyk HD, Adamson PA. Biomaterials in rhinoplasty. Clin Otolaryngol Allied Sci 23:209-217, 1998.
33. Haug RH, Kimberly D, Bradrick JP. A comparison of microscrew and suture fixation for porous high-density polyethylene orbital floor implants. J Oral Maxillofac Surg 51:1217-1220, 1993.
34. Romano JJ, Iliff NT, Manson PN. Use of Medpor porous polyethylene implants in 140 patients with facial fractures. J Craniofac Surg 4:142-147,1993.
35. Rohrich RJ, Lowe JB, Hackney FL, et al. An algorithm for abdominal wall reconstruction. Plast Reconstr Surg 105:202-216, 2000.
36. Eppley BL, Sadove AM, Havlik RJ. Resorbable plate fixation in pediatric craniofacial surgery. Plast Reconstr Surg 100:1-7, 1997.
37. Rohrich RJ. Safety of silicone breast implants: scientific validation/vindication at last. Plast Reconstr Surg 104:1786-1788, 1999.

# 10. Negative Pressure Wound Therapy

Janae L. Maher, Raman C. Mahabir

## DEFINITION

Negative pressure wound therapy (NPWT) is a wound-healing adjunct in which a contact dressing is applied to a wound and sealed with an adhesive drape. Subatmospheric pressure is applied, effectively converting an open wound into a controlled closed wound to prepare the wound bed and accelerate healing or allow for closure.

## MECHANISM OF ACTION

*Largely unknown, but the most common theories are discussed here.*

- **Fluid-based mechanism**
  - Removes excess interstitial fluid which can compromise microcirculation and oxygen delivery, transport of nutrients and waste products, and removal of locally accumulated toxins (proteolytic enzymes, acute phase proteins, metalloproteinases, proinflammatory mediators, and cytokines) in wounds.[1]
- **Mechanical mechanism**
  - Cellular proliferation in response to mechanical tissue stress (tension-stress effect).
  - **Macrostrain:** Negative pressure causes the contact wound dressing to collapse, equally distributing the negative pressure, and the force is transferred to the wound edges, drawing them closer together.[2]
  - **Microstrain:** Tiny pieces of tissue are drawn into a foam contact dressing causing microdeformations and inducing mechanical stress, stimulating angiogenesis and tissue growth.[3]
- **Reduction of bacterial load**[4]

## METHOD OF APPLICATION[5] (Fig. 10-1)

- Place nonadherent contact layer, such as Adaptic (Johnson & Johnson, New Brunswick, NJ) or Xeroform (Covidien, Mansfield, MA), between prepared wound bed and contact dressing, if needed.
- Apply contact dressing.
  - **Open cell foam**
    - **Polyurethane "black" foam**
      - Hydrophobic
      - Average pore size range of 400-600 μm to maximize tissue growth
      - Vast majority of evidence relates to use of this contact dressing
    - **Polyvinyl alcohol "white" foam**
      - Hydrophilic
      - Denser pore distribution, 60-270 μm
      - Useful in areas where rapid rates of granulation tissue are less desirable

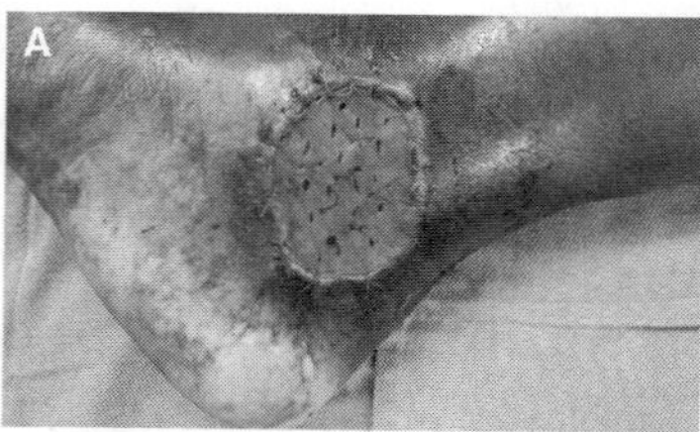


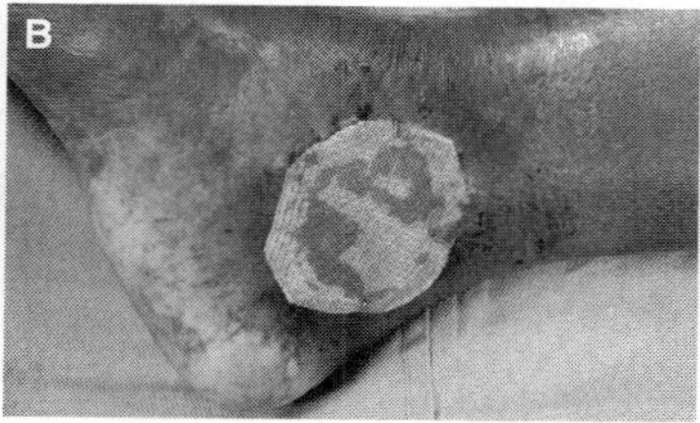


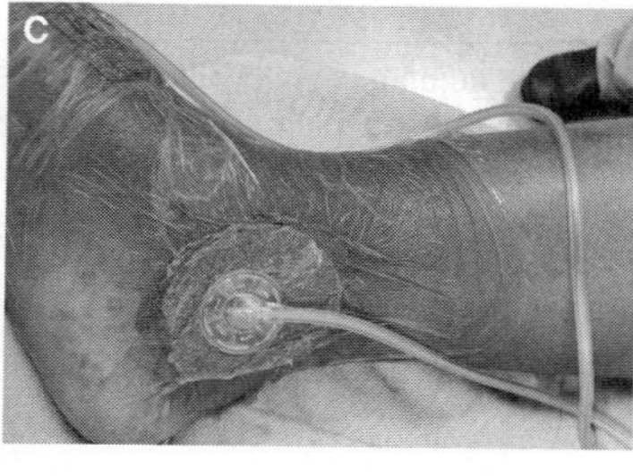


**Fig. 10-1** **A,** Split-thickness skin graft placed on ankle wound. **B,** Nonadherent dressing placed over the skin graft and held in place with a few staples. **C,** NPWT device placed over the split-thickness skin graft and dressing.

- ▸ **Silver-coated sponges**
  - ♦ Decreases odor of wound, probably by decreasing bacterial counts
  - ♦ Recommended in wounds when contamination still present
  - ♦ Contraindicated in patients with silver allergy
- **Gauze**
  - ▸ Easier to apply, because no shape memory[6]
  - ▸ Fewer patients report pain with gauze dressing changes than with foam[7]
- **Honeycombed textiles**
- **Other evidence for contact dressing:**
  - ▸ In vivo evidence shows no difference between gauze and foam for blood flow, wound contraction in small wounds, microdeformation of the wound bed, or pressure transmitted to the wound bed.[8-10]
  - ▸ No clinically observable differences in reduction of wound size, healing time, or time to prepare for grafting.[7,11,12]
  - ▸ Foam is better suited to uniform contractible wounds, and gauze to shallow wounds.
  - ▸ Use of a nonadherent interface or wound contact layer is recommended when using NPWT to bolster skin grafts.

- ■ Seal with adhesive drape.
- ■ Apply subatmospheric pressure.
  - Continuous or intermittent pressure application
    - ▸ Intermittent pressure shown to produce more rapid granulation tissue deposition.
  - Pressure of −50 to −125 mm Hg applied.
    - ▸ **Maximum increase in blood flow seen at −125 mm Hg.**[13]
- ■ Alarm systems are present on some NPWT machine models to increase margin of safety; warn of bleeding, excessive fluid output, and loss of adequate seal.
- ■ Recommended dressing change no less than three times a week for noninfected wounds, more frequently for infected wounds as needed.

- Fluid instillation as an adjunct.
  - Most commonly isotonic solution containing antibiotics or antibacterials.
  - Can be intermittent suction (when the pressure is stopped, the device instills fluid, and when negative pressure is restarted, the fluid is removed into a waste canister) or continuous suction (fluid is instilled at one end of the wound and removed/suctioned at the other).
  - This technique may contribute to infection control.[14-16]

**TIP:** Many surgeons are comfortable transitioning to twice a week dressing changes once the wound is clean and stable.

## INDICATIONS AND PREPARATION

*Wide spectrum of wound types treated with NPWT: chronic, acute, traumatic, and dehisced wounds, partial-thickness burns, ulcers (diabetic, pressure, venous stasis), flaps, and grafts.*

- **Acute wounds** (large soft tissue injuries with compromised tissue, contaminated wounds, hematomas, gunshot wounds)
  - Debride wound of all nonviable tissue.
  - Remove foreign bodies.
  - Obtain hemostasis.
  - Preferably cover vital structures such as major vessels, viscera, and nerves with mobilization of local muscle or soft tissue.
  - If significant contamination suspected or patient has signs of sepsis, change dressings at 24-hour intervals with judicious debridement and appropriate antibiotic coverage.
- **Chronic wounds** (pressure ulcers, long-term dehisced wounds, venous stasis ulcers, vascular and diabetic ulcers)
  - Debride wound of all nonviable tissue.
  - Converts a chronic wound into a quasiacute wound that responds to NPWT closure more rapidly.

**TIP:** NPWT has a wide clinical range of indications for use, so it is important to simply understand contraindications to its use.

## CONTRAINDICATIONS TO NEGATIVE PRESSURE WOUND THERAPY

- Exposed vessels, nerves, and organs
- Malignancy in wound
- Untreated osteomyelitis
- Nonenteric or unexplored fistulas
- Fresh anastomotic site
- Necrotic tissue with eschar present

**TIP:** Some surgeons may cover vessels, nerves, and organs temporarily using either a nonadherent contact layer or a white foam contact dressing on a case-by-case basis.

## TREATMENT GOALS[17]

- **Manage and protect the wound:** Improve fluid management, prevent environmental contamination, and prevent wound desiccation.
- **Prepare wound bed for surgical closure or progress to healing by secondary intention:** Improve granulation tissue formation, manage infection control, and reduce wound size and complexity.
- **Improve patient comfort:** Decrease pain, decrease number of dressing changes, improve patient mobility, and manage wound exudate and odor.
- **Reduce costs:** Shorten time to closure or next additional surgery, prevent wound complications, decrease nursing time, and allow management of wounds as outpatient for faster hospital discharge.
- **Improve outcomes:** Splint wound and prevent postoperative complications.

## CLINICAL APPLICATIONS AND EVIDENCE

### Extremities and Orthopedic Injuries[18-20]

*NPWT has become a first-line treatment for allowing definitive reconstruction to be performed in a stable, clean wound on an elective basis.*

- Allows serial debridement of only obviously nonviable soft tissue and bone, minimizing large, unnecessarily aggressive debridements.
- Removes edema and increases perfusion, giving the injury zone of stasis a chance to survive.
- Viable soft tissue is drawn together so that the wound does not enlarge with edema and retraction.
- Bone is kept in a moist environment, minimizing desiccation.
- Can be placed directly over hardware.
- NPWT can assist after fasciotomies, reducing edema and allowing primary closure sooner than with standard techniques.

### Sternal Infections and Mediastinitis[21,22]

- Many cardiac surgeons use NPWT as primary initial treatment for sternal infections after debridement of nonviable tissue and sternum.
  - **Superficial sternal infections**
    - NPWT allows skin to be opened and superficial infection drained while splinting the chest and minimizing risk of loosening sternal wires.
    - Many patients heal without any additional surgery for closure.
  - **Deep sternal infections**
    - NPWT used primarily as a bridge to allow patient to stabilize or recover following sepsis and the respiratory complications that accompany sternal infection.[23,24]
    - Many place a nonadherent contact layer on the heart first, then cover with sponge; must exercise caution when organs and vessels are exposed.
- In-hospital stay shorter without increase in mortality (Level 1 evidence).
- Fewer painful dressing changes required.
- Chest wall stabilized, decreasing need for paralytic agents and ventilator assistance.
- Rewiring occurs earlier.
- Number of soft tissue flaps needed for closure is decreased.
- Negative mediastinal microbiological cultures achieved earlier.
- C-reactive protein levels decline more rapidly.
- Trend toward higher overall survival rate than those with conventional dressing changes.
- Allows the surgeon to decide whether and when the sternum should be closed.

## Abdominal Wall Defects[18,25,26]

- **Partial-thickness defects:** Some component of the abdominal wall prevents evisceration
  - Depending on size of defect, NPWT is used as primary treatment or as bridge to later definitive treatment when optimal wound conditions exist and the patient is stable systemically.
- **Full-thickness defects:** Abdominal viscera exposed
  - NPWT is used for open abdomen after damage control laparotomy in trauma, decompression for abdominal compartment syndrome, peritonitis, ruptured aneurysm repair.
    - Removes wound contamination and intraabdominal exudates
    - Decreases visceral edema
    - Higher rate of delayed primary closure
    - Minimizes time spent in ICU
    - Decreased ventilator dependence
    - Increased risk of enterocutaneous fistula formation when NPWT placed directly on bowel, therefore a wound contact layer recommended to mitigate this risk
    - Increased rate of survival
- **Enterocutaneous fistula**
  - Initially was a contraindication to NPWT use; now occasionally used as a treatment modality.
  - Low-output fistulas close faster than high-output fistulas

## Pressure Sores and Perineum

- Often used after adequate debridement and initiation of appropriate antibiotics if osteomyelitis is present.
- NPWT is useful because dressing changes in this area are difficult and contamination risk is high.
  - Achieving a seal can be more difficult.

## Diabetic Foot Disease[27-29]

- NPWT used to facilitate healing by secondary intention
  - Decreased wound surface area (Level I evidence)
  - Safe and more effective: Total number of patients with healed ulcers, time to wound closure, overall incidence of limb amputation (Level I evidence)
- Used as a bridge to surgical closure

## Venous Ulcers[30,31]

- As primary treatment, evidence lacking
- As adjunct to skin graft
  - Skin graft preparation time reduced by 58% (Level I evidence)
  - Overall complete healing time reduced by 35% (Level I evidence)
  - Skin graft take 92%; skin graft take without NPWT 67% (Level II evidence)

## Skin Grafting[30-33]

- Sponge contours to surface of recipient site
  - Maintains pressure
  - Minimizes disruption
  - Especially useful in areas such as perineum, axilla, neck, and lower extremity, as well as for large surface area skin grafting such as with burn victims
- NPWT creates a pressure gradient, changing inosculation from a passive process to an active one

- Fenestrations in skin graft allow the NPWT system to actively remove serum and blood from under the graft
- Technique
  - Apply nonadherent contact layer over graft.
  - Apply sponge.
  - Apply continuous −75 to −125 mm Hg pressure for 4-7 days.
- Superior for wound bed preparation (Level I evidence)
- Diminishes loss of split-thickness skin grafts (STSGs) (Level I evidence)
- Shortens hospital stay (Level I evidence)
- Improves appearance of STSGs (Level I evidence)
- Improved chronic leg ulcer graft take of 93%; 67% with standard therapy (Level II evidence)

**TIP:** This technique is also beneficial for accelerating the incorporation of synthetic matrices such as Integra (Integra Life Sciences, Inc., Plainsboro, NJ).

### Grafting Over Bone

NPWT may be used on surgically exposed cranial diploe or other bones by drilling at 1 cm intervals to bleeding level to partially remove the cortex; NPWT accelerates the formation of a viable layer of granulation tissue for later skin grafting.

### Incisional Negative Pressure Wound Therapy[20]

- Used on closed surgical wounds with early signs of inadequate healing or on those located at anatomic sites associated with high complication rates
- Thought to provide continuous evacuation of excessive drainage, thereby avoiding skin irritation and bacterial colonization while reducing edema
- Technique
  - Line incision with thin strips of adhesive dressing just lateral to the suture or staples.
  - Place nonadherent contact dressing over the incision.
  - Cut sponge to the length of the incision and place over the nonadherent dressing, avoiding direct contact with skin.
  - Apply occlusive dressing and pressure of −50 to −125 mm Hg.
  - Discontinue after 2-5 days.

## COMPLICATIONS

- Skin edge erythema, maceration, ulceration
- Mechanical malfunction/failure
- Retained sponge
- Bleeding
- Infection and toxic shock syndrome from partial or incomplete drainage

## COST EFFECTIVENESS[34]

- Time involvement and costs of nursing staff significantly lower for NPWT group in randomized clinical trial with conventional dressings
- Overall costs similar
- Another advantage noted was comfort for the patients and nursing staff with fewer dressing changes

## Key Points

- ✓ Intermittent pressure has been shown to produce more rapid granulation tissue deposition.
- ✓ Maximum increase in blood flow seen at −125 mm Hg.
- ✓ NPWT has a wide clinical range of indications for use, so it is important to simply understand contraindications to its use.
- ✓ NPWT is widely used as a first-line therapeutic modality; however, conclusive, adequately powered, high-level evidence studies confirming its benefits, other than for diabetic foot ulcers and skin grafts, are currently lacking in the literature.
- ✓ NPWT has allowed plastic surgeons to perform definitive reconstructions of acute and chronic wounds on an elective basis, after the patient is medically optimized with a stable, clean wound.

## References

1. Argenta LC, Morykwas MJ. Vacuum-assisted closure: a new method for wound control and treatment: clinical experience. Ann Plast Surg 38:563-576, 1997.
2. Urschel JD, Scott PG, Williams HTG. The effect of mechanical stress of soft and hard tissue repair: a review. Br J Plast Surg 42:182-186, 1988.
3. Plikaitis CM, Molnar JA. Subatmospheric pressure wound therapy and the vacuum-assisted closure device: basic science and current clinical successes. Expert Rev Med Devices 3:175-184, 2006.
4. Morykwas MJ, Argenta LC, Shelton Brown EI, et al. Vacuum-assisted closure: a new method for wound control and treatment: animal studies and basic foundation. Ann Plast Surg 38:553-562, 1997.
5. DeFranzo AJ Jr, Argenta LC. Management of wounds with vacuum-assisted closure. In Pu LLQ, Levine JP, Wei FC, eds. Reconstructive Surgery of the Lower Extremity. St Louis: Quality Medical Publishing, 2013.
6. Jeffery SL. Advanced wound therapies in the management of severe military lower limb trauma: a new perspective. Eplasty 21:e28, 2009.
7. Dorafshar AH, Franczyk M, Gottlieb LJ, et al. A prospective randomized trial comparing subatmospheric wound therapy with a sealed gauze dressing and the standard vacuum assisted closure device. Ann Plast Surg 69:79-84, 2012.
8. Malmsjö M, Ingemansson R, Martin R, et al. Wound edge microvascular blood flow: effects of negative pressure wound therapy using gauze or polyurethane foam. Ann Plast Surg 63:676-681, 2009.
9. Malmsjö M, Ingemansson R, Martin R, et al. Negative-pressure wound therapy using gauze or open-cell polyurethane foam: similar early effects on pressure transduction and tissue contraction in an experimental porcine wound model. Wound Repair Regen 17:200-205, 2009.
10. Borgquist O, Gustafsson L, Ingemansson R, et al. Micro- and macromechanical effects on the wound bed of negative pressure wound therapy using gauze and foam. Ann Plast Surg 64:789-793, 2010.
11. Hu KX, Zhang HW, Zhou F, et al. [A comparative study of the clinical effects between two kinds of negative-pressure wound therapy] Zhonghua Shao Shang Za Zhi 25:253-257, 2009.
12. Fraccalvieri M, Zingarelli E, Ruka E, et al. Negative pressure wound therapy using gauze and foam: histological, immunohistochemical, and ultrasonography morphological analysis of the granulation tissue and scar tissue. Preliminary report of a clinical study. Int Wound J 8:355-364, 2011.
13. Morykwas MJ, Faler BJ, Pearce DJ, et al. Effects of varying levels of subatmospheric pressure on the rate of granulation tissue formation in experimental wounds in swine. Ann Plast Surg 47:547-551, 2001.
14. Kiyokawa K, Takahashi N, Rikimaru H, et al. New continuous negative-pressure and irrigation treatment for infected wounds and intractable ulcers. Plast Reconstr Surg 120:1257-1265, 2007.

15. Timmers MS, Graafland N, Bernards AT, et al. Negative pressure wound treatment with polyvinyl alcohol foam and polyhexamide antiseptic solution instillation in posttraumatic osteomyelitis. Wound Repair Regen 17:278-286, 2009.
16. Giovinco NA, Bui TD, Fisher T, et al. Wound chemotherapy by the use of negative pressure wound therapy and infusion. Eplasty 10:e9, 2010.
17. Birke-Sorensen H, Malmsjö M, Rome P, et al. Evidence-based recommendations for negative pressure wound therapy: treatment variables (pressure levels, wound filler and contact layer)—steps towards an international consensus. J Plast Reconstr Aesthet Surg 64(Suppl):S1-S16, 2011.
18. Argenta LC, Morykwas MJ, Marks MW, et al. Vacuum-assisted closure: state of clinic art. Plast Reconstr Surg 117(7 Suppl):S127-S142, 2006.
19. Runkel N, Krug E, Berg L, et al. Evidence-based recommendations for the use of negative pressure wound therapy in traumatic wounds and reconstructive surgery: steps towards an international consensus. Injury 42(Suppl 1):S1-S12, 2011.
20. Streubel PN, Stinner DJ, Obremskey WT. Use of negative-pressure wound therapy in orthopaedic trauma. J Am Acad Orthop Surg 20:564-574, 2012.
21. Raja SG, Berg GA. Should vacuum-assisted closure therapy be routinely used for management of deep sternal wound infection after cardiac surgery? Interact Cardiovasc Thorac Surg 6:523-528, 2007.
22. Vos RJ, Yilmaz A, Sonker U, et al. Vacuum-assisted closure of post-sternotomy mediastinitis as compared to open packing. Interact Cardiovasc Thorac Surg 14:17-21, 2012.
23. Agarwal JP, Ogilvie M, Wu LC, et al. Vacuum-assisted closure for sternal wounds: a first-line therapeutic management approach. Plast Reconstr Surg 116:1035-1040, 2005.
24. Janis JE. Discussion: Vacuum-assisted closure for sternal wounds: a first-line therapeutic management approach by Agarwal JP, et al. Plast Reconstr Surg 116:1041-1043, 2005.
25. Boele van Hensbroek P, Wind J, Dijkgraaf MGW, et al. Temporary closure of the open abdomen: a systematic review on delayed and primary fascial closure in patients with an open abdomen. World J Surg 33:199-207, 2009.
26. Perez D, Wildi S, Demartines N, et al. Prospective evaluation of vacuum-assisted closure in abdominal compartment syndrome and severe abdominal sepsis. J Am Coll Surg 205:586-592, 2007.
27. Armstrong DG, Lavery LA. Negative pressure wound therapy after partial diabetic foot amputation: a multicenter, randomized controlled trial. Lancet 366:1704-1710, 2005.
28. Blume PA, Walters J, Payne W, et al. Comparison of negative pressure wound therapy using vacuum-assisted closure with advanced moist wound therapy in the treatment of diabetic foot ulcers: a multicenter randomized controlled trial. Diabetes Care 31:631-636, 2008.
29. McCallon SK, Knight CA, Valiulus JP, et al. Vacuum-assisted closure versus saline-moistened gauze in the healing of postoperative diabetic foot wounds. Ostomy Wound Manage 46:28-32,34, 2000.
30. Korber A, Franckson T, Grabbe S, et al. Vacuum assisted closure device improves the take of mesh grafts in chronic leg ulcer patients. Dermatology 216:250-256, 2008.
31. Vuerstaek JD, Vainas T, Wuite J, et al. State-of-the-art treatment of chronic leg ulcers: a randomized controlled trial comparing vacuum-assisted closure (VAC) with modern wound dressings. J Vasc Surg 44:1029-1037, 2006.
32. Llanos S, Danilla S, Barraza C, et al. Effectiveness of negative pressure closure in the integration of split thickness skin grafts: a randomized, double-masked, controlled trial. Ann Surg 244:700-705, 2006.
33. Moisidis E, Heath T, Boorer C, et al. A prospective, blinded, randomized, controlled clinical trial of topical negative pressure use in skin grafting. Plast Reconstr Surg 14:917-922, 2004.
34. Braakenburg A, Obdeijn MC, Feitz R, et al. The clinical efficacy and cost effectiveness of the vacuum-assisted closure technique in the management of acute and chronic wounds: a randomized controlled trial. Plast Reconstr Surg 118:390-397, 2006.

# 11. Lasers in Plastic Surgery

Amanda K. Silva, Chad M. Teven, John E. Hoopman

## BACKGROUND[1]

### Laser Physics

- Light energy, either wave or photon
- Color of light determined by wavelength (distance between two successive light waves)
  - Ultraviolet 200-400 nm
  - Visible 400-750 nm
  - Near-infrared 750-1400 nm
  - Infrared 1400-20,000 nm
- Photon created when excited electron falls back into resting orbit
- If photon collides with excited electron, causes release of another photon, which is *in phase* with the initial photon
- When energy added to system, photons hit mirrors and multiple photons in phase: **L**ight **A**mplification by the **S**timulated **E**mission of **R**adiation (LASER)
- Device components
  - Lasing medium: Solid, liquid, or gas whose electrons are in resting state
  - Pump source: Flashlamp, electricity, or another laser
  - Mirrors: At each end, one mirror only partially reflecting, which allows light to escape tube

### Laser Definitions

- **Laser light characteristics**
  - Coherent: Light is in phase
    - Intense pulsed light is noncoherent
  - Monochromatic: Light is one color
  - Collimated: Tight formation of light
- **Excimer:** Short-lived dimeric or heterodimeric molecule formed from two species, at least one of which is in an electronic excited state
- **Chromophore:** Region in a molecule where an energy difference between two different molecular orbits falls within the range of the visible spectrum (i.e., part of a molecule responsible for its color)
- **Flashlamp:** Produces pump pulses for either free-running or Q-switched lasers

### Laser Properties

- **Wavelength**[2] (Fig. 11-1)
  - The longer the wavelength from visible through near-infrared (400-1400 nm), the deeper the penetration.

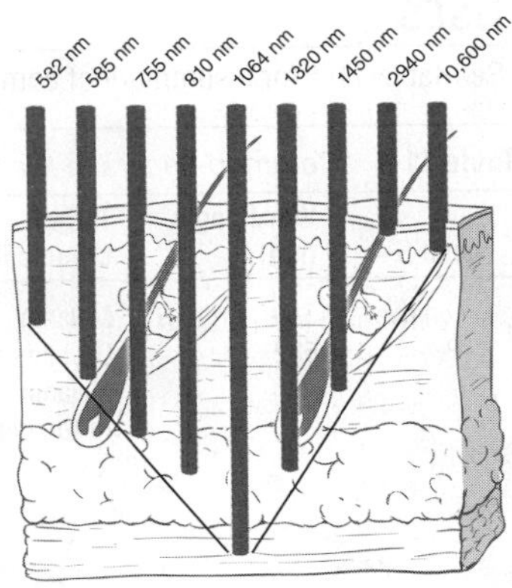


**Fig. 11-1** Absorption length.

- **Spot size**
  - Larger spot size = Achievement of maximum absorption length potential of wavelength
- **Energy density (fluence)**
  - Joules/centimeter squared (J/cm$^2$)
- **Power**
- **Duration of action (pulse width)**
  - Should be less than the target tissue thermal relaxation time (time to dissipate 51% of energy absorbed). *The energy must be introduced to the target faster than it thermally relaxes.*
    - Proportional to the square of the target's diameter in millimeters
      - Shorter (nanosecond to picosecond) range: Tattoo pigment
      - Longer (millisecond to continuous) range: Vasculature
- **Energy delivery modes**
  - Continuous wave: Rarely used anymore, likely to cause scarring
  - Pulsed: Timing to match the size of the target and thermal relaxation time (TRT)
  - Q-switched: Extremely high bursts of energy delivered in short intervals in the nanoscecond and picosecond ranges to target small particles such as melanin and tattoo pigment
    - Cautioned use in patients with rheumatoid arthritis treated with systemic gold

**TIP:** Ideal pulse time is usually half the thermal relaxation time of the target.

### Tissue Effects

- Light is reflected, scattered, transmitted, or absorbed.
- Selective photothermolysis: The science of selectively targeting and heating a singular and specific chromophore with a selected wavelength to a desired temperature
- Energy is converted to thermal energy.
  - At 60°-70° Celsius, tissue coagulates and structural proteins denature.
  - At 100° C, tissue vaporizes.
- Usually requires multiple treatment sessions for desired effect

## USES

See Table 11-1 for a summary of common laser types used in plastic surgery.

**Table 11-1** *Common Lasers in Plastic Surgery*

| Name | Wavelength (nm) | Target Chromophore | Clinical Application | Key Points |
|---|---|---|---|---|
| Green dye | 510 | Melanin | Café-au-lait macules | |
| KTP | 532 | Oxyhemoglobin<br>Melanin<br>Tattoo pigment | Venous and venolymphatic malformations, facial telangiectasias, spider veins, pigmented lesions, tattoo removal, hypertrophic scars and keloids | Nd:YAG sent through frequency-doubling KTP crystal<br>Wider selection of pulse widths<br>Less posttreatment purpura<br>Higher melanin absorption (use in Fitzpatrick I-III)<br>High rate of hyperpigmentation<br>Best for red tattoo inks |

*KTP,* Potassium titanyl phosphate.

| Name | Wavelength (nm) | Target Chromophore | Clinical Application | Key Points |
|---|---|---|---|---|
| Yellow dye | 585, 595 | Oxyhemoglobin | Hemangiomas, port-wine stains, facial telangiectasias, spider veins, hypertrophic scars and keloids | Better for superficial lesions<br>High rate of posttreatment purpura |
| Ruby | 694 | Melanin<br>Tattoo pigment | Pigmented lesions, tattoo removal | |
| Alexandrite | 755 | Oxyhemoglobin<br>Melanin<br>Tattoo pigment | Spider veins, pigmented lesions, hair removal, tattoo removal | Best for green tattoo ink |
| Diode | 800, 810, 940, 980 | Oxyhemoglobin<br>Melanin | Facial telangiectasias, spider veins, pigmented lesion, hair removal, liposuction | |
| Nd:YAG | 1064<br>1320<br>Near-infrared | Oxyhemoglobin<br>Melanin<br>Tattoo pigment | Hemangiomas, venous and venolymphatic malformations, facial telangiectasias, spider veins, pigmented lesions, hair removal, tattoo removal, hypertrophic scars and keloids, liposuction | Deeper penetration (4-8 mm)<br>Near-infrared more poorly absorbed by melanin (safer in Fitzpatrick IV-VI) |
| Fraxel | 1550<br>Infrared | Water | Skin resurfacing | |
| Er:YAG | 2940 | Water | Skin resurfacing | Ablative |
| $CO_2$ | 10,600 | Water | Skin resurfacing | Ablative |

## VASCULAR LESIONS[3] (Table 11-2)

**Table 11-2** *Devices Used to Treat Vascular Lesions*

| Device | Wavelength (nm) | Skin Types | Tan |
|---|---|---|---|
| Pulsed dye | 585-595 | I-III | No |
| KTP | 532 | I-III | No |
| Nd:YAG | 1064 | I-VI | Yes |
| IPL/BBL | 585+ | I-III | No |

*IPL/BBL,* Intense pulsed light/broadband light; *KTP,* potassium titanyl phosphate.

- **Target:** Hemoglobin and oxyhemoglobin
  - Absorption at 418, 532, 577-600, and 700-1100 nm

- **Effects**
  - Damage vessel intima
  - Contract types I and III collagen surrounding vessel
  - Vessel flow stasis
- **Laser types**
  - Potassium titanyl phosphate (KTP) 532 nm
  - Yellow pulsed dye 585 or 600 nm
  - Alexandrite 755 nm
  - Diode 800, 810, 940, 980 nm
  - Neodymium:yttrium-aluminum-garnet (Nd:YAG) 1064 nm
  - Intense pulsed light 400-1300 nm
- **Applications**
  - **Hemangiomas**[4]
    - Lasers: Nd:YAG
    - Effective in early stage, ulcerated (may treat associated pain by coagulation of sensitive nerve endings), and regressed lesions
    - Contraindicated in proliferation phase: Induces ulceration and necrosis
  - **Capillary vascular malformations (port-wine stains)**
    - Lasers: Pulsed yellow dye, intense pulsed light
    - Variables affecting efficacy
      - Age: Children respond better, may begin treatment at age 6 months
      - Color of lesion: Lighter respond better
      - Fitzpatrick criteria skin type: Better in types I-III
      - Anatomic location: Best response in head and neck (except $V_2$ dermatome distribution), worst response in extremities
  - **Venous and venolymphatic malformations**
    - Lasers: Nd:YAG
    - Usually too large for isolated laser therapy, combine with surgical debulking or sclerotherapy
    - Prolonged energy delivery needed for efficacy increases risk of scarring.
      - Lips and oral mucosa more forgiving
    - May place laser intralesionally for deep coagulation
  - **Facial telangiectasias and rosacea**[5]
    - Lasers: KTP (most common), pulsed yellow dye, diode, Nd:YAG
    - Less effective for very small ($<100$ μm) or large ($>300$ μm), or if located on nasal tip or alae
  - **Spider veins**[6]
    - Lasers: KTP, pulsed yellow dye, alexandrite, diode, Nd:YAG (common choice), intense pulsed light
    - Address venous insufficiency first, likely need nonlaser treatments as well
    - Indications
      - Superficial, fine vessels not amenable to cannulation
      - Areas prone to ulceration (i.e., ankle)
      - History of poor response to sclerotherapy
      - Allergy to sclerosing agents

**TIP:** Lasers can be combined for improved results: 532 nm exposure enhances 1064 nm efficacy.

## PIGMENTED SKIN LESIONS[7]

- **Target:** Melanin
  - Absorption throughout visible spectrum, longer wavelengths desired because of isolation from hemoglobin, but melanin absorption decreases as wavelength increases
- **Effects**
  - Melanin fragmented and naturally exfoliated
- **Laser types**
  - KTP 532 nm
  - Q-switched and long pulsed ruby 694 nm
  - Q-switched and long pulsed alexandrite 755 nm
  - Diode 800 nm
  - Q-switched Nd:YAG 1064 nm
  - Erbium:yttrium-aluminum-garnet (Er:YAG) 2940 nm
  - Carbon dioxide ($CO_2$) 10,600 nm
  - Fractionated lasers
  - Intense pulsed light
- **Applications**
  - Lentigines
  - Seborrheic keratoses
  - Ephelides (freckles)
  - Café-au-lait macules
    - High recurrence rate
  - Becker's nevus
    - Brown irregular patch with dark, coarse hair
    - Q-switched ruby slightly more effective for pigment, but long pulsed lasers better for hair removal
  - Melasma
    - Caution with treatment: May worsen and recurrences common
  - Congenital nevi
    - Controversial, some do not recommend because creates difficulty in surveillance for malignant transformation
  - Nevus of Ota: Blue-black, brown, or grey patch in trigeminal nerve distribution
  - Nevus of Ito: Blue-black, brown, or grey patch on shoulder

## HAIR REMOVAL[3,8] (Table 11-3)

**Table 11-3** *Devices Used for Hair Removal*

| Device | Wavelength (nm) | Hair Color | Skin Type | Tan | Currently Used |
|---|---|---|---|---|---|
| Alexandrite | 755 | Dark | I-III | No | Yes |
| Diode | 810 | Dark | I-VI | Yes | Yes |
| Nd:YAG | 1064 | Dark | I-VI | Yes | Yes |
| IPL/BBL | 690+ | Dark | I-III | No | Yes |

*IPL/BBL,* Intense pulsed light/broadband light.

- **Target:** Melanin
- **Laser types**
  - Diode 800 nm
  - Alexandrite 755 nm
  - Nd:YAG 1064 nm
  - Intense pulsed light 4000-1300 nm
    - Best for fair hair
- **Applications**
  - Best on fair skin and dark hair

**TIP:** It is optimal to target during the anagen phase of growth when the most abundant active target is present.

## Tattoo Removal[9]

- **Target:** Tattoo pigments
- **Effects**
  - Q-switched lasers create acoustic waves, which cause mechanical disruption.
  - Pigment fragmented and phagocytized by macrophages
- **Laser types**
  - Q-switched ruby 694 nm
  - Q-switched alexandrite 755 nm
  - Q-switched Nd:YAG 532 nm (KTP)/1064 nm
- **Applications**
  - Avoid in suntanned patients unless using Q-switched Nd:YAG
  - Usually require different laser for different pigments
    - Dark ink (black, blue): All work well, Nd:YAG 1064 nm recommended
    - Green ink: Q-switched alexandrite
    - Red inks (purple, red, brown): Q-switched Nd:YAG (KTP) 532 nm
    - Yellow and orange ink highly resistant to treatment
      - Best absorb light in UV range, which is absorbed by and damages melanocytes, and affects ability of light to penetrate to dermis

## Scars[10]

- **Target:** Oxyhemoglobin
- **Effects**
  - Causes coagulation necrosis
  - Decreases number and proliferation of fibroblasts
  - Increases MMP-13 (collagenase-3) activity
  - Decreases collagen III deposition
- **Laser types**
  - Pulsed yellow dye 585 or 595 nm
  - Nd:YAG 532 (KTP)/1064 nm
- **Applications**
  - Hypertrophic scars
  - Keloids
  - Burn scars: Pulsed yellow dye most common

## SKIN RESURFACING[3,11] (Table 11-4)

**Table 11-4** *Full-Field and Fractional Resurfacing Devices*

| Name | Wavelength (nm) | Ablative | Nonablative | Full Field | Fractional |
|---|---|---|---|---|---|
| $CO_2$ | 10,600 | Yes | No | Yes | Yes |
| Erbium | 2940 | Yes | No | Yes | Yes |
| YSGG | 2790 | Yes | No | Yes | Yes |
| Thulium | 1927 | No | Yes | No | Yes |
| Er:Glass | 1540 | No | Yes | No | Yes |
| Nd:YAG | 1440 | No | Yes | No | Yes |
| Nd:YAG | 1319 | No | Yes | Yes | Yes |
| Nd:YAG | 1064 | No | Yes | Yes | No |

*YSGG,* Yttrium-scandium-gallium-garnet.

- **Target:** Water
- **Effects**
  - Stimulates angiogenesis, neocollagen formation, and regeneration of dermal elastic fibers
  - Can penetrate as deep as upper reticular dermis
  - Less effect on pigmentation abnormalities than other resurfacing modalities
  - Melanocytes retain ability to function: Less hypopigmentation than with peels
  - Effects similar to phenol peel
- **Techniques**
  - **Nonablative**
    - Wound-healing response within the dermis and epidermis via application of heat without creating a traumatic wound
  - **Ablative**
    - Wound-healing response because of induced thermal injury from removal of dermal and epidermal layers
- **Laser types**
  - Fractional 1550 nm
    - Fractional emission of light into microscopic treatment zones, creating small columns of injury to skin in pixilated fashion
    - Degenerated dermal material incorporated into columns of microscopic epidermal necrotic debris and then exfoliated
  - $CO_2$ 10,600 nm, ablative
    - Thermal injury >ablation
    - More tissue contraction
    - Long-lasting results
    - Possible prolonged recovery: 7 days for reepithelialization
    - Increased risk of hypopigmentation and scarring
    - End treatment at junction of whitish-brown reticular dermis and deeper tan, yellow tissue

- Er:YAG 2940 nm, ablative
  - Ablation >thermal injury
  - 13 times greater affinity for water than $CO_2$ laser: More controllable depth of penetration (safer)
  - Can be used in areas with very thin skin (i.e., tip of nose and neck)
  - Possible shorter recovery: 5 days for reepithelialization
  - Less postoperative erythema

- **Applications**
  - Rhytids
  - Dyschromia
  - Atrophic scars (acne)
  - Texture abnormalities
- **Pretreatment**
  - Hydroquinone 4% and tretinoin 0.05% 4-6 weeks pretreatment
    - Stimulates faster healing and prevents posttreatment hyperpigmentation
  - Discontinue oral isotretinoin (Accutane) products 6 months to 1 year before treatment because of increased risk of scarring.
- **Prophylaxis**
  - Antivirals 48 hours before and 7-10 days after in all patients undergoing ablative, and in patients with a history if undergoing nonablative treatment.

> **TIP:** Only oral isotretinoin (Accutane) is contraindicated before laser resurfacing treatment. Tretinoin (Renova, Retin A) does not increase the risk of healing complications.

## LASER LIPOSUCTION[12]

- **Target:** Water and fat
- **Effects**
  - Adipocyte membrane rupture
  - Coagulation of small vessels
  - Coagulation of dermal collagen
- **Laser types**
  - Nd:YAG 1064 nm: Longest track record
  - Diode 980 nm: High-power settings effective on areas with large amounts of fat
  - Nd:YAG 1064/1320 nm: Selective for dermal collagen, potential for skin tightening
- Not enough evidence of increased efficacy compared with standard
- **Hypothesized advantages**
  - Decreased blood loss
  - Collagen tightening
  - Can use in difficult areas (i.e., face, chin, neck, arms)
- **Disadvantages**
  - Longer operative time
  - Equipment cost
  - Steep learning curve
  - Risk of thermal injury (1%)

## COMPLICATIONS

- Normal to develop purpura after treatment with some lasers (i.e., pulsed dye); resolves in 1-2 weeks
- Postinflammatory hyperpigmentation is most common (up to 33%)
  - More common in darker skin types or history of sun exposure
  - Appears 6 weeks to 6 months after treatment
  - Usually transient, but can persist 9 months to 1 year
  - Treat with hydroquinone
- Hypopigmentation: 10%-20%
  - May be caused by melanin absorption with smaller wavelengths; use longer wavelengths in dark-skinned patients
  - Appears as late as 1-2 years after treatment
- Hypertrophic scarring
  - Avoid treatment in patients who have taken oral isotretinoin (Accutane) in past 6 months to 1 year (increased risk).
- Herpes infection: 2%-7% of facial resurfacing patients, even with prophylaxis
  - If outbreak despite prophylaxis, Tzanck smear, cultures, increase dose to zoster levels
- Lid retraction and ectropion
- Paradoxic darkening of tattoos
  - Tattoo pigment ferric oxide oxidized to darker ferrous oxide

> **TIP:** Hyperpigmentation is more common and usually occurs earlier after treatment than hypopigmentation, which can present years later.

## SAFETY[13]

- Recommendations
  - Pretreatment physician evaluation
  - Proper training and accreditation for all personnel using the laser
  - Physicians should perform the more invasive procedures involving $CO_2$ and erbium-type lasers.
  - Some procedures may be performed by a licensed nonphysician, but a physician should be on site. (Requirements vary from state to state; check with local boards.)
- Equipment and setup
  - Operator and patient must wear laser-specific eye protection.
  - Entire orbit of patient should be isolated from laser radiation.
  - Windows must have opaque coverings that correspond to the wavelength being used.
  - Protect patient with wet drapes or metal if using $CO_2$ laser.
  - Use laser-safe endotracheal tube if patient intubated and treating perioral lesions
  - Use lowest possible $FiO_2$ setting, approximately 30% or below, to prevent risk of inhalation or flash burn.
  - Use plume evacuator with lasers that create significant plume (i.e., erbium and $CO_2$ laser) to prevent transmission of virus particles. Ensure ultra-low-penetration air (ULPA) filtration.
  - Cool skin to prevent burns.
    - Ice area immediately before and after procedure.
    - Apply clear, cold gel to treatment area.
    - Use cold sapphire contact handpieces or conductive metal plates.
    - Use continuous-flow cool air (4° C).
    - Apply cryogen spray to skin 10-50 milliseconds before laser exposure.

## Key Points

- ✓ $CO_2$ lasers target water as the chromophore (selective photothermolysis).
- ✓ The most frequent infectious complication associated with resurfacing is a reactivation of the herpes simplex virus (usually occurs within the first postoperative week during the reepithelialization process). Antiviral prophylaxis should be started 1-2 days before and continued for 10-14 days after the procedure.
- ✓ The Q-switched Nd:YAG 1064 nm has the deepest penetration and carries the least risk of hypopigmentation; therefore it is often used for professional tattoo removal.
- ✓ The use of isotretinoin within the last 6 months to 1 year is a contraindication to resurfacing procedures.
- ✓ The current standard of care for removing most unwanted tattoos is to use specific lasers to target the wavelength of the color pigments.
- ✓ A wavelength of 2940 nm (Er:YAG) has the greatest affinity for water. However, $CO_2$ lasers at 10,600 nm have 13 times less affinity for water than Er:YAG lasers.

## References

1. Low DW, Thorne C. Lasers in Plastic Surgery. In Thorne CH, Bartlett SP, Beasley RW, et al, eds. Grabb and Smith's Plastic Surgery, 6th ed. Philadelphia: Lippincott Williams & Wilkins, 2007.
2. Kenkel JM, Farkas JP, Hoopman JE. Five parameters you must understand to master control of your laser/light-based devices. Aesthet Surg J. 2013 Aug 22. [Epub ahead of print]
3. Nahai F. The Art of Aesthetic Surgery: Principles & Techniques, 2nd ed. St Louis: Quality Medical Publishing, 2011.
4. Burns AJ, Navarro JA. Role of laser therapy in pediatric patients. Plast Reconstr Surg 124(1 Suppl):82e-92e, 2009.
5. McCoppin HH, Goldberg DJ. Laser treatment of facial telangiectases: an update. Dermatol Surg 36:1221-1230, 2010.
6. McCoppin HH, Hovenic WW, Wheeland RG. Laser treatment of superficial leg veins: a review. Dermatol Surg 37:729-741, 2011.
7. Polder KD, Landau JM, Vergilis-Kalner IJ, et al. Laser eradication of pigmented lesions: a review. Dermatol Surg 37:572-595, 2011.
8. Haedersdal M, Beerwerth F, Nash JF. Laser and intense pulsed light hair removal technologies: from professional to home use. Br J Dermatol 165(Suppl 3):S31-S36, 2011.
9. Kent KM, Graber EM. Laser tattoo removal: a review. Dermatol Surg 38:1-13, 2012.
10. Parret BM, Donelan MB. Pulsed dye laser in burn scars: current concepts and future directions. Burns 36:443-449, 2010.
11. Perrotti JA, Thorne C. Cutaneous resurfacing: chemical peeling, dermabrasion, and laser resurfacing. In Thorne CH, ed. Grabb and Smith's Plastic Surgery, 6th ed. Philadelphia: Wolters Kluwer/Lippincott Williams & Wilkins, 2007.
12. Fakhouri TM, Kader el Tal A, Abrou AE, et al. Laser-assisted lipolysis: a review. Dermatol Surg 38:155-169, 2012.
13. Rohrich RJ, Burns AJ. Lasers in office-based settings: establishing guidelines for proper usage. Plast Reconstr Surg 109:1147-1148, 2002.

# 12. Anesthesia

**Babatunde Ogunnaike**

## TECHNIQUES OF ANESTHESIA

- General anesthesia
- Regional anesthesia, including peripheral nerve blocks
- Sedation and analgesia (moderate or conscious sedation)

## GENERAL ANESTHESIA

**Objectives:** Amnesia, analgesia, skeletal muscle relaxation, and control of sympathetic responses

### PREOPERATIVE EVALUATION

- Questions that should be answered:
  - Is the patient in optimal health?
  - Can the physical or mental condition be improved before surgery?
- Determine the American Society of Anesthesiologists (ASA) physical status: Overall description of patient status, which correlates with outcomes[1] (Table 12-1)
- No need to order routine preoperative laboratory tests if patient is in optimal medical condition and procedure is minimally invasive
- **Premedication:** Goal is anxiety-free and fully cooperative patient
  - Psychological preparation: Visit by the anesthesiologist
  - Pharmacologic premedication agents
    - Anxiolytics: Benzodiazepines
    - Anticholinergics: Scopolamine, atropine
    - Analgesics: Acetaminophen, nonsteroidal antiinflammatory drugs (NSAIDs), opioids
    - Antiemetics: Ondansetron, scopolamine, droperidol

**Table 12-1** *American Society of Anesthesiologists (ASA) Physical Status Classification*

| Physical Status | Description |
|---|---|
| **Class 1** | Normal, healthy patient |
| **Class 2** | Mild systemic disease with no functional limitations (e.g., diabetes mellitus, hypertension) |
| **Class 3** | Severe systemic disease with functional limitation (e.g., angina pectoris, previous myocardial infarction) |
| **Class 4** | Severe systemic disease that is a constant threat to life (e.g., congestive heart failure, unstable angina, advanced system disease) |
| **Class 5** | Moribund patient not expected to survive without the operation (e.g., head injury with raised intracranial pressure, ruptured aortic aneurysm) |
| **Class 6** | Brain-dead patient for organ retrieval for donor purposes |
| **Emergency surgery (E)** | Any of the above patient classes requiring emergency operation (e.g., normal, healthy patient for surgery is Class 1E) |

## INTRAOPERATIVE MANAGEMENT (Table 12-2)

- **Induction of anesthesia**
  - **Intravenous induction:** Rapid-acting hypnotic agent such as propofol, etomidate, thiopental, ketamine
  - Rapid-sequence induction (RSI)
    - IV agent followed by rapid-acting neuromuscular blocking drug (e.g., succinylcholine, rocuronium) to facilitate tracheal intubation
    - Apply cricoid pressure: Occludes upper esophageal sphincter to prevent regurgitation and aspiration
  - **Inhalation (mask) induction**
    - Used for pediatric patients who are afraid of needle sticks
    - Sevoflurane is the agent of choice
- **Maintenance of anesthesia**
  - **Inhalational maintenance**
    - Gases (nitrous oxide) and volatile agents
    - Volatile agents (vapors): Sevoflurane, desflurane, isoflurane
      - Little or no analgesic effect
      - May be associated with postoperative hepatic dysfunction
  - **Intravenous maintenance:** Continuous intravenous infusion of propofol
  - **Neuromuscular blocking drugs (depolarizing and nondepolarizing)**
    - Allow decreased use of anesthetics
    - Risk of intraoperative awareness with inadequate anesthetic administration
  - **Opioids:** Attenuate sympathetic responses

**Table 12-2** *Intravenous Sedatives, Opioids, and Anesthetics*

| Drug | Dose | Comments |
|---|---|---|
| **Benzodiazepines** | | |
| Midazolam | 0.04-0.08 mg/kg IV or IM;<br>0.4-0.8 mg/kg PO<br>**Induction: 0.2-0.6 mg/kg IV** | No analgesic properties<br>Risk of significant respiratory depression when combined with opioid<br>Reliable anxiolytic and amnestic<br>Anticonvulsant<br>Decrease dose in elderly |
| Diazepam | 0.03-0.1 mg/kg IV or IM<br>0.07-0.15 mg/kg PO<br>**Induction: 0.3-0.6 mg/kg** | PO absorption more reliable than IM<br>No analgesic properties<br>Pain on injection |
| **Opioids** | | |
| Alfentanil | 5-20 μg/kg bolus | May cause skeletal muscle rigidity with large bolus—administer slowly<br>Cardiac and respiratory depressant |
| Fentanyl | 0.5-2 μg/kg bolus | Skeletal muscle rigidity <alfentanil<br>Cardiac and respiratory depressant |
| Remifentanil | 0.05-0.1 μg/kg/min infusion | Rapid onset and offset by ester hydrolysis in plasma<br>Adjustable IV infusion best for sedation |
| Sufentanil | 0.15-0.3 μg/kg | 10× more potent than fentanyl<br>Respiratory depression and bradycardia common<br>Skeletal muscle rigidity |

*CBF,* Cerebral blood flow; *$CMRO_2$,* cerebral metabolic rate for oxygen; *CNS,* central nervous system; *EEG,* electroencephalogram; *ICP,* intracranial pressure; *IM,* intramuscular; *IV,* intravenous; *MAO,* monoamine oxidase; *μg,* microgram; *mg,* milligram; *PO,* per os.

| Drug | Dose | Comments |
|---|---|---|
| **Opioids—cont'd** | | |
| Morphine | 0.05-0.1 mg/kg | Dilute and administer slowly<br>Histamine release—pruritus<br>Biliary spasm $<1\%$ |
| Meperidine | 0.5-1.5 mg/kg | Dilute and administer slowly<br>Atropine-like side effects<br>Normeperidine (active metabolite): CNS stimulant, can cause seizures<br>MAO inhibitor therapy: contraindication |
| **Anesthetics** | | |
| Propofol | 250-500 μg/kg boluses<br>25-100 μg/kg/min infusion<br>**Induction: 2-3 mg/kg IV** | Pain on injection (less pain on injection in larger veins)<br>Motor activity (nonepileptic myoclonia)<br>Anticonvulsant<br>Cardiac and respiratory depressant<br>Bronchodilator<br>Antiemetic<br>Antipruritic<br>Prompt recovery |
| Ketamine | 4-6 mg/kg PO; 2-4 mg/kg IM; 0.25-1 mg/kg IV<br>**Induction: 1-2 mg/kg IV**<br>**5-15 mg/kg IM** | "Dissociative anesthesia" (profound analgesia and amnesia)<br>Maintains respiration<br>Psychomimetic reactions at recovery<br>Significant bronchodilation<br>Increases in oral secretions<br>Cardiovascular (sympathetic) stimulation: Hypertension |
| Etomidate | **Induction: 0.2-0.5 mg/kg** | Induction of hemodynamically unstable patients (minimal cardiovascular depression)<br>Myoclonic movements<br>Anticonvulsant<br>High incidence of nausea and vomiting |
| **Barbiturates**<br>Thiopental<br>Methohexital | **Induction:**<br>**3-5 mg/kg**<br>**1-2 mg/kg** | Very alkaline pH (arterial injection causes severe tissue injury): Spasm and thrombosis<br>Methohexital: Shorter elimination half-life<br>Potent anticonvulsant |

## Current Inhalation Anesthetic Agents

- **Nitrous oxide** (gas): Analgesic properties
  - Diffuses into nitrogen-filled (air-filled) spaces to increase pressure (e.g., tension pneumothorax)
- **Isoflurane:** Very pungent, not suitable for inhalation induction
  - Induces coronary vasodilation (may cause "coronary steal" in patients with coronary artery disease)
- **Desflurane:** Most pungent of all volatile anesthetics
  - Laryngospasm if used for mask induction
  - Very low fat solubility (rapid emergence)
  - Sympathetic stimulation (tachycardia, hypertension) in high doses
- **Sevoflurane:** Sweet-smelling, minimal odor, nonpungent
  - Best for face mask induction of anesthesia
  - Potent bronchodilator

### Neuromuscular Blocking Agents

- **Succinylcholine**
  - Ultrarapid onset, ultrashort duration
  - Rapid hydrolysis by plasma cholinesterase
  - Depolarizes the motor endplate (fasciculation)
  - Triggers malignant hyperthermia
  - Only currently available depolarizing muscle relaxant
- **Vecuronium**
  - Hepatobiliary (75%) and renal (25%) excretion
  - No histamine release
  - No cardiovascular effects
- **Rocuronium**
  - Faster onset, used for RSI
  - Hepatobiliary (70%) and renal (30%) excretion
  - No histamine release
  - No cardiovascular effects
- **Atracurium/cisatracurium**
  - Favorable in hepatic and renal failure (renal and hepatobiliary excretion are insignificant)
  - Spontaneous (Hoffman) degradation in plasma

> **TIP:** Malignant hyperthermia is triggered ONLY by succinylcholine and all volatile anesthetic agents.

## REGIONAL ANESTHESIA

- **Local infiltration anesthesia**
- **Peripheral nerve block**
- **Central neuraxial anesthesia**

## LOCAL ANESTHETICS[2-4] (Table 12-3)

### Mechanism of Action

- Neural conduction is interrupted by inhibiting influx of sodium ions through sodium channels (receptor site) within the neuronal membrane.
- Penetration of nerve membrane requires un-ionized (base) form.
- pKa determines the ratio of ionized to un-ionized local anesthetic.
- The closer the pKa is to the body pH, the faster the onset.
- Stability is enhanced by adjusting pH of solutions to mildly acidic.

### Clinical Characteristics of Nerve Fibers

- There is a differential sensitivity of nerve fibers (myelinated and smaller nerve fibers most affected).
- Sequence of block onset (clinical anesthesia) is reflected in involved nerves.
- Recovery occurs in reverse order.

**Table 12-3** *Classification and Function of Nerve Fibers*

| Fiber Type/Subtype | Diameter (μm) | Conduction Velocity (m/sec) | Function |
|---|---|---|---|
| **A: Myelinated** | | | |
| α-alpha | 12-20 | 80-120 | Proprioception, large motor |
| β-beta | 5-15 | 60-80 | Small motor, touch, pressure |
| γ-gamma | 3-8 | 30-80 | Muscle tone |
| δ-delta | 2-5 | 10-30 | Pain, temperature, touch |
| **B: Myelinated** | 3 | 5-15 | Preganglionic autonomic |
| **C: Unmyelinated** | 0.3-1.5 | 0.5-2.5 | Dull pain, temperature, touch |

*μm,* Micrometer; *m/sec,* meters per second.

## SEQUENCE OF LOCAL ANESTHETIC BLOCKADE (Fig. 12-1; Table 12-4)

- **Sensitivity to local anesthetic blockade is inversely related to nerve fiber diameter.**
- Smaller fibers are preferentially blocked, because the critical length over which an impulse can travel passively is shorter.
- Smaller fibers with shorter critical lengths are blocked more quickly than larger fibers (same reasoning for faster recovery of smaller fibers).

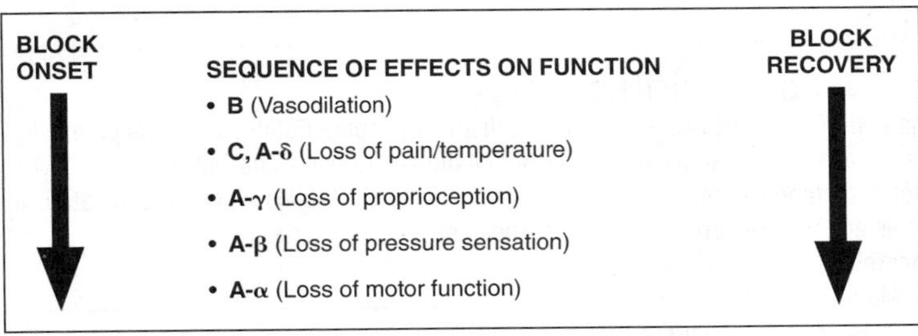


**Fig. 12-1** Sequence of local anesthetic blockade.

**Table 12-4** *Classes of Local Anesthetics*

| Local Anesthetic | Available Concentrations (%) | Max. Dose for Infiltration (mg) | Onset (min) | Duration After Infiltration (min) | Infiltration | Topical Application | Intravenous Regional | Peripheral Block | Epidural | Intrathecal (spinal) |
|---|---|---|---|---|---|---|---|---|---|---|
| **Esters** | | | | | | | | | | |
| Procaine | 1, 2, 10 | 500 | 2-5 | 40-60 | Yes | No | No | Yes | No | Yes |
| Chloroprocaine* | 1, 2, 3 | 600 | 6-12 | 30-60 | Yes | No | No | Yes | Yes | ±Yes |
| Tetracaine | 1 | 20 | >10 | 120-360 | No | Yes | No | No | No | Yes |

*Rarely used for spinal (intrathecal) anesthesia.

*Continued*

**Table 12-4** *Classes of Local Anesthetics—cont'd*

| Local Anesthetic | Available Concentrations (%) | Max. Dose for Infiltration (mg) | Onset (min) | Duration After Infiltration (min) | Infiltration | Topical Application | Intravenous Regional | Peripheral Block | Epidural | Intrathecal (spinal) |
|---|---|---|---|---|---|---|---|---|---|---|
| **Amides** | | | | | | | | | | |
| Lidocaine | 0.5, 1, 1.5, 2 | 300 | 0.5-1.5 | 60-120 | Yes | Yes | Yes | Yes | Yes | Yes |
| Mepivacaine* | 1, 1.5, 2, 3 | 300 | 3-5 | 90-180 | Yes | No | No | Yes | Yes | ±Yes |
| Bupivacaine | 0.25, 0.5, 0.75 | 150 | 5 | 240-480 | Yes | No | No | Yes | Yes | Yes |
| Levobupivacaine | 0.25, 0.5, 0.75 | 150 | 5 | 240-480 | Yes | No | No | Yes | Yes | Yes |
| Ropivacaine | 0.2, 0.5, 0.75, 1 | 200 | 1-15 | 240-480 | Yes | No | No | Yes | Yes | Yes |
| Prilocaine* | 0.5, 1, 2 | 400 | $<2$ | 60-120 | Yes | No | Yes | Yes | Yes | ±Yes |

*Rarely used for spinal (intrathecal) anesthesia.

## ESTER-LINKED (AMINO-ESTERS) (Fig. 12-2)

- Plasma half-life is short because of metabolism by pseudocholinesterase (decreased plasma cholinesterase level or atypical pseudocholinesterase increases half-life).
- Product of metabolism includes paraaminobenzoic acid (PABA), which is associated with allergy.
- Examples are cocaine, procaine, chloroprocaine, and tetracaine.
  - **Cocaine**
    - Mainly used to provide topical anesthesia of upper respiratory tract
    - Good vasoconstrictor
  - **Procaine**
    - Low potency, slow onset, short duration
    - Mainly used for infiltration analgesia
  - **2-chloroprocaine**
    - Most rapidly metabolized local anesthetic (low toxicity potential)
    - Not recommended for intrathecal or intravenous anesthesia
  - **Tetracaine:** Longer duration, more potent, more toxic

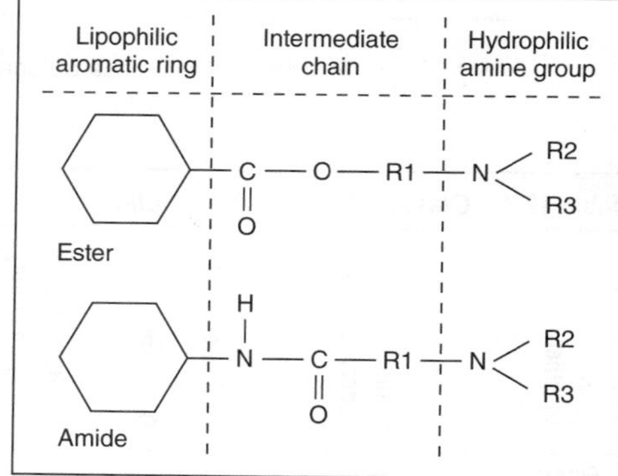


**Fig. 12-2** Ester and amide bonds.

## AMIDE-LINKED (AMINO-AMIDES) (see Fig. 12-2)

- Metabolized in the liver (elimination half-life: 2-3 hours)
- True allergy rare. Multidose vials may contain PABA as preservative, which may cause allergy.
- Examples: Lidocaine, bupivacaine, mepivacaine, prilocaine, etidocaine, dibucaine, ropivacaine, levobupivacaine
  - **Lidocaine**
    - Most commonly used
    - Rapidly absorbed from gastrointestinal and respiratory mucosae
    - Potential neurotoxicity (cauda equina syndrome) with intrathecal (spinal) anesthesia[5,6]
  - **Bupivacaine**
    - Slower onset, longer acting, more cardiotoxic (severe ventricular arrhythmias) than lidocaine
    - Cardiotoxicity enhanced by acidosis, hypercarbia, and hypoxemia
  - **Mepivacaine**
    - Poor topical local anesthetic
    - Longer duration but less vasodilation than lidocaine
  - **Prilocaine**
    - Metabolite (orthotoluidine) causes methemoglobinemia
    - Rapid metabolism
  - **Etidocaine**
    - Long acting
    - Preferential motor blockade often outlasts sensory blockade (a major disadvantage).
  - **Ropivacaine**
    - Long acting
    - Reduced CNS and cardiac toxicity
    - Less motor blockade
  - **Levobupivacaine:** Reduced cardiotoxicity

**TIP:** All amino-amides have the letter "i" in the prefix.

## LIPOSOME-ENCAPSULATED (SUSTAINED-RELEASE) LOCAL ANESTHETICS[7,8]

- Multivesicular liposomes loaded with local anesthetic for local tissue infiltration
- Bupivacaine is the only currently available formulation (aqueous suspension).
- Provides postsurgical analgesia for up to 72 hours, reducing opioid consumption and opioid-related side effects

**CAUTION: Coadministration with any other local anesthetic increases the release of bupivacaine from liposomes and should be avoided.**

**Antiseptics such as chlorhexidine and povidone-iodine disrupt lipid layers, leading to uncontrolled release of bupivacaine.**

## LOCAL ANESTHETIC ADDITIVES

- During manufacturing or just before administration
- Objectives: Shorten onset time, limit absorption, increase intensity of action, stabilize local anesthetic molecule, and inhibit microbial growth

- **Opioids** (morphine, hydromorphone, fentanyl, sufentanil)
  - Improve quality and duration of neuraxial analgesia
  - Risk of delayed respiratory depression with morphine
  - Fentanyl and sufentanil probably act via systemic uptake.
- **Clonidine**
  - Alpha-2 adrenergic agonist
  - Has analgesic effect. Intensifies and prolongs analgesia up to 50% more.
  - Sedation and dry mouth are side effects.
- **Sodium bicarbonate**
  - Speeds onset of blockade
  - Increases percentage of un-ionized fraction of local anesthetic by reducing acidity
  - Dose: 8.4% $NaHCO_3$ (0.1 to 10 ml bupivacaine or 1 to 9 ml lidocaine or mepivacaine)
  - Onset of block faster with lidocaine and mepivacaine than with bupivacaine and ropivacaine

**TIP:** Ropivacaine and bupivacaine may precipitate with the addition of sodium bicarbonate.

- **Epinephrine**
  - Most common concentrations 1:200,000 (5 μg/ml or 1 mg/200 ml) and 1:100,000 (10 μg/ml or 1 mg/100 ml)
  - Makes local anesthetics acidic and less stable by decreasing the nonionized fraction[9]
- **Advantages**
  - Causes vasoconstriction
    - Less vascular absorption
    - Decreases bleeding
  - Shortens time to onset of anesthesia
  - Increases duration of anesthesia
- **Disadvantages**
  - Increases myocardial irritability
    - May cause tachycardia, hypertension, and arrhythmias
    - Use cautiously in patients with known cardiac disease

**TIP:** Local anesthetics that contain epinephrine have red labels or red text.

**CAUTION: Concentrations of epinephrine of 1:200,000 or higher may be detrimental to the survival of delayed skin flaps.**

- **Contraindications**
  - **Absolute**
    - Do not use in penis.
    - Do not use in any skin flap with limited perfusion.
    - Do not use in hand when disease processes potentially involve the digital vessels at the base of the proximal phalanx (e.g., infection or trauma).
  - **Relative (use cautiously)**
    - Hypertension (can worsen)
    - Diabetes (Limited cutaneous perfusion may become severely compromised.)

- Heart disease (Myocardium sensitivity to epinephrine may precipitate ischemia, infarct, or both.)
- Thyrotoxicosis (Epinephrine could trigger a thyroid storm.)
- Certain concomitant uses of drugs

■ **Drug interactions:** The following drug interactions are unlikely with the small volume of local anesthetics used in most cutaneous surgery but have been reported. Caution is indicated when larger doses of local anesthetics with epinephrine are used.
- MAO inhibitors may cause a hypertensive crisis when epinephrine is used, because a pool of available endogenous catecholamines is created.
- Beta-adrenergic blocking agents have been reported to cause a serious hypertension-bradycardia crisis in rare instances because of interaction with epinephrine.

## Epinephrine Use in Digits

- Coinjection of procaine and cocaine (each causes digital infarction when given alone) with epinephrine decades ago created longstanding belief of finger infarction with epinephrine.[10]
- Incidence of finger infarction with elective injection of low-dose epinephrine is remote and unlikely.[11]
- Elective epinephrine use removes the need for tourniquet and reduces need for sedation and general anesthesia for hand surgery (significant cost reduction).[11,12]
- Phentolamine injection (1 mg/ml) decreases the duration of, and reliably reverses, epinephrine-induced vasoconstriction.[13] Nitroglycerin ointment is also useful.
- Injection of different concentrations of epinephrine (1:100,000, 1:10,000, 1:1000) into different fingers leads to spontaneous recovery within 12 hours without use of reversal agent such as phentolamine.[14]

## Recommendations for Epinephrine Use in Digits[10]

- Small amounts of local anesthetics with dilute epinephrine are probably safe for digital infiltration or blocks.
- Use dilute solutions such as 1:200,000 or less.
- Do not perform a circumferential block of the digits.
- Block preferentially at the level of the metacarpal heads rather than the digit.
- Use small needles to prevent injuring the vessels.
- Avoid postoperative hot soaks.
- Buffer the anesthetic to avoid acidic solutions.
- Bandages should not be constrictive or excessively tight.
- Patients should be followed to monitor for prolonged ischemia, which could require reversal with phentolamine injections or nitroglycerin ointment.
- Do not use epinephrine in patients with vasospastic, thrombotic, or extreme medical conditions.

## Mixing Local Anesthetics

- Rationale: Faster onset (e.g., lidocaine) and longer duration (e.g., bupivacaine)
- Mixtures of ester- and amide-linked local anesthetics benefit from different modes of elimination.
- Onset, duration, and potency become less predictable, and there is a risk of drug error.
- It is better to choose concentrations of single agents to achieve desired effects.
- Toxicity is additive with unintentional intravenous administration.

## TOXICITY OF LOCAL ANESTHETICS[15,16]

- Magnitude of systemic absorption depends on dose, site of injection, and presence or absence of vasoconstriction.

### ALLERGIC REACTIONS

- True allergy is rare. Contact (type IV) hypersensitivity is more common with lidocaine.
- Amino-esters more likely to cause allergic reaction because of their metabolism to PABA, a known antigen.
- Methylparaben (preservative in some esters and amides) resembles PABA and may cause allergic reaction.
- Cross-sensitivity does not occur. Ester-allergic patients may receive amide local anesthetics.

### SYSTEMIC TOXICITY (CENTRAL NEURONAL, CARDIOVASCULAR, HEMATOLOGIC SYSTEMS)

- Liver disease increases toxicity of amide-linked local anesthetics.
- Pseudocholinesterase deficiency increases toxicity of ester-linked local anesthetics.

### CENTRAL NERVOUS SYSTEM (CNS) TOXICITY (Fig. 12-3)

- Local anesthetics readily cross blood-brain barrier.
- Features of toxicity are dose dependent.
- Acidosis, decreased protein binding, vasoconstriction, and hyperdynamic circulation increase CNS toxicity.
- CNS depressants (barbiturates, benzodiazepines) and decreased systemic absorption (vasoconstrictive drugs such as epinephrine) decrease CNS toxicity.

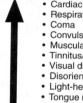

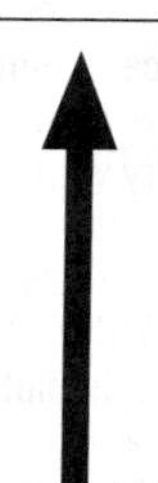
• Cardiac arrest
• Respiratory arrest
• Coma
• Convulsions (grand mal seizures)
• Muscular twitching/spasms
• Tinnitus/auditory hallucinations
• Visual disturbance
• Disorientation
• Light-headedness
• Tongue numbness/metallic taste
• Antiarrhythmic and anticonvulsant at ≤5 μg/ml serum concentration

**Fig. 12-3** Features of local anesthetic toxicity with increasing plasma concentration.

### CARDIOVASCULAR TOXICITY

- Requires higher systemic levels than for CNS
- Bupivacaine (greatest cardiac toxicity): Stronger binding affinity to and slower dissociation from sodium channels
- Sudden cardiovascular collapse: Ventricular arrhythmias resistant to resuscitation

### HEMATOLOGIC TOXICITY

- Methemoglobinemia: Liver metabolism of prilocaine forms orthotoluidine, which oxidates hemoglobin to methemoglobin.[17]
- **Treatment:** Spontaneous reversal or intravenous methylene blue

### MANAGEMENT OF LOCAL ANESTHETIC TOXICITY[18]

- **Prevention:** Frequent syringe aspirations, small test dose, divided doses injection
- **Initial focus:** Supportive treatment
  - Stop further injection of local anesthetic.
  - Airway management: Hyperventilate with 100% oxygen to prevent detrimental effects of hypoxia, hypercarbia, and acidosis that may potentiate toxicity.
  - Seizure suppression: Benzodiazepines (e.g., midazolam) are preferred.
  - Muscle relaxants may help stop movements during seizures.
  - Basic and Advanced Cardiac Life Support (BLS/ACLS) may require prolonged effort (stronger affinity of bupivacaine to cardiac muscle).

- **Intravenous 20% lipid emulsion acts as a binding agent to the local anesthetic.**
- Fluid resuscitation and vasopressor, antiarrhythmic, and inotropic therapy may be needed.

**CAUTION: Do not give cardiac depressant drugs to patients with signs of cardiovascular instability.**

## CHECKLIST TO PREVENT TOXICITY

- Always calculate the maximum allowable dose by weight.
- Mix two anesthetics to increase volume for administration but also decrease total individual local anesthetic given.
- Dilute local anesthetic with saline solution.
- Use solutions with epinephrine whenever possible to increase maximum allowable dosage.
- Always aspirate before injecting to confirm needle tip is not intravascular.

## LOCAL AND REGIONAL ANESTHESIA

### LOCAL INFILTRATION

- Pain on injection may be decreased by:
  - Use of a very small-gauge needle (25- to 30-gauge)
  - Slow administration of local anesthetic
  - Buffering with sodium bicarbonate (except for bupivacaine and ropivacaine)

**TIP:** Deposit local anesthetic just under dermal layers. Deeper administration into adipose tissue (poorly innervated) increases total dose without significant anesthetic or analgesic effect.

- Local infiltration with as high as 1:200,000 epinephrine has no harmful effect on primary skin flap survival.[19]
- Epinephrine in as low a dose as 1:800,000 will provide adequate hemostasis.
- Infected tissues are acidic, decreased amount of un-ionized local anesthetic, less effectiveness

### PERIPHERAL NERVE BLOCK

- Confirm normal coagulation or history of bleeding problems.
- Rule out preexisting neuropathy.
- A catheter may be inserted for continuous infusion.

### INTRAVENOUS REGIONAL ANESTHESIA (BIER BLOCK)

- A large volume of dilute local anesthetic is intravenously injected into an extremity (in proximity to a nerve plexus) after circulatory occlusion by tourniquet.
- Lidocaine 0.5% is most commonly used. Prilocaine 0.5% may also be used.
- Local anesthetic is injected into an exsanguinated limb using double tourniquet. The proximal tourniquet is inflated first and is deflated after inflation of the distal tourniquet over an anesthetized area.
- Duration of block is approximately 2 hours.

**TIP:** Do not deflate the tourniquet before 40 minutes to prevent local anesthetic toxicity.

**TIP:** Watch for systemic signs and symptoms of toxicity caused by a faulty tourniquet.

## Central Neuraxial Block

- **Epidural Anesthesia**
  - It can be performed at any level of the spine (spinal [intrathecal] can only be performed in lumbar region).
  - Segmental sensory block is easier to produce.
  - Epidural catheters allow titration of block for surgery and later administration of dilute local anesthetic and/or opioid solutions for postoperative analgesia.
- **Spinal (Intrathecal) Anesthesia**
  - Local anesthesic is injected into the cerebrospinal fluid (CSF) at the lumbar vertebral level.
  - Smaller volumes of local anesthetic are used.
  - Baricity (density of local anesthetic relative to density of CSF) of the local anesthetic determines its spread (i.e., it is affected by gravity).
  - Example: In the sitting position, hyperbaric local anesthetic solutions spreads caudad, hypobaric solution spreads cephalad, and isobaric solutions have limited spread.
- **Complications of epidural and spinal block**
  - **Postdural puncture headache (PDPH):** More common with inadvertent puncture ("wet tap") with larger epidural needle (17- or 18-gauge Tuohy). Rate of loss of CSF exceeds production—downward displacement of brain with stretch on sensitive supporting structures.
    **Treatment:** Bed rest, fluids, analgesics, and epidural blood patch for resistant headaches
  - **"High spinal" or "total spinal" anesthesia:** Excessive cephalad spread of local anesthetic; results in apnea and loss of consciousness because of ischemia of medullary centers from hypotension or direct effect of local anesthetic on medulla
    **Treatment:** Maintain airway (endotracheal intubation) and circulation with adequate ventilation, vasopressors, and fluid infusion.
  - **Epidural hematoma:** Confirm diagnosis with MRI. Urgent surgical evacuation of hematoma is needed to prevent permanent neurologic damage.[20]
  - **Hypotension:** From sympatholysis resulting in vasodilation
  - **Urinary retention:** Local anesthetic interference with bladder innervations

## TOPICAL ANESTHETICS[19,21] (Table 12-5)

- Qualities of ideal topical anesthetic:
  - Fast acting
  - Easy to apply and remove
  - Nonstaining
  - Nontoxic
  - Does not require occlusion
  - Fast acting with effective anesthesia
  - Minimal systemic absorption

## Sedation and Analgesia (Moderate or Conscious Sedation)

- A drug-induced depression of consciousness during which patients respond purposefully to verbal commands either alone or accompanied by light tactile stimulation
- Allows protective reflexes to be maintained
- Retains the patient's ability to maintain a patent airway independently and continuously
- Permits appropriate responses by the patient
- Drugs titrated in increments rather than large bolus doses
- Continuous infusions superior to intermittent boluses because less fluctuation in drug concentration

**Table 12-5** *Topical Anesthetic Agents*[19]

| Product | Active Ingredient | Vehicle | Occlusive Dressing | Comments |
|---|---|---|---|---|
| **EMLA** | Lidocaine 2.5% and prilocaine 2.5% | Eutectic cream | Required | Anesthetic effect after 60 min |
| **LMX-4; LMX-5** | Lidocaine 4%, 5% | Liposome | Not required | Anesthetic effect after 20-30 min |
| **Betacaine** | Lidocaine 5% | Ointment | Not required | Anesthetic effect after 20-30 min |
| **Betacaine-LA** | Lidocaine, prilocaine, dibucaine, phenylephrine | Petrolatum | Not required | Phenylephrine reduces systemic absorption |
| **Topicaine** | Lidocaine 4%, 5% | Water based | May or may not be used | Anesthetic effect after 30 min<br>5% formulation has shea butter |
| **Tetracaine gel** | Tetracaine 4% | Lecithin gel | Yes | Onset: 30-45 min<br>Longlasting: 4-6 hr |
| **Lidocaine laser ointment** | Lidocaine 30% (compounded) | Ointment | Not required | Onset: 60 min |
| **Viscous lidocaine** | Lidocaine 2%, 5% | Cellulose-based | Not applicable | Onset within 5 min |
| **Cryoanalgesia** | Ice | ± Needlelike probe | Not applicable | Nonpharmacologic<br>Ice itself may cause discomfort |

## Goals of Conscious Sedation

- Facilitate the performance of a procedure
- Control behavior, including anxiety
- Return the patient to a state in which safe discharge is possible

## Candidates

- Patients who are ASA I or II are good candidates for conscious sedation in an office or emergency room setting.
- Infants and elderly patients are good candidates.
- ASA III and IV patients may have conscious sedation, but it should be performed in a well-controlled environment (e.g., operating room) with constant monitoring by anesthesia personnel.

## Documentation of Conscious Sedation Should Include

- Patient consent to procedure (consent required from parent or legal guardian with minors)
- Compliance with fasting precautions that are consistent with accepted norms for general anesthesia when applicable (e.g., no solids during the preceding 6 hours and only clear liquids up to 2 hours before the procedure)
- Medical history
- General health of the patient as noted from a previous physical examination
- Vital signs during the procedure (heart rate, respiratory rate, oxygen saturation)
- Medication used and route administered during the procedure

## Personnel

- A physician responsible for administering the drugs (and possibly treating the patient) and a physician, registered nurse, or nurse anesthetist not involved in the administration of drugs must be present to monitor the patient throughout the procedure.
- When conscious sedation is performed for an emergency room procedure, the emergency room physician is responsible for the conscious sedation orders, because he or she must be immediately available until the patient is alert.

## Intraoperative Monitoring

- Oxygen saturation, pulse rate, blood pressure
- Capnography monitoring of expired carbon dioxide levels (and respiratory pattern and rate) highly recommended
- Documentation of vital signs by appropriate frequency during the procedure (frequency generally determined by type and amount of medication administered, length of the procedure, and general condition of the patient)
- Complete documentation of the procedure, medications, their effects, and any untoward incidents

**TIP:** Patients should be able to cooperate and remain immobile.

## Key Points

- ✓ Routine preoperative laboratory tests are not needed if a patient is in optimal medical condition and the procedure is minimally invasive.
- ✓ Ingestion of clear liquids is permitted up to 2 hours before induction of anesthesia.
- ✓ Desflurane is the most pungent of all volatile anesthetics and causes laryngospasm if used for induction of anesthesia.
- ✓ Ester-linked local anesthetics are more likely to cause allergic response because of their metabolism to PABA, a known antigen.
- ✓ Methylparaben (preservative in some esters and amides) resembles PABA and may cause allergic response.
- ✓ The incidence of finger infarction with elective injection of low-dose epinephrine is remote and unlikely.
- ✓ Liposome-encapsulated bupivacaine provides postsurgical analgesia for up to 72 hours, reducing opioid consumption and opioid-related side effects.
- ✓ The level of sedation during monitored anesthesia care should allow verbal communication to assess the level of sedation and reassure the patient.
- ✓ During sedation and analgesia, it is better to use a combination of drugs to produce adequate amnesia, analgesia, and hypnosis and to reduce the dose of individual drugs and their side effects.
- ✓ Monitoring of expired carbon dioxide levels is highly recommended during conscious sedation.

## REFERENCES


1. Dripps RD. New classification of physical status. Anesthesiology 24:111, 1963.
2. Becker DE, Reed KL. Local anesthetics: review of pharmacological considerations. Anesth Prog 59:90-102, 2012.
3. Butterworth J. Clinical pharmacology of local anesthetics. In Hadzic A, ed. Textbook of Regional Anesthesia and Acute Pain Management. New York: McGraw-Hill, 2007.
4. Moore PA, Hersh EV. Local anesthetics: pharmacology and toxicity. Dent Clin N Am 54:587-599, 2010.
5. Drasner K. Local anesthetic neurotoxicity: clinical injury and strategies that may minimize risk. Reg Anesth Pain Med 27:576-580, 2002.
6. Lee H, Park YS, Cho TG, et al. Transient adverse neurologic effects of spinal pain blocks. J Korean Neurosurg Soc 52:228-233, 2012.
7. Chahar P, Cummings KC. Liposomal bupivacaine: a review of a new bupivacaine formulation. J Pain Res 5:257-264, 2012.
8. Candiotti K. Liposomal bupivacaine: an innovative nonopioid local analgesic for the management of postsurgical pain. Pharmacotherapy 32(9 Suppl):S19-S26, 2012.
9. Thornton PC, Grant SA, Breslin DS. Adjuncts to local anesthetics in peripheral nerve blockade. Int Anesthesiol Clin 48:59-70, 2010.
10. Denkler K. A comprehensive review of epinephrine in the finger: to do or not to do. Plast Reconstr Surg 108:114-124, 2001.
11. Lalonde D, Bell M, Benoit P, et al. A multicenter prospective study of 3110 consecutive cases of elective epinephrine use in the fingers and hand: the Dalhousie Project clinical phase. J Hand Surg Am 30:1061-1067, 2005.
12. Thomson CJ, Lalonde DH, Denkler KA, et al. A critical look at the evidence for and against elective epinephrine use in the finger. Plast Reconstr Surg 119:260-266, 2007.
13. Nodwell T, Lalonde DH. How long does it take phentolamine to reverse adrenaline-induced vasoconstriction in the finger and hand? A prospective randomized blinded study: the Dalhousie Project experimental phase. Can J Plast Surg 11:187-190, 2003.
14. Fitzcharles-Bowe C, Denkler K, Lalonde D. Finger injection with high-dose (1:1,000) epinephrine: does it cause finger necrosis and should it be treated? Hand 2:5-11, 2007.
15. Hadzic A, Vloka JD. Clinical pharmacology of local anesthetics. In Hadzic A, ed. Hadzic's Peripheral Nerve Blocks and Anatomy for Ultrasound-Guided Regional Anesthesia, 2nd ed. New York: McGraw-Hill, 2012.
16. Heavner JE. Pharmacology of local anesthetics. In Longnecker DE, Brown DL, Newman MF, et al, eds. Anesthesiology, 2nd ed. New York: McGraw-Hill, 2012.
17. Hjelm M, Holmdahl MH. Biochemical effects of aromatic amines. Acta Anaesthesiol Scand 2:99-120, 1965.
18. Neal JM, Bernards CM, Butterworth JF, et al. ASRA practice advisory on local anesthetic systemic toxicity. Reg Anesth Pain Med 35:152-161, 2010.
19. Atabey A, Galdino G, El-Shahat A, et al. The effect of tumescent solutions containing lidocaine and epinephrine on skin flap survival in rats. Ann Plast Surg 53:70-72, 2004.
20. Groen RJ, van Alphen HA. Operative treatment of spontaneous spinal epidural hematomas: a study of factors determining postoperative outcome. Neurosurgery 39:494-508, 1996.
21. Amin SP, Goldberg DJ. Topical anesthetics for cosmetic and laser dermatology. J Drugs Dermatol 4:455-461, 2005.

# 13. Photography for the Plastic Surgeon

Amanda Y. Behr, Holly P. Smith

## BASICS OF STANDARDIZED PHOTOGRAPHY

Photographic documentation serves medicolegal functions and has many educational, research, clinical, and marketing applications. It provides a means to assess surgical success or failure and leads to better communication between the patient and physician. It is one of the most useful tools to the plastic surgeon, but it can also be one of the most fallible. If quality and proper standardizations are not maintained, medical photographs can become misleading and unable to provide accurate photographic documentation.

## ELEMENTS OF STANDARDIZED PATIENT PHOTOGRAPHY

A routine standardized procedure saves time, because decisions are determined by existing rules.[1] Standardization requires planning, a systematic approach, adherence to protocols, and attention to detail.[2,3]

- **Use a standardized series** (a predetermined set of photographs per procedure) to ensure that the same views are photographed each time.
- **Use Cardiff scales of reproduction with 35 mm film.**[4]
  - Advocates using a lens with focal length equal to at least twice the diagonal of the image plane to prevent unwanted image distortion
  - Controls magnification and perspective and ensures standardization among photographs taken by different photographers
- **Use a flash or a lighting setup for consistent lighting.**
- **Color management**
  - Use an 18% gray card to balance color.
  - White balance the camera.
- **Attention to detail**
  - Have patient remove jewelry, glasses, and heavy makeup.
  - Keep area clean.
  - Use a background.

## PHOTOGRAPHIC TERMINOLOGY

### APERTURE

Aperture *refers to the size of the adjustable opening (iris) of a lens, which determines the amount of light falling onto the film or sensor.*

- The size of the opening is measured using an f-number or f-stop (e.g., f8, f11).
- Because f-numbers are fractions of the focal length, larger f-numbers represent smaller apertures.
- The smaller the aperture, the greater the depth of field.

## Shutter Speed

Shutter speed *determines how long the iris of the camera is open to expose the film or sensor to light (e.g., a shutter speed of 1/125s will expose the sensor for 1/125th of a second).*

- Electronic shutters act by switching on the light-sensitive photodiodes of the sensor for as long as requested by the shutter speed.

## Depth of Field

*Objects within a certain range behind or in front of the main focus point appear sharp.* Depth of field *refers to the distance between the closest and farthest in-focus area of a photograph (also called the* focal range*).*

- Depth of field is affected by the aperture, subject distance, focal length, and film or sensor format.
- The smaller the aperture, the greater the depth of field.

## Focal Length

Focal length *is the distance in millimeters from the optical center of the lens to the focal point, which is located on the sensor or film.*

- The longer the focal length, the narrower the field of view.
- The shorter the focal length, the larger the field of view.

## Lenses

*Camera lenses are categorized as* ***normal, wide angle,*** *and* ***telephoto,*** *according to focal length and film size.*

- **Normal:** The focal length of a lens is close to the diagonal measurement of the film/sensor's format. For example, 43.27 mm is the length of the diagonal in a 35 mm (35 mm × 24 mm) film plane. The closest equivalent lens is 50 mm. A 50 mm lens has a field of view of 46 degrees.
- **Wide angle:** The focal length is shorter than the film/sensor's diagonal. For example, using a 20 mm lens with a 35 mm film plane is wide angle. A 20 mm lens has a field of view of 94 degrees.
- **Telephoto/long:** The focal length of a lens is longer than the film/sensor's diagonal. For example, using a 105 mm lens with a 35 mm film plane is telephoto. A 105 mm lens has a field of view of 23 degrees.

**NOTE: On some digital cameras an equivalent lens will have a much smaller focal length, because the image sensors are much smaller than 35 mm. The manufacturer may provide a multiplication factor that can be used to assess the focal length in 35 mm terms, or the manual may show the equivalent focal length to the 35 mm focal length.**

## Single Lens Reflex

*A single lens reflex camera of 35 mm or medium format has a system of mirrors that shows the user the image precisely as the lens renders it.*

- Through the Lens (TTL)
  - *A through-the-lens metering system has a light-sensitive mechanism in the camera body that measures exposure from the image light passing through the lens.*

# DIGITAL PHOTOGRAPHY TERMINOLOGY

## Resolution

Resolution *is a measurement of the pixel count of an image, given either as pixels per inch (ppi) or total pixels.*

- Digital cameras capture images using a sensor. The resolution is calculated by multiplying the pixels captured along the width and length of the sensor.
- The amount of resolution needed can be determined by output needs. Images for use on the Internet or for PowerPoint presentations do not need as much resolution as images intended for output to a printer.

**TIP:** Increased resolution is not always better. Match resolution to output needs. The higher the resolution, the larger the file size, and the more storage is needed. This can become costly and slow down software applications and file transfer time.

## Recommended Resolution According to Output

High-resolution retina display devices require higher-resolution images than regular display devices. The simplest solution if images appear pixilated on retina display devices is to double the dimension size of the image (keeping the resolution the same). For example, to display an image at 200 × 300 pixels, use an image that is 400 × 600 pixels. This will increase the file size and may delay download when viewed online. Image size must be weighed against the appearance of the image.

- 72-96 ppi for Internet and e-mail
- 150 ppi for PowerPoint presentations
- 300 ppi for print publications

**TIP:** One way to estimate resolution needed for printing is to multiply the size of the desired image by 300 ppi (the standard for photographic quality) (Table 13-1).

**Table 13-1** *Image Resolution and Megapixel Recommendation*

| Type of Image | Minimum Pixel Dimensions (pixels) | Minimum Effective Resolution (megapixels) |
|---|---|---|
| 4 × 6 web image at 72 ppi | 288 × 432 | 1.4 |
| 4 × 6 print image at 300 ppi | 1200 × 1800 | 2.5 |
| 5 × 7 print image at 300 ppi | 1500 × 2100 | 3.3 |
| 8 × 10 print image at 300 ppi | 2400 × 3000 | 7.6 |

*ppi,* Pixels per inch.

## Camera Sensor

*A camera sensor is similar to a computer chip that senses light focused on its surface. It consists of an array of pixels that collect photons.*

- The two most popular sensors in digital cameras are the charged couple device (CCD) and the complementary metal oxide semiconductor (CMOS).

## Storage Cards

- Storage cards perform the function that film does in conventional cameras. They are removable drives that store captured data.
  - Compact Flash I
  - Secure Digital (SD)
  - Secure Digital High Capacity (SDHC): Larger capacity and speed
  - SD eXtended Capacity (SDXC): Largest capacity and speed
- Compact Flash and Secure Digital are now the dominant types of digital camera memory storage. The most commonly used storage drive at this time is the Secure Digital.
- SD cards look similar, but the higher-capacity cards are not universally supported. Check camera specifications to be sure that the camera supports SDHC and SDXC card formats.
- When recording video or taking large photos in quick succession, it is beneficial to use a higher-speed memory card.

## Image Compression

- It is sometimes necessary to compress image files to reduce file size.
- The larger the resolution of a digital image, the larger the file size, which can make demands on storage.
- Data compression is important if many images need to be stored, or if they are to be published on the Internet.
- There are two compression types
  - **Lossless** does not lose any image data.
  - **Lossy** reduces the image data each time it is saved.

## File Types

- Digital images may be saved as different file types.
  - **JPEG (Joint Photographic Expert Group)**
    - One of the most universally used formats; compatible with browsers, viewers, and image-editing software
    - Lossy compression
    - Considered the best compression file type for photographs
  - **Raw**
    - The unprocessed original image as it comes off the sensor before in-camera processing
    - Similar to a negative in film photography
  - **TIFF (Tagged Image File Format)**
    - Universal image format compatible with most image editing viewing programs
    - Lossless uncompressed format that produces no artifacts commonly seen with other image formats such as JPEG

**TIP:** Although the TIFF and raw formats preserve image quality better, they are not practical for storing many files. Resaving often in a JPEG format degrades an image, which becomes noticeable over time. For images that are resaved often, work from a copy of the image rather than the original.

## PRACTICAL POINTS

- Compact digital camera with removable lens and bounce flash for clinical photos
- Point-and-shoot or compact interchangeable lens camera for operative settings
- 10 or more megapixels
- HD video capability
- Adjustable LCD screen
- Lens to accommodate low light
- Auto vs. manual settings: Use both settings, adjust light mode for optimum photo
- Must have one extra camera battery for backup, two camera batteries total
- Two camera memory cards, 8 GB
- Suggested photo organization software (Adobe Bridge, ACD Systems International)

## WHAT TO LOOK FOR IN A DIGITAL CAMERA

### Camera Types

- Digital single lens reflex (SLR) with interchangeable lenses
- Digital compact point-and-shoot
- Compact interchangeable lens cameras (CILC),[5] four thirds and micro four thirds

### Focus

- Method of focusing and positioning
  - Automatic focus using anatomic regions for positioning
  - Manual focus using set distances and focal lengths

### Sensor Size

- Image sensor size (Fig. 13-1)
  - Converts light from the photographic exposure into a digital representation of the image
  - Sensors contain pixels that capture the image. Larger sensors have larger pixels and can capture better images in lower-light conditions.[5]

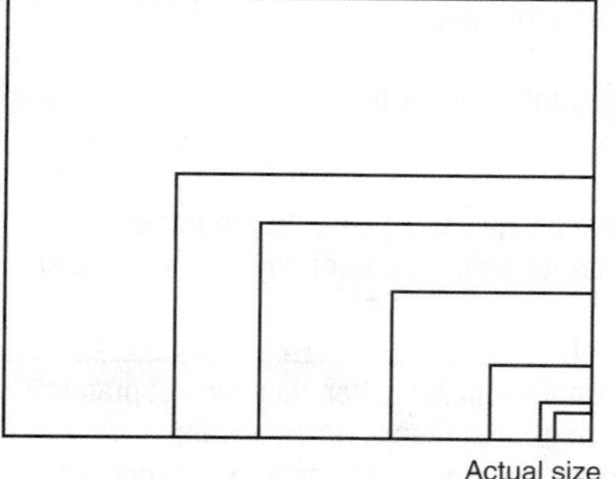


**Fig. 13-1** Comparison of digital camera sensor sizes, which affects quality of digital photographs.

## Digital Versus Optical Zoom

- **Digital zoom** takes a part of the scene and interpolates data to fit on the CCD sensor plane.
  - It mimics a greater zoom without gaining image detail.
  - It often results in a blurry and pixilated image.
- **Optical zoom** changes the amount of the scene falling on the CCD sensor.
  - Information is not interpolated and can be enlarged and cropped with good results.
  - A 33 optical zoom gives a focal length of 35-105 mm, which is the minimum necessary for photographing the face and body.

## Viewfinders

*The viewfinder is the window you look through to compose a scene.*[6]

- Optical viewfinder on a digital compact camera
  - The optical viewfinder is positioned above the camera lens so what you see through the optical viewfinder is different from what the lens projects onto the sensor.
  - This type of sensor has parallax error which can make framing inaccurate when photographing close-ups.
- Optical viewfinder on a digital SLR camera (TTL)
  - These viewfinders use a mirror and a prism to show what the lens will project on the sensor.
    - This type of viewfinder does not have parallax errors.
  - LCD on a digital compact camera (TTL)
  - An LCD shows in real time what is projected onto the sensor by the lens.
  - An LCD does not have parallax errors but does shorten battery life, and it can be difficult to see LCD screens in bright sunlight conditions.
- Electronic viewfinder (EVF) on a digital compact camera (TTL)
  - An electronic viewfinder shows in real time what is projected onto the sensor by the lens.
  - It simulates in an electronic way the effect of the (superior) optical TTL viewfinders found on digital SLRs and does not have parallax errors.
  - EVF allows accurate framing but can shorten battery life.

## Video

- Many consumer cameras come with digital video capability.
- Some cameras offer HD movie mode that allows the capture of high-definition video for display on HD devices.
- Although video resolutions are small and the recording time depends on the size of storage, video can be useful for relaying information between physicians and for media presentations.
- Evaluate the following characteristics: maximum frame size, frame rate, the ability to use external audio (external audio jack), maximum recording time, quality of compression.

## Camera Overall Resolution and Effective Resolution

*Megapixels* is a common measurement to distinguish camera resolution. A megapixel is a million pixels. The resolution measurement is determined by multiplying the length and width in pixels of the image capture or image sensor. Camera advertisers may advertise the camera's overall resolution, which is the total number of pixels on the image sensor. *Effective resolution* is a smaller measurement that is the actual number of pixels used to capture an image (Fig. 13-2). Some of the pixels on the sensor are cropped out of the image to maintain an aspect ratio. It is best to use both measurements when comparing camera resolution.[7]

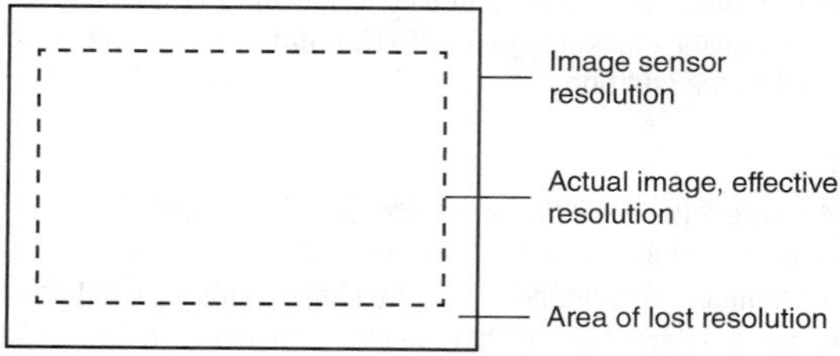


**Fig. 13-2** Effective resolution is the true measure of camera resolution.

## Focal Length and Lenses

The need for a normal, wide-angle, or telephoto focal length is determined based on the required field of view. The focal length of a digital camera is smaller than that of a 35 mm camera, because sensors are smaller than 35 mm. To obtain the 35 mm focal length equivalent, the manufacturer's equivalent of a 35 mm focal length is used, or the provided multiplication factor is multiplied by the digital camera focal length. When choosing a camera with a fixed lens that cannot be removed, the desired focal length must be selected. The focal length for point-and-shoot cameras is measured in terms of zoom factor. A zoom factor of 10× will typically be the equivalent of a 28-200 mm lens. This is variable and requires checking with the manufacturer for specific equivalents.[7]

## Flashes

- On-camera flash
- Hot shoe connection: User has more flash and remote synchronization options
- Flash synchronization port on camera: Multiple flash devices may be added.

**TIP:** A separate bounce flash (with swivel head) with plastic diffuser is recommended in clinical settings for photographs of the face and body. The best results are obtained by angling the head of the flash 45 degrees upward. This will allow the light to diffuse from the ceiling, providing consistent lighting in each photograph without the harsh flattened effect of a straight-on flash.[8]

**NOTE: For clinical settings, a digital SLR camera or CILC with interchangeable, fixed focal length lenses is highly recommended. This allows the distance on the lens to be set and ensures an accurate and reproductive focal length. Choose a set meter on the lens and achieve focus by moving the camera closer to or farther from the subject. This will ensure consistent comparative views when photographing a patient over time.**

**In an operative setting in which comparative views are not a priority, a compact point-and-shoot camera or CILC with a swivel body or a twist LCD provides better flexibility. Cameras with bodies that swivel are especially useful for taking pictures directly over a supine or prone patient.**

## MAGNIFICATION

- The Westminster scales of reproduction established the principle of standardizing clinical photograph magnification.[9] The Cardiff scales of reproduction revised this scale because of the change in size of the average person.[4]
- Focal lengths provided throughout the series are intended for photographing in a clinical setting. They are also intended for 35 mm film and higher-end digital SLR cameras with interchangeable fixed lenses whose CCD sensor is equal in size to 35 mm film.
- If using a camera with a CCD sensor smaller than 35 mm film, the focal length modifier can be determined by dividing the 35 mm plane (43.3 mm) by the digital camera's sensor diagonal. The size of the sensor usually can be found in the camera's literature supplied by the manufacturer. The sensors on most consumer digital cameras are 1.5 times smaller than 35 mm film.
  - For instance, a 50 mm lens used on a digital camera with a focal length modification of 1.5 is equivalent to a 75 mm lens.
- It is important to correct for disparities in focal lengths, because they can make dramatic differences, especially in comparative views[4] (Fig. 13-3).

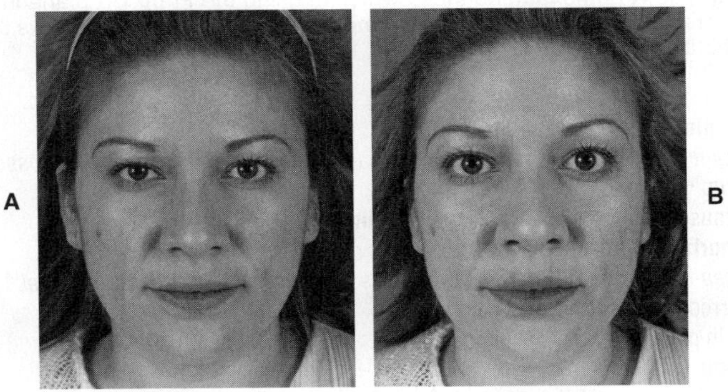


**Fig. 13-3** Image **A** was created using a 105 mm lens 1:10. Image **B** was created with a 50 mm lens 1:10, which shows the lens distortion called a *barrel distortion*.

## INFECTION CONTROL

- In the clinic, maintain barrier control and treat the photographic equipment as a possible contaminant.
- Within the surgical setting, maintain sterility by segregating photographic personnel from the sterile field. Support personnel can be trained to photograph surgery without contaminating the sterile field.[10]

- In a surgical setting, an underwater camera case can be sterilized to allow photographs to be taken within a sterile environment.[11]

## HEAD POSITIONING

The **Frankfort plane** is used as a reference line for correct head positioning for x-ray films and has been used by physicians as a standard for head alignment when photographing the face. Some physicians choose to use the natural horizontal facial plane for alignment[1] (Fig. 13-4).

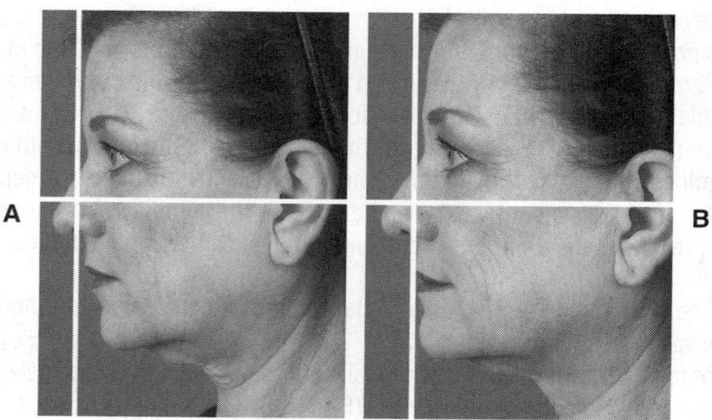


**Fig. 13-4** Image **A** demonstrates the downfall to using the Frankfort plane in which neck retraction overemphasizes the degree of submental soft tissue. Image **B** shows the patient in the natural horizontal facial plane.

- **Frankfort plane**
*Horizontal plane that transverses the top of the tragus (external auditory canal) across the infraorbital rim*[12]
    - Can cause noticeable changes in jaw definition and submental soft tissue[13]
- **Natural horizontal facial line**
*Achieved when the patient looks straight ahead as if looking into a mirror at eye level*[14]
    - Preferred for rhinoplasty surgery
    - Used in patients who have low-set ears[14]
- **Positioning**
    - Anatomically correct (top of head should be nearest the top of photograph)
    - Arms and hands: Exception to anatomic rule
    - Photographs of the location should be taken in addition to close-ups for accurate perspective and proportion.
- **Oblique variables**
    - Some physicians prefer the tip of the nose to touch the side of the far cheek for a rhinoplasty series, whereas others want the dorsum of the nose to visually touch the medial eye (Fig. 13-5).
- **The true lateral**
    - Photographing the head overrotated or underrotated in lateral views is a common mistake (Fig. 13-6) but one that can be corrected easily by viewing straight across both oral commissures[15] (Fig. 13-7).

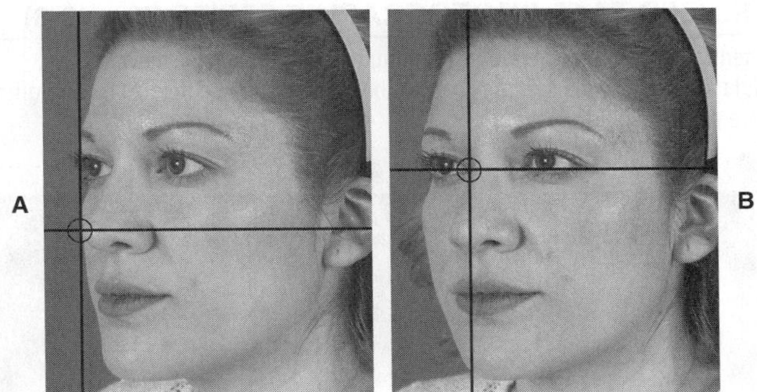


**Fig. 13-5** Oblique view. **A,** Some physicians prefer the tip of the nose to touch the side of the far cheek for a rhinoplasty series. **B,** Others want the dorsum to visually touch the medial eye.

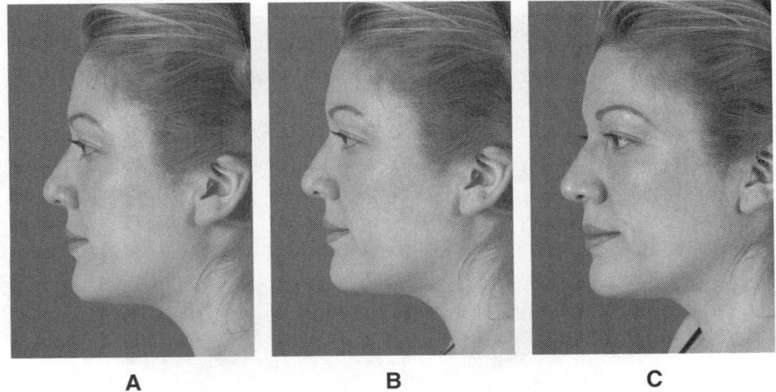


**Fig. 13-6** Lateral view. **A,** Underrotation. **B,** True lateral. **C,** Overrotation.

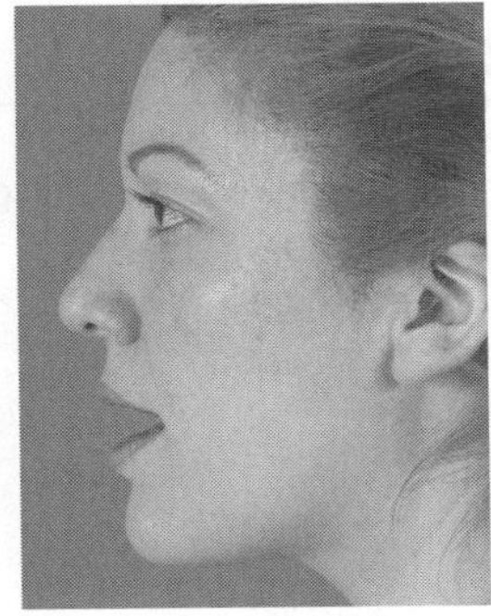

**Fig. 13-7** A true lateral image may be obtained by viewing straight across the two oral commissures to verify correct rotation.

## STANDARDIZED FACE PHOTOGRAPHIC SERIES (Fig. 13-8)

- Careful attention should be given to head tilting that can distort the view.
- It is helpful to check earlobe symmetry from the anterior view to determine straightness of the head before photographing.[14]

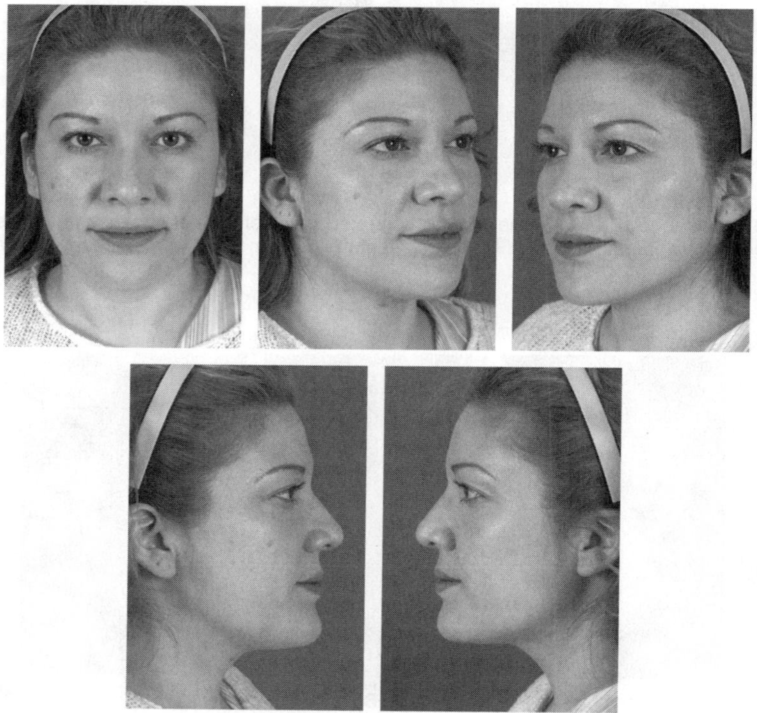

**Fig. 13-8** Overview of standardized face series and set distances. Some of the photographs can be eliminated, depending on the particular procedure performed.

## STANDARDIZED FACE/NECK LIFT SERIES (Box 13-1)

- The contour of the neck can vary greatly depending on head and shoulder positions.
- Make sure that the head is in the standard anatomic position and that the patient is sitting straight.

- Any degree of neck flexion or head retraction can greatly enhance submental fat at the jowl line. Conversely, neck extension can improve the jowl line.[13]
- A full-face series is photographed at 1 m with a 105 mm lens.

**Box 13-1** *KEY POINTS FOR PHOTOGRAPHING FACE AND NECK SERIES (see Fig. 13-8)*

- Photograph vertically.
- Photograph from top of hairline to sternal notch.
- Camera should be parallel with subject and positioned at midpoint of face (usually the nose).
- Ask patient to relax face and to not smile.
- Remove any distracting jewelry or heavily applied makeup.
- Fold down turtlenecks and turn collars away from neck.
- Pull hair back with neutral-colored headband.
- For oblique views, line the radix of the nose to touch the medial part of the opposite eye (see Fig. 13-5).

## SUPPLEMENTAL FACE/NECK VIEWS

- When photographing for a neck or face-lift series, views are typically added to show platysmal banding (teeth gritting), and a reading view accentuates submental fat, as shown in Fig. 13-9.[16]

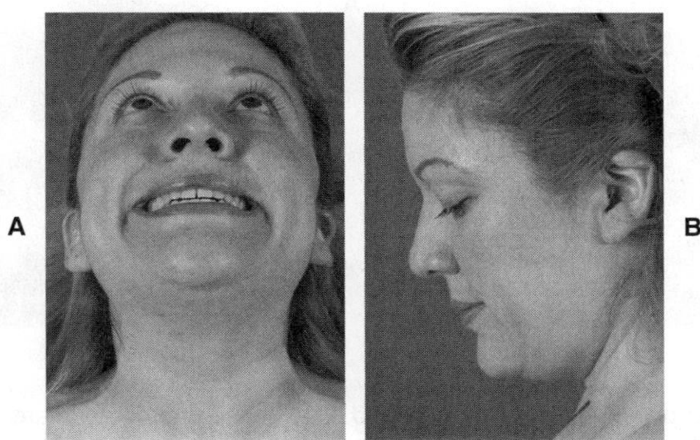


**Fig. 13-9** **A,** View to show platysmal banding (teeth gritting). **B,** A reading view accentuates submental fat.

## STANDARDIZED UPPER BROW/EYE SERIES (Box 13-2; Fig. 13-10)

- When photographing the eyes and brow, pay close attention to lower and upper lid excess, scleral show, ectropion, and upper lid hooding.

**Box 13-2** *KEY POINTS FOR PHOTOGRAPHING BROW AND EYE SERIES*

- Photograph horizontally.
- The close-up of the brow should extend below the lower crease of the lower eyelids to slightly above the hairline (see Fig. 13-10, *A*).
- Ask patient to relax the brow while gazing upward (see Fig. 13-10, *B*).
- Eyes should gaze downward to reveal any excess lower lid fat (see Fig. 13-10, *C*).
- Make sure interpupillary line is horizontal in all views.

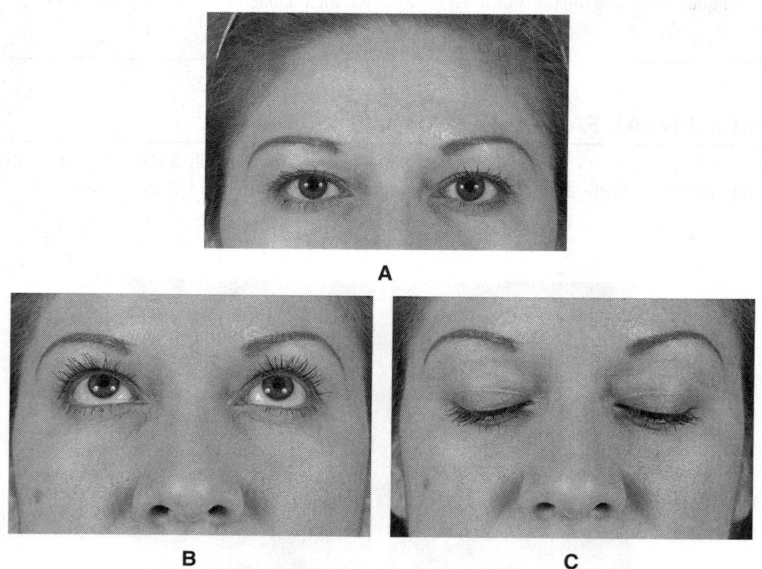

**Fig. 13-10** When photographing the eyes and brow, these photographs are taken in addition to the standard face/neck lift series. Image **A** was photographed at 0.8 m. Images **B** and **C** were photographed horizontally at 0.6 m with a 105 mm lens.

## STANDARDIZED LASER/CHEMICAL PEEL SERIES (Box 13-3; Fig. 13-11)

**Box 13-3** *KEY POINTS FOR PHOTOGRAPHING LASER/CHEMICAL PEEL SERIES*

- Remove heavy makeup.
- Close-up, oblique cheek views are photographed vertically at jaw line to slightly above eyebrow at 0.6 m.
- Lateral photographs taken further back (0.8 m) show tonal changes in the skin, if any, from cheek to jaw to neck.
- For a chemical peel of the chest area, an additional view is taken at 1 m as shown in the bottom of Fig. 13-11.

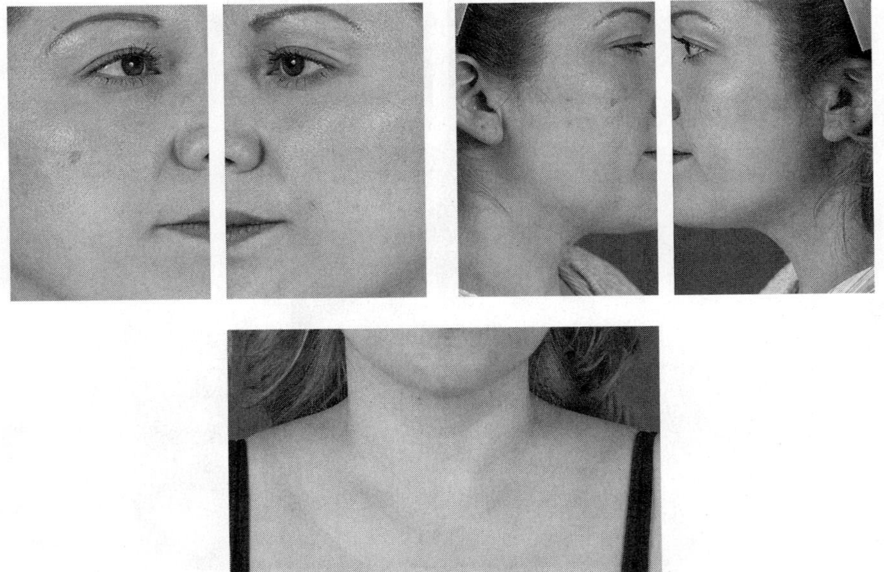

**Fig. 13-11** Laser/chemical peel series. These photographs are taken in addition to the standard face/neck lift series. Close-ups are photographed at 0.6 m and 0.8 m with a 105 mm lens.

## STANDARDIZED LIP SERIES (Box 13-4; Fig. 13-12)

**Box 13-4** *KEY POINTS FOR PHOTOGRAPHING THE STANDARDIZED LIP SERIES*

- Remove lipstick and liners.
- Inferior philtral column should intersect cheek on opposite side in oblique view.
- Lips should be slightly parted and relaxed.

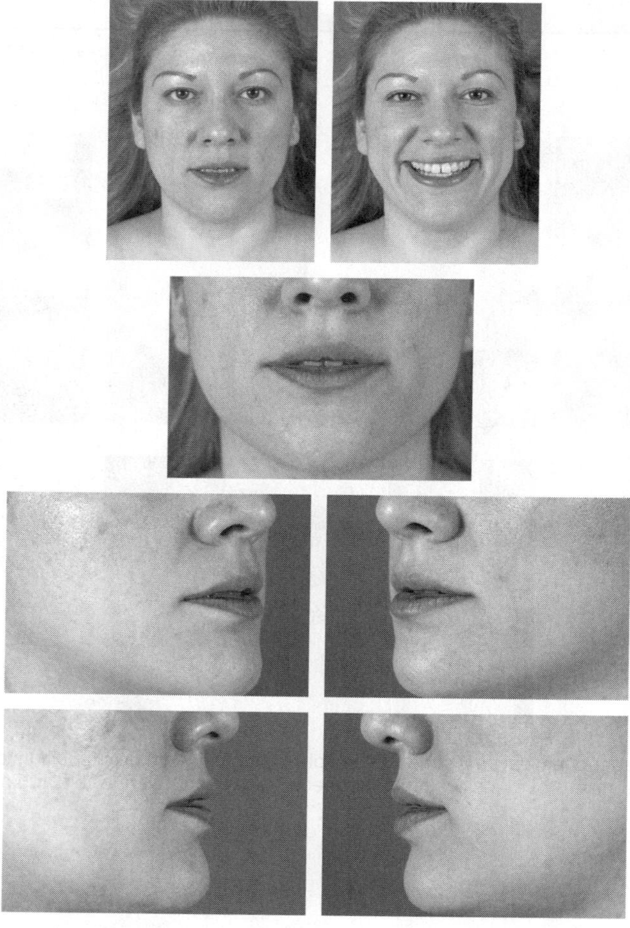

**Fig. 13-12** Complete standardized lip series. Close-ups of the lips are photographed at 0.6 m with a 105 mm lens, whereas the full face is photographed at 1 m.

## STANDARDIZED RHINOPLASTY/FACIAL FRACTURE SERIES (Box 13-5; Fig. 13-13)

- The nose is often one of the most difficult series to photograph.
- It is often necessary to make small adjustments to the series.
- The oblique preference must be decided on before photographing.
- The series can be used for facial fractures and for Mohs' reconstruction using forehead flaps or nasolabial flaps.

**Box 13-5** *Key Points for Photographing the Standardized Rhinoplasty Series*

- Photograph close-up views horizontally.
- Make sure camera is parallel to subject and focused on the midpoint (nose) and that a horizontal line can be drawn through the lower lateral eyes perpendicular to the dorsum.
- Line the tip of the nose between the eyebrows in the full basal view (see Fig. 13-13, *A*). You may need to make adjustments for this view if the patient has low tip projection or a large upper lip that blocks the alar area.
- In the half basal view, set the tip of the nose just below the eyes (see Fig. 13-13, *B*).
- Ask patient to relax face and to not smile.
- Have patient remove distracting jewelry.
- Pull hair back with neutral-colored headband.

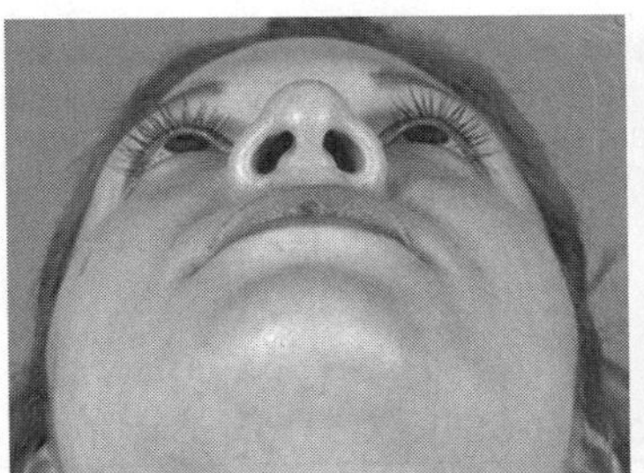

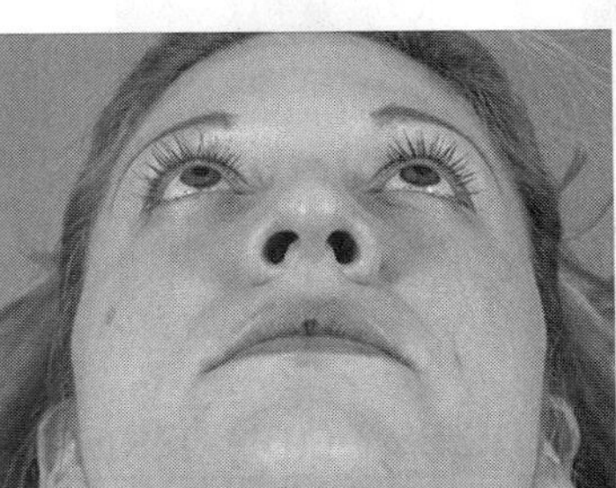

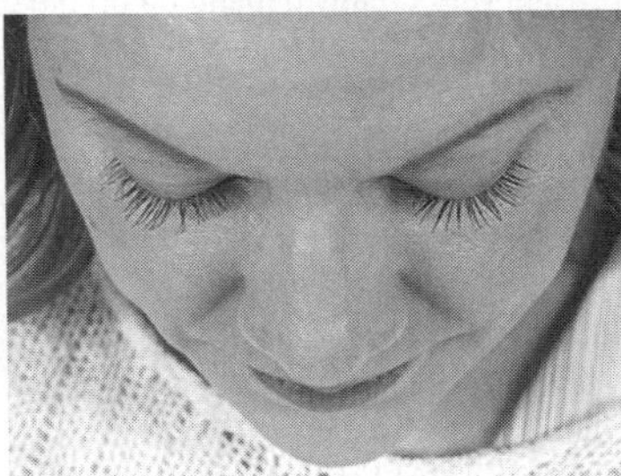

**Fig. 13-13** Standardized rhinoplasty series. These photographs are taken in addition to the standard face/neck lift series. Close-up views are photographed with a 105 mm lens at 0.8 and 0.6 m.

## SUPPLEMENTAL RHINOPLASTY VIEWS

- If a depressor septi release is to be performed, additional lateral and anterior views of the patient smiling are photographed (Fig. 13-14).
- A cephalic view is helpful to show nasal deviations[17] (Fig. 13-15).

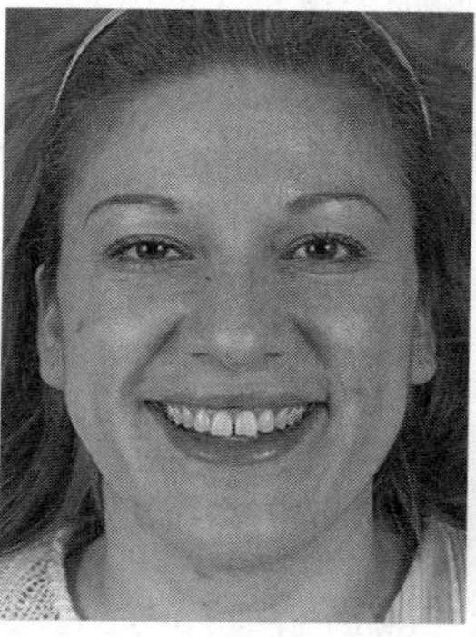
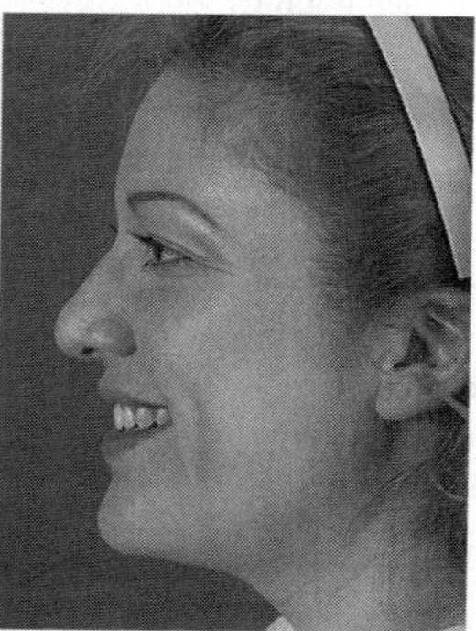

**Fig. 13-14** Additional anterior and lateral views are needed if the patient is having a depressor septi release.

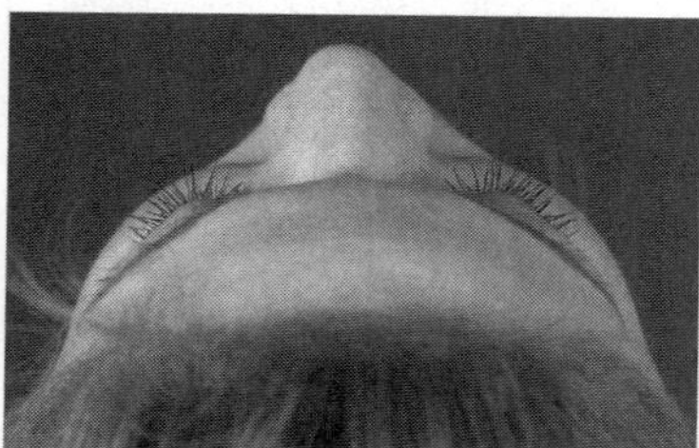

**Fig. 13-15** A cephalic view is helpful to show nasal deviations.

## STANDARDIZED BODY SERIES (Box 13-6; Fig. 13-16)

- Contour and muscle structure can vary greatly depending on the positioning of the feet. Feet should always be parallel, with weight distributed evenly[18] (Fig. 13-17).
- The body is photographed with a 50 mm lens at 1 m.

**Box 13-6** *KEY POINTS FOR PHOTOGRAPHING THE BODY SERIES (Fig. 13-17)*

- Photograph body vertically.
- Ask patient to distribute weight evenly between legs.
- Camera should be parallel with subject and positioned at midpoint of body (usually the abdomen).
- Legs should be set at hip width.
- Set knees straight, feet parallel with each other.
- Hands may be folded across breast area but no higher.
- Have patient relax abdomen.
- Use generic underwear.
- Photograph arms horizontally with elbows bent at 90 degrees and hands forward.
- Have patient remove watch and jewelry.

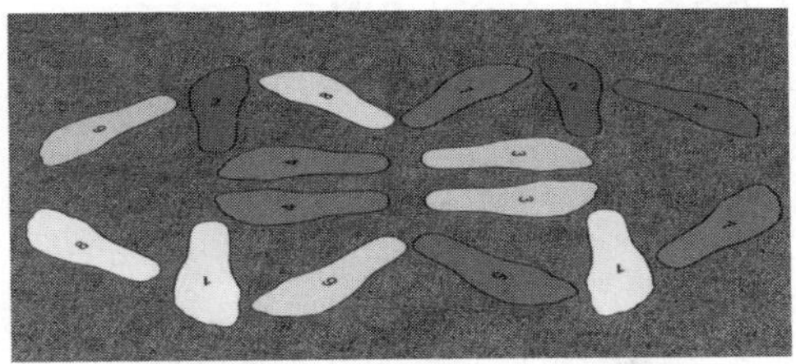

**Fig. 13-16** For ease of positioning, place cut-out feet on the floor for the patient as a standing reference.

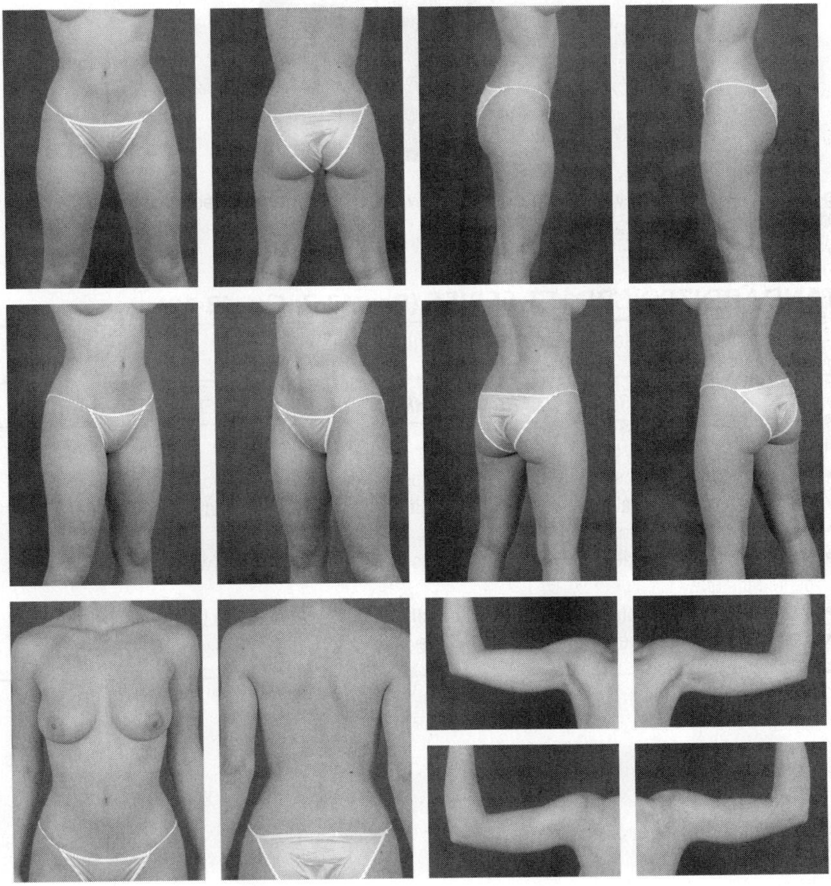

**Fig. 13-17** Standardized body series.

## SUPPLEMENTAL BODY CONTOURING SERIES

- The diver's view is sometimes photographed to evaluate skin laxity[16] (Fig. 13-18).

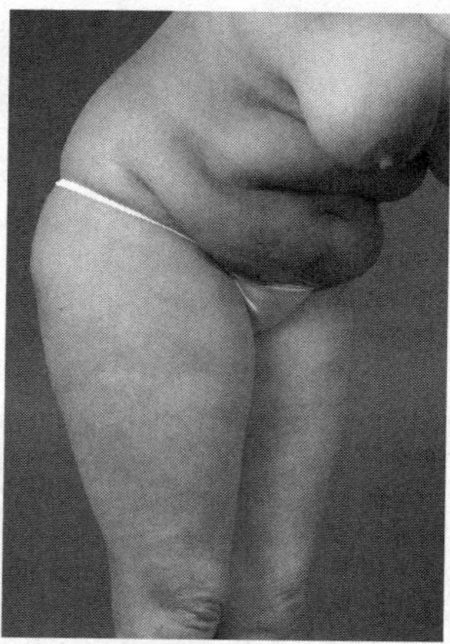

**Fig. 13-18** The diver's view is an oblique view with the patient folded over while relaxing the abdomen.

## STANDARDIZED BREAST SERIES (Box 13-7; Fig. 13-19)

- The breast series is photographed with a 50 mm lens at 1 m.

**Box 13-7** *KEY POINTS FOR PHOTOGRAPHING THE BREAST SERIES*

- Photograph body horizontally.
- Photograph above shoulders and below navel for reference and proportion.
- Camera should be parallel with subject and positioned at midpoint of body (usually the areolae).
- Ask patient to relax shoulders.
- Reductions, mastopexies, and reconstructions should be photographed with arms positioned behind the body.
- The bottom photographs in Fig. 13-19 are specifically for latissimus flap breast reconstruction.
- Have patient remove necklaces, watches, and jewelry.

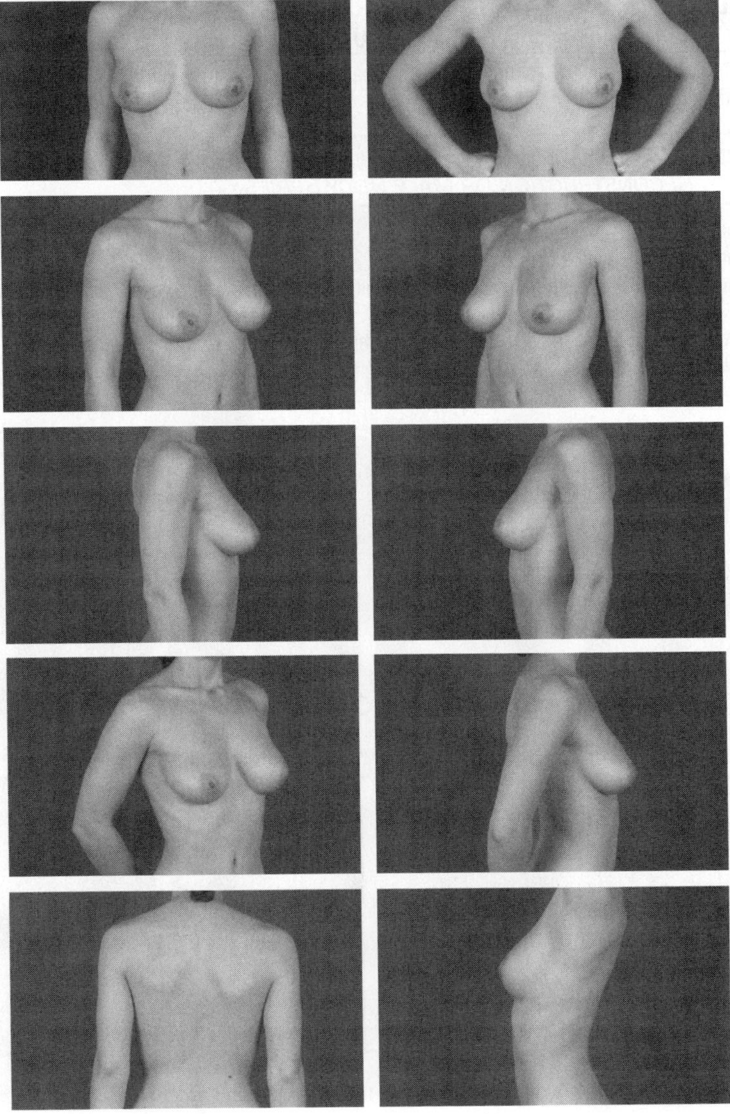

**Fig. 13-19** Standardized breast series.

## STANDARDIZED TRAM BREAST RECONSTRUCTION AND MALE BODY SERIES (Box 13-8; Fig. 13-20)

- The TRAM breast reconstruction series and male body series are photographed at 1 m with a 50 mm lens.

**Box 13-8** *KEY POINTS FOR PHOTOGRAPHING THE TRAM BREAST RECONSTRUCTION OR MALE BODY SERIES*

- Photograph the patient vertically.
- Photograph above shoulders and below navel.
- Camera should be parallel with subject and positioned at midpoint of body (usually the ribcage).
- Ask patient to relax shoulders.
- Position arms behind body in all views except the anterior and posterior.
- Have patient remove jewelry.
- Use generic undergarments.

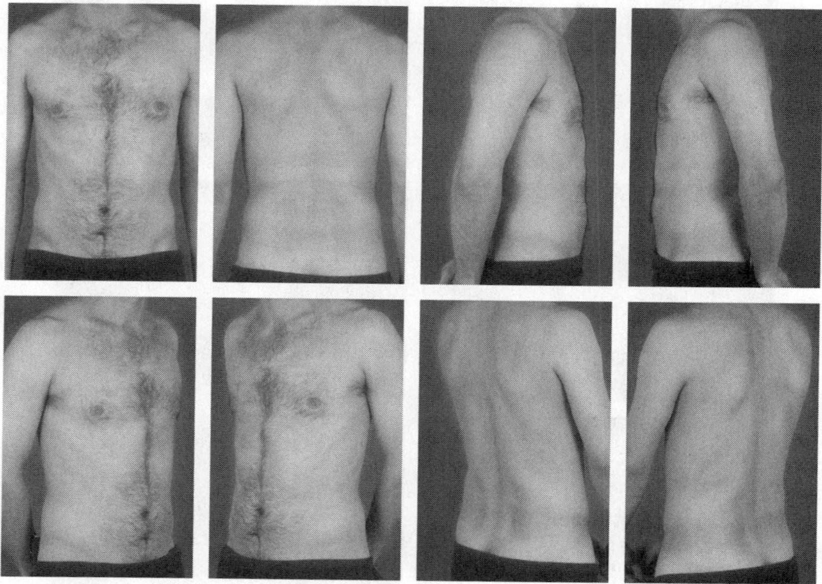

**Fig. 13-20** The male body series and the TRAM breast reconstruction series.

## PHOTOGRAPHING IN THE OPERATIVE SETTING (Boxes 13-9 and 13-10)

Lighting and background can be better controlled when photographing in a clinical setting versus an operative setting.

**Box 13-9** *KEY POINTS FOR KEEPING PHOTOGRAPHS CLEAN*

- Clear any unnecessary information and elements from photographs that may distract or misrepresent what the photograph intends to show.
- Cover unwanted areas with surgical towels.
- Clean blood off patient and clear surgical tools from frame before photographing.
- Have patient remove makeup if photographing the face.

**Box 13-10** *KEY POINTS FOR KEEPING PHOTOGRAPHS GENERIC*

- Use generic undergarments when photographing the body.
- Cover areas of clothing with towels or remove clothing.
- Have patient remove large or distracting jewelry, hats, and sunglasses.
- Cover tattoos if possible.
- Keep a backdrop with you at all times to block out unnecessary people or furniture.
- If it is necessary to have a hand in the photograph, make sure examination gloves are used.
- Remove brand names from rules and equipment if possible.

## THREE-DIMENSIONAL IMAGING

Three-dimensional (3D) scanning allows users to capture a 3D digital model of an object or person by translating physical form into a 3D digital representation called a *point cloud.* Scanners can capture color data as well as 3D form. Some scanning systems can capture 3D form on a timeline to record 3D movement.

- 3D scanners allow the capture of 3D volume models of patients.
- Clinical practice 3D scanning and simulation systems allow clinicians to:
  - Capture 3D data in color.
  - Simulate surgical outcomes.
  - Capture and store preoperative and postoperative 3D images.
  - Compare volumetric data.[19]

## PHOTOGRAPHIC CONSENT/HIPAA COMPLIANCE[17,20]

### PATIENT PHOTOGRAPHY CONSENT AND LEGALITY

- HIPAA, Health Insurance Portability and Accountability Act of 1996
- Patient photographs, videotape, or digital images cannot be released for publication, medical teaching or publicity without a signed consent by the patient or legal representative.
- Patient privacy must be preserved.

### STANDARDS FOR HIPAA COMPLIANCE

Along with keeping your patients generic (see Box 13-10), it is important to maintain anonymity. The following are the standards used for the Health Insurance Portability and Accountability Act (HIPAA). Private or smaller entities may have different requirements.

- **Photographing for treatment**
  - Health care providers may photograph or create audio or video recordings of patients for treatment purposes without obtaining written authorization.

- **Photographing for nontreatment purposes**
  - If a patient agrees to be photographed or recorded for nontreatment purposes, the patient's written authorization must be obtained.
  - Nontreatment purposes that require patient authorization are:
    - Educational lectures and presentations for health care professionals (e.g., CME)
    - Scientific publications for which another authorization is not already on file
    - Patient education materials
    - Use in broadcast, print, or Internet media for educational or public interest purposes
- According to HIPAA, authorizations are not required if all identifiable patient information is removed from the photograph or recording.

**NOTE: Although HIPAA does not require authorization for the use of photographs that have had all identifiable patient information removed, the health care provider may be liable for invasion of privacy. Courts have imposed liability primarily when the provider has exploited the patient for commercial benefit.**[21]

- Identifiable patient information cannot be removed from any full-face or comparable images, which always require authorization.
- A photograph or electronic reproduction is considered to identify a patient if it shows the full face of the patient, or if any of the 19 elements of protected health information are present. These elements are:
  - Name
  - Date of birth
  - Address
  - Telephone number
  - Fax number
  - E-mail address
  - Social Security number
  - Medical record number
  - Account number
  - Driver's license number
  - Credit card number
  - Names of relatives
  - Name of employer
  - Health plan beneficiary number
  - Vehicle or other device serial number
  - Internet universal resource locator (URL)
  - Internet protocol (IP) address
  - Fingerprints or voiceprints
  - Date and time of treatment
- **It is *not* satisfactory to block the eyes.** Recognition of a patient applies to all distinguishing features of the face.[1] HIPAA does not specifically address masking the eyes, but it is strongly recommended to obtain a consent form when using any part of the face for purposes other than treatment.
- As standard practice, even if a patient has a photographic consent for nontreatment purpose on file, always contact the patient before potential nontreatment use.
- Remove or cover any other identifying elements such as jewelry and tattoos.

## Patient Photographic Data Protection

- Use encryption and password protection on any storage device containing patient photographs to prevent unauthorized access in the event of theft or loss. This includes desktop and laptop computers, external storage drives, and mobile devices.
- Do not access patient photographs in public settings. Use a screen guard to prevent unintended viewing of computer screens.

## Patient Photography, Video, and Digital Files for Commercial Use[22]

- Metadata dangers
  - Scrub all commercial photographs for metadata
  - Obtain written assurances from publishers, websites, advertising and marketing entities, and social media outlets stating that metadata will be removed before photos can be shared.

**TIP:** Sometimes metadata can be seen by simply "mousing over" web images—watch out![22]

## Key Points

- ✓ Uniformity and standardization are essential for the production of accurate photographic documentation.
- ✓ Lack of quality can distort clinical findings and lead to misrepresentation of images.
- ✓ Successful patient photography begins with a basic familiarity of both digital and conventional 35 mm photography.
- ✓ Advances in digital photography and 3D surface imaging have led to a variety of options for recording clinical results. Refer to the final output and treatment goals as a guide for choosing the right camera or device.
- ✓ Special attention should be given to legal and ethical issues before undertaking any clinical photography.

## References

1. Grom RM. Clinical and operating room photography. Biomed Photogr 20:251-301, 1992.
2. Roos O, Cederblom S. A standardized system for patient documentation. J Audiov Media Med 14:135-138, 1991.
3. DiBernardo BE, Adams RL, Krause J, et al. Photographic standards in plastic surgery. Plast Reconstr Surg 102:559-568, 1998.
4. Young S. Maintaining standard scales of reproduction in patient photography using digital cameras. J Audiov Media Med 24:162-165, 2001.
5. Long B, ed. Complete Digital Photography, 7th ed. Boston: Course Technology, 2013.
6. Bockaert V. Viewfinder, 2005. Available at *http://www.dpreview.com/glossary/camera-system/viewfinder.*
7. Long B. Choosing a digital camera. In Long B, ed. Complete Digital Photography, 7th ed, 2013. Available at *www.completedigitalphotography.com/CDP7/CDP7-Chapter23-ChoosingADigitalCamera.pdf.*
8. Sheridan P. Practical aspects of clinical photography. I. Principles, equipment and technique. ANZ J Surg 83:188-191, 2013.

9. Williams AR. Clinical and operating room photography. In Vetter JP, ed. Biomedical Photography. Boston: Focal Press, 1992.
10. Sheridan P. Practical aspects of clinical photography. II. Data management, ethics and quality control. ANZ J Surg 83:293-295, 2013.
11. Kao CL, Cheng BC, Lu MS, et al. A simple method for making photographic records under sterile conditions. Ann Thorac Surg 84:2125-2126, 2007.
12. Thomas JR, Tardy ME Jr, Przakop H. Uniform photographic documentation in facial plastic surgery. Otolaryngol Clin North Am 13:367-381, 1980.
13. Sommer DD, Mendelsohn M. Pitfalls of nonstandardized photography in facial plastic surgery patients. Plast Reconstr Surg 114:10-14, 2004.
14. Galdino GM, DaSilva D, Gunter JP. Digital photography for rhinoplasty. Plast Reconstr Surg 109:1421-1434, 2002.
15. Davidson TM. Photography in facial plastic and reconstructive surgery. J Biol Photogr Assoc 47:59-67, 1979.
16. Gherardini G. Standardization in photography for body contour surgery and suction-assisted lipectomy. Plast Reconstr Surg 100:227-237, 1997.
17. LaNasa JJ Jr, Smith O, Johnson CM Jr. The cephalic view in nasal photography. J Otolaryngol 20:443-544, 1991.
18. Williams AR. Positioning and lighting for patient photography. J Biol Photogr Assoc 53:131-143, 1985.
19. Mailey B, Freel A, Wong R, et al. Clinical accuracy and reproducibility of Portrait 3D Surgical Simulation Platform in breast augmentation. Aesthet Surg J 33:84-92, 2013.
20. US Department of Health and Human Services. Standards for privacy of individually identifiable health information (45 CFR parts 160 and 164). Federal Register 65; Dec 28, 2000.
21. Roach WH Jr, ed. Medical Records and the Law. Gaithersburg, MD: Aspen Publishers, 1994.
22. Reisman N. Scrub your commercial photographs for metadata. Plastic Surgery News, American Society of Plastic Surgeons, 2012. Available at *http://psnextra.org/Columns/OLG-June-12.html.*

# Part II

## Skin and Soft Tissue

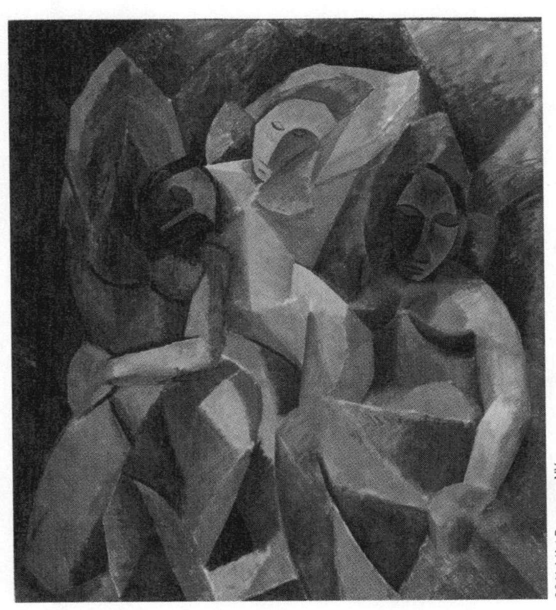

# 14. Structure and Function of Skin

Brian P. Bradow, John L. Burns, Jr.

## GENERAL FUNCTIONS

- **Largest body organ:** 16% total body weight
- **Protection:** UV, mechanical, chemical, thermal, barrier to microorganisms
- **Metabolic:** Vitamin D synthesis
- **Thermoregulation**

## ANATOMY OF SKIN (Fig. 14-1 and Table 14-1)

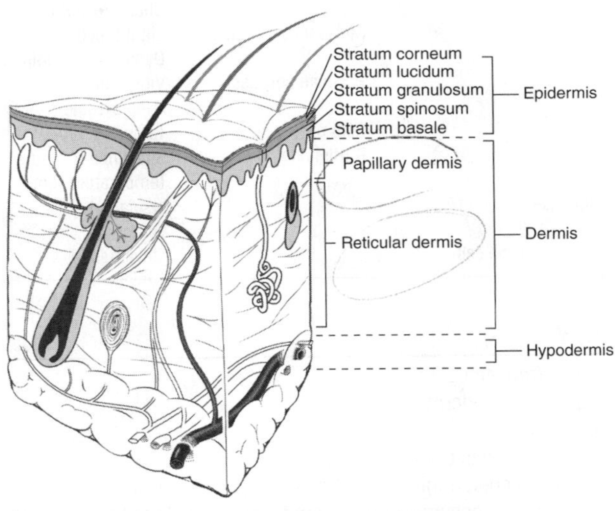


**Fig. 14-1** Layers of the skin with adnexal structures.

**Table 14-1** *Contents of Skin Layers*

| | Cells | Appendages | Function/Responses |
|---|---|---|---|
| Epidermis | Keratinocyte (predominant) | | Protective barrier |
| | Melanocyte | | Pigmentation |
| | | | UV protection |
| | Langerhans cell | | Immunity (antigen presentation) |
| | Merkel cell | | Constant touch and pressure |
| | | | Static two-point discrimination |
| Dermis | Fibroblast | | Collagen/elastic fiber |
| | | | Ground substance |
| | Macrophange | | Scavenger |
| | Mast cell | | Allergic response |
| | | Hair follicle | |
| | | Sebaceous gland | Sebum |
| | | Eccrine sweat gland | Thermoregulation |
| | | Apocrine sweat gland | Sweat |
| | | Naked nerve fiber | Pain |
| | | | Temperature |
| | | | Chemoreceptor |
| | | Meissner's corpuscle | Light touch |
| | | | Dynamic two-point discrimination |
| | | Pacinian corpuscle | Vibration |
| | | | Deep pressure |
| | | Bulb of Krause | Temperature (cold) |
| | | Ruffini ending | Sustained pressure |
| | | | Temperature (hot) |
| Hypodermis | Adipocyte | | Insulation |
| | | | Energy |
| Muscle | Striated muscle cell | | Movement |

## EMBRYOLOGY

- **Epidermis:** Derived from ectoderm
- **Dermis:** Derived from mesoderm
- **Immigrant cells:**
  - Melanocytes: Neural crest origin
  - Merkel cells: Neural crest origin
  - Langerhans cells: Mesenchymal origin (from precursor cells of bone marrow)

## HISTOLOGY[1,2]

### EPIDERMIS (Table 14-2)

- **Thickness**
  - Varies by location, but average approximately 100 μm
  - Compare to 1500-4000 μm for full-thickness skin
  - Palmar skin thickest because of stratum corneum
- **Keratinocyte is the major cell.** Keratinocyte differentiation occurs in 28-45 days, progressing from basal proliferative germinal layer to dead cornified layer.
- **Immigrant cells** (see Embryology above)

**Table 14-2** *Five Layers of Epidermis*

| Layer | Cell Types | Clinical Significance |
|---|---|---|
| Stratum corneum | Nonviable keratinocytes | Responsible for thickness of glabrous skin<br>Exfoliates with use of topical tretinoin |
| Stratum lucidum | Nonviable keratinocytes | |
| Stratum granulosum | Marginally viable keratinocytes | Thickens the most with tissue expansion |
| Stratum spinosum | Viable keratinocytes | |
| Stratum basale | Mitotically active keratinocytes, melanocytes, tactile cells, nonpigmented granular dendrocytes | Origin of various skin cancers |

## DERMIS

- The two layers, **papillary and reticular,** make up an integrated system of cells, fibrous amorphous connective tissue, neurovascular networks, and dermal appendages.
- **Overall thickness**
  - Highly variable
  - Thicker on scalp, back, and feet
  - Thinnest on eyelids
- **Papillary dermis**
  - Begins at basement membrane, which is located at base of epidermis
  - Thickness similar to epidermis (100 μm)
  - High content of type III collagen, less type I
  - Collagenase activity
  - Mature elastic fibers absent
- **Reticular dermis**
  - Papillary dermis to hypodermis
  - Bulk of dermis (2000-2500 μm)
  - Primarily type I collagen organized into large fibers and bundles
  - Contains large, mature, bandlike, elastic fibers that extend between collagen bundles
  - Elastic and collagen bundles progressively larger toward hypodermis
- **Structural components**[3]
  - **Collagen** (Table 14-3)
    - Principle building block of connective tissue
    - A third of total body protein content
    - Provides tensile strength
    - **Ratio (type I:III)**
      - Adult skin: 4:1
      - Immature and hypertrophic scars: 2:1
      - Keloid: 3:1
      - Fetal wound: 1:3
    - Collagen synthesis (Fig. 14-2)
      - Amino acid (AA) chains produced in fibroblast cytoplasm
      - Secreted into extracellular matrix in form of tropocollagen
      - Triple helix configuration formed by binding of three polypeptide alpha chains
      - Disarrayed during relaxation and straight with parallel alignment during stretch

**Table 14-3** *Five Types of Collagen*

| Type | Structure | Distribution |
|---|---|---|
| Type I | Hybrid of two chains<br>Low in hydroxylysine and glycosylated hydroxylysine | Bone<br>Tendon<br>Skin<br>Dentin<br>Ligament<br>Fascia<br>Arteries<br>Uterus |
| Type II | Relatively high in hydroxylysine and glycosylated hydroxylysine | Hyaline cartilage<br>Eye tissues |
| Type III | High in hydroxylysine<br>Contains interchain disulfide bonds | Skin<br>Arteries<br>Uterus<br>Bowel wall |
| Type IV | High in hydroxylysine and glycosylated hydroxylysine<br>May contain large globular regions | Basement membrane |
| Type V | Similar to type IV | Basement membrane |

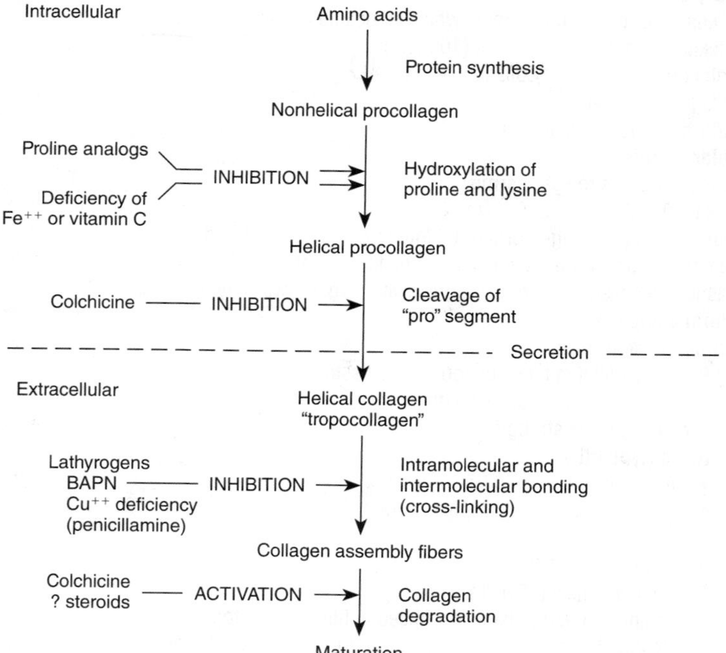


**Fig. 14-2** Collagen synthesis. (*BAPN,* Beta-aminopropionitrile.)

- **Elastin**
  - Sheets of rubberlike material synthesized from fibroblasts
  - Precursor from tropoelastin
  - Polymerizes and interweaves with collagen
  - Fibrillin needed for elastin deposition and fiber formation
  - Confers stretch and elastic recoil
  - Disruption leads to loss of recoil
  - Fibers decrease with aging
- **Ground substance**
  - Amorphous transparent material like semifluid gel
  - Permits metabolite diffusion
  - Composed of glycosaminoglycans in the form of hyaluronic acid and proteoglycans

## VASCULARITY AND CUTANEOUS NERVES (Fig. 14-3)

- Receptor types
  - Mechanoreceptors
    - Touch
    - Pressure
    - Vibration
    - Stretch
  - Thermoreceptors
  - Chemoreceptors
  - Nociceptors (mostly raw/free nerve endings)

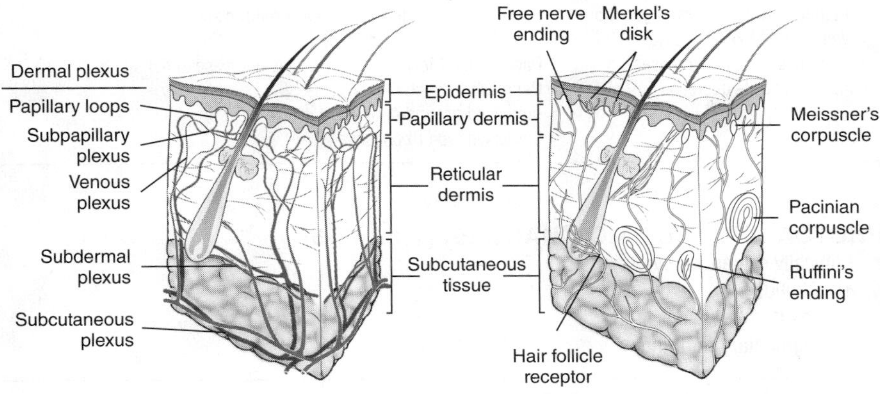


**Fig. 14-3** The vascular plexuses of the integument and cutaneous nerves.

## AGING SKIN[4-6]

### HISTOLOGIC EFFECTS OF AGING (Fig. 14-4 and Table 14-4)

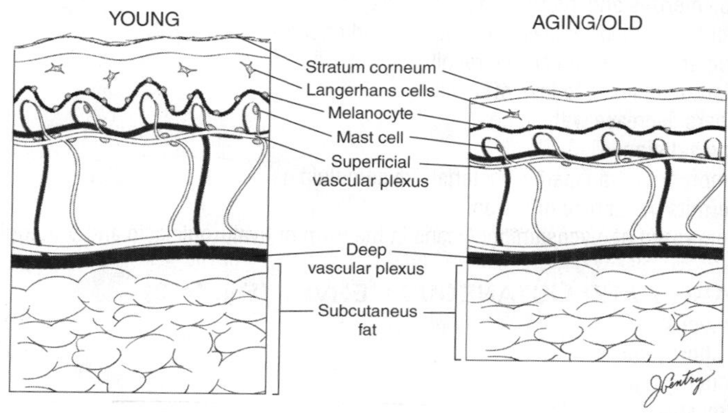


**Fig. 14-4** Histology of aging skin.

**Table 14-4** *Histologic Findings in Aging Skin*

| Epidermis | Dermis |
|---|---|
| Compact laminated stratum corneum | Dermal atrophy |
| Flattened dermal-epidermal junction | Fibroblasts enlarge and decrease mitotic activity |
| Fewer layers of keratinocytes | |
| Melanocyte density decreases | Pacini's and Meissner's corpuscles decrease in density by a third |
| Langerhans cells decrease | Decreased elastic fibers |
| | Increased ground substance |
| | Increased type III collagen |

### PHOTOAGING (ACTINIC CHANGES) (Table 14-5)

- Clinically evidenced by:
  - Rhytids
  - Laxity
  - Pigmentary mottling

**Table 14-5** *Histologic Findings in Photoaging*

| Epidermis | Dermis |
|---|---|
| Atrophic and flat | Dermoelastosis |
| Loss of vertical polarity | *Grenz zone* is characteristic |
| Thick, ragged basement membrane | Increased ground substance |
| Pigmentary mottling | Increased elastic fibers |

## PHYSIOLOGIC EFFECTS OF AGING (Box 14-1)

**Box 14-1** *PHYSIOLOGIC EFFECTS OF AGING*

Cell replacement decreases
Injury response decreases
Barrier function lessens
Chemical clearance worsens
Sensory perception decreases
Immune responsiveness decreases
Thermoregulation worsens
Vascular responsiveness decreases
Sweat production decreases
Vitamin D production decreases

## GENETIC DISORDERS OF THE SKIN[7-15]

### EHLERS-DANLOS SYNDROME (CUTIS HYPERELASTICA)

- Incidence: 1:400,000
- Variable inheritance patterns
- Connective tissue disorder, collagen cross-linking problem
- Hypermobile joints
- Thin, friable, hyperextensive skin predisposing patients to:
  - Poor wound healing, hypertrophic scarring
  - Redundant periocular skin (e.g., epicanthal folds, wide nasal bridge)
  - Ventral hernia

### CUTIS LAXA (ELASTOLYSIS)

- Incidence: Only several hundred cases known worldwide
- Variable inheritance patterns, can also be acquired
- Hypoelastic (degeneration of elastic fibers in the dermis), does not spring back immediately when stretched (hyperextensible)
- Appearance of premature aging
- **Wound healing normal**
- Other associated problems
  - Increased risk of ventral hernia
  - Cardiopulmonary and gastrointestinal issues

### PSEUDOXANTHOMA ELASTICUM

- Incidence: 1:25,000-100,000
- Skin laxity from calcification and degeneration/fragmentation of elastic fibers
  - Variable inheritance patterns
- Cobblestone yellowish plaques characteristic
- **Wound healing normal**
- Ocular and cardiac manifestations

## Progeria (Hutchinson-Gilford Syndrome)

- Incidence: 1:1,000,000
- Autosomal recessive
- Skin laxity, loss of subcutaneous fat
- Poor wound healing
- Growth retardation, premature death
- Craniosynostosis, micrognathia
- Baldness, prominent ears
- Findings similar to premature aging

## Werner's Syndrome (Adult Progeria)

- Rare, autosomal recessive disorder
- Features of premature aging
- Scleroderma-like skin
- Hyperpigmentation and hypopigmentation of skin
- Microangiopathy (contraindication to plastic surgery)
- Diabetes, cataracts
- High-pitched voice, baldness

**TIP:** Avoid rejuvenation surgery for patients with Ehlers-Danlos syndrome and progeria because of wound healing issues.

Rejuvenating surgery is possible for patients with cutis laxa and pseudoxanthoma elasticum.

## Key Points

- ✓ The epidermis is composed of five layers. The two most superficial layers (stratum corneum and stratum lucidum) are made up of nonviable keratinocytes.
- ✓ Collagen provides the tensile strength of the skin.
- ✓ Adult skin contains a 4:1 ratio of type I/type III collagen.
- ✓ Predictable physiologic and histologic skin changes occur with age.
- ✓ Cutis laxa and pseudoxanthoma elasticum are the only congenital skin disorders that are responsive to surgical rejuvenation.

## References

1. Young B, Woodford P, O'Dowd G, eds. Wheater's Functional Histology: A Text and Color Atlas, 6th ed. New York: Churchill Livingstone, 2013.
2. Fawcett DW, Jensh RP. Bloom & Fawcett: Concise Histology, 2nd ed. London: Hodder Arnold, 2002.
3. Gibson T. Physical properties of the skin. In McCarthy JG, ed. Plastic Surgery, vol 1. General Principles. Philadelphia: WB Saunders, 1990.
4. Gilchrest BA. Age-associated changes in the skin. J Am Geriatr Soc 30:139-143, 1982.
5. Gilchrest BA. Aging of the skin. In Soter NA, Baden HP, eds. Pathophysiology of Dermatologic Diseases, 2nd ed. New York: McGraw-Hill, 1991.
6. Savin JA. Old skin. Br Med J 283:1422-1423, 1981.
7. Thorne CH, ed. Grabb and Smith's Plastic Surgery, 6th ed. Philadelphia: Lippincott Williams & Wilkins, 2007.

8. Kumar P, Sethi N, Friji MT, et al. Wound healing and skin grafting in Ehlers-Danlos syndrome. Plast Reconstr Surg 126:214e-215e, 2010.
9. Breighton P, Bull JC. Plastic surgery in the Ehlers-Danlos syndrome. Case Report. Plast Reconstr Surg 45:606-609, 1970.
10. Girotto JA, Malaisrie SC, Bulkely G, et al. Recurrent ventral herniation in Ehlers-Danlos syndrome. Plast Reconstr Surg 106:1520-1526, 2000.
11. Banks ND, Redett RJ, Mofid MZ, et al. Cutis laxa: clinical experience and outcomes. Plast Reconstr Surg 111:2434-2442, 2003.
12. Laube S, Moss C. Pseudoxanthoma elasticum. Arch Dis Child 90:754-756, 2005.
13. Bercovitch L, Patrick T. Pseudoxanthoma elasticum. J Am Acad Dermatol 51:s13-s14, 2004.
14. Thomas WO, Moses MH, Craver RD, et al. Congenital cutis laxa: a case report and review of loose skin syndromes. Ann Plast Surg 30:252-256, 1993.
15. Weinzweig J, ed. Plastic Surgery Secrets Plus. Philadelphia: Elsevier, 2010.

# 15. Basal Cell Carcinoma, Squamous Cell Carcinoma, and Melanoma

Danielle M. LeBlanc, Smita R. Ramanadham, Dawn D. Wells

## BASAL CELL CARCINOMA (BCC)

### DEMOGRAPHICS[1-3]

- **BCC is the most common form of skin cancer.**
  - It is 4-5 times more common than squamous cell carcinoma (SCC).
- More than 2 million cases were diagnosed in 2010, and incidence is rising rapidly.
- 95% of cases occur between 40 and 79 years of age.
- Estimated annual cost in Medicare population is >$400 million.
- Greater than 80% occur in the head and neck.
- *It is the most common malignancy of the eyelid.*[4]

### RISK FACTORS

- Fitzpatrick skin type[5] (Table 15-1)
- Sun exposure
- Advancing age
- Immunosuppression: AIDS, organ transplant medications
  - 13-fold increase in 10-year incidence of nonmetastatic skin cancer in transplant population vs. general population[6]
- Carcinogen exposure: UV and ionizing radiation, arsenic, hydrocarbons[7-9]
- Genetic mutations[3]
  - Mutations in *PTCH* (patched) gene coding for the sonic hedgehog signaling pathway
  - UV-induced mutations in tumor suppressive gene *p53*
  - Mutations in oncogenes *ras* and *fos;* however, role of oncogenesis is unclear
  - **Albinism**[10]
    - Defective production of melanin from tyrosine
      - Type 1: Tyrosinase-related oculocutaneous albinism with affected activity of tyrosinase
      - Type 2: Tyrosinase-positive oculocutaneous albinism with normal tyrosinase activity

**Table 15-1** *Fitzpatrick's Classification of Sun-Reactive Skin Types*

| Skin Type | Color | Reaction to First Summer Exposure |
|---|---|---|
| I | White | Always burn; never tan |
| II | White | Usually burn; tan with difficulty |
| III | White | Sometimes mild burn; tan average |
| IV | Moderate brown | Rarely burn; tan with ease |
| V | Dark brown* | Very rarely burn; tan very easily |
| VI | Black | Do not burn; tan very easily |

*Asian Indian, Asian, Hispanic, or light African descent.

- **Nevoid basal cell syndrome (Gorlin's syndrome)**[1,11]
  - Autosomal dominant inheritance pattern on chromosome 9q22.3-q31
    - Multiple basal cells, odontogenic keratocysts, palmar and plantar pits, calcification of falx cerebri, bifid ribs, hypertelorism, broad nasal root
- **Xeroderma pigmentosum (XP)**
  - Autosomal recessive inheritance pattern
  - Impaired DNA repair mechanism
  - Intolerance to UV radiation
  - Multiple epithelial malignancies

- Premalignant lesions
  - **Nevus sebaceus of Jadassohn**
    - Present at birth on scalp or face
    - Well-circumscribed, hairless, yellowish plaque that becomes verrucous and nodular at puberty
    - **10%-15% malignant degeneration to BCC**

## Recurrence and Metastasis

- Risk factors for recurrence[1,3] (Table 15-2)
  - Depends on size, location (head and neck >trunk and extremity), borders, rate of growth, pathology, neural involvement, history of radiation or immunosuppression
- 30%-50% will recur within 5 years.
- New lesions tend to be same histopathologic type as previous lesion.
- Risk of cutaneous melanoma is increased.
- Metastasis is rare, with less than 0.1% incidence overall to lymph nodes, lungs, and bones.

**Table 15-2** *Risk Factors for Recurrence of BCC and SCC*

| | Low Risk | High Risk |
|---|---|---|
| **Location/size** | <20 mm trunk/ext<br><10 mm cheek, forehead, scalp, neck<br><6 mm central face, genitalia, hands, feet | >20 mm trunk/ext<br>>10 mm cheek, forehead, scalp, neck<br>>6 mm central face, genitalia, hands, feet |
| **Defined borders** | Well-defined | Poorly defined |
| **Primary vs. recurrent** | Primary | Recurrent |
| **Immunosuppression** | – | + |
| **Prior radiotherapy** | – | + |
| **Pathology** | Nodular, superficial, keratotic, infundibulocystic | Morpheaform, sclerosing, micronodular, mixed infiltrative, adenoid,* desmoplastic* |
| **Perineural involvement** | – | + |
| **Rapidly growing*** | – | + |
| **Depth*** | <2 mm, Clark I-III | >2 mm, Clark IV and V |
| **Lymphovascular invasion*** | – | + |
| **Degree of differentiation*** | Well-differentiated | Poorly differentiated |

*SCC only.

## Biology

- Tumors originate from the pluripotential epithelial cells of epidermis and hair follicles (basal keratinocytes) at the dermoepidermal junction.

## Types of BCC[1,4,12-15]

*There are **26** identified subtypes that follow particular histologic patterns*[12] (Fig. 15-1). *Mixed patterns are found in 38.5% of cases.*

- **Nodular**
  - Most common histologic type: 50%-60%
  - Well-defined borders, flesh-colored, pearly nodule with overlying telangiectasias
  - May be ulcerated: Central ulcer surrounded by rolled border; historically called *rodent ulcer*
- **Superficial spreading**
  - 9%-15% of BCCs, second most common type
  - Located in epidermis, no dermal invasion
  - Flat, pink, scaly patches with ulcerations and crusting, usually multiple, on trunk
  - Often mistaken for fungal infection, actinic keratosis, psoriasis, or eczema
- **Micronodular**
  - 15% of BCCs
  - Small rounded nodules of tumor the size of hair bulbs
- **Infiltrative**
  - 7% of BCCs
  - Opaque yellow-white color, blends with surrounding skin
  - Tumor islands of variable size with jagged configuration
- **Pigmented**
  - 6% of BCCs
  - Pigmentation from melanin
  - Often confused with melanoma
- **Morpheaform (sclerosing or fibrosing)**
  - 2%-3% of BCCs, **most aggressive**
  - Typically described by patients as an "enlarging scar" without history of trauma
  - Usually an indurated, flat, or slightly elevated papule or plaque with white to yellow scarlike appearance
  - Rarely ulcerates
  - **High incidence of positive margins after excision**

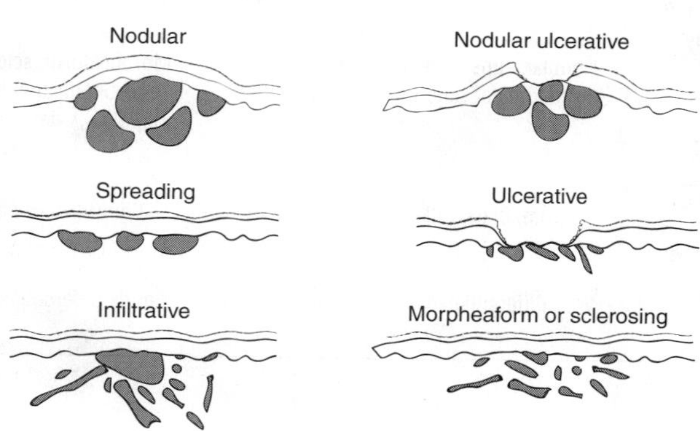


**Fig. 15-1** Histologic types of basal cell carcinoma.

## TREATMENT[3]

*Goal of treatment is cure of tumor with preservation of function and cosmesis.*

- Each case should be treated differently according to size, anatomic location, histologic type, and whether it is primary or recurrent, with low or high risk.
- Treatment modalities include medical, destructive, and surgical excision.
- **Medical**
  - Superficial therapies: Reserved for patients in whom surgery or radiation is contraindicated or impractical.
  - **Imiquimod 5% (Aldara) or 5-fluorouracil**
    - Topical cream
    - Effective for multiple, low-risk superficial BCC and SCC in situ
  - **Radiotherapy (RT):** Option for nonsurgical candidates, reserved for ages >60 years
    - Delivered in fractionated doses involving orthovoltage x-rays or electron beam
    - Criteria expanded to include tumors up to 15 mm in high-risk locations and up to 20 mm in intermediate-risk locations
    - Overall cure rate of primary lesions 92%[16]
    - Avoid in verrucous cancer and genetic conditions predisposing to skin cancer
    - Associated risks of osteitis and skin necrosis
- **Destructive**
  - **Curettage and electrodesiccation (C&E)**[3]
    - Curettage removes visible tumor; electrodesiccation removes residual tumor cells.
    - Use for low-risk tumors.
    - If it is performed based only on appearance of tumor; send tissue for pathology.
    - Avoid use in hair-bearing areas and in tumors that extend into subcutaneous layer.
    - Techniques allow healing by secondary intention.
    - Cure rates are 96%-100% for tumors <2 mm.[17]
    - Overall cure rate is 74%.[16]
  - **Cryosurgery**[18]
    - Cooling tumor cells to −40° C during repetitive freeze-thaw cycles destroys malignant tissue.
    - Techniques are appropriate for small to large nodular and superficial BCC with clearly definable margins (laterally and in depth).
    - They are not indicated for tumors deeper than 3 mm unless thermocouples are used to measure depth of freeze.
    - Contraindications include cold intolerance, morpheaform, recurrent BCC, and cosmetically sensitive areas.
    - Treatment causes prolonged edema (4-6 weeks) and permanent pigment loss.
  - **Laser phototherapy ($CO_2$ laser)**
    - Ablation of BCC is confined to epidermis and papillary dermis.
    - Disadvantages include inability to evaluate surgical margins.
  - **Photodynamic therapy (PDT)**
    - Light-activated photosensitizing drugs (methylaminolevulinate [MAL], porfirmer sodium, topical aminolevulinic acid) create oxygen free radicals that selectively destroy target cells.
    - It is used for premalignant or superficial low-risk lesions.
- **Surgical excision**[3]
  - **Primary surgical excision**
    - Current literature recommends **4 mm margin** for small primary BCC on face or other low-risk lesions.[19]
    - **10 mm margins** are recommended for primary resection of high-risk larger tumors on trunk or extremities.

> **TIP:** If tissue rearrangement or skin grafting is necessary for closure, intraoperative margin assessment is recommended.

- **Mohs micrographic surgery**

Sequential horizontal excision using topographic map of lesion and repeat excision until all positive margins are tumor free
  - Performed under local anesthesia in office
  - Cure rates 99% for primary tumors with significant tissue conservation[20]
  - **Indications**
    - Recurrent tumors
    - Cosmetically sensitive areas (periorbital, periauricular, paranasal)
    - Morpheaform and sclerosing types or aggressive malignant features
    - Poorly delineated margins in scar tissue
    - Other tumor types: Squamous cell with perineural invasion, dermatofibrosarcoma protuberans, microcystic adnexal carcinoma
- **Adjuvant treatment**[3]
  - **RT** recommended for tumors with perineural involvement, positive tissue margins, lymph node involvement in the head and neck
    - Consider in patients with regional disease of trunk and extremities who have undergone lymph node dissections
  - **Vismodegib:** Hedgehog pathway inhibitor
    - For patients in whom all surgical and radiation options for advanced BCC have been exhausted
    - Recently FDA approved
    - Adverse events: muscle spasm, alopecia, taste loss, weight loss, fatigue

*Enrollment in a clinical trial is recommended for residual disease.*

### FOLLOW-UP[3]

- Patients treated for BCC should be observed every 6-12 months with full H&P and complete skin examination.
- Patient education is critical and includes sun protection and self-examination.

## CUTANEOUS SCC

### DEMOGRAPHICS[21,22]

- **SCC is second most common skin cancer after BCC.**
- Incidence in North America is 41:100,000.
- Predilection occurs in sun-exposed regions.
  - Common on face, hands, forearms
  - 60% of all tumors of external ear[4]

### RISK FACTORS

- Fitzpatrick skin type: Types I and II have increased risk
- Sun exposure: Cumulative exposure strongly correlated to SCC
- Carcinogen exposure: Pesticides, arsenic, organic hydrocarbons
- Viral infection: HPV and herpes simplex
- Radiation: Long-term latency between exposure and disease
- Immunosuppression: 253-fold increased risk for SCC in renal transplant patients, more aggressive SCC in these patients because of greater number of tumors and/or tumor behavior

- Chronic wound caused by thermal burn, discoid lupus, fistula tract, osteomyelitis
- Psoralen and ultraviolet A light (PUVA) for psoriasis treatment
- **Premalignant lesions**[4]
  - **Actinic keratosis/solar keratosis**
    - Occur in regions of sun exposure
    - Macular/papular lesions with scaly irregular surface
    - Malignant transformation common
  - **Bowen's disease**
    - In situ demonstrates full-thickness cytologic atypia of keratinocytes with normal basal cells
    - Erythematous plaque with sharp borders and slight scaling
    - **Erythroplasia of Queyrat:** Bowen's disease of the glans penis, vulva, or oral mucosa; malignant transformation in 30%
    - In general, 10% malignant transformation
  - **Leukoplakia**
    - Most common premalignant lesion of oral mucosa
    - Mucosal changes with white patch
    - Malignant transformation 15%
  - **Keratoacanthoma**
    - Smooth dome-shaped mass of squamous cells and keratin grows rapidly over 1-6 weeks and ulcerate with central crusting.
    - Once stabilized, tumors spontaneously regress over 2-12 months and heal with scarring.
    - Keratoacanthoma resembles SCC histologically.
    - Larger or atypical lesions should be treated as SCC.

## RECURRENCE AND METASTASIS[1,3,23]

- Clinical lymphadenopathy with biopsy-proven metastatic disease warrants lymphadenectomy and further imaging for staging.
- Local metastasis occurs to regional nodal basins.
- Distant metastasis occurs by hematogenous dissemination most commonly to the lungs, liver, brain, skin, or bone.
- Metastasis from primary:
  - 2%-5% on trunk
  - 10%-20% on face/extremity
- Three-year cumulative risk of a subsequent SCC after an index SCC is 18%.
- Presence of positive nodes from lesions on an extremity carries dismal 35% 5-year survival despite nodal dissection.

**NOTE: Most SCC-related deaths result from ear lesions.**

- **Predictors of tumor recurrence for SCC**
  - **Degree of cellular differentiation**
    - Well-differentiated: 7% recurrence
    - Moderately differentiated: 23% recurrence
    - Poorly differentiated: 28% recurrence
  - **Depth of tumor invasion:** Increased aggressiveness in SCC deep into reticular dermis or subcutaneous fat
  - **Perineural invasion**
  - **Desmoplastic SCC**

**TIP:** Lymph node examinations are critical.

**CAUTION: All recurrent SCC should be considered to have perineural invasion until proven otherwise.**

**Tumors that penetrate dermis or are thicker than 8 mm are associated with high risk for death.**

## BIOLOGY

- SCC arise from the malpighian or basal layer of epidermis.

## TYPES OF SCC

- All types are histologically similar with irregular masses of squamous epithelium proliferating downward toward dermis.
- Tumor grade is the degree of cellular differentiation and measures the ratio of atypical pleomorphic and anaplastic cells to the normal epithelium.
- **Verrucous**
  - Exophytic and slow growing
  - Common on **palms and soles**
  - Less likely to metastasize
- **Ulcerative**
  - Aggressive with raised borders and central ulceration
  - Commonly metastasizes to regional lymph nodes
- **Marjolin's ulcer**[24]
  - **Typically arise in chronic wounds** (burn scars, fistulas)
  - Burn scars have 2% lifetime malignant degeneration potential.
  - Latency period is proportional to age of injury, but average interim is **32.5 years.**
  - Metastasis to lymph nodes is common.
- **Subungual**
  - Squamous changes involving the **nail bed**
  - Presents as erythema, swelling, and localized pain followed by nodularity and ulceration

## TREATMENT

*Biopsies of suspicious lesions are essential. Treatment modalities include medical, destructive, and surgical excision.*

- **Medical**
  - **Radiation**[25]
    - Cure rate for primary RT is 90%.
    - Reserved for:
      - Debilitated patients who are poor surgical candidates
      - Adjuvant therapy in management of high-stage large tumors
      - Recurrent tumors that require multimodal therapy
    - Brachytherapy recently suggested as an option for SCC management; however, not widely used given requirements for special equipment and expertise[3]
  - **Oral medications**[3]
    - Retinoids have been effective in decreasing the development of precancers and skin cancers in some patients.
    - Disadvantages are increased adverse reactions, decreased therapeutic effects with cessation, teratogenic effects.
  - **Topical**
    - 5-FU excellent for treating premalignant lesions (e.g., actinic keratosis)

- **Chemotherapy**[3]
  - Usually reserved for adjuvant therapy with large tumors, recurrent or metastatic disease.
  - Cisplatin with or without 5-FU produces limited results
  - Cetuximab shown to have tumor regression in one phase II study; low toxicity profile[26]

- **Destructive**
  - **Curettage and electrodesiccation and cryosurgery**
    - Reserved for small superficial lesions
    - Does not produce a surgical specimen for histology and margin analysis
  - **Photodynamic therapy**
    - Better against premalignant lesions
- **Surgical**[3]
  - **Excision**
    - Wide local excision is a good treatment option with 95% cure rate.
    - Most recent recommendations are based on size, grade, location of tumor, and depth of invasion.[1,27]
    - Generally **4-6 mm margins** are recommended.
      - Smaller than 2 cm, grade 1, low-risk region, depth to dermis: >**4 mm margins**
      - Larger than 2 cm, grade 2, 3, or 4, high-risk region, depth to subcutaneous fat: >**6 mm margins**
    - Frozen sections often give false negatives.
  - **Mohs micrographic surgery**
    - 95% cure rate for primary SCC
    - Lower recurrence rates with tissue preservation
    - Five-year recurrence rates for primary cutaneous SCC 3.1% (versus 8.1% for surgical excision, and 10% for RT)[25]
    - Same indications as BCC
  - **Lymphadenectomy**
    - This is indicated for clinically palpable nodes.
    - Fine-needle aspiration (FNA) or open lymph node biopsy may be used to confirm metastatic disease first.
    - Sentinel lymph node dissection (SLND) maps the first node in basin by injection of radiolabeled technetium colloid and local lymphoscintigraphy with blue lymphangiography dye.
      - Determines nodal status of basin with less morbidity than total basin lymphadenectomy
      - Indicated for high-risk SCC without palpable nodes
      - If positive, proceed with lymphadenectomy
    - Elective lymph node dissection (ELND) involves removal of clinically negative nodes from a nodal basin.
      - Technique is indicated for tumor extending to parotid capsule or contiguous nodal drainage basin.

*Radiation with or without concurrent cisplatin therapy is an alternative for those who are not surgical candidates.*

## FOLLOW-UP[3]

- Local disease: H&P, skin and nodal examinations every 3-6 months for 2 years, then every 6-12 months for 3 years, then yearly
- Regional disease: H&P, skin and nodal examination every 1-3 months for 1 year, then every 2-4 months for 1 year, then every 4-6 months for 3 years, and then every 6-12 months for life
- Patient education about sun protection and self-examinations

# MELANOMA

## DEMOGRAPHICS[1,28,29]

- 76,250 new cases diagnosed in 2012
- Incidence is increasing in men more rapidly than any other malignancy as well as in women, other than lung cancer.
- Lifetime risk in 2005 was 1:55, median age at diagnosis is 59 years.
- 82%-85% of patients present with localized disease, 10%-13% with regional disease, and 2%-5% with distant disease.
- 5-year survival rate
  - Localized >1 mm thickness: >50%-90%
- Regional disease, stage III: >20%-70% depending on nodal tumor burden
- Distant disease: generally <10%

## RISK FACTORS[1,29-31]

- **UV exposure**
  - High altitude
  - Extreme southern latitudes (Australia, New Zealand)
- **Age**
  - 50% occur in patients older than 50 years.
- **Prior melanoma**
- **Family history**
  - History is positive in 10% of patients.
  - Risk may be up to 8 times higher depending on number of relatives.
  - Familial melanomas occur at a younger age.
- **Phenotype**
  - Fitzpatrick types I, II
  - Lighter hair color
    - When compared with black hair:
      - **Redhead:** 3.6 times higher
      - **Brunette:** 2.8 times higher
      - **Blond:** 2.4 times higher
- **Sex**[32]
  - Males: 1:49 lifetime risk; more common on trunk and head
  - Females: 1:72 lifetime risk; more common in lower extremity
- **Race**
  - Risk is 10 to 20 times higher for whites than blacks.
  - Prognosis in darker skin is worse because of delayed diagnosis.
- **Other**
  - Higher socioeconomic status yields higher risk.
  - Immunosuppression
- **Predisposing conditions**
  - **Atypical mole syndrome:** B-K mole syndrome, familial atypical multiple-mole melanoma (FAMMM)
    - More than 100 melanocytic nevi measuring 6-15 mm
    - One or more measuring >8 mm
    - One or more with clinically atypical features
    - 10% risk of melanoma
    - Nevi present at birth and increase in number around puberty

- **Dysplastic nevus**
  - Atypical melanocytes with potential for transformation
  - 6%-10% lifetime risk of malignant degeneration
  - Histopathologic diagnosis
  - Clinically indistinguishable from melanoma in situ
- **Congenital nevus:** 6% lifetime risk depending on size
- **Typical moles:** Increased risk if more than 50
- **Melanoma in situ:** Lesions have intraepidermal proliferation with fully developed cellular atypia
- **Xeroderma pigmentosum** (See description in BCC section.)
- **Lentigo maligna**
  - Also known as ***Hutchinson freckle,*** *senile freckle,* or *circumscribed precancerous melanosis*
  - Nonnested proliferation of variably atypical melanocytes and atrophic dermis

## Benign Pigmented Lesions Mistaken for Melanoma[33]

**TIP:** Melanomas are characterized by **ABCD**s: **A**symmetry, **B**order irregularity, **C**olor variation, and **D**iameter more than 6 mm. Pigmented lesions >5-10 mm in diameter are more likely to be malignant than benign.[34]

- **Junctional nevi**
  - Flat, uniform color on palms, soles, genitalia, and mucosa
  - Pale to dark brown
  - Smooth macular and sharply defined
  - Appear usually around ages 4-12 and change little during childhood
- **Compound nevi**
  - Darker and palpable raised border
  - Smooth or rough and can have hair
  - Appear during puberty and fade
  - Halo nevus is compound nevus surrounded by depigmented ring of skin
- **Intradermal nevi**
  - Raised pale papules with pigment in flecks
  - Coarse dark terminal hairs may grow in lesions
  - Occur in second or third decade of life
  - Most commonly found on face and neck
- **Blue nevi**
  - Blue-black lesion <5 mm that remains stable with time
  - Usually found on dorsum of hands or feet, head, neck, buttocks
  - Very rare degeneration potential
- **Spitz nevus**
  - Juvenile melanoma of children and young adults
  - Smooth surface, dome shaped, red or pink
  - Telangiectasias typically are present
  - Most common on head and neck
  - Typically less than 6 mm in diameter
  - Often noticed after rapid change in size or color
  - Proliferation of enlarged spindled/epithelioid melanocytes

- **Lentigo**
  - Pigmented macular lesions with reticulated pattern
  - Most common in middle age from sun exposure
  - Simple lentigo: Common brown/black mole
  - Solar lentigo: Liver spot or age spot
- **Seborrheic keratosis**
  - Multiple, variously colored, raised verrucous papules
  - Most commonly found on **trunk**

**TIP:** Seborrheic keratosis can mimic melanoma.

- **Pyogenic granulomas**
  - Short development course of days to weeks
  - Commonly occurs at site after minor trauma
  - Raised with surrounding inflammation
  - Painless
  - Most common on hands and around mouth
- **Pigmented BCC**

## Melanoma Growth Patterns[4,35,36]

- **Superficial spreading melanoma**
  - Most common: 50%-70%
  - Usually arises from **preexisting nevus**
  - Long horizontal growth phase before vertical growth
  - Typical appearance: Flat junctional nevus, asymmetrical borders, color variegation
- **Nodular melanoma**
  - 15%-30% of all cases
  - Aggressive
  - Typically arises de novo in normal skin
  - More common in men (2:1)
  - 1-2 cm, dome shaped
  - Resembles a blood blister
  - Keeps sharp demarcation because of lack of horizontal growth pattern
  - 5% amelanotic
- **Lentigo maligna**
  - 4%-10% of all cases
  - Least aggressive subtype
  - Clearly related to sun exposure
  - Appearance of skin stain in multiple shades of brown
  - More common in **women**
  - Radial growth phase of precursor lesion (Hutchinson freckle)
  - Transition to vertical growth marks transition to melanoma
- **Acral-lentiginous melanoma**
  - 2%-8% of cases in whites, but 35%-60% of cases in nonwhites
  - **Usually on palms, soles of feet, subungual, or sun-protected sites**
  - Melanonychia: Linear pigmented streak in the nail
  - 3 cm, usually flat with irregular border and multiple color shades
  - Long radial growth phase, transition to vertical growth increases metastatic risk

- **Desmoplastic melanoma**
  - 1% of all cases
  - Propensity for perineural invasion
  - Immunohistochemical stain reactive to S-100 protein
  - High rate of regional lymph node spread
- **Amelanotic melanoma**
  - No pigment by light microscopy
  - Diagnosis by immunohistochemical staining
  - Usually diagnosed in vertical growth phase
- **Noncutaneous melanoma**
  - 2% of all cases
  - Mucosal melanoma
  - Arises on mucosal surfaces
  - Usually large at diagnosis
  - Poor prognosis
- **Ocular melanoma**
  - 2%-5% of all cases
  - Vision interference leads to earlier diagnosis
  - Liver metastases are common

## MELANOMA STAGING[28,37,38]

- Histologic analysis of full-thickness biopsy specimen is categorized by microstaging.
  - **Breslow thickness:** Measurement of tumor thickness in millimeters
  - **Clark's level:** Level determined by histologic invasion through skin layers[37] (Fig. 15-2)
- American Joint Committee on Cancer (AJCC) introduced revised tumor-node-metastasis (TNM) melanoma staging system in 2010[29] (Tables 15-3 and 15-4).
  - **Tumor thickness (Breslow thickness) replaces level of invasion (Clark's level) as the most important prognostic variable of primary tumor invasion that best predicts survival.**
  - Ulceration of the primary tumor (microscopic histopathologic ulceration) upstages the disease to the next highest T substage.
  - Mitotic rate $\geq$1 per mm$^2$ is independently associated with worse disease-specific survival, especially in tumors $\leq$1 mm thick.
  - Number of metastatic lymph nodes replaces the size of lymph nodes in the N stage.
  - Lymphatic mapping data (lymphoscintigraphy) and micrometastatic local regional disease within lymph nodes are incorporated in clinical and pathologic staging.
  - Subcategorization of stage IV metastatic disease is based on anatomic site of the metastasis and elevated serum LDH.

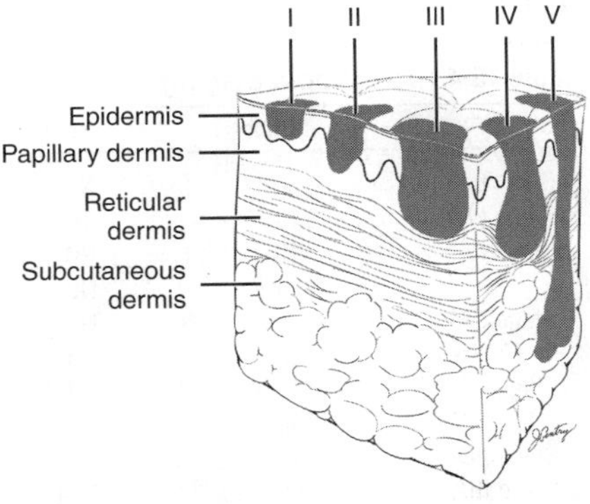

**Fig. 15-2** Levels of tumor invasion according to the Clark microstaging criteria.

**Table 15-3** *AJCC TNM Melanoma Staging Classification, 2010*

| Tumor Classification | Depth of Invasion |
|---|---|
| TX | Primary tumor cannot be assessed |
| Tis | Melanoma in situ |
| T1 | <1.0 mm |
| T2 | 1.01-2.0 mm |
| T3 | 2.01-4.0 mm |
| T4 | >4.0 mm |

NOTE: a and b subcategories of T: a, without ulceration and mitosis $<1/\text{mm}^2$; b, with ulceration or mitoses $>1/\text{mm}^2$.

| Node Classification | |
|---|---|
| NX | Cannot be assessed |
| N1 | One node |
| N2 | Two to three nodes |
| N3 | Four or more nodes, matted, or in transit satellites with metastatic nodes |

NOTE: a, b, and c subcategories of N: a, micrometastasis (diagnosed after sentinel lymph node biopsy); b, macrometastasis (clinically positive nodes); c, in transit satellites without nodes (N2 only).

| Metastatic Classification | |
|---|---|
| M1a | Metastases to skin, subcutaneous, distant nodes |
| M1b | Metastases to lung |
| M1c | Metastases to other viscera or any distant site combined with elevated serum LDH |

**Table 15-4** *Pathologic Staging*

| Stage | Tumor | Node | Metastasis |
|---|---|---|---|
| Stage 0 | Tis | N0 | M0 |
| Stage IA | T1a | N0 | M0 |
| Stage IB | T1b | N0 | M0 |
| | T2a | N0 | M0 |
| Stage IIA | T2b | N0 | M0 |
| | T3a | N0 | M0 |
| Stage IIB | T3b | N0 | M0 |
| | T4a | N0 | M0 |
| Stage IIC | T4b | N0 | M0 |
| Stage IIIA | T(1-4)a | N1a | M0 |
| | T(1-4)a | N2a | M0 |
| Stage IIIB | T(1-4)b | N1a or N2a | M0 |
| | T(1-4)a | N1b, N2b, or N2c | M0 |
| Stage IIIC | T(1-4)b | N1b, N2b, or N2c | M0 |
| | Any T | N3 | M0 |
| Stage IV | Any T | Any N | M1 |

## WORKUP[29]

- Obtain biopsy samples of lesion. Stage patient by evaluating lymph node status and imaging for metastatic disease.
- Obtain biopsy specimens of all suspicious lesions.[29,39-44]
  - 5-7 mm punch biopsy is adequate but may miss thickest portion of tumor.
  - Obtain incisional biopsy for low-suspicion lesion or in cosmetically sensitive regions. Orient incision longitudinally in extremities.
  - Excisional biopsy with 1-3 mm margins is recommended.
  - Shave biopsy forfeits ability to stage on thickness.
  - Full-thickness biopsy is not required in subungual melanoma, because it offers no prognostic information.
  - Evaluate for Breslow thickness, ulceration status, dermal mitotic rate, deep and peripheral margins, microsatellitosis, Clark's level, and desmoplasia.

**TIP:** Avoid cauterizing, because margins may be distorted.

- Imaging[29]
  - Stages I and II: CT scan, PET/CT, MRI generally not recommended unless evaluating specific symptoms
  - Stage III: Can consider imaging, including CT chest, abdomen/pelvis, CT/MRI brain with or without PET/CT
- Physician preference
- CT pelvis in patients with inguinofemoral lymphadenopathy
  - Stage IV: Confirm metastatic disease with FNA or open biopsy. Obtain baseline imaging as above.

## TREATMENT OF MELANOMA[29,39-44]

- **Surgical excision**[45-48]
  - Wide local excision (WLE) with surgical margins based on tumor thickness
    - In situ: 0.5 cm margin
    - <1 mm: 1 cm margin
    - 1-4 mm: 2 cm margin
    - <4 mm: 2 cm margin
  - **Depth of resection should not include fascial layer,** because this increases risk of metastatic disease without improving long-term survival.
  - For subungual melanoma, amputation is recommended proximal to distal interphalangeal joint (or IP joint of thumb).
  - If not a surgical candidate, topical imiquimod or RT can be used for in situ disease or lentigo maligna.
- **Lymph nodes**
  - **Sentinel lymph node biopsy (SLNB)**[49]
    - **Staging procedure, not a therapeutic treatment**
    - Low false-negative rate and complication rate
    - Performed in conjunction with WLE of primary tumor
    - Skip metastasis reported 0%-2%

- **Indications**
  - Stage IB melanoma or stage II
  - 0.76-1 mm thick with ulceration or mitotic rate $\geq 1$ per mm$^2$, or more than 1.0 mm thick[49]
  - In transit stage III if resectable
- No role for elective lymph node dissection if negative SLNB or nonpalpable disease
- **Therapeutic lymph node dissection (LND)**[29,50]
  - Performed for positive SLNB patients or clinically palpable disease (MSLT1)
  - Only potential cure for metastatic nodal disease
  - Poor prognosis for patients with clinically palpable nodes
  - Extent of dissection modified according to the specific basin (i.e., patients with inguinal lymphadenopathy are candidates for pelvic LND if >3 superficial lymph nodes are involved, when superficial lymph nodes are clinically positive, or when Cloquet's node is positive.)
  - In transit disease[29]
  - Resection is mainstay
- Isolation limb perfusion: Melphalan is the most widely used drug.
- Intralesional injection of bacillus Calmette-Guérin (BCG), local ablation therapy, topical imiquimod, or radiation

- **Adjuvant therapy**
  - No adjuvant therapy is so effective that it is routinely recommended.
  - It is more effective against subclinical micrometastases than primary tumors, and against residual disease after removal of gross disease.
  - Patients may benefit by palliation of symptoms and prolongation of life.
    - **Interferon (INF)**
      - Interferon alfa-2b: Recombinant version of naturally occurring leukocyte interferon alfa-2b
      - Low-dose INF: At 5 years, INF was associated with a significant relapse-free survival (RFS) but did not increase overall survival (OS).[45]
      - Intermediate-dose INF: No progression-free survival benefits[29]
      - High-dose INF in stage IIB, IIC, and III patients: Treatment includes 1 month of IV induction followed by 11 months of subcutaneous maintenance INF.
        - Relapse-free survival benefit and OS at a median of 6.9 years. At 12.6 years, there was no difference in OS.[51]
        - Larger follow-up trial showed an RFS advantage but no OS advantage.[29]
        - Pooled analysis confirmed an improvement in RFS in patients with high-risk resected melanoma (stages IIB and III) but not in OS.[52]
      - Appropriate in stage IIB and III patients (regional nodal/in transit metastasis or node-negative patients with primary melanomas deeper than 4 mm)
      - Inappropriate for node-negative patients with nonulcerated lesions <4 mm.
      - Uncertain in patients with ulcerated lesions of intermediate depth (2-4 mm)

**NOTE: INF is a toxic therapy and is not tolerated well by many patients.**

- **Pegylated interferon:** Approved by FDA in 2011[29]
  - Alternative to high-dose INF in completely resected stage III disease with positive nodes, not in transit disease
  - EORTC protocol (18991) trial: Four-year RFS was significantly better in INF group than observation but no effect on OS

- **RT**[29]
  - Rarely indicated as primary treatment of cutaneous melanoma, except lentigo maligna or desmoplastic melanomas
  - Adjuvant RT to nodal bed should be considered if four or more positive nodes, nodes 3 cm or larger, or macroscopic extranodal soft tissue expansion
  - Lower threshold for radiation in cervical lymph node disease following adequate LND
  - Benefit of RT: cervical >axillary >inguinal
  - Can be used as preoperative or postoperative treatment of primary site for patients with inadequate margins, in unresectable lymph node basins, with extensive neurotropism, microsatellitosis, in patients with recurrence after previous excision, or in palliation of metastatic disease especially CNS[53]
- **Chemotherapy**[29]
  - Agents such as dacarbazine (DTIC), temozolomide, cisplatin, vinblastin, carboplatin, paclitaxel as monotherapy or combination therapy
  - Generally palliative only, with some success for regression of tumor burden
  - Overall modest response rates under 20% in first-line and second-line settings
- **Immunotherapy**[29]
  - Ipilimumab, a monoclonal antibody directed to the receptor CTLA-4
    - FDA approval in March 2011 for patients with unresectable metastatic disease
    - Stimulates T-cells, therefore high risk for immune-related reactions
  - Vemurafenib, a BRAF kinase inhibitor
    - For use in stage IV patients with mutation of the intracellular signaling kinase BRAF
    - FDA approval in August 2011 for metastatic or unresectable melanoma
  - Imatinib is for tumors with c-KIT mutations.
  - Interleukin-2 has been approved for stage IV disease.
  - Vaccines have shown disappointing results.[29,54,55]
    - GM2/BCG vaccine, MAGE-A3 protein vaccine: Trial results pending, cultured melanoma cell vaccine (Canvaxin)

## SURVEILLANCE AND RECURRENCE[29,43,56]

- Local recurrence usually occurs within 5 cm of original lesion within 3-5 years, usually resulting from incomplete resection of primary tumor.
- Reports of second primary melanomas are 2%-3.4%.
- Guidelines of follow-up programs include early detection and treatment of recurrent disease.
  - Stage IA-IIA: H&P and skin/nodal examination every 3-12 months for 5 years, then annually
  - Stage IIB-IV: H&P and skin/nodal examination every 3-6 months for 2 years, then every 3-12 months for 3 years, then annually
  - Consider chest radiographs, CT, and/or PET/CT every 3-12 months to screen for recurrent/metastatic disease.
  - Consider brain MRI/CT annually.
  - Routine imaging to screen for asymptomatic disease after 5 years is not recommended.
- Treatment of recurrence
  - Reexcision is the primary treatment of local recurrences.
  - Regional recurrence can also be treated with radiation or chemotherapy.

## Key Points

- ✓ BCC is the most common type of skin cancer.
- ✓ Nodular BCC is the most common histologic subtype.
- ✓ Recommended surgical margins for BCC are usually 4-10 mm depending on the risk for recurrence and location.
- ✓ Erythroplasia of Queyrat is Bowen's disease of the glans penis, vulva, or oral mucosa.
- ✓ Leukoplakia is the most common premalignant lesion of oral mucosa.
- ✓ Most SCC-related deaths are associated with ear lesions.
- ✓ Marjolin's ulcers are SCCs that arise in chronic wounds.
- ✓ Surgical margins for SCCs are usually 4-6 mm, sometimes more.
- ✓ Superficial spreading is the most common growth pattern of melanoma.
- ✓ Acral-lentiginous melanoma usually occurs on the palms and soles and is more common in blacks.
- ✓ Breslow thickness is the most important prognostic variable that predicts survival (melanoma).
- ✓ WLE margins in melanoma are based on tumor thickness.

## References


1. Habif TP, ed. Clinical Dermatology: A Color Guide to Diagnosis and Therapy, 4th ed. St Louis: Mosby–Year Book, 2004.
2. Shanoff LB, Spira M, Hardy SB. Basal cell carcinoma: a statistical approach to rational management. Plast Reconstr Surg 39:619, 1967.
3. Miller S, Alam M, Anderson J, et al. NCCN Guidelines. Clinical practice guidelines in oncology: basal cell and squamous cell skin cancers version 2.2012. Available at *http://www.nccn.org/professionals/physician_gls/f_guidelines.asp#nmsc.*
4. Netscher DT, Leong M, Orengo I, et al. Cutaneous malignancies: melanoma and nonmelanoma types. Plast Reconstr Surg 127:37e, 2011.
5. Fitzpatrick TB. The validity and practicality of sun-reactive skin types I through VI. Arch Dermatol 124:869, 1988.
6. Collett D, Mumford L, Banner NR, et al. Comparison of the incidence of malignancy in recipients of different types of organ: a UK Registry audit. Am J Transplant 10:1889, 2010.
7. Kubasiewicz M, Starzynski Z. Case-referent study on skin cancer and its relation to occupational exposure to polycyclic aromatic hydrocarbons. Pol J Occup Med 2:221, 1989.
8. Hutchinson J. Arsenic cancer. Br Med J 2:1280, 1888.
9. Lever LR, Farr PM. Skin cancers or premalignant lesions occur in half of high-dose PUVA patients. Br J Dermatol 131:215, 1994.
10. Baskurt H, Celik E, Yesiladah G, et al. Importance of hereditary factors in synchronous development of basal cell carcinoma in two albino brothers. Ann Plast Surg 66:640, 2011.
11. Gorlin RJ, Goltz RW. Multiple nevoid basal epithelioma, jaw cysts and bifid ribs: a syndrome. N Engl J Med 262:908, 1960.
12. Jacobs GH, Rippey JJ, Altini M. Prediction of aggressive behavior in basal cell carcinoma. Cancer 49:533, 1982.
13. Bolognia JL, Jorizzo J, Rapini R, eds. Dermatology, vol 2, 2nd ed. St Louis: Mosby-Elsevier, 2012.
14. SEER cancer statistics review, 1973-1995. Bethesda, MD: National Cancer Institute, 1998. National Institute of Health Publication No 98-2789.
15. Pollack SV, Goslen JB, Sheretz EF, et al. The biology of basal cell carcinoma: a review. J Am Acad Dermatol 7:569, 1982.

16. Dubin N, Kopf AW. Multivariate risk score for recurrence of cutaneous basal cell carcinomas. Arch Dermatol 119:373, 1983.
17. Salasche SJ. Curettage and electrodesiccation in the treatment of midfacial basal cell epithelioma. J Am Acad Dermatol 8:496, 1983.
18. Zacarian SA. Cryosurgery of cutaneous carcinomas: an 18-year study of 3,022 patients with 4,228 carcinomas. J Am Acad Dermatol 9:947, 1983.
19. Kimyai-Asadi A, Alam A, Goldberg LH, et al. Efficacy of narrow-margin excision of well-demarcated primary facial basal cell carcinomas. J Am Acad Dermatol 53:464, 2005.
20. Cottel WI, Proper S. Mohs' surgery, fresh tissue technique: our technique with a review. J Dermatol Surg Oncol 8:576, 1982.
21. Vitaliano PP, Urbach F. The relative importance of risk factors in nonmelanoma carcinoma. Arch Dermatol 116:454, 1980.
22. Gallagher RP, Hill GB, Coldman AJ, et al. Sunlight exposure, pigmentation factors, and risk of nonmelanotic skin cancer. II. Squamous cell carcinoma. Arch Dermatol 131:164, 1995.
23. Immerman SC, Scanlon EF, Christ M, et al. Recurrent squamous cell carcinoma of the skin. Cancer 51:1537, 1983.
24. Lawrence EA. Carcinoma arising in the scars of thermal burns. Surg Gynecol Obstet 95:579, 1952.
25. Rowe DE, Carroll RJ, Day CL Jr. Prognostic factors for local recurrence, metastasis, and survival rates in squamous cell carcinoma of the skin, ear, and lip. J Am Acad Dermatol 26:976, 1992.
26. Maubec E, Petrow P, Scheer-Senyarich I, et al. Phase II study of cetuximab as first-line single-drug therapy in patients with unresectable squamous cell carcinoma of the skin. J Clin Oncol 29:3419, 2011.
27. Broadland DG, Zitelli JA. Surgical margins for excision of primary cutaneous squamous cell carcinoma. J Am Acad Dermatol 27:108, 1992.
28. National Cancer Institute. What you need to know about melanoma: information about detection, symptoms, diagnosis, treatment, and other resources. NIH Pub No 02-1563, 2003. Available at *http://www.checkbook.org/sitemap/health/Melanoma/.*
29. Coit D, Andtbacka R, Anker C, et al. NCCN Guidelines. Clinical practice guidelines in oncology: melanoma version 2.2013. Available at *http://www.nccn.org/professionals/physician_gls/f_guidelines.asp#melanoma.*
30. Crombie IK. Racial differences in melanoma incidence. Br J Cancer 40:185, 1979.
31. Devesa SS, Silverman DT, Young JL Jr, et al. Cancer incidence and mortality trends among whites in the United States, 1947-1984. J Natl Cancer Inst 79:701, 1987.
32. National Cancer Institute. Surveillance, Epidemiology, and End Results (SEER) Program. SEER 17 incidence and mortality, 2000-2003, 2006. Available at *http://seer.cancer.gov/csr/1975_2003/results_merged/topic_graph_surv_rates.pdf.*
33. Rhodes AR. Potential precursors of cutaneous melanoma. In Lejeune FJ, Chaudhuri PK, Das Gupta TK, eds. Malignant Melanoma: Medical and Surgical Management. New York: McGraw-Hill, 1994.
34. Elwood JM, Gallagher RP, Hill GB, et al. Pigmentation and skin reaction to sun as risk factors for cutaneous melanoma: Western Canada Melanoma Study. Br Med J 288:99, 1984.
35. Mihm MC Jr, Fitzpatrick TB, Brown MM, et al. Early detection of primary cutaneous malignant melanoma: a color atlas. N Engl J Med 289:989, 1973.
36. Milton GW. Clinical diagnosis of malignant melanoma. Br J Surg 55:755, 1968.
37. McGovern VJ, Mihm MC Jr, Bailly C, et al. The classification of malignant melanoma and its histologic reporting. Cancer 32:1446, 1973.
38. Balch CM, Buzaid AC, Soong SJ, et al. Final version of the American Joint Committee on Cancer staging system for cutaneous melanoma. J Clin Oncol 19:3635, 2001.
39. Balch CM, Buzaid AC. Finally, a successful adjuvant therapy for high risk melanoma. J Clin Oncol 4:1, 1996.

Breslow

40. Kim CJ, Dessureault S, Gabrilovich D, et al. Immunotherapy for melanoma. Cancer Control 9:22, 2002.
41. Morton DL, Wen DR, Wong JH, et al. Technical details of intraoperative lymphatic mapping for early stage melanoma. Arch Surg 127:392, 1992.
42. Gershenwald JE, Fischer D, Buzaid AC. Cutaneous melanoma: clinical classification and staging. Clin Plast Surg 27:361, 2000.
43. Wagner JD, Gordon MS, Chuang TY, et al. Current therapy of cutaneous melanoma. Plast Reconstr Surg 105:1774, 2000.
44. Uren RF, Thompson JF, Coventry BJ, et al. Lymphoscitigraphy in patients with melanoma. In Balch CM, Houghton AN, Sober AJ, et al, eds. Cutaneous Melanoma, 5th ed. St Louis: Quality Medical Publishing, 2009.
45. Khayat D, Rixe O, Martin G, et al; French Group of Research on Malignant Melanoma. Surgical margins in cutaneous melanoma (2 cm versus 5 cm for lesions measuring less than 2.1-mm thick). Cancer 97:1941, 2003.
46. Balch CM, Soong SJ, Smith T, et al. Long-term results of a prospective surgical trial comparing 2 cm vs. 4 cm excision margins for 740 patients with 1-4 mm melanomas. Ann Surg Oncol 8:101, 2001.
47. Cohn-Cedermark G, Rutqvist LE, Andersson R, et al. Long term results of a randomized study by the Swedish Melanoma Study Group on 2-cm versus 5-cm resection margins for patients with cutaneous melanoma with a tumor thickness of 0.8-2.0 mm. Cancer 89:1495, 2000.
48. Veronesi U, Cascinelli N. Narrow excision (1-cm margin). Arch Surg 126:438, 1991.
49. McMasters KM, Noyes RD, Reintgen DS, et. al. Lessons learned from the Sunbelt Melanoma Trial. J Surg Oncol 86:212, 2004.
50. Mortan DL, Thompson JF, Cochran AJ, et al. Al. Sentinel-node biopsy or nodal observation in melanoma. N Engl J Med 355:1307, 2006.
51. Kirkwood JM, Strawderman MH, Ernstoff MS, et al. Interferon alfa-2b adjuvant therapy of high-risk resected cutaneous melanoma: the Eastern Cooperative Oncology Group Trial EST 1684. J Clin Oncol 14:7, 1996.
52. Kirkwood JM, Manola J, Ibrahim J, et al; Eastern Cooperative Oncology Group. A pooled analysis of Eastern Cooperative Oncology Group and intergroup trials of adjuvant high-dose interferon for melanoma. Clin Cancer Res 10:1670, 2004.
53. Hong A, Fogarty G. Role of radiation therapy in cutaneous melanoma. Cancer J 18:203, 2012.
54. Davar D, Tarhini AA, Kirkwood J. Adjuvant therapy for melanoma. Cancer J 18:192, 2012.
55. Yang JC. Melanoma vaccines. Cancer J 17:277, 2011.
56. Brobeil A, Rappaport D, Wells K, et al. Multiple primary melanomas: implications for screening and follow-up programs. Ann Surg Oncol 4:19, 1997.

# 16. Burns

Reza Kordestani, John L. Burns, Jr.

## DEMOGRAPHICS

### INCIDENCE[1]

- 450,000 burn injuries receive medical treatment.
  - 3500 deaths
- High-risk groups: Pediatric, geriatric, and disabled populations

### PROGNOSIS

- Major predictor of mortality: **Age, total body surface area (TBSA), inhalation injury**[1]
  - **Baux score[1]: 50% mortality if age + %TBSA = 110 (Baux score). However, if there is associated inhalation injury, then 50% mortality associated with age + %TBSA = 100 (Baux score)**
- Dramatic decrease in deaths is attributed to prevention, advancements in critical care, and early excision and grafting.[2] However, with improved survival come many more patients with reconstructive and functional needs.

## PATHOPHYSIOLOGY (Table 16-1)

### BURN WOUNDS CLASSIFIED BASED ON DEPTH OF PENETRATION

- Depth depends on: Temperature, source, contact time, skin thickness
- **First degree**
  - Epidermis only
    - Skin erythema, pain
    - Blanches with pressure
    - No blistering
    - Symptoms subside over 2-3 days, epithelium peels at ~day 4.

**Table 16-1** *Burn Tissue Histology*

| Zone | Clinical Finding | Treatment |
|---|---|---|
| Zone of coagulation (necrosis) | Nonviable necrotic tissue in center of burn wound | Excision and grafting |
| Zone of stasis (edema) | Surrounds zone of coagulation, initially viable | Aggressive resuscitation to improve perfusion and prevent transformation to necrosis |
| Zone of hyperemia (inflammation) | Outermost zone, viable | Aggressive resuscitation |

- **Second degree**
  - **Superficial:** Papillary dermis **sparing skin appendages**
    - Painful
    - Blanches with pressure
    - Blistering may be delayed for 12-24 hours after burn.
    - Most heal within 3 weeks via stem cells from **skin appendages** without hypertrophic scarring.
  - **Deep:** Reticular dermis involving **loss of skin appendages**
    - Decreased sensation
    - No capillary refill
    - Blistering
    - Heal in 3-9 weeks, hypertrophic scarring common, usually treated with excision and grafting
- **Third degree**
  - Entire dermis and adnexal structures
    - Blistering absent
    - **Insensate,** leathery consistency
    - Color varies with mechanism of burn.
    - If no intervention, it will demarcate and separate over days to weeks. However, this delays healing and risks infection.
    - Circumferential third-degree burns of extremities may lead to compartment syndrome if muscles become edematous; likewise circumferential chest wall burns may inhibit expansion and breathing.

## CRITERIA FOR TRANSFER TO A BURN CENTER[3]

### INDICATIONS/PATIENT SELECTION

- Partial-thickness burns >10% of TBSA
- Third-degree burns
- Burns involving face, hands, feet, genitalia, perineum, or major joints
- Chemical burns
- Electrical burns
- Any burn with concomitant trauma in which burn poses greatest risk to patient
- Inhalation injury
- Preexisting medical disorders that could affect mortality
- Hospitals without qualified personnel or equipment for care of burned children
- Patients who will require special social, emotional, or rehabilitative intervention

> **TIP:** The criteria for transfer to a burn center are frequently asked on examinations, including boards.

## PREOPERATIVE DIAGNOSIS AND TREATMENT

### FACIAL BURNS[2,4,5]

- Extensive edema formation (blood supply and loose connective tissue): Head elevation
- Eye examination and fluorescein staining for corneal injury before extensive edema
- Ophthalmology consult

## INHALATION INJURY[2,5]

- **Supraglottic injury (thermal/chemical):** Hoarseness, pharyngeal erythema, and edema
- **Infraglottic injury (chemical):** Mental status changes because of hypoxia
- Carboxyhemoglobin (≥10% in CO poisoning)
- Arterial blood gas analysis
- Chest radiographic examination (typically normal initially)
- Bronchoscopy
- Increased resuscitation fluid requirements

## COMPARTMENT SYNDROME

- Pain on passive stretch
- Tense compartments on palpation
- Paresthesias
- Doppler flowmeter
- Compartment testing: **Pressure >30 mm Hg is indication for escharotomy/fasciotomy.** However, decision to operate is usually made on **clinical factors.**

## ELECTRICAL INJURIES[2,5]

- Most sequelae from high-voltage injury (>1000 volts)
- Find contact points
- EKG
- Cardiac monitoring
- Renal function testing
- Tea-colored urine indicates myoglobinuria.
  - Maintain urine output at **75-100 ml/hr** to minimize myoglobin precipitation. Bicarbonate or mannitol may be needed.
- Risk of compartment syndrome in involved extremity

## CHEMICAL BURNS[2,5]

- **Alkali:** Penetrates deeply because of liquefactive necrosis.
  - Copious irrigation
  - Avoid neutralization with weak acids, which causes a hyperthermic reaction.
- **Acids:** Coagulative necrosis limits depth.
  - Copious irrigation
- **Hydrofluoric acid:** Flouride ion binds calcium.
  - Treat topically with calcium gel, intradermal calcium gluconate, or intraarterial calcium gluconate based on severity
- **Phenol:** Coagulative necrosis, can cause systemic derangement (e.g., liver, kidney).
  - Irrigate and treat with polyethylene glycol
- **Phosphorus:** Stain particles with 0.5% copper sulfate or detect with UV light and surgically remove.

**TIP:** These chemical injuries and their treatments are frequently on tests.

## RESUSCITATION: PARKLAND FORMULA

- Burn shock from systemic response typically occurs with >20% TBSA (>15% in pediatric/geriatric patients).
- Burn shock requires resuscitation; otherwise, maintenance fluids may be adequate.

- **4 ml × Weight (kg) × %TBSA burned** (Fig. 16-1)
  - Additional fluid is typically required in concurrent trauma, electrical injury, inhalation injury.
  - Maintenance fluid with D5 ½ NS in addition to resuscitation fluid is required in infants and children.
- **Half of the total amount in lactated Ringer's solution given over the first 8 hours from the time of injury and the second half over the next 16 hours,** with rate adjusted based on hourly urine output

> **TIP:** Adequate volume resuscitation is paramount, because this can preserve the zone of stasis (edema) and prevent further tissue loss.

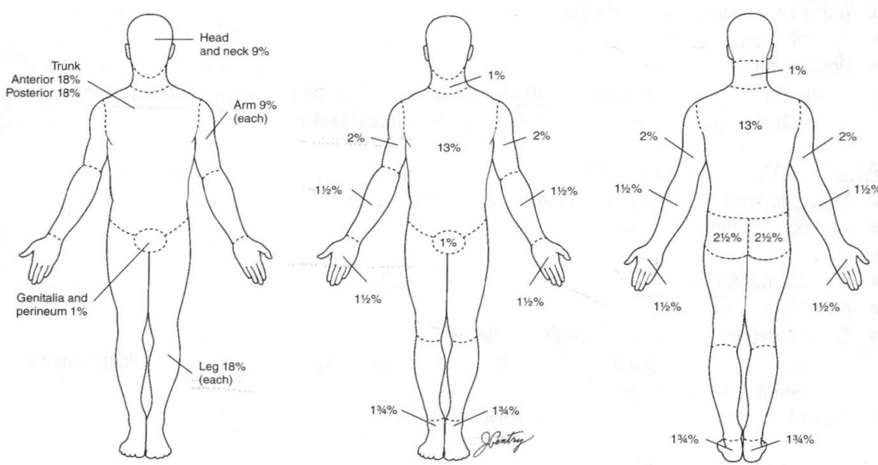


**Fig. 16-1** Calculation of total body surface area.

## OPERATIVE TREATMENT

### Acute-Phase Burn Reconstruction

- Excision[6]
  - Fascial excision results in less blood loss than tangential excision but creates a more severe deformity.
  - The decision on how much to excise during a single setting is determined by the patient's comorbid conditions, blood availability, and the ability to cover the wound.[2]
- Wound coverage[2,7] (Table 16-2)
- Eyelid and oral commissure contractures surgically treated in the acute burn period to prevent exposure keratitis and irreversible damage to dentition
- Aggressive splinting and therapy

> **TIP:** Plan for surgical blood loss of 0.5 ml/cm$^2$ (area of burn excision).

**Table 16-2** *Options for Burn Wound Coverage*

| Temporary | Characteristics | Uses |
|---|---|---|
| Allograft | Cadaveric split-thickness skin graft | **Benchmark for temporary coverage**<br>Lasts 3-4 weeks, until rejection by host |
| Xenograft | Typically porcine skin graft | Application on equivocal superficial vs. deep dermal burn may obviate need for autograft |
| Biobrane (Smith & Nephew, Largo, FL) | Nylon fabric coated with porcine dermal collagen with silicone membrane | Promotes fibrovascular ingrowth<br>Not widely used |
| TransCyte (Smith & Nephew) | Biobrane and cultured human neonate fibroblasts | Not widely used, though used as an adjunct at some burn programs |
| **Permanent** | | |
| Autograft | Epidermis and partial (STSG) vs. entire (FTSG) thickness of dermis | Adheres by imbibition, inosculation, and capillary ingrowth over 5 days |
| • STSG | Secondary contraction >primary contraction<br>May be meshed to cover larger area | More reliable graft take versus FTSG<br>Donor site heals in approximately 10 days-2 weeks depending on thickness of graft |
| • FTSG | Primary contraction (elastic fibers) >secondary contraction | Less reliable graft take versus STSG<br>Donor site closed primarily<br>Typically used for face and hand wound coverage |
| Integra (Integra LifeSciences, Plainsboro, NJ) | Bovine tendon collagen, shark chondroitin-6-sulfate, silicone layer | Forms neodermis in 10 days-3 weeks, then can be covered with thin STSG, which is predominantly epidermis (<0.008 inch), in a second operation<br>Used if insufficient autograft or for treatment of scar contractures |
| AlloDerm (LifeCell, Branchburg, NJ) | Human acellular dermal matrix | Replaces dermis and can be covered with thin STSG, which is predominantly epidermis (<0.008 inch), in one operation<br>Inspect on day 7, when autograft should look white and yellow |
| Cultured epithelial autograft | Sample of patient skin is cultured in lab to produce epithelial cells, which are then attached to petrolatum gauze | Fragile wound coverage given absence of dermal layer<br>When applied over AlloDerm, successful take increases by 40% |

*FTSG,* Full-thickness skin graft; *STSG,* split-thickness skin graft.

## Intermediate-Phase Burn Reconstruction

- Hypertrophic burn scars mature over months to years. In this period, goal of reconstruction is scar modification to promote favorable scar maturation.
  - Depth of initial injury and wound tension determine final scar appearance.
  - Techniques to relieve tension include Z-plasty, releases with grafting, intralesional steroids (used sparingly).
- Aggressive splinting and therapy

## Late-Phase Burn Reconstruction

- Mature burn scars blend into surrounding normal tissue as they become more pliable, less hypertrophic, and less hyperemic.
- Goals of therapy after scar maturation are definitive treatment of remaining functional and aesthetic deformity. Postoperative therapy is critical to outcome in some regions.
- Scars that remain hypertrophic and hyperemic typically are under persistent tension and may be treated with release and laser treatment.[2]
- Each body region presents unique problems that may be best approached at various levels of the reconstructive ladder.
  - **Head and neck:** Eyebrows, eyelids, ears, nose, perioral, scalp[4,8,9,10]
  - **Extremities:** Larger joints of the extremity are important for hand and foot positioning. Assess the entire extremity during operative planning to maximize functional restoration.
  - **Breasts:** Releases with grafting, flaps, tissue expansion, and implant exchange. Obtain symmetry in unilateral burn injury, because a burned breast may not become ptotic over time.[2]

## POSTOPERATIVE TREATMENT

- Systemic antibiotics for suspected infections
  - Culture guided: Sputum, blood, tissue, urine
- Topical antimicrobials (Table 16-3)
- Nutrition
  - Metabolic demands are usually increased 120%-150% in modern burn care setting.[2]
  - Malnutrition results in delayed wound healing, organ failure, compromised immune system.
  - Enteral feeding is preferred to total parenteral nutrition (TPN) because of its trophic effect and decreased complications.
  - Curreri formula is used to calculate caloric needs:
    - 25 kcal/kg/day + 40 kcal/%TBSA/day
    - Dedicate 1.5-2 g/kg/day of protein with additional glutamine supplementation,[2] providing a calorie/nitrogen ratio of 100:1.

**Table 16-3** *Commonly Prescribed Topical Antimicrobials for Burn Wounds*

| Drug | Target Organism | Properties and Side Effects |
|---|---|---|
| Silver sulfadiazine (Silvadene) | Broad spectrum with gram-positive and gram-negative coverage | Transient leucopenia<br>Penetrates eschar poorly |
| Mafenide acetate (Sulfamylon) | Gram-positive | Potent carbonic anhydrase inhibitor<br>Hyperchloremic metabolic acidosis<br>Compensatory hyperventilation<br>Penetrates deeply |
| 0.5% silver nitrate solution | Staphylococcus species and gram-negative aerobes (Pseudomonas) | Hyponatremia<br>Hypokalemia |
| Sodium hypochlorite | Broad spectrum | At 0.025% is bactericidal without inhibiting fibroblasts or keratinocytes |
| Nystatin | Fungus | Powder easily mixed with other antimicrobials |

## COMPLICATIONS

- Care related[2,11]
  - Pneumonia: Most common cause of death in burn patients
  - Sepsis
  - Gastrointestinal complications: Ileus and ulceration
  - Renal failure: Acute tubular necrosis (ATN) from hypoperfusion
  - Shock: Inadequate end-organ perfusion

**TIP:** Signs of sepsis:

1. Hyperventilation
2. Fever or hypothermia
3. Hyperglycemia
4. Obtundation
5. Ileus
6. Hypotension and oliguria

- Surgical
  - Graft loss
  - Burn scar contracture
  - Wound breakdown

**TIP:** Three most common causes of skin graft loss:

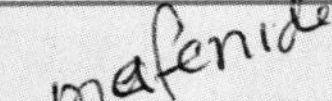


1. Hematoma
2. Infection
3. Shear

### KEY POINTS

- ✓ Decreased sensation occurs with deep second-degree and deeper burns.
- ✓ Know the criteria for admission for burn injuries—they are frequently asked on tests.
- ✓ The Parkland formula is used to calculate initial resuscitation for the first 24 hours after burn injury. The time of injury, not the time of presentation, is used to figure the rate.
- ✓ Silver sulfadiazine can cause leukopenia.
- ✓ Mafenide acetate can cause metabolic acidosis secondary to its inhibition of carbonic anhydrase.

## REFERENCES


1. American Burn Association National Burn Repository Advisory Committee. 2011 National Burn Repository: report of data from 2001-2010. Available at *http://www.ameriburn.org/2011NBRAnnualReport.pdf.*
2. Herndon DN, ed. Total Burn Care, 4th ed. Philadelphia: Saunders-Elsevier, 2012.
3. American College of Surgeons Committee on Trauma. Guidelines for the operation of burn centers. In American College of Surgeons Committee on Trauma, ed. Resources for Optimal Care of the Injured Patient. Chicago, IL: American College of Surgeons, 2006.
4. Feldman J. Facial burns. In McCarthy JG, ed. Plastic Surgery, vol 3. Philadelphia: WB Saunders, 1990.

5. Advanced Burn Life Support Advisory Committee. Advanced Burn Life Support Course: Provider Manual. Chicago, IL: American Burn Association, 2007. Available at *http://ameriburn.org/ABLSProviderManual_20101018.pdf.*
6. Hendon DN, Barrow RE, Rutan RL, et al. A comparison of conservative versus early excision therapies in severely burned patients. Ann Surg 209:547-552, 1989.
7. Kagan RJ, Peck MD, Ahrenholz DH, et al. Surgical management of the burn wound and use of skin substitutes. American Burn Association White Paper. Chicago, IL: American Burn Association, 2009.
8. Brent B. Reconstruction of ear, eyebrow, and sideburn in the burned patient. Plast Reconstr Surg 55:312-317, 1975.
9. Falvey MP, Brody GS. Secondary correction of the burned eyelid deformity. Plast Reconstr Surg 62:564-570, 1978.
10. Grace SG, Brody GS. Surgical correction of burn deformities of the nose. Plast Reconstr Surg 62:848-852, 1978.
11. Tobin MJ. Advances in mechanical ventilation. N Engl J Med 344:1986-1996, 2001.

# 17. Vascular Anomalies

Samer Abouzeid, Christopher A. Derderian, John L. Burns, Jr.

## CLASSIFICATION[1,2] (Fig. 17-1)

- Rapidly involuting congenital hemangioma (RICH)
- Noninvoluting congenital hemangioma (NICH)
- Arteriovenous malformation (AVM)

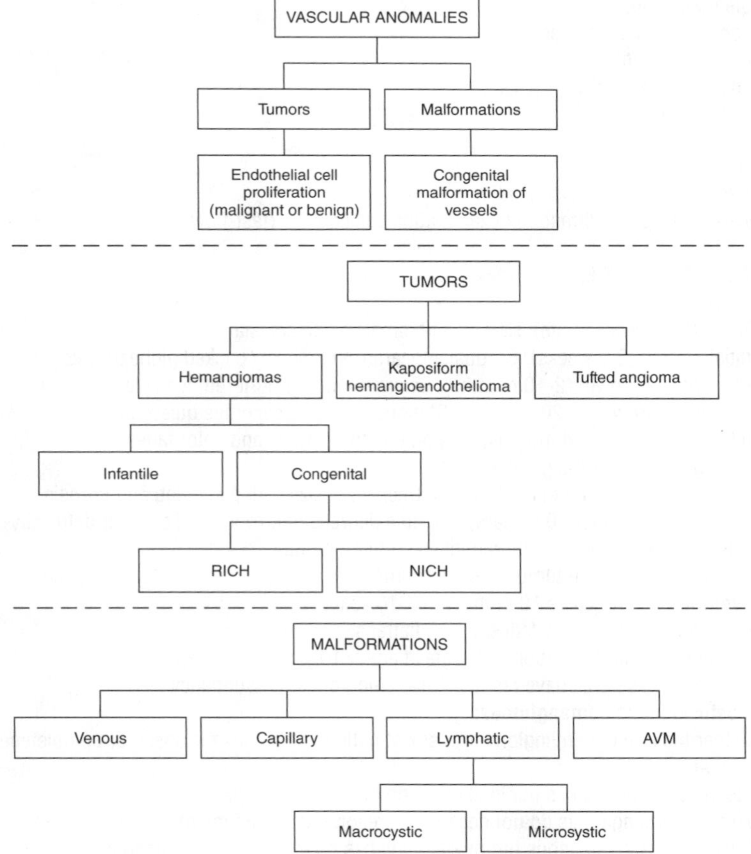


**Fig. 17-1** Classifications. (*AVM,* Arteriovenous malformation; *NICH,* noninvoluting congenital hemangioma; *RICH,* rapidly involuting congenital hemangioma.)

> **TIP:** Accurate terminology is critical for diagnosis and treatment.
>
> Hemangiomas will involute and often do not require surgery.
>
> *Port-wine stain* is a widely accepted term for venous capillary malformation.
>
> *Lymphatic malformation* should be used instead of *cystic hygroma* or *lymphangioma.*

## INFANTILE HEMANGIOMAS[3]

### EPIDEMIOLOGY

- **Most common benign tumors of infancy**
- Incidence: 4%-10% by age 1 year
- More frequent in premature low-birth-weight infants: 23%
- Female/male ratio: 3:1
- 60% occur on head and neck
- 25% occur on trunk
- 15% occur on extremity
- 80% single tumor

### DIAGNOSIS

- By history and physical examination
- If uncertain, Doppler/ultrasound examination will confirm (fast-flow tumor)

### CLINICAL COURSE

- **Appearance**
  - Origin (first weeks of life): Herald spot, small telangiectasia
  - Initial growth (2-5 weeks): Gradual appearance of closely packed pinhead lesions
  - Intermediate growth (2-10 months): Enlargement of bright red, tense lesion
  - Completed growth (6-20 months): Stationary period, becomes quiescent
  - Initial involution (6-24 months): Lesion softens/flattens and color fades.
    - Begins with central graying of skin
  - Intermediate involution (1.5-5 years): Decreased size with blanching and fibrosis
  - Completed involution (0.5 years): Variable degrees of atrophy and contour deformity
  - **Proliferative phase:** Evolution until age 0 to 12 months
    - 80% of maximum tumor size by 3-5 months
  - **Involuting phase:** Lasts 12 months to 7-10 years
    - Tumor shrinks, color fades, lesion flattens.
  - **Involuted phase:** Involution complete at age >10 years
    - 50% of cases will have residual bulk, color, or skin redundancy.
- **Prognostic signs in hemangiomas:**
  - Neither the size of hemangioma nor sex of patient influences the speed or completeness of resolution.
  - Site of hemangioma has minimal effect on final result.
  - Multiple hemangiomas do not necessarily resolve at same time or speed.
  - Presence of subcutaneous tumor elements has no effect on final outcome.
  - Early dramatic growth is not a prognostic sign of resolution.
  - Time of involution is indicative of outcome.
  - Presence of ulceration has no prognostic significance except for scar consequences.

## TREATMENT[4,5]

- **Conservative management:** Total involution occurs in 50% of hemangiomas by 5 years, in 70% by 7 years, and in >90% by 9 years.
- **Propranolol:**
  - Nonselective beta-blocker
  - Blocks noradrenaline increase of VEGF production
  - Effect on renin-angiotensin: Angiotensin-converting enzyme expressed on immature capillaries of proliferating infantile hemangioma
  - Induction of apoptosis and fat development
  - Side effects: Bradycardia, hypotension, hypoglycemia, diarrhea, somnolence
- **Steroids:**
  - In growth phase, oral or intralesional steroids can arrest growth of hemangioma but will not cause regression.
  - If lesion is too large for intralesional, give systemic steroids 3mg/kg/day for 4-8 weeks.
- **Laser:** Pulsed dye and Nd:YAG lasers can be used. Its primary role is in treatment of ulcerated hemangiomas and removing residual color from involuted hemangiomas.
- **Surgery:**
  - Depending on circumstances, surgery is typically delayed until the child is of school age and beginning to experience psychological consequences.
  - Urgent surgery is performed during proliferative phase if lesion threatens important structures or function.
    - **Visual obstruction:** During the first year of life for a period of 1 week can result in deprivation amblyopia or anisometropia
    - **Nasolaryngeal obstruction:** Hemangiomas in a "beard distribution" proliferating in subglottic airway potentially life-threatening; requires aggressive treatment with propranolol, steroids, surgery, or laser
    - **Auditory canal obstruction:** Can result in mild to moderate conductive hearing loss

## COMPLICATIONS

- **Bleeding:** Usually responds to pressure and rarely requires surgical ligation
- **Ulceration:** Most common complication, in <5% of patients
- **Infection:** Rare but more common with intraoral or perianal hemangiomas
- **Kasabach-Merritt syndrome:** Profound thrombocytopenia with kaposiform hemangioendothelioma
- **High-output heart failure:** Associated with very large liver/visceral hemangiomas, usually seen with hemangiomatosis
- **Multiple neonatal hemangiomatosis:** Mortality in infants with multiple neonatal hemangiomatosis is 54%.
- **Skeletal distortion:** Bones are typically deformed by pressure from hemangioma; bony hypertrophy is rarely seen.
- **Emotional/psychological distress:** Children become aware of their deformity around age 5; treatment should be more aggressive at this time.

## ASSOCIATED DISORDERS (Table 17-1)

- **Congenital hemangioma**
  - Fully grown at birth
  - Two clinical forms:
    1. **RICH:** Accelerated after birth involution, disappears at first year of age
    2. **NICH:** Does not involute or respond to pharmacotherapy and needs surgery if problematic

**Table 17-1** *Associated Disorders*

| Disorder | Comments |
|---|---|
| Maffucci's syndrome | Enchondromatosis associated with multiple cutaneous hemangiomas |
| von Hippel-Lindau disease | Hemangiomas of the retina<br>Hemangioblastomas of the cerebellum<br>Commonly associated with cysts of the pancreas, liver, adrenal glands, and kidneys<br>Possible seizures and mental retardation |
| PHACE syndrome | Large facial hemangiomas associated with **p**osterior fossa malformations, **h**emangiomas, **a**rterial anomalies, **c**oarctation of the aorta and other cardiac defects, and **e**ye abnormalities |
| Epithelioid hemangioma | Rare tumor of adulthood with borderline malignant potential |

- **Kaposiform hemangioendothelioma/tufted angioma**
  - Locally aggressive but does not metastasize
  - 1:1 sex ratio
  - Usually >5 cm
  - 50% association with Kasabach-Merritt phenomenon
  - **Evolution:**
    - Enlarges in early childhood
    - Regresses partially after 2 years
  - **Treatment:**
    - Systemic corticosteroids
    - Surgery

## VASCULAR MALFORMATIONS[5-8] (Table 17-2) (Fig. 17-2)

- Structural and morphologic anomalies resulting from faulty embryonic morphogenesis
- **Present at birth, grow proportionately with the child, and do not regress, unlike hemangiomas**

**Table 17-2** *Vascular Malformations*

| Malformation | Comments |
|---|---|
| Port-wine stains | Capillary malformation most commonly seen on the face in trigeminal nerve distribution |
| Venous malformation | Venous anomaly swells in the dependent position |
| Lymphatic malformation | Lymphatic anomaly, frequently infected |
| Arteriovenous malformation | High-flow lesion causes local destruction and can result in heart failure and profound consumptive coagulopathy |

### PATHOGENESIS

- **Three stages**
  1. Capillary network of interconnected blood lakes forms with no identifiable arterial or venous channels.
  2. Venous and arterial channels appear on either side of the capillary network on day 48 of gestation. Errors in this stage could result in vascular malformations.
  3. Vascular channels mature and further differentiate.
- **Development of vascular system is also influenced by autonomic nervous system, which is why port-wine stains often occur along the trigeminal nerve distribution.**

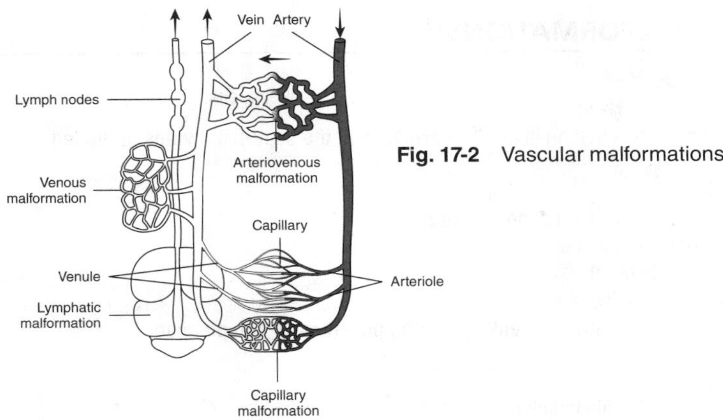


**Fig. 17-2** Vascular malformations.

## CAPILLARY MALFORMATION/PORT-WINE STAINS (Table 17-3)

### EPIDEMIOLOGY

- 0.3% of newborns affected
- Most frequent in the face: 80%
- Can exist everywhere on the body
- If trigeminal ($V_1$-$V_2$) nerve distribution:
  - Sturge-Weber syndrome
  - Sometimes accompanied by ocular and central nervous system disorders
- Female/male ratio: 3:1

### TREATMENT[9,10]

- Photocoagulation with pulsed dye laser (585 nm) and/or Nd:YAG laser
  - Multiple treatments necessary with $V_2$ distribution (responds poorly)
- Combined laser and pharmacologic treatment: Pulsed dye laser and imiquimod (antiangiogenetic agent)
- Ophthalmologic evaluation for glaucoma if $V_1$ lesions
- Left untreated, 70% progress to cobblestoning ectasia.

**Table 17-3** *Syndromes With Port-Wine Stains*

| Syndrome | Comments |
|---|---|
| Sturge-Weber syndrome | Large facial port-wine stain with $V_1$ and commonly $V_2$ trigeminal nerve distribution<br>Associated with leptomeningeal venous malformations and frequent mental retardation |
| Klippel-Trénaunay syndrome | Patchy port-wine stain on an extremity overlying a deeper venous and lymphatic malformation with associated skeletal hypertrophy |
| Parkes Weber syndrome | Similar to Klippel-Trénaunay but distinguished by the presence of an arteriovenous fistula |

## VENOUS MALFORMATIONS[11]

### Epidemiology

- Incidence: 1%-4%
- Most common presentation in adults: **Varicosity of the superficial veins of the leg**

### Diagnosis

- Blue or purple lesions with spongy texture
- Swell in dependent position
- **Deflate when elevated**
- Aching in extremity lesions
- Can be hormone sensitive and enlarge during puberty and with pregnancy

### Treatment

- Many lesions amenable to sclerotherapy
- Extremity aching managed with compression garments, NSAIDs, analgesics
- Laser treatment: Nd:YAG or argon laser
- Surgical resection
- Complications
  - Episodes of thrombosis
  - Localized intravascular coagulation that could evolve into disseminated intravascular coagulation

## LYMPHATIC MALFORMATIONS

### Diagnosis

- Clear cutaneous vesicles signify a dermal lymphatic component in a vascular malformation.
- Soft and compressible
- Often cause **bony overgrowth**

### Pathogenesis

- Combined venous and lymphatic vascular anomalies are frequent.
- Histologic types
  - Macrocystic
  - Microcystic

### Treatment

- Injection with sclerosing agent effective in macrocystic type
- Laser ablation for cutaneous blebs
- Surgery
- Compression
- Corticosteroids and antibiotics for inflammatory episodes

### Complications

- **Frequent infection:** Aggressive antibiotic therapy crucial
- Surgical morbidity high with lymphatic formation of blebs through the surgical area, prolonged draining, slow wound healing, and potential infection
- Recurrence after surgical resection

## ARTERIOVENOUS MALFORMATIONS (AVMs)[4] (Table 17-4)

### Diagnosis

- **Pulsatile high-flow lesion**
- Anatomy and hemodynamics defined by angiography
- MRI useful in determining extent of lesion

### Clinical Aspects

- **Stage 1 (quiescent):** Warm pink to bluish stain
- **Stage 2 (expansion):** Thrill and dilated venous network formation
- **Stage 3 (destruction):** Cutaneous ulcers, necrosis, frequent bleeding
- **Stage 4 (decompensation):** Cardiac decompensation

### Treatment

- Preoperative medical management of any underlying coagulation defect secondary to thrombotic consumption
- Preoperative embolization followed by surgical resection **within 72 hours**
- **Wide local excision because recurrence rates are very high**
- Use of ischemic suture techniques, hypotensive anesthesia, and cardiopulmonary bypass to control bleeding
- Postexcisional reconstruction with flaps often necessary

### Complications

- Consumptive coagulopathy
- Congestive heart failure
- Local destruction of normal anatomy
- Surgical bleeding

**Table 17-4** *Syndromes With Vascular Anomalies*

| Syndrome | Comments |
|---|---|
| Bannayan-Zonana syndrome | Microcephaly, multiple lipomas, multiple vascular malformations |
| Riley-Smith syndrome | Pseudopapilledema, microcephaly, vascular malformations |
| Blue rubber bleb nevus syndrome | Similar to Klippel-Trénaunay syndrome but distinguished by the presence of an arteriovenous fistula |
| Osler-Weber-Rendu disease (hereditary hemorrhagic telangiectasia) | Multiple malformed ecstatic vessels in the skin, mucous membranes, viscera |

## KEY POINTS

- ✓ AVMs frequently require preoperative embolization immediately before surgical resection.
- ✓ Hemangiomas are the most common tumor of infancy and frequently involute spontaneously (general rule: 70% involute by 7 years).
- ✓ Treat hemangiomas nonsurgically unless they involve bleeding, ulceration, or obstruction of an orifice.
- ✓ Vascular malformations are present at birth (in contrast to hemangiomas) and do not regress.
- ✓ Port-wine stains typically affect the area along the distribution of the trigeminal nerve.
- ✓ Venous malformations swell in the dependent position and can be hormone sensitive.
- ✓ Lymphatic malformations often cause bony overgrowth.

## REFERENCES

1. Philandrianos C, Degardin N, Casanova D, et al. [Diagnosis and management of vascular anomalies] Ann Chir Plast Esthet 56:241-253, 2011.
2. Greene AK, ed. Vascular Anomalies: Classification, Diagnosis, and Management. St Louis: Quality Medical Publishing, 2013.
3. Drolet BA, Esterly NB, Frieden IJ. Hemangiomas in children. N Engl J Med 341:173-181, 1999.
4. Folkman J. Successful treatment of an angiogenic disease. N Engl J Med 320:1211-1212, 1989.
5. Greene AK. Management of hemangiomas and other vascular tumors. Clin Plast Surg 38:45-63, 2011.
6. Young AE. Pathogenesis of vascular malformations. In Mulliken JB, Young AE, eds. Vascular Birthmarks: Hemangiomas and Malformations. Philadelphia: WB Saunders, 1988.
7. Kohout MP, Hansen M, Pribaz JJ, et al. Arterio-venous malformations of the head and neck: natural history and management. Plast Reconstr Surg 102:643-654, 1998.
8. Huang JT, Liang MG. Vascular malformations. Pediatr Clin North Am 57:1091-1110, 2010.
9. Greene AK, Orbach DB. Management of arteriovenous malformations. Clin Plast Surg 38:95-106, 2011.
10. Maguiness SM, Liang MG. Management of capillary malformations. Clin Plast Surg 38:65-73, 2011.
11. Greene AK, Alomari AI. Management of venous malformations. Clin Plast Surg 38:83-93, 2011.

# 18. Congenital Nevi

Dawn D. Wells, John L. Burns, Jr., Kendall R. Roehl

## DEMOGRAPHICS

### INCIDENCE[1]

Lesion must be present at birth to be classified as congenital.

- Equal prevalence in males and females
- Occurrence in all races
- One percent incidence in newborns, with greater incidence in blacks (1.8%)
- Giant congenital nevocytic nevi (CNN) (>20 cm): 1:20,000

## CLASSIFICATION

- Classification based on size and clinical appearance (Table 18-1)

**Table 18-1** *Classification of Congenital Nevi*

| Size | Comments |
|---|---|
| Small (<1.5 $cm^2$) | Tan to brown, irregularly shaped maculae or papules with mottled freckling<br>Darken with puberty<br>May become elevated and develop hair |
| Medium (1.5 $cm^2$-20 $cm^2$) | Same properties as small congenital nevi |
| Giant (>20 $cm^2$) | Dark, hairy, with verrucous texture<br>Satellite lesions often present<br>Also called *bathing suit nevi, stocking,* or *coat-sleeve*<br>May extend into the leptomeninges and have associated neurologic manifestations such as epilepsy<br>Those that overlie the vertebral column may be associated with spina bifida or meningomyelocele<br>May be associated with neurofibromatosis |

**TIP:** After birth, CNN grow in proportion to overall increase in body size.

## HISTOPATHOPHYSIOLOGY

### DISTINGUISHING FEATURES

- CNN are usually characterized as nevus cells between collagen bundles located in the deeper dermis, but they may also invade appendages, vessels, and nerves.
- **Acquired nevi** are usually composed of nevus cells limited to papillary and upper reticular dermis and **do not involve skin appendages.**

- Giant CNN have similar histopathology as small and medium nevi, except they may extend into muscle, bone, dura mater, and cranium.
- Nevus cells originate from neural crest melanocytes. Congenital nevi have been found to harbor *N-RAS* mutations.[2]

## NEUROCUTANEOUS MELANOSIS[2]

- *Neuromelanosis* is melanocytic proliferation (benign or malignant, nodular or diffuse) within the leptomeninges and brain parenchyma.
- *Neurocutaneous melanosis* is neuromelanosis associated with CNN.
- When the central nervous system is affected, patients are usually symptomatic by 2 years of age.
- Symptoms are related to increased intracranial pressure (headache, lethargy, recurrent vomiting, and photophobia), hydrocephalus, seizures, cranial nerve palsies, sensorimotor deficits, bowel and bladder dysfunction, and developmental delay.
- Diagnostic image of choice is **MRI;** should be done in first 4 months of life before myelination, which may obscure melanin deposits.
- Little to no treatment except managing intracranial pressure issues.
- If neurologic symptoms are present, prognosis is very poor.

## RISK OF MALIGNANT TRANSFORMATION

The risk of malignant transformation is a controversial topic for which there are many opinions.[3-6]

- Small CNN lifetime risk of melanoma development is 1%-5%.
- Medium CNN lifetime risk of melanoma development is uncertain.
- Small- and medium-sized nevi rarely change into melanoma before puberty.
- **Of giant nevi, 5%-10% result in melanoma, and 50% usually arise between 3 and 5 years.**
- Melanoma development with giant CNN has a poor prognosis.

### CLINICAL FINDINGS

- Rapid increase in size
- Irregularity of border
- Development of asymmetry
- Variation of color within the nevus
- Development of satellite lesions
- Changes in texture

## MANAGEMENT

Management is controversial and is based on risk of malignant transformation, cosmetic appearance, risk of scarring, and psychological issues.

- CNN occurring within the first 2 years of life are called *congenital nevus tardive* and should be managed according to appearance and growth pattern.
- Nongiant nevi should be observed annually for changes. If suspicious, a biopsy should be performed, or the nevi should be removed by prophylactic excision, especially if they are anatomically difficult to monitor (e.g., on the back or scalp).
- Nevi smaller than 1.5 cm not known to be present at birth should be treated like acquired nevi and managed according to their color, growth, and pattern.
- Atypical-appearing CNN should be removed regardless of size.

- Giant CNN should be completely excised as soon as possible.
- Surgical techniques include skin grafts, flaps, tissue expanders, or tissue culture using the patient's own healthy skin.[7-10]
  - **Scalp:** Serial tissue expansion is the modality of choice for larger lesions, and serial excision can be used for smaller lesions.
  - **Face:** Often requires combined tissue expansion and skin grafting (split and full thickness) with careful attention to preserving anatomic structures (such as eyelid, eyebrow, nose, lip, and hairline). Often tissue expansion is used to create larger skin grafts to limit donor scars (e.g., supraclavicular region).
  - **Trunk:** Tissue expansion and flap transposition, usually using abdominoplasty principles anteriorly. Also, expanded free tissue transfers can be used when necessary. Trend is to use less skin grafting in this location.
  - **Extremities:** Challenging because of tissue expansion limitations. Many use expanded full-thickness skin grafts to improve contour, but even these lead to long-term color mismatch/contour deformities. When possible use local flaps (expanded if necessary) and free-tissue transfers to add soft tissue bulk.
- Patients with giant nevi should have imaging studies performed to rule out CNS involvement.
- Other modalities (e.g., laser or curettage) to remove congenital nevi have high recurrence rates.[10]

## DIFFERENTIAL DIAGNOSIS

**The following lesions can sometimes be confused with CNN:**

- **Café au lait spot:** May be present at birth, but usually develops in childhood; well-circumscribed, homogenous color of coffee with milk, oval, completely macular. Often associated with neurofibromatosis.
- **Nevus spilus:** Usually acquired, but some are congenital; tan macula commonly 1-4 cm in diameter and speckled with dark brown papules or maculae 1-6 mm in diameter.
- **Epidermal nevus:** Present at birth or develop in early childhood; tan or brown warty macules or papules, linear array without plaques or hair; most commonly located on extremities.
- **Common acquired nevus:** Few nevi are present in early childhood; may be brown, tan, or skin-colored; round or ovoid lesions.
- **Atypical (dysplastic) nevus:** Occurs during puberty or later; usually more than one color of brown, irregular lesion; usually larger than 6 mm; most commonly found on trunk.
- **Blue nevus:** Usually appears in late adolescence; generally smaller than 1 cm; firm, dark-blue to gray-black, sharply defined round papule; most commonly found on dorsa of hands or feet, head, and neck.
- **Becker's nevus:** Onset at adolescence; lesions commonly found on the shoulders of males in unilateral distribution; color varies from uniformly tan to dark brown; margins usually irregular; hair usually develops after pigmentation; mean size 125 $cm^2$.
- **Halo nevus:** Generally seen in individuals younger than 20 years; appears as white halo around nevus (lymphocytic reaction); most commonly found on upper backs of teenagers.
- **Mongolian spot:** Steel-blue macula present at birth or first few weeks of life in **lumbosacral** area; size ranges from a few centimeters to 20 cm or more; more common in darkly pigmented skin; usually disappears in early childhood.
- **Nevus of Ota:** Onset at birth or less than 1 year and around puberty; especially found in Asians and blacks; blue-brown unilateral periocular macula; size varies from a few centimeters in diameter to lesions covering half the face; **areas follow the distribution of the first two branches of the trigeminal nerve.**

- **Nevus of Ito:** Usually appears at birth; typically found in Asians and blacks; large, blue-brown macula located on posterior shoulder, areas innervated by posterior supraclavicular and lateral cutaneous brachial nerves.
- **Spitz nevus:** Usually appears at birth; also called juvenile melanoma; red or pigmented smooth dome-shaped papule; **telangiectasia** is a frequent finding; average diameter 8 mm; most commonly found on head and neck; recommended excision both diagnostic and therapeutic.
- **Nevus sebaceus:** Onset at birth; solitary yellowish-orange, waxy plaque; usually found on scalp; **potential transformation to basal cell carcinoma (10%-15%),** so excision recommended.

## KEY POINTS

- ✓ Congenital nevi *must* be present at birth.
- ✓ Congenital nevus tardive are nevi that occur within the first 2 years of life.
- ✓ Giant congenital nevi are usually classified as those nevi larger than 20 $cm^2$, covering more than 1% of total body surface area (TBSA), or bigger than the size of a palm.
- ✓ CNN cells invade skin appendages, whereas acquired nevi cells do not.
- ✓ Giant nevi have a malignant transformation rate of 5%-10% (melanoma).
- ✓ Imaging studies are necessary for patients with giant nevi to rule out CNS involvement.
- ✓ Blue nevi commonly occur on the head, neck, and dorsa of hands or feet.
- ✓ A nevus of Ota follows the distribution of $V_1$ and $V_2$.
- ✓ A nevus of Ito is located on the posterior shoulder along the distribution of the posterior supraclavicular and lateral cutaneous brachial nerves.
- ✓ Nevus sebaceous have potential for malignant transformation (10%-15%) (basal cell).

## REFERENCES


1. Bett BJ. Large or multiple congenital melanocytic nevi: occurrence of cutaneous melanoma in 1008 persons. J Am Acad Dermatol 52:793-797, 2005.
2. Alikhan A, Ibrahimi OA, Eisen DB. Congenital melanocytic nevi: where are we now? Part I. Clinical presentation, epidemiology, pathogenesis, histology, malignant transformation, and neurocutaneous melanosis. J Am Acad Dermatol 67:495, 2012.
3. Marghoob AA. Congenital melanocytic nevi: evaluation and management. Dermatol Clin 20:607-616, 2002.
4. Patterson WM, Lefkowitz A, Schwartz RA, et al. Melanoma in children. Cutis 65:269-272, 2000.
5. Rhodes AR, Silverman RA, Harrist TJ, et al. A histologic comparison of congenital and acquired nevomelanocytic nevi. Arch Dermatol 121:1266-1273, 1985.
6. Rhodes AR, Wood WC, Sober AJ, et al. Nonepidermal origin of malignant melanoma associated with a giant congenital nevocellular nevus. Plast Reconstr Surg 67:782-790, 1981.
7. Bauer BS, Vicari FA. An approach to excision of congenital giant pigmented nevi in infancy and early childhood. Plast Reconstr Surg 82:1012-1021, 1988.
8. Gosain AK, Santoro TD, Larson DL, et al. Giant congenital nevi: a 20-year experience and an algorithm for their management. Plast Reconstr Surg 108:622-636, 2001.
9. Bauer B. Discussion: Giant congenital nevi: a 20-year experience and an algorithm for their management. Plast Reconstr Surg 108:632, 2001.
10. Ibrahimi OA, Alikhan A, Eisen DB. Congenital melanocytic nevi: where are we now? Part II. Treatment options and approach to treatment. J Am Acad Dermatol 67:515, 2012.

# PART III

## Head and Neck

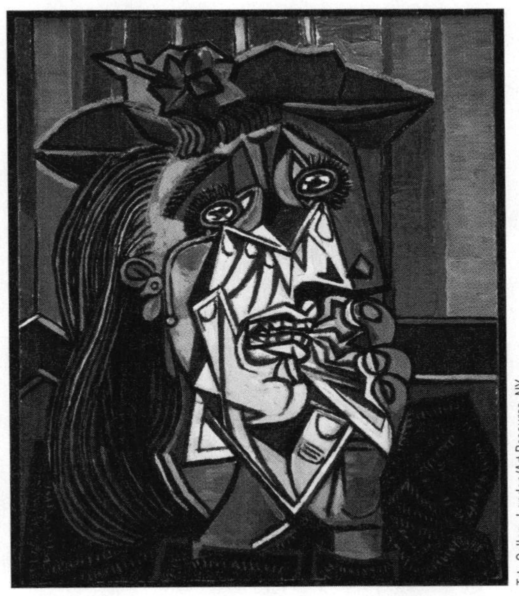

Part III opening art: Picasso, Pablo (1881-1973) © Artist Rights Society (ARS), NY. The Weeping Woman [Femme en pleurs]. 1937. Oil on canvas, 60.8 × 50.0 cm. Tate Gallery, London, Great Britain. Photo Credit: Tate Gallery, London/Art Resource, NY. © 2006 Estate of Pablo Picasso/ARS, New York.

# 19. Head and Neck Embryology

Huay-Zong Law, Thornwell Hay Parker III

## THE BUILDING BLOCKS[1-5]

- **Ectoderm:** Nervous system, skin (epidermis and appendages), and neural crest cells and derivatives
- **Mesoderm:** Bone, cartilage, muscles, connective tissue (dermis), dura mater, heart, vessels, blood, reproductive organs, and genitourinary system
- **Endoderm:** Gastrointestinal and respiratory lining and digestive organ parenchyma

## PHARYNGEAL (BRANCHIAL) STRUCTURES[2-6]

- **Neural crest cells** are uniquely ectodermal in origin but pluripotent.
  - Migrate along cleavage planes, differentiating into connective, muscle, nervous, endocrine, and pigmentary tissues
  - Induce differentiation of the tissue they invade
- **Pharyngeal arches** form from migrating neural crest cells and surrounding pharyngeal endoderm and mesoderm (Fig. 19-1).
- They are different from **somites,** which are mesodermal swellings around the neural tube.
- Each arch is separated by **pharyngeal grooves** on the *external* surface, and **pharyngeal pouches** on the *internal* surface. Grooves and pouches are separated by mesoderm.

**NOTE:** ***Branchia*** **comes from Greek root for** ***gill.*** **Some recent texts prefer the use of** ***pharyngeal*** **to** ***branchial.***

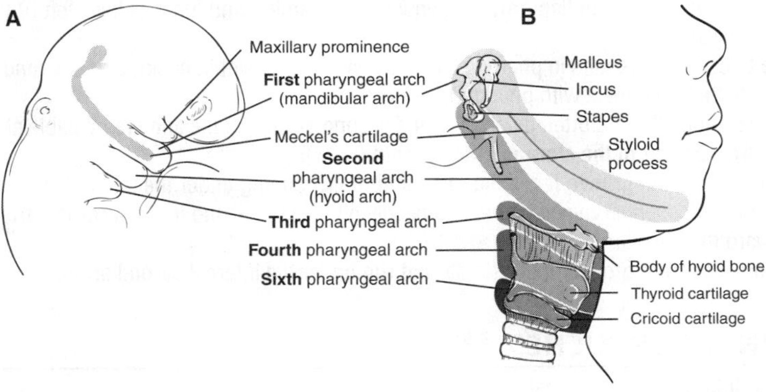


**Fig. 19-1** **A,** Lateral view of pharyngeal arches. **B,** Cartilaginous and bony structures.

## PHARYNGEAL ARCHES[1-5] (Table 19-1)

- Typically **six** arches are described; however, the first four are the most prominent.
- Each arch has four components: nervous, arterial, muscular, and bony.
- Original muscular innervations are maintained despite migration.

**Table 19-1** *Pharyngeal Arch Derivatives*[1-5]

| Arch | Nerve | Artery | Bone | Muscle |
|---|---|---|---|---|
| I | **CN V** | Maxillary | Greater wing of sphenoid, incus, malleus, **maxilla,** zygomatic, temporal (squamous), **mandible** | **Muscles of mastication,** anterior digastric, mylohyoid, tensor tympani, **tensor veli palatini** |
| II | **CN VII** | Stapedial (corticotympanic) | Stapes, styloid process, stylohyoid ligament, lesser horn and upper body of hyoid | **Muscles of facial expression,** posterior digastric, stylohoid, stapedius |
| III | **CN IX** | Common carotid, proximal internal carotid | Greater horns and lower body of hyoid | Stylopharyngeus |
| IV/VI | **CN X** | Aortic arch, right subclavian, origin of pulmonary arteries, ductus arteriosus | Laryngeal cartilages | **Pharyngeal constrictors, levator veli palatini,** palatoglossus, striated upper esophageal muscles, **laryngeal** muscles |

**TIP:** The boldface structures above are usually tested on written examinations.

## PHARYNGEAL GROOVES[2-5]

- **Groove I:** Becomes the **external auditory canal.** The mesoderm becomes the tympanic membrane.
- **Grooves II-IV:** Operculum flap grows downward from arch II and fuses below cleft IV to create the *cervical sinus.*
- Failure to obliterate results in pharyngeal cleft **cysts** (sealed within neck), **sinuses** (end in blind sac), or **fistulas** (connect with pharynx).
  - These anomalies are often detected in the second decade of life and are palpable at the **anterior border of the sternocleidomastoid** (SCM).
  - Anomalies from **groove II are the most common,** running under the middle/lower SCM, over the glossopharyngeal nerve, and between the external and internal carotid arteries toward the tonsillar fossa.
  - Anomalies from groove III are similar but run under the internal carotid artery.

## PHARYNGEAL POUCHES[1-3,5]

- **Pouch I:** Internal auditory canal
- **Pouch II:** Palatine tonsil
- **Pouch III:** Inferior parathyroid and thymus
- **Pouch IV:** Superior parathyroid **(pouch IV migrates above pouch III)**
- **Pouch V:** Ultimobranchial body (thyroid C cells)

## BONE FORMATION[2,4]

- **Intramembranous ossification:** Cartilaginous precursors resorb; mesenchymal cells directly differentiate into osteoblasts without a cartilaginous intermediate.
- **Endochondral ossification:** A cartilaginous template is directly and gradually replaced with a bony matrix.

## CRANIUM[1,2,7]

- **Neurocranium:** Portion of skull encasing and protecting the brain
  - **Membranous neurocranium**
    - Forms via **intramembranous ossification** of neural crest origin
    - Includes paired frontal, squamosal, and parietal bones, and upper occipital bone
  - **Cartilaginous neurocranium (e.g., basicranium)**
    - Forms via **endochondral ossification** of mesodermal origin
    - Includes sphenoid and ethmoid bones, mastoid and petrous temporal bone, and the base of the occipital bone
- **Viscerocranium:** Bones of facial skeleton
  - Forms primarily via **intramembranous ossification** of **pharyngeal arch I,** except for **Meckel's cartilage** (which forms the malleus and mandibular condyles)
- **Growth**
  - Cranial vault grows in response to brain growth.
  - Bone growth proceeds perpendicular to orientation of sutures.
  - **Craniosynostosis:** Sutures fuse prematurely, associated with *FGFR* and *TGFβR,* and *Twist* and *Wnt* pathways (see Chapter 21).
  - **Virchow's law:** After suture fusion, growth proceeds parallel to suture instead of perpendicular.

## FACE[1-7] (Figs. 19-2 and 19-3)

- The face develops from **five prominences:** Frontonasal (1), maxillary (2), and mandibular (2).
- **Frontonasal prominence**
  - Pulled ventrally and caudally, forming the forehead, nasal dorsum, and medial and lateral nasal prominences
  - **Nasal placodes** at lateral aspect of frontonasal complex develop into depressed **nasal pits** initially in contact with the stomodeum, and eventually form the nares.
  - Diverticula of lateral nasal walls extend into bones to form **sinuses** (maxillary at 3 months' gestation, ethmoid at 5 months' gestation, sphenoid 5 months postnatally, frontal 2-6 years postnatally).
  - The **medial nasal prominence** forms the primary palate, midmaxilla, midlip, philtrum, central nose, and septum.
  - The **lateral nasal prominence** forms the nasal alae.
- **Maxillary prominences**
  - These migrate medially to form the secondary palate, lateral maxilla, and lateral lip.
  - This action compresses the medial nasal prominences together, separating the nasal pits and stomodeum (the eventual nasal and oral cavities).
  - The junction with the lateral nasal prominences forms the nasolacrimal groove and nasolacrimal duct system. Failure of fusion produces an **oblique facial cleft** (Tessier number 3).

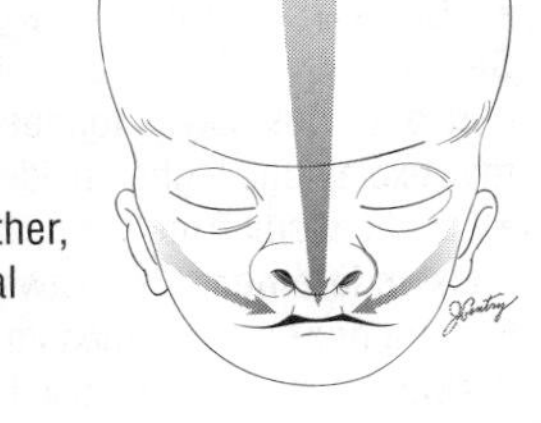

**Fig. 19-2** Migratory pattern of ectomesenchyme to form the facial processes.

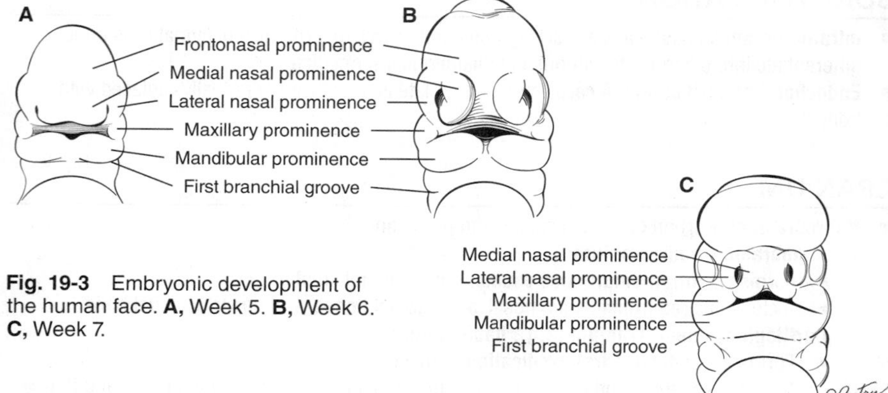


**Fig. 19-3** Embryonic development of the human face. **A,** Week 5. **B,** Week 6. **C,** Week 7.

- **Mandibular prominences** form the mandible, lower lip, and lower face.
- Prominent **growth factors** and **signaling pathways** are important, numerous, and increasingly identified. These include TGFβ, BMP, FGF, SH3, IRF, Wnt, and FOXE1.
  - Teratogens affecting the Sonic hedgehog pathway include retinoids, alcohol, and certain drugs that influence cholesterol synthesis and transport.

## MOUTH[2-5]

- **Stomodeum:** Primitive mouth forms at 3-4 weeks from invagination of ectoderm around buccopharyngeal membrane.
- **Unilateral cleft lips** result from failure of fusion of a medial nasal prominence and a maxillary prominence.
- A cleft at the **lateral oral commissure** results from failure of fusion of maxillary and mandibular prominences (Tessier number 7).
- **Median cleft lips** are rare and result from failure of medial nasal prominences to fuse (Tessier number 0). Central defects of the lower lip and chin similarly result from failure of mandibular processes to merge.

## PALATE[2-7]

- **Primary palate** (5-6 weeks): Medial nasal prominences come together to form the primary palate, midmaxilla, and septum.
  - Clefts result from failure of fusion of medial and lateral palatine processes.
- **Secondary palate** (9-12 weeks): Lateral palatine shelves initially hang vertically but assume a horizontal position as tongue drops with mandibular growth; the right palate drops first, which may explain the higher incidence of clefts on the left side.
  - Clefts result from failure of fusion of lateral palatine process with nasal septum.
- **Incisive foramen:** Lies between the primary and secondary palate
- **Epstein pearls** along median raphe or junction of hard/soft palates result from cystic degeneration of epithelial lining at edges.
- **Nasopalatine duct cysts** at the incisive foramen result from epithelial entrapment at the junction of developing primary/secondary palates.

## THYROID[2-5]

- From endodermal proliferation of **foramen cecum** of tongue. The thyroid descends with a trailing thyroid diverticulum to final position distal to cricoid cartilage.
- **Thyroglossal duct cysts** may form anywhere along this path, presenting as a painless midline neck mass. Infection and rupture may result in sinus or fistula formation.
- **Lingual thyroids** result from failure of descent.

## TONGUE[2-5]

- **Anterior two thirds** originates from pharyngeal arch I and is innervated by the lingual nerve (CN $V_3$).
- **Posterior third** originates from arches III and IV (these overtake arch II) and is innervated by CN IX and X.
- Muscles arise largely from occipital myotomes (CN XII) except for the palatoglossus (CN X).

## EXTERNAL EAR[2-5]

- Forms at interface between pharyngeal arches I and II.
- **Arch I** forms three anterior hillocks (tragus, root of helix, and superior helix).
- **Arch II** forms three posterior hillocks (antitragus, antihelix, and lobule).
- **Groove I** lies between these arches and forms the external auditory canal.

**TIP:** These are frequent test questions.

- The ear develops in the neck region. Arrested growth (microtia) usually results in an inferiorly displaced auricle.

### KEY POINTS

✓ **Arch I**
  - Produces maxillary and mandibular arches
  - Forms muscles of mastication and carries CN V
  - Forms three anterior hillocks: Tragus, root of helix, and superior helix

✓ **Cleft I**
  - Becomes external auditory canal

✓ **Arch II**
  - Forms muscles of facial expression, carries CN VII
  - Forms three posterior hillocks: Antihelix, antitragus, and lobule

✓ **Frontonasal prominence:** Forehead and apex of nose, medial and lateral nasal prominences

✓ **Medial nasal prominence:** Primary palate, midmaxilla, midlip, philtrum, central nose, and septum

✓ **Lateral nasal prominences:** Nasal alae

✓ **Maxillary prominences:** Secondary palate, lateral maxilla, and lateral lip

✓ **Mandibular prominences:** Mandible, lower lip, and lower face

✓ Anomalies of **pharyngeal groove II** are the most common and typically are present over the SCM.

✓ **Pharyngeal pouch III** becomes the **inferior** parathyroid glands, and **pharyngeal pouch IV** becomes the **superior** parathyroid glands.

## REFERENCES


1. Afshar M, Brugmann SA, Helms JA. Embryology of the craniofacial complex. In Neligan PC, ed. Plastic Surgery, 3rd ed. London: Elsevier, 2013.
2. Carlson BM, ed. Human Embryology and Developmental Biology, 4th ed. Philadelphia: Elsevier, 2009.
3. Gosain AK, Nacamuli R. Embryology of the head and neck. In Thorne CH, Bartlett SP, Beasley RW, et al, eds. Grabb and Smith's Plastic Surgery, 6th ed. Philadelphia: Lippincott Williams & Wilkins, 2007.
4. Moore KL, Persaud TV, Torchia MD, eds. The Developing Human: Clinically Oriented Embryology, 9th ed. Philadelphia: Saunders Elsevier, 2008.
5. Sadler TW, ed. Langman's Medical Embryology. Baltimore: Lippincott Williams & Wilkins, 2012.
6. Tepper OM, Warren SM. Craniofacial embryology. In Weinzwig J, ed. Plastic Surgery Secrets Plus, 2nd ed. Philadelphia: Elsevier, 2010.
7. Rice DP. Craniofacial genetics and dysmorphology. In Guyuron B, Eriksson S, Persing J, eds. Plastic Surgery: Indications and Practice. Philadelphia: Saunders Elsevier, 2009.

# 20. Surgical Treatment of Migraine Headaches

Jeffrey E. Janis, Adam H. Hamawy

## DEMOGRAPHICS[1-3]

- Migraine headaches affect 12% of the population.
- Affects over 35 million Americans
- Worldwide lifetime prevalence between 11% and 32%
- Affects one in every four households
- Affects 18% of women and 6% of men
  - Ninth leading cause of disability in women globally
- Cost of medical treatment in United States over $14 billion
- More common than asthma and diabetes combined
- Commonly interferes with daily function
- 112 million collective workdays lost each year
- A third of patients not helped by standard medications

## ETIOLOGIC FACTORS/PATHOPHYSIOLOGY[3]

### Centrally Mediated

- Interictal cortical derangements result in hyperexcitable cortical neurons.
- Periaqueductal gray matter is dysfunctional.

### Peripherally Mediated

- Trigeminal nerve branch irritation causes release of substance P, calcitonin gene–related peptide (CGRP), and neurokinin A in cell bodies.
- Substances travel up nerve, resulting in localized meningitis.
- **Nerve irritation is thought to occur by adjacent muscular, skeletal, fascial, or vascular compression.**

## TRADITIONAL MIGRAINE THERAPY

Combination of avoidance of migraine triggers, prophylactic pharmacologic intervention, abortive therapy, and acute analgesic therapy

### Prophylactic Pharmacotherapy

- Goal: **Reduce frequency and severity** of migraine attacks
- Beta-blockers: Propranolol (Inderal)
- Calcium channel blockers: Verapamil (Covera)
- Antidepressants: Amitriptyline (Elavil), nortriptyline (Pamelor)
- Anticonvulsants: Gabapentin (Neurontin), valproic acid (Depakote), topiramate (Topamax)
- Antihistamines: Diphenhydramine (Benadryl), cyproheptadine (Periactin)

### Abortive Pharmacotherapy

- Goal: **Prevent migraine or stop attack** once it has begun
- Triptans: Tryptamine-based drugs that act on serotonin 5-$HT_{1b}$ and 5-$HT_{1d}$ receptors in cranial blood vessels and nerve endings
  - Sumatriptan (Imitrex)
  - Zolmitriptan (Zomig)
  - Eletriptan (Relpax)
  - Naratriptan (Amerge, Naramig)
  - Rizatriptan (Maxalt)
  - Frovatriptan (Frova)
  - Almotriptan (Axert)
- Inhibit release of several neuropeptides, including CGRP and substance P

### Acute Analgesics

- Goal: Relieve mild to moderate symptoms of migraine after onset
  - Nonsteroidal antiinflammatory drugs (NSAIDs): Ibuprofen, aspirin, diclofenac
  - Acetaminophen (Tylenol)
  - Combination of aspirin, acetaminophen, and caffeine (Excedrin)
    - Combination shown to be as effective as sumatriptan for moderate to severe migraine pain[4]

### Disadvantages of Traditional Treatments

- Must be taken on a regular basis
- Can be expensive, even with insurance
- Time required to take effect
- Can have unacceptable side effects
  - Drowsiness
  - Weight gain
  - Alopecia
  - Difficulty concentrating
  - Contraindicated with some conditions, including pregnancy, heart disease, stroke
  - Do not "cure" the migraine
  - Ineffective in about 30% of patients

## PERIPHERAL TRIGGER ANATOMY

### Frontal Triggers

- **Supraorbital nerve (SON)**
  - Terminal branch of ophthalmic division ($V_1$) of the trigeminal nerve
  - Four branching patterns relative to corrugator muscle[5] (Fig. 20-1)
  - Multiple points of compression
    - Muscular: Corrugator supercilii, depressor supercilii, and procerus
      - Corrugators start 3 mm lateral to midline and end at ~85% of distance to lateral orbital rim (Fig. 20-2).
      - Nerve may branch inside body of corrugators.
    - Bony and fascial: Nerve entrance into brow through **supraorbital foramen** or **tight supraorbital notch,** with compression of nerve as it passes through
      - Fascial band identified in 86% of supraorbital notches
      - Subclassified into three categories[6]

1. **Type I** bands are composed of a simple facial band over a single opening and are most prevalent (51%).
2. **Type II** bands have "partial bony" spicules bridging the neurovascular bundle (30%).
3. **Type III** bands contain a "septum" that can be horizontal (IIIA) or vertical (IIIB) and allow a double passage for the supraorbital neurovascular bundle (Fig. 20-3).

- Vascular: Adjacent supraorbital artery

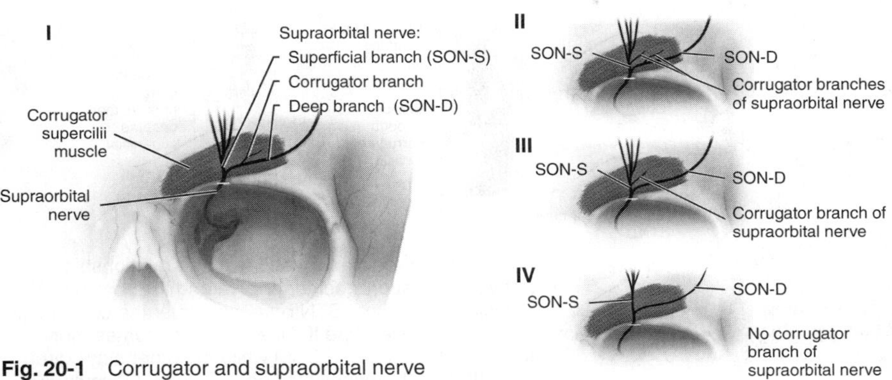


**Fig. 20-1** Corrugator and supraorbital nerve anatomy.

**Fig. 20-2** Comprehensive corrugator supercilii muscle dimensions.

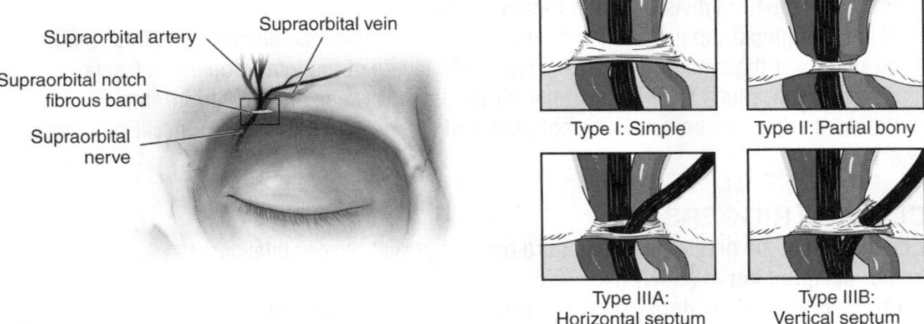


**Fig. 20-3** Bony, fascial, and vascular compression of the supraorbital nerve.

- **Supratrochlear nerve (STN)**[7]
  - Terminal branch of ophthalmic division ($V_1$) of the trigeminal nerve
  - Three branching patterns relative to corrugator muscle (Fig. 20-4)
  - Three points of compression
    1. **Bony:** Nerve entrance into brow through frontal notch or foramen
    2. **Muscular:** Entrance of nerve from the corrugators
    3. **Muscular:** Exit of nerve from the corrugators

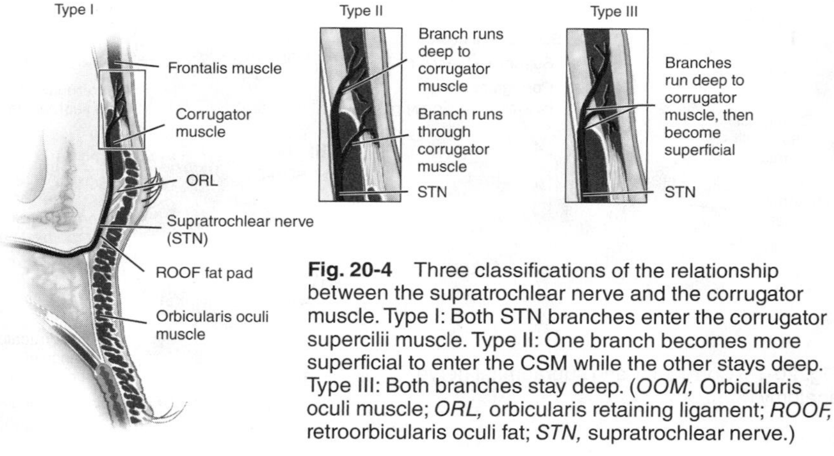


**Fig. 20-4** Three classifications of the relationship between the supratrochlear nerve and the corrugator muscle. Type I: Both STN branches enter the corrugator supercilii muscle. Type II: One branch becomes more superficial to enter the CSM while the other stays deep. Type III: Both branches stay deep. (*OOM,* Orbicularis oculi muscle; *ORL,* orbicularis retaining ligament; *ROOF,* retroorbicularis oculi fat; *STN,* supratrochlear nerve.)

## Temporal Triggers (Fig. 20-5)

- **Zygomaticotemporal branch of the trigeminal nerve**[8]
  - Terminal branch of the maxillary division ($V_2$) of the trigeminal nerve
  - Provides sensation to small area of skin over temple
  - Multiple potential points of compression
    - **Bony:** Exits lateral orbital wall through foramen in the zygomatic bone about 17 mm lateral and 6 mm cephalad to lateral orbital commissure
    - **Muscular:** Long tortuous course through temporalis muscle
    - **Fascial:** Passes through deep temporal fascia
    - **Vascular:** As it crosses under branches of the superficial temporal artery
- **Auriculotemporal nerve**[9,10]
  - Branch of the third division of the trigeminal nerve ($V_3$)
  - Exits through parotid gland, then travels over the temporomandibular joint (TMJ) before dividing over the zygomatic arch and within the layers of the temporoparietal fascia
  - Provides sensation to the tragus, anterior portion of the ear, and posterior temple
  - Potential compression within the soft tissue of the temple by adjacent superficial temporal artery

## Occipital Triggers

- Compression of the greater occipital, third occipital, or lesser occipital nerves
- **Greater occipital nerve (GON)** (Fig. 20-6)
  - Medial branch of the dorsal primary ramus of the second cervical spinal nerve
  - GON trunk exits ~3 cm below and 1.5 cm lateral to the occipital protuberance (Fig. 20-7).
  - Multiple (6) compression points[11]

- **Muscular and fascial entrapments**
  - GON can be compressed as it courses through the semispinalis capitis, obliquus capitis, and trapezius muscles and their investing fascia.
- Occipital artery can cause **vascular** irritation.[12]
  - Occipital artery intersects GON 54% of time.
  - Artery can be helically intertwined or have single crossover with GON.
  - May be primary cause of **occipital neuralgia–related chronic migraine**[13]

- **Lesser and third occipital nerves** can also be a source of pain for patients who have pain more laterally.

## Intranasal Triggers

- Severe septal deviation, bony spurs, concha bullosa, and turbinate enlargement result in mucosal inflammation and pressure on paranasal branches of the trigeminal nerve.
- Often cause retroorbital symptoms and headaches associated with sinuses or weather.

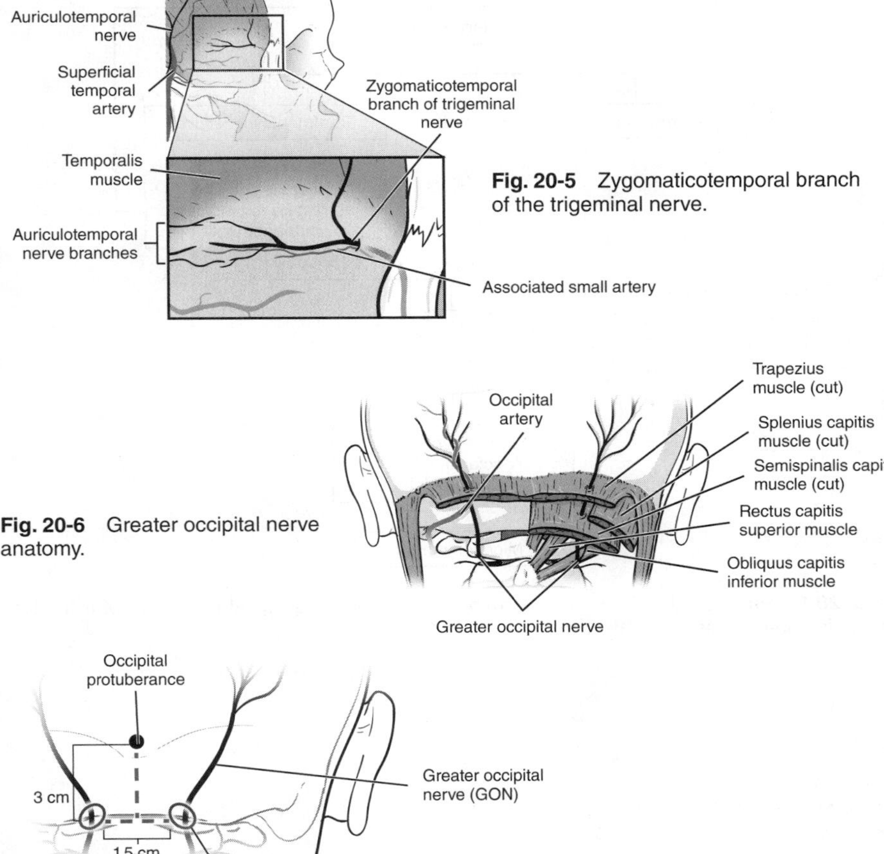


**Fig. 20-5** Zygomaticotemporal branch of the trigeminal nerve.

**Fig. 20-6** Greater occipital nerve anatomy.

**Fig. 20-7** Incision for greater occipital nerve release.

## INDICATIONS/PATIENT SELECTION (Fig. 20-8)

- Established diagnosis of migraines by neurologist
- Failure or intolerance of traditional medication
- Significant disability
- Identifiable supraorbital, temporal, or occipital trigger sites
  - Improved with botulinum toxin A and/or blocks
  - Alternatively, anatomic isolation determined by precise constellation of symptoms[14] (Box 20-1)
- Anatomic intranasal septal pathology causing compression of trigeminal nerve branches

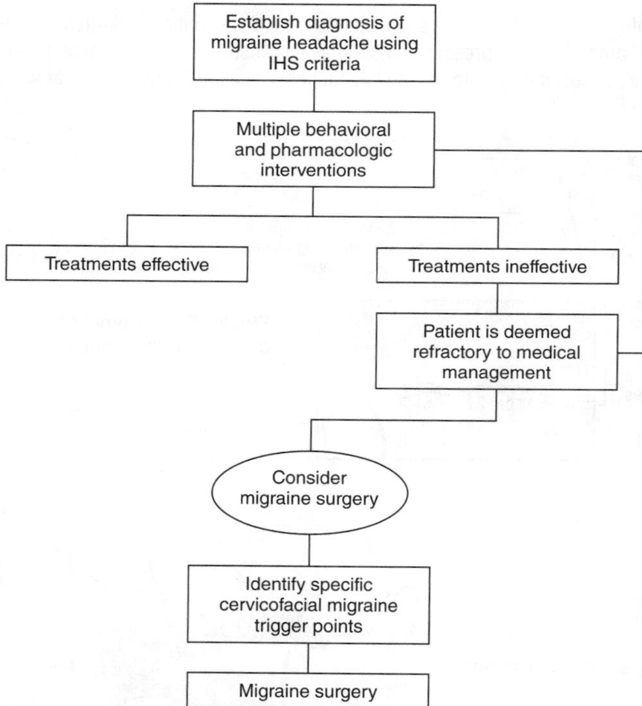


**Fig. 20-8** Practice algorithm for determining the need for surgical treatment of refractory migraine headaches.

**Box 20-1** *Constellation of Symptoms Related to Different Migraine Headaches*

**Frontal Migraine Headache**

Pain starts above eyebrows and usually in the afternoon.
Strong corrugator muscle activity causes deep frown lines on animation and repose.
Points of emergence of supraorbital and supratrochlear nerves from the corrugator muscle or the foramen are tender to touch.
Patients commonly have eyelid ptosis on affected side at the active pain.
Pressure on sites may abort the MH during initial stages.
Application of cold or warm compresses on sites can reduce or stop the pain.
Pain is usually imploding in nature.
Stress can trigger frontal MH.

**Temporal Migraine Headache**

Pain starts in temple area approximately 17 mm lateral and 6 mm cephalad to the lateral canthus.
Patients usually wake up in the morning with pain after clenching or grinding their teeth all night.
Pain is associated with tenderness of the temporalis or masseteric muscle.
Dental facets may be worn.
Rubbing or pressing the exit point of the zygomaticotemporal branch of the trigeminal nerve from the deep temporal fascia can stop or reduce the pain.
Application of cold or warm compresses may reduce or stop the pain.
Pain is characterized as *imploding.*
Stress can trigger temporal MH.

**Rhinogenic Migraine Headache**

Pain starts behind the eye.
Patient commonly wakes up with pain in the morning or at night.
MH can be triggered by weather changes.
Rhinorrhea can accompany pain on the affected side.
MH can be related to nasal allergy episodes.
Menstrual cycles can trigger rhinogenic MH.
Pain is usually described as *exploding.*
Concha bullosa, septal deviation with contact between the turbinates and septum, septa bullosa, and Haller's cell can be seen on CT.

**Occipital Migraine Headache**

Pain starts at the point of exit of the greater occipital nerve from the semispinalis capitis muscle (3.5 cm caudal to occipital tuberosity and 1.5 cm off midline).
Pain has no specific starting time.
Patients may have a history of whiplash.
Neck muscles are usually tight.
Heavy exercise can trigger occipital MH.
Compression can stop the pain in the early stage.
This point is tender in later stages.
Application of cold or heat may result in some improvement in pain.
Stress can trigger occipital MH.

*MH,* Migraine headache.

## CONTRAINDICATIONS

- Relative
  - Known neurologic or medical condition that causes headaches
  - Pregnancy and nursing
- Absolute
  - Failure of chemodenervation *and* absence of intranasal pathology

## PREOPERATIVE WORKUP

- Have patient maintain headache journal to establish baseline and identify trigger sites.
- Identify trigger sites by constellation of symptoms.
- Confirm supraorbital, temporal, and occipital triggers by injection of botulinum toxin A or blocks.
- Confirm intranasal trigger by exclusion of other sites. Perform intranasal examination and CT to confirm pathology.

## BOTULINUM TOXIN A

- Botox (Allergan, Irvine, CA) approved by FDA in 2010 for treating chronic migraine.
- Causes muscular paralysis by preventing release of acetylcholine at the neuromuscular junction
- **Acts as an effective test to confirm suspected trigger sites**
- **Triggers systematically injected based on symptoms and physical examination**[3,15] (Fig. 20-9)
  - Efficacy is measured and tracked with log.
  - Injection and improvement of one site may unmask other triggers.
  - *Improvement* is defined as 50% reduction in intensity or frequency of migraines in 4 weeks.
- Patients who improve are considered for surgery.

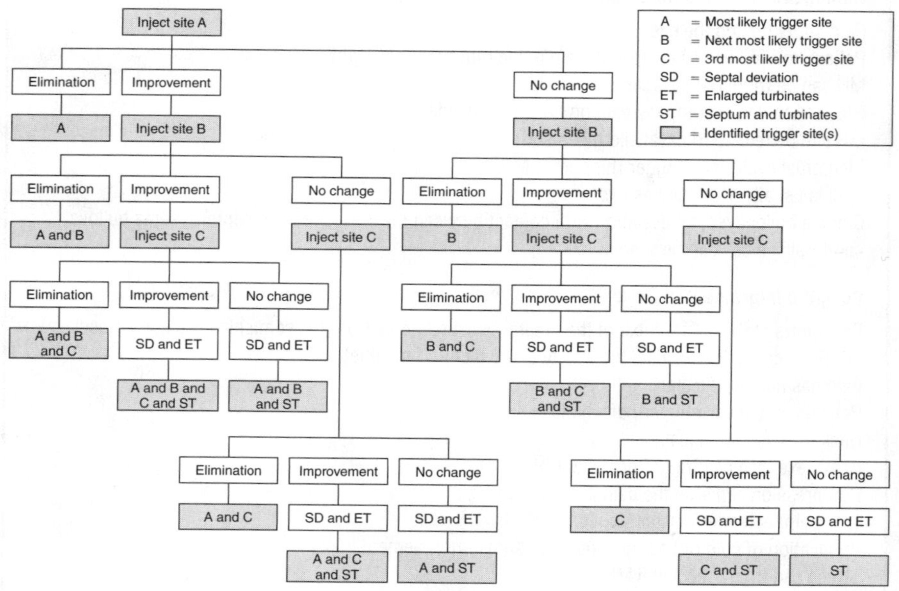


**Fig. 20-9** Algorithm for identification of migraine trigger sites by botulinum toxin injection.

## LOCAL NERVE BLOCK

- Local anesthetic: Combination of lidocaine and bupivacaine to effectively treat acute, active migraine
- Results in immediate but short-term relief of symptoms
- Works by anesthetizing the target nerve, not the muscle compressing it
- May be effective in identifying triggers that Botox misses, such as the auriculotemporal nerve

## SURGICAL MANAGEMENT[2]

### Corrugator Resection and Supraorbital Foraminotomy

- When indicated for frontal headaches[16]
- **Objective:** Complete resection of corrugators and relief of all external compression points to adequately release the trunk and all branches of the SON and STN
- Can be performed using a transpalpebral or endoscopic approach
  - Endoscopic approach attributed to higher success rates possibly because of better visualization of the corrugator muscle and supraorbital foramen[17]
- Similar to brow-lift procedures using same approaches

### Zygomaticotemporal Nerve Avulsion

- **Objective:** Removal of nerve so that it is not subject to compression by temporalis muscle
- Endoscopic approach
- Consequences minimal: Usually a temporary loss of small area (2.5 $cm^2$) of sensation on parietal scalp

### GON Release and Fat Flap Transposition

- **Objective:** Decompress the GON by releasing pressure from adjacent structures
- Approached through a 4 cm posterior midline incision
- GON identified before partial resection of semispinalis capitis and trapezius fascial bands along its course
- Ligation/resection of occipital artery, if applicable
- Subcutaneous, inferiorly based adipose flap elevated and placed under the GON to protect it and reduce recurrence

### Septoplasty and Inferior Turbinate Resection or Outfracture

- Remove deviated septum or spurs.
- Relieve intranasal contact points.
- Reduce size of inferior turbinates, if needed.
- Treat concha bullosa, if present.

## COMPLICATIONS

- Paresthesias of the temple, frontoparietal, or occipital scalp
- Alopecia at incision sites
- Injury to temporal branch of the facial nerve
- Nasal dryness
- Hollowing of temples
- All complications are usually temporary and short lasting.

## OUTCOMES[18,19]

- >80% of patients who have surgery reported **improvement,** defined as >50% improvement in symptoms and frequency.
- 57% reported **complete elimination** of migraine when all trigger points were addressed.
- Outcomes were shown to be persistent after 5 years if they were present at 1 year.
- Factors associated with successful outcome:
  - Older age of patient at migraine onset
  - Fewer baseline migraines per month
  - Daily use of over-the-counter migraine medications
  - Surgery on the frontal and temporal trigger sites
  - Surgery on all four trigger sites
- Factors associated with worse outcome:
  - History of head or neck injury
  - Increased intraoperative bleeding
  - Single or only two operative sites, inadequately treating all triggers

### Key Points

- ✓ Migraines affect 12% of the population and are more common in women.
- ✓ Migraines that respond poorly to traditional treatments can be effectively managed by surgical intervention.
- ✓ Chronic migraine should be diagnosed and medically managed by a neurologist before surgery is considered.
- ✓ Trigger sites are identified by locating the onset with constellation of symptoms or by injection of botulinum toxin A or blocks to determine the response and improvement.
- ✓ Intranasal pathology can be located by physical examination and CT.
- ✓ Retrobulbar symptoms can be caused by septonasal pathology and treated with septoplasty and turbinate resection.
- ✓ Systematic assessment to diagnose and treat all trigger sites is essential for successful elimination of headaches.

## References


1. Hu XH, Markson LE, Lipton RB, et al. Burden of migraine in the United States: disability and economic costs. Arch Intern Med 159:813, 1999.
2. Guyuron B, Reed D, Kriegler J, et al. A placebo-controlled surgical trial of the treatment of migraine headaches. Plast Reconstr Surg 124:461, 2009.
3. Guyuron B, Eriksson E, Persing JA, eds. Plastic Surgery: Indications and Practice. Philadelphia: Saunders Elsevier, 2009.
4. Goldstein J, Silberstein SD, Saper JR, et al. Acetaminophen, aspirin, and caffeine versus sumatriptan succinate in the early treatment of migraine: results from ASSET trial. Headache 45:973, 2005.
5. Janis JE, Ghavami A, Lemmon JA, et al. The anatomy of the corrugator supercilii muscle. II. Supraorbital nerve branching patterns. Plast Reconstr Surg 121:233, 2008.
6. Fallucco M, Janis JE, Hagan RR. The anatomical morphology of the supraorbital notch: clinical relevance to the surgical treatment of migraine headaches. Plast Reconstr Surg 130:1227, 2012.
7. Janis JE, Hatef DA, Hagan R, et al. Anatomy of the supratrochlear nerve: implications for the surgical treatment of migraine headaches. Plast Reconstr Surg 131:743, 2013.

8. Janis JE, Hatef DA, Thaker H, et al. The zygomaticotemporal branch of the trigeminal nerve. II. Anatomic variations. Plast Reconstr Surg 126:435, 2010.
9. Janis JE, Hatef DA, Ducic I, et al. Anatomy of the auriculotemporal nerve: variations in its relationship to the superficial temporal artery and implications for the treatment of migraine headaches. Plast Reconstr Surg 125:1422, 2010.
10. Chim H, Okada HC, Brown MS, et al. The auriculotemporal nerve in etiology of migraine headaches: compression points and anatomical variations. Plast Reconstr Surg 130:336, 2012.
11. Janis JE, Hatef DA, Ducic I, et al. The anatomy of the greater occipital nerve. II. Compression point topography. Plast Reconstr Surg 126:1563, 2010.
12. Janis JE, Hatef DA, Reece EM. Neurovascular compression of the greater occipital nerve: implications for migraine headaches. Plast Reconstr Surg 126:1996, 2010.
13. Ducic I, Felder JM, Janis JE. Occipital artery vasculitis not identified as a mechanism of occipital neuralgia-related chronic migraine headaches. Plast Reconstr Surg 128:908, 2011.
14. Liu MT, Armijo BS, Guyuron B. A comparison of outcome of surgical treatment of migraine headaches using a constellation of symptoms versus botulinum toxin A to identify trigger sites. Plast Reconstr Surg 129:413, 2012.
15. Kung TA, Guyuron B, Cederna PS. Migraine surgery: a plastic surgery solution for refractory migraine headache. Plast Reconstr Surg 127:181, 2011.
16. Chepla KJ, Oh E, Guyuron B. Clinical outcomes following supraorbital foraminotomy for treatment of frontal migraine headaches. Plast Reconstr Surg 129:656e, 2012.
17. Liu MT, Chim H, Guyuron B. Outcome comparison of endoscopic and transpalpebral decompression treatment for frontal migraine headaches. Plast Reconst Surg 129:1113, 2012.
18. Guyuron B, Kriegler J, Davis J, et al. Five-year outcome of surgical treatment of migraine headaches. Plast Reconstr Surg 127:603, 2011.
19. Larson K, Lee M, Davis J, et al. Factors contributing to migraine headache surgery failure and success. Plast Reconstr Surg 128:1069, 2011.

# 21. Craniosynostosis

Carey Faber Campbell, Christopher A. Derderian

## DEFINITION

*Premature fusion of one or more cranial sutures.*[1]

### INCIDENCE

1:2500 live births[2]

## NORMAL PHYSIOLOGY

- **Normal cranial growth**
  - Growth responds to increasing brain and CSF volume
    - Brain size triples by 1 year
    - Quadruples by 2 years
    - Approximates 85% adult growth by 3 years of age
    - Near adult size at age 6-10[3]
  - Normal skull growth occurs through two mechanisms
    - *Sutural growth:* Perpendicular to sutures
    - *Appositional growth:* Bone resorption on the inner surface and deposition on the outer surface of the skull.
- **Normal suture anatomy** (Fig. 21-1)[4]
- **Normal suture fusion**
  - **Metopic:** 6 to 8 months[5]
  - **Sagittal:** 22 years
  - **Coronal:** 24 years
  - **Lambdoidal:** 26 years
- **Normal fontanelle closure**
  - **Posterior fontanelle:** 3-6 months
  - **Anterior fontanelle:** 9-12 months

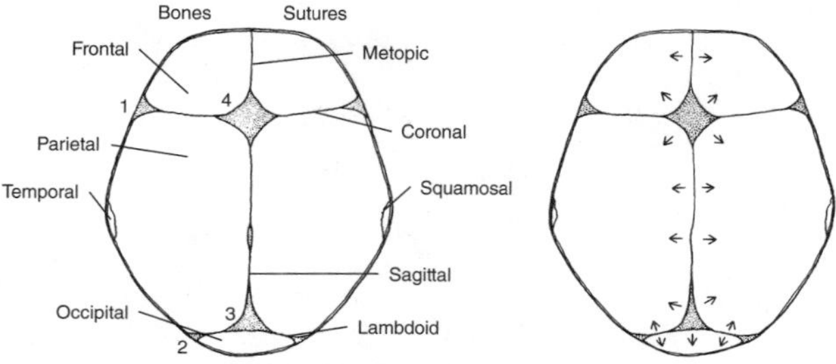


**Fig. 21-1** Cranial sutures in the human fetus. Premature closure produces growth restriction perpendicular to the line of the suture and compensatory overgrowth parallel to it.

## ETIOLOGIC FACTORS AND PATHOPHYSIOLOGY

### Virchow's Law

***Premature suture fusion results in cranial growth predominately parallel to sutures (rather than perpendicular).***

### Theories of Suture Closure

- **Cranial base**
  - Synostoses result from abnormal tension exerted by cranial base through the dura.
  - Theory does *not* account for isolated synostoses.
- **Intrinsic suture biology**
  - Synostoses result from the osteoinductive properties of dura mater, which contains osteoblast-like cells.
- **Extrinsic factors**
  - Synostoses result from extrinsic forces or systemic disease.
    - In utero compression or ischemic event
    - Hydrocephalus decompression
    - Abnormal brain growth (e.g., microcephaly)
    - Systemic pathology (e.g., hypothyroidism or rickets)

### Genetics[6]

- 21% genetic
  - Causes:
    - Chromosomal abnormalities (15%)
    - Mutations in FGFR2 (32%)
    - FGFR3 (25%)
    - TWIST1 (19%)
    - EFNB1 (7%)
- 67% nonsyndromic
- 11.5% other syndromes
- Causative mutations found in 11% multisuture, 37.5% bilateral coronal, and 17.5% unilateral coronal craniosynostosis

## INDICATIONS FOR TREATMENT[7]

- To prevent or treat elevated intracranial pressure (ICP)
- To address skull deformity to aid in normal social interactions
- Early suture closure may **decrease intracranial volume and restrict brain growth (Cephalocranial disproportion)** causing elevated intracranial pressures (>15 mm Hg).
  - Elevated ICP is not solely attributed to cephalocranial disproportion.
  - Additional causes of increased ICP in syndromic craniosynostosis:
    - Intracranial venous congestion
    - Hydrocephalus
    - Upper airway obstruction
  - Intracranial volume can be increased as in Apert syndrome: The intracranial volume is within normal range at birth but increases to greater than 3 standard deviations above normal after 3.5 months of age,[8] but still 83% incidence of elevated ICP.
- More affected sutures correlates with increased intracranial pressures (ICP).[9]
  - **13%** incidence of increased ICP with **isolated** synostosis
  - **42%** incidence of increased ICP with **multiple** suture nonsyndromic synostoses

- **Signs of elevated ICP:**
  - Morning headache, irritability, recurrent emesis, difficulty sleeping
  - Mental impairment/neuropsychiatric disorders
  - Change in developmental curve
  - Optic atrophy and vision loss
  - Documented elevated ICP (but there is no universal definition of elevated ICP in children)
- **Chiari malformation:** Downward displacement of cerebellar tonsils through foramen magnum.
  - In craniosynostosis: Believed to be secondary to hindbrain growth in a posterior fossa of inadequate volume
  - 70% of patients with Crouzon's syndrome, 82% with Pfeiffer syndrome, 100% kleeblattschädel
  - May cause noncommunicating hydrocephalus
- More involved sutures correlate with increased mental impairment.
  - Neurodevelopmental injury: Gradual, irreversible, and difficult to detect

## DIAGNOSIS AND EVALUATION

- **History and physical examination**
  - No movement at sutures
  - Palpable ridges from thickening of closed sutures
  - Bulging fontanels (Volcano sign)
  - **Abnormal cranial morphology,** predictable changes in head shape from closure of sutures (Fig. 21-2), orbital rim relationship to cornea, abnormal/asymmetrical facial features
- **ICP Monitoring**
  - **Direct intraparenchymal monitoring** (benchmark, but invasive; multiple risks)
    - No consensus on timing, frequency, duration, or normal ICP value in children
  - **Radiographic films**
    - Anteroposterior (AP), lateral, and Townes projection; C-spine (for associated C-spine anomalies)
      - *Harlequin sign* seen on AP view in coronal synostoses
      - "Thumb printing" or "copper beating" from pressure of gyri on inner table; low specificity
  - **Fundoscopic examination:** Papilledema (98% specific in all ages; only 22% sensitive under age 8; 100% sensitive over age 8)[10]
  - **Transorbital ultrasound:** Measures optic nerve sheath diameter, which increases with increased ICP
  - **Visual evoked potentials:** Measures latency time of average encephalographic response to visual stimuli; compared to baseline; prolonged latency correlates with axonal injury and elevated ICP
- **Imaging studies**
  - **CT scan**
    - Not required but commonly used for preoperative planning
    - Used routinely in syndromic synostoses
    - Three-dimensional imaging to better define suture fusion, abnormal morphology, and intracranial volume
    - Allows for monitoring for hydrocephalus, Chiari malformation, and other bone/brain abnormalities commonly seen in some syndromes
  - **MRI**
    - Usually unnecessary
    - Used for select syndromes (Apert syndrome or Pfeiffer syndrome) with suspicion of anomalous venous drainage or other CNS pathology

## CLASSIFICATION (IN ORDER OF INCIDENCE)[11,12] (Fig. 21-2)

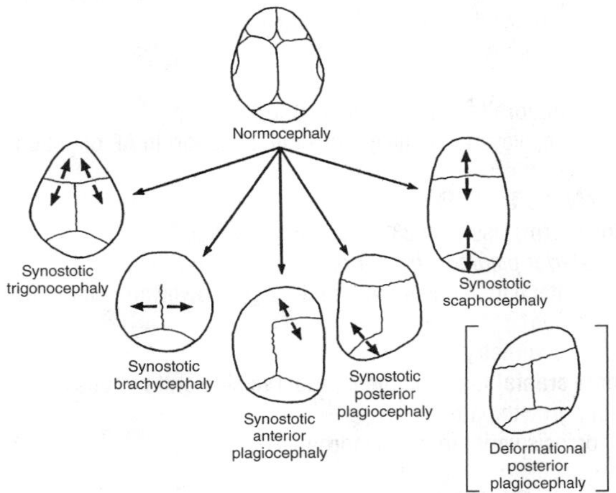


**Fig. 21-2** Skull shapes and affected sutures in craniosynostosis.

### SAGITTAL SYNOSTOSIS

- **Incidence:** 40%-50% of craniosynostosis
- **Morphology:** *Scaphocephaly;* also called *dolichocephaly;* "boat-shaped"
  - Increased AP diameter and decreased biparietal width
  - Frontal bossing and occipital coning
- Male/female ratio: 4:1

### METOPIC SYNOSTOSIS

- **Incidence:** 23%-28% of craniosynostosis[13,14]
- **Morphology:** *Trigonocephaly,* "keel shaped, triangular"
  - Spectrum of deformities ranging from isolated metopic ridge to the most severe keel-shaped forehead
  - Bitemporal narrowing, hypotelorism, bilateral supraorbital retrusion, medially slanted lateral orbital rims, epicanthal folds
  - Intracranial findings: Omega sign, hard diagnosis by angle of pterygium to nasion
  - Anterior cranial base increased in the AP dimension
- **ICP elevation:** 4%-10%

### UNILATERAL CORONAL SYNOSTOSIS

- **Incidence:** 13%-20% of isolated craniosynostosis
- **Morphology:** *Anterior plagiocephaly*
  - Ipsilateral frontal flattening and contralateral frontoparietal bossing
  - Ipsilateral occipitoparietal flattening, ipsilateral temporal fossa convexity
  - **Harlequin deformity:** Lack of descent of greater wing of the sphenoid (also ipsilateral)
  - Recessed supraorbital, lateral, and inferior rim; shallow orbit
  - Root of nose constricted and deviated to ipsilateral side
  - Anteriorly displaced ipsilateral glenoid fossa causes the chin to point to contralateral side
  - Cranial base short in AP direction

## Bilateral Coronal Synostosis

- **Incidence:** 5%-10% of isolated craniosynostosis (many cases of bilateral coronal synostosis once thought to be nonsyndromic are likely familial)[15]
- **Morphology:** *Brachycephaly*
  - Broad, flat forehead
  - Recession of supraorbital ridges with bulging forehead
  - Wide cranial base, elevation in height of skull, but short in AP direction

## Lambdoid Synostosis

- **Incidence:** Rarest form, less than 3% of craniosynostosis
- **Morphology:** *Posterior plagiocephaly or occipital plagiocephaly*
  - Ipsilateral occipital flattening and **mastoid bulge,** downward cant of the posterior skull base to the affected side
  - Variable facial asymmetry
  - **Larger middle cranial fossa on the unaffected side** and petrous ridge angle (typical compensatory growth pattern)[16]
  - Bilateral synostosis very rare nonsyndromically

## Deformational Plagiocephaly

**Table 21-1** *Anatomic Features That Differentiate Synostotic and Deformational Frontal Plagiocephaly*

| Anatomic Feature | Synostotic | Deformational |
|---|---|---|
| Ipsilateral superior orbital rim | Up | Down |
| Ipsilateral ear | Anterior and high | Posterior and low |
| Nasal root | Ipsilateral | Midline |
| Ipsilateral cheek | Forward | Backward |
| Chin deviation | Contralateral | Ipsilateral |
| Ipsilateral palpebral fissure | Wide | Narrow |
| Anterior fontanel deviation | Low contralateral | High none |

- **Incidence:** 1:300 in the general population
- No functional sequelae

> **TIP:** Often mistaken for lambdoidal or coronal plagiocephaly
> - Head assumes parallelogram configuration
> - Ipsilateral occipital flattening and frontal bossing
> - Ear displaced anteriorly

- **Not craniosynostosis,** but deformation secondary to external forces
  - **Supine positioning:** American Academy of Pediatrics recommends infants sleep supine to lessen risk of sudden infant death syndrome (SIDS); this has led to an increasing incidence of deformities.
  - **Rotational forces:** Torticollis, vertebral abnormalities, and visual field deficits may all cause preferential rotation and unequal pressure on the occiput.

## Other Morphologic Variants

- **Turricephaly:** Excessive skull height and vertical forehead from untreated brachycephaly
- **Oxycephaly:** Pointed head; forehead retroverted and tilted back; from pansynostosis
- **Kleeblattschädel (cloverleaf deformity):** Secondary to synostosis of all sutures except squamosal suture

## Syndromic Craniosynostosis[1,7,17,18]

- **Crouzon syndrome** (Fig. 21-3)
  - Described by French neurologist Crouzon in 1912
  - **Autosomal dominant; FGFR2** (multiple mutations); variable expression; common to have increased penetrance in child than parent
  - **Incidence:** 1:25,000 (most common syndromic craniosynostosis)
  - **Intracranial:** Hydrocephalus, ICP elevation in 65%, 72% type I Chiari malformation
  - **Cranial/upper face:** Bicoronal synostosis most common; usually brachycephalic but scaphocephaly, trigonocephaly, cloverleaf deformity, and normocephalic described
  - **Orbits:** Exorbitism may cause exposure conjunctivitis/keratitis; herniation of globe (rare)
  - **Midface hypoplasia;** anterior open bite, class III malocclusion; narrow and high arched palate
  - **Extremities:** No common limb anomaly (defining feature)
  - **Other:** Conductive hearing loss

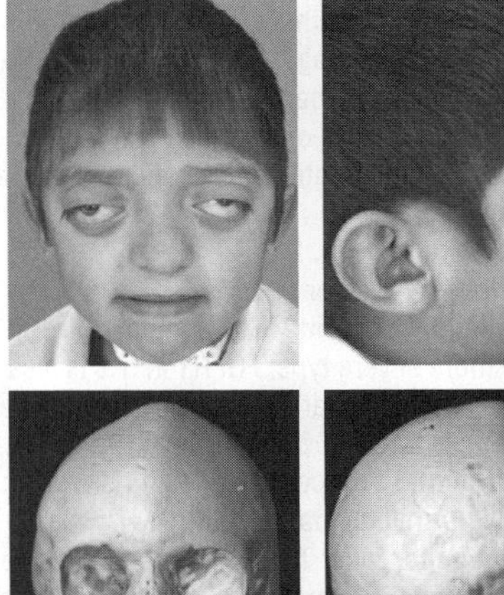

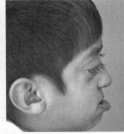

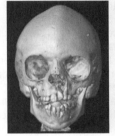

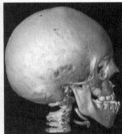

**Fig. 21-3** A 6-year-old boy with untreated Crouzon syndrome showing exorbitism, midface hypoplasia, pancraniosynostosis, and an anterior open bite.

- **Apert syndrome (Fig. 21-4)**
  - Described by Apert in 1906
  - **Autosomal dominant,** most cases are sporadic
  - **Incidence:** 1:100,000-1:160,000

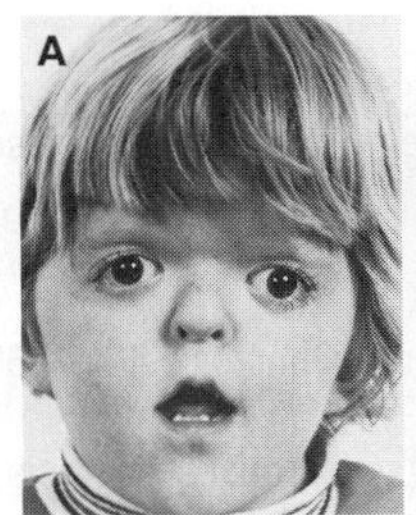

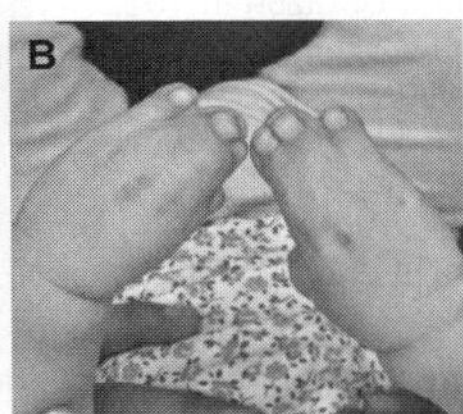

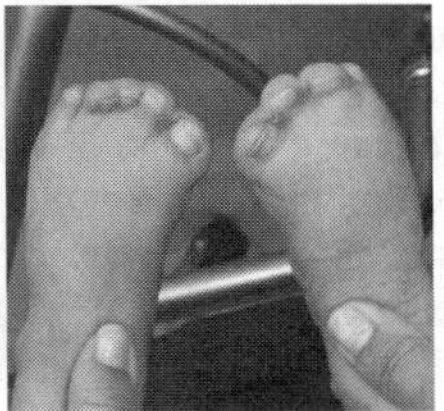

**Fig. 21-4** **A,** 6-year-old child with Apert syndrome. **B,** Complex syndactyly is characteristic of Apert syndrome.

- **Intracranial:** ICP elevation in 83% with average age of onset 18 month,[19] ventriculoperitoneal (VP) shunts may be needed, some develop normal intelligence (70% have decreased IQ)
- **Cranial/upper face:** Bicoronal synostoses with significant turribrachycephaly, enlarged anterior fontanel, bitemporal widening, occipital flattening
- **Orbits:** Exorbitism, downslanting palpebral fissures, and mild hypertelorism
- **Midface:** Hypoplasia (more severe than in Crouzon's syndrome), parrot beak deformity; high arch or cleft palate, anterior open bite, class III malocclusion which may result in airway compromise needing tracheostomy
- **Extremities (defining):** Complex syndactyly of hands and feet (usually second through fourth fingers and toes)
- **Other:** Acne in 70% of adolescents
- 35% of patients treated successfully for elevated ICP develop a second episode 3.33 years later on average

■ **Pfeiffer syndrome (Fig. 21-5)**
- Described by Pfeiffer in 1964
- **Autosomal dominant:** FGFR2 mutation in 95% of patients and is the more severe type; FGFR1 in 5% is less severe and has features more similar to Crouzon's syndrome
- **Incidence:** 1:100,000 live births
- **Intracranial:** Hydrocephalus, high risk for Chiari malformation, usually normal mental status
- **Cranial/upper face:** Turribrachycephaly; bicoronal synostoses
- **Orbits:** Shallow, **exorbitism,** hypertelorism, downslanting palpebral fissures, strabismus
- **Midface: Hypoplasia,** nose turned down with low nasal bridge (parrot beak); class III malocclusion with anterior open bite that may result in airway compromise and tracheostomy
- **Extremities: Broad thumbs and halluces,** mild cutaneous syndactyly (second and third fingers, second through fourth toes)
- **Other:** Frequently have obstructive sleep apnea (OSA) and require tracheostomy
- Cohen classification system[20]:
  - *Type I:* Classic (61%) with bicoronal synostosis, exorbitism, and midface hypoplasia
  - *Type II:* Moderate, kleeblattschädel cloverleaf (25%)
  - *Type III:* Most severe (14%)
- Undergo an average of 2.5 cranial vault procedures, 1.6 neurosurgical procedures, 3.5 other procedures; often need permanent tarsorrhaphies[21]

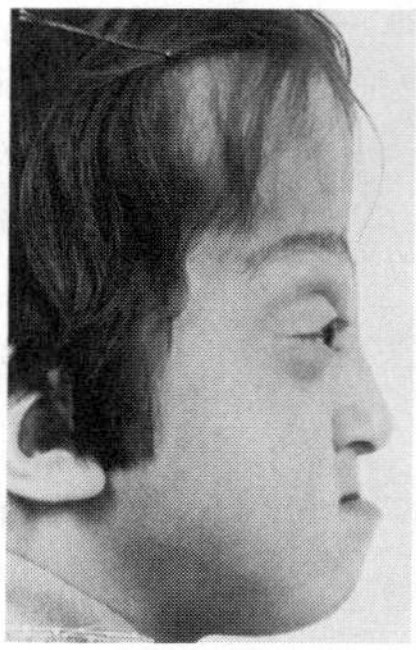

**Fig. 21-5** A 5-year-old child with Pfeiffer syndrome.

■ **Saethre-Chotzen syndrome**
- Described by Saethre in 1931 and Chotzen in 1932
- **Autosomal dominant,** variable expression; **TWIST-1** gene mutation on chromosome 7p21 causing dysregulated bone deposition
- **Incidence:** 1:25,000-1:50,000
- Mental status usually normal
- **Cranial/upper face:** Asymmetrical brachycephaly; bicoronal synostosis 45%-76%, unicoronal synostosis 18%-27%,[22] **low frontal hairline**
- **Orbits: Ptosis** of eyelids, findings typical of bicoronal and unicoronal synostosis
- **Ears: Prominent crus helicis** extending throughout the conchal bowl
- **Midface:** Facial asymmetry, deviated nasal septum, narrow palate, less common midface hypoplasia

- **Extremities:** Partial syndactyly, short stature
- **Other:** 40% risk of elevated ICP after initial cranial vault expansion, high reoperation rate 42%-65%

- **Muenke syndrome**
  - **Genotype** described by Muenke in 1996: pro250Arg mutation in FGFR3 on chromosome 4p[23]
  - **Autosomal dominant,** variable expression (not all patients with Muenke syndrome have craniosynostosis)
  - **Incidence:** 1:10,000, may be present in 10% of unicoronal and bicoronal synostosis previously thought to be nonsyndromic
  - Developmental delay
  - **Cranial/upper face:** Coronal suture craniosynostosis (sexual dimorphism: males 37% bicoronal versus 29% unicoronal; females 58% bicoronal versus 20% unicoronal)[24]
  - **Midface:** Uncommon to have hypoplasia
  - **Extremities:** Thimble-like middle phalanges
  - **Other: Sensorineural hearing loss** bilaterally; few extracranial manifestations
  - Reoperation rate for elevated ICP is five times more common than for those without the mutation

## TREATMENT

- Multidisciplinary team approach
  - Plastic surgeon, neurosurgeon, oral surgeon/dentist/orthodontist, ear/nose/throat surgeon, ophthalmologist, speech therapist, pediatrician, geneticist, child psychologist, nurses

## SURGERY

- Intracranial correction of recessed forehead and supraorbital region in adults described by Tessier in 1967[25]

### GOALS

- Expand intracranial volume
- Reduce risk of developing increased ICP to allow normal brain growth
- Normalize head shape and appearance

### TIMING

- Controversial
- Approach to treatment is significantly different for nonsyndromic than for syndromic patients
  - Syndromic patients: Much higher risk for elevated ICP and repeat intracranial procedures, decreased growth potential
  - Single-suture nonsyndromic patients usually require only a single open vault procedure, whereas syndromic patients require two or three procedures on average
- Major risk in young patients is the volume of blood loss given their small circulating blood volume (70-80 cc/kg)
- Usually treat craniosynostosis between 6 months and 1 year of age, but earlier if pansutural involvement or elevated ICP
- **Early surgery (6-12 months of age):**
  - **Pros:**
    - Bones are malleable
    - Less compensatory growth has occurred
    - Spontaneously heal defects (younger than 11 months) and regenerate bone faster

- **Cons:**
  - Large volume of growth remains, resulting in high likelihood of recurrence
- **Later surgery (after 12 months of age):**
  - **Pros:**
    - Bones are stronger and can hold fixation better
    - More growth has occurred, resulting in decreased severity of recurrence
  - **Cons:**
    - Bones are more difficult to shape
    - Bony defects are less likely to close spontaneously
    - More compensatory growth to address

## SYNDROMIC CRANIOSYNOSTOSIS TECHNIQUES[1,7]

- General timeline
  - Urgent decompression for elevated ICP: Strip craniectomy (<3 months)
  - Suture release, cranial vault remodeling, cranial vault distraction, upper orbital reshaping/advancement (4-12 months)
    - When staged, usually perform posterior vault expansion first in syndromic patients because:
      - Greater volume increase per millimeter of advancement
      - Decreases compensatory anterior growth
      - Allows delay of anterior cranial vault remodeling to a later age
      - Decompressive effects in patients with Chiari malformation
  - Midface (LeFort III ± I): 6-12 years
  - LeFort I ± mandible: 14-18 years
- Surgery in the first year of life
  - **Posterior cranial vault remodeling**
    - Greater change per millimeter of advancement than anterior vault remodeling
    - Useful in severe turricephaly and occipital flattening
    - Single-stage procedures historically complicated by problems with healing and propensity to relapse from weight of head on construct. Outcomes improved with resorbable plate systems.
  - **Posterior vault expansion with distraction osteogenesis**[26,27]
    - **Pros:**
      - Maintains vascularity of bone flap
      - Provides new, vascularized bone
      - Limits dead space
      - Expands soft tissue envelope
      - Greater intracranial volume gain than single-stage procedures
      - Improvement in cerebellar anatomy
      - Decreased operative time
      - Still need fronto-orbital advancement for correction of retrusive brow, but can be delayed to a later age
    - **Cons:**
      - Need for second procedure to remove device
      - Potential device complications
      - Longer treatment time
    - Technique: In prone position for posterior cranial vault exposure; coronal incision; posterior craniotomy performed with maintenance of dural attachments; barrel staves with out-fracture on inferior occipital segment

- Two distraction devices placed in parasagittal, collinear positions with uniform parallel vectors dictated by skull shape; distracter arms exit anterior scalp (Fig. 21-6)
- Start distraction 72 hours postoperatively, 1 mm/day with range of 20-35 mm; consolidation phase for approximately 8 weeks before removal
- Weekly plain film radiography and then CT after removal of devices

- **Fronto-orbital advancement (FOA)**
  - Goals:
    - Expand intracranial volume
    - Reshape vault and advance frontal bone
    - Advance supraorbital bar for globe protection and aesthetic improvement
  - Technique: Coronal incision, frontal craniotomy, removal of frontal bone, bandeau harvested and shaped; advancement of the bandeau, which is secured with cranial bone graft and resorbable plates or sutures (Fig. 21-7)

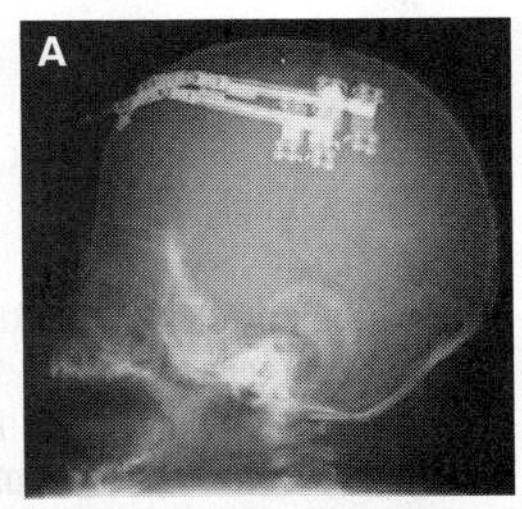


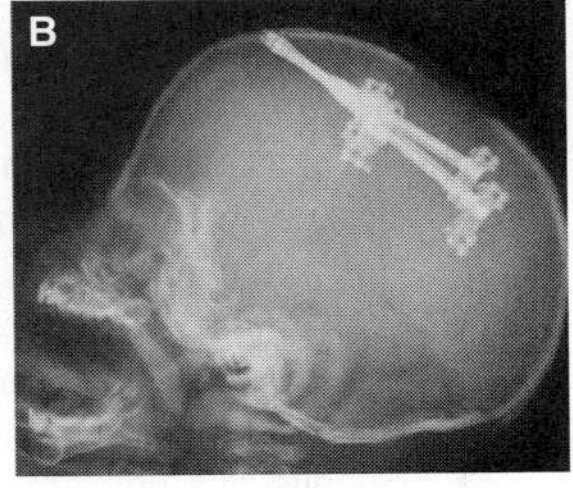


**Fig. 21-6** The progress of distraction osteogenesis is followed by weekly radiographs. **A,** Start of activation. **B,** End of activation.

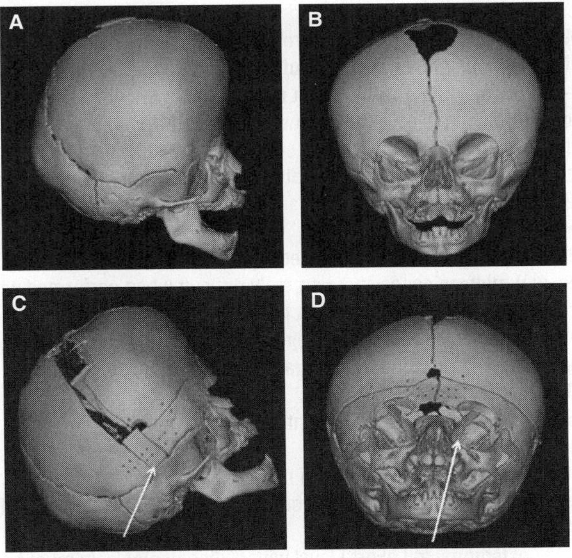


**Fig. 21-7** Fronto-orbital advancement. **A** and **B,** Preoperative. **C,** A cranial bone graft buttresses the forward advancement of the bandeau, fixed with an absorbable plate. **D,** Cranial bone graft struts can be seen bridging the cut edges of the orbital roof, providing additional AP stability to the advanced bandeau.

- Overcorrection of the forehead and supraorbital bar to account for decreased growth potential
- 20% of patients will have persistent cranial defects if no bone graft is used; particulate bone graft from endocortex can be used to fill defect with 95% closure of defects[28]
- Often used as initial procedure only if ocular protection needed; otherwise performed after posterior vault distraction

- **Postoperative care for open cranial vault procedures**
  - Observation in ICU for 24-48 hours
  - Close monitoring: Neurologic examination every 2 hours; hematocrit and sodium every 6 hours for 24 hours
  - Transfusions commonly given if hematocrit falls below 21
  - Parents instructed to guard against head trauma, but otherwise may hold and lay child down as usual
- **Complications**
  - Bleeding: Most require transfusions; large surface area of raw bone bleeds most during the first 24 hours
  - Venous air embolism
  - Infection: Although postoperative fever is very common, it does not warrant extensive workup unless other clinical signs of infection[29]
  - Cerebrospinal fluid leak: Check intraoperatively with Valsalva maneuver

■ **Surgery in childhood: Midface/LeFort III advancement**
- Timing is controversial: 4-7 years old or delay surgery until skeletal maturity (unless airway obstruction or exorbitism)
  - Early: Psychosocial benefits and improved quality of life; risk of malocclusion recurrence
- **LeFort III (midface advancement) craniofacial disjunction**
  - Single-stage procedure or **distraction osteogenesis** (most common)
  - Advance midface alone or with supraorbital bar and frontal bone flaps in monobloc procedure (when supraorbital rim-to-cornea relationship already correct)
  - Distraction is preferred method for both LeFort III and monobloc because of decreased morbidity and significantly larger advancements associated with gradual expansion over single-stage procedure.
  - Facial bipartition may be used to correct hypertelorism, down-slanting palpebral fissures, and midface concavity (extremely difficult when performed with LeFort III)
  - Transition from class III to class II occlusion
  - Primary goal is to get appropriate projection of zygoma and restore orbital volume

■ **Surgery in adolescence/adulthood: Orthognathic and contouring**
- **Orthognathic surgery**
  - Team approach with dentist, orthodontist, craniofacial surgeon
  - Orthodontics to optimize bite
  - Correct malocclusion associated with midface hypoplasia and anterior open bite
  - Surgery may be indicated following completion of maxillary and mandibular growth (age 14-18)
    - Usually osteotomy at LeFort I level with sliding genioplasty must be customized to patient
- **Facial contouring**
  - Correct any remaining contour irregularities by smoothing irregularities, bone grafts, resuspending soft tissue

## Nonsyndromic Craniosynostosis Techniques

- **Scaphocephaly: Extended strip craniectomy or open calvarial vault reconstruction**
  - Extended strip craniectomy with helmet
    - Primarily used for isolated sagittal synostoses when less than 4 months of age
    - Open versus endoscopic approaches: Endoscopic meant to minimize scalp incision, blood loss, operative time, recovery[30]
    - Wedge ostectomies made adjacent to coronal and lambdoid sutures allow for transverse expansion
    - Helmet molding applied postoperatively for up to 18 months
  - Spring-assisted cranioplasty
    - Uses continuous force generated by a spring across an osteotomy, strip craniectomy, or patent suture
    - Primarily for sagittal synostosis (but can be used in any of the symmetrical patterns of craniosynostosis)
    - Requires second procedure for device removal, little control of expansion rate/distance and opposing forces
  - Open cranial vault reconstruction: May stage reconstruction into anterior and posterior stages
    - Posterior 2/3 reconstruction only: Patients with sagittal synostosis are shown to normalize their forehead shape if an isolated posterior-middle vault expansion is performed, avoiding FOA[31]
    - Anterior and posterior vault reconstruction in two stages
    - Total vault reconstruction in one stage (rare)
    - Clamshell: In children less than 1 year old, clamshell craniotomy with interleaving barrel-stave osteotomies may be used[32]
- *Plagiocephaly and brachycephaly:* Bifrontal craniotomy, fronto-orbital advancement repositioning frontal bar, recontouring frontal bone, barrel staves
- *Trigonocephaly:* Overcorrection of frontal dysmorphology and bitemporal constriction with bifrontal craniotomy, frontal reshaping and expansion of supraorbital bar and frontal bone flaps with interpositional bone graft, wedge osteotomies, bone grafting[33] (Fig. 21-8)
- *Lambdoid craniosynostosis:* Biparieto-occipital craniotomies, occipital switch, and contouring

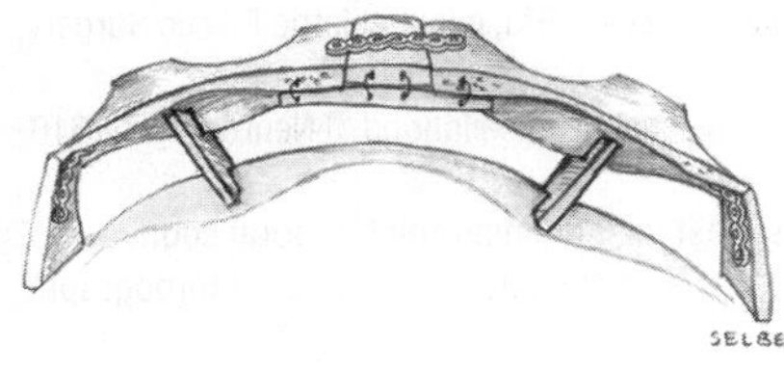


**Fig. 21-8** Fronto-orbital advancement with or without midline graft for treatment of trigonocephaly. Technique involves transverse expansion of the supraorbital bar using an interpositional bone graft with resorbable fixation of the closing wedge osteotomy, calvarial bone placed posterior to the interposition bone graft, and inlay bone strut to orbital roof.

## Fixation

- Hardware
  - Wires/sutures
  - Titanium screws and plates
  - Absorbable hardware (most common)

## Grafts

- Autologous bone grafts
  - Split calvarial: Usually parietal bone split ex vivo
  - Split rib: Leave periosteum intact for rib regeneration; harder to mold and increased resorption

- Iliac wing
- Particulate bone graft
- ■ Methylmethacrylate: Resin
- ■ Hydroxyapatite: Calcium phosphate, which is 70% of human bone
- ■ Preformed ceramics or moldable nonceramic (but small pores for vascular ingrowth)

## Key Points

- ✓ Brain size triples by 1 year and quadruples by 2 years.
- ✓ Incidence of non-syndromic synostosis by suture:
  - Sagittal (40%-50%): Leads to scaphocephaly
  - Metopic (20%-28%): Leads to trigonocephaly
  - Unicoronal (13%-20%): Leads to anterior plagiocephaly
  - Bicoronal (5%-10%): Leads to brachycephaly/turribrachycephaly
  - Lambdoid (<3%): Leads to posterior plagiocephaly with trapezoid configuration and mastoid bulge
- ✓ Deformational plagiocephaly
  - Parallelogram configuration
  - Anterior displacement of ear
- ✓ Syndromes
  - Crouzon syndrome: Normal extremities
  - Apert syndrome: Complex severe syndactyly, acne, common mental impairment
  - Pfeiffer syndrome: Broad thumbs/halluces, usually no mental impairment
  - Saethre-Chotzen syndrome: Low hairline and eyelid ptosis, prominent crus helices
  - Muenke syndrome: Common cause of unicoronal and bicoronal craniosynostosis with high reoperation rate; family history common

## References


1. Derderian CA, Bartlett SP. Craniosynostosis Syndromes. In Thorne C, ed. Grabb and Smith's Plastic Surgery, 7th ed. Philadelphia: Lippincott Williams & Wilkins, in press.
2. Knoll B, Persing JA. Craniosynostosis. In Bentz ML, Bauer BS, Zuker RM, eds. Pediatric Plastic Surgery, 2nd ed. St Louis: Quality Medical Publishing, 2008.
3. Sgouros S, Hockley AD, Golden JH, et al. Intracranial volume change in childhood. J Neurosurg 91:610-616, 1999.
4. Weinzweig J, Kirschner RE, Farley A, et al. Metopic synostosis: defining the temporal sequence of normal suture fusion and differentiating it from synostosis on the basis of computed tomography images. Plast Reconstr Surg 112:1211-1218, 2003.
5. Carson BS, Dufresne CR. Craniosynostosis and neurocranial asymmetry. In Defresne CR, Carson BS, Zinreich SJ, eds. Complex Craniofacial Problems. New York: Churchill Livingstone, 1992.
6. Wilkie AO, Byren JC, Hurst JA, et al. Prevalence and complications of single-gene and chromosomal disorders in craniosynostosis. Pediatrics 126:e391-e400, 2010.
7. Derderian C, Seaward J. Syndromic craniosynostosis. Semin Plast Surg 26:64-75, 2012.
8. Gosain AK, McCarthy JG, Glatt P, et al. A study of intracranial volume in Apert syndrome. Plast Reconstr Surg 95:284-295, 1995.
9. Renier D, Sainte-Rose C, Marchac D, et al. Intracranial pressure in craniostenosis. J Neurosurg 57:370-377, 1982.
10. Tuite GF, Chong WK, Evanson J, et al. The effectiveness of papilledema as an indicator of raised intracranial pressure in children with craniosynostosis. Neurosurgery 38:272-278, 1996.

11. Persing JA. MOC-PS(SM) CME article: management considerations in the treatment of craniosynostosis. Plast Reconstr Surg 121:1-11, 2008.
12. Cohen MM Jr, MacLean RE. Anatomic, genetic, nosologic, diagnostic, and psychosocial considerations. In Cohen MM Jr, MacLean RE, eds. Craniosynostosis: Diagnosis, Evaluation, and Management, 2nd ed. New York: Oxford University Press, 2000.
13. Beckett JS, Chadha P, Persing JA, et al. Classification of trigonocephaly in metopic synostosis. Plast Reconstr Surg 130:442e-447e, 2012.
14. Selber J, Reid RR, Chike-Obi CJ, et al. The changing epidemiologic spectrum of single-suture synostosis. Plast Reconstr Surg 122:527-533, 2008.
15. Bastidas N, Mackay DD, Taylor JA, et al. Analysis of the long-term outcomes of nonsyndromic bicoronal synostosis. Plast Reconstr Surg 130:877-883, 2012.
16. Smartt JM Jr, Elliott RM, Reid RR, et al. Analysis of differences in the cranial base and facial skeleton of patients with lambdoid synostosis and deformational plagiocephaly. Plast Reconstr Surg 127:303-312, 2011.
17. Katzen JT, McCarthy JG. Syndromes involving craniosynostosis and midface hypoplasia. Otolaryngol Clin North Am 33:1257-1284, 2000.
18. Agochukwu NB, Solomon BD, Muenke M. Impact of genetics on the diagnosis and clinical management of syndromic craniosynostosis. Childs Nerv Syst 28:1447-1463, 2012.
19. Marucci DD, Dunaway DJ, Jones BM, et al. Raised intracranial pressure in Apert syndrome. Plast Reconstr Surg 122:1162-1168, 2008.
20. Cohen MM Jr. Pfeiffer syndrome update, clinical subtypes, and guidelines for differential diagnosis. Am J Med Genet 45:300-307, 1993.
21. Fearon JA, Rhodes J. Pfeiffer syndrome: a treatment evaluation. Plast Reconstr Surg 123:1560-1569, 2009.
22. Foo R, Guo Y, McDonald-McGinn DM, et al. The natural history of patients treated for TWIST1-confirmed Saethre-Chotzen syndrome. Plast Reconstr Surg 124:2085-2095, 2009.
23. Bellus GA, Gaudenz K, Zackai EH, et al. Identical mutations in three different fibroblast growth factor receptor genes in autosomal dominant craniosynostosis syndromes. Nat Genet 14:174-176, 1996.
24. Honnebier MB, Cabiling DS, Hetlinger M, et al. The natural history of patients treated for FGFR3-associated (Muenke-type) craniosynostosis. Plast Reconstr Surg 121:919-931, 2008.
25. Tessier P. The definitive plastic surgical treatment of the severe facial deformities of craniofacial dysostosis: Crouzon's and Apert's disease. Plast Reconstr Surg 48:419-442, 1971.
26. Derderian CA, Barlett SP. Open cranial vault remodeling: the evolving role of distraction osteogenesis. J Craniofac Surg 23:229-234, 2012.
27. Derderian CA, Bastidas N, Bartlett SP. Posterior cranial vault expansion using distraction osteogenesis. Childs Nerv Syst 28:1551-1556, 2012.
28. Greene AK, Mulliken JB, Proctor MR, et al. Primary grafting with autologous cranial particulate bone prevents osseous defects following fronto-orbital advancement. Plast Reconstr Surg 120:1603-1611, 2008.
29. Hobar PC, Masson JA, Herrera R, et al. Fever after craniofacial surgery in the infant under 24 months of age. Plast Reconstr Surg 102:32-36, 1998.
30. Barone CM, Jimenez DF. Endoscopic craniectomy for early correction of craniosynostosis. Plast Reconstr Surg 104:1965-1973, 1999.
31. Khechoyan D, Schook C, Birgfeld CB, et al. Changes in frontal morphology after single-stage open posterior–middle vault expansion for sagittal craniosynostosis. Plast Reconstr Surg 129:504-516, 2012.
32. Smyth MD, Tenenbaum MJ, Kaufman CB, et al. The "clamshell" craniotomy technique in treating sagittal craniosynostosis in older children. J Neurosurg(4 Suppl)105:245-251, 2006.
33. Selber J, Reid RR, Gershman B, et al. Evolution of operative techniques for the treatment of single-suture metopic synostosis. Ann Plast Surg 59:6-13, 2007.

# 22. Craniofacial Clefts

Samer Abouzeid, Christopher A. Derderian, Melissa A. Crosby

## EMBRYOLOGY[1]

- 3-8 weeks: Facial development occurs [2] (Fig. 22-1).
  - 3-4 weeks:
    - Frontonasal prominence of forebrain results in nasal and olfactory placodes that become medial and lateral processes.
      - **Medial nasal process:** Nasal tip, columella, philtrum, and premaxilla
      - **Lateral nasal process:** Nasal ala
    - Mandibular arch bifurcates to form mandibular and maxillary processes that move toward midline to form lower mouth and upper portions of the mouth, respectively.
  - 5-6 weeks:
    - Nasal processes enlarge, migrate, and coalesce in midline to unite with maxillary process to form upper lip. Growth of midface is completed when coalescence occurs.

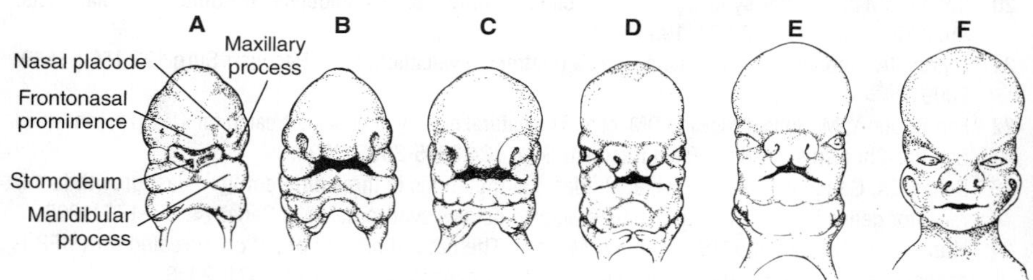


**Fig. 22-1** Embryonic development of the human face. **A,** 4-week embryo. **B,** 5-week embryo. **C,** 6-week embryo. **D,** 6½-week embryo. **E,** 7-week embryo. **F,** 8-week embryo.

## PATHOGENESIS

### THEORIES

- **Classic**[3,4]
  - Facial processes fail to fuse.
  - Face forms as maxillary processes meet and coalesce with paired globular processes beneath the nasal pits.
  - Epithelial contact is established, and mesodermal penetration completes fusion to form lip and hard palate.
  - Cleft forms when process is disrupted.
- **Mesodermal penetration**[5-7]
  - Face consists of a bilaminar ectodermal membrane with epithelial seams that demarcate major processes.
  - Mesenchyme migrates into double wall of ectoderm to penetrate and smooth out seams.
  - Dehiscence occurs and cleft is produced if penetration fails and epithelial walls are unsupported.

## CLASSIFICATION[1,7-9] (Figs. 22-2 through 22-6)

- **Anatomic:** A number is assigned to each malformation according to its position relative to midline.[8]
- **Embryologic:** Craniofacial skeleton develops along a helical course symbolized by the letter *S* (not commonly used as a classification system).[10]

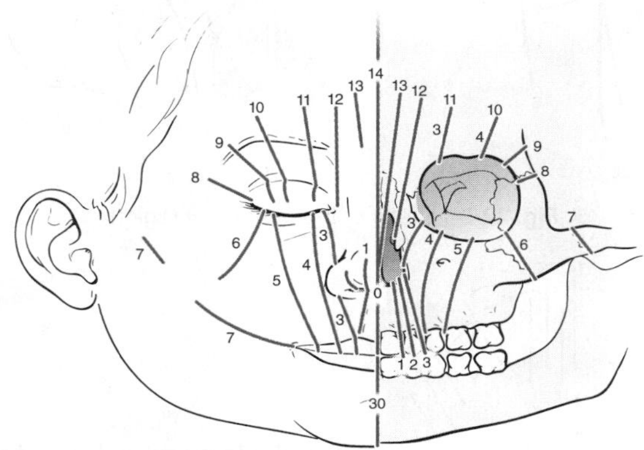

**Fig. 22-2** Tessier classification of clefts. Paths of various clefts on the face *(left);* location of the clefts on the facial skeleton *(right).*

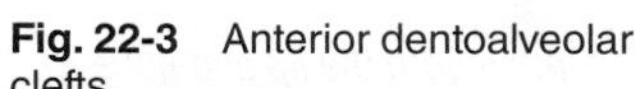

**Fig. 22-3** Anterior dentoalveolar clefts.

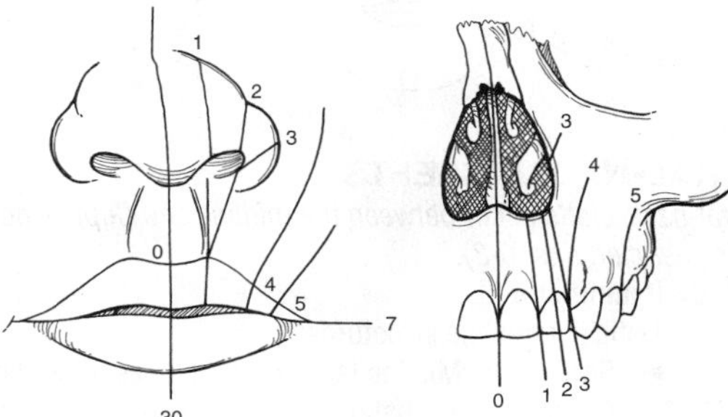

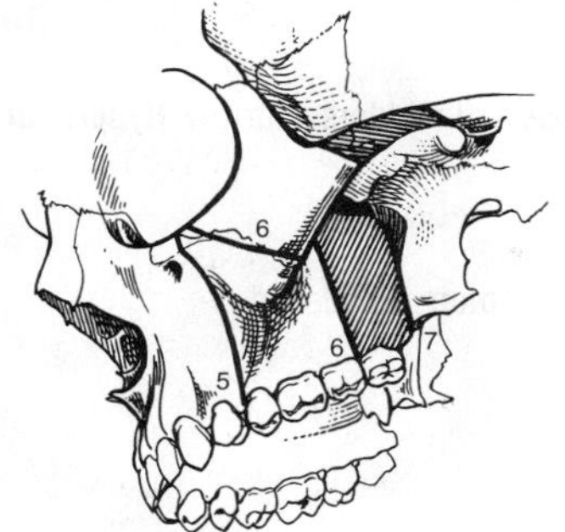

**Fig. 22-4** Posterior dentoalveolar clefts.

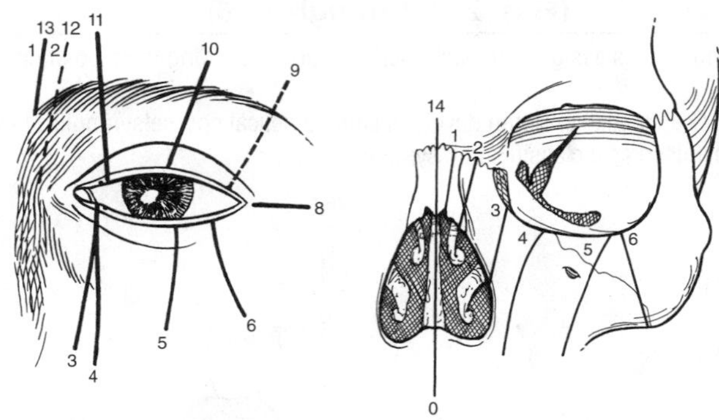


**Fig. 22-5** Clefts of the periorbital region.

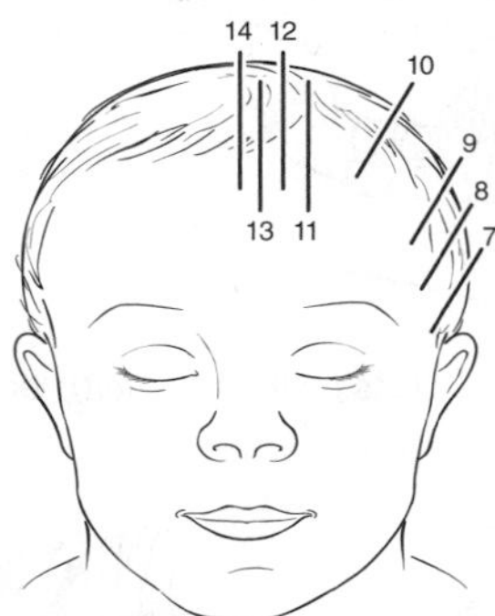


**Fig. 22-6** Temporal and cranial clefts.

## ORAL-NASAL CLEFTS

*Oral-nasal clefts occur between the midline and Cupid's bow, disrupting both the lip and nose (Tessier cleft nos. 0-3).*

- **Cleft number 0**
  - Deficient midline structures:
    - Soft tissue: Midline facial cleft includes upper lip/nose, leading to **hypotelorism** (holoprosencephaly).
    - Skeletal involvement: Premaxilla is absent with secondary palate cleft and partial to total absence of nasal bones.
  - Excess midline structures:
    - Soft tissue: Duplicated frenulum and bifid nose and middorsal furrow. **Hypertelorism.**
    - Skeletal involvement:
      - Diastema of the upper incisors
      - Keel-shaped maxillary alveolus
      - Nasal maxillary process, nasal bones, and septum broadened
  - Can continue as cleft number 14

- **Cleft no. 1**
  - Soft tissue:
    - Pattern is similar to that of cleft lip and palate.
    - Cleft through lateral margin of Cupid's bow progresses into nose, typically causing notching of dome and soft triangle but may extend medially to a malpositioned medial canthus.
  - Skeletal involvement:
    - Cleft separates nasal floor from piriform and the nasal bone from the frontal process of the maxilla.
    - Cleft passes between central and lateral incisor.
  - Classified as nasoschizis (subtype of nasal dysplasia)
  - Can continue as cleft number 13
- **Cleft no. 2**
  - Soft tissue:
    - Originates at lateral margin of Cupid's bow and extends into the alar rim lateral to dome
    - Ala typically hypoplastic and soft tissue of nose is flattened
    - Medial canthus displaced but lacrymal duct not involved
  - Skeletal involvement:
    - Cleft through lateral incisor extends into piriform aperture.
    - Nasal ala is hypoplastic.
  - Extremely rare
  - Can extend as cleft number 12
- **Cleft no. 3**
  - Common
  - Unilateral or bilateral with equal distribution
  - Soft tissue:
    - Originates from lateral margin of Cupid's bow and extends across the alar through the frontal process of the maxillary process; extends through the nasolacrimal duct and into lacrimal groove
    - Alar base usually superiorly displaced and the nose foreshortened
    - Lacrimal system often blocked with anomalous drainage onto the cheek
    - Colobomas of lower eyelid
    - Globe malpositioned inferiorly and laterally; risk of corneal desiccation if no soft tissue deficiency
  - Skeletal involvement:
    - Direct communication of oral, nasal, and orbital cavities
    - Between lateral incisor and canine
  - Can continue as cleft number 10 or 11

## ORAL-OCULAR CLEFTS

*These clefts connect the oral and orbital cavities without disrupting the integrity of the nose. They occur lateral to Cupid's bow, extend through soft tissue of the cheek and maxillary process, and are called* meloschisis *(Tessier cleft numbers 4-6).*

- **Cleft number 4**
  - One of most disruptive and complicated clefts
  - Unilateral, bilateral, or combined with other clefts
  - Soft tissue:
    - Begins **lateral to Cupid's bow** between commissure of mouth and philtral crest, passes onto cheek **lateral to nasal ala,** and curves into lower eyelid to terminate medial to punctum
    - Lower canniculus usually disrupted along with most of the inferior supporting structures to the eye
    - Colobomas
    - Medial canthal ligament and lacrimal apparatus usually intact
  - Skeletal involvement:
    - Nose displaced superiorly especially in bilateral cases
    - Begins between lateral incisor and canine teeth; extends onto anterior surface of maxilla lateral to piriform aperture, medial to infraorbital foramen; medial and inferior portions of orbital wall disrupted
- **Cleft number 5**
  - **Rarest of oral-ocular clefts**
  - Soft tissue:
    - Begins medial to oral commissure and courses along cheek lateral to the nasal ala
    - Terminates in the lateral half of the lower eyelid
  - Skeletal involvement:
    - Begins lateral to the canine
    - Courses **lateral to infraorbital foramen** and terminates in lateral aspect of orbital rim and floor
    - Lateral orbital wall possibly thickened and greater sphenoid wing abnormal
- **Cleft number 6**
  - Includes incomplete forms of Treacher Collins syndrome
  - Transition between oral-ocular and lateral facial clefts
  - Ear normal
  - Zygomaticomaxillary cleft
  - Soft tissue:
    - Cleft is a vertical furrow extending from oral commissure to lateral lower eyelid.
    - Lateral palpebral fissure is pulled downward and lateral canthus follows, causing antimongoloid slant.
    - This creates an appearance of ectropion and colobomas of the lower eyelid.
  - Skeletal involvement:
    - Choanal atresia is common.
    - Cleft is connected to the inferior orbital fissure.
    - Zygoma is hypoplastic.
    - Anterior cranial fossa is narrowed.

## LATERAL FACIAL CLEFTS

*These include Tessier cleft numbers 7-9, Treacher Collins syndrome, Goldenhar's syndrome, hemifacial microsomia, and necrotic facial dysplasia.*

- **Cleft number 7**
  - ***Most common of all craniofacial clefts,*** often accompanies craniofacial microsomia
  - Males affected more frequently than females
  - 10% bilateral
  - Occurs in 1-6 of 8000 births in sporadic fashion
  - Has been postulated that cleft is a result of **disruption of stapedial artery** in embryogenesis
  - Variable degrees of soft tissue deformity
  - Middle ear, zygoma, maxilla, and mandible affected
  - Paresis of CN V and CN VII common
  - Soft tissue:
    - Begins at oral commissure and varies from a mild broadening to a complete fissure
    - Extends laterally toward the ear, ceasing at anterior border of masseter muscle
    - Ear deformity varies from a skin tag to a complete microtic ear.
  - Skeletal involvement:
    - Cleft passes through the pterygomaxillary junction.
    - Posterior maxilla and ramus (condyle and coronoid) are hypoplastic.
    - Zygomatic body is also severely hypoplastic and displaced.
    - Cranial base is asymmetrical.
    - Open bite or crossbite is seen.
  - Involves orbit, mandible, ear, soft tissue, and facial nerve
- **Cleft number 8**
  - Rare: Almost always exists in combination with another rare cleft
  - Isolated largely to orbital area
  - Soft tissue:
    - Coloboma of the lateral commissure with absence of the lateral canthus
  - Skeletal involvement:
    - Involves frontozygomatic suture
    - Zygoma hypoplastic or absent and lateral orbital wall missing
    - Continuity of the orbit and temporal fossa
  - Associated with Goldenhar's syndrome
- **Cleft number 9**
  - Extremely rare
  - May be accompanied by encephaloceles
  - Soft tissue:
    - Lateral third of upper eyelid and brow abnormalities (hallmarks)
    - Microphthalmia (rare)
    - CN VII palsy to the forehead and upper eyelid
  - Skeletal involvement:
    - Hypoplastic greater wing of the sphenoid causes posterior displacement of lateral orbital rim.
    - Dimension of anterior cranial fossa is reduced.

## Treacher Collins Syndrome (Fig. 22-7)

- **Bilateral combination of Tessier cleft numbers 6-8**
- Described by Treacher Collins in 1900
- **Autosomal dominant** with incidence of 1:10,000 live births
- Change in gene on chromosome 5
- Includes coloboma and retraction of lower lid (antimongoloid slant), with hypoplasia of lower lid lashes
- Upper lid redundant in lateral half and gives false impression of ptosis
- Lateral canthus displaced inferiorly
- Absence of zygomatic arch
- Hypoplasia of temporalis muscle
- Ear malformations
- Abnormalities of hairline, including tongue-shaped processes extending toward cheeks
- Absence of lateral inferior orbital rim
- Hypoplasia of malar bones and mandible
- Airway management priority in newborn because of narrow pharyngeal diameter and mandibular shortening

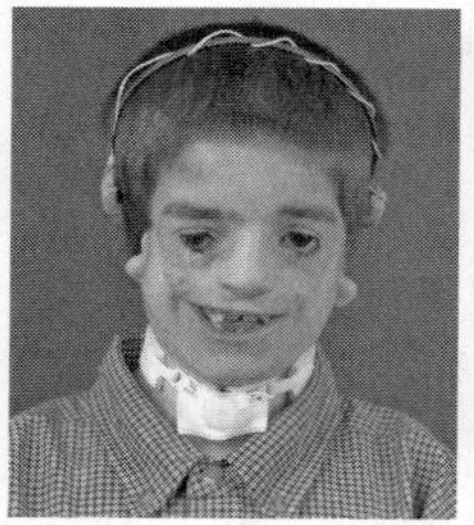
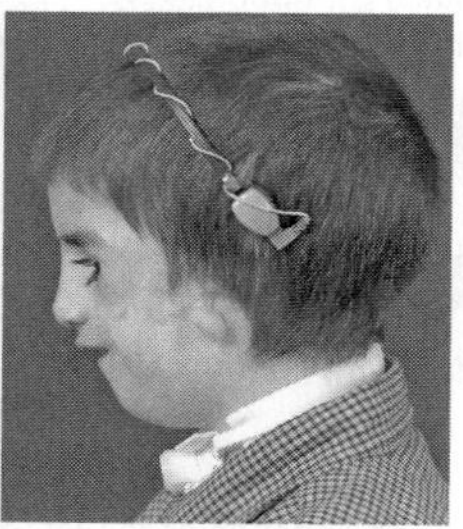

**Fig. 22-7** Patient with Treacher Collins syndrome and tracheostomy for airway management.

## Goldenhar's Syndrome

- Sporadic occurrence
- Prominent frontal bossing
- Low hairline
- Mandibular hypoplasia
- Low-set ears
- Colobomas of upper eyelid
- Epibulbar dermoids
- Bilateral anterior accessory auricular appendages (Fig. 22-8)
- Vertebral abnormalities

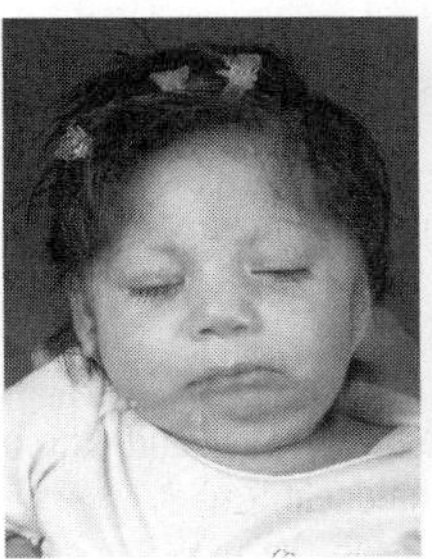
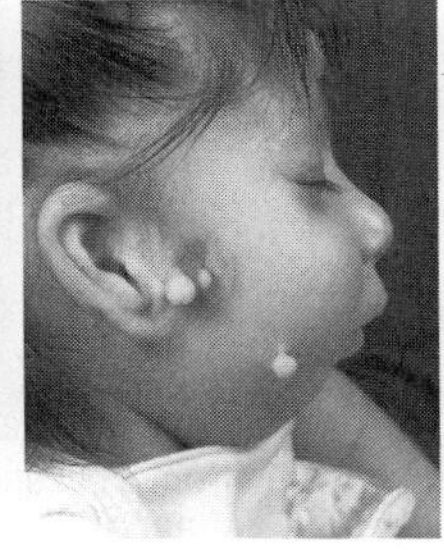
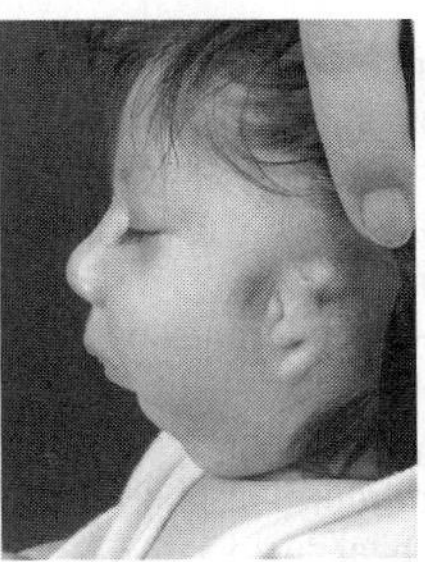

**Fig. 22-8** Patient with Goldenhar's syndrome demonstrating anterior accessory auricular appendages.

## Cranial Clefts

*Clefts extend superiorly from the lateral orbit to the midline and proceed through the frontal bone and often into the base of the cranial vault.*

- **Cleft number 10**
  - Corresponds to cranial branch of cleft number 4
  - Soft tissue:
    - Begins at middle third of upper eyelid and eyebrow
    - Coloboma in mid-upper lid and irregular retracted central brow
  - Skeletal involvement:
    - Cleft at middle orbital rim just lateral to supraorbital foramen
    - Encephalocele common, and hypertelorism from inferolateral rotation of orbit
    - Anterior cranial base distortion
- **Cleft number 11**
  - Found in combination with cleft number 3
  - Soft tissue:
    - Medial third of upper eyelid and brow with a coloboma
    - Disruption extends to hairline
  - Skeletal involvement:
    - Extensive pneumatization of ethmoid cells produces hypertelorism/encephalocele.
    - Cranial base is normal.
- **Cleft number 12**
  - Extension of cleft number 2
  - Soft tissue:
    - Cleft lies medial to the medial canthus, which is displaced laterally.
    - Colobomas extend to the root of the eyebrow.
    - Paramedian frontal hairline projects downward.
  - Skeletal involvement:
    - Orbital hypertelorism and telecanthus from increased dimension of ethmoidal cells
    - Frontal and sphenoid sinuses pneumatized
    - Lies lateral to the cribriform plate, which is normal
    - Anterior and middle cranial fossas enlarged

- **Cleft number 13**
  - Extension of cleft number 1
  - Soft tissue:
    - Paramedian frontal encephalocele located between nasal bone and frontal process of maxilla
    - V-shaped frontal hair projection
  - Skeletal involvement:
    - Hypertelorism from widening of cribriform plate olfactory groove and ethmoid cells
    - Cribriform plate displaced inferiorly by frontal encephalocele
    - Orbital dystopia
- **Cleft number 14**
  - Midline facial clefts accompany central nervous system abnormalities
  - Extension of cleft number 0
  - If true cleft, see herniation of intracranial contents, resulting in arrest of normal migration of orbit
  - Life expectancy severely limited
  - Like cleft number 0, may produce agenesis or overabundance of tissue
  - Soft tissue:
    - Abundance:
      - Hypertelorism
      - Midline encephalocele
      - Long midline frontal hairline
    - Agenesis:
      - Holoprosencephaly: Hypotelorism, microcephaly, severe CNS abnormalities
      - Cyclopia
      - Malformation of the forebrain proportional to degree of facial deformity
  - Skeletal involvement:
    - Medial frontal defect leads to an encephalocele
    - Midline structures bifidity: crista galli, perpendicular plate of ethmoid
    - Cribriform plate caudally displaced up to 20 mm
    - Harlequin deformity of orbits from the upslanting of the anterior cranial fossa
- **Cleft number 30**
  - Soft tissue:
    - There is a notch in the lower lip.
    - Anterior tongue can be bifid and attached to the mandible by a dense fibrous band.
  - Skeletal involvement:
    - Cleft between the central incisors extends into mandibular symphysis.
    - Hyoid bone may be absent.
    - Thyroid cartilage is incompletely formed.

# RECONSTRUCTION

## MULTIDISCIPLINARY APPROACH

- Initially focuses on soft tissue closure, with excision of all scars within clefts until normal tissue is reached, followed by meticulous layered closure of soft tissue
- Skeletal reconstruction often necessary but delayed until child is older

## GOALS

- Functional correction of macrostomia
- Soft tissue reconstruction of eyelid to prevent globe exposure
- Separation of the confluent oral, nasal, and orbital spaces
- Aesthetic correction of deformity

## KEY POINTS

✓ The most common craniofacial cleft is number 7.
✓ Treacher Collins syndrome involves Tessier cleft numbers 6-8.
✓ Goldenhar syndrome is associated with Tessier cleft number 8.
✓ Know the Tessier diagram and location of each cleft relative to midline.

## REFERENCES


1. Hunt JA, Hobar PC. Common craniofacial anomalies: facial clefts and encephaloceles. Plast Reconstr Surg 112:606-616, 2003.
2. Kawamoto HK Jr. Rare craniofacial clefts. In McCarthy JG, ed. Plastic Surgery, vol 4. Cleft Lip and Palate and Craniofacial Anomalies. Philadelphia: WB Saunders, 1990.
3. Carstens M. Development of the facial midline. J Craniofac Surg 13:129-187, 2002.
4. David DJ, Moore MH, Cooter RD. Tessier clefts revisited with a third dimension. Cleft Palate J 26:163-184, 1989.
5. Kawamoto HK Jr. The kaleidoscopic world of rare craniofacial clefts: order out of chaos (Tessier classification). Clin Plast Surg 3:529-572, 1976.
6. Argenta LC, David LR. Craniofacial clefts and other related deformities. In Achauer BM, Eriksson E, Kolk CV, eds. Plastic Surgery: Indications, Operations, and Outcomes. St Louis: Mosby–Year Book, 2000.
7. Hunt J, Flood J. Craniofacial anomalies II: syndromes and surgery. Sel Read Plast Surg 3(25), 2002.
8. Tessier P. Anatomical classification of facial, cranio-facial, and latero-facial clefts. J Maxillofac Surg 4:69-92, 1976.
9. Bentz ML, Bauer BS, Zuker RM. Principles and Practice of Pediatric Plastic Surgery. St Louis: Quality Medical Publishing, 2008.
10. Van der Meulen JC, Mazzola R, Vermey-Keers C, et al. A morphogenetic classification of craniofacial malformations. Plast Reconstr Surg 71:560-572, 1983.

# 23. Distraction Osteogenesis

**Christopher A. Derderian, Samer Abouzeid,**
**Jeffrey E. Janis, Jason E. Leedy**

## DEFINITION

**Distraction osteogenesis (DO)** generates vascularized bone between the cut ends of an osteotomy or corticotomy by gradually separating them from one another using a specialized fixation device.

## PHYSIOLOGY

- Takes advantage of the body's innate ability to heal bone and accommodate soft tissue expansion
- Success depends on several factors:
  - Vascularity and quality of the tissues
  - Stability of the distraction device
  - Time delay between osteotomy and initiation of distraction (latency)
  - Rate and frequency of distraction

### Bone

- DO generates vascularized bone with normal cortical and medullary features.
- A **generate** develops, which is akin to a callus.
- Unlike in a callus, the collagen fibers in the generate are organized parallel to the vector of distraction.
- The generate has three distinct histologic zones and two transitional zones[1] (Fig. 23-1).

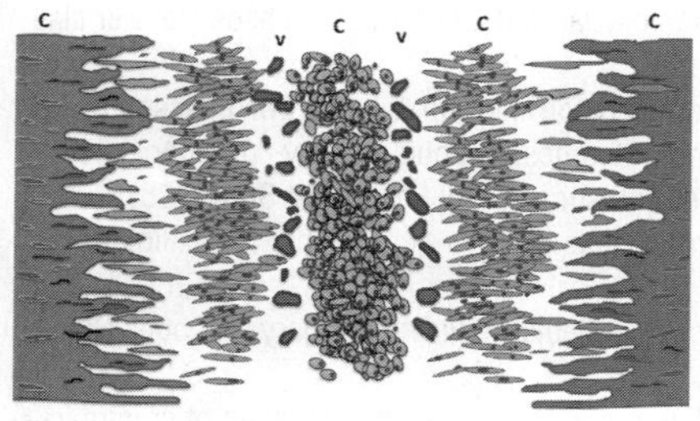


**Fig. 23-1** Five zones and four transition areas are present in the generate during the activation phase of DO: a central zone of proliferating mesenchymal cells *(C),* two paracentral zones, and two zones where mature bone meets the generate. The four transitional areas comprise two areas of vasculogenesis *(v)* and two mineralization fronts.

1. Central zone: Cellular proliferation
2. Transitional zone of vasculogenesis
3. Paracentral zone: Parallel orientation of collagen fibers with osteoid production
4. Transitional mineralization front: Primary mineralization found with bone spicule formation
5. Mature bone zone: Progressive calcification of primary mineralization front with formation of cortical and cancellous elements

- During the consolidation phase, the less mature central portions of the generate mature and merge with the mineralizing fronts for union.
- **Bone formed through the process of DO is indistinguishable from natural mature bone.**

## SOFT TISSUE

- The skin, subcutaneous tissue, nerves, vasculature, and muscles elongate in response to the alterations in mechanical load produced by elongation of the bone (tissue histogenesis).
- This provides gradual expansion of the soft tissue envelope and maintains this expansion during consolidation.
- Results in:
  - Less blood loss
  - Decreased infection rate
  - Reduction of dead space
  - Lower incidence and degree of relapse from soft tissue recoil than common single-stage procedures with bone grafts

## DISTRACTION PROCESS[2]

- **Osteotomy or corticotomy**
  - Usually osteotomy created through cortical and medullary bone that attempts to minimize periosteal stripping while protecting nerves
- **Application of distraction device**
- **Latency:** Period between osteotomy and commencement of distraction
  - Depends on patient age: Neonates requiring mandibular distraction for Pierre Robin sequence can range from 0 to 72 hours; 5-7 days for most patients
  - Allows osteocyte precursor cell migration and proliferation and initiation of angiogenesis in the maturing clot found between the cut bone ends. Clot serves as substrate for production of a generate.
  - ***Rate:*** Millimeters of distraction per day
    - Neonates and infants can tolerate 2-4 mm of mandibular distraction per day
    - Patients older than 1 year: Usually 1 mm/day
      - Too slow leads to premature ossification
      - Too fast results in fibrous union
  - ***Rhythm:*** Number of times per day the distractor is activated
    - The more highly fractionated the rhythm (many very small movements), the better the volume and quality of generate; however, for practicality, the rate is divided between 2 and 4 turns/day.
- **Activation phase:** Period of active distraction and production of the generate
- **Consolidation phase:** Begins when desired length of distraction is achieved and activation ends
  - Length of time is case dependent, but usually is 6-8 weeks for mandibular distraction.
  - Distractor is left in place and serves as a rigid fixation device, which is critical to achieve union.
  - Although radiographs are useful for checking device stability and tracking areas of clinical interest as they move in space, **there is often no radiographic evidence of bone in the zone of distraction at the time of device removal.** Occasionally a faint outline of the generate can be seen, but visibility is not necessary for safe device removal (Fig. 23-2).

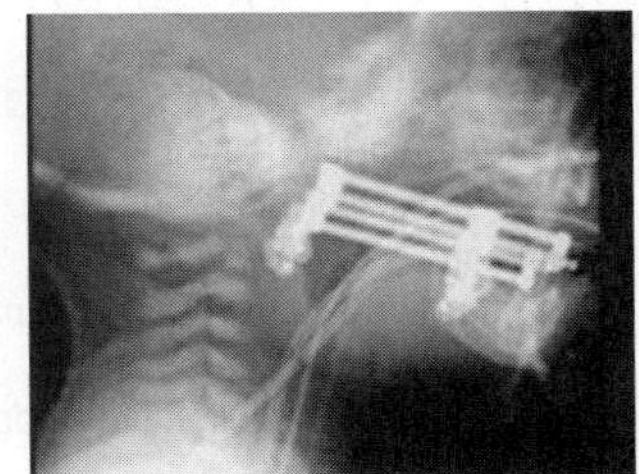

**Fig. 23-2** Radiographs can be used to check new bone quality during the consolidation phase of mandibular distraction.

## INDICATIONS FOR DISTRACTION

- **Mandibular lengthening**
  - Hemifacial microsomia
  - Micrognathia
  - Airway compromise in newborn secondary to micrognathia
- **LeFort I advancement**
  - For large anterior movements (>1 cm)
  - Particularly useful for clefts with significant class III malocclusion from maxillary hypoplasia, when soft tissues are less compliant and often require large movements
- **LeFort III/monobloc advancement**[3,4]
  - Most commonly used for patients with syndromic craniosynostosis who have severe midface hypoplasia and exorbitism
- **Posterior cranial vault distraction**[5]
  - Recently introduced for expanding the posterior vault in syndromic bicoronal craniosynostosis (see Chapter 21).

## DISTRACTION DEVICES

### EXTERNAL (Fig. 23-3)

- Percutaneous pins fixed to either a uniplanar or multiplanar mandibular distraction device or rigid external distraction (RED) halo device to control the distraction segments
- **Advantages**
  - Easier to apply and remove
  - Better control of segments: Can employ multiple vectors and change vectors during distraction
- **Disadvantages**
  - It is socially stigmatizing for the patient.
  - Device may become dislodged.
  - Percutaneous pin-site scars may require revision.

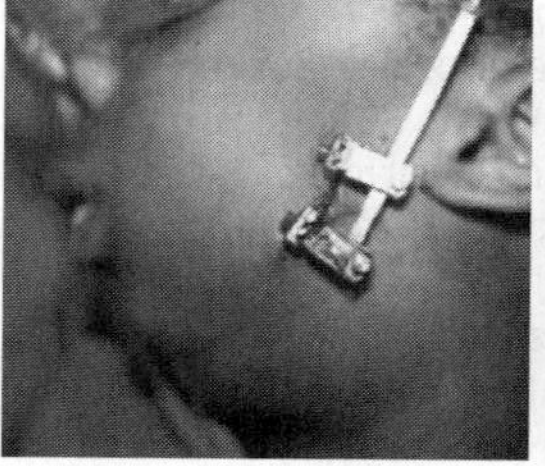
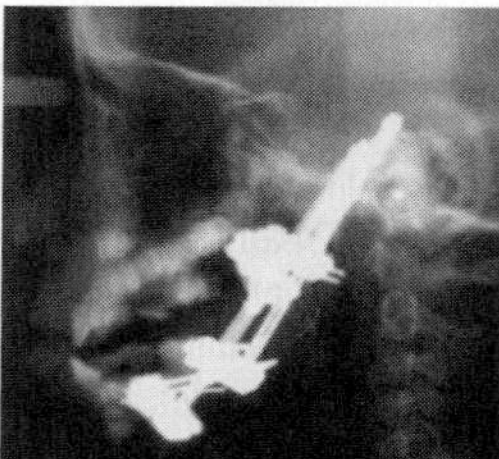

**Fig. 23-3** External distraction device.

### INTERNAL (Fig. 23-4)

- Internal (buried) distraction devices placed directly on bone
- **Advantages**
  - Minimizes cutaneous scarring
  - Less stigmatizing
  - Less likely to become dislodged
- **Disadvantages**
  - Committed to single vector determined at the time of placement
  - More difficult to apply
  - Open procedure using anesthesia required for removal

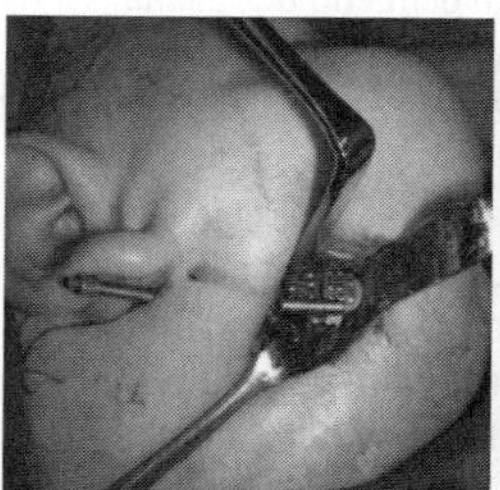
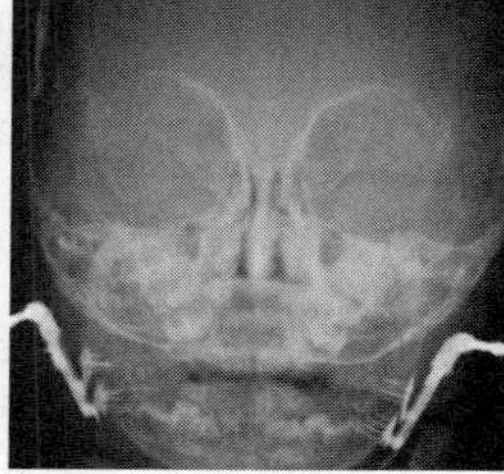

**Fig. 23-4** Internal distraction device.

### Resorbable

- Hybrid devices will likely be available soon, but are not yet widely used.

## MANDIBULAR DISTRACTION

### Goals

- Achieve proper occlusion.
- Restore normal dimensions to the mandible, which normalizes the relationship of the tongue base to the airway.
- Transport distraction may be used to reconstruct the temporomandibular joint.

### Operative Technique

1. Gain adequate exposure of mandible through a Risdon or intraoral incision.
2. Identify proposed osteotomy site based on preoperative imaging.

> **TIP:** Typically the osteotomy is not completed until after the distraction device is secured, because mobility of the ramus after completion makes device application significantly more difficult.

- L-shaped or straight vertical osteotomy on ramus to give horizontal advancement
  - Can make C-shaped osteotomy to exclude coronoid process (and pull from temporalis) from anterior segment (Fig. 23-5)
- Oblique osteotomy on lower ramus to give both horizontal and vertical advancement
- Horizontal osteotomy on ramus to give vertical lengthening (not commonly used)

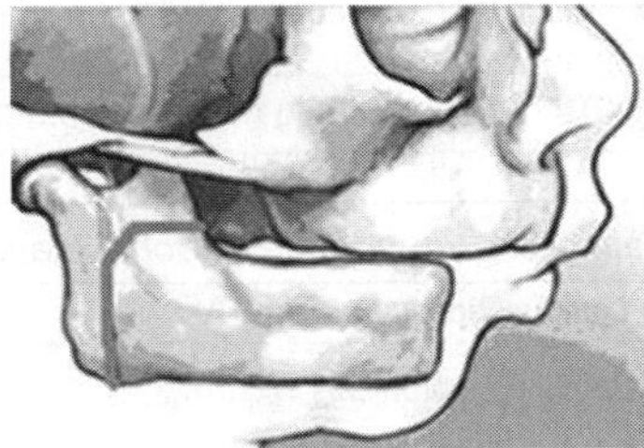

**Fig. 23-5** C-shaped osteotomy of the mandible.

> **TIP:** Avoid disruption of tooth buds and the inferior alveolar nerve by using preoperative dental examinations, radiographs, and CT scans.

3. Place the distraction device and confirm that vectors are correct and collinear if bilateral.
4. Complete the osteotomies and confirm completion by activating the distraction device.
5. Perform closure.

## MIDFACE/MAXILLARY DO

### Goals

- **Achieve class I functional occlusion**
- **Correct midface retrusion**
  - Useful if more than 1 cm of advancement is desired, because a gradual process with distraction allows soft tissues to adapt better than if advancement is performed immediately.
- **Improve aesthetic appearance**

## Operative Technique

1. Gain adequate exposure of midface/maxilla through a gingivobuccal incision and/or a coronal incision, if necessary.
2. Identify proposed osteotomy site based on preoperative imaging (LeFort I, II, or III).

**TIP:** Again, always avoid tooth bud disruption!

3. Ensure completion of osteotomy/disjunction by rotating the alveolar or midface segment in three planes.
4. Place the distraction device.
5. Perform closure.

## COMPLICATIONS/TECHNICAL ERRORS[6] (Table 23-1)

- Infection
- Nerve (inferior alveolar) injury
- Fibrous or nonunion
- Premature consolidation
- Tooth bud disruption
- Inappropriate vector

**TIP:** Bone grafting may be required if distraction failure occurs.

**Table 23-1** *Incidence of Complications in Craniofacial Distraction Osteogenesis*

| Complication | Frequency (%) |
|---|---|
| Compliance problems | 4.7 |
| Hardware failure | 4.5 |
| Device dislodgement | 3.0 |
| Premature consolidation | 1.9 |
| Pain that prevents distraction | 1.0 |
| Fibrous nonunion | 0.5 |
| Inappropriate vector (single-vector device) | 8.8 |
| Inappropriate vector (multivector device) | 7.2 |
| Pin tract infection | 5.2 |

## Key Points

✓ DO involves osteotomy, latency, activation, and consolidation phases.
✓ Device selection and treatment strategy are patient and situation specific.
✓ The beneficial effects of gradual expansion of the soft tissue envelope that accompanies distraction include less blood loss, decreased infection rate, dead space reduction, larger advancements, and decreased incidence and degree of relapse than with single-stage advancements.

## REFERENCES

1. Yu JC, Fearon J, Havlik RJ, et al. Distraction osteogenesis of the craniofacial skeleton. Plast Reconstr Surg 114:1E-20E, 2004.
2. McCarthy JG, Stelnicki EJ, Mehrara BJ, et al. Distraction osteogenesis of the craniofacial skeleton. Plast Reconstr Surg 107:1812-1827, 2001.
3. Fearon JA. Halo distraction of the Le Fort III in syndromic craniosynostosis: a long-term assessment. Plast Reconstr Surg 115:1524-1536, 2005.
4. Bradley JP, Gabbay JS, Taub PJ, et al. Monobloc advancement by distraction osteogenesis decreases morbidity and relapse. Plast Reconstr Surg 118:1585-1597, 2006.
5. Derderian CA, Bastidas N, Bartlett SP. Posterior cranial vault expansion using distraction osteogenesis. Childs Nerv Syst 28:1551-1556, 2012.
6. Mofid MM, Manson PN, Robertson BC, et al. Craniofacial distraction osteogenesis: a review of 3278 cases. Plast Reconstr Surg 108:1103-1114, 2001.

# 24. Cleft Lip

Bridget Harrison

## DEMOGRAPHICS

- Cleft lip and/or palate (CL/P) has a **variable racial distribution**[1]
  - High: Asians, approximately 2:1000
  - Intermediate: Whites, approximately 1:1000
  - Low: Blacks, approximately 0.5:1000
- **CL/P more frequent in males (2:1),** but no significant sex difference for cleft lip alone.
- **Left unilateral CL/P is the most common configuration.**
  - Left/right/bilateral: 6:3:1
  - Unilateral clefts are six times more common than bilateral clefts
- 10% of all infants with cleft lip and palate have an associated syndrome[2]

**TIP:** Cleft lip with or without cleft palate is the most common craniofacial abnormality.

## EMBRYOLOGY AND ANATOMY

### Facial Development

- The face forms from five facial primordia: Frontonasal prominence, bilateral maxillary prominences, and bilateral mandibular prominences.
  - Frontonasal prominence: Forehead, nose, and top of the mouth
  - Maxillary prominences: Lateral sides of the mouth
- Failure of **medial nasal process to contact maxillary process** results in cleft lip.[3] (Fig. 24-1)
- Lip formation occurs during weeks 4-7 of gestation.

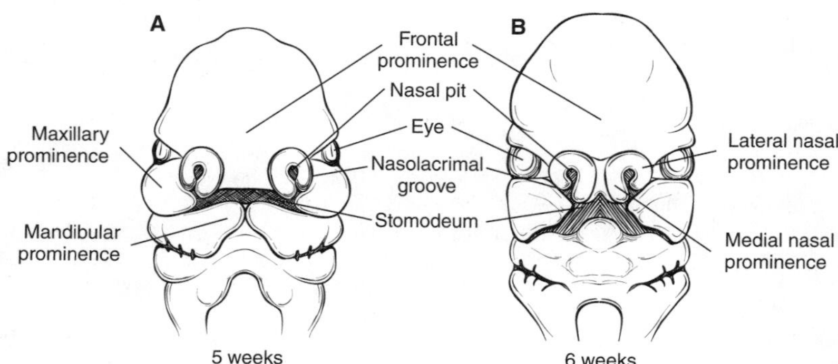


**Fig. 24-1** **A,** Five-week embryo. **B,** Six-week embryo. The frontonasal and medial nasal prominences fuse to form the intermaxillary segment. Failure of these structures to fuse results in cleft lip deformity.

## Normal Upper Lip Anatomy

- **Surface landmarks**
  - **Philtral columns:** Bilateral vertical bulge created by dermal insertion of orbicularis oris fibers
  - **Philtral dimple:** Concavity between columns created by relative paucity of muscle fibers
  - **White roll:** Prominent ridge just above cutaneous-vermilion border
  - **Vermilion:** Red mucosal portion of the lip divided into dry (keratinized) and wet (nonkeratinized); widest at the peaks of Cupid's bow
  - **Red line:** Junction between the dry and wet vermilion mucosa
  - **Cupid's bow:** Curvature of the central white roll; two lateral peaks are the inferior extension of the philtral columns
  - **Tubercle:** Vermilion fullness at central inferior apex of Cupid's bow
- **Muscles**
  - **Orbicularis oris:** Fibers decussate in midline and insert into dermis of opposite philtral column
    - **Deep portion:** Functions as a sphincter; continuous fibers pass from commissure to commissure across midline and extend deep to vermilion
    - **Superficial portion:** Functions in speech and facial expressions
  - **Levator labii superioris:** Inserts inferiorly on white roll; contributes to peaks of Cupid's bow and functions to elevate lip
- **Blood supply and innervation**
  - **Arterial supply:** Bilateral superior labial arteries
  - **Sensory:** Trigeminal nerve ($V_2$)
  - **Motor:** Facial nerve (VII)

## Cleft Lip Anatomy[4]

The severity of the anatomic deformity is highly variable and depends on whether the cleft is complete or incomplete.

> **TIP:** A slight notch in the vermilion may be the only sign of an incomplete cleft.

- Cleft lip results in projection and outward rotation of the premaxilla and retropositioning of the lateral maxillary segment.
- Orbicularis oris muscle in lateral lip element ends at margin of the cleft and inserts into the alar wing.
  - There is hypoplasia and disorientation of the pars marginalis (part of the orbicularis oris).
- Philtrum is short.
- Vermilion width is decreased on the medial side of the cleft and increased laterally.
- Bilateral cleft:
  - Two deep clefts separate prolabium from paired lateral elements.
  - Prolabium has no Cupid's bow, no philtrum or philtral columns, and no orbicularis.
  - Lateral lip element muscle fibers run parallel to cleft edges toward alar bases.

> **TIP:** The muscle does not typically cross the cleft unless the bridge is at least one third the height of the lip.[5]

- **Simonart's band**
  - Residual skin bridge spanning upper portion of cleft lip

## Cleft Nasal Deformity (Fig. 24-2)[6]

- Attenuated lower lateral cartilage
- Nasal tip and nostrils asymmetrical
- Cleft side inferior turbinate hypertrophic
- Alar base displaced laterally, posteriorly, and sometimes inferiorly
- Deficient vestibular lining on cleft side
- Columella shorter on cleft side
- Caudal septum deviated to noncleft side

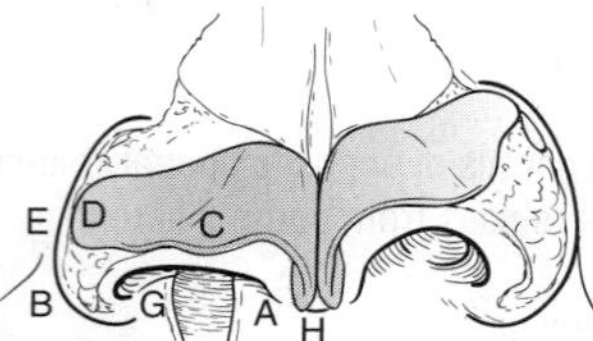


**Fig. 24-2** Unilateral cleft nasal deformity. *A,* Nasal tip deviated. *B,* Alar cartilage displaced caudally. *C,* Angle between medial and lateral crura more obtuse. *D,* Buckling in the lateral crura. *E,* Flattened alar facial angle. *G,* Widened nostril floor. *H,* Columella and anterior caudal septal border deviated. Not shown: Deficiency in bony development, and posterior septum convex on cleft side causing varying degrees of obstruction.

# ETIOLOGIC FACTORS AND PATHOPHYSIOLOGY[2,7]

## Genetic Factors

- No single gene has been identified as the universal culprit of CL/P.
- **Isolated cleft palate is genetically distinct from isolated cleft lip with or without cleft palate.**
- A positive family history increases the likelihood of recurrence (Table 24-1).
- Maternal age <20 or >39 may increase the incidence of CL/P.

**TIP:** A parent affected by CL/P has a 3% to 5% risk of having an affected child.

**Table 24-1** *Risk of Familial Recurrence in Cleft Lip With or Without Cleft Palate*

| Risk of Familial Recurrence | Percent |
|---|---|
| 1 affected parent | 3-5 |
| 1 affected child | 4 |
| 2 affected children | 9 |
| Affected parent and affected child | 17 |
| Monozygotic twins | 40-50 |
| Dizygotic twins | 5 |
| Affected niece or nephew | 1 |
| Affected cousin | 0.5 |

## Environmental Factors

- Phenytoin increases rate of cleft formation 10-fold.
- Infants exposed to anticonvulsants have an increased risk of isolated cleft lip.
- Smoking during the first trimester increases the risk of CL/P.
- Folic acid plays a role in the prevention of CL/P.

# EVALUATION

## Treatment Planning

- Multidisciplinary team approach
  - Requires evaluation by a team, including:
    - Audiologist
    - Geneticist
    - Neurosurgeon
    - Otolaryngologist
    - Pediatrician
    - Plastic surgeon
    - Speech-language pathologist
    - Dentist

## Classification

- Unilateral or bilateral
- Complete or incomplete
  - **Complete clefts:** Extend through lip into nasal floor
  - **Incomplete clefts:** Nasal sill intact
  - **Microform cleft:** Also known as forme fruste
    - Vertical furrow or scar
    - Vermilion notch
    - White roll imperfection
    - Varying degree of vertical lip shortness
- Kernahan striped Y logo sometimes used for diagrammatic representation of CL/P

**TIP:** Microform (forme fruste) cleft lip has three components: Small notch in vermilion, band of fibrous tissue running from edge of red lip to nostril floor, and a deformity of the ala on the side of the notch.

## Feeding

- Infants with isolated cleft lip can usually be fed by breast or regular bottle.
- The presence of a cleft palate prevents the creation of adequate suction.
- Effective nipple is soft and has a cross-cut or several holes.
  - Haberman nipple
    - One-way valve separates nipple from bottle.
  - Squeezable cleft palate nurser (Mead Johnson)
    - Long cross-cut nipple on soft squeeze bottle.
  - Pigeon nipple
    - Long cross-cut nipple on soft squeeze bottle.

**TIP:** Infants with isolated cleft lip are usually able to feed on their own.

## TREATMENT (Table 24-2)

### INTRAUTERINE REPAIR

- CL/P can be detected by prenatal 2D or 3D ultrasound in the second trimester, although accuracy varies, depending on the gestational age and ultrasound technology.
- Intrauterine repair was encouraged by findings of scarless healing in fetal ectoderm.
- Modeled by Hedrick in the fetal lamb model[8]
- More recent advances use fetoendoscopy to reduce fetal membrane trauma.
- Major risks include preterm labor.
- Not currently a standard of care because of high risks.

**Table 24-2** *Cleft Lip Repair*

| Procedure | Age |
|---|---|
| Cleft lip repair | 3 mo |
| Tip rhinoplasty | |
| Tympanostomy tubes | |
| Palatoplasty | 9-18 mo |
| T-tube placement | |
| Speech evaluation | 3-4 yr |
| Velopharyngeal insufficiency workup and surgery | 4-6 yr |
| Alveolar bone grafting | 9-11 yr |
| Nasal reconstruction | 12-18 yr |
| Orthognathic surgery | Completion of mandibular growth (>16 yr) |

### NASOALVEOLAR MOLDING

- **Goals**
  - Align and approximate alveolar segments
  - Correct malposition of nasal cartilages
  - Elongate columella
- **Active** appliances use hard acrylic plate and controlled forces, including extraoral traction.
  - **Latham** device: Two-piece maxillary splint retained by pins
    - Requires surgical procedure to place and remove
- **Passive** appliances use molding plates that are gradually altered as positing improves.

### LIP ADHESION

- Pressure from closed lip to move maxillary segments closer together
- Convert complete cleft lip into an incomplete cleft lip
- Performed at 1-2 months of age
- May feed immediately after procedure
- Indications may include wide unilateral complete clefts and poorly aligned maxillary segments
- Reduction in lip/nasal deformity and facilitation of definitive closure
- Scar formation may interfere with subsequent repair and risk dehiscence

## Gingivoperiosteoplasty

- **Goals**
  - Eliminate nasoalveolar fistulas
  - Support alar base
- 60% of patients who underwent nasoalveolar molding and gingivoperiosteoplasty did not require secondary bone grafting[9]
- Has not been shown to impair maxillary growth
- Performed at time of primary repair or in conjunction with lip adhesion

**TIP:** Presurgical orthopedics followed by periosteoplasty and lip adhesion (POPLA).

## Methods of Unilateral Cleft Lip Repair

- **Rose-Thompson**
  - Straight-line repair
  - May be useful in microform clefts and repair of vermilion notching
- **Triangular flap repair**
  - Popularized by Tennison[10] and Randall[11]
  - Utilizes single Z-plasty at vermilion-cutaneous margin
- **Quadrangular flap repair**
  - Introduced by Hagedorn, modified by LeMesurier[12]
- **Rotation-advancement**
  - Introduced by Millard[13] in 1955
  - Rotates medial lip element downward and fills resulting defect with lateral lip
  - Places scar along the proposed philtral column
  - Most commonly used method of unilateral repair
  - Criticisms include technical difficulty in wide clefts, wide soft tissue undermining, and tension across nostril sill

## Marking a Unilateral Cleft Lip

- Marks may be made with methylene blue dye on pointed end of cotton swab
- **Key points to be marked**[7]
  - Peak of Cupid's bow on normal (noncleft) side
    - Made at junction of red vermilion and normal skin
  - Low point of Cupid's bow
  - Peak of Cupid's bow on cleft side
    - Can use distance between previous two points to mark proposed peak
  - Midpoint of columella
  - Lateral bases of columella
  - Inset of alar base
  - Proposed peak of Cupid's bow on lateral lip element
    - Made at junction of red vermilion and normal skin
  - Low point of Cupid's bow

## Millard Rotation-Advancement Repair (Fig. 24-3)[14]

- Cutaneous incisions are made through rotation and advancement flaps with No. 15c, 15, or 67 Beaver knife blade.
- Mucosal incisions are made with No. 11 blade in submucosal plane.
- **C flap,** *or columellar flap,* is triangle of skin beginning inferiorly at high point of Cupid's bow.
  - Has been used to close nasal sill or lengthen columella
- **M flap,** *for mucosa or medial,* is rectangular flap of mucosa off medial lip element.
  - Used to line gingivobuccal sulcus following release of oral mucosa

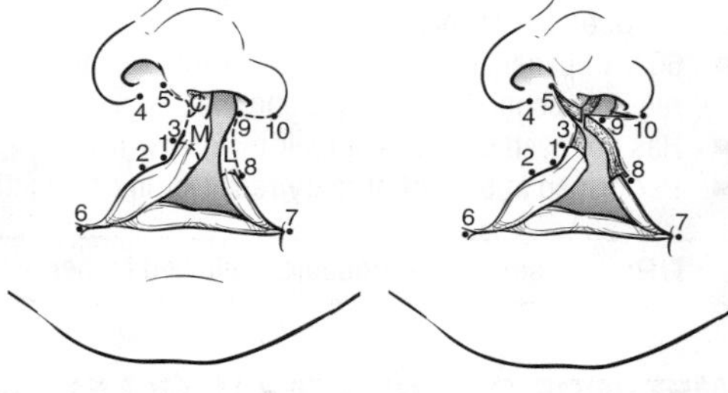

**Fig. 24-3** Rotation-advancement unilateral cleft lip repair and primary nasal repair (Byrd modification of Millard technique).

- **L flap,** *for lateral,* is superiorly based flap of mucosa on lateral lip element.
  - Used to line lateral nasal vestibule
- Skin and mucosa are elevated off orbicularis muscle.
- Muscle is released from abnormal attachments to nose, columella, nasal sill, and alar base.
- Incising gingivobuccal sulcus bilaterally releases soft tissues off maxilla.
- Dissection performed from medial and lateral incisions using small tenotomy scissors is performed over lower lateral cartilages, nasal tips, and onto nasal dorsum.
- Nasal reconstruction may be performed beginning with sutures extending from one alar base to the other.
- **Closure begins with internal structures and proceeds to external, accessible ones.**
- L flap is sutured into defect of lateral wall of nasal vestibule.
- Lateral gingivobuccal sulcus is closed.
- M flap is used to close medial sulcus.
- Orbicularis oris muscle is approximated with vicryl sutures.
- Lip is closed after **inferior rotation** of rotation flap and **medial advancement** of advancement flap.
- Superior defect is closed with C flap.
- A **Noordhoff flap** is a triangular flap of dry mucosa taken from lateral lip element and rotated into incision along wet-dry junction of medial lip element to provide additional bulk.

## Techniques for Primary Cleft Rhinoplasty[15,16]

- Nasal extensions of presurgical maxillary orthopedic device may help mold cartilage.
- Nasal ala must be completely released during cleft lip repair.
- Distal midvault and tip are widely dissected.
- Sutures are placed from lateral alar base to opposite stable footplate.
- Mattress sutures through lower lateral cartilage are used to correct alar webbing.
- **Tajima suture** (Fig. 24-4)[17]
  - Infracartilaginous inverted U incision made on cleft side
  - Suture placed through caudal cleft side lower lateral cartilage to contralateral upper lateral cartilage
  - Supports lower lateral cartilage
- **McComb suture** (Fig. 24-5)[18]
  - Placed from the skin to the middle genu of the lower lateral cartilage on the cleft side and tied over a bolster

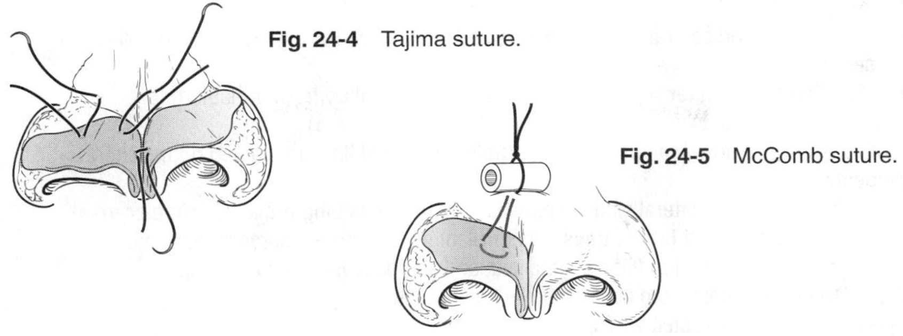

**Fig. 24-4** Tajima suture.

**Fig. 24-5** McComb suture.

## BILATERAL CLEFT LIP REPAIR[19] (Fig. 24-6)

- Philtral flap is marked 3-4 mm wide between peaks of Cupid's bow and 2 mm wide at columellar-labial junction.
- Philtral flap is created from central skin of prolabium.

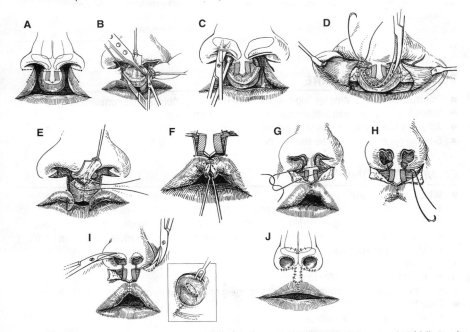

**Fig. 24-6** Bilateral complete cleft lip repair. **A,** Markings for one-stage repair of bilateral complete cleft lip and nasal deformity. **B,** Dissection of the orbicularis oris muscle in lateral labial element. **C,** Exposure of lower lateral cartilages through rim incision. **D,** Completion of bilateral gingivoperiosteoplasty and trimming redundant premaxillary vermilion-mucosa. **E,** Apposition of orbicular muscle; uppermost suture is placed through periosteum overlying anterior nasal spine. **F,** Construction of Cupid's bow and median tubercle. **G,** Placement of interdomal mattress suture. **H,** Insertion of mattress sutures to suspend lower lateral cartilage overlapping upper lateral cartilage. **I,** Narrowing interalar dimension with cinch suture. **J,** Trimming tip of alar flaps and securing the bases to underlying muscle and maxillary periosteum.

- **Millard Repair**
  - Cupid's bow and central tubercle are created from white roll and vermilion of lateral lip segments.
  - **Modified Manchester repair** uses white roll and vermilion from prolabium for reconstruction of Cupid's bow and tubercle.[20,21] (Table 24-3)
- Proposed Cupid's bow peak points and vermilion/mucosal line are marked on the lateral labial elements.
- Philtral flap is incised, lateral skin deepithelialized and remaining prolabial skin discarded.
  - Millard used **banked forked flaps** from prolabium for future columellar lengthening.
- Lateral white line–vermilion flaps are incised, and alar base flaps are elevated.
- Orbicularis is dissected from lateral labial elements.
- Nasal floor is reconstructed with bilateral mucosal flaps.
- Orbicularis is closed and philtral flap is inset.

**Table 24-3** *Comparison of Modified Manchester and Millard Repairs for Bilateral Cleft Lips*

| | Modified Manchester | Millard |
|---|---|---|
| Central vermilion | Reconstructed from prolabium | Reconstructed from lateral lip elements |
| Lateral prolabium | Discarded | Banked as forked flaps |
| Orbicularis | Not reconstructed | Reconstructed in repair |

## POSTOPERATIVE CARE

- Immediate postoperative feeding may be allowed and does not increase complications.[22,23]
- Wound may be cleansed with cotton swab and half-strength $H_2O_2$.
- Although used by some surgeons postoperatively, arm restraints are generally unnecessary.[24]
- Silicone gel sheeting may be started after 1 week and used for 6-8 weeks.

## COMPLICATIONS[25]

- **Whistling deformity**
  - Central vermilion deformity more common after bilateral cleft lip repair
  - Presents as notching or inadequate vermilion with exposure of central incisors in repose
  - If excess vermilion present lateral to defect or in buccal sulcus, V-Y advancement can fill defect
  - May require Abbé flap
- **Short lip**
  - More frequent after Millard repair
  - Can be corrected with rerotation/advancement or V-Y advancement from nostril sill
- **Long lip**
  - More frequent after LeMesurier or triangular flap repair
  - Requires full-thickness excision below nostril sill
- **Widened lip scar**
  - May be evidence of inadequate orbicularis continuity
- **Lip landmark abnormalities**
  - May be corrected with elliptical excision or Z-plasty

## KEY POINTS

- ✓ The incidence of CL/P varies according to race, whereas the incidence of cleft palate does not.
- ✓ Evaluation of patient with cleft lip begins with description of defect, determination of associated anomalies, and appropriate consultations.
- ✓ Presurgical nasoalveolar molding can optimize primary repair of the cleft lip and nose.
- ✓ Primary cleft nasal repair is commonly incorporated into primary lip repair.
- ✓ The best treatment for secondary deformities is accurate primary cleft lip repair.
- ✓ Correction of secondary deformities is optimally performed after cessation of facial growth.

## REFERENCES


1. Wantia N, Rettinger G. The current understanding of cleft lip malformations. Facial Plast Surg 18:147-153, 2002.
2. Merritt L. Part 1. Understanding the embryology and genetics of cleft lip and palate. Adv Neonatal Care 5:64-71, 2005.
3. Bentz M, Bauer B, Zuker R. Principles and Practice of Pediatric Plastic Surgery. St Louis: Quality Medical Publishing, 2008.
4. Burt JD, Byrd HS. Cleft lip: unilateral primary deformities. Plast Reconstr Surg 105:1043-1055, 2000.
5. Cardoso AD. [New technique for repair of hairlip] Rev Paul Med 42:127-131, 1953.
6. Spira M, Hardy SB, Gerow FJ. Correction of nasal deformities accompanying unilateral cleft lip. Cleft Palate J 7:112-123, 1970.
7. LaRossa D, Donath G. Primary nasoplasty in unilateral and bilateral cleft nasal deformity. Clin Plast Surg 20:781-791, 1993.
8. Harling TR, Stelnicki EJ, Hedrick MH, et al. In utero models of craniofacial surgery. World J Surg 27:108-116, 2003.
9. Santiago PE, Grayson BH, Cutting CB, et al. Reduced need for alveolar bone grafting by presurgical orthopedics and primary gingivoperiosteoplasty. Cleft Palate Craniofac J 35:77-80, 1998.
10. Tennison CW. The repair of unilateral cleft lip by the stencil method. Plast Reconstr Surg 9:115-120, 1952.
11. Randall P. A triangular flap operation for the primary repair of unilateral clefts of the lip. Plast Reconstr Surg Transplant Bull 23:331-347, 1959.
12. LeMesurier AB. The quadrilateral Mirault flap operation for hare-lip. Plast Reconstr Surg 16:422-433, 1955.
13. Millard DR. A radical rotation in single harelip. Amer J Surg 95:318-322, 1958.
14. Byrd HS. Unilateral cleft lip. In Aston SJ, Beasley RW, Thorne CHM, eds. Grabb and Smith's Plastic Surgery, 5th ed. Philadelphia: Lippincott-Raven, 1997.
15. Byrd HS, Salomon J. Primary correction of the unilateral cleft nasal deformity. Plast Reconstr Surg 106:1276-1286, 2000.
16. Millard D Jr. Earlier correction of the unilateral cleft lip nose. Plast Reconstr Surg 70:64-73, 1982.
17. Tajima S, Maruyama M. Reverse-U incision for secondary repair of cleft lip nose. Plast Reconstr Surg 60:256-261, 1977.
18. McComb H. Primary correction of unilateral cleft lip nasal deformity: a 10-year review. Plast Reconstr Surg 75:791-797, 1985.
19. Mulliken JB. Bilateral cleft lip. Clin Plastic Surg 31:209-220, 2004.

20. Millard DR. Closure of bilateral cleft lip and elongation of columella by two operations in infancy. Plast Reconstr Surg 47:324-331, 1971.
21. Broadbent TR, Woolf RM. Bilateral cleft lip repairs: review of 160 cases, and description of present management. Plast Reconstr Surg 50:36-41, 1972.
22. Cohen M. Immediate unrestricted feeding of infants following cleft lip and palate repair. Br J Plast Surg 50:143, 1997.
23. Jackson IT, Beal B. Early feeding after cleft repair. Br J Plast Surg 50:217, 1997.
24. Tokioka K, Park S, Sugawara Y, et al. Video recording study of infants undergoing primary cheiloplasty: are arm restraints really needed? Cleft Palate Craniofac J 46:494-497, 2009.
25. Garza JR, Futrell JW. Secondary deformities of the cleft lip and nose. In Bentz M, ed. Pediatric Plastic Surgery. New York: McGraw-Hill, 1997.

# 25. Cleft Palate

Marcin Czerwinski, Amanda A. Gosman

## EMBRYOLOGY

### PRIMARY PALATE

- The lip, nostril sill, alveolus, and hard palate **anterior** to the incisive foramen
- The medial and lateral nasal prominences of the frontonasal process migrate and fuse with the maxillary prominence to form the primary palate during weeks 4-7 of gestation.
- The median palatine process forms by the fusion of the bilateral medial nasal prominences.

### SECONDARY PALATE

- The hard palate **posterior** to the incisive foramen and the soft palate
- Migration and fusion of the lateral palatal processes of the maxillary prominence form the secondary palate between weeks 5 and 12 of gestation.
- At 8 weeks of gestation the lateral palatal processes are vertical and then rotate into horizontal positions, fusing from anterior to posterior as the tongue takes an inferoposterior position within the oral cavity.

### PATHOGENESIS

- Interruption of the migration or fusion of these processes may result in a cleft of the palate.
- Clefts of the lip and/or palate (CL/P) and isolated palatal clefts (CPO) are pathogenetically distinct. CL/P is thought to occur secondary to failure of mesodermal penetration.[1,2] CPO is thought to occur secondary to failure of epithelial fusion.[3,4]
- The right lateral palatal process becomes horizontal before the left process, increasing the risk of a cleft at the latter location.

## ANATOMY

### HARD PALATE SKELETAL ANATOMY

- **Primary palate (anterior to incisive foramen)**
  - Premaxillary portion of maxilla
- **Secondary palate (posterior to incisive foramen)**
  - Palatine processes of maxilla
  - Palatine processes of palatine bone

## Soft Palate (Velum) Muscular Anatomy (Fig. 25-1)

- **Levator veli palatini (LVP)**
  - Originates from petrous portion of temporal bone and eustachian tube; passes inferior to musculus uvulae and joins opposite side LVP to form a muscular sling in the intermediate 40% of velar length
  - Function: Elevates and lengthens velum posteriorly
- **Tensor veli palatini (TVP)**
  - Originates from spine and scaphoid fossa of sphenoid bone and eustachian tube; travels around pterygoid hamulus, giving rise to palatal aponeurosis, and joins opposite side TVP in anterior 25% of the soft palate
  - Function: Opens the eustachian tube, may serve as an anterior insertion point for LVP, palatopharyngeus, and musculus uvulae
- **Palatopharyngeus**
  - Arises from superior pharyngeal constrictor muscle and thyroid cartilage, passes through posterior tonsillar pillar, and inserts into posterior border of hard palate, palatal aponeurosis, and LVP
  - Function: Depresses soft palate; elevates and constricts oropharynx
- **Palatoglossus**
  - Originates from the tongue, passes through anterior tonsillar pillar, and inserts into fibers of LVP
  - Function: Depresses and pulls soft palate anteriorly
- **Musculus uvulae** (the only intrinsic muscle of the soft palate)
  - Originates from palatine aponeurosis and reaches an indistinct termination at the base or within the substance of the uvula
  - Bulk of the muscle resides in the middle 40% of the nasal side of the soft palate.
  - Function: Upward movement and shortening of the uvula; creates a "bulge" (levator eminence, velar knee) on the nasal side of the soft palate

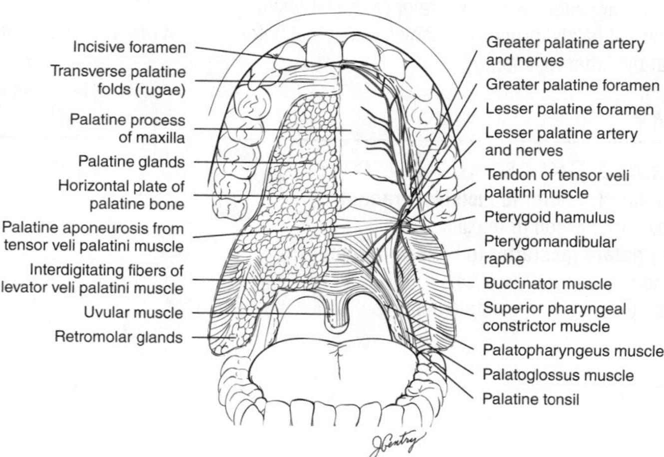


**Fig. 25-1** Anatomy of the normal palate.

- **Superior pharyngeal constrictor**
  - Originates from the posterior pharyngeal raphe and courses downward and forward to insert into the pterygoid hamulus, lateral pterygoid plate, pterygomaxillary ligament, mandible, and floor of the mouth
  - Function: Mesial movement of the lateral pharyngeal wall
- **Salpingopharyngeus**
  - Originates from posterior surface of the end of the eustachian tube and terminates within palatopharyngeus muscle
  - Function: Does not contribute to velopharyngeal (VP) closure
- **Stylopharyngeus**
  - Originates from the styloid process of the temporal bone and inserts between the fibers of the superior and middle pharyngeal constrictors
  - Function: Does not contribute to VP closure

## Blood Supply and Innervation

- **Hard palate**
  - Greater palatine artery (from the maxillary artery, via the descending palatine artery) and greater palatine nerve (CN V) pass through the greater palatine foramen, providing dominant hard palate supply.
  - Nasopalatine artery (from the maxillary artery, via the sphenopalatine artery) and nasopalatine nerve (CN V) communicate with the greater palatine artery and nerve at the incisive foramen to supply the premaxilla.
  - Anterior superior alveolar artery (from the maxillary artery, via the infraorbital artery) and posterior superior alveolar artery (from maxillary artery directly) supply the anterior and posterior alveoli, respectively.
- **Soft palate**
  - Ascending pharyngeal (from the external carotid artery) and ascending palatine arteries (from facial artery) provide principal velar blood supply.
  - Lesser palatine artery (from the maxillary artery, via the descending palatine artery) and lesser palatine nerve (CN V) pass through the lesser palatine foramen.
  - All muscles of the velum are innervated by the pharyngeal plexus (CN IX, CN X, and contributions from CN XI), **except for the TVP, which is supplied by CN V.**

**TIP:** The following question is typically asked on written examinations: Which muscle of the velum is not innervated by the pharyngeal plexus, and what is its innervation?

## Cleft Palate Anatomy[5] (Fig. 25-2)

- Varying degrees of cleft anomaly exist, from a bifid uvula to a complete overt bilateral cleft of the palate with associated alveolar and lip clefts.
- Muscular abnormality is confined to the portion that is within the palate, with normal extrinsic velar portions.[6]
  - Fibers of musculus uvulae, medial fibers of palatopharyngeus and LVP insert into fibrous tissue along the medial border of the velar cleft.
  - Lateral fibers of palatopharyngeus insert into palatal aponeurosis and medial border of the cleft of the hard palate.
  - TVP fibers (palatal aponeurosis) and palatoglossus insert along posterior border of hard palate.
- The muscle fibers are often hypoplastic with corresponding thicker connective tissue layer occupying the muscular bed.[7]

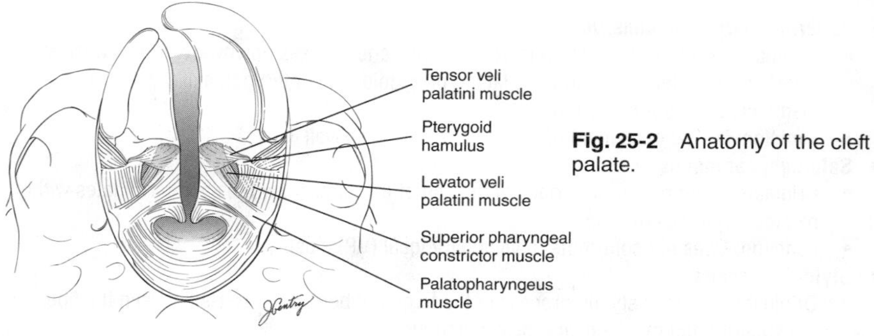


**Fig. 25-2** Anatomy of the cleft palate.

## CLEFT CLASSIFICATION

Kernahan and Stark developed a cleft classification system based on embryologic development and later proposed a symbolic striped-Y classification based on it.[8,9] Smith's modification of the latter system accurately describes cleft varieties using an alphanumeric system[10] (Fig. 25-3).

- Clefts of primary palate (lip and premaxilla) only
  - Unilateral (R or L)
    - Total
    - Subtotal
  - Median
    - Total (premaxilla absent)
    - Subtotal (premaxilla rudimentary)
  - Bilateral
    - Total
    - Subtotal
- Clefts of the secondary palate only
  - Total
  - Subtotal
  - Submucous (triad of bifid uvula, zona pellucida, hard palatal notch)
- Clefts of primary and secondary palates
  - Unilateral (R or L)
    - Total
    - Subtotal

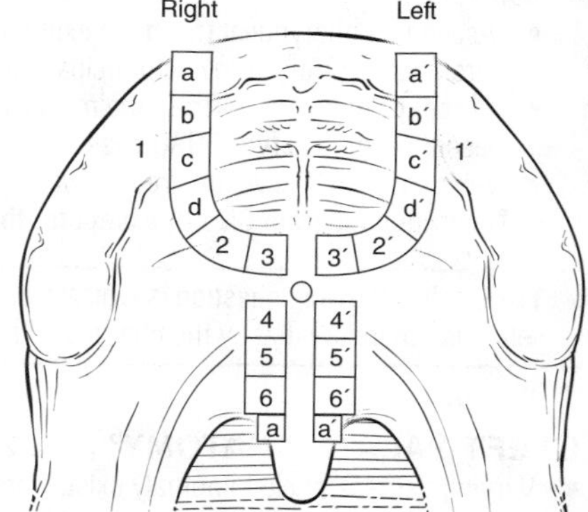


**Fig. 25-3** Smith modification of the Kernahan striped-Y classification. Boxes are shaded to indicate the extent of the cleft. The *circle* represents the incisive foramen. All right-sided clefts are designated by numerals without prime, and left-sided clefts are designated by numerals with prime. Incomplete cleft lips vary from microform to one to two thirds, and these are classified as *a-c* or *a′-c′* for right and left, respectively. Lips with Simonart's band are classified as *d*. The alveolus is documented as *2* or *2′*. The palate anterior to the incisive foramen and posterior to the alveolus is documented as *3* or *3′*. The secondary palate, lying posterior to the incisive foramen, is subdivided into three segments based on the anatomic segments involved in the cleft. *4* denotes a cleft up to the palatine process of the maxillary bone, *5* is a cleft up to the palatine process of the palatine bone, *6* is a cleft including the soft palate only, and *a* is a submucous cleft.

- Median
  - Total (premaxilla absent)
  - Subtotal (premaxilla rudimentary)
- Bilateral
  - Total
  - Subtotal

# EPIDEMIOLOGY

## Overall Incidence of Oral Clefts

- Cleft lip, with or without cleft palate, and isolated cleft palate are genetically and epidemiologically distinct
  - 1:750 live births (46% CL/P, 33% CPO, 21% CL)[11]
  - Bifid uvula: 2% of the population[12]

## Racial Distribution[13]

- CL/P
  - Asians: 2:1000
  - Whites: 1:1000
  - Blacks: 0.5:1000
- CPO
  - 0.5:1000 births, equal in all races

## Gender Distribution

- Male/female CL/P: 2:1
- Male/female CPO: 1:2

## Positional Distribution

- Left/right/bilateral CL/P: 6:3:1

## Familial Distribution[14]

- CL/P
  - Normal parents (with or without a family history of CL/P), one child with CL/P: Frequency of CL/P in next child is 4%
  - Normal parents, two children with CL/P: Risk for next child is 9%
  - Parent with CL/P, no affected children: Risk for next child is 4%
  - Parent with CL/P, one child with CL/P: Risk for next child is 17%
  - Risk of CL/P in siblings increases with severity of deformity (bilateral greater than unilateral)[15]
    - Child with unilateral CL: Risk of CL/P for next child is 2.5%
    - Child with bilateral CL and CP: Risk of CL/P for next child is 5.7%
- CPO
  - Normal parents, one child with CP: Frequency of CP in next child is 2%
  - Normal parents, family history of CP, one child with CP: Risk for next child is 7%
  - Normal parents, two children with CP: Risk for next child is 1%
  - Parent with CP, no affected children: Risk for next child is 6%
  - Parent with CP, one child with CP: Risk for next child is 15%

## ASSOCIATED ANOMALIES

### Nonsyndromic Clefts

Nonsyndromic clefts are characterized by one or multiple anomalies that are the result of a single initiating event or primary malformation.

- Incidence of isolated associated anomalies
  - CL/P: 7%-14%[15] (bilateral >unilateral), CPO 17%[16]
- Robin sequence (RS) is the most common associated anomaly.[17]
  - Triad includes **micrognathia/retrognathia, glossoptosis, and airway obstruction.** CP is a common but not essential finding.
  - When present, the palatal cleft is typically very wide and U-shaped, compared with the V-shaped cleft of the palate without RS.

### Syndromic Clefts

Syndromic clefts are characterized by more than one malformation involving more than one developmental field, occurring together at least 15%-20% of the time. More than 300 syndromes include a palatal cleft.

- Incidence[15]
  - CL/P: 13.8%
  - CP: 41.8%
- Common syndromes
  - **Stickler syndrome:** 25% of syndromic CP[18]
    - Autosomal dominant
    - Mutation in gene for type 2 collagen
    - RS, ocular malformations, hearing loss, and arthropathies
  - **Velocardiofacial (Shprintzen's) syndrome:** 15% of syndromic CP[18]
    - Autosomal dominant with variable expression
    - 22q11 "CATCH 22" chromosomal deletion (diagnose with fluorescence in situ hybridization [FISH])
    - **Cardiovascular abnormalities,** abnormal facies, developmental delay
  - **Van der Woude syndrome:** 19% of syndromic CL/P and CP[15]
    - Autosomal dominant with 70%-100% penetrance
    - CL/P or CP and **lower lip pits**

## ETIOLOGIC FACTORS

### Genetic Factors

The genetic contribution to nonsyndromic oral clefts is estimated to be 20%-50%. Remaining percentages are attributed to environmental or gene-environment interactions.[19]

- **Nonsyndromic CP**
  - Mode of inheritance likely a recessive single-gene model, several interacting loci, or both[20,21]
- **Nonsyndromic CL/P**
  - Combination of multiple interacting major genes and multifactorial inheritance[22,23]

### Environmental Factors

- **Maternal smoking:** Inconsistent data associated with increased risk of clefts
- **Maternal alcohol and caffeine ingestion:** Not associated with increased risk of isolated oral clefts[24]
- **Maternal corticosteroid use:** Associated with increased risk of CL/P and CP[25]

- **Teratogens (e.g., alcohol, anticonvulsants, retinoids):** Associated with multiple malformations, which may include oral clefts but not associated with isolated oral clefts
- **Folic acid and multivitamin supplements:** Lower incidence of CL/P births[26] when taken by pregnant women with family history of CL/P
- **High altitude:** Increased relative risk of CL/P[27]
- **Parental age:** Increased incidence of CL/P if both parents older than 30 years, paternal age more significant than maternal age

## MANAGEMENT

### INITIAL EVALUATION

Initial evaluation should be performed shortly after birth and focuses on airway, feeding, presence of concomitant anomalies, and presentation of a management plan to the family.

- **Airway compromise is rare** in the absence of associated anomalies (most commonly RS).
  - Evaluation
    - Degree of respiratory compromise (respiratory rate and effort, continuous pulse oximetry, serial ABGs, polysomnography)
    - Pathogenesis of respiratory compromise (degree of micrognathia/retrognathia, ± relief with Muller maneuver, laryngotracheobronchoscopy)
  - Treatment depends on cause. Options include:
    - Lateral/prone positioning
    - Tongue-lip adhesion
    - Mandibular distraction osteogenesis
    - Tracheotomy
    - Nasopharyngeal airway and endotracheal intubation may provide temporary support in patients who failed positioning before operative intervention.
- **Feeding:** Presence of a cleft palate prevents the generation of negative pressure necessary for adequate suction. Most patients require assistance through the use of nipples with large cross-cut fissures, squeezable bottles, or palatal obturator.
  - Early consultation with a feeding specialist is essential to ensure appropriate parental teaching, provide feeding supplies, and monitor weight gain.
- **Middle ear function:** Incidence of otitis media in patients with cleft palate is 97%.[28] Incidence of hearing loss is 50%.[29] Eustachian tube dysfunction may be related to abnormal insertion of velopharyngeal musculature and oronasal reflux leading to tube irritation.
  - Early myringotomy tube placement may be associated with improved hearing and speech outcomes.[30]

Full interdisciplinary cleft team evaluation is usually performed after discharge. Each team should be accredited by the American Cleft Palate–Craniofacial Association and must include a pediatrician, plastic surgeon, pediatric otolaryngologist, audiologist, speech pathologist, pediatric dentist, orthodontist, oral surgeon, developmental psychologist, social worker, and geneticist.

### SURGERY

- **Goals**
  - Construction of normal palatal anatomy is accomplished by closure of oral and nasal mucosae to divide the oral and nasal cavities and to provide a potential space for alveolar bone graft placement; repositioning of LVP muscles from a posteroanterior to a lateromesial course to create an intact velopharyngeal sphincter
  - Minimization of growth disruption is achieved by surgical dissection of only as much as required to achieve normal palatal anatomy.

- **Timing**
  - Early (<12 months) repair is important to facilitate normal speech development. Some studies also note improved middle ear function.[31]
  - Late (>12 months) repair allows greater uninterrupted maxillary growth
  - *Optimal time for repair is controversial.* Most favor early palatal closure, because facial growth imbalance correction is recommended in most at skeletal maturity, using orthodontic techniques or orthognathic surgery. Correction of compensatory articulations caused by persistent velopharyngeal insufficiency is difficult. Presence of an associated abnormality increases the risk for postoperative airway compromise and may delay the traditional repair time.
- **Techniques—soft palate**
  - ***Intravelar veloplasty***[32,33]: LVP and palatopharyngeus complex is freed from its abnormal insertion, cut free from tensor aponeurosis, dissected off the nasal and oral mucosae, and reoriented transversely to construct the velopharyngeal sphincter. Several variations of the technique exist.[34]
  - ***Double opposing Z-plasty***[35]: Two Z-plasties based on cleft midline are designed from oral and nasal surfaces of the soft palate. Anteriorly based flaps contain only mucosa, and posteriorly based flaps contain mucosa and LVP. As the nasal mucosal flaps are transposed, the levator sling is reoriented transversely. Lengthening according to the Z-plasty principle is achieved. Repositioning of the musculus uvulae in an oblique direction renders this technique not completely anatomic (Fig. 25-4).
- **Techniques—hard palate:** Soft palate construction is required in conjunction with the below techniques to allow optimal speech outcomes.
  - ***Von Langenbeck palatoplasty***[36,37]: Bilateral, bipedicled, mucoperiosteal flaps are elevated and sutured in the midline (Fig. 25-5).
  - ***Bardach two-flap palatoplasty***[37,38]: Bilateral mucoperiosteal flaps based on greater palatine arteries are elevated and sutured in the midline (Fig. 25-6).
  - ***Veau-Wardill-Kilner V-Y pushback palatoplasty***[39-41]: Bilateral mucoperiosteal flaps based on greater palatine arteries are elevated and closed in a V-Y fashion to lengthen the palate (Fig. 25-7).
  - **Palatoplasty adjuncts**
    - Wide cleft closure: Vomer flaps[42](Fig. 25-8), oral mucosa flap islandization with greater palatine foramen osteotomy, lateral nasal mucosa relaxing incisions, staged early soft palate with late hard palate closure
    - Adult cleft palate closure: A primary pharyngeal flap may be indicated to improve speech outcomes.

## Postoperative Care

- **Immediate**
  - Airway monitoring is particularly important in infants with RS.
    - Continuous pulse oximetry is needed.
    - Avoidance of oversedation is important in preventing respiratory compromise. Treatment is targeted at its cause.
  - Analgesia
    - A combination of nonnarcotic and narcotic analgesia may be important in reducing pain, nausea, and respiratory compromise.
  - Adequate oral intake should be ensured.
    - A soft diet is begun shortly postoperatively. Intravenous hydration is important during period of poor/absent oral intake.
    - No hard objects should be inside the mouth.

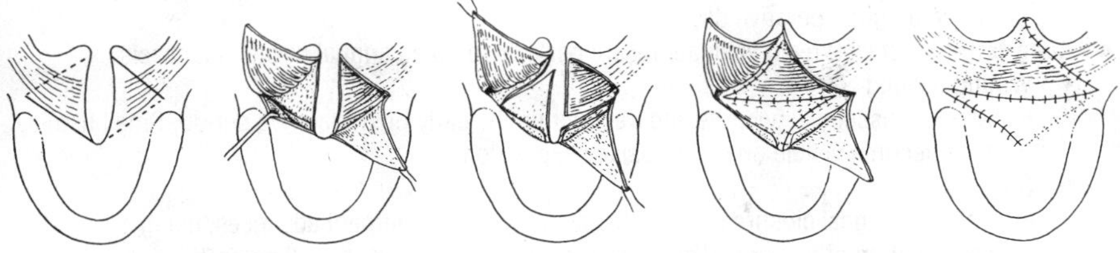

**Fig. 25-4** Furlow's double opposing Z-plasty palatoplasty technique.

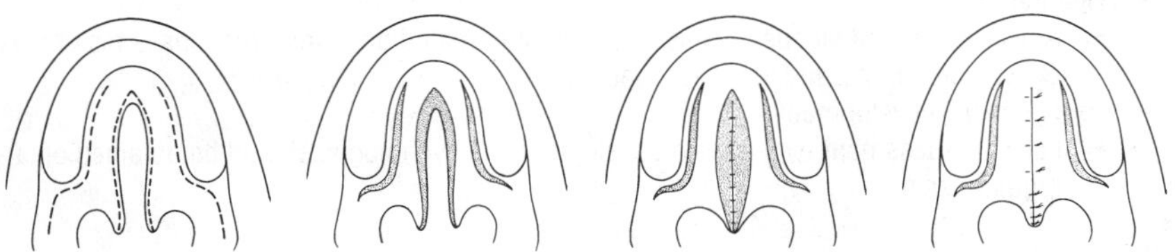

**Fig. 25-5** Von Langenbeck palatoplasty.

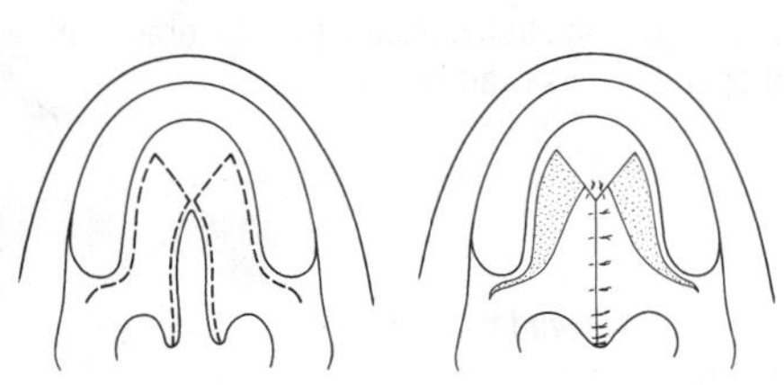

**Fig. 25-6** V-Y pushback palatoplasty (Veau-Wardill-Kilner).

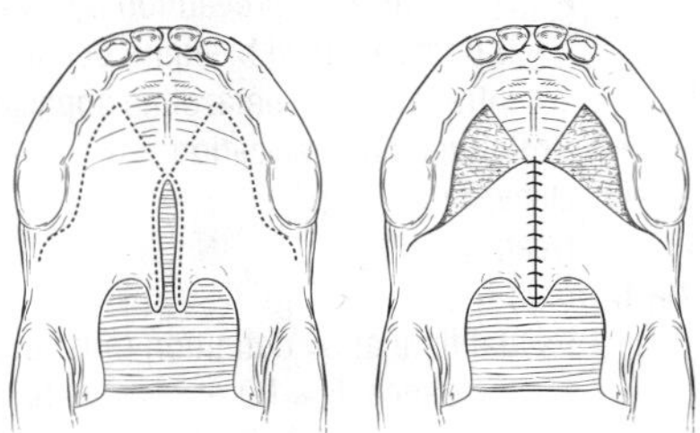

**Fig. 25-7** Two-flap palatoplasty.

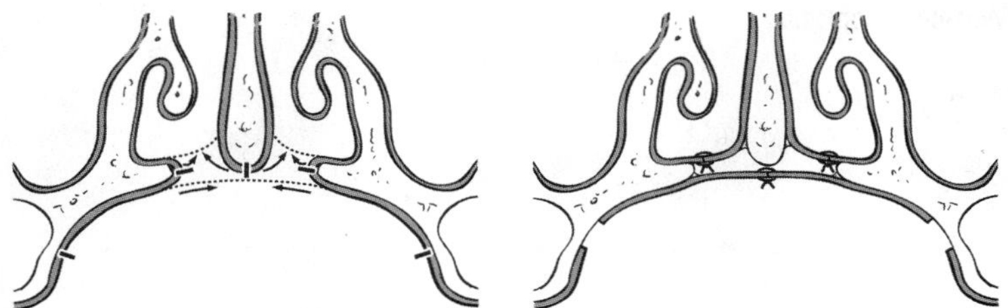

**Fig. 25-8** Bilateral, superiorly based vomer flaps.

- Discharge criteria
  - Adequate airway protection, analgesia, and oral intake are required. Most patients leave home on postoperative day 1.
- **Long-term:** Most cleft team evaluations are performed on an annual or biannual basis.
  - Wound healing
    - Most dehiscences become apparent within the early postoperative period. Small fistulas may become visible only after palatal expansion.
  - Speech
    - Velopharyngeal closure is evaluated as speech development advances, using a combination of perceptual and instrumental assessment (see Chapter 26).
  - Maxillary growth
    - Three-dimensional development of the maxilla may be assessed using a combination of facial photographic and cephalometric analysis and occlusal evaluation.
  - Hearing
    - A hearing test, otoacoustic emissions, and automated brainstem responses may be used to evaluate middle and inner ear function.
  - Psychosocial development
    - Formal assessment by a trained developmental psychologist should be obtained on a regular basis.

## COMPLICATIONS

- **Acute**
  - Airway compromise
  - Bleeding
    - Intraoperative prevention by assurance of complete hemostasis is the best approach. If postoperative bleeding occurs, treatment options include sustained digital pressure, intranasal oxymetazoline application, and operative exploration.
  - Prolonged hospitalization
  - Dehydration
  - Death (0.5%)[43]
- **Chronic**
  - Palatal fistula: By definition must occur posterior to incisive foramen
    - Incidence: 5%-60%, most at hard–soft palate junction
    - Risk factors: Cleft width, staged palatal repair, reoperation
    - Treatment: Usually only if symptomatic, options include re-repair, turnover-rotation lining flaps, FAMM flap(s), tongue flap, radial forearm free flap, palatal obturator
  - Velopharyngeal dysfunction
  - Malocclusion: Anterior underjet, posterior crossbite
  - Midface hypoplasia

## KEY POINTS

- ✓ CL/P is genetically, embryologically, and anatomically distinct from isolated CP.
- ✓ If the greater palatine artery pedicle is accidentally divided when performing a unipedicled palatal flap repair, then the flap usually survives off of the posterolateral supply from the lesser palatine, ascending pharyngeal, and ascending palatine arteries.
- ✓ The tensor veli palatini is the only muscle in the velum not supplied by the pharyngeal plexus. It is supplied by the trigeminal nerve (CN V).
- ✓ Associated anomalies and syndromes are more common with isolated CP than with CL/P. RS is the most common anomaly associated with CP.
- ✓ Optimal management of patients with cleft palate requires an interdisciplinary team.
- ✓ Speech and hearing outcomes are best with early palate repair. Facial growth is best with late palate repair.

## REFERENCES


1. Pohlmann FE. Die embryonale Metamorphose der Physiognomie und der Mundkohle des Katzenkopfes. Morphol Sb 41:617, 1910.
2. Veau V. Harelip embryo 21-23 mm long. Ztschr Anat Entscklng 108:459, 1938.
3. Dursey E. Zur Entwicklungsgeschichte des Kopfes des Menschen und der Hohren Wirbeltheire. Tübingen: H Lauppschen, 1869.
4. His W. Unsere Koerperform und des Physiologische Problem ihrer Entstohung. Leipzig: Verlag von Vogel, 1874.
5. Ross RB, Johnston MC. Cleft Lip and Palate. Baltimore: Williams & Wilkins, 1972.
6. Latham RA, Long RE Jr, Latham EA. Cleft palate pharyngeal musculature in a five month old infant: a three dimensional histologic reconstruction. Cleft Palate J 17:1-16, 1980.
7. Fara M, Dvorak J. Abnormal anatomy of the muscles of palatopharyngeal closure in cleft palates. Plast Reconstr Surg 46:488-497, 1970.
8. Kernahan DA, Stark RB. A new classification for cleft lip and cleft palate. Plast Reconstr Surg 22:435-441, 1958.
9. Kernahan DA. The striped-Y: a symbolic classification for cleft lip and palate. Plast Reconstr Surg 47:469-470, 1971.
10. Smith AW, Khoo AK, Jackson IT. A modification of the Kernahan "Y" classification in cleft lip and palate deformities. Plast Reconstr Surg 6:1842-1847, 1998.
11. Sadove AM, van Aalst AJ, Culp JA. Cleft palate repair: art and issues. Clin Plast Surg 31:231-241, 2004.
12. Lindemann G, Riss B, Severin I. Prevalence of cleft uvula among 2732 Danes. Cleft Palate J 14:226-229, 1977.
13. Sullivan W. Cleft lip with or without cleft palate in blacks: an analysis of 81 patients. Plast Reconstr Surg 84:406-408, 1989.
14. Fraser F. Etiology of cleft lip and palate. In Grabb WC, Rosenstein SW, Bzoch KR, eds. Cleft Lip and Palate: Surgical, Dental, and Speech Aspects. Boston: Little Brown, 1971.
15. Jones MC. Facial clefting: etiology and developmental pathogenesis. Clin Plast Surg 20:599-606, 1993.

16. Morris HL, Bardach J, Ardinger H, et al. Multidisciplinary treatment results for patients with isolated cleft palate. Plast Reconstr Surg 92:842-851, 1993.
17. Hagberg C, Larson O, Milerad J. Incidence of cleft lip and palate and risks of additional malformations. Cleft Palate Craniofac J 35:40-45, 1998.
18. Coleman JR Jr, Sykes JM. The embryology, classification, epidemiology, and genetics of facial clefting. Facial Plast Surg Clin North Am 9:1-13, 2001.
19. Marazita ML, Mooney MP. Current concepts in the embryology and genetics of cleft lip and palate. Clin Plast Surg 31:124-140, 2004.
20. Christensen K, Mitchell LE. Familial recurrence-pattern analysis of nonsyndromic isolated cleft palate: a Danish Registry study. Am J Hum Genet 58:182-190, 1996.
21. Carinci F, Pezzetti F, Scapoli L, et al. Genetics of nonsyndromic cleft lip and palate: a review of international studies and data regarding the Italian population. Cleft Palate Craniofac J 37:33-40, 2000.
22. Carreno H, Paredes M, Tellez G, et al. Association of non-syndromic cleft lip and palate with microsatellite markers located in 6p. Rev Med Chil 127:1189-1198, 1999.
23. Chung CS, Bixler D, Watanabe T, et al. Segregation analysis of cleft lip with or without cleft palate: a comparison of Danish and Japanese data. Am J Hum Genet 39:603-611, 1986.
24. Natsume N, Kawai T, Ogi N, et al. Maternal risk factors in cleft lip and palate: a case control study. Br J Oral Maxillofac Surg 38:23-25, 2000.
25. Carmichael SL, Shaw GM. Maternal corticosteroid use and risk of selected congenital anomalies. Am J Med Genet 86:242-244, 1999.
26. Tolarova M, Harris J. Reduced recurrence of orofacial clefts after periconceptional supplementation with high dose folic acid and multivitamins. Teratology 51:71-78, 1995.
27. Castilla EE, Lopez-Camelo JS, Campana H. Altitude as a risk factor for congenital anomalies. Am J Med Genet 86:9-14, 1999.
28. Dhillon R. The middle ear in cleft palate children pre and post palatal closure. J Roy Soc Med 81:710-713, 1988.
29. Hubbard TW, Paradise JL, McWilliams BJ, et al. Consequences of unremitting middle-ear disease in early life. Otologic, audiologic, and developmental findings in children with and without cleft palate. N Engl J Med 312:1529-1534, 1985.
30. Yules RB. Current concepts of treatment of ear disease in cleft palate children and adults. Cleft Palate J 12:315-322, 1975.
31. Watson DJ, Rohrich RJ, Poole ME, et al. The effect on the ear of late closure of the cleft hard palate. Br J Plast Surg 39:190-192, 1986.
32. Kriens OB. An anatomical approach to veloplasty. Plast Reconstr Surg 43:29-41, 1969.
33. Marsh JL, Grames LM, Holtman B. Intravelar veloplasty. Cleft Palate J 26:46-50, 1989.
34. Andrades P, Espinosa-de-los-Monteros A, Shell DH IV, et al. The importance of radical intravelar veloplasty during two-flap palatoplasty. Plast Reconstr Surg 122:1121-1130, 2008.
35. Furlow L. Cleft palate repair by double opposing Z-plasty. Plast Reconstr Surg 78:724-738, 1986.
36. Lindsay WK. Von Langenbeck palatorrhaphy. In Grabb WC, Rosenstein SW, Bzoch KR, eds. Cleft Lip and Palate: Surgical, Dental, and Speech Aspects. Boston: Little Brown, 1971.
37. Randall P, LaRossa D. Cleft palate. In McCarthy JG, ed. Plastic Surgery. Philadelphia: WB Saunders, 1990.
38. Bardach J. Presented at the Fifth International Congress on Cleft Palate and Related Craniofacial Anomalies, Monte Carlo, Monaco, Sept 1985.
39. Kilner TP. Cleft lip and palate repair technique. St Thomas Hosp Rep 2:127, 1937.
40. Wardill WE. The technique of operation for cleft palate. Br J Surg 25:117, 1937.

41. Afifi GY, Kaidi AA, Hardesty RA. Cleft palate repair. In Evans GR, ed. Operative Plastic Surgery. New York: McGraw Hill, 2000.
42. Nguyen PN, Sullivan PK. Issues and controversies in the management of cleft palate. Clin Plast Surg 20:671-682, 1993.
43. Grabb W. General aspects of cleft palate surgery. In Grabb WC, Rosenstein SW, Bzoch KR, eds. Cleft Lip and Palate: Surgical, Dental, and Speech Aspects. Boston: Little Brown, 1971.

# 26. Velopharyngeal Dysfunction

Marcin Czerwinski

## TERMINOLOGY

- **Velopharyngeal function**[1,2]
  - **Velopharyngeal dysfunction (VPD):** Any abnormal velopharyngeal function, regardless of cause
  - **Velopharyngeal insufficiency:** VPD caused by any structural abnormality at the level of velum or pharyngeal wall
  - **Velopharyngeal incompetence:** VPD caused by impaired neuromotor control of the velum or pharyngeal wall
  - **Velopharyngeal mislearning:** VPD not caused by structural or neuromotor abnormalities
- **Speech**[3,4]
  - **Nasal emission:** Nasal increase in airflow, occurs mostly during production of pressure consonants (plosives [p, b, t, d, k, g], fricatives [f, v, s, z, sh, th], affricates [ch, j])
  - **Hypernasality/hyponasality:** Increased/decreased reverberation of nasally escaping air in a confined postnasal space, occurs mostly during production of vowels
  - **Nasal rustle/turbulence:** Distinct fricative sound on the voiced pressure consonants b, d, g
  - **Grimace:** Aberrant facial muscle movement, produced by attempt to inhibit abnormal nasal airflow by constricting the nares
  - **Nasal substitution:** VPD during production of an oral consonant with appropriately positioned articulators converts it into its nasal equivalent (b becomes m, d becomes n)
  - **Compensatory articulation:** Production of plosives or fricatives despite VPD by inappropriately positioned articulators, closure occurs at glottal or pharyngeal level
  - **Sibilant distortion:** Production of sounds s, z with incorrect tongue placement, often results from malocclusion

## ANATOMY

- **Static anatomy**[5] (see Chapter 25) (Fig. 26-1)
- **Dynamic anatomy**
  - Normal velopharyngeal function involves composite movements of the velum posterosuperiorly, posterior pharyngeal wall ventrally (diffusely or as a well-defined shelf [Passavant's ridge]), and lateral pharyngeal wall mesially, which produces closure of the velopharyngeal port.
  - Closure patterns[6] (Fig. 26-2) indicate the predominant moving component of the velopharyngeal sphincter.[7]
    - Coronal
    - Sagittal
    - Circular
    - Circular with Passavant's ridge
    - Bow tie
  - In VPD, intermittent or pervasive incomplete closure of the velopharyngeal port occurs because of inadequate movement of one or more of its components.

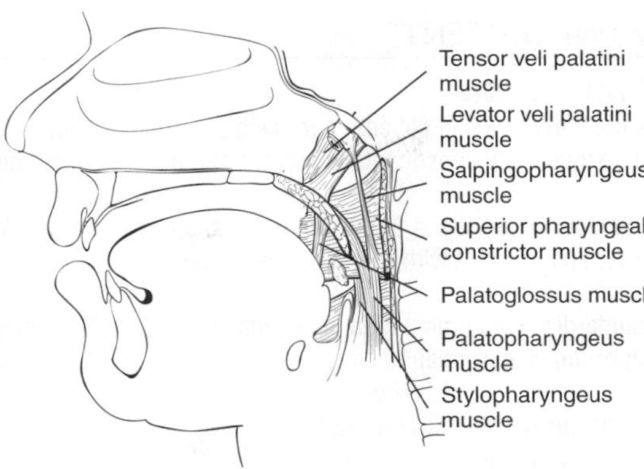


**Fig. 26-1** Sagittal view of the normal adult palate showing the relationships of the levator palatini, the uvula, and the palatoglossus and palatopharyngeus muscles within and beyond the palate. The adjacent superior pharyngeal constrictor muscle is also shown.

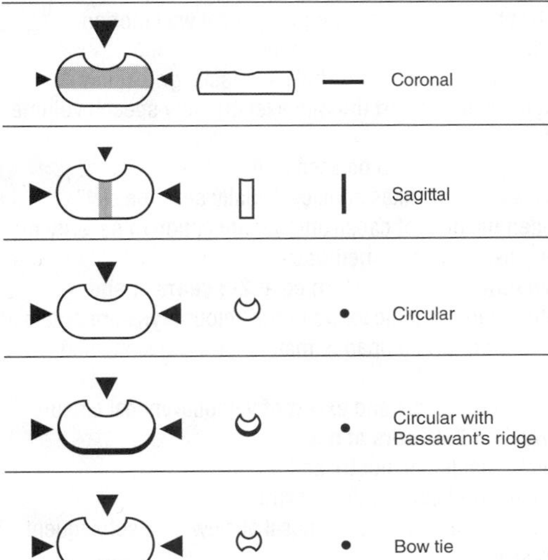


**Fig. 26-2** Bird's-eye view of the velopharynx illustrating directional movements of the representative closure.

## CAUSES

- **Cleft palate**
  - Unrepaired, short, immobile (extensive scar, inadequate velar construction) palate
  - Palatal fistula
  - Midface advancement in patients with prior borderline VPD
- **Noncleft palate**[8]
  - Neuromotor impairment: Congenital or acquired neuromuscular condition (traumatic brain injury [TBI], myasthenia gravis [MG], cerebral palsy [CP])
  - Underlying syndrome (velocardiofacial, VATER, Klinefelter, Turner)
  - Mislearning: Phoneme-specific nasal emission
  - Postadenoidectomy, tonsillar hypertrophy
  - Other: Extensive use of wind-blowing instruments

# MANAGEMENT

## EVALUATION

Evaluation of VPD in patients born with an orofacial cleft begins as soon as articulation of at least some intact oral consonants is present and patient cooperation permits.

This typically begins at 2-3 years of age and must be performed in conjunction with a trained speech pathologist with extensive cleft experience.

Standardized documentation, as suggested by the Multidisciplinary Task Force on Velopharyngeal Reporting, is essential.[9]

- **Intraoral examination**
  - Occlusion
  - Palate: Completeness of repair, length, movement, signs of submucous cleft palate
  - Pharynx: Presence of tonsillar hypertrophy, lateral/posterior pharyngeal wall motion
- **Perceptual speech evaluation:** Allows identification of VPD presence
  - Presence of nasal emission, hypernasality, nasal rustle/ turbulence, facial grimacing, compensatory articulations. Other signs include short utterance length, low speech volume, weak or omitted pressure consonants.
  - Provocative samples and spontaneous speech should be assessed.
    - "Pink puppy," "blue bunny," "sixty-six," "Katy likes cookies," "Sally sees the sky"
- **Instrumental VPD assessment:** Allows identification of cause and quantification of severity of VPD. May be subdivided into **acoustic** and **aerodynamic** methods.
  - **Multiview videofluoroscopy (aerodynamic):** Can be performed at **2-3 years of age**
    - Static and dynamic frontal and lateral radiographic views of the velopharynx are obtained after the patient swallows a small amount of radiopaque material; during sustained production of "ee."
    - This allows semiquantitative assessment of type and extent of velopharyngeal closure.
  - **Nasometry (acoustic):** Can be performed at **3-4 years of age**
    - Air pressure transducers are inserted inside one nostril and mouth; a pneumotachograph (flowmeter) is inserted inside other nostril.
    - This allows measurement of oral and nasal air pressure, nasal airflow, and subsequent calculation of velopharyngeal port size.
    - Port size: $<10\ mm^2$ = normal airflow; 10-20 $mm^2$ = mild, moderate hypernasality; $>20\ mm^2$ = severe hypernasality[1]
  - **Nasoendoscopy (aerodynamic):** Can be performed at **4-5 years of age**
    - Nasopharyngoscope is inserted inside the nostril to observe velopharyngeal port closure during speech.
    - This allows qualitative assessment of closure pattern and port size.
  - **MRI:** An adjunct to VPD evaluation
    - MRA is used to define neck vascular anatomy before surgical intervention in patients with velocardiofacial and DiGeorge syndromes.
    - This may define velar muscular anatomy.[10]

## TREATMENT

- **Nonsurgical treatment**
  - **Speech therapy:** Indicated in treatment of intermittent VPD and initial treatment of pervasive VPD. Length of attempted therapy may be shorter in cases of continued pervasive VPD.
    - Techniques include sucking and blowing exercises, electrical and tactile stimulation, biofeedback, articulation therapy.
  - **Prosthetic management:** Indicated in cases of failed speech therapy when surgery is contraindicated (high risk of airway obstruction, family refusal)[11]
    - Palatal lift: Used with long, supple vela and normal velar length/nasopharyngeal depth ratio with neuromotor dysfunction
    - Velopharyngeal obturator: Used with short, scarred vela and decreased velar length/nasopharyngeal depth ratio
    - Lift-orator (combination): Used when elevation of velum alone is insufficient
- **Surgical treatment:** Indicated in cases of failed speech therapy
  - Algorithm
    - Many recommend choosing a treatment option based on location of velopharyngeal port closure deficiency.
      - Minimal circular gap: Furlow double-opposing Z-plasty/intravelar veloplasty (IVV)
      - Moderate circular gap or sagittal gap: Pharyngeal flap
      - Large circular, coronal, or bow tie gap: Sphincter pharyngoplasty

**NOTE: A recent meta-analysis, however, refutes the effectiveness of this theoretical approach and suggests the superiority of a pharyngeal flap.[12]**

  - Preoperative adjuncts:
    - Hypertrophied tonsils and adenoids should be removed at least 3 months preoperatively, because their presence can prevent posterior tonsillar pillar elevation or their sufficiently high insertion. Postoperative adenoid hypertrophy may lead to airway obstruction following a pharyngeal flap insertion.
  - Options
    - **Furlow double-opposing Z-plasty/IVV**
      - See chapter 25 for details.
    - **Sphincter pharyngoplasty**[6] (Fig. 26-3): Lateral pharyngeal wall muscle and mucosa are elevated and inset into posterior and/or lateral pharyngeal walls at the level of proposed velopharyngeal port closure. Variables include principal muscle elevated, level of inset, adjunctive use of a small pharyngeal flap, unilateral/bilateral design:
      - **Hynes**[13]**:** Bilateral superiorly based salpingopharyngeus muscles with overlying mucosa are elevated and attached to posterior pharyngeal wall.
      - **Orticochea**[14]**:** Bilateral superiorly based palatopharyngeus muscles with overlying mucosa are elevated and attached in an overlapped fashion to posterior pharyngeal wall, with tips covered by an inferiorly based posterior pharyngeal flap.
      - **Jackson and Silverton**[15]**:** Bilateral superiorly based palatopharyngeus muscles with overlying mucosa are elevated and attached in an overlapped fashion to posterior pharyngeal wall, with tips covered by a superiorly based posterior pharyngeal flap.
      - **Moore**[16]**:** Bilateral superiorly based salpingopharyngeus muscles with overlying mucosa are elevated and attached to posterior surface of the velum.

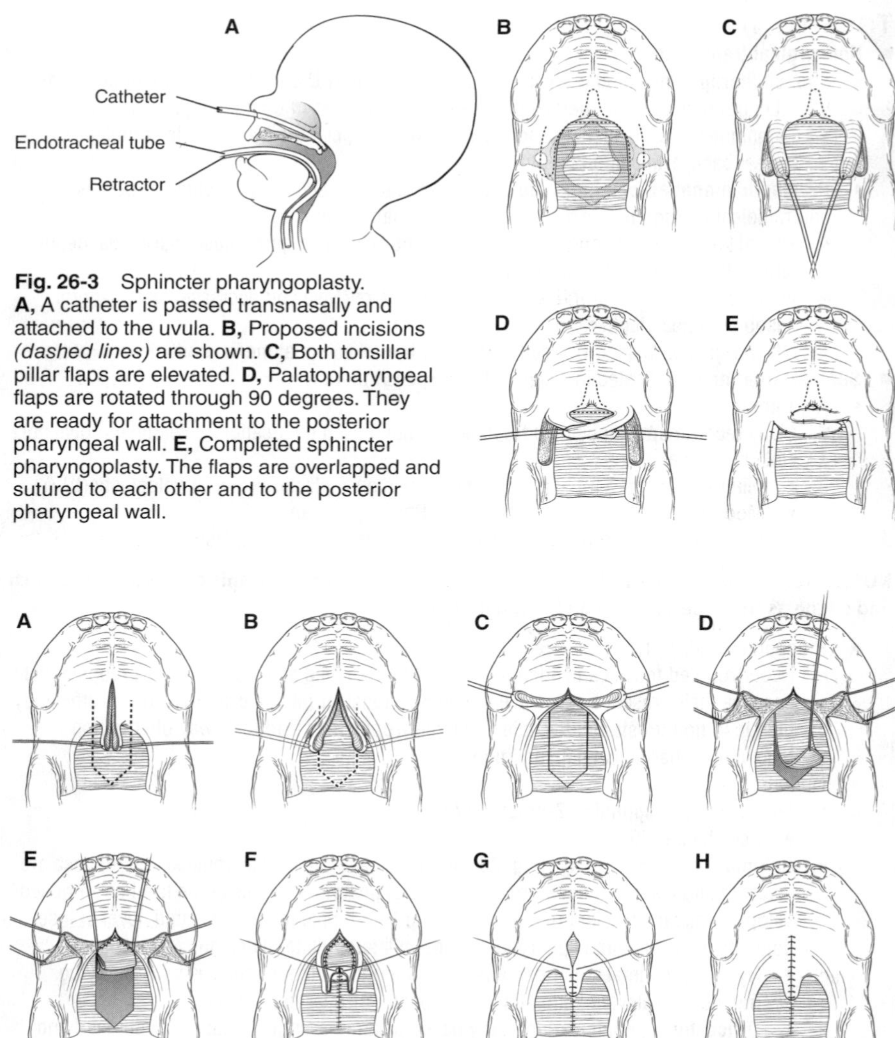


**Fig. 26-3** Sphincter pharyngoplasty. **A,** A catheter is passed transnasally and attached to the uvula. **B,** Proposed incisions *(dashed lines)* are shown. **C,** Both tonsillar pillar flaps are elevated. **D,** Palatopharyngeal flaps are rotated through 90 degrees. They are ready for attachment to the posterior pharyngeal wall. **E,** Completed sphincter pharyngoplasty. The flaps are overlapped and sutured to each other and to the posterior pharyngeal wall.

**Fig. 26-4** Posterior pharyngeal flap. **A,** Sutures are placed bilaterally in the soft palate to enhance visualization. A midline incision divides the soft palate to the posterior nasal spine. **B,** Soft palate flaps are retracted. **C,** An incision is made along the dotted line on the posterior pharyngeal wall down to the prevertebral fascia. A pharyngeal flap is created. A book flap incision that will line the lateral ports with mucous membrane is then made bilaterally on the nasal surface of the soft palate. **D,** The pharyngeal flap is plotted with indelible ink and elevated to the prevertebral fascia. Two soft palate flaps are opened laterally. **E,** The free inferior edge of the pharyngeal flap is sutured to the posterior edge of the soft palate. **F,** Sutures are placed between the pharyngeal flap and the nasal edges of the soft palate. The raw surfaces arising from the origin of the pharyngeal flap are closed by simple approximation of tissue. **G,** Two flaps from the soft palate used to cover the raw tissue of the pharyngeal flap are sutured to the base of the pharyngeal flap. **H,** The oral side of the soft palate is sealed to conceal the pharyngeal flap.

- **Posterior pharyngeal flap**[6] (Fig. 26-4): Posterior pharyngeal wall (mucosa and pharyngeal constrictor muscle) is elevated and inset into the soft palate. Variables include superior/inferior/lateral flap basis, flap width, use of nasal lining flaps, level of flap inset:
  - **Schoenborn**[17]: Inferiorly based posterior pharyngeal flap, superiorly based posterior pharyngeal flap
  - **Hogan**[18]: Superiorly based posterior pharyngeal flap, lined with nasal mucosal flaps from posterior soft palate
  - **Schprintzen**[19]: Superiorly based posterior pharyngeal flap, lined with nasal mucosal flaps from posterior soft palate, width of flap based on lateral pharyngeal wall motion
  - **Kapetansky**[20]: Bilateral, transversely based pharyngeal flaps
- **Posterior pharyngeal wall augmentation:** Variety of materials, including cartilage, fascia, fat, silicone, Teflon, Proplast have been placed behind the posterior pharyngeal wall mucosa. The success of this technique has been limited and the complication rate high.

### Postoperative Care

- Airway monitoring: Particularly important in infants with Robin sequence (RS)
  - Continuous pulse oximetry
  - Avoidance of oversedation is important in preventing respiratory compromise. Treatment is targeted at its cause.
- Analgesia
  - Combination of nonnarcotic and narcotic analgesia may be important in reducing pain, nausea, and respiratory compromise.
- Assurance of adequate oral intake
  - Soft diet is begun shortly postoperatively. Intravenous hydration is important during period of poor/absent oral intake.
  - Emphasize that no hard objects should be inside the mouth.
- Discharge criteria
  - Adequate airway protection, analgesia, and oral intake are required. Most patients go home on postoperative day 1.

## COMPLICATIONS

- Sleep-disordered breathing, acute obstructive sleep apnea (OSA)
- Dehiscence with persistent VPD
- Hyponasality
- Injury to anomalous internal carotid artery

### Key Points

- ✓ VPD may be caused by velopharyngeal insufficiency, velopharyngeal incompetence, or velopharyngeal mislearning and has both cleft and noncleft causes.
- ✓ Perceptual evaluation allows identification of VPD; instrumental evaluation allows quantification of size and location of the velopharyngeal port opening.
- ✓ Speech therapy is typically the first method of VPD treatment. A superiorly based, lined posterior pharyngeal flap appears to be the most effective treatment method for velopharyngeal insufficiency.
- ✓ Acute OSA is a potentially life-threatening complication of VPD surgery.

## REFERENCES


1. Trost-Cardamone JE. Coming to terms with VPI: a response to Loney and Bloem. Cleft Palate J 26:68-70, 1989.
2. D'Antonio LL. Evaluation and management of velopharyngeal dysfunction: a speech pathologist's viewpoint. Probl Plast Reconstr Surg 2:86-111, 1992.
3. Kummer AW. Cleft Palate and Craniofacial Anomalies: Effects on Speech and Resonance, 2nd ed. Clifton Park, NY: Thomson Delmar Learning, 2008. CA: Singular Press, 2001.
4. Wyatt R, Sell D, Russel J, et al. Cleft palate speech dissected: a review of current knowledge and analysis. Br J Plast Surg 49:143-149, 1996.
5. Mathes S, ed. Plastic Surgery, vol 4, 2nd ed. Pediatric Plastic Surgery. Philadelphia: Saunders Elsevier, 2006.
6. Bentz ML, Bauer BS, Zuker RM, eds. Principles and Practice of Pediatric Plastic Surgery. St Louis: Quality Medical Publishing, 2008.
7. Croft CB, Schprintzen RJ, Rakoff SJ. Patterns of velopharyngeal valving in normal and cleft palate subjects: a multi-view videofluoroscopic and nasoendoscopic study. Laryngoscope 91:265-271, 1981.
8. Goudy S, Ingraham C, Canady J. Noncleft velopharyngeal insufficiency: etiology and need for surgical treatment. Int J Otolaryngol 2012:Article ID 296073, 2012.
9. Golding-Kushner KJ, Argamaso RV, Cotton RT, et al. Standardization for the reporting of nasopharyngoscopy and multiview videofluoroscopy: a report from an International Working Group. Cleft Palate J 27:337-347, 1990.
10. Kao DS, Soltysik DA, Hyde JS, et al. Magnetic resonance imaging as an aid in the dynamic assessment of the velopharyngeal mechanism in children. Plast Reconstr Surg 122:572-577, 2008.
11. Riski JE, Gordon D. Prosthetic management of neurogenic velopharyngeal incompetency. N C Dent J 62:24-26, 1979.
12. Collins J, Cheung K, Farrokhyar F, et al. Pharyngeal flap versus sphincter pharyngoplasty for the treatment of velopharyngeal insufficiency: a meta-analysis. J Plast Reconstr Aesthet Surg 65:864-868, 2012.
13. Hynes W. Pharyngoplasty by muscle transplantation. Br J Plast Surg 3:128-135, 1950.
14. Orticochea M. Construction of a dynamic muscle sphincter in cleft palates. Plast Reconstr Surg 41:323-327, 1968.
15. Jackson IT, Silverton JS. The sphincter pharyngoplasty as a secondary procedure in cleft palates. Plast Reconstr Surg 59:518-554, 1977.
16. Moore FT. A new operation to cure nasopharyngeal incompetence. Br J Surg 47:424-428, 1960.
17. Schoenborn K. Uber eine neue methode der staphylorrhaphie. Verh Dtsch Ges Chir 4:235-239, 1886.
18. Hogan VM. A clarification of the goals in cleft palate speech and introduction of the lateral port control pharyngeal flap. Cleft Palate J 10:331-345, 1973.
19. Schprintzen RJ, Lewin ML, Croft CB, et al. A comprehensive study of pharyngeal flap surgery: tailor made flaps. Cleft Palate J 16:46-55, 1979.
20. Kapetansky DI. Bilateral transverse pharyngeal flaps for repair of cleft palate. Plast Reconstr Surg 52:52-54, 1973.

# 27. Microtia

**Danielle M. LeBlanc, Kristin K. Constantine**

## DEMOGRAPHICS

- Incidence: 0.76-2.35 per 10,000 births[1]
- Male predominance: 2:1
- More common in Asians (Japanese) and Hispanics than whites
- Relatively higher incidence rate (0.1%) among Navajos[2]
- Estimated ratio of right/left/bilateral: 5:3:1
- Maternal parity effect seen, with increased risk noted at more than four pregnancies, especially with anotia (most severe form)[3,4]

## EMBRYOLOGY[4]

- **First (mandibular)** and **second (hyoid)** branchial arches are responsible for auricular development[1] (Fig. 27-1).
- During sixth week, external ear begins to develop around the dorsal end of the first branchial cleft. The ear arises from six buds of mesenchyme in the first and second branchial arches, known as the *six hillocks of His.*
- Mandibular arch (first): Hillocks 1-3
- Hyoid arch (second): Hillocks 4-6
- The **lobule** is the last component of the external ear to form.
- Failure of development or adverse effects within 6-8 weeks of gestation lead to clinical variations of microtia. Popular theories include:
  - **Teratogens:** Accutane, retinoic acid, thalidomide
  - **Ischemia:** Decreased blood supply in utero
  - **Genetic:** Syndromic causes
- Later insults in gestational development cause less severe auricular deformities.

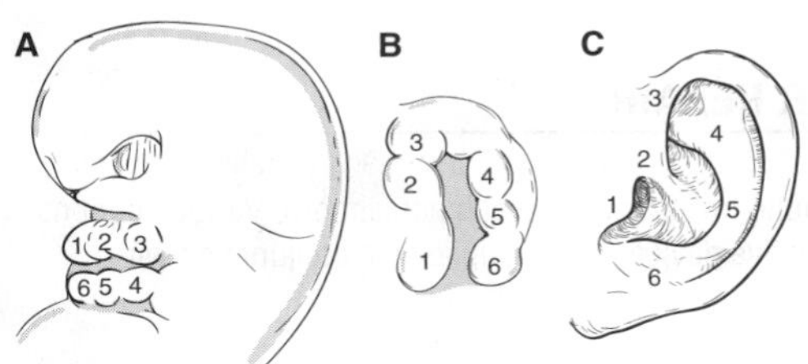


**Fig. 27-1** Embryology of the external ear. **A,** Hillock formation in an 11 mm human embryo. **B,** Hillock configuration in a 15 mm embryo at 6 weeks of gestation. **C,** Adult auricle with hillock derivations.

## ASSOCIATED ABNORMALITIES

**Middle ear** and **external auditory canal (EAC)** defects are commonly associated, although there is no correlation between the severity of the external defect and middle ear function. Defects in hearing are **80%-90% conductive** and **10%-15% sensorineural**.[5]

### CAUSES OF HEARING DEFECTS

- Ossicular chain disruption (fusion/hypoplasia of malleus, incus)
- Absence of ossicles
- Aural atresia[6]
  - Stenosis of EAC: High risk of canal cholesteatoma
  - EAC atresia
  - Likelihood of achieving significant hearing improvement is determined by CT using Jahrsdorfer's criteria
    - Scores >7/10 associated with better hearing outcomes with surgery
- Variable degrees of auricular malformation seen in syndromes
  - Branchial arch syndromes
  - Goldenhar's syndrome
  - Treacher Collins syndrome
  - Oculoauriculovertebral dysplasia
  - Facial nerve abnormalities
  - Cleft lip/palate
  - Hemifacial microsomia: Spectrum of malformations of structures derived from the first and second branchial arches[7,8]
    - Mandibular hypoplasia and unilateral or bilateral microtia

**TIP:** Isolated microtia is the mildest form of hemifacial microsomia.[1,9,10]

### OTHER MALFORMATIONS ASSOCIATED WITH MICROTIA AND ANOTIA[1]

- 30%: Facial clefts and cardiac defects
- 14%: Anophthalmia/microphthalmia
- 11%: Limb reduction defects or renal malformations
- 7%: Holoprosencephaly

## INDICATIONS FOR AURICULAR REPAIR

- **Primary goal**
  - Improvement of acoustic function (sound localization, speech perception): Various options of hearing aids, bone-anchored conductive devices, or canalplasty in conjunction with auricular reconstruction[11]
- **Secondary goals**
  - Speech
  - Social acceptance
  - Emotional development

## TIMING OF AURICULAR RECONSTRUCTION

### PRIMARY FACTORS INFLUENCING TIMING[1]

- **Age of external ear maturity**
  - 85% of ear development is attained by age 4.
  - Ear width continues to grow until age 10.
- **Availability of adequate donor rib cartilage**
  - Usually adequate by age 5-6
- **School age and psychological factors of peer ridicule**
- **Need for middle ear surgery**
  - Auricular reconstruction is commonly performed **before** middle ear surgery when possible.
  - If otologic surgery is performed first, the otologist must coordinate with the plastic surgeon to establish:
    - Canal position
    - Vascular axis of flaps
    - Location of incisions used in auricular reconstruction
  - Most hearing deficits (especially in bilateral microtia) are treated with **conductive hearing aids.** Osseointegrated or bone-anchored devices must be placed to achieve good coaptation and avoid surgical incision sites.
- **Different techniques** are more appropriate for different ages to achieve optimal reconstruction. The classic autogenous cartilage technique continues to predominate today compared with alloplastic methods.[12,13]
  - **Brent technique:** Wait until **age 4-6,** allowing for ear maturity and appropriate school age.
  - **Nagata technique:** Wait until **age 10,** or when **chest circumference at xyphoid is 60 cm,** to allow additional cartilage for use in integrated tragal reconstruction.

## PREOPERATIVE WORKUP

Microtia patients are evaluated by a plastic surgeon and otologist within the first 12 months of life and then are seen annually until they are of an optimal age for reconstruction.

- **Family history** of syndromes, genetic counseling
- **Complete physical examination**
  - Evaluation of ear structure
  - Evaluation of facial symmetry, animation, and dental occlusion
- **Diagnostic studies**
  - Complete **audiometric testing** to determine **conductive versus sensorineural defect**
  - **Temporal bone imaging**
    - **High-resolution CT scan** for evaluating **middle ear ossicles** and cleft to help plan future otologic surgery
    - **MRI** to determine **course of facial nerve,** which can be displaced—especially in absence of pneumatized mastoid[14]
    - Rule out the presence of **cholesteatoma** (squamous epithelium trapped in middle ear), present in 4%-7% of atretic ears.[4]

## CLASSIFICATION

Many attempts have been made to classify microtia based on embryologic development and severity of deformity.[14] Current system (Nagata,[15] Tanzer[16]) divides categories **based on surgical correction** of the deformity.

- **Anotia:** Absence of auricular tissue
- **Lobular type:** Remnant ear with lobule and helix but without concha, acoustic meatus, or tragus
- **Conchal type:** Remnant ear and lobule with concha, acoustic meatus, and tragus
- **Small conchal type:** Remnant ear and lobule with small indentation of concha
- **Atypical microtia:** Cases that do not fall into the previous categories

## TREATMENT OPTIONS

### AUTOGENOUS COSTAL CARTILAGE GRAFT

- **Tanzer**[16]
- Remains best long-term reconstructive option
- Modified by Brent and Nagata (see pp. 297 and 298)
- Shortcomings
  - Donor site morbidity and postoperative sequelae (pulmonary)
  - Chest wall deformity
  - Number of staged procedures

### SILASTIC FRAMEWORK (DOW CORNING, MIDLAND, MI)

- **Cronin**[17]
- Excellent aesthetic appearance
- No donor site morbidity
- Discontinued because of:
  - Spontaneous extrusion
  - Susceptibility to minor trauma
  - Unacceptable long-term failure rates

### POROUS POLYETHYLENE IMPLANT (MEDPOR; POREX SURGICAL, NEWNAN, GA)

- **Reinisch**[18]
- Good short-term aesthetic results and extrusion rates
- No long-term data available

### PROSTHETIC/OSTEOINTEGRATED RECONSTRUCTION

- Limited by available technology and skill of anaplastologist
- Variable cost depending on quality
- Lifespan/durability depends on age of patient.
- Excellent alternative for patients with poor local tissue or high operative risk
  - Failed autogenous reconstruction
  - Trauma
  - Radiation
  - Cancer
  - Elderly patient

## Tissue Engineering

- Scaffolding remains a critical component of successful engineering.
- Nonhuman experimental chondrocyte studies have yielded de novo neocartilage that can be rendered into shapes.[19]

# MOST COMMONLY USED TREATMENT TECHNIQUES

## Brent Technique[20-22]

**Four-stage reconstruction** beginning at **4-6 years of age**

- **Stage I:** A high-profile ear framework is fabricated from contralateral costochondral rib cartilage of synchondrosis of the sixth to eighth ribs and placed in a subcutaneous pocket at the posterior/inferior border of the ear vestige[20] (Fig. 27-2).
- **Stage II:** Lobule transposition occurs several months after framework.
- **Stage III:** Projection of the construct is performed through an incision along the margin of the rim. The posterior capsule is elevated, and projection is stabilized by a wedge of banked costal cartilage placed subfascially. Polyethylene blocks may also be used as a wedge. The retroauricular skin is advanced to minimize visible scarring, and a split-thickness graft (harvested from hip) is used to cover the posterior defect and is secured with a tie-over bolster.
- **Stage IV:** Tragus construction, conchal excavation, and symmetry adjustment. The tragus is fashioned from composite graft from contralateral conchal vault, or in bilateral cases using an anteriorly based conchal flap with cartilage support.

**NOTE: Recently Brent[21] incorporated a tragal component in his initial framework to decrease the total number of stages.**

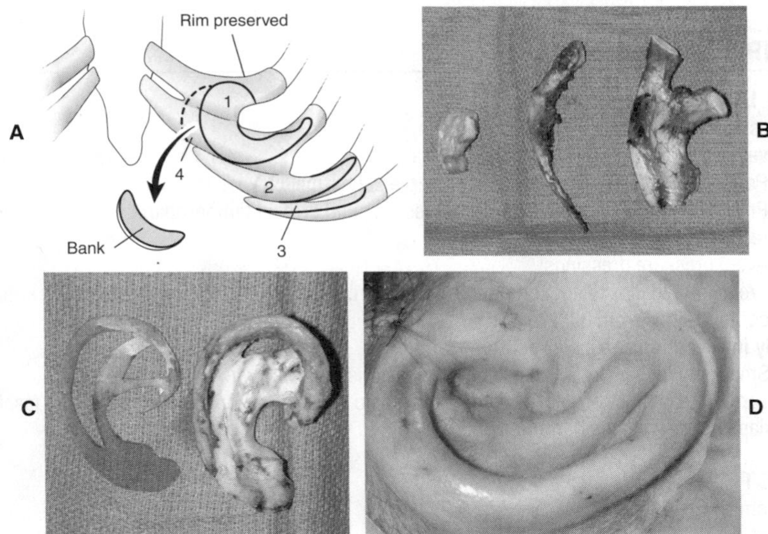


**Fig. 27-2** **A,** Rib cartilages used for total ear construction. *1,* Synchondrotic block used for body of framework; *2,* floating rib used for helix; *3,* strut used for tragus; *4,* extra cartilage wedge to be banked for use during elevation procedure. **B,** Synchondrosis of ribs seven and eight and floating rib. **C,** Autogenous cartilage framework construct with contralateral acetate template. **D,** Subcutaneous placement of cartilaginous framework.

### Nagata Technique[15,23]

Involves **two stages** starting at about **age 10.** Several modifications are involved, depending on the type of microtia present.

- **Stage I: Ipsilateral** rib cartilage high-definition framework from the **sixth through ninth ribs,** leaving most of the perichondrium in situ to minimize chest wall deformity. Framework is constructed **with a tragal component** and placed in a subcutaneous pocket through a W-shaped flap. The lobule is transposed in this stage.
- **Stage II:** Framework elevation staged at 6 months. Additional cartilage is harvested from the fifth rib through previous incision to use as wedge, and temporoparietal fascia flap is elevated and tunneled subcutaneously to cover posterior cartilage grafts. After advancement of retroauricular skin, the remaining defect is covered with skin graft (split thickness from occipital scalp) and secured with bolster.

## POSTOPERATIVE CARE

- **Hemostasis and skin coaptation**
  - Closed suction drain: Brent[20-22] advocates silicone catheter and red-top vacuum tube system to prevent skin necrosis from pressure dressing.
  - Tie-over bolster: Nagata[15] advocates bolster secured for 2 weeks.
- **Monitoring**
  - Frequent postoperative monitoring is imperative for the detection of infection, hematoma, or exposure.
- **Limit activity**
  - To protect framework
  - 3-6 week restriction of sports because of chest wall donor site

## COMPLICATIONS

### Skin Loss

- Rates are variable, depending on technique.
- **Prevention strategy is best.**
  - Perform meticulous dissection to preserve subdermal plexus.
  - Prevent injury to superficial temporal vessels, and protect temporoparietal fascia salvage resource.
  - Avoid pressure dressings.
  - Brent[22] noted closed suction drains instead of compression bolster decreased skin-related complications from 33% to 1%.
- **Early intervention can save the framework.**[20]
  - Small skin loss (<1 cm) may be managed conservatively with local wound care.
  - Larger areas must be debrided and exposed construct covered with local skin and fascia flaps to prevent loss of framework.

### Infection

- Uncommon (<0.5%)[22]
- Arises from:
  - Construct exposure
  - External ear pathogens

- Typical presentation
  - Erythema
  - Edema
  - Subtle fluctuance or drainage
- Rarely presents as pain or fever
- Prevention
  - Meticulous preoperative cleaning of external ear
  - Understanding and recognition of middle ear pathology (otitis/cholesteatoma)
- Treatment: Immediate antibiotic irrigation of flap

### HEMATOMA

- Condition is rare (0.3%) but devastating.
- **Early recognition is vital.**
- Treatment is immediate drainage.

### CHEST WALL DONOR SITE COMPLICATIONS

- **Pneumothorax** (rate unknown)
  - May require intraoperative catheter to evacuate air
- **Atelectasis**
  - Improved with infusion pumps of local anesthetics
- **Chest wall deformity rates vary by age**
  - Up to 64% at age 10 or younger
  - 20% in older children
  - Reduced by amount of perichondrium left intact at donor site
- **Hypertrophic scar**
  - Important to consider for placing donor site incision in inframammary fold with female patients

## LONG-TERM COMPLICATIONS

- **Suture extrusion**
  - Minor
  - Treatment is excision.
- **Cartilage resorption rates**
  - Rates variable
  - Require regrafting if framework shape altered
  - Avoid placing new cartilage in scarred bed; avoid tight sutures
- **Low hairline complications**
  - Can be prevented
    - Preoperative laser treatment
    - Intraoperative destruction of follicles
  - Native skin always preferable to skin graft
- **Relative size discrepancy**
  - Brent[22] noted trend in growth rates of reconstructed ears
    - 48%: Same
    - 41.6%: Larger
    - 10.3%: Smaller

## Key Points

✓ The first and second branchial arches are responsible for auricular development.
✓ Ear reconstruction is usually undertaken when the patient is at least 6 years old.
✓ Autogenous ear reconstruction (with costal cartilage) is the classic preferred method of reconstruction.
✓ A temporoparietal fascia flap can be used for soft tissue coverage over the underlying autogenous framework.

## References

1. Beahm EK, Walton RL. Auricular reconstruction for microtia. I. Anatomy, embryology and clinical evaluation. Plast Reconstr Surg 109:2473, 2002.
2. Aase JM, Tegtmeier RE. Microtia in New Mexico: evidence of multifactorial causation. Birth Defects Orig Artic Ser 13:113, 1977.
3. Harris J, Kallen B, Robert E. The epidemiology of anotia and microtia. J Med Genet 33:809, 1996.
4. Kelly PE, Scholes MA. Microtia and congenital aural atresia. Otolaryngol Clin N Am 40:61, 2007.
5. Llano-Rivas I, Gonxales-del Angel A, del Castillo V, et al. Microtia: a clinical and genetic study at the National Institute of Pediatrics in Mexico City. Arch Med Res 30:120, 1999.
6. Shonka DC Jr, Livingston WJ III, Kesser BW, et al. The Jahrsdorfer grading scale in surgery to repair congenital aural atresia. Arch Otolaryngol Head Neck Surg 134:873, 2008.
7. Ongkosuwito EM, van Neck JW, Wattel E, et al. Craniofacial morphology in unilateral hemifacial microsomia. Br J Oral Maxillofac Surg, 2012 Nov 29. [Epub ahead of print]
8. Chowchuen B, Pisek P, Chowchuen P, et al. Craniofacial microsomia: goals of treatment, staged reconstruction and long-term outcome. J Med Assoc Thai 94(Suppl 6):S100, 2011.
9. Bennun RD, Mulliken JB, Kaban LB, et al. Microtia: a microform of hemifacial microsomia. Plast Reconstr Surg 76:859, 1985.
10. Figueroa AA, Friede H. Craniovertebral malformations in hemifacial microsomia. J Craniofac Genet Dev Biol Suppl 1:167, 1985.
11. Lipan MJ, Eshraghi AA. Otologic and audiology aspects of microtia repair. Semin Plast Surg 25:273, 2011.
12. Sivayoham E, Woolford TJ. Current opinion on auricular reconstruction. Curr Opin Otolaryngol Head Neck Surg 20:287, 2012.
13. Im DD, Paskhover B, Staffenberg DA, et al. Current management of microtia: a national survery. Aesthetic Plast Surg 37:402, 2013.
14. Rogers BO. Microtic, lop, cup and protruding ears: four directly inheritable deformities? Plast Reconstr Surg 41:208, 1968.
15. Nagata S. A new method for total reconstruction of the auricle for microtia. Plast Reconstr Surg 92:187, 1993.
16. Tanzer RC. Total reconstruction of the external ear. Plast Reconstr Surg 23:1, 1959.
17. Cronin TD. Use of a Silastic frame for total and subtotal reconstruction of the external ear: preliminary report. Plast Reconstr Surg 37:399, 1966.
18. Reinisch J. Microtia reconstruction using a polyethylene implant: an eight year surgical experience. Presented at the Seventy-eighth Annual Meeting of the American Association of Plastic Surgeons, Colorado Springs, CO, May 1999.

19. Walton RL, Beahm EK. Auricular reconstruction for microtia. II. Surgical techniques. Plast Reconstr Surg 110:234, 2002.
20. Brent B. Technical advances in ear reconstruction with autogenous rib cartilage grafts: personal experience with 1200 cases. Plast Reconstr Surg 104:319, 1999.
21. Brent B. Modification of the stages in total reconstruction of the auricle: I to IV (discussion). Plast Reconstr Surg 93:267, 1994.
22. Brent B. Auricular repair with autogenous rib cartilage grafts: two decades of experience with 600 cases. Plast Reconstr Surg 90:355, 1992.
23. Achauer BM, Eriksson E, Guyuron B, et al. Plastic surgery: indications, operations, and outcomes. St Louis: Mosby–Year Book, 2000.

# 28. Prominent Ear

Jeffrey E. Janis, Adam Bryce Weinfeld

## NORMAL EAR ANATOMY[1-6] (Fig. 28-1)

- Lateral skin is dense, adherent, and thin.
- Medial skin is loose, fibrofatty, and thick.
- By the third year of life, the ear has attained 85% of its adult size.
- Ear width reaches its mature size in boys at 7 years and in girls at 6 years.
- Ear length matures in boys at 13 years and in girls at 12 years.
- The older a person becomes, the stiffer and more calcified the cartilage.
- Cartilage is much floppier and more malleable in neonates.

**TIP:** Nonoperative correction of some congenital ear anomalies can be performed by molding if initiated within the first 72 hours of life to take advantage of cartilage malleability, which results from circulating maternal hormones. Early molding intervention can employ splinting, taping, and gluing techniques to create the desired auricular shape.

## EMBRYOLOGIC ORIGINS

- **Mandibular branchial arch (first):** Anterior hillock—contributes the tragus, root of helix, and superior helix only (upper third of ear)
- **Hyoid branchial arch (second):** Posterior hillock—contributes the rest (antihelix, antitragus, lobule) (lower two thirds of ear)
- Ear begins to protrude from developing face at approximately 3-4 months of gestation.

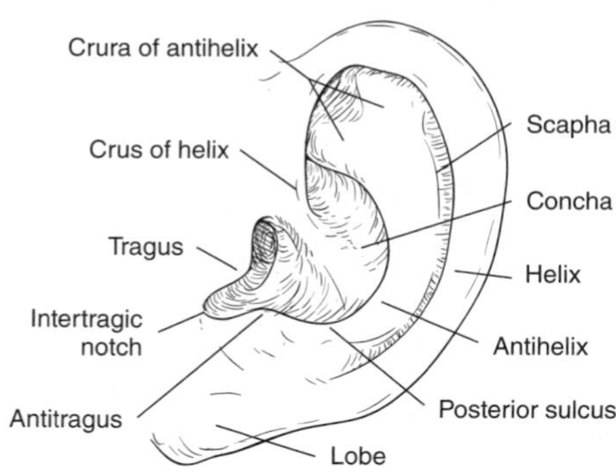


**Fig. 28-1** Anatomy of the external ear.

## VASCULARITY[7] (Fig. 28-2)

- Terminal branches of the external carotid artery
- Posterior auricular artery
- Superficial temporal artery

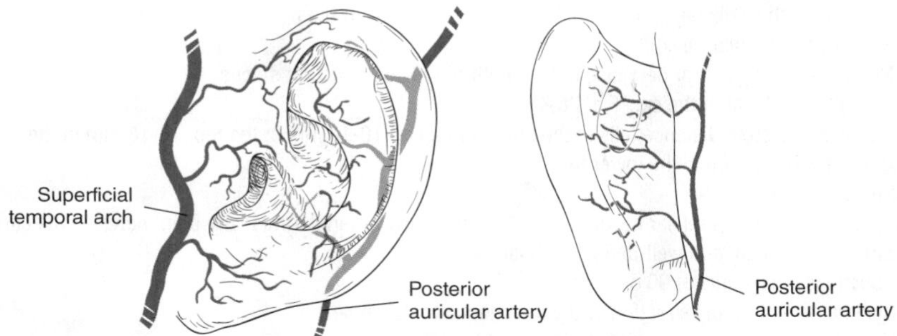


**Fig. 28-2** Vascularity of the ear.

## INNERVATION[7] (Fig. 28-3)

### Auriculotemporal Nerve

- Branch of the trigeminal nerve
- Provides sensitivity to the tragus and crus helicis

### Great Auricular Nerve

- Separates into anterior and posterior divisions
- Branch of the cervical plexus (C2-3)
- Supplies rest of ear
- Auricular branches of the vagus (Arnold's nerve)
- Supplies the external acoustic meatus

### Lesser Occipital Nerve

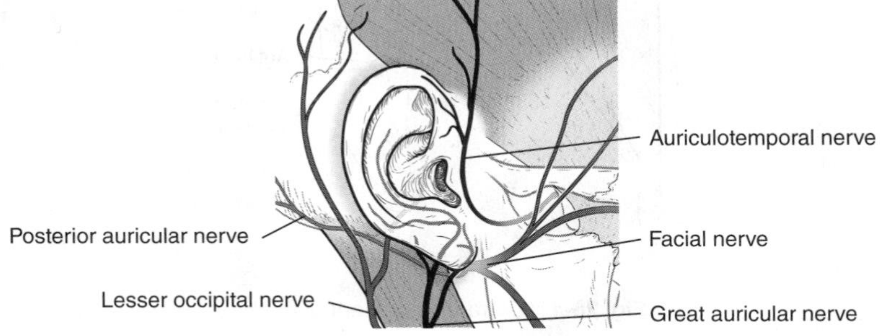


**Fig. 28-3** Innervation of the ear.

## NORMAL EAR AESTHETIC PROPORTIONS[4,8,9] (Box 28-1)

**Box 28-1** *BASIC GOALS OF OTOPLASTY*

- Correction of all upper-third protrusion
- Visibility of the helix beyond the antihelix when viewed from the front
- Smooth and regular helix
- No marked distortion or decrease in the depth of the postauricular sulcus
- Correct placement of the ear (Fig. 28-4)

The helix-to-mastoid distance falls in the normal range of 10-12 mm at the top, 16-18 mm in the middle, and 20-22 mm in the lower third.

- Bilateral symmetry

The position of the lateral ear border to the head matches within 3 mm at any point between the ears.

- Smooth, rounded, and well-defined antihelical fold
- Conchoscaphal angle of 90 degrees
- Conchal reduction or reduction of the conchomastoidal angle
- Helical rim that projects laterally farther than the lobule

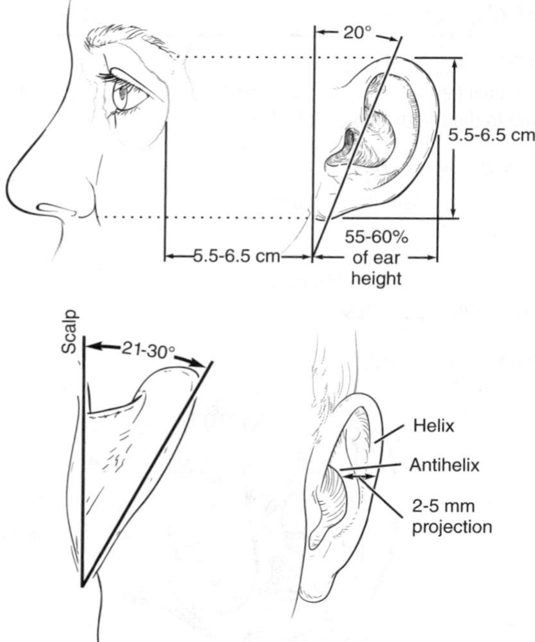


**Fig. 28-4** Correct placement of ear.

## EPIDEMIOLOGY[10]

- Relatively common, with an incidence in whites of about 5%
- Autosomal dominant trait
- Despite benign physiologic consequences, numerous studies attest to the psychological distress, emotional trauma, and behavioral problems this deformity can inflict on children.[5,11-13]
- Commonly caused by a combination of two defects:
  1. Underdevelopment of antihelical folding
  2. Overdevelopment of the conchal wall

## PREOPERATIVE EVALUATION

The following should be assessed[14]:

- Degree of antihelical folding
- Depth of the conchal bowl
- Plane of the lobule and deformity, if present
- Angle between the helical rim and the mastoid plane
- Quality and spring of the auricular cartilage
- Assess presence of other exacerbating and correctable anomalies/variations.

## MAJOR ANATOMIC CHARACTERISTICS

1. Poorly defined antihelical fold
2. Conchoscaphal angle >90 degrees
3. Conchal excess (can be determined by placing medial pressure along helical rim)

## EXACERBATING ANOMALIES/VARIATIONS

1. Stahl's ear
2. Darwin's tubercle
3. Mastoid prominence

## NONSURGICAL TREATMENT[2,3]

- Molding techniques initiated within the first 72 hours of birth
  - Takes advantage of circulating maternal hormones that result in more pliable and malleable cartilage
  - Perform continuously for 6-8 weeks
  - May avoid surgical treatment
  - Options: Splinting (custom vs. commercially available [EarWell; Beacon Medical, Naperville, IL]), taping, and gluing

## GOALS OF SURGICAL TREATMENT[15]

- All traces of protrusion in the upper third of the ear must be corrected. (Some remaining protrusion in the middle or lower portions may be acceptable, provided that the top is thoroughly corrected; but the reverse does not hold true.)
- From the front view, the helix of both ears should extend beyond the antihelix (at least down to the midear and preferably all the way down).
- The helix should have a smooth and regular line throughout.
- Treat Darwin's tubercle when present.

- The postauricular sulcus should not be marked, decreased, or distorted.
- The ear should not be placed too close to the head, especially in boys. (Posterior measurement from the outer edge of the helix to skin of the mastoidal region should be 10-12 mm in the upper third, 16-18 mm in the middle third, and 20-22 mm in the lower third.)
- The positions of the two ears (i.e., the distances from the lateral borders to the head) should match fairly closely—**to within 3 mm at any given point.**

## TIMING OF SURGERY

- Timing depends on a rational approach based on auricular growth and age of school matriculation.
- Because the ear is nearly fully developed by age 6-7 years, correction may be performed by this time.
  - In 76 patients who underwent cartilage excision otoplasty for prominent ears, Balogh and Millesi[16] demonstrated that auricular growth was not halted after a 7-year mean follow-up.
  - Given that growth retardation is unlikely, surgery can be performed at a younger age, as young as 5, if a child demonstrates a maturity level sufficient to cooperate with postoperative instructions and restrictions.

## SURGICAL TECHNIQUES

### MOST COMMON

- Mustarde[17]: Cartilage molding
- Furnas[18]: Cartilage molding
- Converse and Wood-Smith[19]: Cartilage breaking

### OTHERS

- Stenstroem[20]: Cartilage scoring
- Chongchet[21]: Cartilage scoring

**NOTE: Cartilage scoring techniques are based on the observation that cartilage curls away from a cut surface, which has been attributed to "interlocked stresses" that are released when the perichondrium is incised.**[22,23]

> **TIP:** Antihelical fold scoring should be performed on the ear's lateroanterior surface. Narrow otobraders can be introduced into subcutaneous pockets on the lateroanterior surface from medial/posterior access via small transcartilage fenestrations. This maneuver prevents anterior incisions and/or total auricular degloving for the purpose of lateroanterior exposure.

### MUSTARDE TECHNIQUE[7] (Fig. 28-5)

- Used to correct upper-third deformities, most often a poorly defined antihelical fold
- Technique (scaphaconchal sutures):
  - Press medially on the ear and mark the concha and outer portion of the antihelical fold with a methylene blue–dipped 25-gauge needle (full thickness to tattoo the postauricular skin).
  - Mark the postauricular skin excision between the marks.
  - Excise the skin and carry incision down to raw cartilage.
  - Place permanent mattress sutures (clear nylon or Mersilene full thickness) through the cartilage along the tattooed marks, making sure to capture the anterior perichondrium without piercing the anterior skin.

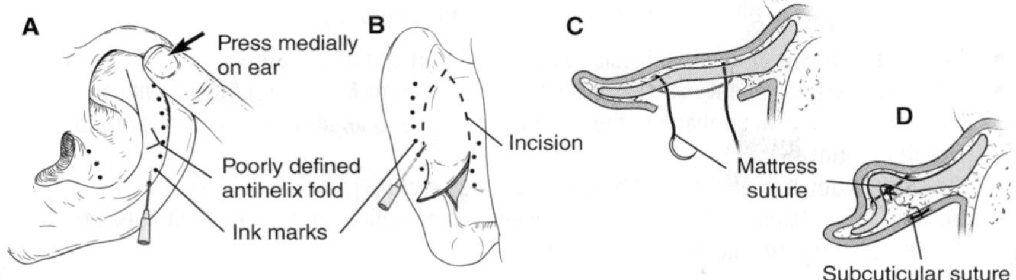


**Fig. 28-5** The Mustarde technique. **A,** Several pairs of ink marks are made on the concha and outer aspect of the antihelix. **B,** Several 23-gauge needles dipped in ink are used to transfer the ink marks to the postauricular skin. **C,** The skin excision is carried down to cartilage. After hemostasis is obtained, several sutures are placed through the full thickness of cartilage. Usually two or three well-placed sutures are all that are required. **D,** The sutures are tied simultaneously. A subcuticular 4-0 nylon suture is used for closure.

- Tie sutures down to effect (may require "floating" sutures).
- Close and dress with compression dressing of choice.
- Patient should wear elastic ski band continuously for 3 weeks and avoid strenuous activity.

**CAUTION: Watch for iatrogenic narrowing of the external auditory canal.**

## FURNAS TECHNIQUE[7] (Fig. 28-6)

- Used to correct deformities of the upper two thirds of the ear, most often conchal excess
- Can be combined with other techniques (e.g., Mustarde technique for correcting an absent antihelical fold)
- Technique (conchamastoid sutures):
  - Perform a postauricular skin excision down through perichondrium to raw cartilage.
  - Dissect medially and laterally to expose the postauricular muscles and ligaments.

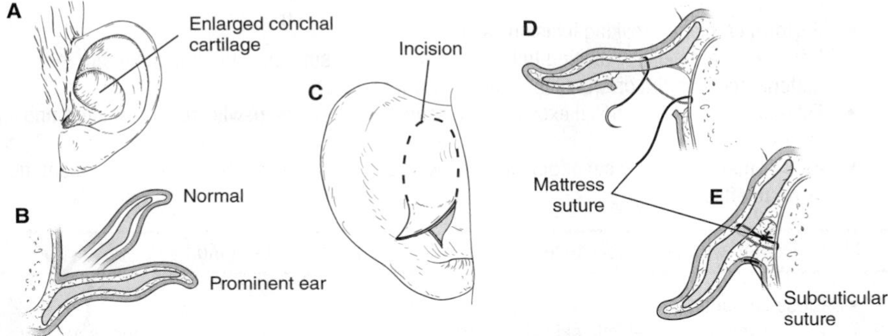


**Fig. 28-6** The Furnas technique. **A,** The Furnas technique is best used for patients with prominence of the superior two thirds of the ear. **B,** The deeply cupped and enlarged conchal cartilage of the prominent ear is contrasted with normal conchal cartilage in cross-section. **C,** An ellipse of skin is excised in the postauricular sulcus, exposing the posterior auricular muscles and ligaments. These are divided and resected. **D** and **E,** Several mattress sutures are used to attach conchal cartilage to the mastoid fascia. The mattress sutures should be placed through the full thickness of conchal cartilage. The sutures are tied simultaneously.

**CAUTION: Avoid injuring branches of the great auricular nerve.**

- Resect a segment of mastoid fascia to expose underlying periosteum.
- Place several permanent mattress sutures (clear nylon or Mersilene) full thickness through the conchal cartilage to the mastoid fascia/periosteum (capturing the anterior perichondrium).
- Tie sutures down to effect (may require "floating" sutures).
- Mastoid fascia flaps have recently been used in conjunction with suture techniques to bolster posterior/medial conchal repositioning.[24]
- Close and bolster.
- Patient should wear elastic ski band continuously for 3 weeks and avoid strenuous activity.

## Converse–Wood-Smith Technique

- A **cartilage-breaking technique,** rather than cartilage-molding technique, as in the previous examples
- Useful when treating the stiffer cartilage of young adults and adults
- Useful for correcting more severe prominent ear deformities (e.g., when entire ear is involved)
  - Conchal excess
  - Loss of antihelical fold
  - Increased conchoscaphal angle
- Drawbacks
  - Secondary sharp ridging
  - Contour irregularities
- Technique:
  - Press helix medially against the scalp.
  - Mark the superior rim of the triangular fossa, the upper border of the superior crus, and the junction of the helix and scapha.
  - Mark the full length of the conchal rim.
  - Transpose these marks to the postauricular skin using full-thickness punctures with methylene blue–dipped 25-gauge needles.
  - Demarcate the area of postauricular skin resection and excise. Dissect down to raw cartilage.
  - Perform cartilage-breaking incisions sharply.
  - Reform the antihelix by placing full-thickness mattress sutures with permanent suture material (clear nylon or Mersilene) and tie down to effect.
  - Estimate amount of conchal excess by pressing inward on the newly created antihelix and excise.
  - Approximate the newly cut edges of the concha and antihelix with permanent suture and tie down to effect.

**TIP:** Do not evert edges, because doing so will cause permanent ridging.

- Close and bolster.
- Patient should wear elastic ski band continuously for 3 weeks and avoid strenuous activity.

## CORRECTION OF LOBULE PROMINENCE (LOWER THIRD) (Fig. 28-7)

- Corrected using the modified fishtail excision (Wood-Smith)[25]
- Technique:
  - Mark a "V extension" from the inferior aspect of the postauricular incision used for correction of prominent ear deformity (e.g., Mustarde, Furnas).
  - Transpose the marking to the mastoid skin while the ink is still fresh, forming a mirror image pattern in the shape of a fishtail.
  - Excise along the demarcated line.
  - Close and dress.
- Alternative technique: Posterior dissection of antitragus via inferior portion of postauricular incision followed by antitragus retrorepositioning and suture anchorage to inferior concha. Improves acute angle between tragus and antitragus which is often an anatomic factor contributing to lobular prominence (Fig. 28-8).

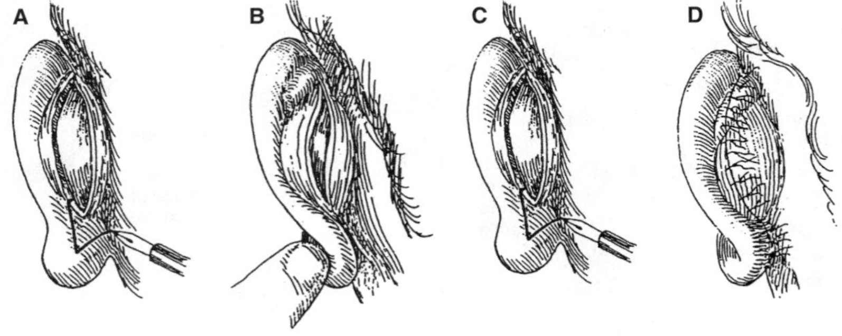


**Fig. 28-7** Modified fishtail excision. **A,** A V extension of the posterior auricular incision is drawn on the posterior surface of the lobule. **B,** While the ink is still wet, the lobule is pressed against the mastoid skin. **C,** The mirror impression of the V is transposed to the mastoid skin. All skin within the borders of the modified fishtail design is excised. **D,** Closure is performed with a running 4-0 nylon suture.

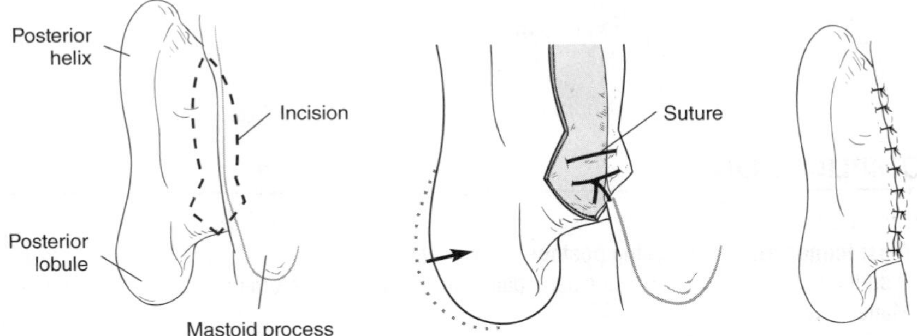


**Fig. 28-8** Alternative technique.

## Adjunctive Techniques for Specific Findings

- **Darwin's tubercle:** A pointed thickening at the junction of the upper and middle third of the helix in approximately 10% of all patients. Full-thickness excision of the excess skin and cartilage can be performed so inconspicuous scar at the transition from lateroanterior to medioposterior. Improves helical contour and further reduces apparent prominence (Fig. 28-9).
- **Stahl's ear:** The presence of the third and/or horizontal superior crus with a pointed upper helix. Results in upper- and middle-third prominence. A variety of techniques exist, including combination approaches.[26] Because of high relapse rate, the upper pole prominence at a minimum should be addressed.
- **Mastoid prominence:** Soft tissue between the concha and mastoid can be resected to mitigate the effect of a prominent mastoid on the projection of the concha. Alternatively, a burr can be used to carefully remove mastoid cortical bone.

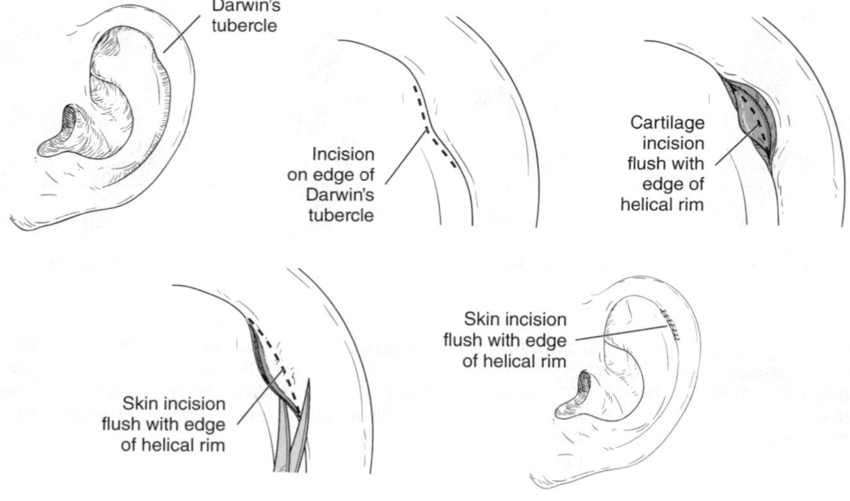


**Fig. 28-9** Darwin's tubercle.

# COMPLICATIONS[27]

## Hematoma

- **Most immediate and pressing postoperative problem**
- If sudden onset of persistent, unilateral pain, then suspect hematoma
- Management
  - Dressing removal, suture removal, and evacuation of clot
  - Reapplication of dressings with mild compression
  - To operating room for reexploration and hemostasis, if active

## Infection

- Rare
- Usually from *Staphylococcus* or *Streptococcus,* occasionally *Pseudomonas*
- **Sulfamylon** useful in preventing spread of infection and chondritis
- Long-term problem is from infection

## Chondritis

- Surgical infection requiring prompt reexploration and excision of necrotic cartilage

## Late Deformity

- Usually manifests within 6 months of surgery
- More often operator dependent than technique dependent
- Tan[28] found:
  - 24% of patients undergoing the Mustarde technique required "reoperation."
  - 10% of patients undergoing the Stenstroem technique required "reoperation."
    - Reason: Presence of sutures resulted in sinuses and wound infection in 15% of cases.
  - Cartilage-breaking techniques (e.g., Luckett, Converse, and Wood-Smith) leave more "sharp edges" and "contour irregularities" than do non-cartilage-breaking techniques (e.g., Mustarde and Stenstroem).

**TIP:** "Break the ring of cartilage" to prevent telephone ear deformity.

## Key Points

- ✓ Ear cartilage is very malleable immediately after birth, and deformities can sometimes be corrected nonsurgically through molding techniques.
- ✓ Otoplasty for prominent ear deformities usually is performed around age 6-7 years (5 years of age is acceptable when patient compliance is predicted).
- ✓ The three typical deformities that make up the prominent ear deformity are a poorly defined antihelical fold, a conchoscaphal angle >90 degrees, and/or conchal excess.
- ✓ There are three approaches to treating a prominent ear: cartilage scoring, cartilage molding, and cartilage breaking.
- ✓ Hematoma and infection are rare but need to be treated immediately and aggressively.
- ✓ The most common long-term complication is recurrence of the deformity, which is technique and surgeon dependent.

## References


1. Allison GR. Anatomy of the external ear. Clin Plast Surg 5:419, 1978.
2. Tan ST, Abramson DL, MacDonald DM, et al. Molding therapy for infants with deformational auricular anomalies. Ann Plast Surg 38:263, 1997.
3. Tan ST, Shibu M, Gault DT. A splint for correction of congenital ear deformities. Br J Plast Surg 47:575, 1994.
4. Farkas LG, Posnick JC, Hreczko TM. Anthropometric growth study of the ear. Cleft Palate Craniofac J 29:324, 1992.
5. Adamson JE, Horton CE, Crawford HH. The growth pattern of the external ear. Plast Reconstr Surg 36:466, 1965.
6. Janis JE, Rohrich RJ, Gutowski KA. Otoplasty. Plast Reconstr Surg 115:60e-72e, 2005.

7. Aston SJ, Beasley RW, Throne CH, eds. Grabb and Smith's Plastic Surgery, 6th ed. Philadelphia: Lippincott Williams & Wilkins, 2007.
8. Farkas LG. Anthropometry of normal and anomalous ears. Clin Plast Surg 5:401, 1978.
9. Ha RY, Trovato MJ. Plastic surgery of the ear. Sel Read Plast Surg 11(R3):1, 2011.
10. Adamson PA, Strecker HD. Otoplasty techniques. Facial Plast Surg 11:284, 1995.
11. Campobasso P, Belloli G. [Protruding ears: the indications for surgical treatment] Pediatr Med Chir 15:151, 1993.
12. Bradbury ET, Hewison J, Timmons MJ. Psychological and social outcome of prominent ear correction in children. Br J Plast Surg 45:97, 1992.
13. Macgregor FC. Ear deformities: social and psychological implications. Clin Plast Surg 5:347, 1978.
14. Ellis DA, Keohane JD. A simplified approach to otoplasty. J Otolaryngol 21:66, 1992.
15. McDowell AJ. Goals in otoplasty for protruding ears. Plast Reconstr Surg 41:17, 1968.
16. Balogh B, Millesi H. Are growth alterations a consequence of surgery for prominent ears? Plast Reconstr Surg 89:623, 1992.
17. Mustarde JC. The correction of prominent ears using mattress sutures. Br J Plast Surg 16:170, 1963.
18. Furnas DW. Correction of prominent ears by conchamastoid sutures. Plast Reconstr Surg 42:189, 1968.
19. Converse JM, Wood-Smith D. Technical details in the surgical correction of the lop ear deformity. Plast Reconstr Surg 31:118, 1963.
20. Stenstroem SJ. A natural technique for correction of congenitally prominent ears. Plast Reconstr Surg 32:509, 1963.
21. Chongchet V. A method of antihelix reconstruction. Br J Plast Surg 16:268, 1963.
22. Gibson T, Davis W. The distortion of autogenous cartilage grafts: its cause and prevention. Br J Plast Surg 10:257, 1958.
23. Fry HJ. Interlocked stresses in human nasal septal cartilage. Br J Plast Surg 19:276, 1966.
24. Szychta P, Stewart KJ. Comparison of cartilage scoring and cartilage sparing techniques in unilateral otoplasty: a 10-year experience. Ann Plast Surg, 2012 Dec 4. [Epub ahead of print]
25. Wood-Smith D. Otoplasty. In Rees T, ed. Aesthetic Plastic Surgery. Philadelphia: WB Saunders, 1980.
26. Weinfeld AB. Stahl's ear correction: synergistic use of cartilage abrading, strategic Mustarde suture placement, and anterior anticonvexity suture. J Craniofac Surg 23:901, 2012.
27. Furnas DW. Complications of surgery of the external ear. Clin Plast Surg 17:305, 1990.
28. Tan KH. Long-term survey of prominent ear surgery: a comparison of two methods. Br J Plast Surg 39:270, 1986.

# 29. Facial Soft Tissue Trauma

James B. Collins, Raman C. Mahabir, Jason K. Potter

## DEMOGRAPHICS

- No gender difference[1]
- Mean age of injury is 28 years[1]

## GENERAL

- The face has five primary functions considered in soft tissue trauma.
  1. Protect the central nervous system
  2. House specialized sensory organs (olfaction, gustation, vision, balance, hearing, and touch)
  3. Initiate digestion
  4. Facilitate respiration
  5. Express emotion

## ETIOLOGIC FACTORS

- Injuries result from motor vehicle collisions, assault, wild and domestic animal attacks, falls, self-infliction, and recreational activities.[1,2]

## CLASSIFICATION

- Abrasion: Scraped area of skin
- Laceration: Jagged cut or tear
- Avulsion: Tearing resulting in an area of skin lifted off the underlying tissue
- Crush: Damage caused by compression
  - Often results in greater tissue injury
- Miscellaneous
  - Gunshot wound (GSW)
    - Substantial soft tissue injury may warrant early intubation.
    - Soft tissue deficits are often minimal.
  - Bite
    - Associated with polymicrobial infections
      - *Eikenella corrodens* and S*treptococcus viridans* in human bites[3]
      - *Pasteurella canis* in canine bites[4]
      - *Pasteurella multicoda* in feline bites[4]

**TIP:** Infections are most common after feline bites because of the deep, puncture-type wounds and virulent bacteria.

## INITIAL EVALUATION

Thorough assessment is essential to fully diagnose the extent of injury and provide appropriate treatment. Particular attention should be given to the mechanism of injury and quality of the wound.

- Patients with a significant mechanism of injury may have associated critical injuries (e.g., intracranial hemorrhage and cervical spine fractures).[5]
  - Mandatory evaluation consistent with Advanced Trauma Life Support guidelines.
- Careful attention is given to soft tissue injuries near specialized facial structures.
  - Lacrimal apparatus
  - External auditory meatus
  - Facial nerve
  - Parotid duct
- Infusion of local anesthetic may aid examination.

**TIP:** Motor and sensory innervation is evaluated before anesthetic is administered.

## MANAGEMENT

- Anatomic realignment is critical to minimize deformity.
- Wounds should be closed as soon as the patient is stabilized.
  - Infectious risk increases the longer a wound is open.[6]
  - The rich vascularity of the head and neck increases resistance to infection.[7-9]
  - Desiccation is prevented with saline-soaked gauze before closure.

### BLEEDING

- The vascularity of the region can lead to **significant blood loss** from lacerations.
  - However, facial bleeding is an unusual cause of hypovolemic shock.
  - Consider other critical injuries for shock.
- Hemorrhage can usually be controlled with local pressure.

**CAUTION: Avoid blind clamping to prevent iatrogenic injury to specialized structures.**

- Use suction, packing, and irrigation to identify bleeding vessels.

**TIP:** Epinephrine may improve visibility through vasoconstriction.

### IRRIGATION AND DEBRIDEMENT

- Irrigation and removal of foreign bodies from wounds is **essential** before closure to reduce the risk of infection.
  - Debris that is not removed from the dermis can result in permanent (traumatic) tattooing.
- All devitalized tissue is removed with sharp debridement.
  - Conserve specialized tissue whenever possible (e.g., nose, periorbital region, lips, ears, and hair-bearing skin).

**TIP:** The vascularity of the face allows surprisingly small portions of tissue to survive.

- Wounds with gross contamination and foreign bodies must be debrided and receive appropriate prophylaxis.

## Repair

- **General**
  - Avoid local flaps in the acute setting, in particular in wounds with crush components, until the extent of the devitalized tissue has declared itself.
  - Layered closure is preferred to relieve tension but may increase the risk of subsequent infection in a dirty wound.

> **TIP:** Select sutures small enough to minimize the risk of tissue damage and suture marks, but strong enough to avoid wound dehiscence. Often 5-0 and 6-0 sutures fit these criteria for the face and eyelid, respectively.

- **Abrasions**
  - Partial-thickness loss
    - Antibiotic ointment while wounds are open
    - Lotion (moisturizer) as wounds epithelialize
  - Full-thickness loss
    - Dressing changes until stable wound
    - Closure with local flaps or skin graft
- **Lacerations/avulsions**
  - Ensure closure of dead space.
  - Layered closure should approximate skin, muscle, and fascia without tension.
  - Place sutures carefully to prevent strangulation of tissues.

> **TIP:** Consider the use of surgical drains to eliminate dead space.

> **TIP:** Drains may be fashioned from 21-gauge butterfly catheters and red-top tubes. Small perforations are made in the distal end of the tubing (<50% of the diameter of the tube to prevent the catheter breaking in vivo). The needle is inserted into the red-top tube using its negative pressure for suction. Tubes are changed every 2-3 hours or when half full.

> **TIP:** Healing by secondary intention is useful only for small defects in depressed areas of the face (i.e., alar/cheek groove). Generally, secondary intention will result in an inferior final appearance compared with other reconstructive options.

- **Bite wounds**
  - These may be loosely closed primarily after aggressive irrigation and debridement.[9]
  - Extended-spectrum beta-lactam (amoxicillin/clavulanate) or fluoroquinolone antibiotics are appropriate for commonly associated organisms.[3]
  - Rabies immunoglobulin and vaccination should be considered if the animal cannot be located and tested.

## Medications

- Prophylactic antibiotics may provide benefit in grossly contaminated wounds, immunocompromised patients, open fractures, wounds contaminated with oral secretion, and with delayed wound closure.[10]

- **Tetanus**
  - Risk factors include time since injury (>6 hours), depth of injury (>1cm), mechanism of injury (crush, burn, GSW, puncture), presence of devitalized tissue, and contamination (grass, soil, saliva, retained foreign body).
  - See Table 29-1[11,12] for recommendations.

**Table 29-1** *Tetanus Recommendations*

| | Tetanus Prone | | Not Tetanus Prone | |
|---|---|---|---|---|
| **History of Immunization** | **Tetanus Toxoid*** | **Tetanus Ig†** | **Tetanus Toxoid** | **Tetanus Ig** |
| Unknown or incomplete | 0.5 ml | 250 U | 0.5 ml | No |
| Complete + booster >10 years ago | 0.5 ml | 250 U | 0.5 ml | No |
| Complete + booster >5 years ago | 0.5 ml | No | No | No |
| Complete + booster <5 years ago | No | No | No | No |

*Tetanus and diphtheria toxoid (Td) 0.5 ml IM.
†Tetanus immune globulin (TIG) 250 units IM.

## SPECIAL ANATOMIC CONSIDERATIONS

Also see specific chapters for further details.

### SCALP

- Associated with subgaleal undermining and avulsion injuries
- Layered closure
  - Galea is approximated with interrupted absorbable suture.
  - Epidermis is approximated with absorbable monofilament suture or staples.

**TIP:** Staples may cause less alopecia on the scalp than other forms of closure.[13,14] Cautery should be used with caution for similar reasons.

### FOREHEAD

- Lacerations may injure the temporal (frontal) branch of the facial nerve or the frontalis muscle directly, causing brow ptosis[15] (Fig. 29-1).
- Layered closure
  - Frontalis is repaired with interrupted absorbable suture.
  - Skin is closed with interrupted nonabsorbable monofilament suture.

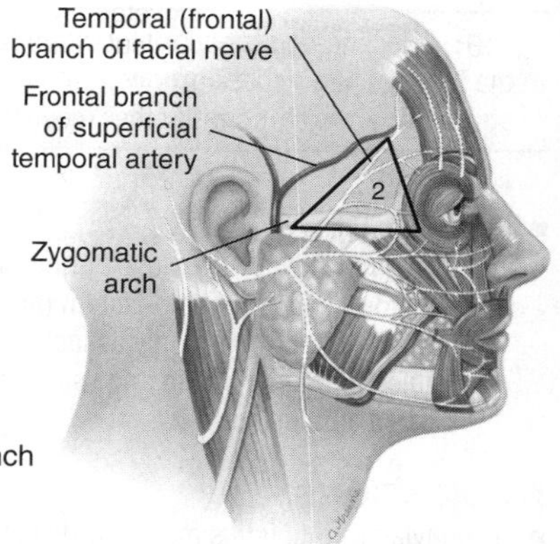

**Fig. 29-1** Course of the temporal branch of the facial nerve above the zygoma.

**TIP:** Scars in the forehead often heal without a significant deformity even when lacerations are oriented in opposition to the relaxed skin tension lines.

## Eyebrow

- Relatively unique structure that is difficult to replace
  - Preserve with minimal debridement.
- Layered closure
  - Dermis is repaired with interrupted absorbable suture.
  - Epidermis is closed with interrupted nonabsorbable monofilament suture.

## Eyelid

- Evaluation is required for injury to the septum and levator, because levator disruption may result in ptosis if not repaired.
- Avoid placing suture adjacent to the cornea to prevent abrasions.
- **Evert palpebral borders to prevent notching.**
- Perform layered closure for lacerations through the lid margin.
  - Use nonabsorbable monofilament sutures to repair the tarsus and skin.

> **TIP:** Select a nonabsorbable suture with minimal inflammatory reaction, and place the knots close to the gray line to prevent corneal irritation and contact.

## Lacrimal Apparatus[16] (Fig. 29-2)

- Tears drain into puncta of the medial upper and lower lids.
  - Injury is associated with medial lid lacerations (most commonly lower lid).
  - If concerned, cannulate puncta with lacrimal probe to identify laceration.
- Treatment includes:
  - Direct repair over lacrimal stent (e.g., Crawford tubes), maintained in place for 4 weeks.
  - Dacryocystorhinostomy may be necessary if cannulation is impossible and injury results in problematic epiphora.

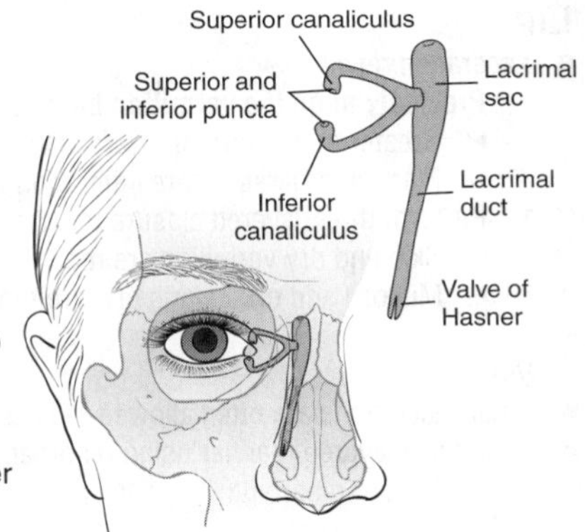


**Fig. 29-2** The lacrimal system is made up of superior and inferior canaliculi that coalesce into the common canaliculus. This empties into the lacrimal sac, which drains into the nose through the lacrimal duct. The upper system is composed of the superior/inferior puncta through the common canaliculus, and the lower system consists of the lacrimal sac and duct.

## Ear

- Cartilaginous injury
  - Debride cartilage stripped of perichondrium.
  - Nonstructural injuries to the cartilage do not need to be repaired and may be excised if nonviable.
- Circumferential external auditory canal lacerations
  - Stent to prevent stenosis.
- Hematomas
  - These result in permanent, thickened fibrosis (cauliflower deformity).
  - Drain and bolster skin flaps and consider through-and-through sutures.
- Layered closure with eversion to prevent notching of the ear folds
  - Skin and cartilage can be repaired with nonabsorbable monofilament sutures.

**TIP:** Hematomas may be drained through a cartilaginous window when a laceration or incision presents itself on the opposite side of the ear.

## NOSE

- Evaluate and repair the **three lamellae of the nose.**
  1. Skin and soft tissue: Absorbable suture in the deep dermis, and nonabsorbable in the skin
  2. Cartilaginous framework: Monofilament nonabsorbable suture
  3. Mucosa: Absorbable suture
- Septal hematomas
  - Intranasal examination is necessary for identification.
  - Treatment involves incising mucosa and packing the nose to prevent reaccumulation.

## SALIVARY GLANDS

- May result in sialocele or cutaneous fistula if not treated
- Parotid gland
  - Parotid duct is located opposite the **second maxillary molar**[16] (Fig. 29-3).
  - Evaluate by stenting Stensen's duct intraorally with a 24-gauge angiocatheter.
    - Extravasation of saline after infusion indicates an injury.
    - Parotid duct lacerations are repaired with microsurgical techniques.
      - Direct repair over Silastic stents may provide benefit.
- Submandibular gland
  - Lacerations should be marsupialized to the floor of the mouth.

## LIP

- Laceration repair
  - **Precisely align the vermilion border.**
    - Greater than 1 mm of discrepancy is noticeable at conversational distance.[17]
    - Mark landmarks before infiltration with local anesthetic.
  - Perform three-layered closure (skin, orbicularis oris, mucosa).
    - Skin and dry vermilion are repaired with nonabsorbable suture.
    - Mucosa and orbicularis oris are repaired with absorbable suture.

## TONGUE

- Small lacerations are often allowed to heal by secondary intention.
- Repair in a layered manner using resorbable sutures.

## NERVES

- **Assess nerve function before anesthetic is administered (facial and trigeminal nerves).**
- Facial nerve lacerations
  - Nerve stimulators may be used **up to 72 hours** after injury.
    - After 72 hours the distal nerve end may not stimulate.
  - Repair with microsurgical technique.
    - *Injuries medial to the lateral canthus or oral commissure may be too small to repair.*

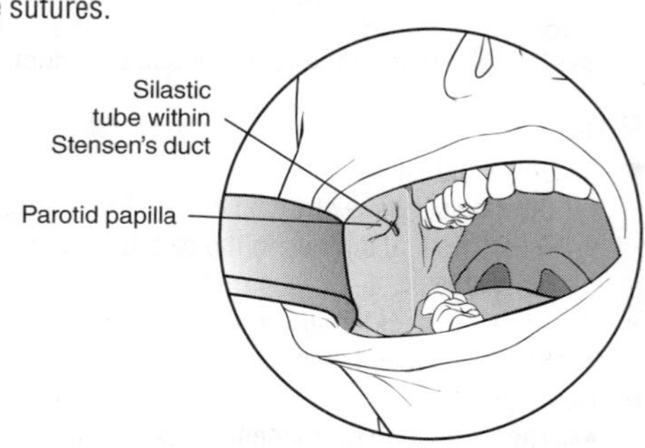


**Fig. 29-3** Method for diagnosing an injury to Stensen's duct.

## POSTOPERATIVE CARE

- Routine wound care is required to prevent desiccation.
  - Apply antibiotic ointment to wounds until epithelialized, then apply lotion.
- Sutures removed at:
  - 5-7 days for the face and neck
  - 2-3 weeks for the scalp

**TIP:** Remove sutures at the earliest time to prevent skin reaction and permanent scarring.

## COMPLICATIONS/OUTCOMES

- Hypertrophic scarring
- Hyperpigmentation
  - Associated with sun exposure up to 1 year after injury
  - Requires sun avoidance, including protective clothing and sunscreen
- Scar contracture resulting in deformation of normal anatomy and possibly functional deficits
- Alopecia
  - May be associated with excessive use of cautery and traumatic tissue handling[18]

### KEY POINTS

✓ Careful hemostasis is required, with attention to blood loss from vascularity of the face.
✓ Perform adequate irrigation and debridement.
✓ Debride conservatively particularly in specialized areas of the face.
✓ It may be possible to primarily close bite wounds to the face after aggressive irrigation and debridement.
✓ Avoid local flaps in acute settings.
✓ Evaluate ears for hematoma.
✓ Meticulous approximation of anatomic structures is critical, with particular attention to the vermilion border.
✓ All structures are closed in layers with obliteration of dead space.
✓ The parotid duct needs to be evaluated.
✓ Facial nerve lacerations should be repaired within 72 hours of injury.

## REFERENCES


1. Gassner R, Tuli T, Hächl O, et al. Cranio-maxillofacial trauma: a 10 year review of 9,543 cases with 21,067 injuries. J Craniomaxillofac Surg 31:51-61, 2003.
2. Gassner R, Tuli T, Hächl O, et al. Craniomaxillofacial trauma in children: a review of 3,385 cases with 6,060 injuries in 10 years. J Oral Maxillofac Surg 62:399-407, 2004.
3. Talan DA, Abrahamian FM, Moran GJ, et al. Clinical presentation and bacteriologic analysis of infected human bites in patients presenting to emergency departments. Clin Infect Dis 37:1481-1489, 2003.
4. Talan DA, Citron DM, Abrahamian FM, et al. Bacteriologic analysis of infected dog and cat bites. N Engl J Med 340:85-92, 1999.
5. Mithani SK, St-Hilaire H, Brooke BS, et al. Predictable patterns of intracranial and cervical spine injury in craniomaxillofacial trauma: analysis of 4786 patients. Plast Reconstr Surg 123:1293-1301, 2009.
6. Waseem M, Lakdawala V, Patel R, et al. Is there a relationship between wound infections and laceration closure times? Int J Emerg Med 5:32, 2012.

7. Adalarasan S, Mohan A, Pasupathy S. Prophylactic antibiotics in maxillofacial fractures: a requisite? J Craniofac Surg 21:1009-1011, 2010.
8. Hollander JE, Singer AJ, Valentine SM, et al. Risk factors for infection in patients with traumatic lacerations. Acad Emerg Med 8:716-720, 2001.
9. Stefanopoulos PK. Management of facial bite wounds. Oral Maxillofac Surg Clin North Am 21:247-257, 2009.
10. Abubaker AO. Use of prophylactic antibiotics in preventing infection of traumatic injuries. Oral Maxillofac Surg Clin North Am 21:259-264, 2009.
11. Centers for Disease Control and Prevention (CDC). Deferral of routine booster doses of tetanus and diphtheria toxoids for adolescents and adults. MMWR Morb Mortal Wkly Rep 50:418,427, 2001.
12. Update on adult immunization. Recommendations of the Immunization Practices Advisory Committee (ACIP). MMWR Recomm Rep 40(RR-12):1-94, 1991.
13. Ritchie AJ, Rocke LG. Staples versus sutures in the closure of scalp wounds: a prospective, double-blind, randomized trial. Injury 20:217-218, 1989.
14. Brickman KR, Lambert RW. Evaluation of skin stapling for wound closure in the emergency department. Ann Emerg Med 18:1122-1125, 1989.
15. Seckel BR, ed. Facial Danger Zones: Avoiding Nerve Injury in Facial Plastic Surgery, 2nd ed. St Louis: Quality Medical Publishing, 2010.
16. Marcus JR, ed. Essentials of Craniomaxillofacial Trauma. St Louis: Quality Medical Publishing, 2012.
17. Thorne CH, Beasley RW, Aston SJ, et al, eds. Grabb & Smith's Plastic Surgery, 6th ed. Philadelphia: Lippincott Williams & Wilkins, 2007.
18. Papay FA, Stein J, Luciano M, et al. The microdissection cautery needle versus the cold scalpel in bicoronal incisions. J Craniofac Surg 9:344-347, 1998.

# 30. Facial Skeletal Trauma

**Jason K. Potter, Adam H. Hamawy**

## GENERAL

- **Trauma** is the number one cause of death in individuals <40 years of age.
- Death from injury accounts for 80% of all deaths among teens and young adults.
- Traumatic injury is the number one cause of lost workforce productivity.
- Approximately 1.7 million head injuries occur annually in the United States.
- Alcohol is a contributing factor in almost 50% of head injuries.
- A review of the Maryland Shock Trauma Registry (1986-1994) reported that 11% of trauma patients (2964 of 25,758) sustained maxillofacial fractures requiring subspecialty intervention.[1,2]

## EPIDEMIOLOGY

- Applied force and facial injury
  - Severity of injury is a function of energy delivered. Kinetic energy: $K = mv^2$
  - Moving object strikes head or moving head strikes static object.
- Variables affecting type and severity of injury
  - **Area of strike:** Specific anatomic location that receives energy
  - **Resistant force:** Resultant movement of head
  - **Angulation of strike:** More severe injury with perpendicular delivery of energy than with tangential delivery

## CLASSIFICATION

### ASSAULT

- Interpersonal violence is an increasing cause of facial fractures.
- Males 18-25 years old are typically attacked by unknown assailants.
- Females are typically attacked by known assailants.
- 40% of ER visits result from assault.
  - 30% present with fracture, 80% of these involve facial bone.
- Elevated blood alcohol is reported in 50% of incidents.
- Incidence ranking: **Nasal > mandible > zygoma > midface**

### MOTOR VEHICLE COLLISION

- Males 18-25 years old
- Associated with more severe trauma
- Frequently involves midface structures (nose, zygoma, maxilla)
- Overall reduction in number of injuries by >30% as a result of modernized auto safety systems such as seatbelts, air bags, and improved engineering.
  - Seat belt laws: Incidence of facial injury reduced from 21% to 6% in 2 years

## FALLS

- Bimodal age group
  - Toddlers
  - Elderly
- Hands-out fall: Fractures of zygoma and lateral face
- No-hands fall: Fractures of central face and dentoalveolar structures

## WAR

- Maxillofacial involvement in 26% of all battle injuries[3]
  - Percentage of maxillofacial combat injuries is increasing compared to wars in the previous century because of modern protective armor.
- The blast mechanism of midface fractures sustained in the battlefield has a high complication rate with associated multiple open fractures, complex lacerations, and associated injuries.[4] Modern high-velocity weapon injuries of head and neck are frequently fatal.

## SPORTS

- Relatively low incidence because of mouth guards and protective headgear

# CLINICAL SIGNIFICANCE

- Facial skeleton provides anterior protection for the cranium.
- Facial appearance is highly valued by most cultures.
- Maxillofacial region is associated with a number of important functions of daily life: Seeing, smelling, eating, breathing, and talking.
- Maxillofacial injuries may occur as isolated injuries or as part of polytrauma[5] (Table 30-1).
- In general, maxillofacial injuries are a low priority in the management of polytrauma patients but are addressed in the Advance Trauma Life Support (ATLS) tertiary survey.
  - Although they can be bloody, they are rarely the sole cause of shock.
  - Exceptions that can lead to life-threatening or irreversible injury:
    - Life-threatening hemorrhage
    - Loss of airway
    - Cervical spine injury
    - Neurologic injury

**Table 30-1** *Prevalence of Concomitant Injuries in Patients With Panfacial Fracture*

| Injury Type | Prevalence (%) |
|---|---|
| Intracranial injury/hemorrhage | 18 |
| Abdominal organ injury | 16 |
| Pneumothorax | 13 |
| Pulmonary contusion | 13 |
| Cervical spine fracture | 13 |
| Rib/sternum fracture | 11 |
| Lower extremity fracture | 11 |
| Upper extremity fracture | 11 |
| Pelvic fracture | 8 |
| Noncervical spine fracture | 8 |

## LONG-TERM PHYSICAL IMPAIRMENT

- A direct relationship has been demonstrated between severity of injury and work disability in patients with complex facial fractures.[2]
  - These patients reported higher incidence of somatic complaints than general trauma patients.
  - Residual cranial nerve deficits, facial numbness, persistent facial pain, headaches, and sinus problems were unrelated to severity of injury.

## PATIENT EVALUATION

### DETAILED HISTORY (Table 30-2)

- **Method of injury:** Include mechanism and specifics for severity of injury (e.g., assault with weapon delivers more force than fists alone).
- **Location of injury**
- **Time of injury:** Length of time from injury to presentation
- **Loss of consciousness**
- **Subjective complaints**
  - Double vision
  - Loss of vision
  - Hearing loss
  - Otorrhea or rhinorrhea
  - Malocclusion
- Inquire about **environmental considerations** that may affect management: Chemical, agricultural, or farm injuries.
- **Preexisting conditions**
  - Many patients who present to the ER for facial trauma have been there before.

**TIP:** Preexisting enophthalmos or malocclusion can mislead and result in significant waste of resources if appropriate inquiries are not made.

**Table 30-2** *Subjective Complaints Suggestive of Craniomaxillofacial Injury*

| Complaint | Suggestive of |
|---|---|
| Diplopia | Orbital fracture |
| Numbness of the cheek/maxillary teeth | Zygomaticomaxillary fracture (infraorbital nerve) |
| Numbness of the chin | Mandible fracture (mental nerve) |
| Malocclusion | Mandible or maxillary fracture |
| Visual change/blindness | Orbital fracture, globe injury |
| Loss of hearing or otorrhea | Temporal bone fracture |
| Rhinorrhea | Cribriform fracture, frontal sinus fracture |
| Trismus | Mandible or zygomatic arch fracture |

- **Identify potentially devastating injuries**
  - **Loss of airway**
    - May result from massive edema or loss of anterior support of the tongue, resulting in obstruction at the level of the hypopharynx
    - Bleeding may cause significant airway visualization challenges.
    - Severe injuries to the midface and mandible can result in structural distortion and subsequent airway obstruction.
      - Patients usually refuse to lie down in an attempt to maintain airway patency.

**TIP:** Be wary of loss of airway in patients with multiple fractures of the anterior mandible.

    - **Four indications for tracheotomy**[6]
      1. Acute airway obstruction and failed endotracheal intubation
      2. Expected prolonged mechanical ventilation
      3. Multiple facial fractures associated with basilar skull injuries
      4. Destruction of nasal anatomy associated with facial fractures
  - **Life-threatening hemorrhage**
    - **Internal maxillary artery** most common source associated with facial fractures
    - **Management**
      - Posterior nasal and oropharyngeal packing after securing airway
      - Immediate reduction of fractures
      - Consideration of angiography and selective embolization for stable patients or ligation of external carotid for hemodynamically unstable patients
  - **Cervical spine injury**
    - 15%-20% of all cervical spine injuries are associated with facial bone fractures. Conversely, 1%-4% of all facial injuries are associated with cervical spine injury.[7]
    - Most important: Diagnosis of cervical spine injury is delayed in 10%-25% of patients when associated with facial injury.

**CAUTION: Spinal precautions should be used with every patient.**

  - **Neurologic injury**
    - Estimated 1.6 million brain injuries annually in the United States
    - 60,000 deaths; 70,000-90,000 cases of permanent neurologic disability[8]
    - 13-75 times greater risk of death from neurologic injury with any middle or upper facial fracture compared with isolated mandibular fracture[7]
    - **Risk for intracranial injury**
      - Presence of skull fracture implies transmission of a large force.
      - Incidence of intracranial injury, with loss of consciousness, is 1.3%-17.2%.[9]
      - Incidence increases with a Glasgow Coma Score (GCS) <15 and longer unconsciousness.
      - **Closed head injury (CHI) occurs in 17.5% of patients with facial fractures.**[10]
      - Midfacial fractures are more often associated with CHI than mandible fractures.[9]
      - Patterns of facial fractures tend to be more severe in patients with CHI.[10]
    - **Classification of neurologic injury**
      - **Primary injury** is the initial injury and the cause of presentation.

- **Secondary injury** is a result of damage to neurons because of systemic physiologic responses to the initial injury.
  - **Hypotension** and **hypoxia** are the major causes of secondary injury.

## PHYSICAL EXAMINATION

Examination of the maxillofacial complex is a detailed process that requires an organized approach to prevent omission of key elements. Before beginning, patients should be cleansed of all dried blood and dirt that may obscure underlying injury.

### INSPECTION

- Thoroughly assess all areas of the head and neck for contusions, lacerations, edema, hematomas, asymmetries, or obvious deformities.
- Inspect pupils for symmetry and reaction to light; inspect the external auditory canal for lacerations and tympanic membrane for rupture, hemotympanum, or otorrhea. This information should help guide the physical examination.

### PALPATION

- Begin in the frontal region.
  - Palpate the frontal process, orbital rims, nasal bones, and zygomas.

> **TIP:** Bimanual, bilateral palpation helps identify side to side differences that may indicate fractures.

  - Note any step-offs, crepitus, or gross deformity.
- Palpate in the region of lacerations or contusion for underlying fracture.
- Proceed intraorally and run fingers along the zygomaticomaxillary (ZM) buttresses, noting step-offs, ecchymosis, or lacerations.
  - Note gingival lacerations and determine whether all teeth are present and nonmobile.
- Place the nondominant hand on the nasal dorsum and, using the dominant hand, grasp the anterior maxilla (dentition) and assess for mobility.
- Grasp the mandible bimanually and assess for mobility along its length.
- Note ecchymosis on the floor of mouth.
- Assess occlusion.
- Palpate cervical spine and note tenderness or step-offs.

### EVALUATE CRANIAL NERVES II-XII (see Chapter 32).

**NOTE: Determine whether paresthesias or functional deficits are present.**

## DIAGNOSTIC IMAGING

- **For diagnostic purposes, patients with abnormal findings during physical examination should have CT of the maxillofacial complex in both axial and coronal planes.**
- CT is the benchmark for middle and upper facial fractures.[11]

- Plain films are not necessary for evaluation of midfacial fractures (unlike mandibular fractures) when CT is available.
- Reconstructed coronal images are not of acceptable quality and should only be tolerated when patient positioning for coronal imaging is precluded by cervical spine precautions.
- Two-dimensional CT is more accurate in assessing orbital floor and medial orbital wall fractures. Three-dimensional CT is better for evaluating complex LeFort and palatal fractures. Ideally both are used for assessment and planning.[12]

## TIMING OF OPERATIVE INTERVENTION

- Prevention or minimization of secondary injury is of primary importance.[13]
- Initial management of head-injured patients should be similar to that for polytrauma patients without head injury, focusing on control of hemorrhage and restoration of perfusion.
- Maintenance of **cerebral perfusion pressure (CPP) >70 mm Hg** is required during the preoperative, perioperative, and postoperative periods.
- Brain injury increases with inadequate resuscitation and with operative procedures that allow hypotension or low CPP.
- Treatment protocol is based on each patient's clinical assessment and treatment needs.

## FIXATION MATERIALS

- Basic understanding of bone healing demonstrates necessity for adequate fixation.
  - Early techniques relied on wire fixation and "bone carpentry" with interdigitating cuts.
  - Plate fixation provides rigid stability and effectively bridges deficits without significant loss of structural strength.
- **Metallic plates**
  - Titanium and titanium alloys provide strength to allow stability for healing and are easily contoured in the operating room to allow adequate coaptation of bone fragments.
    - They are not subject to fibrous encapsulations and are resistant to corrosion.
    - Titanium is the predominant metallic material used in craniofacial systems.
  - Vitallium is more difficult to contour and shape.
    - Used often in mandibular fixation
    - Alloy of cobalt, chromium, and molybdenum
  - Stainless steel plates have been used historically.
- **Bioabsorbable plates**
  - Lack the strength of metallic materials
  - Increased size of plates and screws and higher profile than metallic implants to compensate for strength discrepancy
  - Polymers are radiolucent and do not interfere with diagnostic imaging.
  - Bioabsorbable polymers include polyglycolic acid (Bionix Medical Technologies, Toledo, OH), poly-L-lactic acid (PLLA) (Bionix; Zimmer, Warsaw, IN), polyglyconate and polyglycolic/poly-L-lactic acid (LactoSorb; Walter Lorenz Surgical, Jacksonville, FL), and poly-L-lactide/co-D,L-lactide (MacroPore; MacroPore Biosurgery, San Diego, CA; Synthes, West Chester, PA).
  - Properties, including strength and resorption time, vary between materials.
  - Primarily used in pediatric craniofacial fixation to prevent impact on skull growth and internal migration of permanent implants, which can occur with metallic implants.

- **Screws**
  - Drilling should be performed carefully at low speeds (<1000 rpm) and with irrigation to minimize thermal injury to surrounding bone.
  - Screw fixation is accomplished by tapping a predrilled hole or using **self-tapping screws.**
  - **Self-tapping screws**
    - Opposing vertical cutting blades at the tip
    - More time efficient and use less instruments
    - Recommended in thin bones of the midface
  - **Self-drilling screws**
    - Most common type of screw
    - Tapering shaft with a continuous thread from tip to head
    - Require pilot hole to begin

## FRONTAL SINUS FRACTURES

- **The frontal bone requires the greatest force of any facial bone to fracture;** it can withstand 800-1600 pounds of force[14] (Fig. 30-1).
- The sinus is contained within the frontal bone and drains beneath the **middle meatus** into the nasal cavity through the **nasofrontal ducts.**
- The sinus is not present at birth; development begins at about age 2 years and reaches adult size at about age 12 years.
- The sinus is not identifiable radiographically until about **age 8 years.**
- Two indications for treatment are cosmesis and obstruction of normal sinus drainage.

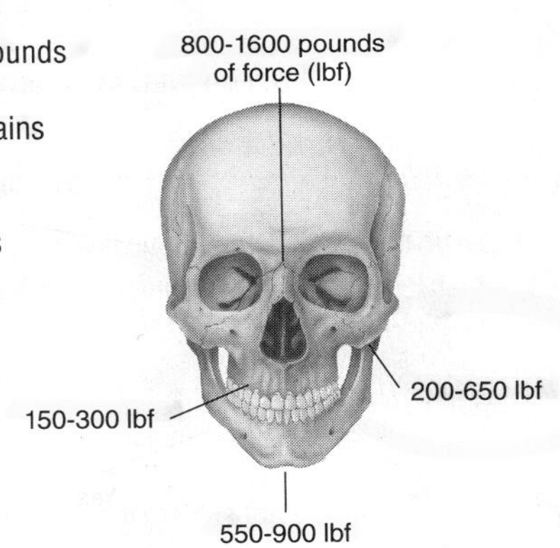


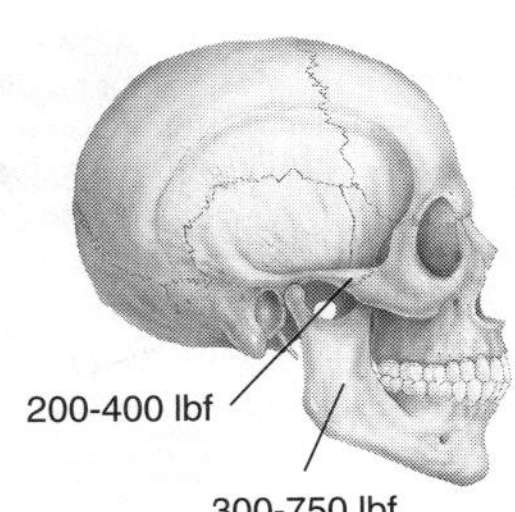


**Fig. 30-1** The forces (measured in pounds) necessary to fracture the frontal sinus are two to three times greater than those needed to fracture the zygoma, maxilla, or mandible.

### Clinical Presentation

- Upper face edema and ecchymosis
- Palpable deformity of frontal bone
- Laceration of forehead
- Paresthesias of supraorbital or supratrochlear nerves
- Cerebrospinal fluid (CSF) rhinorrhea
  - Occurs with dural laceration in region of cribriform plate or adjacent to posterior table fractures
  - Diagnostic laboratory confirmation with β-transferrin test
  - *Ring test* for bedside evaluation
- Globe displacement (forward and inferiorly)
  - May occur when orbital roof is involved

### Imaging

- **CT scans are required.**
- **Evaluate for:**
  - Involvement of anterior and or posterior tables
  - Degree of posterior table displacement or comminution
  - Pneumocephalus

- Level of injury relative to superior orbital rim
- Associated injuries

■ Direct evidence of ductal injury cannot be obtained from CT.

■ Only isolated anterior table fractures and transverse linear fractures through both tables, but above level of sinus floor, are assumed to have no associated duct injury.[15]

## MANAGEMENT

■ **Treatment is based on:**

- Contour deformity secondary to displacement of anterior table
- Presence of CSF leakage
- Likelihood of nasofrontal duct obstruction
- Degree of displacement or comminution of posterior table

■ Surgical access is provided through a coronal flap or existing lacerations.

■ The coronal flap should be elevated in the **subgaleal plane** to allow easy and atraumatic elevation of a pericranial flap, when needed.

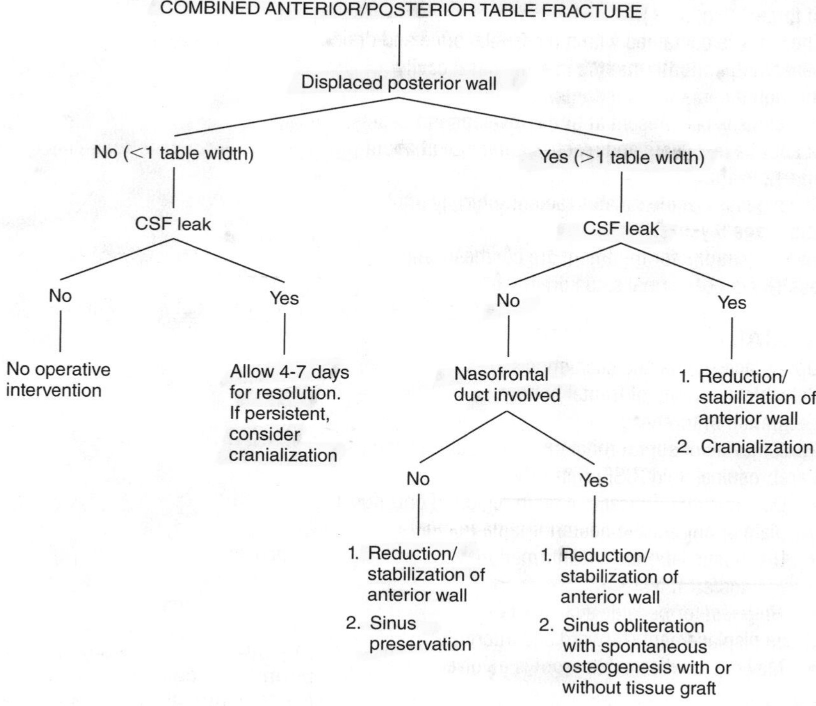


**Fig. 30-2** Management algorithm for combined anterior and posterior table fracture.

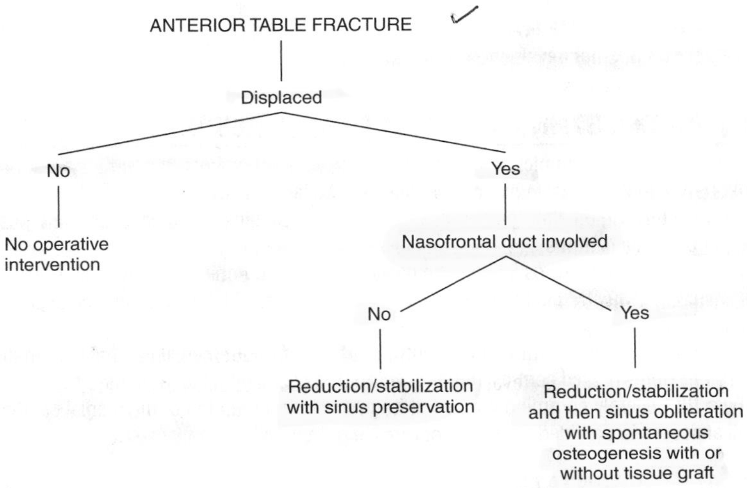


**Fig. 30-3** Management algorithm for anterior table fracture.

- **Open reduction with internal fixation (ORIF) of anterior table**
  - Reserved for isolated anterior table fractures without involvement of nasofrontal duct
  - Used when there is no associated CSF leakage
  - Fixation provided with low-profile miniplates
- **Sinus obliteration**
  - Indicated for fractures of anterior table combined with involvement of nasofrontal ducts
  - Used when posterior table displacement minimal and no CSF leakage
  - Sinus mucosa completely removed with rotary burrs, and obstructed ducts obliterated by grafts
  - Obliteration performed with fat grafts, pericranial flap, spontaneous osteogenesis, or bone grafts

**TIP:** Methylene blue can be placed in the sinus before burring to ensure complete removal of the mucosa.

**TIP:** It is not advisable to obliterate the sinus with bone cement because of complications from infection.

- **Cranialization**
  - Indicated for fractures of anterior table combined with involvement of **CSF leakage, significant displacement, or comminution of posterior table**
  - Procedure performed in conjunction with neurosurgery
  - Posterior table removed, remaining mucosa removed, ducts obliterated, nasal cavity isolated from cranial cavity by interposition of pericranial flap along floor of anterior cranial fossa
  - Anterior table reconstructed as for posterior table
  - Algorithm for management presented in Figs. 30-2 and 30-3.[16]

### Pediatric Considerations

- None; frontal sinus not developed in children

## NASOORBITAL ETHMOID (NOE) FRACTURES

- Fractures of the NOE complex represent the most problematic fractures to repair and probably result in the most noticeable postinjury change in facial appearance.
- Fractures in this region alter the soft tissue–bony relationships of the nasal dorsum, nasoorbital valley, and medial canthus.
- By definition, these fractures involve the nasal and ethmoid bones of the medial orbit.
- **Markowitz classification** is based on the central fragment, which bears the medial canthal tendon[17,18] (Fig. 30-4).
  - **Type I:** A single, noncomminuted, central fragment without medial canthal tendon disruption
  - **Type II:** Comminuted central fragment without medial canthal tendon disruption
  - **Type III:** Severely comminuted central fragment with disruption of the medial canthal tendon
- Surgical access is provided through a coronal approach or existing lacerations.

### Clinical Presentation

- Telecanthus: Sometimes **not** present in monobloc type I fracture
- Loss of dorsal nasal projection
- Periorbital edema or ecchymosis
- Step-offs at orbital rims
- Subconjunctival hemorrhage

### Imaging

- CT is diagnostic.
- Axial and coronal images are required for complete evaluation, and three-dimensional CT can be very helpful.
- Assess for comminution in region of medial canthi, degree of orbital involvement, degree of posterior nasal displacement, and possible frontal sinus involvement.

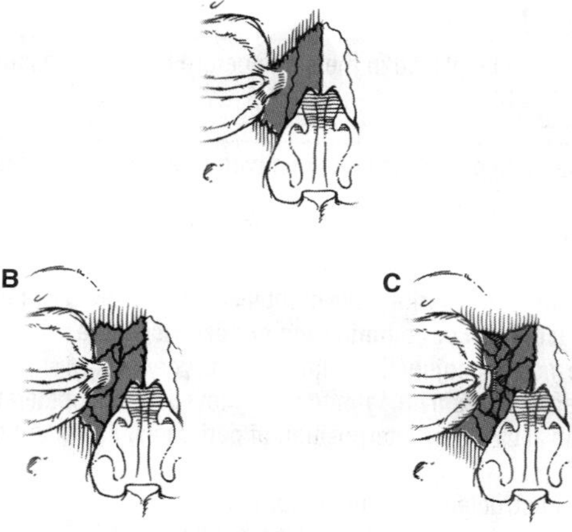


**Fig. 30-4** Classification of NOE fractures. **A,** Type I, **B,** type II, **C,** type III.

### TREATMENT

Treatment is directed at reconstituting the intercanthal relationship, nasal projection, and internal orbital structures.[17,19]

- Wide exposure is provided through coronal flap.
- Bony structures are reduced and stabilized with low-profile miniplates.
- Cranial bone grafts are harvested to reconstruct nasal projection.
- Canthal tendons are reconstructed with transnasal wiring.
- Minimal hardware should be placed in nasoorbital valley to reduce bulk.
- Soft tissues of nasoorbital valley should be redraped with bolsters or thermoplastic nasal splints; if this is not done, the region thickens, creating an uncorrectable deformity.

### PEDIATRIC CONSIDERATIONS

- Nasal reconstruction is aimed at reduction and stabilization.
- Dorsal nasal bone grafts should be reserved for severe injuries and older children.
- **Resorbable fixation systems** are used when feasible.
- The septum is a major growth center of the face, and parents should be counseled about potential growth disturbances.

## NASAL FRACTURES

- Nasal fractures are t**he most common fractures of facial bones.**
- They often occur in isolation or as part of a complex fracture pattern.

**TIP:** During examination, determine whether an NOE component is present.

- Posttraumatic deformity of the nose is common after treatment and reported in up to 50% of patients.
  - Can be minimized by accurate diagnosis and reduction during a thorough external and internal nasal examination
- Septal fractures frequently are undiagnosed and untreated, resulting in late deformity.

**CAUTION: It is essential to identify septal hematomas and provide timely drainage to prevent late destruction of the septum.**

### CLINICAL PRESENTATION

- Nasal deformity
- Nasal edema
- Laceration
- Epistaxis
- Crepitus
- Tenderness
- Septal deviation
- Septal hematoma

### IMAGING

- Nasal fractures usually can be diagnosed clinically at the initial setting or once edema resolves.
- CT for isolated injuries is unnecessary and is a poor use of resources.
- Standard radiographs are of limited value.

## TREATMENT[16] (Figs. 30-5 through 30-7)

- Anatomic reduction of nasal bones and septum is needed to prevent late deformity.
- Algorithm for management is presented in Fig. 30-5.[20]

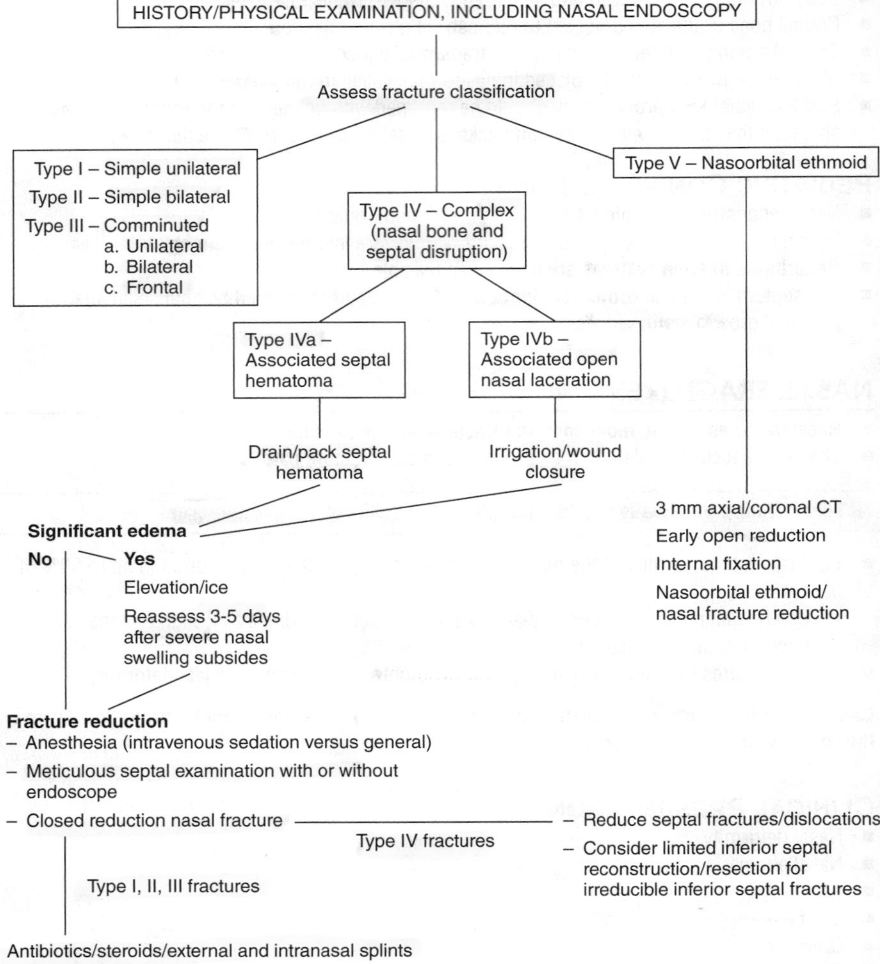


**Fig. 30-5** Nasal fracture algorithm delineating trauma classification and respective treatments.

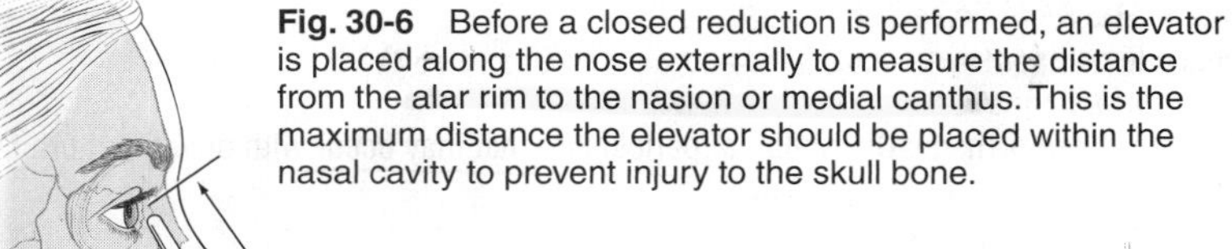

**Fig. 30-6** Before a closed reduction is performed, an elevator is placed along the nose externally to measure the distance from the alar rim to the nasion or medial canthus. This is the maximum distance the elevator should be placed within the nasal cavity to prevent injury to the skull bone.

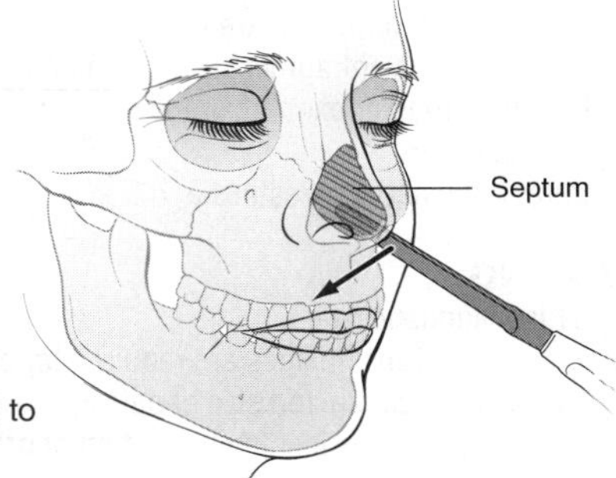


**Fig. 30-7** A Goldman elevator is used to reposition the septum in the midline.

## ORBITAL FRACTURES[21] (Fig. 30-8)

- Fractures of the bony orbit may occur alone or as part of complex facial fractures.
- The bony orbit consists of **seven** individual bones that vary significantly in thickness.
- The thinnest region is along the medial wall (*lamina papyracea* of the ethmoid bone).
- Isolated fractures may occur (without associated fracture of orbital rim) of the floor and medial wall.
  - These are postulated to occur either from increased pressure that develops within the orbit (from posterior displacement of orbital tissues) or when deformation of the orbital bones occurs from a blow, resulting in fractures of thin portions of the floor without fracture of the orbital rim.[21]
- Without treatment, **dystopia** (vertical globe malposition) or **enophthalmos** (posterior malposition) occurs.
  - **Dystopia** results from the loss of bony support maintaining globe position.
  - **Enophthalmos** results from two factors.
    1. Fractures of the orbit increase intraorbital volume and disrupt the fine ligamentous system within the periorbita.
    2. When healing occurs, periorbital soft tissue assumes a spherical shape that has a smaller volume than its previous conical shape.

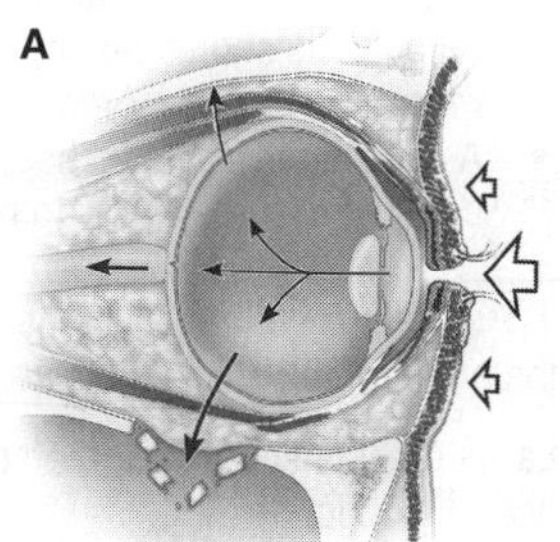


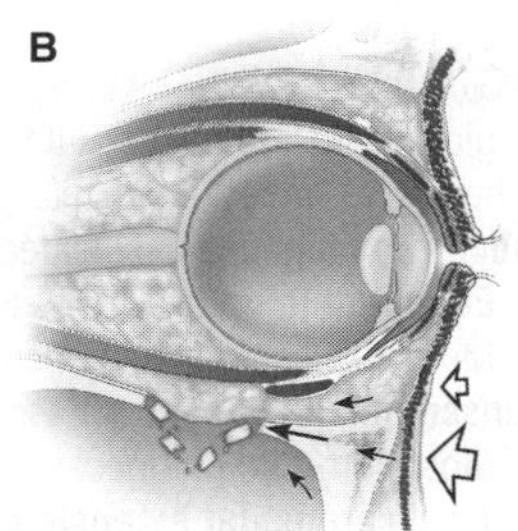


**Fig. 30-8** Mechanism of injury from orbital blowout fractures. **A,** Hydraulic theory. **B,** Bone conduction theory.

**TIP:** In other words, a smaller volume in a larger orbit results in enophthalmos.

## Clinical Presentation

- Periorbital edema or ecchymosis
- Step-offs at orbital rims
- Subconjunctival hemorrhage: Disruption of periosteum that may occur with or without orbital fracture
- Limited eye excursions
  - True entrapment is rare in adults and usually is a result of edema.
  - In children entrapment of recti must be treated promptly or ruled out.
- Enophthalmos or exophthalmos
- Diplopia
- Infraorbital nerve paresthesia

## Imaging

- CT is diagnostic.
- Axial and coronal images are required for complete evaluation.
- Assess for location and size of defect.
- Soft tissue images identify herniation of orbital contents and possible entrapment.

## Treatment

- The goal of treatment is to restore orbital contours and volume.
- A decision to operate should be based on size of defect and presence of enophthalmos or diplopia.
  - All patients should be observed during the 2 weeks after injury to assess development or resolution of symptoms (enophthalmos or diplopia) as edema resolves.
  - A decision to operate should be made during this interval, because cicatricial healing will compromise the ability to restore premorbid orbital position later.

**TIP:** In general, defects smaller than 1 cm do not require operative treatment unless enophthalmos or diplopia persists at 2 weeks.

Large defects should be treated regardless of symptoms, because enophthalmos is likely to occur[18,22] (Fig. 30-9).

## Surgical Approaches

- Surgical access to the orbital floor is provided through subtarsal, transconjunctival (with or without canthotomy), subciliary, or transcaruncular incisions.
- **Subciliary incisions** associated with highest incidence of complications[23]
  - **Ectropion in up to 14% of cases**
  - Most successfully managed with conservative therapy
- **Transconjuctival approach** associated with lowest complication rate (4.4%).
  - Most common complication is entropion in up to 1.5%.
  - **Transcaruncular extension** of the transconjunctival approach allows access to the medial wall; above the level of the canthus.
- **Subtarsal incisions** allow direct access to orbital floor while theoretically preserving innervation of the pretarsal orbicularis oculi.
  - Complication rate of up to 9.7%
  - Hypertrophic or visible scarring rate of up to 3.4%
- A **coronal incision** is an alternative approach that allows wide access to the medial orbital wall.

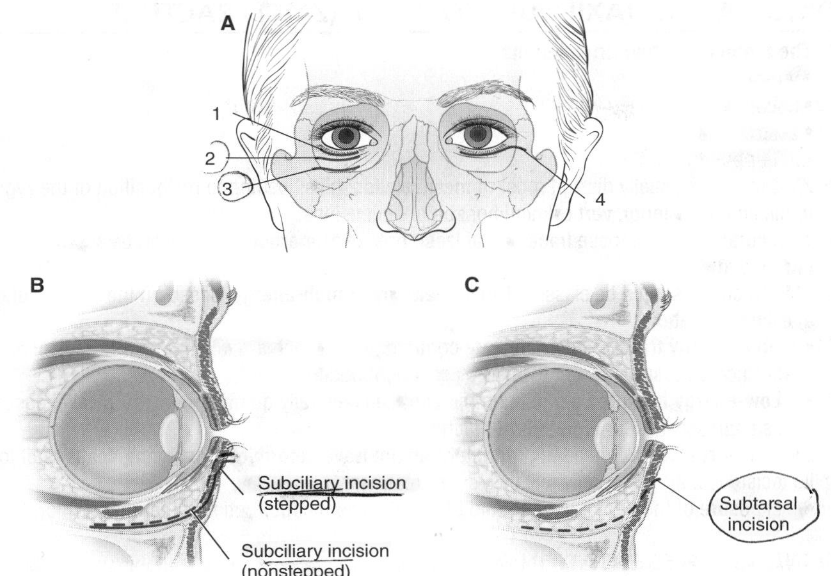


**Fig. 30-9** **A,** Transconjunctival approaches to the inferior orbit: *1,* subciliary, *2,* subtarsal, *3,* infraorbital, and *4,* extended subciliary. NOTE: The infraorbital approach is not recommended. **B,** Sagittal view of the level of the subciliary lower eyelid approach. **C,** Sagittal view of the level of the subtarsal lower eyelid approach.

## Implant Materials

- Many materials are available for reconstruction of the orbital walls.[24]
  - Resorbable implants are ideal for pediatric or small defects ($<$3 cm).
    - Autogenous bone
    - Poly-L-lactide
    - Poly-D-lactide
    - Trimethylene carbonate
    - Polyglycolide
  - Nonresorbable Implants
    - Titanium mesh
    - Polyethylene (Mylar)
    - Porous polyethylene (Medpor; Porex Surgical, Newnan, GA)
    - Nylon sheets (SupraFoil; S. Jackson, Inc., Alexandria, VA)
    - Composite titanium/porous polyethylene

## Pediatric Considerations

- Pediatric bone is more likely to deform and recoil after fracture and may result in **muscle entrapment.**
  - This represents a relatively emergent situation, because true entrapment leads to ischemia and necrosis of the muscle, with further movement dysfunction.
  - 62% of patients with true entrapment present with pain from eye movement or nausea and vomiting.
- **Use resorbable fixation systems when feasible.**

## ZYGOMATICOMAXILLARY COMPLEX (ZMC) FRACTURES

- **The zygoma has four articulations.**
  - Frontal
  - Maxillary
  - Sphenoid
  - Temporal
- ZMC fractures usually disrupt most of these relationships, leading to malposition of the zygoma in the anteroposterior, vertical, and horizontal dimensions.
- To accurately reduce these fractures, at least three of four articulations must be assessed intraoperatively.
- ZMC fractures should be classified as **low-energy** or **high-energy,** based on the comminution at each articulation.
  - **High-energy fractures** demonstrate comminution at each articulation; therefore they require surgical exposure of each to ensure accurate reduction.
  - **Low-energy fractures** are noncomminuted and generally do not require surgical exposure as aggressive as for high-energy fractures.
- ZMC fractures, when treated appropriately, do not leave deformities, and complications of lower lid incisions may be the only telltale sign of treatment.
  - Exposure of the orbital floor should be for planned reconstruction rather than exploration.[25]

### CLINICAL PRESENTATION

- Malar flattening
- Step-offs at orbital rims, zygomatic arch, ZM buttress
- Enophthalmos or dystopia
- Infraorbital paresthesia
- Trismus
- Downward-sloping palpebral fissure

### IMAGING

- CT is diagnostic.
- Axial and coronal images are required for complete evaluation.
- **Assess for:**
  - Degree of comminution (high- or low-energy)
  - Medial or lateral rotation of zygoma
  - Anteroposterior projection of zygoma
  - Position of lateral orbital wall
  - Need for reconstruction of orbital floor

### TREATMENT

Treatment usually requires open reduction and stabilization with internal fixation. Occasionally, minimally displaced injuries may be stable after initial reduction and do not need fixation.

- **Low-energy injuries**[26]
  - These injuries are usually exposed intraorally at the ZM buttress and using an upper blepharoplasty incision.
  - The upper lid incision allows visualization of the zygomaticofrontal (ZF) and zygomatic-osphenoid (ZS) articulations.
  - **The ZS articulation is the most important to assess for reduction.**

**TIP:** A Carroll-Girard screw can provide three-dimensional control of the segment for reduction.

- Initial stabilization of the ZF with a malleable miniplate sets the vertical height and allows continued manipulation of the segment in anteroposterior and horizontal dimensions.
- Perform ZM articulation fixation.
- Additional fixation may be placed along the ZS articulation.
- Lower lid incisions and exposure of the floor are not needed to assess reduction with exposure of ZF, ZM, and ZS articulations and should be reserved for reconstruction of the floor, when indicated.

- **High-energy injuries**
  - Require wide exposure through coronal flap to include exposure of the temporal articulation
  - More frequently require reconstruction of the orbital floor
  - After wide exposure, resuspension of malar soft tissues critical to prevent malar ptosis and soft tissue deformity
- An algorithm for management is shown in Fig. 30-10.[26]

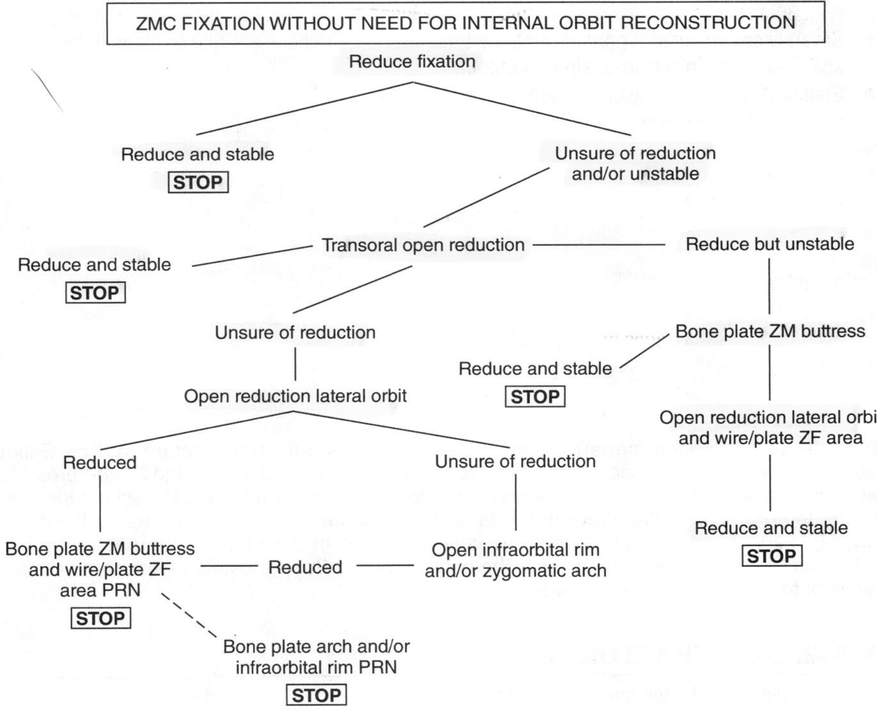


**Fig. 30-10** Treatment algorithm for ZMC fractures.

## Pediatric Considerations

**CAUTION: Permanent dentition development is at risk when fixation screws are placed at the ZM buttress.**

- **Resorbable fixation systems are used when feasible.**

# ZYGOMATIC ARCH FRACTURES

Fractures of the zygomatic arch are almost a purely aesthetic concern, except in rare instances when the fracture segment impedes mandibular excursion by interfering with the coronoid process.

## Clinical Presentation

- Palpable deformity
- Contour deformity
- Trismus

## Treatment

- Uncomplicated fractures can be elevated using **Gillies approach** through a temporal incision[18] (Fig. 30-11).
- Severely comminuted zygomatic arch fractures may require bone grafting or mandibular adaption plates to restore aesthetic contour.[27]
- Stabilization is generally unnecessary.

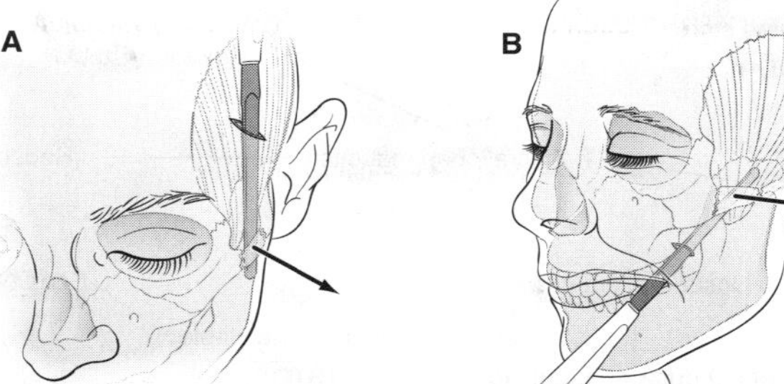


**Fig. 30-11** Reduction maneuvers for an isolated zygomatic arch fracture. **A,** The Gillies approach involves a 2 cm incision placed 2 fingerbreadths above the helix and 2 fingerbreadths anterior. A blunt elevator is placed beneath the deep layer of deep temporal fascia, superficial to the temporalis muscle allowing the tip of the elevator to pass behind the arch without risking injury to the frontal branch of the facial nerve. **B,** In the intraoral approach (Keen), a 1 to 2 cm incision is made laterally in the buccal sulcus. Subperiosteal elevation allows the elevator to be placed behind the arch.

# MAXILLARY FRACTURES

- The maxilla constitutes most of the midface skeleton.
- It contains the maxillary sinus and dentition.
- **Three major buttresses provide strength** (Fig. 30-12).
  1. Nasomaxillary
  2. Zygomatic
  3. Pterygomaxillary

**TIP:** These regions also provide the best quality bone for using rigid fixation.

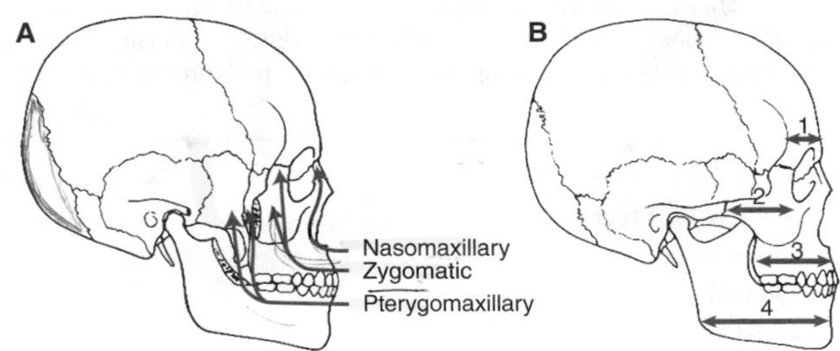


**Fig. 30-12** **A,** Facial buttresses responsible for vertical support: Nasomaxillary, zygomatic, and pterygomaxillary. **B,** Anteroposterior buttresses: *1,* frontal, *2,* zygomatic, *3,* maxillary, and *4,* mandibular.

## Classification

- **Dentoalveolar**
  - Involves teeth and supporting osseous structure
- **LeFort I** (Fig. 30-13, *A*)
  - Separates tooth-bearing maxilla from midface
  - Extends from piriform aperture posteriorly through the nasal septum, lateral nasal walls, anterior maxillary wall, through the maxillary tuberosity or pterygoid plates
  - Upper jaw clinically mobile
- **LeFort II** (Fig. 30-13, *B*)
  - Pyramidal fracture
  - Extends through frontonasal junction along medial orbital wall, usually passing through inferior orbital rim at the ZM suture; continues posteriorly through tuberosity or pterygoid plates
  - Upper jaw and nasal bones clinically mobile as solitary unit
- **LeFort III** (Fig. 30-13, *C*)
  - Craniofacial disjunction
  - Extends through frontonasal junction along medial orbital wall and inferior orbital fissure and out lateral orbital wall

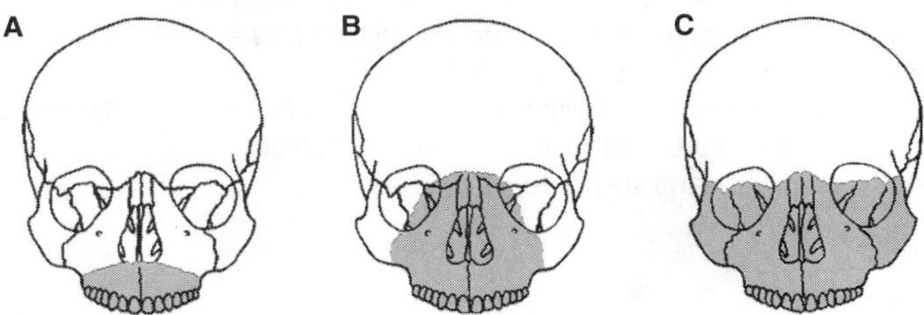


**Fig. 30-13** LeFort midfacial fractures. **A,** LeFort I fracture separating the inferior portion of the maxilla in horizontal fashion, extending from the piriform aperture of the nose to the pterygoid maxillary suture area. **B,** LeFort II fracture involving separation of the maxilla and nasal complex from the cranial base, zygomatic orbital rim area, and pterygoid maxillary suture area. **C,** LeFort III fracture (i.e., craniofacial separation) is complete separation of the midface at the level of the NOE complex and ZF suture area. It extends through the orbits bilaterally.

- Fractures through pterygoid plates at high level
- Clinically, simultaneous mobility at maxilla and nasofrontal and ZF regions

**TIP:** This system provides a good description of injury. However, these injuries usually result in multiple fracture patterns and rarely occur in isolation, making the system clinically less useful.

## Clinical Presentation

- Facial edema
- Periorbital ecchymosis
- Epistaxis
- Malocclusion: Anterior open bite secondary to posteroinferior displacement of maxilla
- Tenderness during palpation at buttresses
- Crepitus
- Mobility of maxilla
- Palpable step-offs

## Imaging

- CT is diagnostic.
- Axial and coronal images are required for complete evaluation.
- **Assess:**
  - Degree of comminution
  - Presence of sagittal fracture component
  - Fracture through pterygoid plates
  - Level(s) of injury

## Treatment

- Treatment for isolated maxillary fractures is directed at **restoring normal premorbid occlusion.**
- Patients with dentoalveolar fractures require stabilization of the dentoalveolar segment with an arch bar for 4-6 weeks.
- During the ensuing weeks, referral to a dentist is appropriate for endodontic evaluation of avulsed teeth in the segment.
- Patients with LeFort-type fractures require open reduction and rigid fixation.
- Closed reduction and maxillomandibular fixation (MMF) are **not** appropriate, because they lead to facial lengthening by downward forces transmitted by the mandible.
- Arch bars should be applied to both dental arches and the fractures exposed using a maxillary circumvestibular incision from first molar to first molar.
- The maxillary segment is mobilized with Rowe disimpaction forceps or similar instruments.
- Once adequate mobility is present to allow passive reduction of the fracture, the segment is manually reduced and the jaws are placed into MMF.

> **TIP:** Placing the jaws into MMF without providing passive reduction of the maxillary segment unseats mandibular condyles from their fossa and results in malocclusion when MMF is released and condyles return to their natural position.

- Occasionally there is a nonreducible maxillary fracture (i.e., unable to obtain premorbid occlusion).
  - This may require a LeFort I level osteotomy to correct the deformity at the time of fracture repair.
  - Fixation of fractures is provided by 1.5-2.0 mm miniplates on stable bone, usually at the region of the piriform (nasomaxillary buttress) or ZM buttress.

### Pediatric Considerations

- Treatment considerations are the same as for adults but may be technically more difficult.
  - Arch bars are difficult to place in pediatric patients because of mixed dentition, missing teeth, and unfavorable dental anatomy of the primary teeth.
  - Difficulty in placing fixation systems is encountered because of developing tooth buds.
- Panoramic radiographs should be obtained to locate developing permanent dentition.

## PANFACIAL FRACTURES

Panfacial fractures are fractures of the upper and midfacial skeleton associated with fractures of the mandible (see Chapter 31). This represents a particularly difficult clinical situation, because there is no stable reference from which to begin reduction of fractures.

> **TIP:** In general, treatment should proceed systematically from top to bottom, bottom to top, and back to front.

- Anatomic reconstruction of the mandible should be performed initially to provide a stable base from which to reconstruct the midface.
  - If bilateral condyle fractures are present, at least one intact condyle should be reconstructed to provide appropriate vertical height relationships for the midface.
- Anteroposterior reconstruction of the zygomas should be reestablished to provide accurate facial projection.
- Reconstruction then proceeds inferiorly from the stable frontal process to the level of the maxilla.
- Fixation across the LeFort I level is the last area to be stabilized.
- Because of the severity of these injuries, some degree of malreduction inevitably will occur.
- By reestablishing the major determinants of facial form early (mandibular base, vertical height, anteroposterior projection), subtle malreductions may be tolerated at the LeFort I level above the dentition[18] (Fig. 30-14).

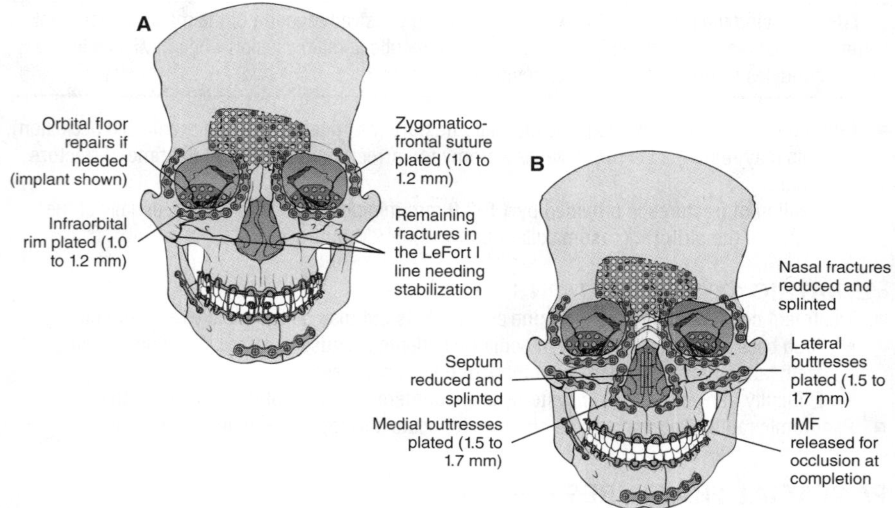


**Fig. 30-14 A,** The final facial width is set by plating across the infraorbital rims, which moves the malar eminences centrally. The orbital rims are now stabilized circumferentially. The orbital floors and walls can be repaired with bone grafts or alloplastic implants. The ZF pivot wires can be exchanged for low-profile titanium plates if desired. **B,** The frontal and upper midface are completed, and the two lower subunits are joined with intermaxillary fixation (IMF). All that remains is plating along the LeFort I line to finalize fixation. The condyles are seated, and the lower units are rotated up to reduce at the LeFort I line. The medial and lateral buttresses are plated. The IMF is released, occlusion is checked, and wire or elastic IMF is reapplied. Nasal and septal fractures are reduced and splinted.

## ASSOCIATED CONDITIONS

### TEMPORAL BONE TRAUMA

- **Signs**
  - Otorrhea
  - Facial palsy
  - Hemotympanum
  - **Battle's sign:** Bruising over mastoid process that appears 24-48 hours after injury
- **Fracture patterns**
  - Longitudinal
    - Accounts for 80%-90% of temporal bone fractures
    - Bilateral in 8%-29% of patients
    - Facial nerve injury in 20% of patients
    - Hearing loss in 67% of patients
  - Transverse
    - Facial nerve injury in 40% of patients
    - Hearing loss in 100% of patients
- **Complications**
  - Facial nerve paresis
    - Paresis occurs in 10%-50% of temporal bone fractures, most commonly with transverse type.

- **Management**
  - Surgery is not indicated for incomplete palsy.
  - Immediate paresis does not usually resolve and is an indication for exploration.
  - Delayed paresis generally has a good prognosis, and exploration is indicated when electrical evidence indicates nerve degeneration.
- Hearing loss
  - Tos[28] studied 248 temporal bone fractures.
    - 26 (10%) were transverse, with 100% having total hearing loss.
    - 222 (90%) were longitudinal, with 67% having hearing loss.
    - Patients with sensorineural hearing loss did not improve.
    - Patients with conductive hearing loss (CHL) eventually improved, except when ossicular chain disruption was present.
  - **CHL present for longer than 2 months suggests ossicular chain disruption and requires exploration.**
- Vestibular dysfunction
  - Nystagmus suggests vestibular injury.
  - Peripheral vestibular nystagmus occurs with vertigo.
  - Spontaneous nystagmus in head-neutral position is pathologic.
  - **Fast component beats away from injured ear.**
  - Finding horizontal nystagmus that is greater with eyes closed suggests peripheral injury.
  - Management is supportive; prognosis is generally good, with most recovering in 6 months.
- CSF leakage
  - CSF otorrhea occurs in 25% of temporal bone fractures.
  - Onset generally occurs within 24 hours.
  - Most close spontaneously in 24 hours.

## Ophthalmic Consequences

- Ocular injuries are reported to be as high as 30% after orbital trauma.[2]
- **Only two ocular emergencies require treatment within minutes.**
  1. Chemical burns
  2. Central retinal artery occlusion
- **Anterior segment trauma**
  - Corneal abrasion
    - Cornea reepithelializes in 1 day under a patch.
    - Use of steroids or topical anesthetic is contraindicated.
  - Iridodialysis: Avulsion from the iris root
  - Traumatic mydriasis
    - Pupillary sphincter rupture produces a widely, permanently dilated pupil.
    - The pupil does not react to direct or consensual stimuli.
  - Hyphema
    - Blood in the anterior chamber is most readily visible with a handheld light.
    - Document visual acuity and height of hyphema.
    - 3%-30% of patients will rebleed in 3-5 days, making prognosis worse.
    - Complications include corneal pigment staining, anterior synechia, and glaucoma.
    - Management focuses on prevention of rebleed: Elevate head of bed, encourage bed rest, and give atropine drops to decrease iris movement.
- **Posterior segment trauma**
  - Vitreous hemorrhage: Vision returns with resolution.
  - Scleral rupture
    - 18% associated with orbital fracture

  - Repair indicated to prevent hypotonia or fibrous ingrowth
  - Retinal detachment
  - Optic nerve avulsion

- **Sympathetic ophthalmia**
  - Bilateral granulomatous inflammation of uvea that usually occurs as complication of penetrating trauma or intraocular surgery
  - Pathogenesis unknown but thought that privileged intraocular antigens, exposed to regional lymph nodes after injury, stimulate cell-mediated response against eye
  - Exact incidence unknown, but estimated at 0.19% with trauma
  - Nontraumatized eye inflamed within 1 year of injury: 65% within 2 months; 80% within 3 months
  - Prevention: Enucleation of severely traumatized, sightless eye within 2 weeks of injury
  - Treatment difficult: If inflammation in sympathizing eye, outcome generally not improved by enucleation of traumatized eye

- **Traumatic optic neuropathy (TON)**

*TON is a traumatic loss of vision without external or initial ophthalmoscopic evidence of injury to the eye or its nerve.*

  - Etiologic factors
    - Direct injury to globe
    - Retinal vascular occlusion
    - Orbital compartment syndrome
    - Injury to proximal neural structures
  - TON may occur without any fracture because of deceleration forces acting within the fixed intracanalicular portion of optic nerve.
  - The only objective finding is the presence of a relative afferent pupillary defect.
  - Optic atrophy will appear weeks later.
  - Improvement in visual acuity may occur in 30%-50% of patients.
  - Treatment includes:
    - Observation
    - High-dose steroids
      - Use of steroids has been extrapolated from the Second National Acute Spinal Cord Injury Study,[29] in which patients with spinal injury treated early with high-dose steroids demonstrated increased neurologic function at 6 weeks.
    - Surgical decompression
    - In 2003 prospective study showed improvement with combined therapy protocol of corticosteroids and surgical decompression.[30]

- **Superior orbital fissure syndrome (SOFS)**
  - Incidence is about 1 out of 130 patients with LeFort II, III, or zygomaticoorbital fractures.
  - Diagnosis is by clinical presentation.
  - Components
    - Oculomotor nerve
      - Trochlear nerve
      - Abducens nerve
      - Trigeminal nerve (lacrimal, frontal, nasociliary branches)
      - Ophthalmic vein
    - **Signs**
      - Ipsilateral ptosis of upper lid
      - Proptosis
      - Ophthalmoplegia

- Anesthesia in distribution of $V_1$
- Dilation and fixation of ipsilateral pupil

▸ **Treatment**

- Operative reduction of fractures results in improvement or resolution.
- Recovery time is reported as 4.8-23 weeks.[31]
- Role of steroids is unclear.

■ **Orbital apex syndrome**

- Syndrome presents **similarly to SOFS,** but also with **loss of vision** because of optic nerve involvement at the orbital apex.

■ **Traumatic carotid–cavernous sinus fistula**

- Fracture results in laceration or tear in arterial wall, allowing blood to shunt from the internal carotid artery to the cavernous sinus. Signs and symptoms may develop several days after the initial injury.
- Signs
  - Proptosis
  - Ocular bruit
  - Marked injection and chemosis of affected eye
  - Ophthalmoplegia of CNs III, IV, or VI
  - Dilated ophthalmic vein on CT of orbit
- Diagnosis is provided by angiography.
- **Prognosis is generally good** and not life threatening.
  - Fistula may close spontaneously, commonly after angiography.
  - Ischemic events may occur secondary to steal phenomena or embolism.
- Treatment includes surgical ligation of carotid artery or interventional placement of coils to obliterate the fistula.

## Key Points

✓ Many patients presenting to the ER have been there before; remember to identify preexisting conditions.

✓ Before examination, patients should be cleaned of all dried blood and dirt that may obscure underlying injuries.

✓ Reconstructed coronal imaging should be accepted only when formal coronal CT scans are precluded by cerebrospinal injury.

## References


1. American College of Surgeons. National Trauma Data Bank Annual Reprot 2012. Available at *http://www.facs.org/trauma/ntdb/pdf/ntdb-annual-report-2012.pdf.*
2. Girotto JA, MacKenzie E, Fowler C, et al. Long-term physical impairment and functional outcomes after complex facial fractures. Plast Reconstr Surg 108:312-327, 2001.
3. Hale RG, Hayes DK, Orloff G, et al. Maxillofacial and neck trauma. In Savitsky E, Eastridge B, eds. Combat Casualty Care: Lessons Learned from OEF and OIF. Falls Church, VA: Borden Institute, 2012.
4. Kittle CP, Verrett AJ, Wu J, et al. Characterization of midface fractures incurred in recent wars. J Craniofac Surg 23:1587-1591, 2012.
5. Follmar KE, DeBruijn M, Baccarani A, et al. Concomitant injuries in patients with panfacial fractures. J Trauma 63:831-835, 2007.
6. Hackl W, Fink C, Hausberger K, et al. The incidence of combined facial and cervical spine injuries. Trauma 50:41-45, 2001.
7. Marik PE, Varon J, Trask T. Management of head trauma. Chest 122:1-21, 2002.

8. Plaisier BR, Punjabi AP, Super DM, et al. The relationship between facial fractures and death from neurologic injury. J Oral Maxillofac Surg 58:708-712, 2000.
9. Cheung DS, Kharasch M. Evaluation of the patient with closed head trauma: an evidence based approach. Emerg Med Clin North Am 17:9-23, 1999.
10. Haug RH, Savage JD Likavek MJ, et al. A review of 100 closed head injuries associated with facial fractures. J Oral Maxillofac Surg 50:218-222, 1992.
11. Winegar BA, Murillo H, Tantiwongkosi B. Spectrum of critical imaging findings in complex facial skeletal trauma. Radiographics 33:3-19, 2013.
12. Jarrahy R, Vo V, Goenjian HA, et al. Diagnostic accuracy of maxillofacial trauma two-dimensional and three-dimensional computed tomographic scans. Plast Reconstr Surg 127:2432-2440, 2011.
13. Giannoudis PV, Veysi VT, Pape HC, et al. When should we operate on major fractures in patients with severe head injuries? Am J Surg 183:261-267, 2002.
14. Nahum AM. The biomechanics of maxillofacial trauma. Clin Plast Surg 2:59-64, 1975.
15. Stanley RB, Becker TS. Injuries of the nasofrontal orifices in frontal sinus fractures. Laryngoscope 97:728-731, 1987.
16. Rohrich RJ, Hollier LH. Management of frontal sinus fractures: changing concepts. Clin Plast Surg 19:219-232, 1992.
17. Markowitz BL, Manson PN, Sargent L, et al. Management of the medial canthal tendon in nasoethmoid orbital fractures: the importance of the central fragment in classification and treatment. Plast Reconstr Surg 87:843-853, 1991.
18. Marcus JR, Erdmann D, Rodriguez ED, eds. Essentials of Craniomaxillofacial Trauma. St Louis: Quality Medical Publishing, 2012.
19. Ellis E III. Sequencing treatment for naso-orbito-ethmoid fractures. J Oral Maxillofac Surg 51:543-558, 1993.
20. Rohrich RJ, Adams WP. Nasal fracture management: minimizing secondary nasal deformities. Plast Reconstr Surg 106:266-273, 2000.
21. Waterhouse N, Lyne J, Urdang M, et al. An investigation into the mechanism of orbital blowout fractures. Br J Plast Surg 52:607-612, 1999.
22. AO North America. Review of surgical approaches to the cranial skeleton, 2010. Available at *www.aona.org*.
23. Ridgway EB, Chen C, Colakoglu, et al. The incidence of lower eyelid malposition after facial fracture repair: a retrospective study and meta-analysis comparing subtarsal, subciliary, and transconjunctival incisions. Plast Reconstr Surg 124:1578-1586, 2009.
24. Potter JK, Ellis E III. Biomaterials for reconstruction of the internal orbit. J Oral Maxillofac Surg 62:1280-1297, 2004.
25. Ellis E III, Reddy L. Status of internal orbit after reduction of zygomaticomaxillary fractures. J Oral Maxillofac Surg 62:275-283, 2004.
26. Ellis E III, Kittidumkerng W. Analysis of treatment for isolated zygomaticomaxillary complex fractures. J Oral Maxillofac Surg 54:386-400, 1996.
27. Buck DW Jr, Heyer K, Lewis VL Jr. Reconstruction of the zygomatic arch using a mandibular adaption plate. J Craniofac Surg 20:1193-1196, 2009.
28. Tos M. [Practura ossi temporalis. The course and sequelae of 248 fractures of the temporal bones] Ugeskr Laeger 133:1449-1456, 1971.
29. Bracken MB, Shepard MJ, Collins WF, et al. A randomized, controlled trial of methylprednisolone or naloxone in the treatment of acute spinal-cord injury: results of the Second National Acute Spinal Cord Injury Study. N Engl J Med 322:1405-1411, 1990.
30. Rajiniganth MG, Gupta AK, Gupta A, et al. Traumatic optic neuropathy: visual outcome following combined therapy protocol. Arch Otolaryngol Head Neck Surg 129:1203-1206, 2003.
31. Levin LA, Beck RW, Joseph MP, et al. The treatment of traumatic optic neuropathy. The International Optic Nerve Trauma Study. Opthalmology 106:1268-1277, 1999.

# 31. Mandibular Fractures

**Jason K. Potter, Lance A. Read**

## ETIOLOGIC FACTORS

### Two Most Common Causes

- Assault
- Motor vehicle collisions (MVCs)

### Other Causes

- Gunshot wounds
- Falls
- Sports injuries

## LOCATION OF FRACTURE

Mandibular fractures are usually described by **location,** which affects the appropriate treatment.

- **Dentoalveolar:** A fracture without disruption of the underlying osseous structures of the mandible and only involving the tooth-bearing area
- **Condyle:** Any fracture that affects the condylar process of mandible; further classified as intracapsular, extracapsular, or neck
- **Coronoid:** Any fracture that affects the coronoid process
- **Ramus:** Region superior to the gonial angle up to the sigmoid notch
- **Angle:** Region of the gonial angle, extending to the region of the third molar
- **Body:** Any fracture that extends from the alveolar process through the inferior border and occurs in the region between the mental foramen and the distal aspect of the second molar
- **Parasymphysis:** Any fracture that extends from the alveolar process to the inferior border that occurs between the mental foramen and the distal aspect of the lateral incisor
- **Symphysis:** Any fracture that runs from the alveolar process to the inferior border of the mandible and occurs in the region of the incisors in a vertical or near-vertical direction[1]

## INCIDENCE BY LOCATION[2] (Fig. 31-1)

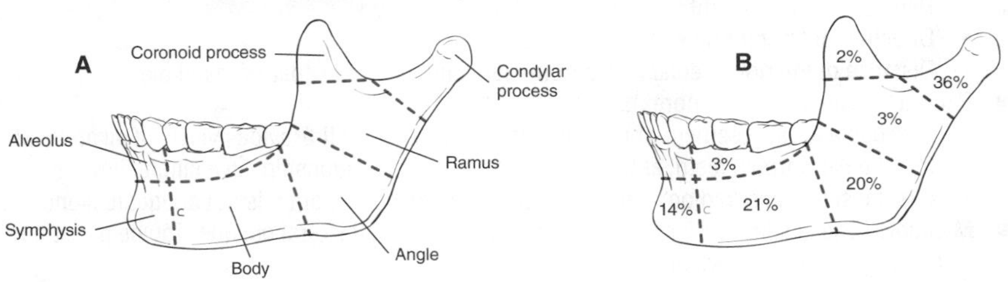


**Fig. 31-1** **A,** Anatomic regions of the mandible. **B,** Frequency of fractures in those regions.

- **Ranking:** Angle > symphysis > body > condyle > coronoid > ramus
- **Assault** most commonly results in **angle** fractures.
- **MVCs** most commonly result in **body** fractures.
- 50% of mandibular fracture cases involve multiple sites.

## PATIENT EVALUATION

Any patient who presents with facial trauma requires a *complete* head and neck trauma evaluation (see Chapters 30 and 31).

### PHYSICAL EXAMINATION

- Inspect occlusion.
  - Evaluate for presence of anterior or posterior open bite in centric occlusion.
  - Evaluate for deviation of mandible upon opening.
- Perform bimanual examination of the mandible to assess mobility and tenderness.
- Palpate condyles, both preauricularly and with finger in external auditory canal, during excursion to elicit tenderness and assess translation.
- Evaluate the lingual and buccal aspects for evidence of trauma.
- All teeth should be accounted for and assessed for mobility.[3]
- Document the presence of mental nerve paresthesias.

**TIP:** Tongue blades should be used to retract the tongue and cheeks for complete inspection.

**TIP:** Ecchymosis in the floor of the mouth is pathognomonic for mandibular fractures.

**TIP:** Deviation of the chin may suggest condyle fracture.

**TIP:** Mental nerve paresthesia suggests fracture along the interosseous component of the inferior alveolar nerve.

### RADIOGRAPHIC EVALUATION[4]

- Obtain two views of each region of the mandible and inspect for the following:
  - Evidence of fractured mandible
  - Fractured teeth
  - Presence of teeth in the line of fracture
  - Degree of displacement
  - Direction of fracture (linear versus oblique)
  - Distance of inferior alveolar nerve from teeth and inferior border of mandible
- Panoramic radiograph (Panorex):
  - Invaluable for assessment of mandibular trauma because it provides views of all areas of mandibular corpus, teeth, and inferior alveolar nerve relationships in a single film
  - It is the single best radiograph for screening the mandible, but it is not adequate alone.
- Mandible series includes PA skull, lateral skull, right and left lateral oblique, Towne projection, and submentovertex views.
- CT images are superior to plain films for mandibular fractures in the acute care setting.

> **TIP:** Occasionally, because of the presence of cervical collars, adequate plain films are not possible and CT images are necessary.

## GENERAL MANAGEMENT

### ABCs

- Initial management always begins with Advanced Trauma Life Support (ATLS) protocols.[5]
- Treatment of mandibular fractures may be delayed up to 2 weeks, with appropriate oral and systemic antibiotic prophylaxis for critically injured patients.

### ANTIBIOTICS

- **All patients with mandibular fractures should receive penicillin-based antibiotics (clindamycin if allergic to penicillin) prophylactically, from presentation to fracture reduction.**
  - This practice reduced the incidence of postoperative infection to **6%,** compared with 50% in patients not receiving prophylactic antibiotics.[6]
- Use of postoperative antibiotics has not been shown to affect the incidence of postoperative infection.[7,8]

> **TIP:** Oral chlorhexidine reduces bacterial counts in the oral cavity in the presence of open fractures.

### TEETH IN THE LINE OF FRACTURE[9]

- Fractures that contain teeth within the line of fracture are considered *open* because of the communication of the fracture with the gingival sulcus and periodontal attachment.[10,11]
- Routine use of antibiotics and internal fixation allows preservation of most teeth within the line of fracture.
- **Five indications for teeth removal**
  1. Grossly mobile teeth showing evidence of periapical pathology or advanced periodontal disease
  2. Partially erupted third molars with associated dental pathology (cysts or periocoronitis)
  3. Teeth prevent fracture reduction
  4. Fractured roots
  5. Exposed root apices
- Nonrestorable teeth may be retained if removal would compromise accurate reduction of the fracture.
- Complete bony impactions typically require removal of large bony surfaces that otherwise would assist in reduction. These should be removed only when necessary.[10,11]

## METHODS OF FIXATION

The mandible and muscles of mastication represent a complex biomechanical system that is beyond the scope of this text (Fig. 31-2). Simply stated, two main trajectories of stress are present within the mandible: **tension and compression.**

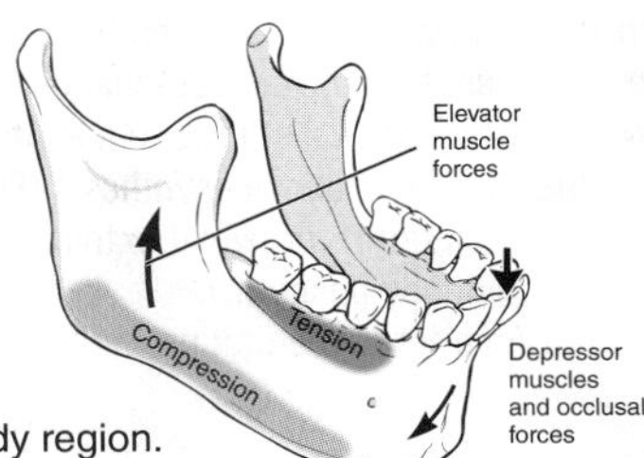


**Fig. 31-2** Functional forces acting across the intact mandibular angle or body region.

Neutralization of these stresses is necessary to achieve stability. Two fundamentally different systems have been advanced for the treatment of mandibular fractures.

- **AO/Association for the Study of Internal Fixation (AO/ASIF)**
  - This system typically requires the use of large, bulky plates.
- **Champy system**[12]
  - Smaller, nonrigid plating system is used to neutralize unfavorable tensile forces, while allowing transmission of more favorable compression forces.
  - A single 2.0 locking miniplate along Champy's line of ideal osteosynthesis with four 8 mm locking monocortical screws plus 1 week of maxillomandibular fixation (MMF) is a reliable and effective treatment modality in selected cases[12,13] (Fig. 31-3).

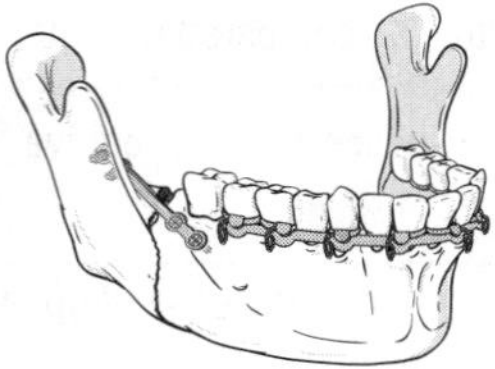

**Fig. 31-3** Plating of an angle fracture with the Champy technique. The fracture is reduced, and a four-hole monocortical miniplate is placed along the external oblique ridge posteriorly with extension onto the buccal surface anteriorly.

## AO/ASIF

- The AO/ASIF was established in 1958 to define conditions for the highest-quality bone surgery. It presented **four conditions** that must be met to accomplish this goal.
  1. Anatomic reduction of fragments
  2. Functionally stable fixation of the fragments
  3. Atraumatic operating technique
  4. Early, active, pain-free mobility
- **Methods of fixation**
  - **Tension band and stabilization plate:** A small plate is placed at the alveolar border to neutralize tensile forces; a larger plate is placed at the inferior border to neutralize compression and torsional stresses.
  - **Reconstruction plate:** A large plate is placed at the inferior border when segmental loss or comminution precludes placement of tension band; a single plate neutralizes tensile, compression, and torsional stresses.

### Champy System

This system advocates the use of monocortical miniplates. It originally was introduced by Michelet in 1967 and was later validated by Champy.[14]

- It is based on the concept that *only tensile stresses are harmful to fracture healing* (Fig. 31-4).
- In biomechanical studies to identify transmission of strains to the mandible, Champy defined the lines of ideal osteosynthesis (Fig. 31-5).
  - Posterior or proximal to the first premolar, a single plate is effective when placed in the midbody position.
  - Anterior to the first premolar, two plates are used, 4-5 mm apart.

**TIP:** This system requires bone to bone abutment of fracture segments and is not applicable to comminuted fractures or situations of segmental bone loss.

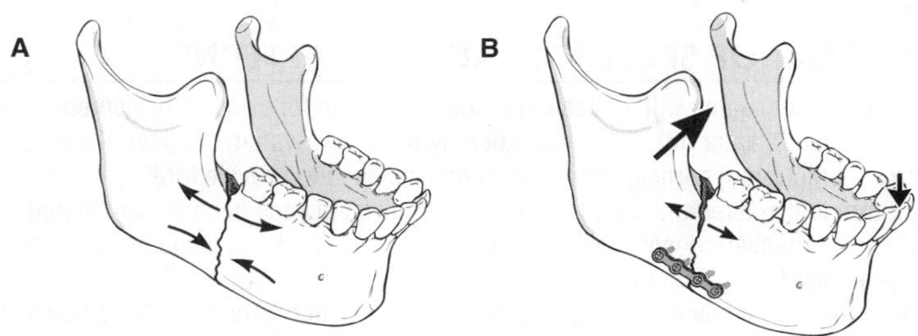


**Fig. 31-4 A,** Fractured mandibular angle. *Arrows* indicate functional forces that lead to tension superiorly and compression inferiorly. **B,** Application of a small plate inferiorly results in the formation of a gap superiorly.

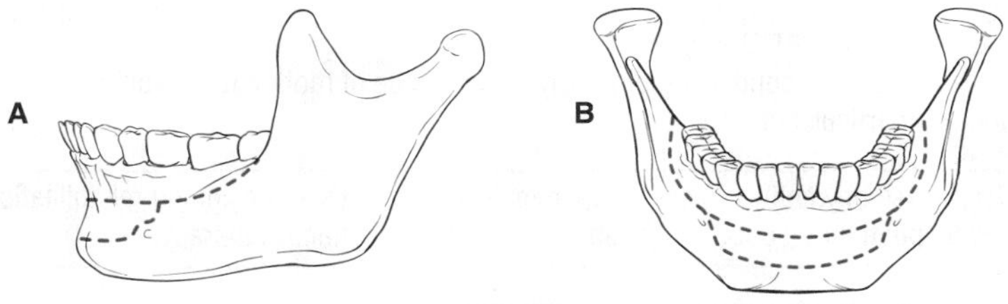


**Fig. 31-5 A-B,** Champy's lines of osteosynthesis.

## DEFINITIONS OF STABILITY

- **Rigid (absolute) stability**
  - No movement occurs across the fracture gap.
  - Rigid stability is an ideal therapeutic principle, but no fixation provides absolute stability in all dimensions of a system as dynamic as the mandible.
- **Functional stability**
  - Movement is possible across the fracture gap but is balanced by external forces and remains within limits that allow the fracture to progress to union.
- **Load-sharing stability**
  - Functional stability is achieved by the fixation system in conjunction with stabilizing forces provided by anatomic abutment of noncomminuted fracture segments.
- **Load-bearing stability**
  - Functional stability, provided solely by the fixation system, is accomplished only by reconstruction plates.

## IMPORTANCE OF STABILITY

- Primary bone healing is possible only in a stable system.
- Mobility leads to bone resorption and fibrous tissue ingrowth.
- When mobility is present, any internal device promotes resorption and infection.

## MANAGEMENT OF SPECIFIC FRACTURE PATTERNS

- Operative treatment begins with extraction of indicated teeth followed by placement of arch bars, MMF screws (see Chapter 32), or a SmartLock Hybrid MMF System (Stryker, Kalamazoo, MI).
- MMF screws or intraoral cortical bone screws may be used to provide MMF. Self-tapping screws, 2 mm in diameter and 8 mm in length, are placed in each quadrant at the junction of the attached and unattached mucosa. Without incisions, screws are advanced between the canine and first premolar taking care to avoid tooth roots.[15]
- 22-gauge embrasure wires may be used as alternatives to arch bars and MMF screws in selected cases.
- Another alternative to arch bars is the SmartLock System with self-drilling locking screws and a plate design to eliminate the need for interdental wiring.
- All fractures are exposed and reduced before MMF is placed.
- Once reduction is confirmed, MMF is placed and fracture fixation proceeds.

### CONDYLE FRACTURES

Fractures of the mandibular condyle require early, active range of motion to rehabilitate the temporomandibular articulation.[16]

> **TIP:** Regardless of whether closed or open techniques are used, beginning rehabilitation in the immediate postinjury period is probably the single most effective therapy.

- **Frequently treated by closed reduction techniques**
  - Difficulty with surgical access, risk to the facial nerve, and small fracture segments prevent widespread use of open reduction with internal fixation (ORIF) techniques.[17]
- **Condyle fracture without malocclusion**
  - This fracture may be treated by soft diet and close observation.
  - If malocclusion develops (usually a deviation to the affected side with contralateral posterior open bite), arch bars should be placed and occlusion controlled with elastics.[17]
- **Condyle fracture with malocclusion**
  - **Closed reduction**
    - Arch bars are placed, and occlusion is controlled with elastics.
      - This is usually possible with a single, class II elastic on the affected side.

> **TIP:** Placement of MMF is *not* always necessary; it may lead to stiffness and fibrosis within the masticatory apparatus, which inhibits rehabilitation.

  - **ORIF**
    - ORIF is necessary when:
      - Condylar segment is displaced and interferes with translation.
      - Condyle is displaced into the middle cranial fossa.

- Combination of bilateral mandibular condyle fractures and midface fractures exist (must reestablish posterior vertical height).
- A normal, reproducible occlusion cannot be established.

### Angle Fractures

**Fractures of the mandibular angle are notorious for being associated with the highest complication rate of any single region of the mandible.**

- ORIF techniques have complication rates equal to those of nonrigid techniques (requiring MMF).[16]

> **TIP:** Surgical access is provided through intraoral approaches, with the assistance of transbuccal trocar when necessary.

### Body Fractures

Fractures of the mandibular body may be treated with either miniplate techniques or reconstruction plates.

- Miniplates are easier to adapt and place but are useful only in noncomminuted fractures, when accurate abutting of fracture segments provides *load-sharing.*
- Reconstruction plates are more difficult to adapt and place but may be used with comminuted fractures and when *load-bearing* fixation is necessary.

> **TIP:** Always consider the location of root apices and the inferior alveolar nerve in this region of the mandible. Use intraoral access.

### Symphysis Fractures

Symphysis fractures may be treated with miniplates or reconstruction plates and are frequently amenable to lag screws.

- Because of torsional forces generated at the symphysis, **two points of fixation are required,** except when using reconstruction plates.
- Intraoral access is preferred.

## SPECIAL CONSIDERATIONS

### Multiple Fractures

- With multiple fractures, the mandible has a tendency to flare outward, which if not corrected and firmly stabilized, results in facial widening and significant deformity.[18]
- More rigid fixation systems should be used to prevent widening.

### Edentulous Fractures

Lack of dentition, small bone stock, and poor bone quality compromise the accuracy of reduction and the healing capacity.

- The Chalmers J Lyons Academy study of edentulous mandibular fractures demonstrated the effectiveness of transfacial approaches to improve reduction and use of reconstruction plates to aid bony union in these situations.[19]
- Application of miniplates or closed reductions using patient's dentures are not recommended.
- In severely atrophic mandibles, bone grafting at the fracture site may be necessary in the acute setting.

## Pediatric Patients

- Stability of arch bars is compromised by unfavorable height of contour associated with primary teeth or missing teeth (mixed dentition stage).
  - This can affect the quality of immobilization provided by MMF.[1,20]
- The presence of developing tooth buds requires selective use of internal fixation to prevent injury.
  - Monocortical screw placement and miniplates can be used cautiously.[1,20]
- Condyle fractures in the pediatric population must be followed very closely, because they can lead to ankylosis and growth disturbances.
  - Start rehabilitation as early as possible.
- The favorable healing potential of children usually allows removal of MMF after 2-3 weeks, compared with 4-6 weeks in adults.
  - Prolonged MMF can significantly compromise rehabilitation.

## Key Points

- ✓ At least two radiographic views of each region of the mandible are required to evaluate injury effectively (mandible series or panoramic radiograph plus selected views).
- ✓ The proper treatment sequence is (1) exposure of all fractures, (2) reduction of all fractures, (3) placement of MMF, and (4) fixation of fractures.
- ✓ MMF must be removed and occlusion reassessed after application of hardware. If the patient is to remain in MMF, it may be reapplied after proper reduction is confirmed.
- ✓ Restoration of preexisting occlusion must be precise in patients treated with internal fixation. Occlusal discrepancies that are present intraoperatively cannot be expected to resolve in the postoperative period.
- ✓ Most patients, especially those with fractures of the condylar process, require closely monitored physical therapy to rehabilitate the masticatory apparatus.

## References


1. Miloro M, Ghali GE, Larsen PE, et al, eds. Peterson's Principles of Oral and Maxillofacial Surgery, vol 1, 3rd ed, 2012.
2. Aston SJ, Beasley RW, Thorne CH, eds. Grabb and Smith's Plastic Surgery, 6th ed. Philadelphia: Lippincott-Raven, 2007.
3. Ellis E III, Miles BA. Fractures of the mandible: a technical perspective. Plast Reconstr Surg 120(7 Suppl 2):S76-S89, 2007.
4. Kuang AA, Lorenz HP. Fractures of the mandible. In McCarthy JG, Galiano RD, Boutros SG, eds. Current Therapy in Plastic Surgery. Philadelphia: Saunders Elsevier, 2006.
5. American College of Surgeons. PHTLS: Basic and Advanced Prehospital Trauma Life Support, 7th ed. St Louis: Mosby-Elsevier, 2011.
6. Kyzas PA. Use of antibiotics in the treatment of mandible fractures: a systematic review. J Oral Maxillofac Surg 69:1129-1145, 2011.
7. Miles BA, Potter JK, Ellis E III. The efficacy of postoperative antibiotic regimens in the open treatment of mandibular fractures: a prospective randomized trial. J Oral Maxillofac Surg 64:576-582, 2006.

8. Abubaker AO, Rollert MK. Postoperative antibiotic prophylaxis in mandibular fractures: a preliminary randomized, double-blind, and placebo-controlled clinical study. J Oral Maxillofac Surg 59:1415-1419, 2001.
9. Chidyllo SA, Marschall MA. Teeth in the line of a mandible fracture: which should be performed first, extraction or fixation? Plast Reconstr Surg 90:135-136, 1992.
10. Schnieder SS, Stern M. Teeth in the line of mandibular fractures. J Oral Maxillofac Surg 29:107-109, 1971.
11. Gerbino G, Tarello F, Fasolis M, et al. Rigid fixation with teeth in the line of mandibular fractures. Int J Oral Maxillofac Surg 23:182-186, 1997.
12. Kelamis JA, Rodriguez ED. Mandible fractures. In Marcus JR, Erdmann D, Rodriguez ED, eds. Essentials of Craniomaxillofacial Trauma. St Louis: Quality Medical Publishing, 2012.
13. Chritak A, Lazow SK, Berger JR. Transoral 2.0-mm locking miniplate fixation of mandible fractures plus 1 week of maxillomandibular fixation: a prospective study. J Oral Maxillofac Surg 63:1737-1741, 2005.
14. Throckmorton GS, Ellis E, Hayasaki H. Masticatory motion after surgical or non-surgical treatment for unilateral fractures of the mandibular condylar process. J Oral Maxillofac Surg 62:127-138, 2004.
15. Fabio R, Amedeo T, Alessandro D, et al. An audit of mandible fractures treated by intermaxillary fixation using intraoral cortical bone screws. J Craniomaxillofac Surg 33:251-254, 2005.
16. Barry CP, Kearns GJ. Superior border plating technique in the management of isolated mandibular angle fractures: a retrospective study of 50 consecutive patients. J Oral Maxillofac Surg 65:1544-1549.
17. Blitz M, Notarnicola K. Closed reduction of the mandibular fracture. Atlas Oral Maxillofac Surg Clin North Am 17:1-13, 2009.
18. Ellis E, Tharanon W. Facial width problems associated with rigid fixation of mandibular fractures. J Oral Maxillofac Surg 50:87-94, 1992.
19. Bruce RA, Ellis E III. The second Chalmers J Lyons Academy study of fractures of the edentulous mandible. J Oral Maxillofac Surg 51:904-911, 1993.
20. Stacey DH, Doyle JF, Mount DL, et al. Management of mandible fractures. Plast Reconstr Surg 117:48e-60e, 2006.

# 32. Basic Oral Surgery

Jason K. Potter, Karthik Naidu

## ANATOMY

### Divisions of the Head

- **Neurocranium:** Upper portion of head; responsible for housing and protecting the brain
- **Visceral cranium:** Lower portion of head; associated with visceral functions of breathing, smelling, eating, talking; may be subdivided into five regions
  1. Orbital region
  2. Infratemporal/temporal fossa
  3. Nasal region
  4. Maxilla (upper jaw)
  5. Mandible (lower jaw)

### Cranial Nerves (Table 32-1)

### Blood Supply

- Arterial supply to the **neurocranium** is provided through the **internal carotid system** and **vertebral system.**
- **Visceral cranium** is chiefly supplied by the **external carotid system.**
  - Midline structures of the forehead and midface receive dual vascularity from both the external and internal systems.
- Venous drainage is provided by the **internal jugular vein.**
  - Major drainage contributions from the face are provided by:
    - Facial vein
    - Retromandibular vein
    - External jugular vein

### Muscle Groups[1]

- **Six major muscle groups in the head assist with functions of the visceral cranium.**
  1. Orbital muscles
     - Include both *intrinsic* and *extrinsic* muscles
       - **Intrinsic muscles:** Associated with controlling light into the eye and lens control; the ciliary muscle, dilator, and constrictor pupillae
       - **Extrinsic muscles:** Responsible for eye movement; the superior rectus, inferior rectus, medial rectus, lateral rectus, superior oblique, and inferior oblique
  2. Masticatory muscles
     - Include the temporalis, medial and lateral pterygoids, and masseter muscles
     - Responsible for lower jaw movement
  3. Muscles of facial expression
     - Major muscles: The frontalis, orbicularis oculi and oris, zygomaticus major and minor, levator labii, depressor labii, buccinator, mentalis, and platysma

**Table 32-1** *Cranial Nerves*

| Number | Name | Type | Foramen | Innervation | Function |
|---|---|---|---|---|---|
| I | Olfactory | Sensory | Cribriform plate | Nasal mucous membrane | Sense of smell |
| II | Optic | Sensory | Optic foramen | Retinas | Sense of sight |
| III | Oculomotor | Motor | Superior orbital fissure | Superior rectus, inferior rectus, medial rectus, inferior oblique, and the ciliary and sphincter pupillae muscles | |
| IV | Trochlear | Motor | Superior orbital fissure | Superior oblique muscle | |
| V | Trigeminal | Motor/ sensory | | | |
| | • Ophthalmic division ($V_1$) | | • Superior orbital fissure | | • Sensation to upper third of face |
| | • Maxillary division ($V_2$) | | • Foramen rotundum | | • Sensation to midportion of face |
| | • Mandibular division ($V_3$) | | • Foramen ovale | | • Sensation to lower face<br>Motor supply to muscles of mastication |
| VI | Abducens | Motor | Superior orbital fissure | Lateral rectus | |
| VII | Facial | Motor/ sensory | Styloid foramen | | Taste to anterior two thirds of tongue (through chorda tympani)<br>Motor supply to muscles of facial expression |
| VIII | Acoustic | Sensory | Internal acoustic meatus | | |
| | • Cochlear division | | | • Organ of Corti | • Sense of hearing |
| | • Vestibular division | | | • Semicircular canals | • Sense of equilibrium |
| IX | Glossopharyngeal | Motor/ sensory | Jugular foramen | Parotid gland | Sensation to oropharynx<br>Motor supply to muscles of pharynx |
| X | Vagus | Motor/ sensory | Jugular foramen | Pharyngeal plexus | Sensation to larynx, trachea, and other aerodigestive mucous membranes<br>Motor supply to muscles of larynx and levator veli palatini, palatoglossus, and palatopharyngeus |
| XI | Accessory | Motor | Jugular foramen | Sternocleidomastoid and trapezius muscles | |
| XII | Hypoglossal | Motor | Hypoglossal canal | Muscles of tongue | |

4. Tongue muscles
   - **Intrinsic muscles** responsible for changing the shape of the tongue include the superior and inferior longitudinal muscles, transversus, and verticalis.
   - **Extrinsic muscles** responsible for gross tongue movements include the genioglossus, hyoglossus, styloglossus, and palatoglossus muscles.
5. Pharynx muscles
   - Include the superior, middle, and inferior pharyngeal constrictors
6. Larynx muscles
   - Located within the larynx; associated with speech production

## Oral Cavity

- Extends from the oral aperture to the palatoglossal fold
- Important anatomic structures within the oral cavity:
  - **Wharton's ducts:** Salivary ducts for the submandibular and sublingual salivary glands on the floor of the mouth
  - **Stensen's ducts** (Fig. 32-1): Salivary ducts for the parotid gland located on the buccal mucosa across from and at the level of the maxillary second permanent molar. An easily discernible papilla is often present.

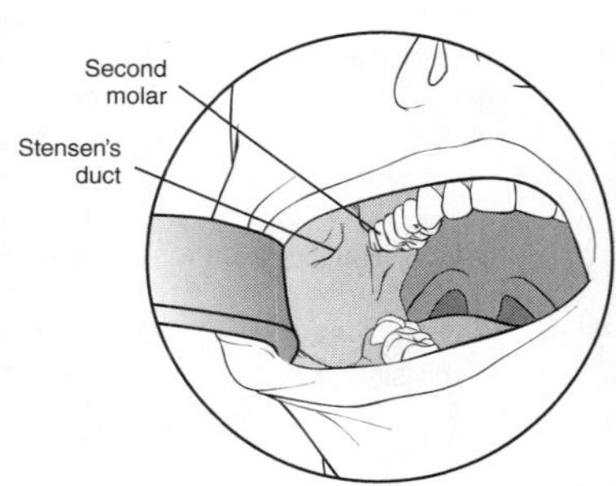


**Fig. 32-1** Stensen's duct.

## Dentition

- **Pediatric (primary/deciduous) dentition:** 20 teeth
  - 4 incisors, 2 canines, 4 molars per arch
  - No premolars in pediatric dentition
  - Pediatric dentition referenced by letter,[2] beginning with the upper right second molar to upper left second molar (A-J) and continuing with the lower left second molar to lower right second molar (K-T) (Figs. 32-2 through 32-4)
- **Mixed dentition:** Variable
  - Marked by the eruption of the first adult tooth (commonly the mandibular first molar) and concluded by exfoliation of the last pediatric tooth

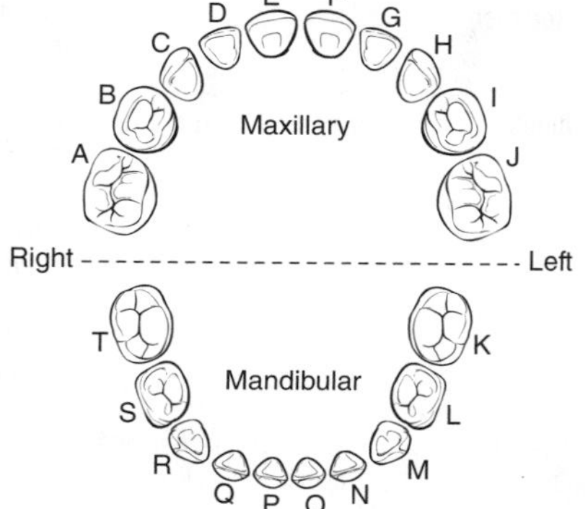


**Upper teeth**
F. Central incisor
G. Lateral incisor
H. Canine (cuspid)
I. First molar
J. Second molar

**Lower teeth**
K. Second molar
L. First molar
M. Canine (cuspid)
N. Lateral incisor
O. Central incisor

**Fig. 32-2** Primary (pediatric) dentition.

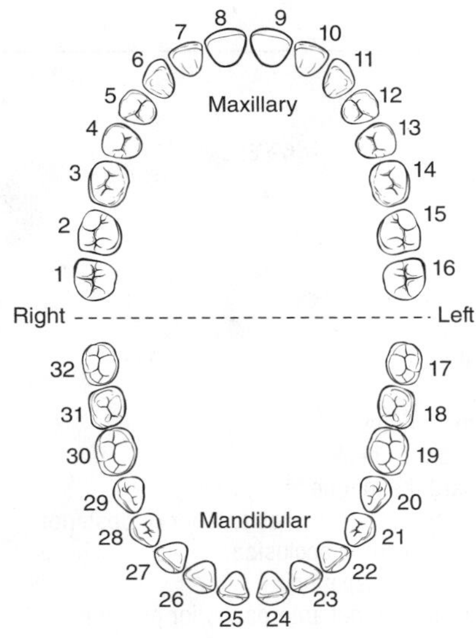


**Upper teeth**
9. Central incisor
10. Lateral incisor
11. Canine (cuspid)
12. First premolar (first bicuspid)
13. Second premolar (second bicuspid)
14. First molar
15. Second molar
16. Third molar (wisdom tooth)

**Lower teeth**
17. Third molar (wisdom tooth)
18. Second molar
19. First molar
20. Second premolar (second bicuspid)
21. First premolar (first bicuspid)
22. Canine (cuspid)
23. Lateral incisor
24. Central incisor

**Fig. 32-3** Secondary (adult) dentition.

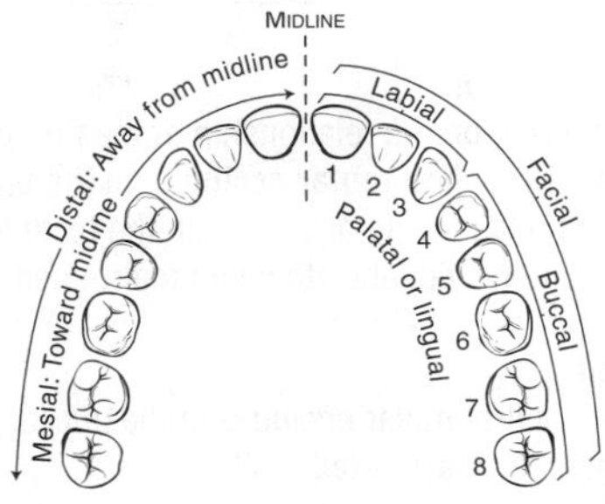


**Fig. 32-4** Dental relationships.

- **Adult (secondary/permanent) dentition:** 32 teeth
  - 4 incisors, 2 canines, 4 premolars, 6 molars per arch
  - Adult dentition referenced by number, beginning with the upper right third molar to upper left third molar (1-16) and continuing with the lower left third molar to lower right third molar (17-32)
  - Supernumerary teeth referenced by adding 50 to the number of the corresponding adult tooth (1-32)
- **Eruption sequence**[3]
  - **First molars:** 6-7 years
  - **Incisors:** 6-9 years
  - **Canines:** 9-12 years
  - **First premolars:** 10-11 years
  - **Second premolars:** 11-12 years
  - **Second molars:** 11-13 years
  - **Third molars:** 17-21 years
- Adult maxillary canines erupt later than the adjacent lateral incisors and first premolars, occasionally resulting in malpositioning.

## DENTAL TERMNINOLOGY

- **Occlusal:** Functional surface of the tooth
- **Apical:** Toward the root tip
- **Incisal:** Occlusal surface of anterior teeth
- **Mesial:** Toward the midline
- **Distal:** Away from the midline
- **Buccal:** Toward the cheek
- **Lingual:** Toward the tongue (mandibular)
- **Palatal:** Toward the palate (maxillary)
- **Overbite:** Amount of vertical overlap of incisal edges
- **Overjet:** Amount of horizontal overlap of incisal edges
- **Proclined:** Anterior tooth angulated toward the lip
- **Retroclined:** Anterior tooth angulated toward the tongue
- **Buccal version:** Posterior tooth angulated toward the cheek
- **Lingual version:** Posterior tooth angulated toward the tongue
- **Crossbite:** Horizontal malrelationship of teeth; may be classified as anterior or posterior
- **Open bite:** Occlusal surfaces not in contact when in centric occlusion
- **Centric occlusion:** Occlusion of teeth in maximal intercuspation
- **Centric relation:** Occlusion of teeth with condyle in its most anterosuperior position

## MALOCCLUSION

*Occlusion* refers to the relationship of teeth to one another.

- Edward H. Angle first described classes of malocclusion.
- Angle hypothesized that normal occlusion was based on the relationship of the first permanent molars so that the **mesiobuccal cusp of the maxillary first molar occludes in the buccal groove of the mandibular first molar.** When this relationship occurs, with the teeth located along a smoothly curving line of occlusion without individual teeth being malrotated or malposed, the patient has *normal occlusion.*
- Angle described **three classes of malocclusion.**

  **Class I:** The mesiobuccal cusp of the maxillary first molar occludes in the buccal groove of the mandibular molar, **but teeth are malposed or malrotated.**

**NOTE: Class I malocclusion is not normal occlusion.**

  **Class II:** The mandibular molar is *distally* positioned relative to the maxillary molar.

  - Two divisions describe the relationship of the incisor.

    **Division I:** Excessive overjet with normal angulation of incisor

    **Division II:** Incisor retroclined to some degree, resulting in less overbite and increased overjet

  **Class III:** The mandibular molar is *mesially* positioned relative to the maxillary molar.

## LOCAL ANESTHESIA

- Local anesthesia of the intraoral structures and facial soft tissues may be provided by regional nerve blocks or infiltration in the area of interest.
- In general, for anesthesia of the teeth, nerve blocks should be performed for mandibular dentition, because mandibular bone density in most areas precludes diffusion of local anesthetic.
- Diffusion occurs easily across the thin maxillary bone to provide dental anesthesia.

**TIP:** Routine bending of anesthetic needles should be avoided; separated needles may be difficult to retrieve.[4]

**TIP:** A local anesthetic needle used to anesthetize an infected site should not be subsequently used for nerve blocks or infiltration in additional sites.

## NERVE BLOCKS

### INFRAORBITAL[5] (Fig. 32-5)

- The infraorbital branch of $V_2$ can be palpated as it exits its foramen approximately 4-7 mm below the inferior orbital rim, along a line dropped from the medial edge of the limbus.
- Several milliliters of local anesthetic may be deposited at the foramen using either an intraoral or extraoral approach.
  - Intraorally, the lip is stretched to make the mucosa taut at the depth of the anterior maxillary vestibule. The needle is inserted at the depth of the vestibule to the level of the foramen. If aspiration is negative, anesthetic is deposited.
  - Extraorally, the foramen is palpated, and the needle is inserted at the superior aspect of the nasolabial fold at an angle to the foramen. If aspiration is negative, anesthetic is deposited.
- An infraorbital nerve block provides anesthesia of lip, medial cheek, lower lid, lateral nose, and buccal gingival to the second premolar.
- Provides dental anesthesia to nearby teeth by diffusion

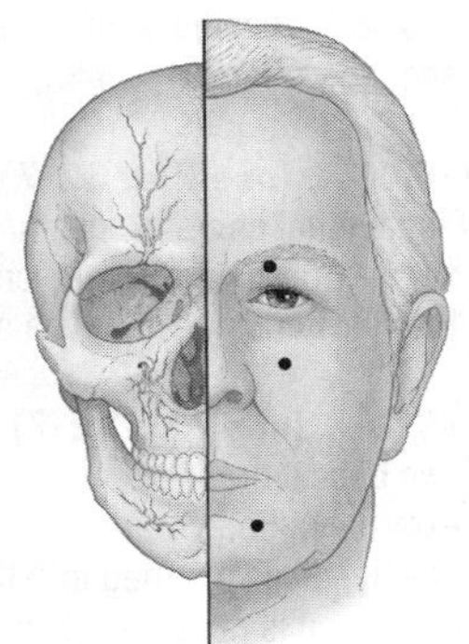

**Fig. 32-5** The infraorbital nerve.

### GREATER PALATINE[5] (Fig. 32-6)

- Foramen is located halfway between the teeth and palatal midline at about the second molar.
- Foramen is palpable as a soft depression in this location on the hard palate. If aspiration is negative, local anesthetic (1-2 ml) is deposited.
- Provides anesthesia of the palatal mucosa to the first premolar on its respective side

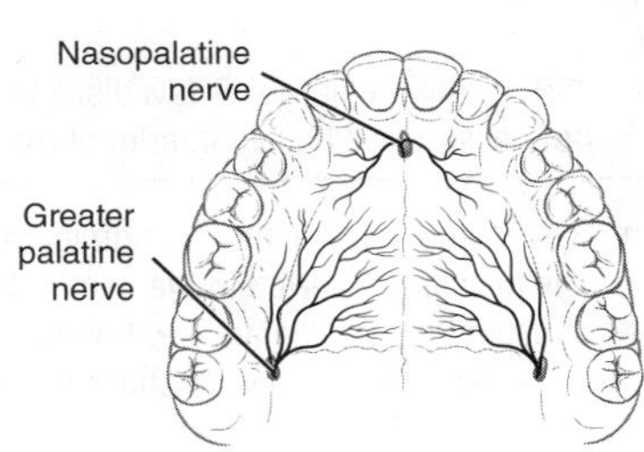


**Fig. 32-6** The greater palatine nerve.

### NASOPALATINE/INCISIVE (see Fig. 32-6)

- Foramen is located at the midline approximately 5-7 mm behind the maxillary incisors.
- If aspiration is negative, local anesthetic (0.5-1 ml) is deposited.
- Provides anesthesia of the palatal mucosa from canine to canine

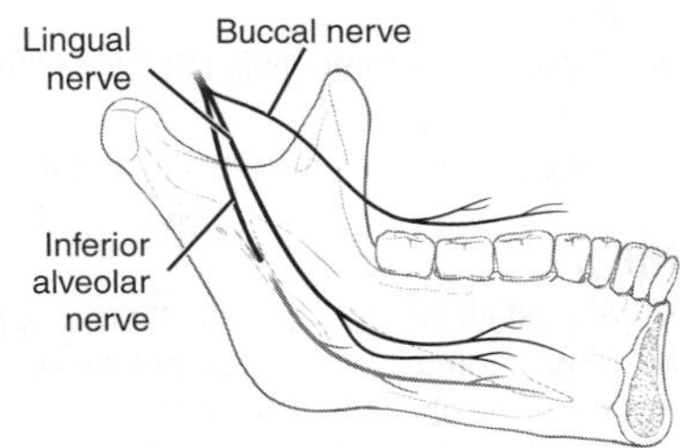


**Fig. 32-7** The inferior alveolar nerve.

### INFERIOR ALVEOLAR[5] (Fig. 32-7)

- The inferior alveolar nerve enters the mandibular foramen on the medial ramus approximately 5-10 mm above the mandibular occlusal plane and 15-20 mm posterior to the anterior border of the ramus.

- With the patient's mouth open wide, the most medial aspect of the anterior surface of the ramus is palpated with the contralateral thumb.
- The needle is inserted at a 45-degree angle to the ramus, entering at least 10 mm above the level of the occlusal plane (it is more effective to be higher than lower) and immediately adjacent to the anteromedial edge of the ramus.
- The needle is inserted until contact is made with bone. If aspiration is negative, several milliliters of anesthetic are injected.
- Provides anesthesia of the entire mandibular hemidentition and buccal mucosa anterior to the second premolar

### Lingual (see Fig. 32-7)

- The lingual nerve is anesthetized during the inferior alveolar nerve block by withdrawing the needle approximately 0.5 cm and depositing 1-2 ml of solution.
- Provides anesthesia of the entire lingual mucosa and respective half of the tongue

### Buccal (see Fig. 32-7)

- The buccal branch of $V_3$ is anesthetized as it crosses the anterior border of the ramus along the external oblique ridge.
- The needle is inserted into the retromolar mucosa over the anterior surface of the ramus. If aspiration is negative, several milliliters of solution are deposited.
- Provides anesthesia of the buccal mucosa and gingiva anteriorly to the region of the first premolar

### Mental

**TIP:** The mental nerve is a distal branch of the inferior alveolar nerve. Therefore this block is not necessary when an inferior alveolar nerve block has been performed.

- The mental nerve exits through its foramen below the second premolar. The lip is stretched, and the needle is inserted to the depth of the vestibule in this location.
- If aspiration is negative, several milliliters of solution are deposited.
- Provides anesthesia of the buccal mucosa and gingiva anterior to the first premolar

## ODONTOGENIC INFECTIONS[6]

- Range from localized without systemic manifestations to diffuse, systemic, life-threatening infections
- Death from odontogenic infections still occurs today, usually from loss of airway or mediastinal involvement.
- Accurate evaluation of patient and involved fascial spaces are requisite to proper management.

### Microbiology

- Almost all odontogenic infections are **polymicrobial.**
- Most common organisms include aerobic gram-positive cocci, anaerobic gram-positive cocci, and anaerobic gram-negative rods.
- **Approximately 60% of infections are mixed aerobic-anaerobic.** Important pathogens include *Streptococcus, Peptostreptococcus, Prevotella, Porphyromonas,* and *Fusobacterium.*

## Pathogenesis

- Odontogenic infections arise from two major sources:
  1. **Periapical infection secondary to pulpal necrosis** leads to bacterial invasion in the periapical tissues.
  2. **Periodontal infection secondary to deep periodontal pockets** allows bacterial invasion in the surrounding tissue.
- **Periapical infection is the most common.**
  - From the periapical tissues the infection may erode through cortical bone into the facial soft tissues.
  - Location of infection is determined by the relationship of muscle attachments to the location of cortical perforation.
  - Example: A periapical infection of a mandibular premolar that erodes through the lingual cortical bone will result in infection of the sublingual space, because the mylohyoid attachment is inferior to the root apex, whereas the same process involving the second molar would present as a submandibular space infection, because the molar root apices lie below the level of the mylohyoid attachment.

## PRINCIPLES OF THERAPY

Standard history and physical examination should always be performed on all patients. Particular consideration should be given to the following:

### Determine Severity of Infection

- Signs of systemic involvement should be sought from the physical examination.
- Vital signs are reviewed for pyrexia, tachycardia, or hypotension (ominous).

**CAUTION: Inability to control secretions or maintain a patent airway may indicate impending loss of airway and a need for emergent intervention.**

- **Trismus** may be the only indication of parapharyngeal space infection. Clinician should take appropriate measures to thoroughly inspect the oropharynx.
- The source of infection should be identified (with assistance of panoramic radiography) and adjacent fascial spaces examined directly for involvement.

### Assess Patient's Host Defense System[7]

- Patients with a medical history significant for conditions that produce immunodeficiency, such as diabetes, HIV, corticosteroid/chemotherapy usage, malnutrition, substance abuse, chronic renal disease, or other disease processes, require more aggressive management.

### Surgically Drain Infection

- Odontogenic infections should be treated by specialists trained in their management (when appropriate).
- The most important intervention after assessment and establishment of a secure airway is drainage of the infection and removal of the source.

### Administer Appropriate Antibiotic Coverage

- *All odontogenic infections should be cultured and tested for aerobic and anaerobic growth.*
- Empiric therapy is begun with penicillin or clindamycin for allergic patients.
- Severe infections may require increased coverage for gram-negative and anaerobic bacteria.
- Antibiotic therapy should be guided by culture results.

## ARCH BARS

- **Arch bars are used to:**
  - Stabilize dentoalveolar fractures
  - Provide stable base from which to institute maxillomandibular fixation
  - Control occlusion in the posttraumatic period
- Difficulty in placing arch bars depends on the age of the dentition (primary versus secondary or mixed), presence of partial edentulism, and extent of active dental decay.
- Arch bars are usually placed from first molar to first molar.
- With mandibular fractures, arch bars ideally extend **two teeth proximal and distal to a fracture line** when possible.
- 25-gauge circumdental wires are used to secure the arch bar to each tooth.
- **Conventionally, wires are always:**
  - Twisted **clockwise** to tighten
  - Passed occlusal to the arch bar in the interproximal region of fractures to prevent the wire from interfering with reduction
  - Passed occlusal to the arch bar on the distal aspect of the last tooth and adjacent to edentulous spans
- Wires are typically applied from midline to posterior to prevent redundancy within the arch bar.
- Gauze director may be used to ensure circumdental wire placement below the height of contour of each tooth.
- **Proper occlusion and fracture reduction must be established before complete tightening of the circumdental wires within the quadrant of the fracture to prevent maintenance of malreduction by the arch bar.**
  - This is facilitated by tightening the wires in the fracture segment after reducing the fracture and establishing maxillomandibular fixation.
  - An alternative to arch bars is the SMARTLock System (Stryker Craniomaxillofacial, Kalamazoo, MI), with self-locking screws and a plate design to eliminate the need for interdental wiring.

## DENTOFACIAL DEFORMITIES[8]

- Treatment is an integrated orthodontic-surgical process.
- Deformities characterized by a skeletal discrepancy between mandible, maxilla, and skull base, or some combination thereof
- Simple orthodontics do not correct the effects of malrelationship on facial balance but may camouflage malocclusion through creation of dental compensations.
- When skeletal elements are present, the surgeon should be involved early in treatment planning to coordinate orthodontic-surgical therapy.
- Orthodontic treatment proceeds to eliminate dental compensations and to level and align arch forms in anticipation of surgical correction of skeletal component.

## DENTAL EVALUATION

### IDENTIFY

- Transverse and anteroposterior discrepancies
- Open bites
- Tooth width discrepancies
- Excess arch curvatures (curves of Spee and Wilson) (Fig. 32-8)
- Occlusal canting

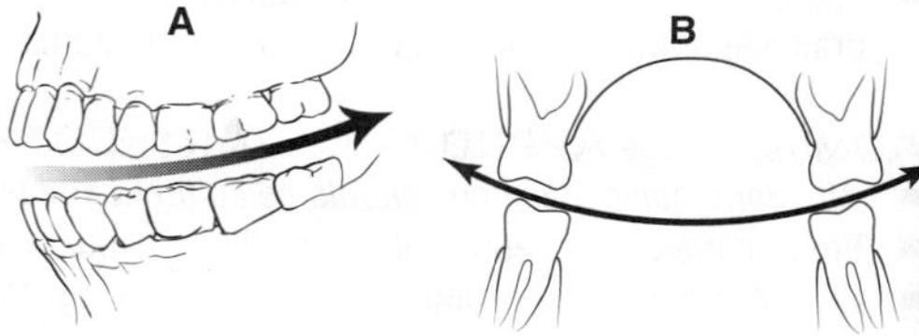


**Fig. 32-8** **A,** Curve of Spee. **B,** Curve of Wilson.

## CEPHALOMETRIC EVALUATION

- Allows standardized measurements from lateral cephalometric radiographs to determine the relationship between the skull base, maxilla, and mandible
- Measurements evaluate dentofacial proportions and clarify anatomic basis of deformity.
- Should be used for diagnostic purposes but should not be the sole basis for planning surgery
- Surgical decisions should be based on aesthetic evaluation of the face after considering the cephalometric diagnosis.
  - Example: Patients with mild to moderate "cephalometrically" defined mandibular prognathism are usually best treated with maxillary advancement and not mandibular setback[9,10] (Fig. 32-9; Boxes 32-1 and 32-2).

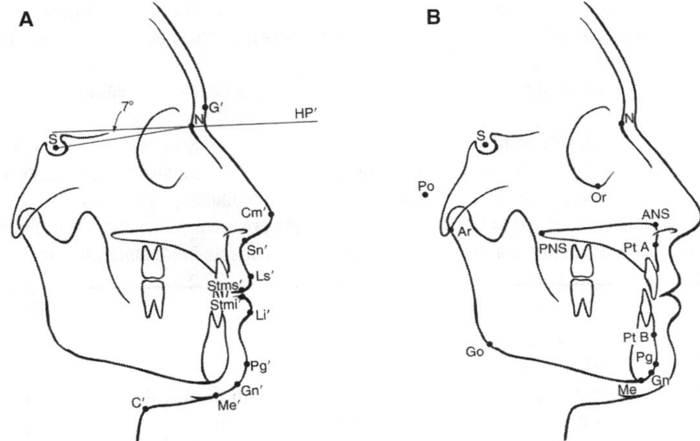


**Fig. 32-9** **A,** Cephalometrics for soft tissue landmarks. **B,** Cephalometrics for hard tissue landmarks.

**Box 32-1** *CEPHALOMETRIC LANDMARKS (SOFT TISSUE)*

| | |
|---|---|
| G′ | Soft tissue glabella: Most prominent point in the midsagittal plane of the forehead |
| Cm′ | Columella point: Most anterior point on the columella of the nose |
| Sn′ | Subnasale: Point at which the nasal septum merges with the upper cutaneous lip and the midsagittal plane |
| Ls′ | Labrale superius: Mucocutaneous border of the upper lip in the midsagittal plane |
| Li′ | Labrale inferius: Mucocutaneous border of the lower lip in the midsagittal plane |
| Pg′ | Soft tissue pogonion: Most anterior point of the soft tissue chin |
| HP′ | Horizontal plane: A plane drawn 7 degrees above the sella-nasion (S-N) plane, from which perpendicular lines are drawn to measure vertical soft tissue distances |
| Stms′ | Stomion superius: Lowermost point of the vermilion of the lower lip |
| C′ | Cervical point: Innermost point between the submental area and where the neck begins its vertical position |
| Me′ | Soft tissue menton: Lowest point on the contour of the soft tissue chin |
| Gn′ | Soft tissue gnathion: Constructed midpoint between soft tissue pogonion and soft tissue menton; located at the intersection of subnasale to soft tissue pogonion line and the line from C′ to Me′ |

**Box 32-2** *CEPHALOMETRIC LANDMARKS (HARD TISSUE/BONY TISSUE)*

| | |
|---|---|
| S | Sella: Center of the pituitary fossa—sella turcica |
| N or Na | Nasion: Most anterior point at the junction of the nasal and frontal bones in the midsagittal plane |
| Po | Porion: Most superior point of the external auditory meatus |
| O or Or | Orbitale: Lowest point on the inferior bony border of the left orbital cavity as viewed from the lateral aspect |
| ANS | Anterior nasal spine: Most anterior tip of the maxillary nasal spine |
| PNS | Posterior nasal spine: Midline tip of posterior spine of hard palate in the midsagittal plane |
| P or Pg | Pogonion: Most anterior point on the contour of the mandibular symphysis |
| Pt A | Point A: Deepest midpoint on the maxillary alveolar process between anterior nasal spine and the crest of alveolar ridge |
| Pt B | Point B: Deepest midpoint on the alveolar process between the crest of the ridge and pogonion |
| Me | Menton: Lowest point on the contour of the mandibular symphysis |
| Gn | Gnathion: Most anteroinferior point on the chin contour constructed point, determined by bisecting the angle formed by the facial and mandibular planes |
| Ar | Articulare: Junction of the basisphenoid and the posterior of the condyle of the mandible |
| Go | Gonion: Point at the angle of the mandible that is directed most inferiorly and posteriorly |

### AESTHETIC EVALUATION

- Includes frontal and profile evaluations, which are divided into evaluation of the upper, middle, and lower facial thirds in the vertical and horizontal dimensions
- **Balance** of these regions is the goal.

## GENERAL DIAGNOSES

### MAXILLARY EXCESS

- May occur in the anteroposterior, vertical, or transverse dimensions
- **Vertical excess facial features include:**
  - Elongation of lower third
  - Narrow nasal base
  - Excessive incisal and gingival show
  - Lip incompetence
- May be associated with anterior open bite (apertognathia)
- Anteroposterior excess characteristically has class II malocclusion with protrusion of maxillary incisors and convex facial profile.
- **Primary surgical correction involves LeFort I osteotomy.**
- Segmental maxillary surgery can be performed for more complex deformities.

### MAXILLARY DEFICIENCY

- May occur in the anteroposterior, vertical, or transverse dimensions

- **Facial features include:**
  - Deficiency of infraorbital/paranasal regions
  - Inadequate upper tooth show
  - Short lower third
  - Deficient upper lip
- **Primary surgical correction involves LeFort I osteotomy.**
- Segmental maxillary surgery can be performed for more complex deformities.
- Bone grafting may be required depending on the magnitude and vector of movement.

### MANDIBULAR EXCESS (PROGNATHISM)

- Typically demonstrates class III molar and canine relationship and reverse overjet of the incisors
- **Facial features include** prominent lower third.
- **Primary correction may involve maxillary advancement or mandibular setback, depending on the facial analysis.**
- Mandibular setback is provided through bilateral sagittal split osteotomies (BSSO) or intraoral vertical ramus osteotomies (IVRO).
- IVRO has the disadvantage of requiring maxillomandibular fixation.
- The likelihood of inferior alveolar nerve injury is significantly higher with BSSO.

### MANDIBULAR DEFICIENCY (RETROGNATHISM)

- Typically demonstrates class II molar and canine relationship
- May demonstrate excess overjet or deep bite
- **Facial features include:**
  - Retruded position of chin
  - Acute labiomental fold
  - Abnormal lip posturing
  - Short thyromental distance
- **Primary surgical treatment involves mandibular advancement using BSSO.**

## STABILITY OF CORRECTION

- Relapse may occur after correction of dentofacial deformities.[11]
- The factors that have the most influence on stability appear to be which jaw is being moved, the direction of movement, and the distance of movement.
- **Orthodontic factors**
  - Inadequate removal of dental compensations
  - Inadequate leveling of dental arches
  - Presurgical orthodontic correction of skeletal transverse discrepancies
- **Surgical factors**
  - Inaccurate positioning of proximal mandibular segment and condyles
  - Inadequate fixation
  - Idiopathic condylar resorption

## Key Points

- ✓ Muscles of mastication include the temporalis, medial pterygoid, lateral pterygoid, and masseter.
- ✓ Stensen's duct is located adjacent to the maxillary second permanent molar.
- ✓ Children have 20 teeth (primary/deciduous dentition).
- ✓ Adults have 32 teeth (secondary/permanent dentition).
- ✓ Adult dentition is numbered 1-32, starting with the upper right third molar and ending with the lower right third molar.
- ✓ Angle class I malocclusion is *not* necessarily normal occlusion.

## References


1. Hollinshead WH, ed. Anatomy for Surgeons: The Head and Neck, 3rd ed. Philadelphia: Lippincott Williams & Wilkins, 1982.
2. Marcus JR, Erdmann D, Rodriguez ED, eds. Essentials of Craniomaxillofacial Trauma. St Louis: Quality Medical Publishing, 2012.
3. Fuller JL, Denehy GE, Schulein TM, eds. Concise Dental Anatomy and Morphology, 4th ed. Iowa City: University of Iowa College of Dentistry, 2001.
4. Malamed SF, ed. Handbook of Local Anesthesia, 6th ed. Philadelphia: Elsevier, 2013.
5. Ellis E III, Kittidumkerng W. Analysis of treatment for isolated zygomaticomaxillary complex fractures. J Oral Maxillofac Surg 54:386, 1996.
6. Topazian RG, Goldberg MH, Hupp JR, eds. Oral and Maxillofacial Infections, 4th ed. Philadelphia: WB Saunders, 2002.
7. Miloro M, Ghali GE, Larsen P, et al, eds. Peterson's Principles of Oral and Maxillofacial Surgery, 3rd ed. Shelton, CT: People's Medical Publishing House USA, 2012.
8. Epker BN, Stella JP, Fish LC, eds. Dentofacial Deformities: Integrated Orthodontic and Surgical Approach, vol 1, 2nd ed. St Louis: Mosby, 1995.
9. Evans G, ed. Operative Plastic Surgery. New York: McGraw-Hill, 2000.
10. Ferraro JW, ed. Fundamentals of Maxillofacial Surgery. New York: Springer-Verlag, 1997.
11. Proffit WR, Turvey TA, Phillips C. The hierarchy of stability and predictability in orthognathic surgery with rigid fixation: an update and extension. Head Face Med 3:21, 2007.

# 33. Principles of Head and Neck Cancer: Staging and Management

Kristin K. Constantine, Michael E. Decherd, Jeffrey E. Janis

## INCIDENCE/ETIOLOGIC FACTORS

- Head and neck malignancy: 78,000 cases annually (7% of all cancers)
- Cancer deaths: 17,500 annually (4% of all cancers)
- **Squamous cell carcinoma (SCC) is the most common**, accounting for >90% of all head and neck cancers.
- Alcohol and tobacco have a synergistic effect: 15-fold increased incidence over nonusers (squamous cell cancer)
- Male predominance more than 2:1
- Other factors include consumption of betel nuts and smoked fish, exposure to wood dust (nasopharyngeal), and human papillomavirus (HPV).

## PRESENTATION

- Persistent sore throat, otalgia, hoarseness, epistaxis, or nasal obstruction
- Dysphagia/odynophagia or shortness of breath
- Weight loss, fatigue
- Painless neck mass, CN palsy, facial pain/numbness

## EXAMINATION/WORKUP

- Full head and neck examination, including cranial nerves, ear/external auditory canal (EAC), scalp; oral and laryngeal with indirect mirror laryngoscopy or flexible fiberoptic laryngoscopy

> **TIP:** Tumors occupying the deep lobe of the parotid/parapharyngeal space can be clinically appreciated during oral examination as an intraoral swelling.

- Labs: Complete blood cell count, electrolytes, liver function tests
- Imaging: Chest radiography, CT of neck and chest with contrast

> **TIP:** Radiographic criteria for nodal metastasis include nodes >1 cm and the presence of central necrosis.

- MRI: Consider for nasopharyngeal, paranasal sinus, infratemporal fossa, parotid, parapharyngeal, or skull base tumors
- PET: Indicates tissues with increased metabolic rate; useful for metastatic evaluation, monitoring for recurrence, and evaluation of an unknown primary
- Fine-needle aspiration (FNA):
- Consider tissue diagnosis in any neck mass present for >2 weeks in smokers >40 years old.

- Excisional biopsy may increase dermal metastasis of SCC.
- Excisional biopsy is needed to determine tumor architecture if FNA suggests lymphoma.
- Send to pathology fresh for flow cytometry
- Panendoscopy with biopsy
- Direct laryngoscopy, rigid esophagoscopy, bronchoscopy
- **Unknown primary:** Malignant neck node with no obvious source
  - Management is controversial.
  - Consider performing:
    - PET scan: Identifies areas to perform directed biopsies
    - Tonsillectomy
    - Biopsies of nasopharynx (Rosenmüller's fossae in particular) and base of tongue

## LEVELS OF THE NECK[1-5] (Fig. 33-1)

**TIP:** The levels of the neck are different from the trauma zones of the neck.

### Level I

- Lymph node groups: Submental and submandibular
- Level Ia: Submental triangle
  - Boundaries: Anterior bellies of the digastric muscle and the hyoid bone
- Level Ib: Submandibular triangle
  - Boundaries: Body of the mandible, anterior and posterior belly of the digastric muscle (includes the submandibular gland, preglandular/postglandular lymph nodes, and prevascular/postvascular lymph nodes [relative to facial vein and artery]).

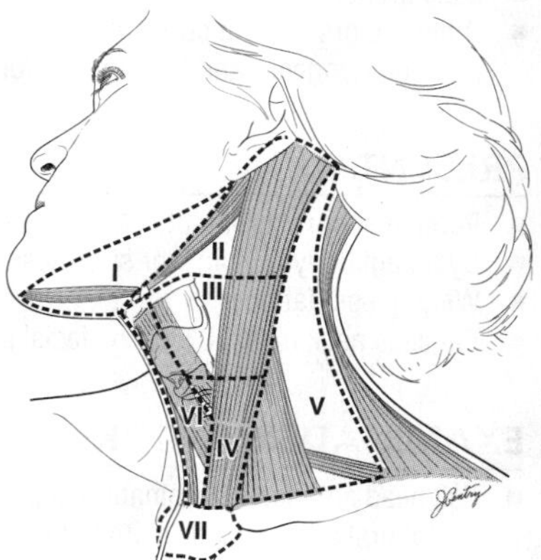

**Fig. 33-1** Levels of the neck.

### Level II

- Lymph node groups: Upper jugular
- Boundaries
  - Anterior: Lateral border of the sternohyoid muscle
  - Posterior: Posterior border of the sternocleidomastoid (SCM) muscle
  - Superior: Skull base
  - Inferior: Level of the hyoid bone (clinical landmark); carotid bifurcation (surgical landmark)
- Level IIa and IIb arbitrarily designated anatomically by splitting level II with the spinal accessory nerve (CN XI)

### Level III

- Lymph node groups: Middle jugular
- Boundaries
  - Anterior: Lateral border of the sternohyoid muscle
  - Posterior: Posterior border of the SCM muscle
  - Superior: Hyoid bone (clinical landmark); carotid bifurcation (surgical landmark)
  - Inferior: Cricothyroid notch (clinical landmark); omohyoid muscle (surgical landmark)

### LEVEL IV

- Lymph node group: Lower jugular
- Boundaries
  - Anterior: Lateral border of the sternohyoid muscle
  - Posterior: Posterior border of the SCM muscle
  - Superior: Cricothyroid notch (clinical landmark), omohyoid muscle (surgical landmark)
  - Inferior: Clavicle
- Level IVa: Lymph nodes that lie along the internal jugular vein but immediately deep to the sternal head of the SCM muscle
- Level IVb: Lymph nodes that lie deep to the clavicular head of the SCM muscle

### LEVEL V

- Lymph node groups: Posterior triangle
- Boundaries
  - Anterior: Posterior border of the SCM muscle
  - Posterior: Anterior border of the trapezius muscle
  - Inferior: Clavicle
- Level Va: Lymphatic structures in the upper part of level V that follow the spinal accessory nerve
- Level Vb: Nodes that lie along the transverse cervical artery
  - Anatomically the division between the two level V subzones is the inferior belly of the omohyoid muscle.

### LEVEL VI

- Lymph node groups: Anterior compartment
- Boundaries
  - Lateral: Carotid sheath
  - Superior: Hyoid bone
  - Inferior: Suprasternal notch

### LEVEL VII

- Lymph node groups: Upper mediastinal
- Boundaries
  - Lateral: Carotid arteries
  - Superior: Suprasternal notch
  - Inferior: Aortic arch

## CLASSIFICATION[6]

The American Joint Committee on Cancer (AJCC) sets the standards for cancer staging. Cancers of the head and neck are divided into the following categories and subsites.

1. **Lip and oral cavity**
   - Mucosal lip: From junction of vermilion border with skin to portion of the lip in contact with opposing lip
   - Buccal mucosa: Membranous lining of inner cheeks/lips from pterygomandibular raphe forward
   - Upper/lower alveolar ridge
   - Retromolar trigone
   - Floor of mouth: Bounded by inferior alveolar ridges and tongue; contains opening of submandibular (Wharton's) and sublingual ducts

- Hard palate: Bounded by superior alveolar ridges and junction of soft palate
- Oral tongue (anterior two thirds): From circumvallate papillae anteriorly; includes tip, lateral border, dorsum, undersurface

2. **Pharynx**
   - Nasopharynx: From posterior choanae to free border of soft palate; includes vault, lateral walls, posterior wall
   - Oropharynx: From plane of superior surface of soft palate to superior surface of hyoid; includes base of tongue, inferior soft palate/uvula, anterior/posterior tonsillar pillars, glossotonsillar sulci, pharyngeal walls
   - Hypopharynx: From superior border of hyoid to lower border of cricoids; includes piriform sinuses, lateral and posterior walls, postcricoid region
3. **Larynx**
   - Supraglottis: Suprahyoid epiglottis, infrahyoid epiglottis, aryepiglottic folds, arytenoids, false vocal cords
   - Glottis: True vocal cords, anterior/posterior commissures
   - Subglottis: Lower boundary of glottis to cricoid cartilage
4. **Paranasal sinuses**
   - Maxillary sinus
   - Nasal cavity: Septum, floor, lateral wall, vestibule
   - Ethmoid sinus
5. **Major salivary glands**
   - Parotid
   - Submandibular
   - Sublingual
6. **Thyroid**
7. **Mucosal melanoma of the head and neck**

- The staging system uses the TNM method (tumor, nodes, metastasis).
  - **T:** 1-4
  - **N:** 0-3
  - **M:** 0-1 (may vary by tumor)

**TIP:** TNM is clinically more useful than stage. Even though a T3N0 and a T1N1 tumor are both stage III, they behave differently and may be treated differently.

- The prefix **p** or **c** is used to designate how the stage is assigned (**p**athologic or **c**linical).
  - **Pathologic staging, if available, supersedes clinical staging.**
- Designators applied: **m,** multiple tumors; **y,** following multimodal therapy; **r,** recurrent tumors; and **a,** at autopsy.
- Biologic factors:
  - Perineural or perivascular invasion
  - Extracapsular spread (ECS)
    - Indicates a more aggressive tumor
    - Should be considered for radiation even if other criteria not met
- **Tumor grade does not have significant prognostic significance.**
- **Tumors should not be restaged.**
  - Example: The stage of a patient who initially is M0 but who is diagnosed with pulmonary metastasis 6 months later is not changed to M1.

## TUMOR STAGING: AJCC 7TH EDITION, 2010[6]

- **T: Extent of primary tumor**
  - **Lip and oral cavity**
    - Tx: No available information on primary tumor
    - T0: No evidence of primary tumor
    - Tis: Carcinoma in situ
    - T1: Greatest diameter of primary tumor $\leq$2 cm
    - T2: Greatest diameter of primary tumor $>$2 cm but $\leq$4 cm
    - T3: Greatest diameter of primary tumor $>$4 cm
    - T4a: Moderately advanced local disease:
      - Lip: Invades through cortical bone, inferior alveolar nerve, floor of mouth, skin of face
      - Oral cavity: Invades adjacent structures only (cortical bone of mandible/maxilla, deep extrinsic muscles of tongue—genioglossus, hyoglossus, palatoglossus, styloglossus—maxillary sinus, skin of face)
    - T4b: Very advanced local disease that invades masticator space, pterygoid plates, skull base; encases internal carotid artery
  - **Nasopharynx**
    - T1: Tumor confined to nasopharynx
    - T2: Parapharyngeal extension
    - T3: Involves skull base or paranasal sinuses
    - T4: Intracranial extension, involves cranial nerves, hypopharynx, orbit, infratemporal fossa/masticator space.
  - **Oropharynx**
    - T1: Greatest diameter of tumor $<$2 cm
    - T2: Tumor 2-4 cm in greatest dimension
    - T3: Tumor $>$4 cm in greatest diameter or extension to lingual epiglottis
    - T4a: Moderately advanced local disease:
      - Tumor invades larynx, tongue, medial pterygoid, hard palate, mandible
    - T4b: Very advanced local disease:
      - Invades lateral pterygoid, pterygoid plates, lateral nasopharynx, skull base; encases internal carotid artery
  - **Larynx**
    - Supraglottis:
      - T1: Tumor limited to one subsite of supraglottis with normal vocal cord mobility
      - T2: Invades more than one adjacent subsite without fixation of larynx
      - T3: Limited to larynx with vocal cord fixation and/or invades postcricoid space, preepiglottic space, paraglottic space, inner cortex of thyroid cartilage
      - T4a: Invades through thyroid cartilage and/or tissues beyond larynx
      - T4b: Invades prevertebral space; encases internal carotid artery, mediastinal structures
    - Glottis:
      - T1a: Tumor limited to one vocal cord with normal mobility
      - T1b: Tumor involves both true vocal cords with normal mobility
      - T2: Extends to supraglottis or subglottis and/or impairs vocal cord mobility
      - T3: Limited to larynx with vocal cord fixation, invasion of paraglottic space, inner cortex of thyroid cartilage
      - T4a: Invades through outer cortex of thyroid cartilage and/or tissues beyond larynx
      - T4b: Invades prevertebral space; encases carotid artery, mediastinal structures

- Subglottis:
  - T1: Limited to subglottis
  - T2: Extends to vocal cords
  - T3: Limited to larynx with vocal cord fixation
  - T4a: Invades cricoid or thyroid cartilage or tissues beyond larynx
  - T4b: Invades prevertebral space, mediastinal structures; encases carotid artery
- Major salivary glands:
  - T1: Tumor ≤2 cm in greatest dimension without extraparenchymal extension
  - T2: Tumor 2-4 cm without extraparenchymal extension
  - T3: Tumor >4 cm and/or extraparenchymal extension
  - T4a: Moderately advanced disease that invades skin, mandible, ear canal, or facial nerve
  - T4b: Very advanced disease that invades skull base, pterygoid plates, or encases internal carotid artery

■ **N: Regional lymph nodes**[6,7]

- Single greatest influence on survival is **presence of nodal metastasis.**
- Nodal staging system is generally the same for upper aerodigestive tumors (except nasopharynx) (Fig. 33-2).
  - Nx: Nodes cannot be assessed
  - N0: No nodes containing metastasis
  - N1: A single ipsilateral node metastasis, ≤3 cm in diameter
  - N2a: A single ipsilateral positive node 3-6 cm in diameter
  - N2b: Multiple positive ipsilateral nodes <6 cm in diameter
  - N2c: Bilateral or contralateral positive nodes <6 cm in diameter
  - N3: Nodes >6 cm in diameter

**NOTE: Older designations such as fixed nodes and matted nodes are no longer used.**

■ **M: Distant metastasis**

- M0: No distant metastasis
- M1: Distant metastasis

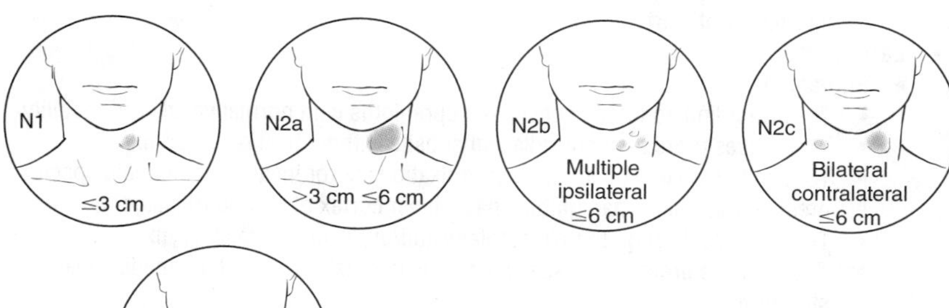


**Fig. 33-2** The nodal staging system is generally the same for upper aerodigestive tumors (except those of the nasopharynx).

## TREATMENT OF THE NECK[8-10]

### GENERAL PRINCIPLES

- Clinical N0 neck options (depends on primary tumor)
  - Observation and serial examinations
  - Neck dissection
  - Radiation
- With clinical N1 neck, comprehensive treatment of neck nodes usually required, either with neck dissection and adjuvant radiotherapy or with primary radiation to 6500 Gy.

### NECK DISSECTION[11-25]

- **Indications**
  - Clinically or radiologically positive lymph nodes
  - Large or rapidly growing tumors, extraglandular extension, facial nerve palsy
  - Aggressive tumors
    - SCC
    - Adenoid cystic
    - Malignant mixed
    - High-grade mucoepidermoid
    - Adenocarcinoma
- **Radical neck dissection (RND)** removes:
  - Lymph nodes in levels I through V
  - SCM muscle
  - Internal jugular vein
  - Spinal accessory nerve (CN XI)
- **Modified radical neck dissection (MRND)**
  - Preserves some or all nonlymphatic structures
  - Type I: Spares CN XI
  - Type II: Spares internal jugular vein and CN XI
  - Type III (functional/Bocca): Spares SCM, internal jugular vein, and CN XI
- **Selective neck dissection**
  - Removes only selected high-risk nodal levels (e.g., levels II through IV)
  - Usually performed on N0 necks
- **Extended neck dissection**
  - Removes more than a standard neck dissection (e.g., the carotid artery)
  - Can still be a modified radical or radical

## SALIVARY TUMORS[26,27]

- **Salivary gland tumors usually require operative intervention.**
- Most salivary gland tumors are in the parotid (80%), submandibular (10%-15%), and sublingual or minor salivary glands (5%-10%).
  - Parotid: 80% benign; 20% malignant
  - Submandibular: 50% benign; 50% malignant
  - Sublingual: 40% benign; 60% malignant
  - Minor salivary: 25% benign; 75% malignant

> **TIP:** The smaller the gland, the higher the incidence of malignancy.

- *All preauricular masses are considered to be of parotid origin unless proven otherwise.*

## Pediatric Salivary Gland Neoplasms

- **Vascular neoplasms are most common.**
- Hemangiomas
  - Present at birth, typically involute by age 5
  - Most common parotid tumor in children
- Lymphangiomas
  - Present in first year of life, rarely involute
  - Consider surgery or sclerosing agents (OK-432).
- **Pleomorphic adenoma is the most common solid tumor.**
- 50% of solid salivary neoplasms are malignant in children.
  - Mucoepidermoid carcinoma is most common.

## Most Common Benign Neoplasms

- **Pleomorphic adenoma**
  - **Most common solid benign tumor (70%)**
  - Most frequently presents as asymptomatic mass in the tail of the parotid
  - Rare facial nerve involvement
  - Parapharyngeal space/deep lobe involvement (10%) may present with intraoral swelling
    - Transoral resection has a higher recurrence rate.
  - Recur if they are shelled out of parotid gland or are incompletely excised
    - If recur then usually reappear as multicentric nodular tumor implants in extraglandular tissue (with increased risk to the facial nerve)
    - 30% recurrence rate for enucleation alone
  - Histology: Myoepithelial component with spindle-shaped cells, epithelial component with variable patterns (solid, trabecular, cystic, papillary), and stromal component with myxoid, chondroid, fibroid, or osteoid components
  - Treatment
    - Superficial parotidectomy with facial nerve preservation for superficial lobe tumors
    - Total parotidectomy for those involving deep lobe
    - Radioresistant
- **Warthin's tumor** (papillary cystadenoma lymphomatosum)
  - **Second most common benign salivary tumor of the parotid**
  - Usually found in male smokers over age 50
  - 10% bilateral, 10% multicentric
  - Technetium 99m uptake because of high mitochondrial content on oncocytes
  - Histology: Biphasic layers—epithelial component with papillary architecture and lymphoid component with mature lymphocytes and germinal centers; cystic spaces abundant
  - Treatment: Superficial or deep parotidectomy with facial nerve preservation

## Most Common Malignant Neoplasms

- **Mucoepidermoid carcinoma**
  - **Most common malignant tumor of the parotid in children and adults**
  - Low grade: Often indolent presentation
    - Translocation t(11;19)
  - High grade: Can be very aggressive
    - Solid sheets of tumor cells
    - Poor prognosis

- **Adenoid cystic carcinoma**
  - **Most common malignant tumor in the submandibular and minor salivary glands**
  - Palate most common site in oral cavity
  - Usually firm, asymptomatic mass
  - Can spread perineurally and metastasize systemically
  - Does not tend to metastasize to cervical lymph nodes
  - Frequently invades extraglandular tissues by direct extension
  - Can recur after many years of disease-free survival
  - Must be followed at regular intervals for life; obtain chest radiographs every year
  - Histology:
    - Cribriform type: Characteristic Swiss-cheese pattern; best prognosis
    - Tubular type: Low grade
    - Solid type: High grade
- **Low-grade malignancies**
  - Low-grade mucoepidermoid
  - Acinic cell carcinoma
- **High-grade malignancies**
  - High-grade mucoepidermoid
  - Adenoid cystic carcinoma
  - SCC
  - Adenocarcinoma
  - Carcinoma ex-pleomorphic adenoma
  - Undifferentiated
- **Malignant mixed tumor**
  - Can develop spontaneously, but many are thought to arise in long-standing benign mixed tumors
  - Aggressive
  - Tend to metastasize early

## SEVEN INDICATIONS FOR ADJUVANT RADIOTHERAPY

1. High-grade malignancies
2. Residual disease
3. Recurrent disease
4. Invasion of adjacent structures/extraglandular extension
5. Close or positive margins
6. Perineural invasion
7. T3 or T4 parotid malignancies

### GENERAL TIPS

- Supraglottic cancers have high rates of occult metastasis and need some form of treatment for the neck (neck dissection or radiation).
- Neck specimens that show greater than N1 disease, or N1 disease that has biologic factors (such as perineural invasion), should be considered for postoperative radiotherapy.
- Bilateral sacrifice of internal jugular veins is survivable but has substantially increased morbidity.
- Postradiation surgery has many more complications.
- Have a low threshold for performing a perioperative tracheotomy.
- Communication is crucial! Talk about a plan in detail ahead of time, because the surgeon who performs the resection may be able to take measures to preserve vessels for free flaps.

- Laryngectomy patients will swallow better if either a pharyngeal plexus neurectomy or cricopharyngeal myotomy is performed at the time of surgery. They will also speak better if using esophageal or tracheoesophageal speech.
- Consider a G-tube early for nutritional support.
- Be very aggressive with delirium tremens prevention postoperatively if there is any suspicion.
- Use high-output drains (especially with the left neck [but possible in the right]) in the early postoperative period or with feeding—be aware of potential chylous fistula.
- Be aware of early spiking fevers as an indicator of pharyngeal fistula.
- First feeding should be with dye before drains are removed to check for fistula (and may help determine aspiration).

## Key Points

- ✓ The single greatest effect on survival is the presence of nodal metastasis.
- ✓ Alcohol and tobacco are predisposing factors for head and neck malignancy.
- ✓ The levels of neck dissection are not the same as the trauma zones of the neck.
- ✓ Mucoepidermoid carcinoma is the most common malignant salivary tumor.
- ✓ Pleomorphic adenoma is the most common benign salivary tumor.
- ✓ Warthin's tumors can be bilateral.

## References


1. Lindberg R. Distribution of cervical lymph node metastases from squamous cell carcinoma of the upper respiratory and digestive tracts. Cancer 29:1446-1449, 1972.
2. Martin H, DelValle B, Ehrlich H, et al. Neck dissection. Cancer 4:441-499, 1951.
3. Medina JE. A rational classification of neck dissections. Otolaryngol Head Neck Surg 100:169-176, 1989.
4. Medina JE, Weisman RA. Management of the neck in head and neck cancer. Part 1. Otolaryngol Clin North Am 31:585-686, 1998.
5. Medina JE, Weisman RA. Management of the neck in head and neck cancer. Part 2. Otolaryngol Clin North Am 31:759-856, 1998.
6. Edge SB, Byrd DR, Compton CC, et al, eds. American Joint Committee on Cancer Staging Handbook, 7th ed. New York: Springer, 2010.
7. Candela FC, Shah J, Jacques DP, et al. Patterns of cervical node metastases from squamous carcinoma of the larynx. Arch Otolaryngol Head Neck Surg 116:432-435, 1990.
8. Johnson JT, Myers EN. Cervical lymph node disease in laryngeal cancer. In Silver CE, ed. Laryngeal Cancer. New York: Thieme, 1991.
9. Kraus DH, Rosenberg DB, Davidson BJ, et al. Supraspinal accessory lymph node metastases in supraomohyoid neck dissection. Am J Surg 172:646-649, 1996.
10. Million RR. Elective neck irradiation of TXN0 squamous carcinoma of the oral tongue and floor of mouth. Cancer 34:149-155, 1974.
11. Anderson PE. The role of comprehensive neck dissection with preservation of the spinal accessory nerve in the clinically positive neck. Am J Surg 168:499-502, 1994.
12. Bocca E, Pignataro O. A conservation technique in radical neck dissection. Ann Otol Rhinol Laryngol 76:975-987, 1967.
13. Pignataro O, Sasaki CT. Functional neck dissection: a description of operative technique. Arch Otolaryngol 106:524-527, 1980.

14. Byers RM, Wolf PF, Ballantyne AJ. Rationale for elective modified neck dissection. Head Neck 10:160-167, 1988.
15. Hoffman HT. Surgical treatment of cervical node metastases from squamous carcinoma of the upper aerodigestive tract: evaluation of the evidence for modifications of neck dissection. Head Neck 23:907-915, 2001.
16. Jaehne M, Ussmüller J, Kehrl W. [Significance of sternocleidomastoid muscle resection in radical neck dissection] HNO 44:661-665, 1996.
17. Robbins TK, Medina JE, Wolfe GT, et al. Standardizing neck dissection terminology: official report of the Academy's Committee for Head and Neck Surgery and Oncology. Arch Otolaryngol Head Neck Surg 117:601-605, 1991.
18. Spiro RH, Strong EW, Shah JP. Classification of neck dissection: variations on a new theme. Am J Surg 168:415-418, 1994.
19. Suen JY, Goepfert H. Standardization of neck dissection nomenclature [editorial]. Head Neck Surg 10:75-77, 1987.
20. Shah JP. Patterns of lymph node metastases from squamous carcinomas of the upper aerodigestive tract. Am J Surg 160:405-409, 1990.
21. Sharpe DT. The pattern of lymph node metastases in intra-oral squamous cell carcinoma. Br J Plast Surg 34:97-101, 1981.
22. Talmi YP, Hoffman HT, Horowitz Z, et al. Patterns of metastases to the upper jugular lymph nodes (the "submuscular recess"). Head Neck 20:682-686, 1998.
23. Teknos TN, Coniglio JU, Netterville JL. Guidelines to patient management. In Bailey BJ, ed. Head and Neck Surgery: Otolaryngology, 2nd ed. Philadelphia: Lippincott Williams & Wilkins, 1998.
24. Cotter CS, Stringer SP, Landau S, et al. Patency of the internal jugular vein following modified radical neck dissection. Laryngoscope 104:841-845, 1994.
25. Crile G. Excision of cancer of the head and neck. J Am Med Assoc 47:1780-1786, 1906.
26. Thackray A, Lucas R, eds. Tumors of the Major Salivary Glands. Atlas of Tumor Pathology, Series 2. Washington, DC: Armed Forces Institute of Pathology, 1974.
27. Witt R. Salivary gland diseases. In Lee KJ, ed. Essential Otolaryngology: Head & Neck Surgery, 10th ed. New York: McGraw-Hill, 2012.

# 34. Scalp and Calvarial Reconstruction

Jason E. Leedy, Smita R. Ramanadham, Jeffrey E. Janis

## APPLIED ANATOMY[1-6]

### SCALP LAYERS (Fig. 34-1)

- Mnemonic: **SCALP**
  - **S** *(skin):* Measures 3-8 mm thick (3 mm at vertex, 8 mm at occiput)[7]
  - **C** *(subcutaneous tissue):* Vessels, lymphatics, and nerves found in this layer
  - **A** *(aponeurotic layer):* Strength layer, continuous with frontalis and occipitalis muscles
  - **L** *(loose areolar tissue):* Also known as subgaleal fascia and innominate fascia; provides scalp mobility; contains emissary veins
  - **P** *(pericranium):* Tightly adherent to calvarium

### CRANIUM LAYERS

- External table
- Diploic space
- Internal table
- Epidural space
- Dura mater
- Subdural space

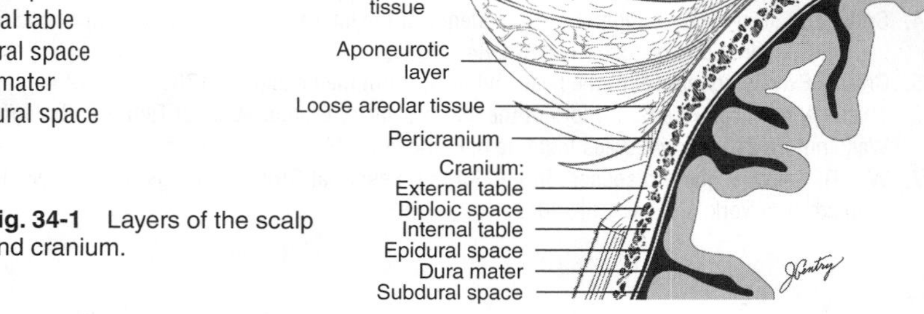


**Fig. 34-1** Layers of the scalp and cranium.

### VASCULARITY (Fig. 34-2)

Arterial branches and venae comitantes of the **internal and external carotid systems** are divided into **four distinct vascular territories.**

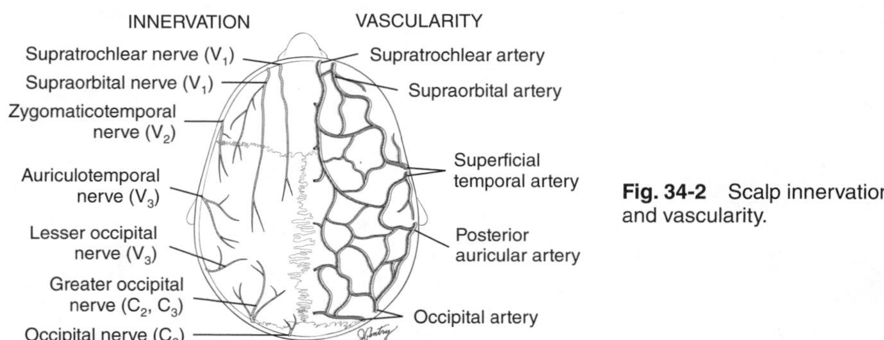


**Fig. 34-2** Scalp innervation and vascularity.

**TIP:** Extensive collateralization of these vascular territories allows total scalp replantation based on a single vascular anastomosis.

- **Anterior territory**
  - **Supraorbital and supratrochlear arteries** (terminal branches of the internal carotid system)
    - Supraorbital artery arises through supraorbital notch or groove, which is located in line with the medial limbus.
    - Supratrochlear arteries arise more medially, usually in plane with the medial canthus.
- **Lateral territory** (largest territory)
  - **Superficial temporal artery** (terminal branch of the external carotid system)
    - Bifurcates at the superior helix of the ear into **frontal** and **parietal** branches
- **Posterior territory**
  - Cephalad to the nuchal line: **Occipital arteries**
  - Caudal to the nuchal line: Perforating branches of the trapezius and splenius capitis muscles
- **Posterolateral territory** (smallest territory)
  - **Posterior auricular artery:** A branch of the external carotid system

## INNERVATION (see Fig. 34-2)

- **Sensory**

Supplied by branches of the three divisions of the trigeminal nerve, cervical spinal nerves, and branches from the cervical plexus

- **Supraorbital nerve**[8]
  - **Superficial division**
    - Pierces the frontalis muscle on the forehead and supplies the skin of the forehead and anterior hairline region
  - **Deep division**
    - Runs superficial to the periosteum to the level of the coronal suture, where it pierces the galeal aponeurosis, approximately 0.5-1.5 cm medial to the superior temporal line, to innervate the frontoparietal scalp
- **Supratrochlear nerve**[9]
  - Terminal branch of $V_1$
  - Smaller than supraorbital nerve
  - Supplies sensation to lower forehead, conjunctiva, upper eyelid skin
- **Zygomaticotemporal nerve**[10]
  - Branches from the maxillary division of the trigeminal nerve
  - Supplies a small region lateral to the brow up to the superficial temporal crest
- **Auriculotemporal nerve**[11]
  - Branches from the mandibular division of the trigeminal nerve
  - Supplies the lateral scalp territory
- **Greater and lesser occipital nerves**[12-14]
  - Branch from the dorsal rami of the cervical spinal nerves and the cervical plexus, respectively
  - Innervate the occipital territory
  - Greater occipital nerve emerges from semispinalis muscle approximately 3 cm below occipital protuberance and 1.5 cm lateral to midline[12]

- **Motor**
  - **Frontal branch of facial nerve (also called temporal branch)**
    - Supplies the frontalis muscle
    - See Chapters 29, 37, and 80 for anatomic location

- **Posterior auricular branch of facial nerve**
  - ▸ Supplies the anterior and posterior auricular muscles, occipitalis muscle
- **Lymphatics**[15]
  - Network is subdermal and subcutaneous and is in association with medium-sized blood vessels.
  - The scalp is devoid of lymph nodes and therefore has no barriers to lymphatic flow.
  - System drains toward the parotid gland, preauricular and postauricular regions, upper neck, and occiput.

## SKIN BIOMECHANICS[16]

Skin biomechanics are important for understanding tissue expansion reconstruction of the scalp.

- **Stress relaxation:** Property of skin that decreases the amount of force necessary to maintain a fixed amount of skin stretch over time
- **Creep:** Skin property whereby skin gains surface area when a constant load is applied
  - As force is applied to a leading skin edge, tissue thickness decreases from extrusion of fluid and mucopolysaccharides, realignment of dermal collagen bundles, elastic fiber microfragmentation, and mechanical stretching of the skin.

## GOALS OF SCALP RECONSTRUCTION[17,18]

- Tension-free closure of defect
- Maintenance of motor and sensory function when possible
- Maintenance of contour
- Maintenance of brow symmetry and hairline
- Protection of cranium/dura/brain

**TIP:** Place scars along relaxed skin tension lines.[17]

**TIP:** Ensure negative margins before definitive oncologic reconstruction.

## PRINCIPLES OF SCALP RECONSTRUCTION

- **Replace tissue with like tissue.**
  - Use adjacent scalp for reconstruction if possible.
  - **Incorporate at least one main-named scalp vessel into flaps.**
  - **Consider using scalp tissue from the parietal region** where scalp mobility is the greatest because of the superficial temporal fascial gliding over the deep temporal fascia.
  - **Only debride devitalized tissue in acute repair of traumatic defects,** because robust vascularity of the scalp may allow recovery of marginal tissues.
- **Consider tissue expansion.**[19,20]
  - It is useful when local tissue rearrangements are inadequate for reconstruction because of the size of the defect, traumatized local tissue, unacceptable rearrangement of hair patterns, or distortion of the hairline.
  - During the expansion process, exposed bone can be covered temporarily with split-thickness skin grafts either after burring of the outer table or coverage with pericranial flaps.
  - As expansion increases, hair density can decrease.

- **Approximately 50% of the scalp can be reconstructed with tissue expansion before alopecia becomes a significant issue.**

**CAUTION: Avoid expansion in irradiated or infected scalp.**

**TIP:** Local anesthetic with dilute epinephrine decreases intraoperative skin edge bleeding and can be used to hydrodissect the subgaleal plane.

**Minimize the use of hemostatic clips and electrocautery on cut edges of the scalp** to prevent potential follicular damage and subsequent iatrogenic alopecia.

**Score the galea perpendicular to the direction of desired tissue gain to prevent** injury to the scalp arteries that lie superficial to the galea. Scoring in 1 cm increments will gain 1.67 mm for each relaxing incision.

Closure requires **approximation of the galea,** because it is the strength layer.

Skin grafts are a viable option for coverage for all locations; however, they require a vascularized bed. If pericranium is not intact, burring of the outer cortex causes bleeding needed for granulation tissue.

Healing by secondary intention provides acceptable aesthetic results and will not cause significant contractures.

## GUIDELINES FOR RECONSTRUCTION[18]

Reconstructive options vary depending on the defect's cause, location, and size. An algorithmic approach is useful.

### ANTERIOR DEFECTS (Fig. 34-3)

- **Location:** The area posterior to the anterior hairline and anterior to the plane of the superficial temporal vessels in front of the root of the helix
- **Principles:** Re-creation of the anterior hairline without derangement of native hairline or creation of dog-ears in cosmetically sensitive areas; undermining of forehead for greater tissue gain without derangement of brow symmetry or position.

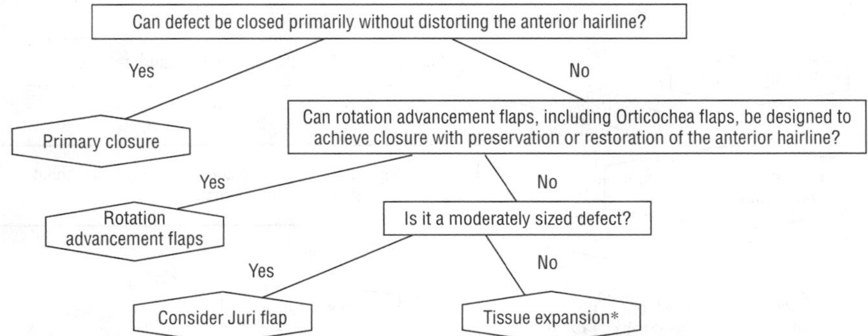


**Fig. 34-3** Algorithm for reconstruction of anterior defects.

- **Small defects (<2 cm$^2$)**
  - Primary closure after undermining
  - Advancement flaps based on subcutaneous pedicles
  - Small rotation advancement flaps
- **Moderate defects (2-25 cm$^2$)**
  - V-Y flaps, V-Y-S flaps, subcutaneous pedicled flaps, rotation advancement flaps
  - Anterior hairline reconstruction: Temporoparietaloccipital flaps or the lateral scalp flap, as described for correction of male pattern baldness
- **Large defects (>25 cm$^2$)**
  - Temporoparietaloccipital flaps
  - Large rotation advancement flaps with back-grafting of the donor site to restore anterior hair and move the defect (incision usually needs to be 4-6 times the size of defect[19])
  - **Orticochea flaps**
    - Two flaps for reconstructing the defect, each based off the superficial temporal vessels, and one large flap based off the occipitals to fill the donor defect
    - Can result in significant alopecia and unnatural hair orientation
- **Tissue expansion**

## Parietal Defects (Fig. 34-4)

- **Location:** Parietal scalp territory (generally supplied by superficial temporal vessels)
- **Principles:** Defects in the parietal scalp are amenable to local tissue rearrangement as a result of high scalp mobility in this region. They are less likely to have exposed bone because of the underlying temporalis muscle and fascia. Avoid sideburn displacement.
- **Small defects (<2 cm$^2$)**
  - Primary closure
  - V-Y flaps, subcutaneous pedicled flaps, and rhomboid flaps possible for temporal sideburn reconstruction
- **Medium defects (2-25 cm$^2$)**
  - Rotation advancement flaps
  - Bilobed flaps

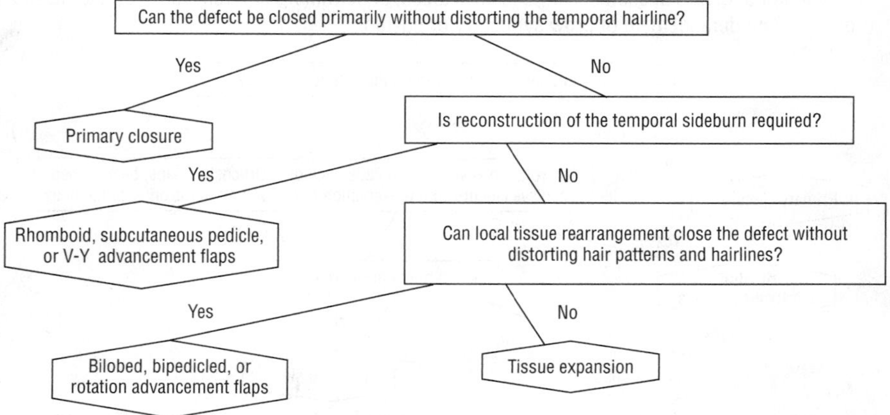


**Fig. 34-4** Algorithm for reconstruction of parietal defects.

- **Large defects (>25 cm$^2$)**
  - **Tissue expansion** is often the only technique available for satisfactory reconstruction.
  - Large bipedicled frontooccipital flaps with large areas of back-grafting have been described but are best reserved for single-stage reconstruction when excellent cosmesis is not required.

## Occipital Defects (Fig. 34-5)

- **Location:** Posterior scalp
- **Principles:** Region of moderate scalp mobility amenable to local tissue transfer; may require restoration or preservation of the occipital hairline
- **Small defects (<2 cm$^2$)**
  - Primary closure
- **Medium defects (2-25 cm$^2$)**
  - Rotation advancement flaps: Dissection carried over the trapezius and splenius capitis muscles to provide increased tissue gain
- **Large defects (>25 cm$^2$)**
  - Larger rotation flaps
  - **Orticochea flaps**[21] (Fig. 34-6)
    - These are classically described for reconstruction of the occipital scalp.
    - Three-flap technique improves flap vascularity over the four-flap technique and decreases postoperative alopecia and wound complications.

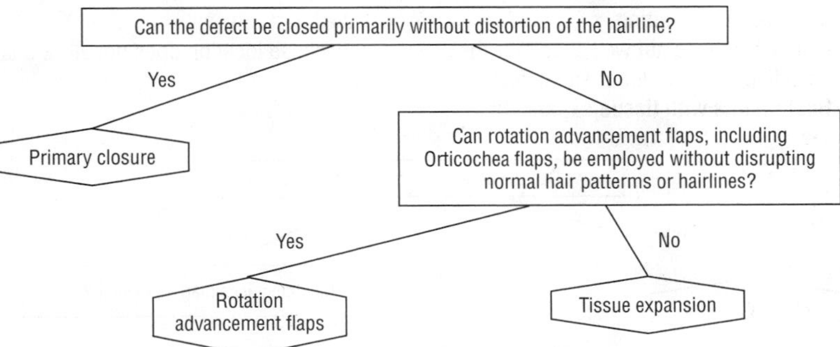


**Fig. 34-5** Algorithm for reconstruction of occipital defects.

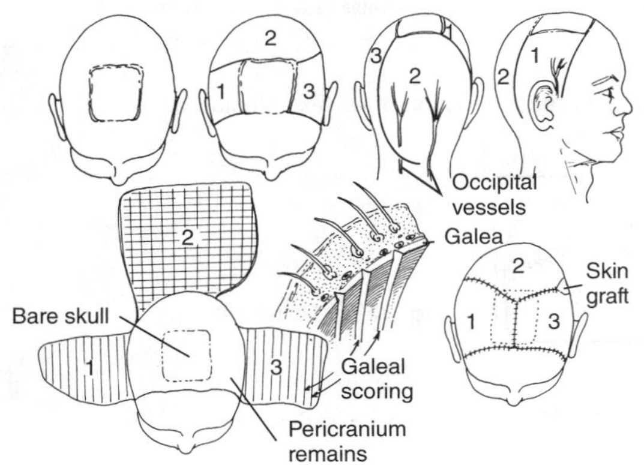


**Fig. 34-6** Orticochea three-flap technique.

**TIP:** Tissue expansion routinely gives a superior result.

Pedicled myocutaneous flaps can be used for lower occipital or temporal defects (i.e., latissimus dorsi, pectoralis, trapezius flaps[19])

## VERTEX DEFECTS (Fig. 34-7)

- **Location:** Central scalp
- **Principles:** Area of limited scalp mobility; requires extensive undermining and recruitment of tissue from the more mobile regions; characteristic whorl pattern of hair growth should be preserved
- **Small defects (<2 cm²)**
  - Primary closure after subgaleal dissection; up to 4 cm wide described
  - Pinwheel flaps and adjacent rhomboid flaps particularly suited to reconstructing whorl pattern[19] (Fig. 34-8)
- **Medium defects (2-25 cm²)**
  - Pinwheel and rhomboid flaps less useful but possible alternatives
  - Double-opposing rotation advancement flaps with incisions parallel to the hairline to prevent distortion; can decrease incision length, because recruitment is from both sides
  - Rotation advancement from the occiput with back-grafting of the donor site
- **Large defects (>25 cm²)**
  - Large rotation flaps that require almost complete scalp undermining and galeal scoring and possible back-grafting
  - Orticochea flaps **not** well suited for these defects, because location does not allow a large third flap to cover donor site defect
  - **Best results with tissue expansion**

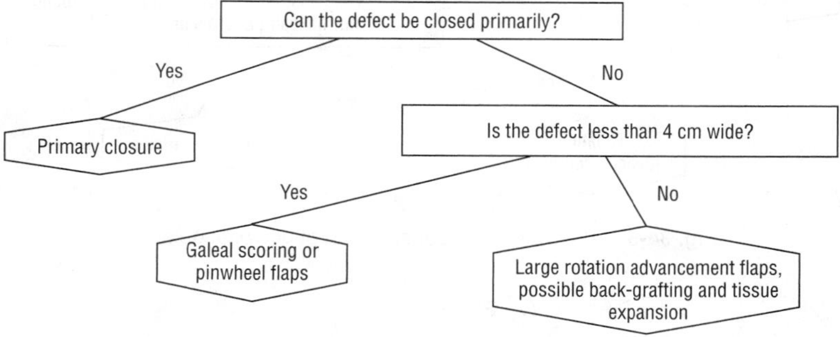


**Fig. 34-7** Algorithm for reconstruction of vertex defects.

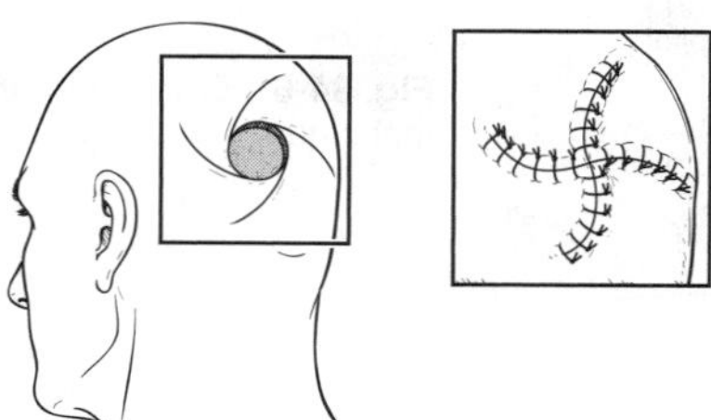

**Fig. 34-8** Pinwheel flap.

### Near-Total Defects[22-26]

- **Free tissue transfer:** Latissimus dorsi muscle, omentum, radial forearm fasciocutaneous, anterolateral thigh
  - Muscle flaps atrophy and contour well to skull over time; however, they can thin excessively and may result in exposed bone.
  - Viability is increased especially in the setting of radiation.
  - Risk of cerebrospinal fluid fistula or leak or alloplastic extrusion is decreased.
- **Serial tissue expansion**
- **Integra** (Integra LifeSciences, Plainsboro, NJ) followed by skin grafting

> **TIP:** Integra is associated with decreased morbidity and mortality and decreased operative time. It can add soft tissue bulk and contour and can be beneficial in oncologic reconstruction when margins are pending.[26]

### Hair Replacement[19]

- This is performed in the secondary setting.
- Recently, **follicular unit grafting** has become popular.
- Incisional split graft is preferred over punch grafting, because it is associated with increased vascularity and density of follicles.

## CALVARIAL RECONSTRUCTION[28-35]

The goal is to provide protection for the brain and maintain normal calvarial shape.

### Surgical Options

- **Autogenous tissue:** Preferred option. Benefits include its biocompatibility, resistance to infection, and increased strength; however, it can be associated with difficulty in contouring, resorption, donor site availability, and morbidity.
  - **Split calvarial bone graft: Parietal bone** preferred because of increased thickness and absence of underlying venous sinuses
  - **Split rib graft:** If periosteum left intact, the rib should regenerate
- **Alloplastic materials:** Benefits include its unlimited supply and lack of donor site morbidity; however, it does not integrate with recipient site bone, is associated with increased infections, and can be costly and brittle.
  - It can be biodegradable or nonbiodegradable.
  - Options include methylmethacrylate, titanium mesh, hydroxyapatite, acrylic, and polyetheretherketone (PEEK).
- Tissue engineering can provide autologous bioengineered alternatives for calvarial reconstruction in the future.

> **TIP:** Computer-designed prefabrication can decrease operative time and aid in contouring and insetting.

## Key Points

- ✓ Scalp avulsions usually occur in the subgaleal plane.
- ✓ The scalp is highly vascularized and can be replanted from a single artery.
- ✓ Most scalp mobility occurs over the parietal region because of the temporoparietal fascia.
- ✓ Galeal scoring can aid in achieving primary closure or decreasing the size of the defect for further reconstruction.
- ✓ Avoid distortion of the hairline and brow position.
- ✓ Consider tissue expansion to achieve coverage with like tissue with acceptable scar placement.

## References


1. Abdul-Hassan HS, von Drasek Ascher G, Acland RD. Surgical anatomy and blood supply of the fascial layers of the temporal region. Plast Reconstr Surg 77:17-28, 1986.
2. Tolhurst DE, Carstens MH, Greco RJ, et al. The surgical anatomy of the scalp. Plast Reconstr Surg 87:603-612, 1991.
3. Williams PL, Warwick R, eds. Gray's Anatomy, 36th British ed. Philadelphia: WB Saunders, 1980.
4. Anson BJ, McVay CB, eds. Surgical Anatomy, 6th ed. Philadelphia: WB Saunders, 1984.
5. Anderson JE, ed. Grant's Atlas of Anatomy, 8th ed. Baltimore: Williams & Wilkins, 2011.
6. Last RJ, ed. Anatomy, Regional and Applied, 12th ed. London: Churchill Livingstone, 1979.
7. Preis FW, Urzola V, Mangano A, et al. Subtotal scalp reconstruction after traumatic avulsion: a technical note. J Craniofac Surg 18:650-653, 2007.
8. Janis JE, Ghavami A, Lemmon JA, et al. The anatomy of the corrugator supercilii muscle revisited. Part 2. Supraorbital nerve topography. Plast Reconstr Surg 121:233-240, 2008.
9. Janis JE, Hatef DA, Hagan R, et al. Anatomy of the supratrochlear nerve: implications for the surgical treatment of migraine headaches. Plast Reconstr Surg 131:743-750, 2013.
10. Janis JE, Hatef DA, Thakar H, et al. The zygomaticotemporal branch of the trigeminal nerve. Part 2. Anatomic variations. Plast Reconstr Surg 126:435-442, 2010.
11. Janis JE, Hatef DA, Ducic I, et al. Anatomy of the auriculotemporal nerve: variations in its relationship to the superficial temporal artery and implications for the treatment of migraine headaches. Plast Reconstr Surg 125:1422-1428, 2010.
12. Mosser SW, Guyuron B, Janis JE, et al. The anatomy of the greater occipital nerve: implication for the etiology of migraine headaches. Plast Reconstr Surg 113:693-697, 2004.
13. Janis JE, Hatef DA, Ducic I, et al. The anatomy of the greater occipital nerve. Part 2. Compression point topography. Plast Reconstr Surg 126:1563-1572, 2010.
14. Dash K, Janis JE, Guyuron B. The lesser and third occipital nerves and migraine headaches. Plast Reconstr Surg 115:1752-1758, 2005.
15. Earnest LM, Byrne PJ. Scalp reconstruction. Facial Plast Surg Clin N Am 13:345-353, 2005.
16. Jackson IT. General considerations. In Jackson IT, ed. Local Flaps in Head and Neck Reconstruction, 2nd ed. St Louis: Quality Medical Publishing, 2007.
17. Angelos PC, Downs BW. Options for the management of forehead and scalp defects. Facial Plast Surg Clin N Am 17:379-393, 2009.
18. Leedy JE, Janis JE, Rohrich RJ. Reconstruction of acquired scalp defects: an algorithmic approach. Plast Reconstr Surg 116:54e-72e, 2005.
19. Lee S, Rafii AA, Sykes J. Advances in scalp reconstruction. Curr Opin Otolaryngol Head Neck Surg 14:249-253, 2006.

20. Manders ER, Graham WP, Schenden MJ, et al. Skin expansion to eliminate large scalp defects. Ann Plast Surg 12:305-312, 1984.
21. Arnold PG, Rangarathnam CS. Multiple-flap scalp reconstruction: Orticochea revisited. Plast Reconstr Surg 69:605-613, 1982.
22. Lutz BS, Wei FC, Chen HC, et al. Reconstruction of scalp defects with free flaps in 30 cases. Br J Plast Surg 51:186-190, 1998.
23. Pennington DG, Stern HS, Lee KK. Free-flap reconstruction of large defects of the scalp and calvarium. Plast Reconstr Surg 83:655-661, 1985.
24. Chicarilli ZN, Ariyan S, Cuono CB. Single-stage repair of complex scalp and cranial defects with the free radial forearm flap. Plast Reconstr Surg 77:577-585, 1986.
25. Davidson SO, Capone AC. Scalp reconstruction with inverted myocutaneous latissimus free flap and unmeshed skin graft. J Reconstr Microsurg 27:261-266, 2011.
26. Labow BI, Rosen H, Pap SA, et al. Microsurgical reconstruction: a more conservative method of managing large scalp defects? J Reconstr Microsurg 25:465-474, 2009.
27. Komorowska-Timek E, Gabriel A, Bennett D, et al. Artificial dermis as an alternative for coverage of complex scalp defects following excision of malignant tumors. Plast Reconstr Surg 115:1010-1017, 2005.
28. Freund RM. Scalp, calvarium and forehead reconstruction. In Aston SJ, Beasley RW, Thorne CH, eds. Grabb and Smith's Plastic Surgery. Philadelphia: Lippincott Williams & Wilkins, 1997.
29. Shestak KC, Ramasastry SS. Reconstruction of defects of the scalp and skull. In Cohen M, ed. Mastery of Plastic and Reconstructive Surgery, vol 2. Philadelphia: Lippincott Williams & Wilkins, 1994.
30. Elliott LF, Jurkiewicz MJ. Scalp and calvarium. In Jurkiewicz MJ, Mathes SJ, Krizek TJ, et al, eds. Plastic Surgery: Principles and Practice. St Louis: CV Mosby, 1990.
31. Marchac D. Deformities of the forehead, scalp, and cranial vault. In McCarthy JG, ed. Plastic Surgery. Philadelphia: WB Saunders, 1990.
32. Sood R. Scalp and calvarial reconstruction. In Achauer BM, Eriksson E, Kolk CV, et al, eds. Plastic Surgery: Indications, Operations, and Outcomes, vol 3. St Louis: Mosby–Year Book, 2000.
33. Hanasono MH, Goel N, Demonte F. Calvarial reconstruction with polyetheretherketone implants. Ann Plast Surg 62:653-655, 2009.
34. Chim H, Schantz J. New frontiers in calvarial reconstruction: integrating computer-assisted design and tissue engineering in cranioplasty. Plast Reconstr Surg 116:1726-1741, 2005.
35. Ducic Y. Reconstruction of the scalp. Facial Plast Surg Clin N Am 17:177-187, 2009.

# 35. Eyelid Reconstruction

Jason K. Potter, Adam H. Hamawy

## EYELID ANATOMY[1]

- The eyelids protect the eye from injury and excessive light and prevent desiccation of the cornea (Fig. 35-1).
- The eyelids consist of **two lamellae** separated by the orbital septum:
  1. **Outer lamella:** Skin and orbicularis oculi muscle
  2. **Inner lamella:** Tarsal plate, medial/lateral canthal tendons, capsulopalpebral fascia, and conjunctiva

**NOTE: The orbital septum is sometimes referred to as the *middle lamella.***

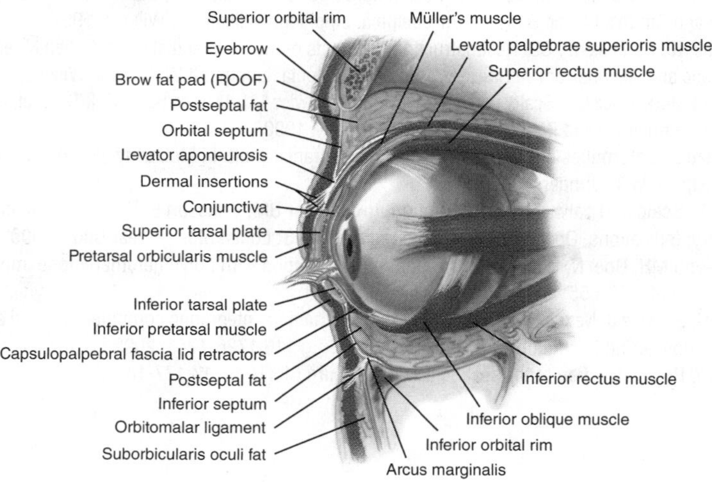


**Fig. 35-1** Anatomy of the eyelid.

### SKIN

- **Eyelid skin is the thinnest in the body,** measuring 0.3 mm in some areas.
- Surgical incisions within the skin of the eyelid generally heal with almost imperceptible scarring.

### ORBICULARIS OCULI (Fig. 35-2)

- Encircles the periorbital region
- Primary constrictor of the lids

- Innervated by the facial nerve (CN VII); runs on deep surface of the muscle
- **Pretarsal fibers:** Lie over region of tarsal plate
  - Responsible for involuntary blink, lower lid tone, and lacrimal pumping mechanism
- **Preseptal fibers:** Overlie orbital septum
  - Assist with blink
- **Orbital fibers:** Overlie orbital rims
  - Responsible for eyelid squeezing, forceful closure, and animated eyelid movements

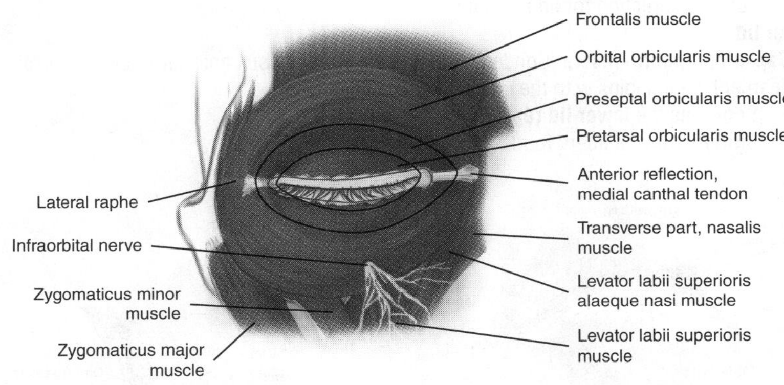


**Fig. 35-2** Muscular anatomy of the periorbital region.

## Orbital Septum (Palpebral Pigment)

- Dense fibrous membrane attached to periosteum of orbital rim; extends through lid to join tarsus
- Separates orbital contents from periorbital soft tissues

## Tarsal Plate

- Located adjacent to lid margin
- Approximately 1-2 mm thick and 25 mm long
- Laterally, tarsi become joined fibrous condensations and form canthal tendons
- **Upper lid**
  - Approximately 12-15 mm in vertical height
  - Superior margin: Attachment site for Müller's muscle and levator aponeurosis
- **Lower lid**
  - Approximately 4-10 mm in vertical height
  - Inferior margin continuous with capsulopalpebral fascia

## Conjunctiva

- Mucosal layer adjacent to the surface of eye
  - **Palpebral portion** lines inner surface of eyelid.
  - **Bulbar portion** lines sclera.

## Eyelid Retractors[2] (Fig. 35-3)

- **Upper lid**
  - Müller's muscle: Innervated by the sympathetic nervous system
    - Arises from inferior surface of the levator and inserts onto superior edge of the tarsus
    - *Loss of Müller's muscle function results in 2-3 mm of ptosis.*
  - Levator palpebrae superioris: Innervated by the superior division of CN III
    - Originates from the lesser wing of the sphenoid, above the optic foramen, and extends forward to insert onto the superior edge of the tarsus
    - Whitnall's ligament serves as fulcrum to redirect the vector of pull from horizontal to superior direction for lid retraction.
- **Lower lid**
  - **Capsulopalpebral fascia:** Condensation of fibroelastic tissue anterior to Lockwood's ligament, which joins with the inferior tarsus
    - Serves as the **lower lid retractor**
    - Smooth muscle fibers found in this condensation

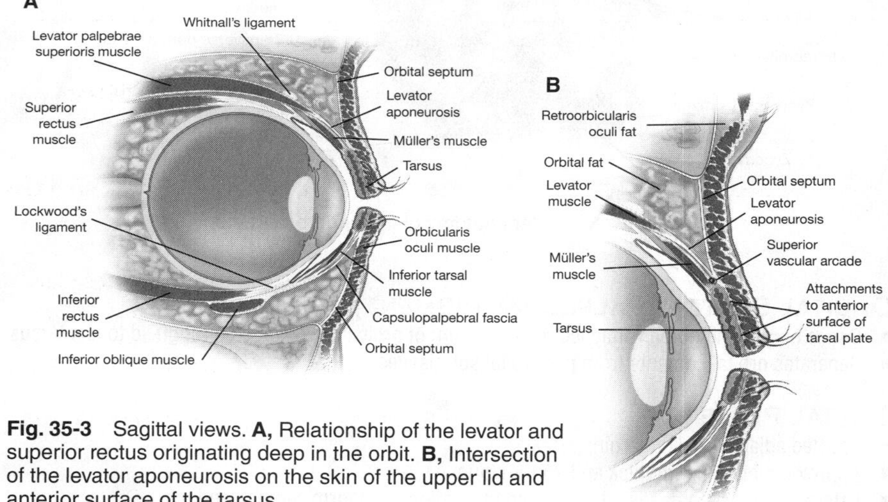


**Fig. 35-3** Sagittal views. **A,** Relationship of the levator and superior rectus originating deep in the orbit. **B,** Intersection of the levator aponeurosis on the skin of the upper lid and anterior surface of the tarsus.

## Blood Supply (Fig. 35-4)

- The **marginal and peripheral arcades** in the supratarsal space and between Müller's muscle and levator aponeurosis provide primary blood supply to the upper lids. They are ~2-3 mm from the lid margin. In the lower lid the arcade travels in the infratarsal space along the lower tarsal border.
- Contributions are made from both the external and internal carotid systems.
- The **upper lid** is supplied primarily by **branches of the ophthalmic artery.**
- The **lower lid** is supplied primarily by **branches of the facial artery.**

## Innervation

- Sensory innervation is provided by the **trigeminal nerve**.
  - The **upper lid** is supplied by the **first division ($V_1$).**
  - The **lower lid** is supplied by the **second division ($V_2$).**

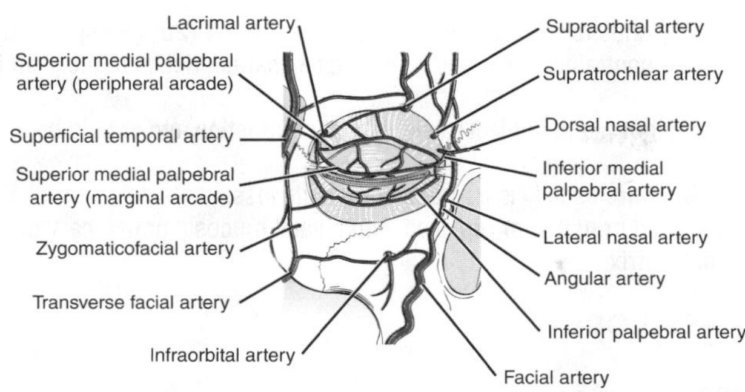


**Fig. 35-4** Arterial supply to the upper lid.

## GENERAL PRINCIPLES[3,4]

Eyelid reconstruction requires thorough assessment of involved structures and estimation of the amount of missing lid tissue.

- Selection of appropriate reconstructive technique is based on **partial- versus full-thickness loss** and, more important, the **amount of missing tissue.**
- *Lid tissue is best reconstructed with lid tissue* for optimal aesthetic outcome.

**CAUTION: Use techniques that borrow tissue from the upper lid cautiously, because the upper lid makes significant contributions to lid function and protection.**

- Defects of up to **30%** of the lid usually can be closed **primarily.**
- Defects of **30%-50%** usually can be closed directly with addition of a **lateral canthotomy and cantholysis.**
- Defects of **50%-75%** usually can be closed with **myocutaneous advancement flaps.**
- Defects >**75%** generally require bringing **tissue from the opposite lid or adjacent regions** (cheek, temporal, forehead).
- Newly reconstructed lids should be adequately anchored by canthal fixation or direct closure of eyelid margin to curtail postoperative sequelae.

## DEFECTS

### PARTIAL-THICKNESS LOSS

- **Skin**
  - Loss of skin may be closed primarily or replaced with full-thickness skin grafts (FTSGs).
  - **FTSGs** are indicated to prevent excessive graft contraction.
  - **Skin from the contralateral lid** is the best source for a thickness match. Alternatively, postauricular skin may be used.

**TIP:** It is imperative not to create tension on the lid with primary closure, because this leads to ectropion.

- **Conjunctiva**
  - Conjunctiva is best replaced by advancement of an **adjacent sliding transconjunctival flap.** When this is not possible, grafting is necessary.
    - ▸ **Buccal or nasal mucosa** provides adequate donor graft.

- Nasal mucosa tends to contract less than buccal mucosa (20% versus 50%).
- Skin grafts are contraindicated, because surface characteristics of the graft irritate the cornea.
- Grafts of conjunctiva are subject to significant contraction and should be avoided.

- **Tarsus**
  - Loss of tarsal structure usually is part of a composite loss.
  - It should be repaired primarily or replaced with palatal mucosal grafts, cartilage grafts, or acellular dermal matrix.

## FULL-THICKNESS LOSS

- **Upper lid**
  - **Direct closure**
    - Defects up to 25%-30% of the lid may be closed primarily[5] (Fig. 35-5).
    - In older patients with significant laxity, 40% defects may be closed similarly.
    - When significant tension is present, lateral canthotomy and cantholysis may provide additional laxity for closure.
    - Precise approximation of tarsal plate is critical for proper lid "skeletal" support.
  - **Flap reconstruction**[6] (Table 35-1)
    - **Tenzel semicircular flap**
      - Combining lateral canthotomy and cantholysis with a laterally based myocutaneous flap allows closure of defects of up to 60% of the upper lid[5] (Fig. 35-6).

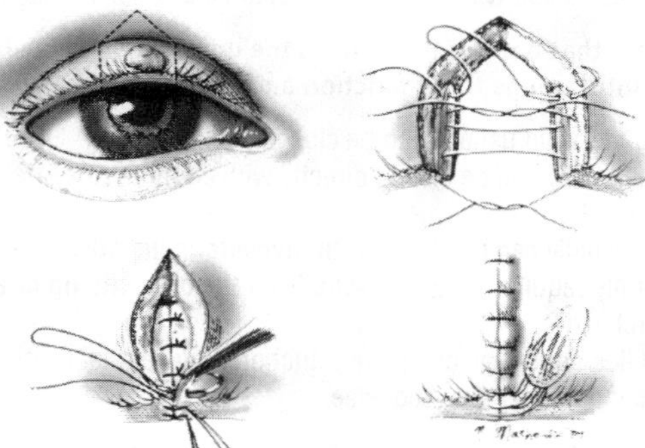

**Fig. 35-5** Upper lid full-thickness excisions must be meticulously repaired in layers to avoid postoperative notching.

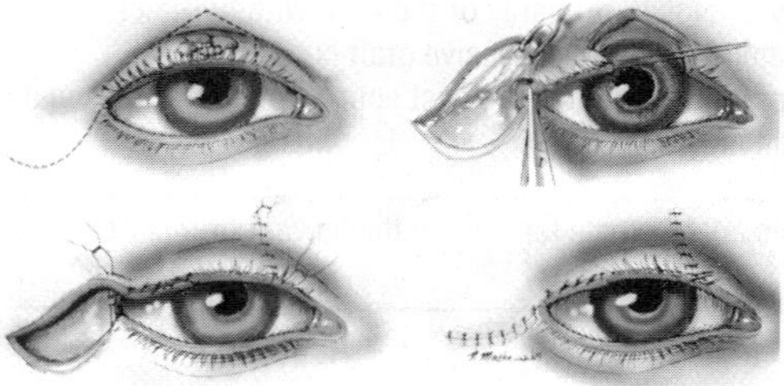

**Fig. 35-6** The semicircular rotation flap, or Tenzel flap, is used for defects of 40%-60% of the upper eyelid. Lateral canthotomy is required to rotate the flap and lateral remaining lid margin.

**Table 35-1** *Indications, Advantages, and Disadvantages of Different Flaps Used for Eyelid Reconstruction*

| | Indications | Advantages | Disadvantages |
|---|---|---|---|
| **Flaps for Upper Eyelid Reconstruction** | | | |
| Direct closure | Defects of 20%-30% of upper lid | Lash continuity | Ptosis possible with tight closure |
| Sliding tarsoconjunctival flap | Medial or lateral posterior lamella defects | One-step procedure<br>Composite flap (tarsus and conjunctiva) | No lash restoration<br>Requires anterior lamella coverage |
| Bridge (Cutler-Beard) flap | Full-thickness defects of the entire upper lid | Reconstruction of total upper lid defects | Two-stage procedure<br>No lash restoration<br>Risk of lower lid ectropion<br>Need for tarsal replacement |
| Lower lid–sharing (Mustarde) flap | Broad, shallow, full-thickness marginal defects of 30%-60% of the upper lid | Lash continuity | Two-stage procedure<br>May need Tenzel flap to close donor site |
| Semicircular rotation (Tenzel) flap | Anterior lamella defects of up to 60% of the eyelid | Reconstruction of large anterior lamella defects | No lash restoration<br>Requires posterior lamella coverage |
| Temporal (Fricke) flap | Anterior lamella defects of the entire upper lid | Reconstruction of large anterior lamella defects | Two-stage procedure<br>Donor skin very thick<br>Risk of frontal branch lesion |
| **Flaps for Lower Eyelid Reconstruction** | | | |
| Direct closure | Defects of 20% of the lower lid | Lash continuity | Ectropion possible with tight closure |
| Advancement tarsoconjunctival (modified Hughes) flap | Posterior lamella defects of the entire lower lid | Reconstruction of large posterior lamella defects; composite flap (tarsus and conjunctiva) | Two-stage procedure<br>Requires anterior lamella coverage |
| Tarsoconjunctival (Hughes) flap | Large, shallow, posterior lamella defects of the lid | Reconstruction of large posterior lamella defects<br>Composite flap (tarsus and conjunctiva) | Two-stage procedure<br>Requires anterior lamella coverage |
| Semicircular rotation (Tenzel) flap | Anterior lamella defects of up to 60% of the eyelid | Reconstruction of large anterior lamella defects | No lash restoration<br>Requires posterior lamella coverage |
| Vertical myocutaneous cheek lift | Broad shallow defects of the anterior lamella | One-stage procedure<br>Natural result | Requires anterior lamella coverage<br>Risk of lower lid malposition<br>No lash restoration |
| Tripier flap | Anterior lamella defects of the entire lower lid | Reconstruction of large anterior lamella defects of the lower lid<br>Thin donor skin | Two-stage procedure<br>Requires posterior lamella coverage<br>Distal part of the unipedicled flap may be unreliable |
| Rotation cheek (Mustarde) flap | Deep vertical defects of the entire lower lid | Reconstruction of large anterior lamella defects of the lower eyelid | Thick donor skin<br>Risk of lower lid malposition<br>Requires posterior lamella coverage |
| Temporal (Fricke) flap | Anterior lamella defects of the entire lower lid | Reconstruction of large anterior lamella defects | Two-stage procedure<br>Donor skin very thick<br>Risk of frontal branch lesion<br>Requires posterior lamella coverage |

- **Cutler-Beard flap**[5] (Fig. 35-7)
  - Two-stage procedure
  - Entails advancement of a full-thickness lower lid flap passed beneath the lower lid margin and sutured into the defect
  - Lacks support at the lid margin and requires cartilage grafting between the conjunctiva and muscle layers
  - Flap division performed at 3-6 weeks
- **Lid-sharing flap (Mustarde pedicled flap)**[2] (Fig. 35-8)
  - Used for defects of the central upper lid
  - Flap divided about week 6 and donor site closed primarily
- **Temporal forehead flap (Fricke flap)**
  - When adequate lid tissue is unavailable for donor tissue, temporally based flaps may be useful.
  - Tissue quality is thicker and less ideal; it should be reserved for special circumstances[2] (Fig. 35-9).

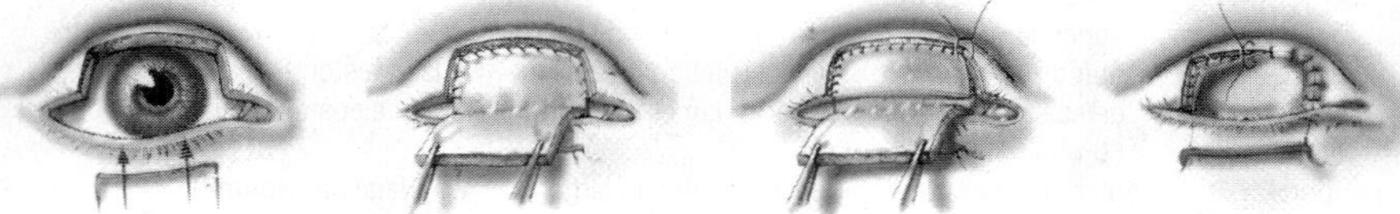

**Fig. 35-7** The bridge flap, or Cutler-Beard flap, is used for total upper lid reconstruction. The flap is a biplanar flap passed under the lower lid margin.

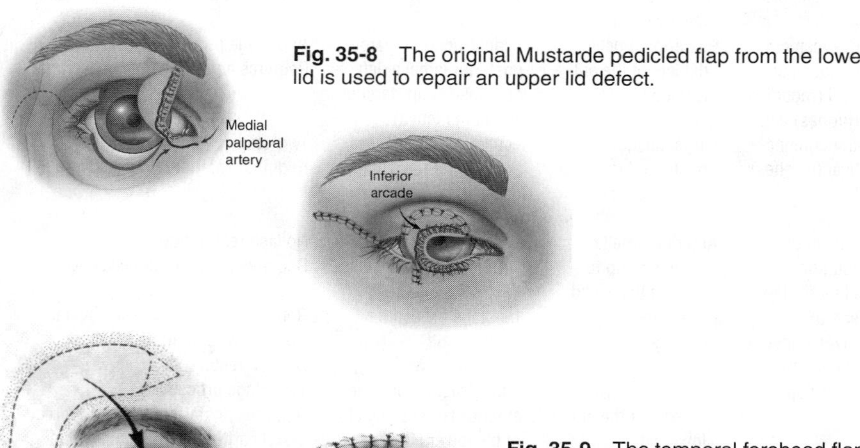


**Fig. 35-8** The original Mustarde pedicled flap from the lower lid is used to repair an upper lid defect.

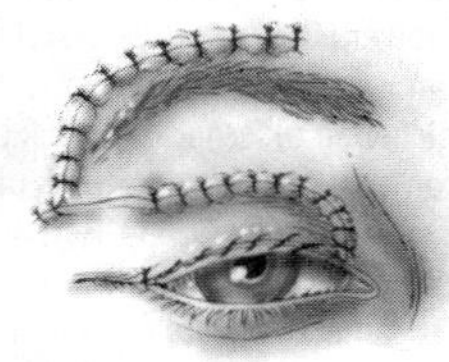

**Fig. 35-9** The temporal forehead flap, or Fricke flap, is a transposition flap from above the eyebrow, used for total upper lid reconstruction.

- **Paramedian forehead flap**[5] (Fig. 35-10)
  - Useful for extensive defects
  - Can be lined with mucosal grafts and cartilage, with delayed placement when needed for lid margin support

■ **Lower lid**

- **Direct closure**
  - Defects of up to 25%-30% of the lid may be closed primarily.
  - In older patients with significant laxity, 40% defects may be closed similarly.

**TIP:** When significant tension is present, lateral canthotomy and cantholysis may provide additional laxity for closure.

- **Flap reconstruction** (see Table 35-1)
  - **Tripier flap**[4] (Fig. 35-11)
    - Myocutaneous flap used for partial-thickness coverage of lower lid
    - Originally described as a bipedicled flap; may be based on a single pedicle

**TIP:** Defects that extend past the pupil usually require a bipedicled technique to prevent distal necrosis.

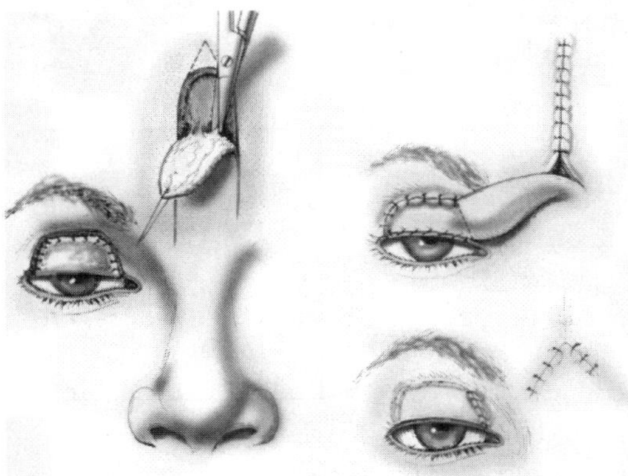

**Fig. 35-10** A forehead flap can be used for total upper lid reconstruction, combined with a mucosal graft for a lining against the cornea.

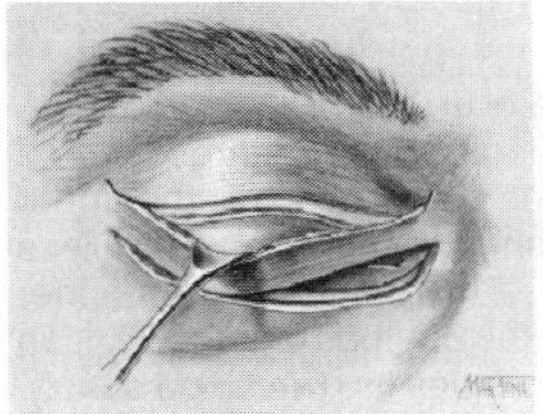

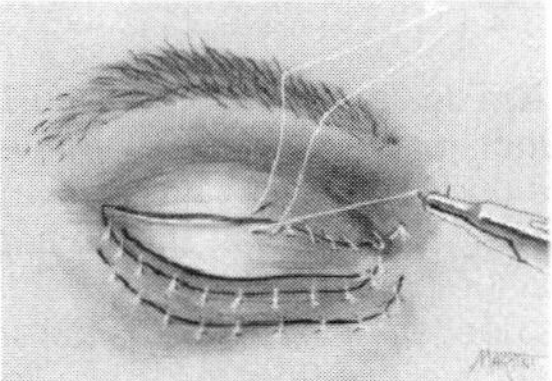

**Fig. 35-11** Lower eyelid reconstruction with a modified bipedicled myocutaneous (Tripier) flap from the upper lid. The flap pedicles are incorporated into the wound.

- **Tenzel semicircular flap** (Fig. 35-12)
  - Combine lateral canthotomy and cantholysis with a laterally based myocutaneous flap for closure of defects of up to 60% of the upper lid.
  - Additional support may be provided with periosteal flap, cartilage, or other homologous graft.
- **Hughes tarsoconjunctival flap**[2,8] (Fig. 35-13)
  - Two-stage procedure; transfers conjunctival lining and a small portion of the superior tarsus for subtotal or total lower lid reconstruction.
  - Skin coverage provided by flap or FTSG; flap divided at 4-6 weeks

**Fig. 35-12** Repair of a lower lid defect with a myocutaneous semicircular flap. The *shaded area* represents the skin-muscle tissue that usually needs to be resected to approximate lid edges after the flap has been rotated.

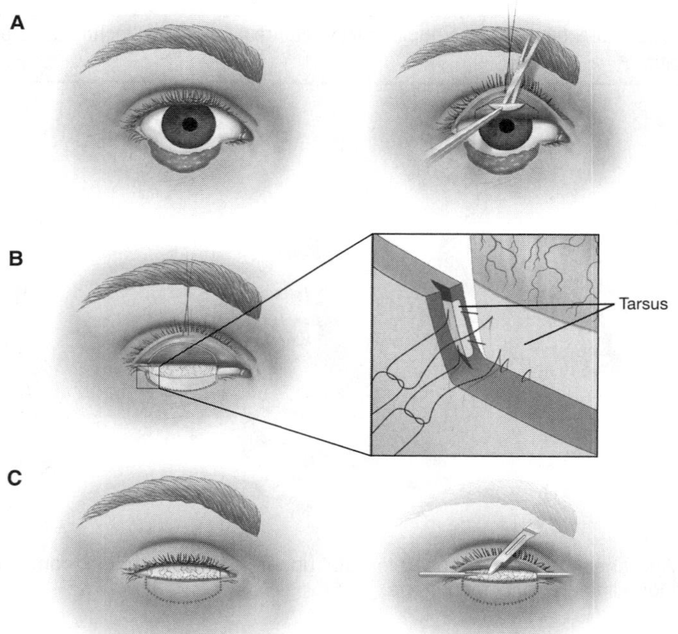


**Fig. 35-13** Tarsoconjunctival flap. **A,** The flap is elevated from the everted upper lid, closer to the margin than the free tarsoconjunctival graft. At least 4 mm of tarsus at the margin should be spared to preserve stability of the upper lid. (The original Hughes procedure split the upper lid at the margin, which produced upper lid trichiasis.) **B,** The flap should be as free of Müller's muscle as possible and sutured into the posterior lamellar defect. If tarsus remains on either edge, edge-to-edge approximation is needed. If the defect is toward the canthus, canthal fixation is needed. **C,** Because the tarsoconjunctival flap from the upper lid includes its own blood supply, an FTSG can be used on its surface. A blepharoplasty or cheek-lift myocutaneous flap can be used if enough tissue is available. Separation usually takes place at 3 weeks, when the flap gains a new blood supply. Separation may be needed later if an FTSG is used.

- **Cheek advancement flap (classic Mustarde)**[1] (Fig. 35-14)
  - Useful for total lower lid reconstruction
  - To prevent lid retraction, critical to provide tension-free mobilization of tissue into targeted site and lateral canthal fixation

**TIP:** Elevation of a thin flap is helpful.

- **Locoregional flaps**
  - If adequate quality lid tissue unavailable, use regional soft tissues
  - Ideal quality tissue not provided because of thickness (Fig. 35-15)

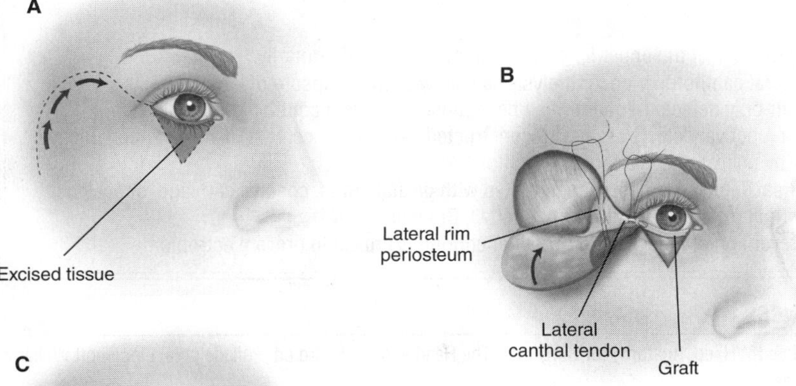


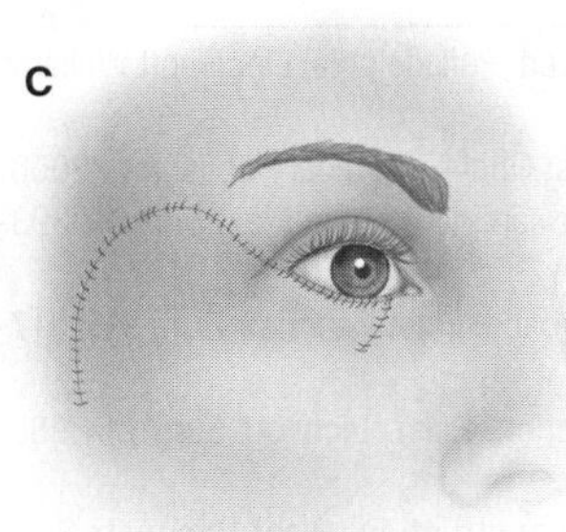


**Fig. 35-14** Classic Mustarde procedure. **A,** An anterior lamellar rotation flap is needed, which requires extension in front of the ear and undermining over the malar area. **B,** The steps include a posterior lamellar lining of nasal chondromucosa and lateral flap fixation. **C,** The flap is rotated to cover the anterior lamellar defect.

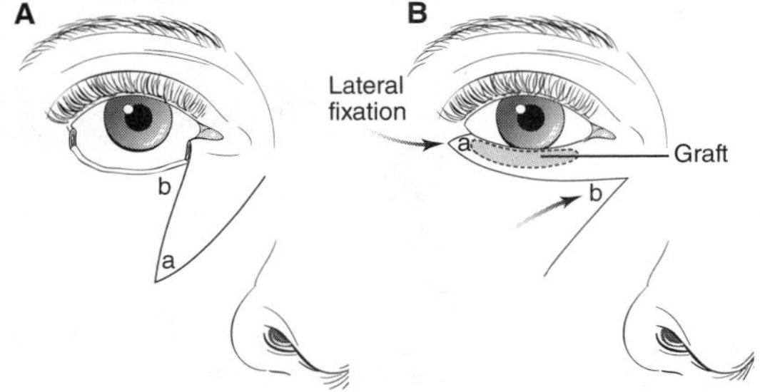


**Fig. 35-15** Full-thickness reconstruction of lower lid with transposition nasolabial flap. **A,** Lower lid defect and outline of transposition flap for the nasolabial area. **B,** The nasolabial flap has been transposed to form the outer surface of the lower lid. The flap is lined with a free mucous membrane–like graft.

## Flap Tissue Anchoring Techniques

- **Lateral canthal anchoring: Direct fixation to periosteum for flap support**
  - **Most common technique**
  - **Essential for lateral-based flap reconstruction of lower lid**
  - Drill-hole fixation useful for additional reinforcement
- **Medial canthal anchoring:** More difficult because of lack of substantial bone
  - Posterior fixation behind lacrimal sac essential for proper lid apposition
  - Direct fixation to local connective tissue
  - Transnasal wire fixation may be necessary when periosteum insufficient

**CAUTION: Care must be taken to prevent injury to the lacrimal ductal system.**

### Key Points

- ✓ Up to 30% of the upper lid or lower lid can be closed primarily.
- ✓ Lateral canthotomy or cantholysis can allow primary closure of larger defects.
- ✓ Skin-only defects frequently can be reconstructed with contralateral eyelid skin.
- ✓ Conjunctival defects are best reconstructed using advancement of adjacent conjunctiva or by buccal or nasal mucosal grafts.
- ✓ Tarsal defects are best reconstructed with palatal grafts, conchal cartilage, or acellular dermal matrix (e.g., AlloDerm; LifeCell, Branchburg, NJ).
- ✓ Prevention of tension with proper anchoring is critical to prevent ectropion.

## References

1. Hollinshead WH, ed. Anatomy for Surgeons: The Head and Neck, 3rd ed. Philadelphia: Lippincott Williams & Wilkins, 1982.
2. McCord CD, Codner MA, eds. Eyelid & Periorbital Surgery. St Louis: Quality Medical Publishing, 2008.
3. Putterman AM. Reconstruction of the eyelids following resection for carcinoma. Clin Plast Surg 12:393-410, 1985.
4. Spinelli HM, Gelks GW. Periocular reconstruction: a systematic approach. Plast Reconstr Surg 91:1017-1024, 1993.
5. DiFrancesco LM, Codner MA, McCord CD. Upper eyelid reconstruction. Plast Reconstr Surg 114:98e-107e, 2004.
6. Codner MA, McCord CD, Mejia JD, et al. Upper and lower lid reconstruction. Plast Reconstr Surg 126:231e-245e, 2010.
7. Levine MI, Leone CR Jr. Bipedicled musculocutaneous flap repair of cicatricial ectropion. Ophthal Plast Reconstr Surg 6:119-121, 1990.
8. Rohrich RJ, Zbar RI. The evolution of the Hughes tarsoconjunctival flap for lower eyelid reconstruction. Plast Reconstr Surg 104:518-522, 1999.

# 36. Nasal Reconstruction

**Fadi C. Constantine, Melissa A. Crosby**

## ANATOMY[1,2] (Fig. 36-1)

- Divided into thirds based on underlying skeletal structure (also called *vaults*)
  - **Proximal:** Lies over nasal bones
  - **Middle:** Lies over upper lateral cartilages
  - **Distal:** Includes nasal tip with paired alae over membranous septum
    - **Columella:** Supported by the medial crura of alar cartilages

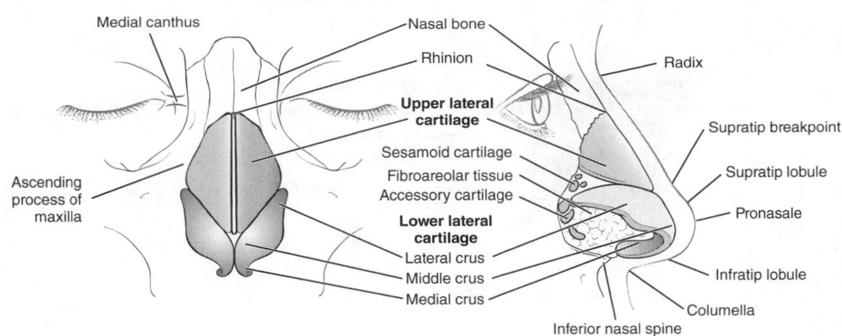


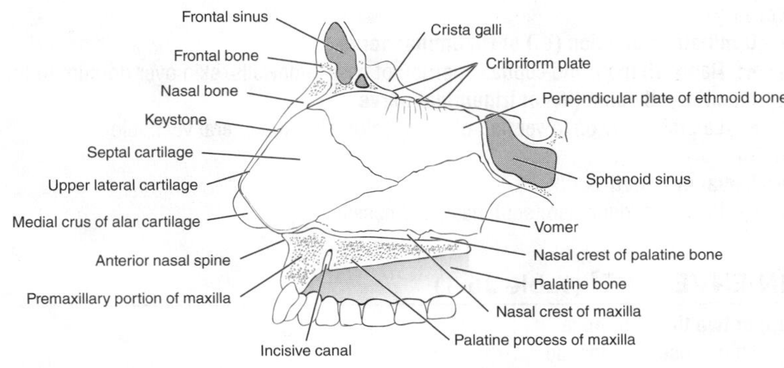


**Fig. 36-1** Nasal anatomy.

## Blood Supply (Fig. 36-2)

- **Arterial**
  - **Angular artery (branch of facial artery):** Lateral surface of caudal nose
  - **Superior labial artery:** Nasal sill, nasal septum, and base of columella
  - **Dorsal nasal branch of ophthalmic artery:** Axial arterial network for dorsal and lateral nasal skin
  - **Infraorbital branch of internal maxillary artery:** Dorsum and lateral sidewalls of nose
- **Venous**
  - Venous drainage parallels arterial supply.

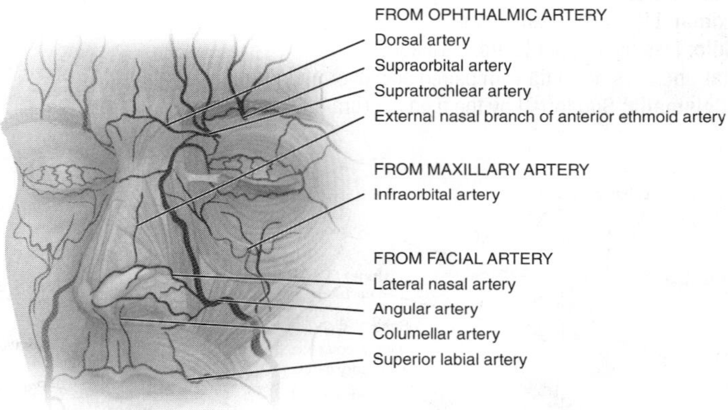


**Fig. 36-2** Blood supply.

## Innervation

- **Sensory**
  - **Ophthalmic division ($V_1$) of trigeminal nerve**
    - Radix, rhinion, and cephalic portion of nasal sidewalls, skin over dorsum to tip
  - **Maxillary division ($V_2$) of trigeminal nerve**
    - Lateral tissue on lower half of nose, columella, and lateral vestibule
- **Motor**
  - **Facial nerve VII**
    - Procerus, depressor septi nasi, and nasalis

## SKIN ENVELOPE[3] (Table 36-1)

- **Upper two thirds of nose**
  - Thin, loose, and mobile
  - Few sebaceous glands
- **Lower third of nose**
  - Thick, less mobile
  - Most sebaceous glands
- **Zone of thin skin:** Dorsum and columella
- **Zone of thick skin:** Nasal tip and ala

**Table 36-1** *Skin Thickness by Location*

| Location | Thickness (μm) |
|---|---|
| Nasal dorsum | 1300 |
| Nasal lobule | 2400 |
| Postauricular | 800 |
| Supraclavicular | 1800 |
| Submental | 2500 |
| Nasolabial | 2900 |

# DEFECT ANALYSIS

## ASSESSMENT OF DEFECT

- **Location**
- **Depth**
  - Skin and soft tissue coverage
  - Cartilage and bone
  - Lining
- **Dimensions of defect**

## GOALS OF RECONSTRUCTION

- Maintain airway patency
- Replace missing layers with similar tissue
- Minimize morbidity
- Optimize aesthetics

## AESTHETIC SUBUNITS OF THE NOSE (BURGET AND MENICK)[4-7] (Fig. 36-3)

**TIP:** Not all authors believe in aesthetic subunit reconstruction.

- **Rules for Reconstruction**
  - If a defect occupies more than 50% of a subunit, enlarge defect to incorporate entire subunit and reconstruct it as a whole.
    - Menick states, ". . . if the scar is placed between topographic subunits, where it follows the normal lighted ridges and shadowed valleys of the nasal surface, it will be taken for normal."[6]
  - Use undamaged contralateral subunit as the reconstructive model.
  - Divide large defects into multiple defects.
- **Controversy**
  - Others disagree with Burget and Menick and adhere to defect-only reconstruction[8,9]

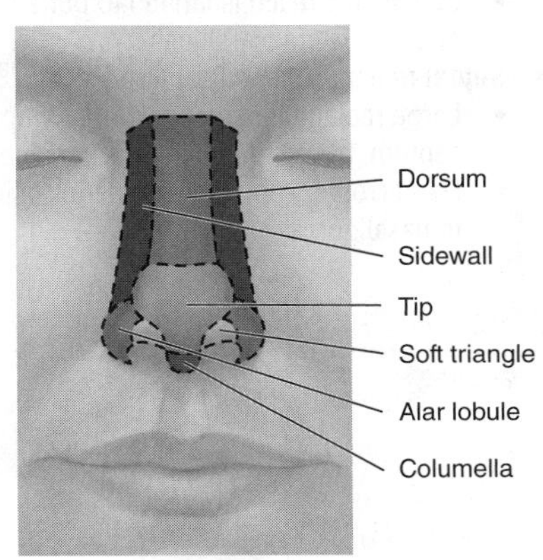


**Fig. 36-3** Aesthetic subunits of the nose.

- Rohrich et al[9] advocate six core principles for nasal reconstruction:
  1. Maximal conservation of native tissue is advised.
  2. Reconstruction of the defect, *not the subunit,* is advised.
  3. Complementary ablative procedures, such as primary dermabrasion, enhance the final result and decrease the number of revision procedures.
  4. Primary defatting is safe in nonsmokers and decreases the number of revision procedures.
  5. The use of axial pattern flaps is preferred.
  6. Good contour is the aesthetic endpoint.

## LINING RECONSTRUCTION

**TIP:** Lining reconstruction is the most critical aspect of reconstruction.

- **Turn-in nasal flap**[10]
  - Flap hinged on the outer cicatricial edge and flipped over to span defect
- **Folded extranasal flap**
  - Can be forehead, nasolabial, or superiorly based upper lip flap turned in
- **Skin graft to forehead flap**
  - Skin graft applied to undersurface of forehead flap
  - May include cartilage
  - Hard palate mucosa can also be used.
- **Septal door flap (de Quervain)**[11,12] (Fig. 36-4)
  - Septal mucosa is removed ipsilateral to defect, and appropriately sized flap of septal cartilage is dissected.
  - Septal door is then made on a dorsal hinge toward the reconstructive side so that septal mucosa on far side bridges the wound and lines the airway.
  - Caudal flap reach is limited to border of upper lateral cartilages.

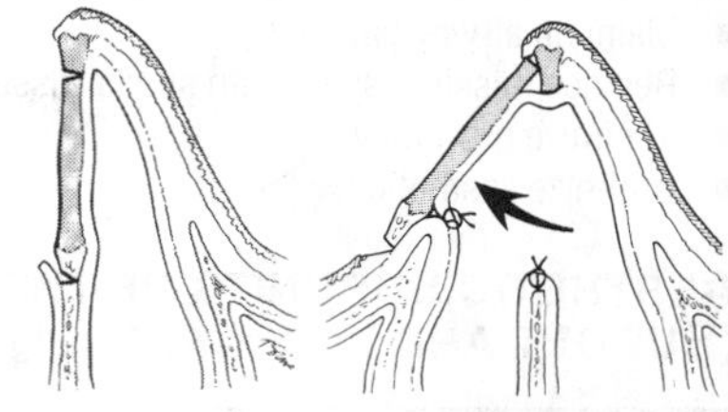

**Fig. 36-4** Septal door flap.

- **Septal mucoperichondrial flap (Gillies**[13] **and Burget and Menick**[6,14]**)** (Fig. 36-5)
  - Large rectangle of mucosa or a composite of mucosa and perichondrium is elevated from septum, based on the septal branch of superior labial artery.
  - Flap pivots on an anterior-inferior point near nasal spine and folds outward to furnish lining to nasal domes.

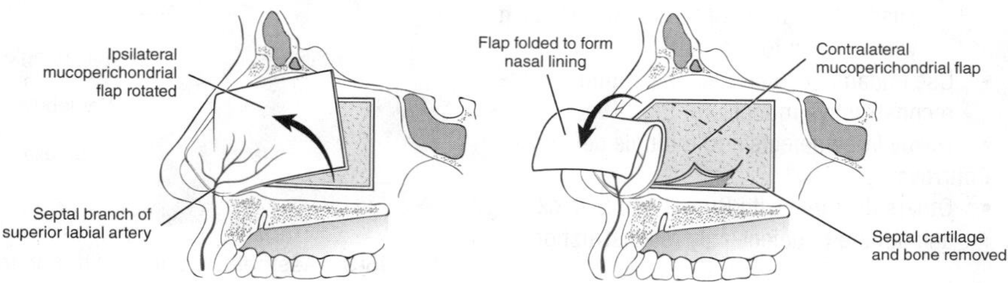


**Fig. 36-5** Septal mucoperichondrial flap.

- **Mucosal advancement flap (Burget and Menick)**[5,14] (Fig. 36-6)
  - Bipedicled mucosal advancement flap is based medially on remaining septum and laterally at the piriform aperture.
  - Flap is based on the lateral floor of vestibule and advanced medially to resurface small lining defects of nasal ala.

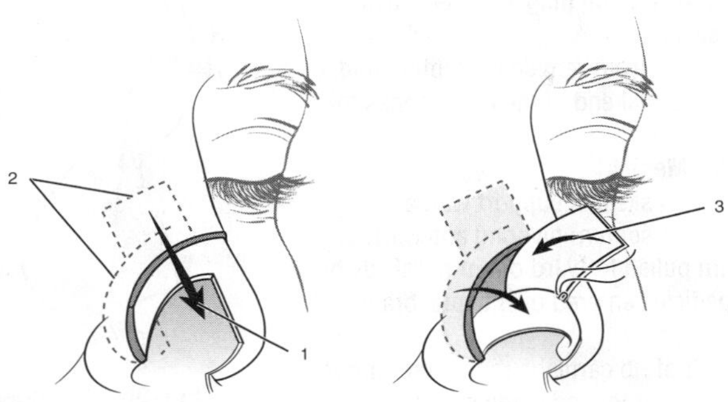


**Fig. 36-6** The entire tip subunit is excised. A bipedicled flap is elevated, based medially on the septum and laterally on the vestibule. This is then advanced distally and sutured down to form alar and medial nasal lining.

- **Septal pivot flap**[15] (Fig. 36-7)
  - Can be used to provide dorsal cartilage support
  - With the flap rotated anteriorly, more than required for support alone, there will be an excess of mucosal lining when the flap is finally shaped.
  - Can fold the excess mucosa outward to provide vault lining bilaterally

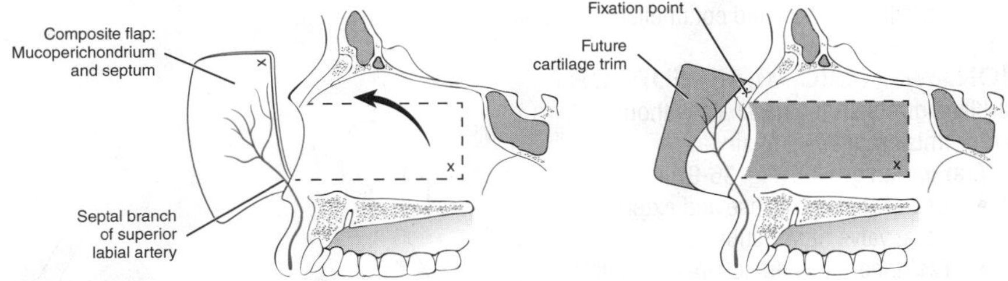


**Fig. 36-7** The residual septum within the piriform aperture can be transposed on bilateral septal branches of the superior labial artery at the nasal spine to provide modest dorsal support and lining to the midvault and part of the ala.

## SKELETAL/CARTILAGINOUS SUPPORT

### Basic Information

- Nasal bone widest at nasofrontal suture (14 mm) and narrowest at nasofrontal angle (10 mm)
- Nasal bone thickest superiorly at nasofrontal angle (6 mm) and progressively becomes thinner toward tip
- Screws for fixation placed usually 5-10 mm below nasofrontal angle, where bone is 3-4 mm thick

## Midline Support

- **Strut technique (Gillies)**[13]
  - Longitudinal piece of bone or cartilage seated on the nasal radix with extension along the dorsum to the tip where it is bent sharply to rest on the anterior nasal spine
- **Hinged septal flap (Millard)**[16,17] (Fig. 36-8)
  - L-shaped flap of septum hinged superiorly to augment nasal angle
  - Septal flap carved from remaining septum and hinged on the caudal end of the nasal bones to pivot upward
- **Septal pivot flap (Menick)**[15]
  - Lining and dorsal skeletal support with a composite flap of septum pivoting anteriorly
  - Entire septum pulled forward out of nasal cavity on narrow pedicle centered over septal branch of superior labial artery
  - Cantilever graft of rib cartilage rongeured through hard tissues of septum and wired to nasal bones

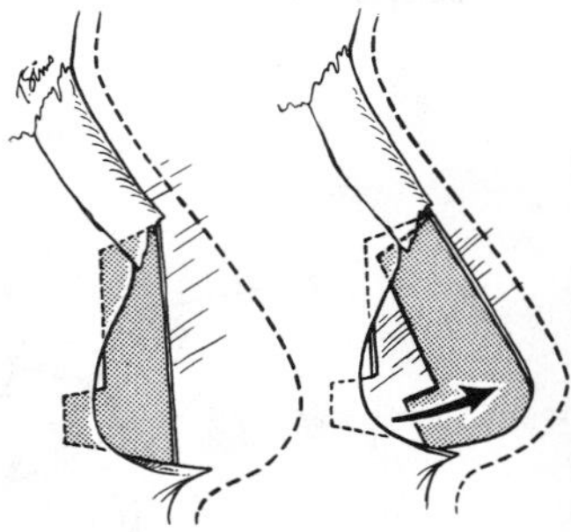

**Fig. 36-8** Hinged septal flap.

- **Cantilever graft (Converse[18] and Millard[19])**
  - Longitudinal piece of bone extends along dorsum down to tip
  - Graft either secures to frontal bone, nasal bones, or both
  - May use osteocartilaginous rib segment

## Anatomic Alar Support

- **Anatomic alar grafts**
  - Use autogenous cartilage grafts that are anatomically shaped and bent to resemble normal lateral crura and fixed to the residual medial crura or columella strut.
  - Proposed advantages over extraanatomic grafts are improved alar rim correction with less nostril distortion and columellar retraction.

## Nonanatomic Alar Support

Cartilage grafts stiffen nasal ala without compromising patency of airway.

- **Alar batten graft**[20] (Fig. 36-9)
  - Used for alar collapse and external nasal valve obstruction
  - Fashioned to span collapse, usually caudal to existing lateral third of lateral crus, and extend to piriform aperture
  - Placed cephalad to alar rim and therefore limited in use for correcting alar rim retraction

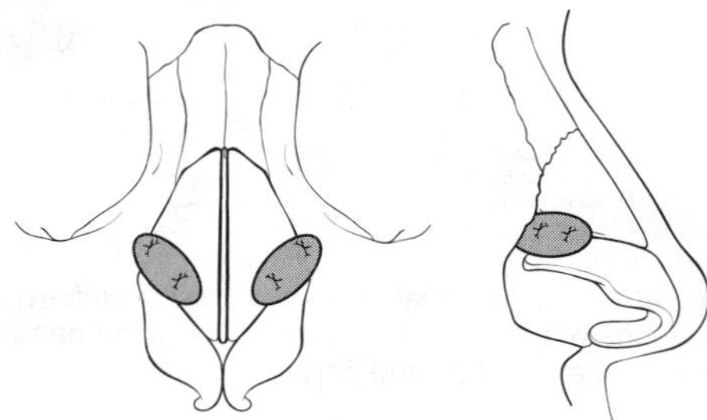

**Fig. 36-9** Alar batten graft.

- **Lateral crural strut graft**[20] (Fig. 36-10)
  - Autogenous cartilage graft placed between the deep surface of the lateral crus and the vestibular skin, and sutured to the crus
  - Measures 3-4 mm wide and 20-25 mm long
  - Lateral end of strut extends to piriform rim and positioned caudal to the alar groove and accessory cartilages
  - Used for alar rim retraction and lateral crural malposition

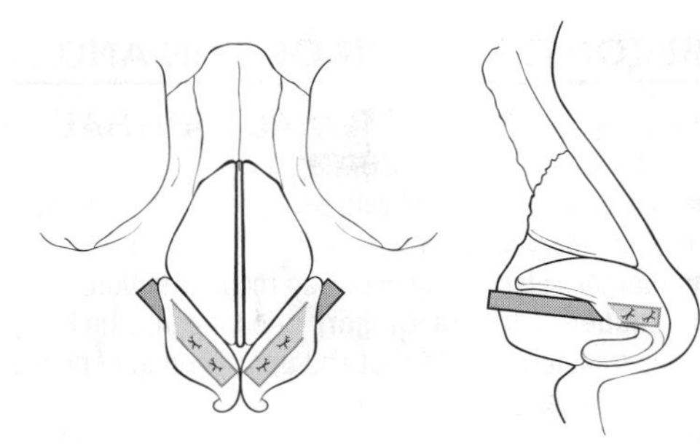

**Fig. 36-10** Lateral crural strut graft.

- **Alar spreader graft**[20] (Fig. 36-11)
  - Corrects pinched-tip deformities and alar or internal nasal valve collapse
  - Bar-shaped or triangular graft inserted between the vestibular surface and the undersurface of the remaining lateral crura to force the crura apart

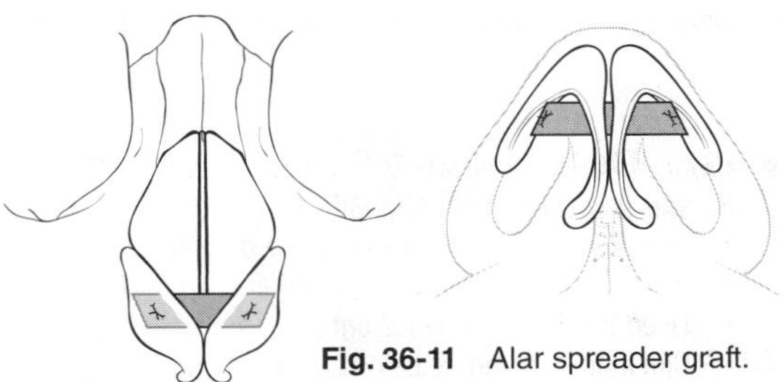

**Fig. 36-11** Alar spreader graft.

- **Alar contour graft**[20] (Fig. 36-12)
  - Autogenous cartilage buttress inserted through an infracartilaginous incision into an alar-vestibular pocket inferior and lateral to rim of the crus
  - Reestablishment of a normally functioning external nasal valve and aesthetically pleasing alar contour

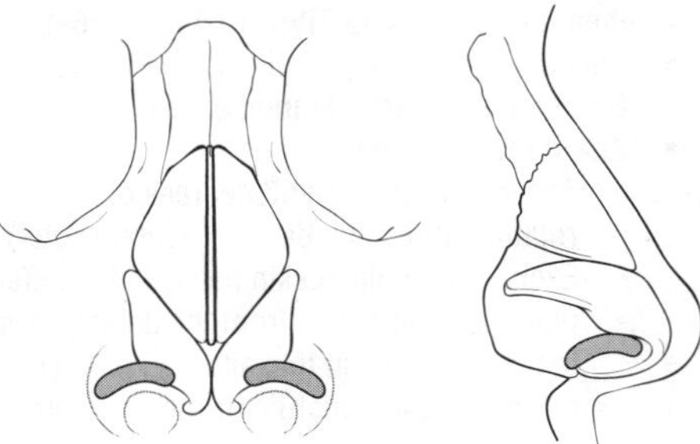

**Fig. 36-12** Alar contour graft.

## ALLOPLASTS

All are used in combination with autogenous tissue.

- **Vitallium or titanium mesh** for dorsal framework
  - Advantages: Pliable, easily stabilized to dorsal and lateral nasal walls, readily accessible
  - Disadvantages: Implant exposure and infection
- **Porous polyethylene** (***Medpor;*** Porex Surgical, Newnan, GA) available as a strut or sheet
  - Advantages: Incorporated into tissue, readily accessible
  - Disadvantages: Multiple implants required, implant exposure, infection

# RECONSTRUCTION OF SKIN AND SOFT TISSUE[17,21]

## GLABELLA AND MEDIAL CANTHAL DEFECTS[22] (Fig. 36-13)

- Defects <1 cm heal with best aesthetic result by secondary intention.
- Larger defects may need flap reconstruction.
- **Glabellar flap (McGregor)**[23]**:** redundant skin in glabella is transferred onto root and upper bridge of nose to repair defects in this area.

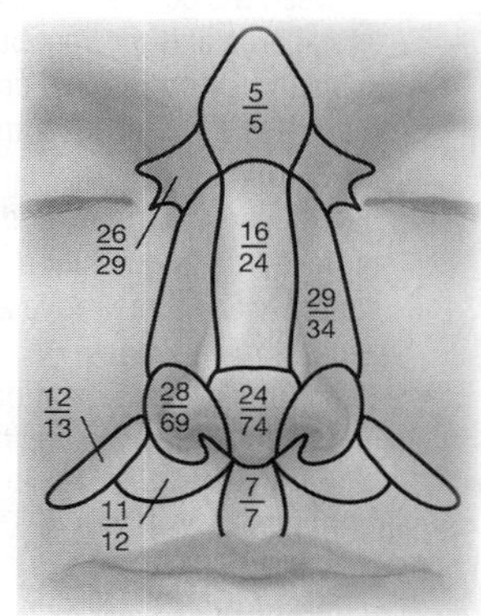


**Fig. 36-13** Nasal and paranasal defects allowed to heal by secondary intention. The denominator is the total number of patients in that subunit; the numerator is the number of patients who achieved a cosmetically acceptable result.

## NASAL DORSUM AND SIDEWALLS

- **Banner flap (Elliot)**[17,24] (Fig. 36-14)
  - Transverse narrow triangular flap of skin from the nasal dorsum adjacent to defect
  - Used for defects 0.7-1.2 cm in diameter
  - Can lengthen and place on side opposite defect, which increases flap reach and elevates nostrils to achieve symmetry
- **Bilobed flap (Esser and Zitelli)**[25-27] (Fig. 36-15)
  - Bilobed flap is flap of choice for defects 0.5-1.5 cm in **thick-skinned areas.**
  - **Zitelli modification**
    - Allow no more than 50 degrees of rotation for each lobe (100 degrees total).
    - Excise a triangle of skin between the defect and the pivot point before rotation (the pivot point lies one radius from the defect); design the flap as large as the nose allows; place the second lobe in thin and loose skin of sidewall or upper dorsum (avoid placing it close to the alar margin or medial canthus).

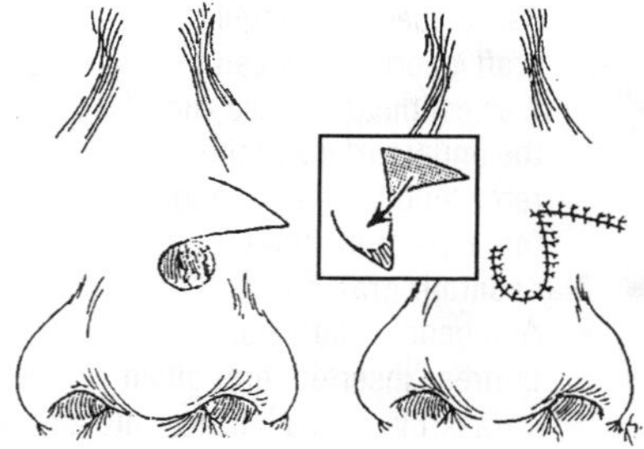

**Fig. 36-14** Banner flap.

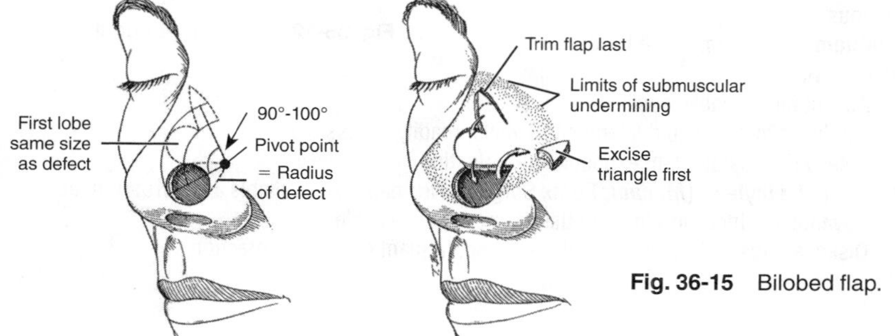


**Fig. 36-15** Bilobed flap.

- Undermine widely just above the perichondrium and periosteum.
- Make diameter of first lobe equal to that of the defect; reduce width of second flap to allow easy donor site closure (but make sure it closes the defect of the first donor).

- Generally, use a laterally based design for defects of the tip, but a medial design for lobule defects.
- Position the pivot away from the alar margin and lower lid to prevent distortion.

- **Dorsal nasal flap (Rieger)**[28]
  - Based laterally and elevated on angular arteries
  - Entire skin of nasal dorsum rotated and advanced caudally
  - For defects of lobule less than 2 cm in diameter, 1 cm away from alar rim, and above tip-defining points
  - Can place superior incision across root of nose, concealed in radix crease[22]
- **Axial frontonasal flap (Marchac and Toth)**[29]
  - Based on vessels emerging at level of inner canthus
  - Pedicle is back-cut to a narrow vascular stalk near medial canthus.
  - Glabellar portion is redundant as flap is rotated, and Burow's triangles are used to equalize two sides of Y closure.
- **Axial nasodorsum flap**
  - Combines pedicle of the nasalis flap with dorsal nasal branches of the ophthalmic artery to encompass territory similar to frontonasal flap
  - Whole nasal dorsal skin elevated and transferred inferiorly for reconstruction of lobule
  - Burow's triangles cut above eyebrows to increase downward mobility
- **Nasalis flap (Rybka)**[30]
  - Sliding nasalis myocutaneous flap from the upper alar crease with approximately 1.25 cm advancement to repair small defects of lateral tip
- **Cheek advancement flap**
  - Used for replacement of nasal sidewall, especially in elderly patients
  - Up to 2.5 $cm^2$ of paranasal and cheek areas can be advanced with primary closure of donor site.
- **Nasolabial flap**[31] (Fig. 36-16)
  - Superiorly or inferiorly based
  - Good for alar reconstruction and lateral nasal wall
  - May need cartilage graft for alar support
  - Can design as transposition flap in single stage

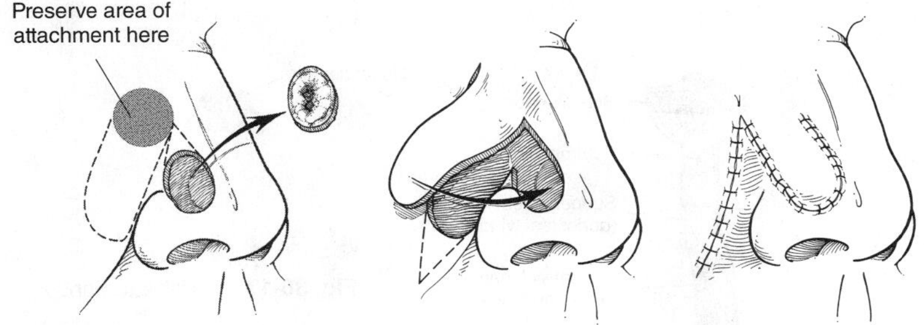


**Fig. 36-16** Nasolabial flap.

- **Turnover flap (Spear et al)**[32]
  - Flap of nasolabial skin on a subcutaneous pedicle based at piriform aperture
  - Flap turned 180 degrees and rotated at a right angle to its base to furnish lining for nostril
  - Folded on itself to provide external cover
  - Donor site closed primarily
- **Sliding flap**
  - Splitting of dorsal nasal skin from nasal lining and rotation
  - Advancement of nasolabial tissue onto lower nose
  - Incisions placed at junction of aesthetic subunits to hide scars
- **Forehead flap**[33] (Fig. 36-17)
  - Most useful flap for tip, lobule, subtotal, and total nasal reconstruction
  - Midline or paramedian based on **supratrochlear** or **supraorbital** vessels from one or both sides
  - **Supratrochlear artery:** Axial vessels in flap are noted to continue into the transverse limb for a short distance.
    - Superficial branch reliably travels 4 cm above the supraorbital rim, and small subcutaneous vessels travel approximately 1 cm across the transverse limb.[34]
  - 2.5-3.0 cm can be taken from central forehead with primary closure.
  - Can orient obliquely if patient's forehead is less than 3 cm along hairline or into hair-bearing scalp for 1.5 cm; use with caution in smokers
  - Flap is usually left for 3-4 weeks before division and inset (because of delay theory).
    - Menick uses a **three-stage technique** with minimal thinning in the first stage and cartilage placement and aggressive thinning during the second stage.

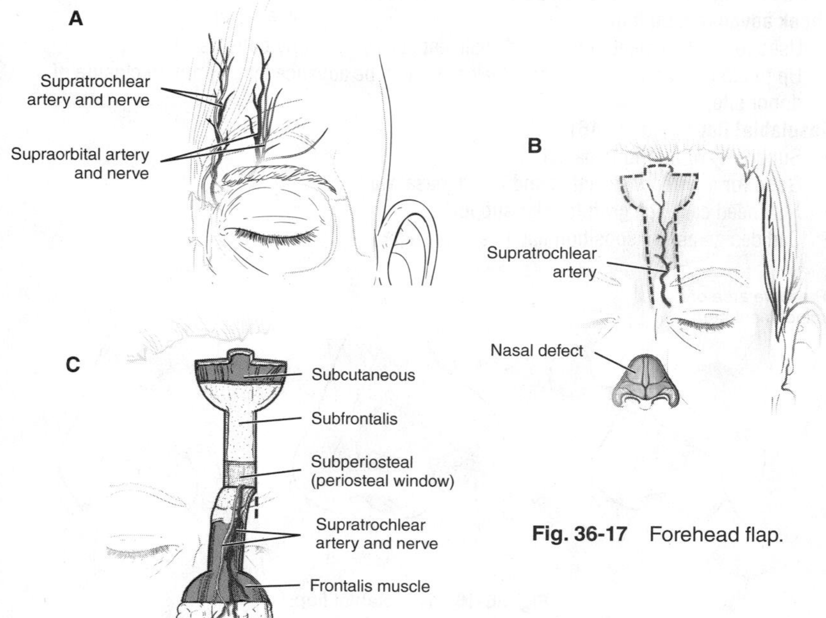


**Fig. 36-17** Forehead flap.

**TIP:** Base forehead flap off vessels contralateral to defect to decrease arc of rotation and subsequent pedicle kinking.

- **Expanded forehead flap**
  - Place expanders and stretch tissue over weeks or intraoperatively.
  - Problems occur with prelaminating nose and unpredictable rebound contraction.
  - Main indication is to expand lateral forehead skin to allow primary closure in large paramedian flaps.
- **Gull-winged flap (Millard)**[35]
  - Modification of forehead flap combines generous amount of skin distally for extensive lobular reconstruction; pedicle is only 1 inch wide
  - "Wings" lie transversely on forehead, and scars are hidden in natural skin creases.
- **Up and down flap (Gillies)**[36]
  - Reconstruction of entire nasal lobule is possible.
  - Flap is longer and wider than paramedian forehead flap.
  - Donor site cannot be closed primarily.
- **Scalping flap (Converse)**[37,38] (Fig. 36-18)
  - Repair of total or near-total defects
  - Elevated through a coronal incision just behind the superficial temporal artery, extending to a skin paddle in the contralateral forehead
  - Frontalis muscle not carried in the distal end of flap, but remainder of pedicle dissected in subgaleal plane
  - Donor site on forehead closed with full-thickness skin graft
  - Scalp defect dressed with nondesiccating dressing or interim split-thickness skin graft

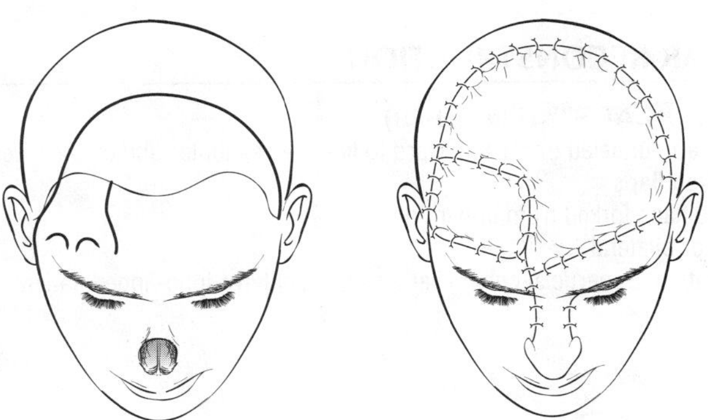

**Fig. 36-18** Scalping flap.

- **Sickle flap (New)**[39]
  - Donor site in lateral forehead
  - Randomly vascularized so requires delay
  - Problems with pedicle kink and crossing over eyelid
  - Multiple modifications but outcomes poor with any method

- **Frontotemporal flap (Schmid[40] and Meyer[41])**
  - Tubular flap with an internal supraciliary pedicle carrying lateral forehead skin with embedded ear cartilage to tip of nose or ala
  - Narrow horizontal pedicle courses above brow from glabella to temple
  - Young patients with low hairlines
- **Temporomastoid flap (Loeb[42] and Hunt[43])**
  - Also called the **Washio flap**[44]
  - Carries postauricular skin as flap based on superficial temporal arteries
  - Allows thin (auricular) and thick (mastoid) skin transfer
  - Ample hairless skin for complete nasal coverage
  - Auricular cartilage availability
  - No flap delay
  - No visible facial scars

### Nasal Tip, Alae, and Lower Third

- **Skin grafting is an appropriate option with the following conditions.**[45]
  - Superficial defects
  - Diameter <1cm
  - Nonsmokers
  - Color-matched donor sites (forehead skin is an excellent match)
  - Liberal dermabrasion starting at 6 weeks to optimize final contour and color match
- **Chondrocutaneous composite grafts**
  - Small through-and-through defects of alar rim
  - Donor site ear
  - Maximum safe size is 1.5 cm

## COLUMELLAR RECONSTRUCTION

### Nasolabial Flaps[46] (Fig. 39-19)

- Bilateral flaps are tunneled or rolled inward to line the vestibules and create a central post.
- **Upper lip forked flaps**
  - Transverse flaps forked from upper lip
  - Unilateral or bilateral
  - Best indication: Superficial columellar loss in an elderly, long-lipped patient

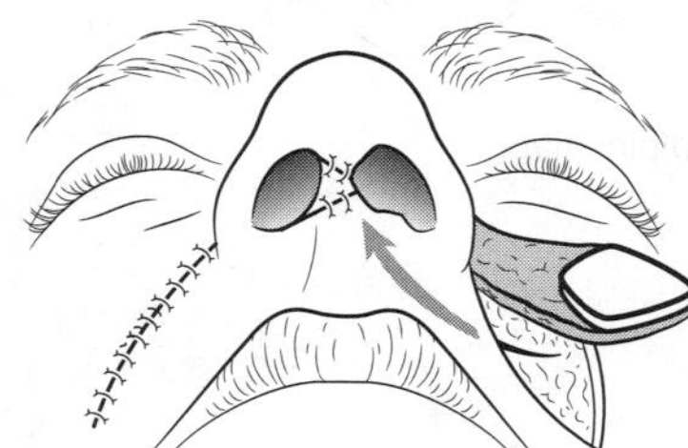

**Fig. 36-19** Bilateral nasolabial flaps.

- **Vestibular flaps (Mavili and Akyurek)**[47]
  - Transfer of internal nasal vestibular skin flap combined with bilateral labial mucosa flaps
  - No external scars
- **Forehead flap**
  - Millard prefers extension of forehead flap to reconstruct columella
- **Chondrocutaneous grafts (Paletta and Van Norman)**[48]
  - Auricular composite grafts

## SOFT TRIANGLE RECONSTRUCTION[50]

Of all nine subunits, **the soft triangle is perhaps the most challenging to re-create** because of its geographically distant location on the nose, as well as its complex shape, which is essentially quadrilateral with both convex and concave curvatures.

- **Define Defect → Reconstruct** (Fig. 36-20)
  - Type I: Defect with skin intact, but with soft tissue and mucosal lining defects
  - Type II: Defect includes surrounding structures with mucosa intact, but with absent soft tissue and overlying skin
  - Type III: Defect with adjacent structures, including a complete mucosal, soft tissue, and skin defect.

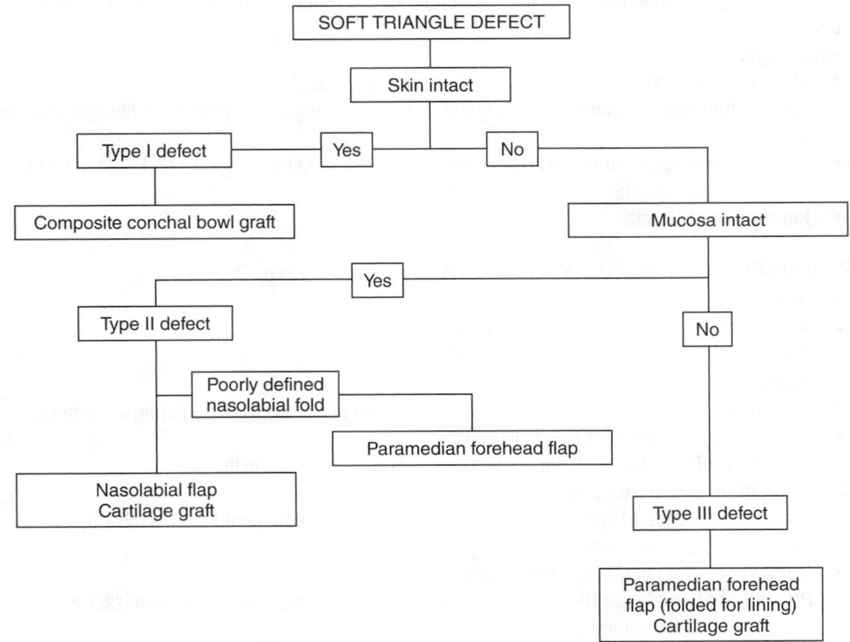


**Fig. 36-20** Algorithm for the treatment of soft triangle defects.

## TOTAL NASAL RECONSTRUCTION

**TIP:** Nose may be prefabricated using cartilage and lining under forehead flap or other large flap.

- **Free flaps:** Used only when forehead flap not available
  - Radial forearm free flap (can be prefabricated)
  - Serratus anterior free flap
  - Dorsalis pedis free flap
  - Postauricular free flap
  - Helix free flap
  - Deltopectoral free flap

## RHINOPHYMA[50]

From Greek *rhis* meaning nose and *phyma* meaning growth.

Sebaceous hyperplasia of nasal skin with bulbous enlargement of nose and erythematous skin

- Twelve times more common in men than women
- Typical patient is white male in his sixties.
- Represents a severe form of **acne rosacea,** but **has no true association with alcohol intake.**
- Malignant degeneration into basal cell carcinoma higher in these patients; reported 15%-30% but likely lower
- Four Stages:
  - **First (prerosacea):** Frequent facial flushing with increased vascularity
  - **Second (vascular rosacea):** Thickened skin, telangiectasias, and persistent facial erythema or erythrosis
  - **Third (acne rosacea or inflammatory rosacea):** Erythematous papules and pustules of the forehead, glabella, malar region, nose, and chin
  - **Fourth: Rhinophyma**

### TREATMENT: TYPICALLY FOR STAGES 1-3[49] (Fig. 36-21)

- **Nonsurgical**
  - Avoidance of sun exposure with UVA/UVB protection
  - Good skin hygiene
  - Tetracycline
  - Topical tretinoin; may irritate skin and could worsen erythema by stimulating angiogenesis
  - Isotretinoin; avoidance of skin irritation
  - Metronidazole topical (Metrogel; Galderma Laboratories, Ft. Worth, TX)
- **Surgical: Mainstay of treatment for stage 4**
  - Tangential excision of skin and hypertrophic appendages using cold knife excision, dermaplaning, or dermabrasion
  - $CO_2$ laser can be helpful for hemostasis.
  - Placement of nondesiccating, bacteriostatic dressings to promote reepithelialization
  - Outcomes similar among excision methods
  - Important to send tissue samples to pathology to rule out cancer

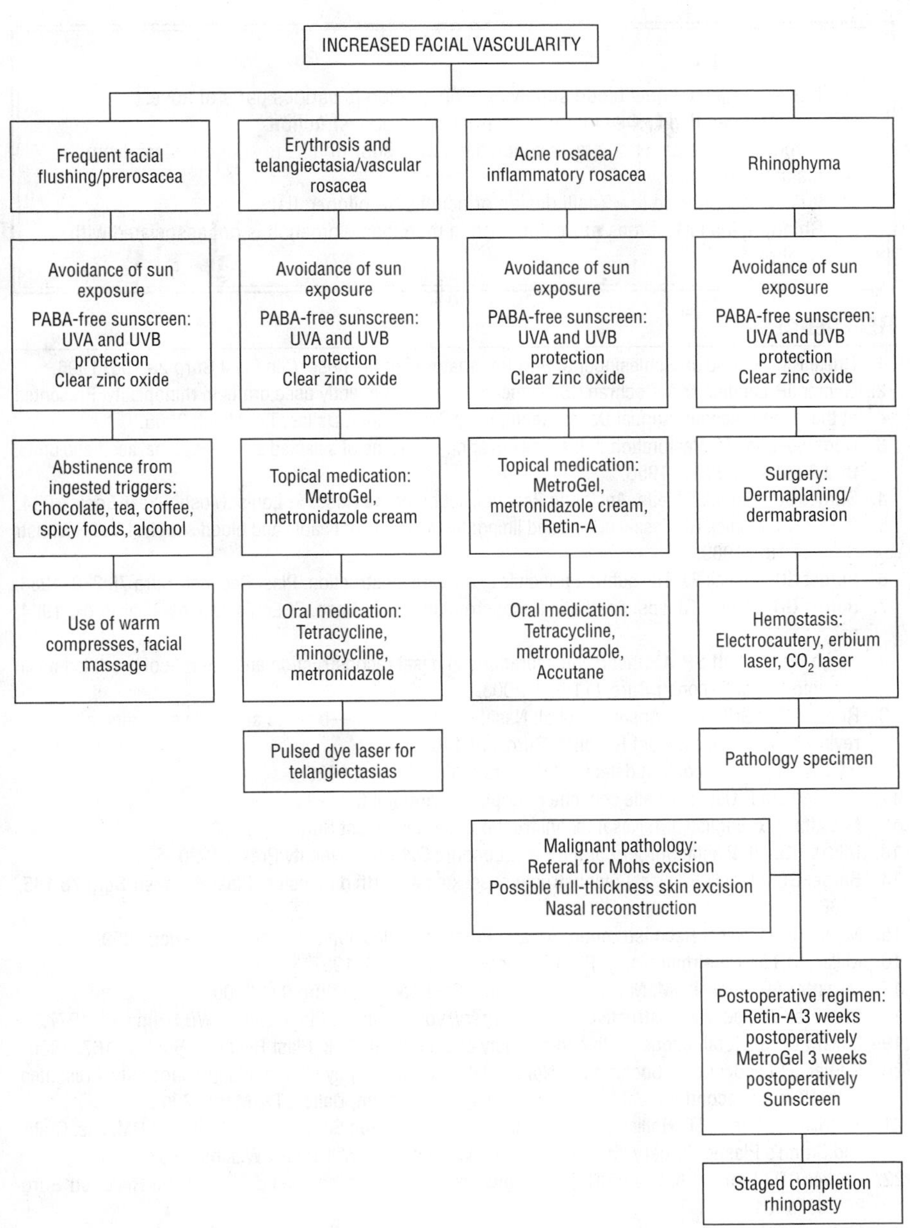


**Fig. 36-21** Algorithm for the treatment of rosacea and rhinophyma.

## Key Points

- ✓ It is essential to know blood supply and innervation to various parts of nose.
- ✓ The forehead flap is the workhorse for nasal tip reconstruction.
- ✓ Forehead flap dissection starts subcutaneous to subfrontalis to subperiosteal, from distal to proximal.
- ✓ It is important to follow Zitelli design principles for bilobed flaps.
- ✓ Rhinophyma is 12 times more common in men than women; it is not associated with alcohol.

## References


1. Oneal RM, Beil RJ Jr, Schlesinger J. Surgical anatomy of the nose. Clin Plast Surg 23:195, 1996.
2. Gunter JP, Landecker A, Cochran CS. Nomenclature for frequently used grafts in rhinoplasty. Presented at the Twenty-second Annual Dallas Rhinoplasty Symposium, Dallas, TX, March 2005.
3. González-Ulloa M. Restoration of the face covering by means of selected skin in regional aesthetic units. Br J Plast Surg 9:212, 1956.
4. Burget GC, Menick FJ, eds. Aesthetic Reconstruction of the Nose. St Louis: Mosby–Year Book, 1994.
5. Burget GC, Menick FJ. Nasal support and lining: the marriage of beauty and blood supply. Plast Reconstr Surg 84:189, 1989.
6. Burget GC, Menick FJ. The subunit principle in nasal reconstruction. Plast Reconstr Surg 76:239, 1985.
7. Burget GC, Menick FJ, eds. Aesthetic Reconstruction of the Nose. St Louis: Mosby–Year Book, 1994, p 7.
8. Singh DJ, Bartlett SP. Aesthetic considerations in nasal reconstruction and the role of modified nasal subunits. Plast Reconstr Surg 111:639, 2003.
9. Rohrich RJ, Griffin JR, Ansari M, et al. Nasal reconstruction—beyond aesthetic subunits: a 15-year review of 1334 cases. Plast Reconstr Surg 114:1405, 2004.
10. Ivy RH. Repair of acquired defects of the face. JAMA 84:181, 1925.
11. de Quervain F. Ueber patielle seitliche rhinoplstik. Zentralbl Chir 29:297, 1902.
12. Muzaffar AR, English JM. Nasal reconstruction. Sel Read Plast Surg 9:9, 2000.
13. Gillies HD, ed. Plastic Surgery of the Face. London: Oxford University Press, 1920.
14. Burget GC, Menick FJ. Nasal reconstruction: seeking a fourth dimension. Plast Reconstr Surg 78:145, 1986.
15. Menick F, ed. Nasal Reconstruction: Art and Practice. Philadelphia: Saunders Elsevier, 2009.
16. Millard DR Jr. Hemirhinoplasty. Plast Reconstr Surg 40:440, 1967.
17. Muzaffar AB, English JM. Nasal reconstruction. Sel Read Plast Surg 9:5, 2000.
18. Converse JM, ed. Reconstructive Plastic Surgery, vol 2, 2nd ed. Philadelphia: WB Saunders, 1977.
19. Millard DR Jr. Total reconstructive rhinoplasty and a missing link. Plast Reconstr Surg 37:167, 1966.
20. Gunter JP, Landecker A, Cochran CS. Nomenclature for frequently used grafts in rhinoplasty. Presented at the Twenty-second Annual Dallas Rhinoplasty Symposium, Dallas, TX, March 2005.
21. Rohrich RJ, Barton FE, Hollier L. Nasal reconstruction. In Aston SJ, Beasley RW, Thorne HM, eds. Grabb and Smith's Plastic Surgery, 5th ed. Philadelphia: Lippincott Williams & Wilkins, 1997.
22. Becker GD, Adams LA, Levin BC. Nonsurgical repair of perinasal skin defects. Plast Reconstr Surg 88:768, 1991.
23. McGregor IA, ed. Fundamental Techniques of Plastic Surgery and Their Surgical Applications. Edinburgh: Livingston, 1960, p 160.

24. Elliot RA Jr. Rotation flaps of the nose. Plast Reconstr Surg 44:147, 1969.
25. Esser JF. Gestielte lokale nasenplastik mit zweizipfligen lappen, deckung des sekundaren defektes vom ersten zipfel durch den zweiten. Dtsch Z Chir 143:385, 1918.
26. Zitelli JA. The bilobed flap for nasal reconstruction. Arch Dermatol 125:957, 1989.
27. Burget GC, Menick FJ, eds. Aesthetic Reconstruction of the Nose. St Louis: Mosby–Year Book, 1994, p 136.
28. Rieger RA. A local flap for repair of the nasal tip. Plast Reconstr Surg 40:147, 1967.
29. Marchac D, Toth D. The axial frontonasal flap revisited. Plast Reconstr Surg 76:686, 1985.
30. Rybka FJ. Reconstruction of the nasal tip using nasalis myocutaneous sliding flaps. Plast Reconstr Surg 71:40, 1983.
31. Rohrich RJ, Barton FE, Hollier L. Nasal reconstruction. In Aston SJ, Beasley RW, Thorne HM, et al, eds. Grabb and Smith's Plastic Surgery, 5th ed. Philadelphia: Lippincott Williams & Wilkins, 1997, p 518.
32. Spear SL, Kroll SS, Romm S. A new twist to the nasolabial flap for reconstruction of lateral alar defects. Plast Reconstr Surg 79:915, 1987.
33. Rohrich RJ, Barton FE, Hollier L. Nasal reconstruction. In Aston SJ, Beasley RW, Thorne HM, et al, eds. Grabb and Smith's Plastic Surgery, 5th ed. Philadelphia: Lippincott Williams & Wilkins, 1997, p 520.
34. Reece E, Schaverien M, Rohrich R. The paramedian forehead flap: a dynamic anatomical vascular study verifying safety and clinical implications. Plast Reconstr Surg 121:1956, 2008.
35. Millard DR Jr. Reconstructive rhinoplasty for the lower half of a nose. Plast Reconstr Surg 53:133, 1974.
36. Gillies HD. The development and scope of plastic surgery (The Charles H. Mayo Lectureship in Surgery, Fourth Lecture). Bull Northwestern Univ Med Sch 35:1, 1935.
37. Converse JM. New forehead flap for nasal reconstruction. Proc R Soc Med 35:811, 1942.
38. Rohrich RJ, Barton FE, Hollier L. Nasal reconstruction. In Aston SJ, Beasley RW, Thorne HM, et al, eds. Grabb and Smith's Plastic Surgery, 5th ed. Philadelphia: Lippincott Willliams & Wilkins, 1997, p 521.
39. New GB. Sickle flap for nasal reconstruction. Surg Gynecol Obstet 80:497, 1945.
40. Schmid E. Uber die haut-knorpel-transplantationen aus der ohrmuschel und ihre funktionelle und asthetische bedeutung gei der dechung von gesichtsdefekten. Fortschr Kiefer-Gesictschir 7:48, 1961.
41. Meyer R. Aesthetic refinements in nose reconstruction. Aesthetic Plast Surg 24:241, 2000.
42. Loeb R. Temporo-mastoid flap for reconstruction of the cheek. Rev Lat Am Chir Plast 6:185, 1962.
43. Hunt HL, ed. Plastic Surgery of the Head, Face, and Neck. Philadelphia: Lea & Febiger, 1926.
44. Washio H. Retroauricular temporal flap. Plast Reconstr Surg 43:162, 1969.
45. McCluskey PD, Constantine FC, Thornton JF. Lower third nasal reconstruction: when is skin grafting an appropriate option? Plast Reconstr Surg 124:826, 2009.
46. Muzaffar AB, English JM. Nasal reconstruction. Sel Read Plast Surg 9:24, 2000.
47. Mavili ME, Akyurek M. Congenital isolated absence of nasal columella: reconstruction with an internal nasal vestibular skin flap and bilateral labial mucosa flaps. Plast Reconstr Surg 106:393, 2000.
48. Paletta FX, Van Norman RT. Total reconstruction of the columella. Plast Reconstr Surg 30:322, 1962.
49. Constantine FC, Lee MR, Sinno S, et al. Soft tissue triangle reconstruction. Plast Reconstr Surg 131:1045-1050, 2013.
50. Rohrich RJ, Griffin JR, Adams WP. Rhinophyma: review and update. Plast Reconstr Surg 110:860, 2002.

# 37. Cheek Reconstruction

Chantelle M. DeCroff, Raman C. Mahabir,
David W. Mathes, C. Alejandra Garcia de Mitchell

## ANATOMY

- **Soft tissue**
  - **Subcutaneous musculoaponeurotic system (SMAS):** Underlies the subcutaneous tissue and skin of the cheek and is continuous with the temporoparietal fascia, galea, and platysma. Typically, motor nerves are deep to, and sensory nerves are superficial to, the SMAS
- **Musculature**
  - Inferior portion of the obicularis oculi
  - Zygomaticus major and minor
  - Levator labii superioris alaeque nasi and superioris alaeque nasi
  - Masseter
  - Buccinator
- **Blood supply**
  - End branches of the **external carotid artery**
    - Facial
    - Superficial temporal
  - Venous drainage mirrors arterial supply
- **Sensory innervation**
  - Maxillary and mandibular divisions of the trigeminal nerve
    - Infraorbital
    - Zygomaticofacial
    - Buccal (includes oral mucosa)
    - Mental
    - Auriculotemporal
    - Great auricular
- **Motor innervation**
  - Branches of the facial and trigeminal nerves
- **Lymphatic drainage** to parotid and submandibular nodes

## AESTHETIC UNITS OF THE CHEEK

The cheek is divided into three overlapping aesthetic zones (Fig. 37-1)[1,2]

### ZONE 1: SUBORBITAL

- **Medial boundary:** Nose-cheek junction and nasolabial fold
- **Lateral boundary:** Anterior edge of the sideburn
- **Inferior boundary:** Gingival sulcus
- **Superior boundary:** Lower eyelid (see Chapter 35)

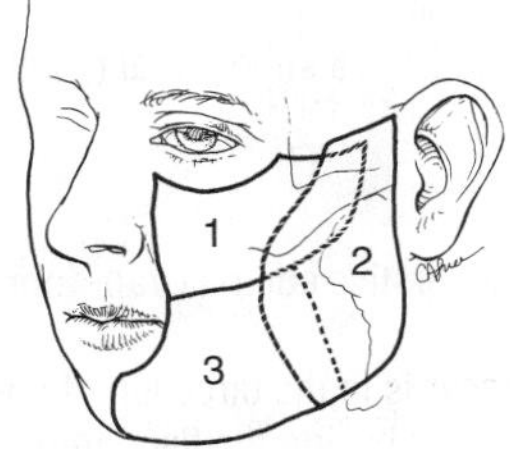


**Fig. 37-1** Three overlapping zones of the cheek aesthetic unit.

- **Can be subdivided into three subunits**
  - **A subunit:** Skin medial to a line drawn perpendicular to the lateral edge of the eyebrow
  - **B subunit:** Skin lateral to a line drawn perpendicular to the lateral edge of the eyebrow
  - **C subunit:** Skin of the lower eyelid up to its junction with the cheek skin

### Zone 2: Preauricular

- Superolateral junction of the helix and cheek
- Medially across sideburn to malar eminence
- Inferiorly to the angle of the mandible

### Zone 3: Buccomandibular

- Includes the lower cheek area and oral lining (in full-thickness defects)
- Inferior to suborbital area
- Anterior to the preauricular zone

> **TIP:** Zones 1 and 2 can be reconstructed with cervicofacial flaps, whereas zone 3 typically cannot.

## RECONSTRUCTIVE OPTIONS[3-6]

### Defect Analysis

- Analysis of the defect or anticipated defect
  - Simple: Skin and subcutaneous tissues
  - Complex: Muscle, facial nerve, parotid gland and duct, mucosa, bone
- Anatomic reconstruction of all layers when possible
  - Facial nerve reconstruction (see Chapter 42)
  - Contour revisions may be necessary for complex reconstructions (see below)

### Zone 1: Suborbital

- **Primary closure**
  - Smaller lesions can be closed with an elliptical excision typically oriented in the direction of natural relaxed skin tension lines (RSTLs)
  - Care must be taken not to distort structures, such as the lower lid
- **Skin grafts**
  - **Split-thickness** grafts can be used for temporary closure, but they often result in significant distortion, contracture, and/or scarring if used for definitive coverage
  - **Full-thickness** skin grafts provide better long-term results
    - Best donor sites are preauricular, postauricular, supraclavicular

- Templates of the defect ensure adequate size and shape
- Skin grafts used for defects with depth >5 mm often have a suboptimal result[7]
- Can look like a "patch" permanently

■ **Local flaps** (smaller defects, <4 cm)
- Rotation, advancement, transposition flaps, V-Y
- Ideally, design is **inferiorly based** to minimize postoperative edema (trap-door effect)
- **Rhomboid flaps** (Fig. 37-2)[2]
  - The flap should be designed so that donor site scar is in the direction of the RSTLs
  - Need to balance the goals of scars in the RSTLs and having the flap inferiorly based (Fig. 37-3)
  - Defect can be circular[8]—increases versatility of rhomboid design
  - Angle should be **60 degrees**

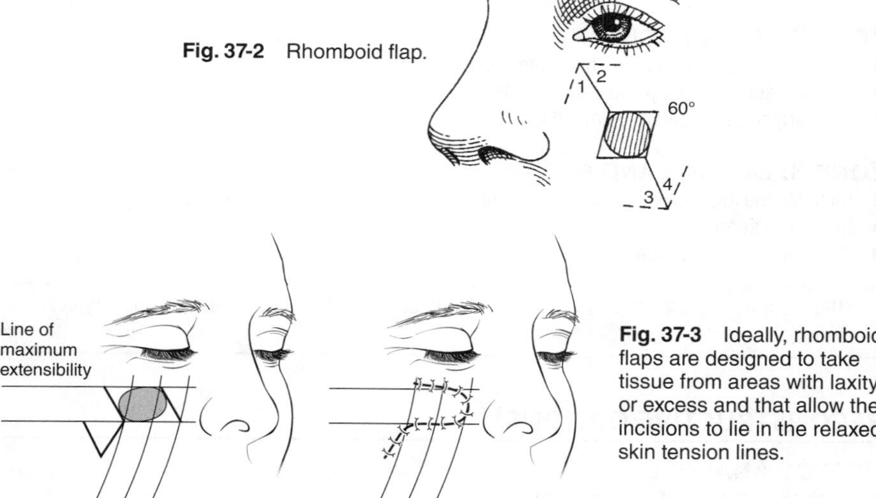


**Fig. 37-2** Rhomboid flap.

**Fig. 37-3** Ideally, rhomboid flaps are designed to take tissue from areas with laxity or excess and that allow the incisions to lie in the relaxed skin tension lines.

- **Bilobed flaps** (Fig. 37-4)[9]
  - Originally described with 90 degrees between the two flaps
  - **Zitelli modification** is recommended (reduces angle between two flaps)
  - Flap divides tension between the two advancement lobes
  - Best used for moderate to large central defects where the remaining lateral preauricular skin is used in the primary flap, and posterior auricular or cervical skin is used for secondary flap
  - Disadvantage: Multiple scars
- **Forehead flap**

**TIP:** Use a pinch test to make sure the donor defect of the secondary flap can be closed primarily.

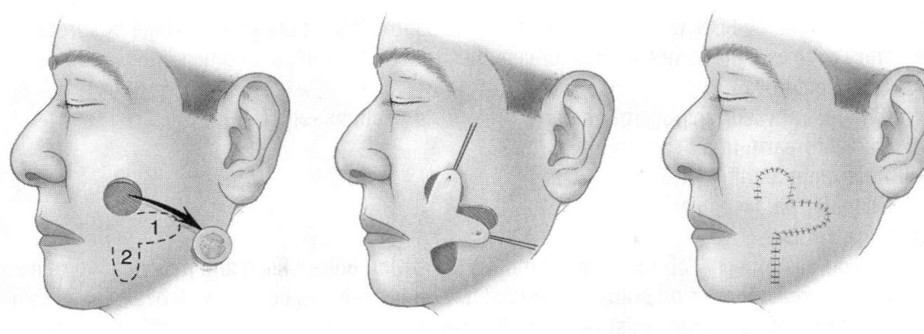


**Fig. 37-4** Bilobed flap.

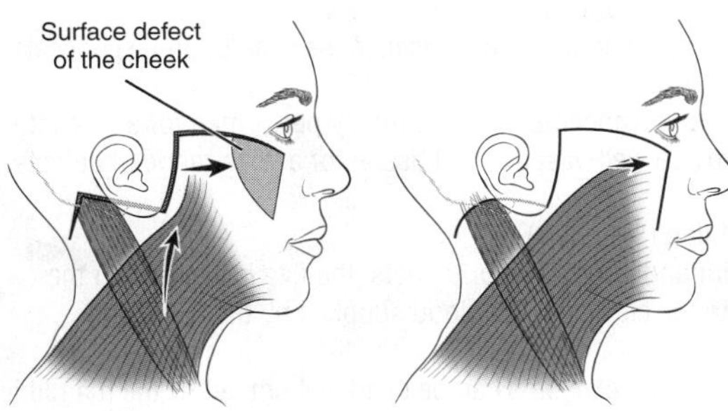


**Fig. 37-5** Cervicofacial flap.

- **Local flaps** (larger defects >4 cm)
  - **Cervicofacial flap** (Fig. 37-5)
    - Large surface defects of the cheek can be repaired.[10]
    - Local flaps bring tissue of excellent color, texture, hair, and contour match to the cheek.
    - Dissection can be carried posteriorly along the mastoid hairline to create a generous-sized, rotation-advancement flap; extensive undermining prevents excess tension at the suture lines.
    - Dog-ear deformities may be created with larger flaps and should be excised.

**TIP:** To prevent ectropion, anchor sutures to the periosteum along the zygomatic arch and inferolateral orbital rim. Also, consider performing a lateral canthopexy if there is any question.[11]

    - Because of the tenuous vascularity of the distal aspect of cervicofacial flaps, especially in smokers, most authors recommend a **deep-plane cervicofacial advancement** (inclusion of the platysma) to reconstruct the malar, lateral orbit, and temporal regions.[12]
- **Tissue expansion (TE)**[13]
  - TE offers the best color and texture match with the least number of additional incisions.
  - Custom-made expanders are often needed in the cheek and two or more expanders may be needed.
  - Orient the incision for expander placement perpendicular to the axis of the defect.
  - Choose an expander with length and width at least as large as the defect.
  - Fill TE intraoperatively to safest maximum level to reduce hematoma and seroma formation.
  - Delay expansion for about 2 weeks postoperatively, then fill expander at least once per week.

- Overexpand by 30% to 50% to overcome flap contraction at the second stage of surgery.
- Incise the capsule as needed to increase the stretch of the expanded flap, but avoid capsulectomy.

- **Free flaps:** For resurfacing larger defects or entire sub-units
  - Radial forearm free flap (FRFF)
  - Anterolateral thigh (ALT)
  - Scapular/parascapular
- **Salvage options**
  - Temporalis muscle flap (will leave temporal hollowing unless filled and may need to remove arch for reach); graft on cranial bone (will take, but often has poor quality healing and thin coverage that does not resist radiation therapy well)

## Zone 2: Preauricular

- **Primary closure:** Skin laxity in this region often allows for primary closure
- **Full-thickness skin grafts:** Better tolerated in this zone, because they can often be concealed
- **Local flaps**
  - Skin laxity can often be utilized for advancement as commonly performed for a face lift.
  - Extension onto the neck can provide well-vascularized tissue for a wide range of defects.
- **Regional flaps**
  - **Anteriorly based cervicofacial flap** (Fig. 37-6)
    - This flap is used for posterior and large anterior defects; the flap is elevated in the subcutaneous plane down to the clavicle, with blood supplied by the facial and submental arteries.[14]
    - To avoid deep plane dissection, the platysma can be divided 4 cm below the mandible.
    - Platysma can be incorporated into the flap, which enhances vascularity.
    - Donor site may require skin grafting.
  - **Cervicopectoral flap**
    - For larger defects (6-10 cm)
    - Includes skin from anterior chest
    - Includes platysma muscle and deltoid/pectoral fascia
    - Brings blood supply from anterior thoracic perforators from the internal mammary artery
  - **Submental flap**
    - Perforator flap based on branches of the facial artery
    - Hair-bearing status is an issue in men (although radiation when necessary will ameliorate this)
- **Tissue expansion:** Similar to zone 1

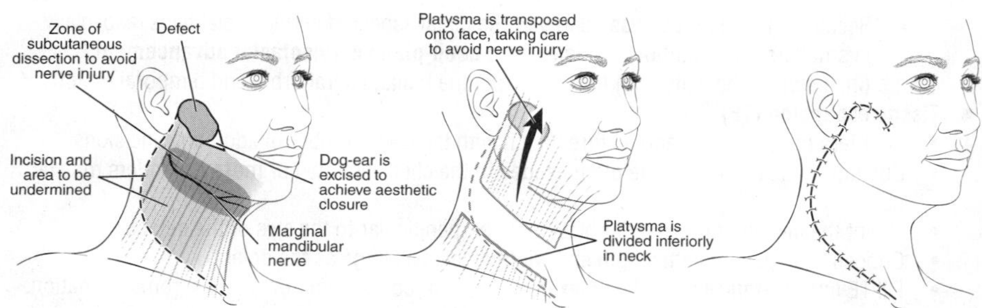


**Fig. 37-6** Anteriorly based cervicofacial flap.

- **Free flaps:** Similar to zone 1
- **Salvage flaps:** Temporalis muscle, deltopectoral flap (best used in a delayed fashion), pectoralis major muscle/myocutaneous flap, trapezius myocutaneous flap, latissimus dorsi flap

## Zone 3: Buccomandibular

**NOTE: Reconstruction may require cheek skin as well as lining and lip**

- **Lining:** If required, it is important to obtain a water-tight closure
  - Hemitongue flap based on axial lingual artery
  - Turnover or hinge flaps: Donor site must be covered by another tissue source
  - Buccal fat-pad flap
  - Masseter crossover
  - Facial artery myomucosal (FAMM) flap
  - Submental flap
  - Can skin graft on back of a well-vascularized flap (or prelaminate if time is not an issue)
  - Two skin paddle free flaps, using one for lining and one for the external surface (e.g., ALT with skin perforators)
- **Primary closure:** Typically less skin laxity and significant distortion of surrounding structures
- **Full-thickness skin graft:** Tends to look like a patch
- **Local flaps**
  - Rotation, advancement, transposition, rhomboid, V-Y, bilobed
  - W-plasty or Z-plasty may help camouflage the scar crossing the mandibular border
- **Regional flaps**
  - Inferiorly based advancement flap[15]
  - Submental flap
  - Deep plane composite flaps: High risk of nerve injury[16]
- **Tissue expansion:** Similar to zone 1
- **Free flaps** (defects usually >10 cm or full thickness): Fasciocutaneous flaps are typically the best match (FRFF, ALT, scapular/parascapular, lateral arm)
- **Salvage flaps:** Deltopectoral flap, pectoralis major muscle/myocutaneous flap (Fig. 37-7), trapezius myocutaneous flap, latissimus dorsi flap, internal mammary artery perforator (IMAP) flap may reach lower defects

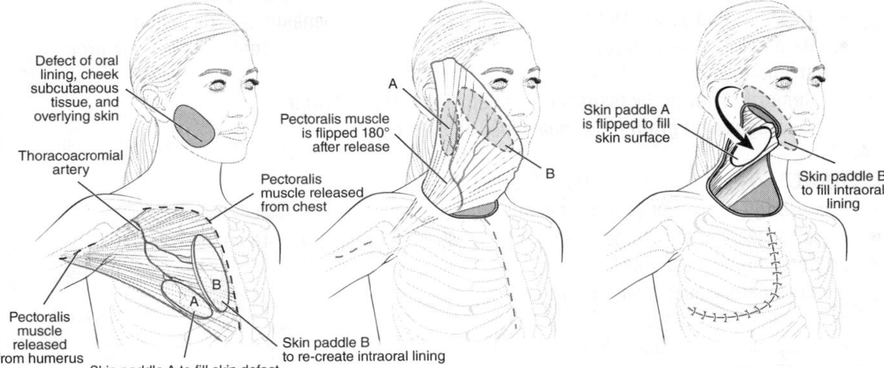


**Fig. 37-7** Pectoralis major flap with two skin paddles: one for the intraoral defect and one for the cutaneous defect. (Although this was a common flap in years past, it is now mostly used as a salvage option.)

## CONTOUR DEFECTS

- **Associated with:**
  - Romberg's disease
  - Scleroderma
  - Facial lipodystrophy
  - First or second branchial arch syndrome
  - Significant facial trauma
  - Tumor extirpation
  - Radiation-induced atrophy

### RECONSTRUCTIVE OPTIONS

- **Injectable fillers**
  - Both temporary and permanent injectable fillers are available
  - Good for minor contour defects, but morbidity increases with volume
- **Dermal and dermal-fat grafts**[17]
  - Much of the fat is reabsorbed, but some bulk persists
- **Autologous fat grafts** (see Chapter 89)
- **Local flaps**
  - Use of the platysma has been described
  - Deepithelialized flaps
  - Buccal fat[18]
- **Free tissue transfer**
  - Deepithelialized fasciocutaneous flaps: FRFF, ALT, scapular/parascapular

### REVISION PROCEDURES

- Now the **standard of care** in free tissue transfer reconstruction and are discussed before the initial procedure
- Applicable to nearly all free flap reconstructive patients, regardless of the initial indication for surgery
- Standardized surgical approach helps optimize aesthetic outcomes[19]
  - All revisions performed **more than 6 months** after initial procedure
  - **Flap debulking** by liposuction, sharp debridement, and/or curetting with more removed at the jawline; precise surface contouring with the addition of a microdebrider
  - **Treat the flap as SMAS** tissue regarding plication, suspension, and resection
  - **Release tethered scars,** and **overcorrect** oral commissure, canthal region, nasofrontal junction
  - **Support lower lid** by resuspending flap high on lateral orbit
  - **Autologous fat grafting** for final small adjustments

### COMPLEX RECONSTRUCTION

- **Restoration of the bony contour** is important for maintaining facial symmetry
- Typically seen in large tumor ablation or substantial trauma, but are uncommon
- **Osteocutaneous free flaps**
  - Scapular/parascapular flap with bone
  - Osteocutaneous fibula
  - Deep circumflex iliac artery
  - FRFF with bone

- **Large defects**
  - Frequently involve the maxilla, palatal, orbital, and/or nasal bony constructs that require planned multiple-stage reconstruction
  - A combination of local flaps, muscle flaps, free tissue transfers, nerve grafts, and bone grafts or osseous flaps may be used

## KEY POINTS

✓ For the novice or the expert, there are two outstanding texts with detailed coverage and extensive images for local flaps in the head and neck. One of the two is a must if these defects are to be part of your practice.[9,20]
✓ Rebuild or resurface entire units.
✓ Use the contralateral side as a guide.
✓ Use exact templates to design flaps.
✓ If possible, avoid vertical incisions anterior to a line drawn perpendicular to the lateral canthus.
✓ Hide scars in blepharoplasty incisions, face-lift incisions, nasolabial fold, or RSTL.
✓ Avoid ectropion by anchoring the flap to the underlying periosteum, and consider lateral canthopexy.

## REFERENCES


1. Cabrera RC, Zide BM. Cheek reconstruction. In Aston SJ, Beasley RW, Thorne HM, eds. Grabb and Smith's Plastic Surgery, 5th ed. Philadelphia: Lippincott Williams & Wilkins, 1997.
2. Zide BM. Deformities of the lips and cheeks. In McCarthy JR, ed. Plastic Surgery. Philadelphia: WB Saunders, 1990.
3. Dobratz EJ, Hilger PA. Cheek defects. Facial Plast Surg Clin North Am 17:455-467, 2009.
4. Menick FJ. Reconstruction of the cheek. Plast Reconstr Surg 108:496-505, 2001.
5. Mureau MA, Hofer SO. Maximizing results in reconstruction of cheek defects. Clin Plastic Surg 36:461-476, 2009.
6. Rapstine ED, Knaus WJ, Thornton JF. Simplifying cheek reconstruction: a review of over 400 cases. Plast Reconstr Surg 129:1291-1299, 2012.
7. Wagner J. Reconstructive considerations in the surgical management of melanoma. Surg Clin North Am 83:187-230, 2003.
8. Quaba AA, Sommerlad BC. "A square peg into a round hole": a modified rhomboid flap and its clinical application. Br J Plast Surg 40:163-170, 1987.
9. Jackson IT. Local Flaps in Head and Neck Reconstruction, 2nd ed. St Louis: Quality Medical Publishing, 2007.
10. Juri J, Juri C. Advancement and rotation of a large cervicofacial flap for cheek repairs. Plast Reconstr Surg 64:692-696, 1979.
11. Jelks GW, Jelks EB. Prevention of ectropion in reconstruction of facial defects. Clin Plast Surg 28:297-302, 2001.
12. Crow ML, Crow FJ. Resurfacing large cheek defects with rotation flaps from the neck. Plast Reconstr Surg 58:196-200, 1976.
13. Wieslander JB. Tissue expansion in the head and neck: a 6-year review. Scand J Plast Reconstr Hand Surg 25:47-56, 1991.
14. Kaplan I, Goldwyn RM. The versatility of the laterally based cervicofacial flap for cheek repairs. Plast Reconstr Surg 61:390-393, 1978.

15. Kroll SS, Reece GP, Robb G, et al. Deep-plane cervicofacial rotation-advancement flap for reconstruction of large cheek defects. Plast Reconstr Surg 94:88-93, 1994.
16. Al-Shunnar B, Manson PN. Cheek reconstruction with laterally based flaps. Clin Plast Surg 28:283-296, 2001.
17. Leaf N, Zarem HA. Correction of contour defects of the face with dermal and dermal-fat grafts. Arch Surg 105:715-719, 1972.
18. Kim JT, Naidu S, Kim YH. The buccal fat: a convenient and effective autologous option to prevent Frey syndrome and for facial contouring following parotidectomy. Plast Reconstr Surg 125:1706-1709, 2010.
19. Haddock NT, Saadeh PB, Siebert JW. Achieving aesthetic results in facial reconstructive microsurgery: planning and executing secondary refinements. Plast Reconstr Surg 130:1236-1245, 2012.
20. Baker S. Local Flaps in Facial Reconstruction, 2nd ed. St Louis: Mosby-Elsevier Health Sciences, 2007.

# 38. Ear Reconstruction

Christopher M. Shale, Amanda A. Gosman,
Edward M. Reece

## ANATOMY

### CARTILAGINOUS FRAMEWORK: THREE TIERS[1]

1. Conchal complex
2. Antihelix-antitragus complex
3. Helix-lobule complex

### BLOOD SUPPLY[2] (Fig. 38-1)

- **Posterior auricular artery** *(dominant blood supply)*
  - Supplies anterior and posterior surface of the auricle
  - Perforators enter ear at medial aspect of triangular fossa, cymba conchae, cavum conchae, helical root, and earlobe
- **Superficial temporal artery**
  - Supplies lateral surface of the auricle
  - Interconnections between posterior auricular and superficial temporal arteries allow perfusion from each system alone
- **Occipital artery**
  - Supplies posterior auricular skin in approximately 7% of population
- **Venous drainage**
  - Posterior auricular veins (drain into external jugular system)
  - Superficial temporal vein
  - Retromandibular veins

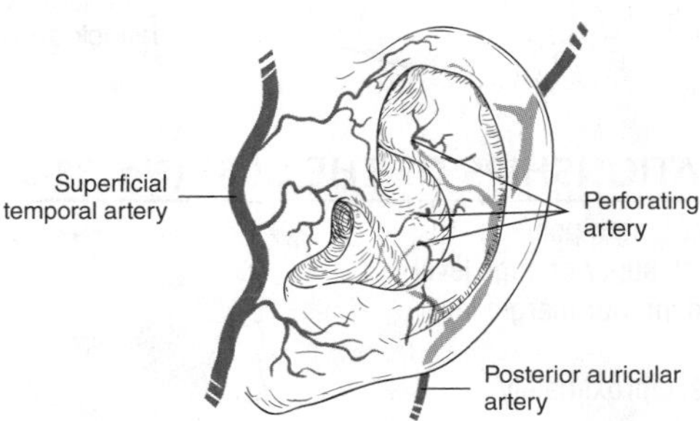


**Fig. 38-1** Anterior ear vasculature.

## NERVOUS SYSTEM[1,3]

- **Great auricular nerve** ($C_2$-$C_3$)
  - Supplies lower lateral portion and inferior cranial surface of ear
- **Auriculotemporal nerve** ($V_3$)
  - Supplies superior lateral surface and anterior superior surface of external acoustic meatus
- **Lesser occipital nerve** ($C_2$-$C_3$)
  - Supplies superior cranial surface of ear
- **Arnold's nerve** (CN VII, CN XI, CN X)
  - Auricular branch of vagus nerve (CN X) that receives contributions from facial nerve (CN VII) and glossopharyngeal nerve (CN IX)
  - Supplies posterior inferior external auditory canal and meatus, and inferior conchal bowl
  - Mediates clinical phenomena, such as referred otalgia, from other structures within the head and neck, and the initiation of coughing during manipulation of the ear canal

**TIP:** Most of the external ear can be anesthetized readily with a ring block of local anesthetic around the ear. The exception is the concha and the posterior auditory canal, which are innervated by Arnold's nerve.

## LYMPHATIC DRAINAGE[4,5] (Fig. 38-2)

- Drainage correlates with six embryologic hillocks.
  - The **tragus, root of the helix,** and **superior helix** arise from **first** branchial arch (anterior hillocks 1-3) and drain to parotid nodes.
  - The **antihelix, antitragus,** and **lobule** arise from **second** branchial arch (posterior hillocks 4-6) and drain to cervical nodes.

A

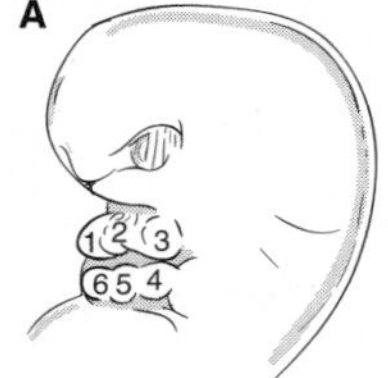


B

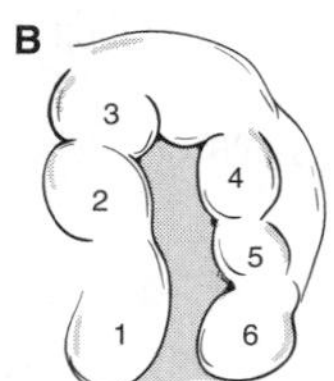


C

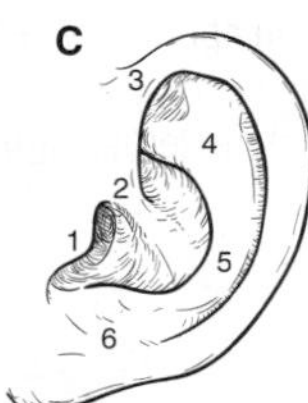


**Fig. 38-2** Embryology of the external ear. **A,** Hillock formation in an 11 mm human embryo. **B,** Hillock configuration in a 15 mm embryo at 6 weeks of gestation. **C,** Adult auricle with hillock derivations.

## AESTHETIC RELATIONSHIPS OF THE EAR[6] (Fig. 38-3)

- Ear is located one ear-length posterior to lateral orbital rim, with superior edge level with lateral brow and inferior margin level with ala of nose.
- Height of adult ear is approximately 5.5-6.5 cm.
- Width is approximately 55% of its length.
- Lateral protrusion of the helix is 1-2 cm from the scalp.
- Average incline from the vertical is 21-25 degrees.

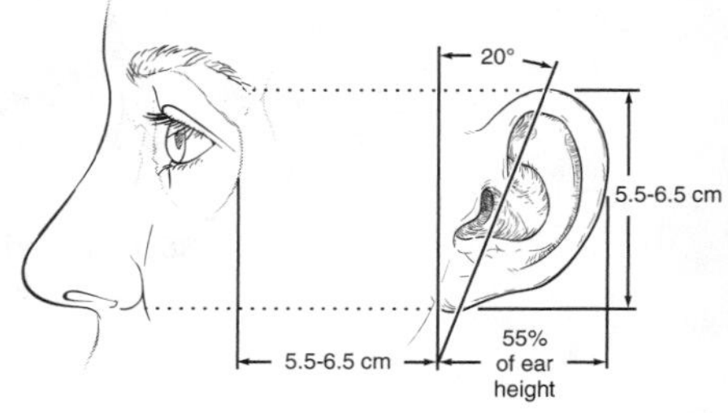


**Fig. 38-3**

- The long axis tilts posteriorly 20 degrees on average, but there is much variability.
- Projection from mastoid to helix:
  - Superior: 10-12 mm
  - Middle: 16-18 mm
  - Inferior: 20-22 mm

## ACQUIRED DEFORMITIES

### TRAUMA AND ACUTE MANAGEMENT

- **Human and animal bites**
  - **Dog bites** in children are the **most common** bite injury.
  - **Infection** is the most common complication of bites (1.6%-30%).[7,8]
  - Treat with conservative debridement, loose closure, and immediate antibiotic prophylaxis.
    - *Pasteurella multocida* is the most common pathogen in **dog** and **cat bites.**
    - *Viridans* group streptococci are most common pathogens in **human bites.**
    - Both can be treated with amoxicillin/clavulanate.
- **Blunt trauma**
  - **Hematomas** are the most common complication.
    - **Treat with immediate hematoma evacuation and compressive bolster dressing.**
  - **Cauliflower ear** deformity occurs after a subperichondrial hematoma surrounding devascularized cartilage. This results in fibrosis, and the formation of new cartilage is distorted by the scarred and restricting perichondrium.

**TIP:** A method for bolster dressings involves Xeroform gauze doubled over, positioned anteriorly and posteriorly over the wound, and held in place with through-and-through permanent sutures to help close off the potential space.

- **Lacerations, avulsions, and amputations**
  - Cleanse with minimal debridement and use skin-only closure for clean lacerations. Suturing the cartilage is not recommended.
  - Close skin when delayed reconstruction is planned.
  - Partial skin avulsions can be reattached when underlying perichondrium is present.
  - Small avulsed ear pieces (<1.5 cm) that are clean should be reattached within 6 hours as a composite graft, especially in children.
  - Large open areas where immediate closure is not feasible: Clean, debride, and perform dressing changes with bacitracin ointment and with Xeroform gauze to avoid desiccation before definitive reconstruction.
- **Thermal injury**
  - **Frostbite:** Manage with rapid rewarming, using warm saline-soaked dressings and antibiotics (fluoroquinolones).
    - Use of heparin or dextran can limit thrombosis and tissue loss.[7]
  - **Burns:** Manage with mafenide acetate (Sulfamylon) cream, noncompressive dressings, and conservative debridement of eschar after demarcation.
    - *Pseudomonas* infections are the most common cause of suppurative eschar.

## TUMORS

- **Benign**
  - **Keloid**
    - A fibroproliferative disorder of the skin that grows beyond the boundaries of the original wound and has thick eosinophilic collagen bundles.[9]
      - Earlobe is the most common site.
      - Ear piercing is the most common cause.
      - Risk factors: Race, trauma (or traumatic surgical technique), tension on wound closure, wound infections, and foreign body reactions.[9]
    - **Demographics**
      - Race: 15 times more frequent in patients with darker skin than those with lighter skin, with a 6%-16% incidence in African populations.[9,10]
      - Age: Highest incidence is in the second decade of life.[7]
    - **Treatment**
      - Simple excision alone has a recurrence rate of 45%-100%, and is reserved for smaller lesions; larger, more complicated lesions are treated in combination with adjuvant therapies.[7,9,10]
      - Intralesional corticosteroid injections can decrease symptoms and flatten keloids, but recurrence rates range from 9%-50%.[7]
      - Corticosteroid injections, combined with surgical excision, have a recurrence rate of 0%-100%.[7]
      - Excision followed by radiation has a success rate of 67%-98%.[9,10]
      - Radiation alone has a response rate of 10%-94%, but it should be reserved for lesions resistant to other treatment methods because of potential morbidity from radiation.[7]
      - Cryotherapy can be used alone or with intralesional steroid injection.[9,10]
      - Silicone dressings applied to keloids can decrease the volume of the lesion.
      - Continuous silicone dressing and pressure after surgical excision (24 hours a day for 3 months) can prevent keloid formation in up to 85% of cases.[7]
  - **Chondrodermatitis nodularis chronica helicis**[11,12]
    - Painful, chronic inflammatory, nodular, cystic, or ulcerative lesion; most commonly seen on the superior pole of the helix
    - More common in men, 4:1 male to female ratio
    - Frequently mistaken for malignant skin tumor; pain with pressure can help differentiate from malignancy
    - Complete excision of the lesion and underlying cartilage
    - Recurrence rate: 11%-31% after excision[11]

**TIP:** One frequently sees test questions on chondrodermatitis nodularis chronica helicis.

**TIP:** Prevent recurrence by ensuring adequate postoperative pressure relief, avoiding sharp corners during excision, and using pressure-relief foam pillows for the ears.

- **Malignant**
  - External ear is the site of 6% of all skin cancers and of 10% of skin cancers in the head and neck.
  - **Squamous cell carcinomas are the most common** (50%-60%).
    - The average rate of cutaneous metastasis is 11%, compared with 2% from other primary sites.[7]

- Basal cell carcinomas are the second most common (30%-40%).
- Melanomas are present in 1%-2% of malignant ear lesions.

# RECONSTRUCTIVE ALGORITHM

## Auricular Defect Classification

- **Partial-thickness**
- **Full-thickness** defects classified according to location
  - Helical rim
  - Superior, middle, and inferior third of auricle
  - Lobule

## Partial-Thickness Defects

- **Perichondrium intact**
  - Cover with skin graft taken from contralateral postauricular region.
- **Perichondrium missing**
  - Wedge excision is made (<1.5 cm defect).
  - Preauricular or postauricular flaps are rotated, advanced, or tunneled through cartilage into defect.
- Two bipedicle flap technique, based on posterior skin and advanced anteriorly[13]

> **TIP:** For partial thickness defects, with or without missing perichondrium in noncritical support areas (such as the conchal bowl), excision of the cartilage will leave the bare area of the postauricular skin as a well-vascularized recipient site for a full-thickness skin graft. Be sure to use bolster dressings with through-and-through stitches to stabilize the graft.

## Full-Thickness Defects

- **Helical rim**
  - **Small defects** (<2 cm)
    - Contralateral composite graft (<1.5 cm defect)
    - **Antia-Buch procedure**[14] (Fig. 38-4)
      1. Incision is made in helical sulcus through anterior skin and cartilage; posteromedial skin is undermined.
      2. Helix is advanced into defect, based on posterior skin flap.
      3. Defects up to 2 cm can be closed by advancing the helix in both directions and creating V-Y advancement of crus helicis.
    - **Chondrocutaneous rotation flaps,** inferiorly based on the antihelix, antitragus, or lobule, are used for defects of the middle and lower helix.[15] Defects up to 5 cm can be closed by including a lobule advancement flap and scapha resection.[16]

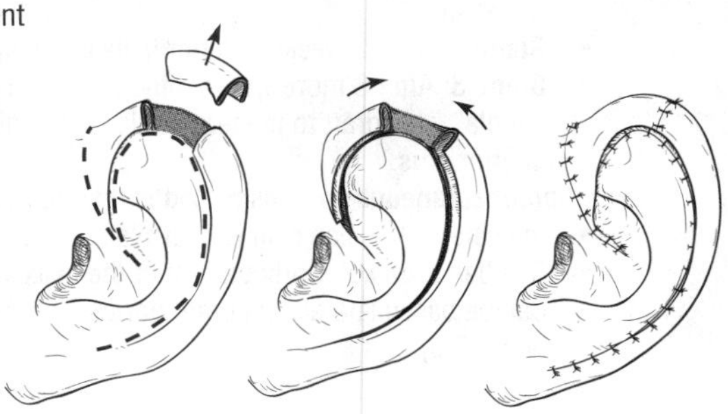

**Fig. 38-4** The Antia-Buch procedure of helical rim advancement.

- **Large defects** (>2 cm)
  - **Auricular cartilage grafts** are covered by preauricular flap or staged postauricular pocket flap.[17]
  - **Converse's tunnel technique**[18] (Fig. 38-5): A prefabricated composite flap is created in two stages.
    - **Stage 1:** Contralateral auricular cartilage strut graft is tunneled under postauricular skin adjacent to helical defect.
    - **Stage 2:** After 3 weeks, the anteriorly based skin flap and underlying cartilage strut are inset into helical rim.
  - **Tubed-pedicle flaps** from the postauricular skin or cervical skin are created and transferred in three stages.
    - **Stage 1:** Elevation and tubing of flap is created in postauricular or cervical skin with direct closure of donor site.
    - **Stage 2:** After 3 weeks, the inferior end of tube is divided and inset into inferior helical rim.
    - **Stage 3:** After 3 more weeks, superior end of tube is divided and transferred to superior helical rim.
    - Treatment may require delayed insertion of a cartilage graft to support rim and correct drooping flap after transfer and healing are completed.

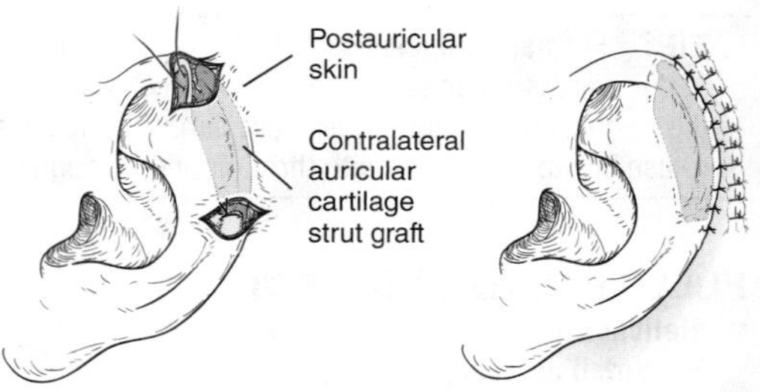


**Fig. 38-5** Converse's tunnel technique. Contralateral auricular cartilage strut graft is tunneled under postauricular skin adjacent to helical defect. Anteriorly based skin flap and underlying cartilage strut are inset into helical rim as a composite flap after 3 weeks.

- **Superior third defects**
  - **Small defects** (<2 cm)
    - Auricular reduction is used with Tanzer's excision patterns and primary closure[19] (Fig. 38-6).
  - **Large defect** (>2 cm)
    - **Contralateral auricular cartilage graft** is used with preauricular banner flaps.[20]
    - **Valise handle** technique is used for bipedicled chondrocutaneous flap.[21]
      - **Stage 1:** Contralateral auricular cartilage graft is implanted subcutaneously adjacent to defect.
      - **Stage 2:** After 3 weeks, inferior helix is transposed to cartilage graft.
      - **Stage 3:** After 3 more weeks, bipedicled composite flap is elevated as a "valise handle"; skin graft to posterior sulcus to achieve projection of helix and definition of inferior crus.
    - **Chondrocutaneous composite flap** is rotated from conchal bowl.
      - Indicated when flap skin is unavailable for coverage of cartilage graft.
      - Can be based anteriorly on root of the helix as described by Davis[15,18] (Fig. 38-7).
      - Can be based laterally on outer border of helix as described by Orticochea[22] (Fig. 38-8).

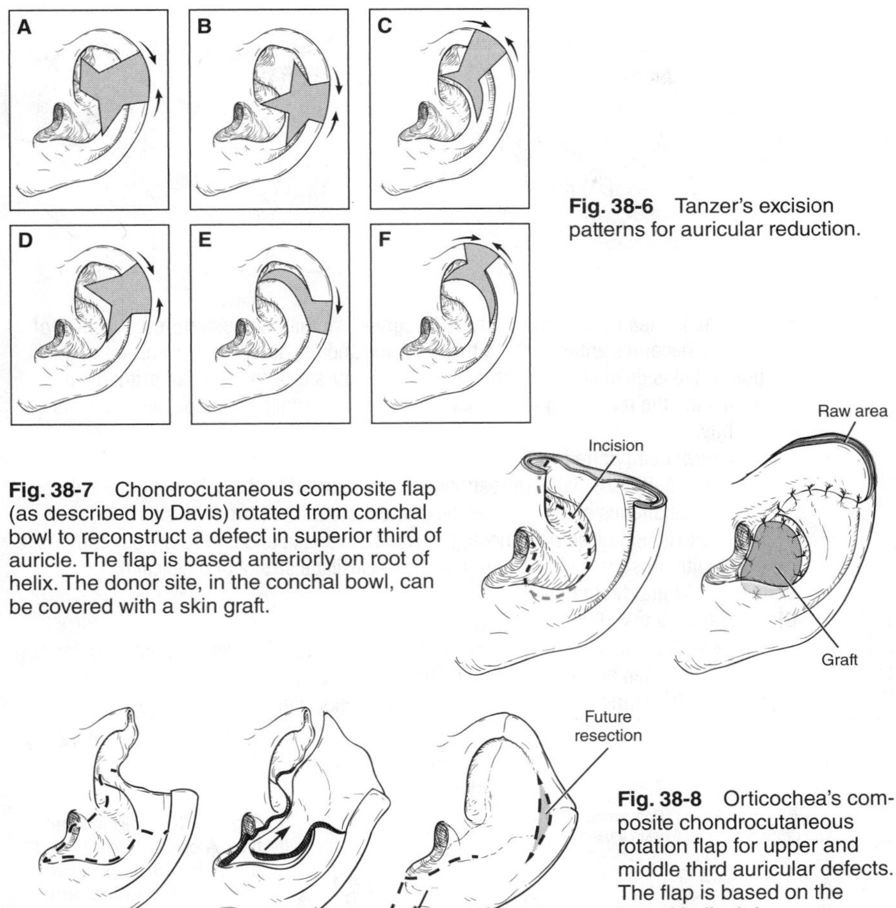


**Fig. 38-6** Tanzer's excision patterns for auricular reduction.

**Fig. 38-7** Chondrocutaneous composite flap (as described by Davis) rotated from conchal bowl to reconstruct a defect in superior third of auricle. The flap is based anteriorly on root of helix. The donor site, in the conchal bowl, can be covered with a skin graft.

**Fig. 38-8** Orticochea's composite chondrocutaneous rotation flap for upper and middle third auricular defects. The flap is based on the lateral helical rim.

- ▸ **Costal cartilage graft,** covered by temporoparietal or mastoid fascia flap and skin graft, may be needed for very large defects or when residual tissues are inadequate for reconstruction.

- ■ **Middle third defects**
  - **Small defects** (<2 cm)
    - ▸ Auricular reduction using Tanzer's excision patterns and primary closure[19]
  - **Larger defects** (>2 cm)
    - ▸ **Rotated postauricular island flap: "Flip-flop" flap (Fig. 38-9)**[23,24]
      - ♦ For conchal defects, a postauricular island flap is elevated that includes the skin, a portion of the postauricular muscle, and fascia and is based off the posterior auricular artery; if there is no defect in the conchal cartilage, one is created to allow passage of the flap anteriorly to fill the defect.

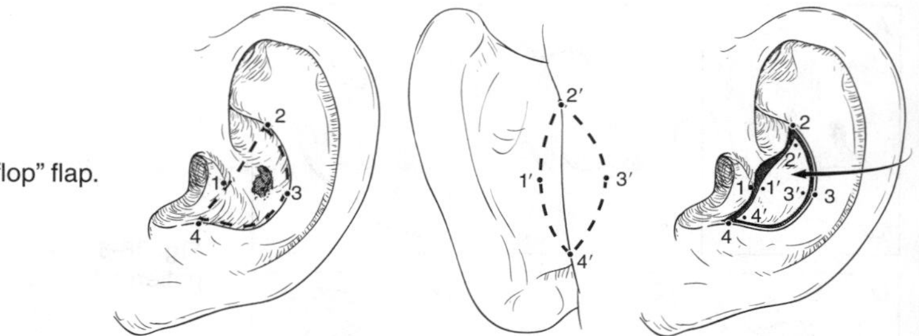


**Fig. 38-9** "Flip-flop" flap.

- The flap is then rotated anteriorly 180 degrees, so that the posteriormost aspect of the flap becomes anterior along the antihelix, and the anteriormost portion of the donor flap is deep in the conchal bowl; the donor site is then closed primarily by advancing the remaining postauricular skin, which shallows the posterior sulcus slightly.
- **Contralateral composite graft**
  - If there is sufficient viable retroauricular skin adjacent to the defect, a contralateral chondrocutaneous composite can be grafted to that retroauricular skin.
  - Graft take is optimized by removing retroauricular skin and cartilage from composite graft, with preservation of anterior skin and cartilage strut along helical rim.[21]
- **Converse's tunnel technique**[18]
- **Dieffenbach's flap**[18] (Fig. 38-10)
  - **Stage 1:** Contralateral auricular cartilage graft is sutured to defect; postauricular skin is elevated, then advanced over cartilage graft to fill defect.
  - **Stage 2:** Postauricular skin flap is divided 3 weeks later.

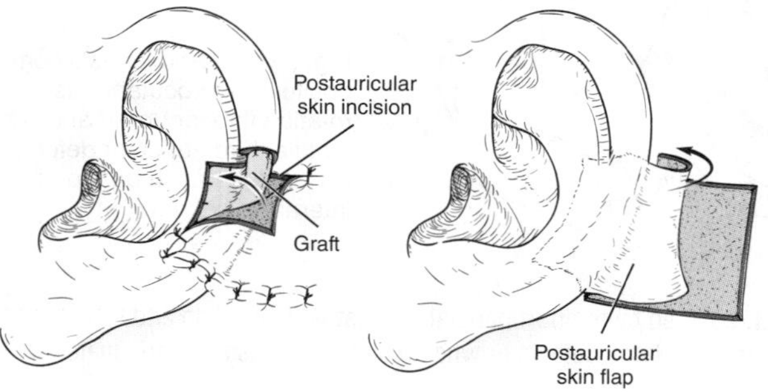


**Fig. 38-10** Dieffenbach's flap. A contralateral auricular cartilage graft is sutured to defect and covered with postauricular skin flap. The postauricular skin flap is divided 3 weeks later.

- **Inferior third defects**
  - Superiorly based flaps are doubled over with subcutaneous cartilage graft for contour and support.
  - Valise handle technique for bipedicled chondrocutaneous flaps can be modified for lower defects to achieve definition of posterior conchal wall.[21]
- **Earlobe defects and deformities**
  - Composite graft from contralateral lobule.
  - Postauricular flap is transposed and sutured to superiorly based anterior skin flap.[25]

- Chondrocutaneous flaps from the postauricular surface can be rotated inferiorly, based on a subcutaneous pedicle, to reconstruct the anterior surface of the lobule; the posterior surface of the lobule can be reconstructed with a local retroauricular skin flap.[26]
  - The inclusion of conchal cartilage prevents scar contracture.
  - The donor defect is closed primarily by advancing retroauricular skin.
- **Cleft earlobe reconstruction**
  - Make a wedge excision and everted closure.
  - Use a Z-plasty closure to prevent notching.
  - A thin flap from the edge of the cleft can be rolled into superior aspect of wedge repair immediately after repair of cleft to preserve skin-lined channel for earring use.[27]

## Replantation and Banking

- **Replantation**[28]
  - The **superficial temporal artery** or **posterior auricular artery** must be available for microvascular anastomosis to consider replantation.
  - Even if a venous anastomosis is performed, often to the superficial temporal vein, **leech therapy** is almost always required; replantation can be done without venous anastomosis, using just leech therapy, but this has a higher risk for partial flap/ear loss.
  - Successful replantation yields a superior aesthetic result compared with secondary reconstruction.[28]
- **Banking of ear cartilage**
  - Traumatized ear cartilage can be banked under temporoparietal fascia, postauricular skin, or volar forearm; the success of banking is inconsistent.
  - **Mladick's pocket principle for banking ear cartilage**[29]
    - Dermabrasion is used to remove the epidermis from the avulsed ear.
    - Cartilage is reapplied to the remaining ear and banked under a postauricular skin pocket.
    - The graft is left in place for 3 weeks and will reepithelialize when exposed.
  - **Baudet's fenestration technique**[30]
    - Posterior skin of the amputated part is removed, and fenestrations are made in avulsed auricular cartilage to increase the vascular recipient area.
    - The amputated portion is reattached, and exposed cartilage is covered with a postauricular skin flap.
    - The flap is divided after 3 months, and a skin graft is applied.

**TIP:** The temporoparietal fascia flap should be preserved for secondary reconstruction; its use for *acute* coverage of replanted cartilage is *not* recommended.

## Total Ear Reconstruction

- Options for total ear reconstruction include use of a framework covered with either a free or pedicled temporoparietal fascial flap and skin graft, or tissue-expanded periauricular skin; the underlying framework can either be sculpted costal cartilage or a prefabricated Medpore implant (Porex Surgical, Newnan, GA).
  - For costal cartilage frameworks, the **contralateral costal synchondrosis (ribs 6-8)** is preferred.
  - The cartilage is flexible in children, and the helical rim can be created by attaching a separate carved piece of rib cartilage to the framework.
  - The cartilage is stiff in adults, and the framework, including the helical rim, is best carved en bloc, because cartilage does not tolerate bending.
  - The framework should be based on a **template from the contralateral ear** to match size and contour.

- Successful microvascular reconstruction of the ear, with prefabricated composite flaps, has been reported.[31,32]
- In instances where the patient is not interested, or is not a candidate for ear reconstruction osteointegrated implants are an option; they provide stable insertion points for a prosthetic ear.

## KEY POINTS

✓ The blood supply of the auricle is provided by an intercommunicating network from the posterior auricular and superficial arteries. Either artery can perfuse the entire auricle through this network.

✓ Arnold's nerve is the auricular branch of the vagus nerve (CN X) and receives contributions from the facial nerve (CN VII) and glossopharyngeal nerve (CN IX). It mediates clinical phenomena, such as the initiation of coughing during manipulation of the ear canal and referred otalgia from other structures within the head and neck.

✓ Suturing the cartilage is not recommended when repairing a clean laceration of the ear. Skin-only suturing is sufficient and reduces the risk of secondary deformity.

✓ Chondrodermatitis nodularis chronica helicis is a benign tumor that should be completely excised to definitively exclude any malignant skin tumor and reduce the risk of recurrence.

✓ The most effective treatment for keloids is multimodality therapy, such as excision followed by radiation.

✓ To facilitate a logical approach to reconstruction, ear defects should be classified according to location and extent of tissue loss.

✓ Replantation of an avulsed auricle yields the best aesthetic result.

## REFERENCES

1. Allison GR. Anatomy of the external ear. Clin Plast Surg 5:419-422, 1978.
2. Park C, Lineaweaver WC, Rumley TO, et al. Arterial supply of the anterior ear. Plast Reconstr Surg 90:38-44, 1992.
3. Brent B. Reconstruction of the auricle. In McCarthy JG, ed. Plastic Surgery, vol 3. Philadelphia: WB Saunders, 1990.
4. Songcharoen S, Smith RA, Jabaley ME, et al. Tumors of the external ear and reconstruction of defects. Clin Plast Surg 5:447-457, 1978.
5. Beahm EK, Walton RL. Auricular reconstruction for microtia: part 1. Anatomy, embryology, and clinical evaluation. Plast Reconstr Surg 109:2473-2482, 2002.
6. Farkas L. Anthropometry of normal and anomalous ears. Clin Plast Surg 5:401-412, 1978.
7. Elsahy N. Acquired ear defects. Clin Plast Surg 29:175-186, 2002.
8. Talan DA, Citron DM, Abrahamian FM, et al. Bacteriologic analysis of infected dog and cat bites. N Engl J Med 340:85-92, 1999.
9. Ogawa R. The most current algorithms for the treatment and prevention of hypertrophic scars and keloids. Plast Reconstr Surg 125:557-568, 2010.
10. Lorenz P, Bari AS. Scar prevention, treatment, and revision. In Neligan PC, Gurtner GC. Plastic Surgery, 3rd ed. Philadelphia: Saunders-Elsevier, 2013.
11. Wagner G, Liefeith J, Sachse MM. Clinical appearance, differential diagnoses, and therapeutical options of chondrodermatitis nodularis chronica helicis Winkler. J Dtsch Dermatol Ges 9:287-291, 2011.
12. Zuber TJ, Jackson E. Chondrodermatitis nodularis chronica helicis. Arch Fam Med 8:445-447, 1999.

13. Elsahy N. Reconstruction of the ear after skin and perichondrium loss. Clin Plast Surg 29:187-200, 2002.
14. Antia NH, Buch VI. Chondrocutaneous advancement flap for the marginal defect of the ear. Plast Reconstr Surg 39:472-477, 1967.
15. Davis JE. Reconstruction of the upper third of the ear with a chondrocutaneous composite flap based on the crus helix. In Milton E, Tanzer RC, eds. Symposium on Reconstruction of the Auricle. St Louis: CV Mosby, 1974.
16. Butler CE. Single-stage reconstruction of middle and lower third helical rim defects using chondrocutaneous helical rim and lobular advancement flaps and a scaphal reduction cartilage graft. Plast Reconstr Surg 122:463-467, 2008.
17. Lavasani L, Leventhal D, Constantinides M, et al. Management of acute soft tissue injury to the auricle. Facial Plast Surg 26:445-450, 2010.
18. Aguilar EA. Traumatic total or partial ear loss. In Evans GR, ed. Operative Plastic Surgery. New York: McGraw-Hill, 2000.
19. Tanzer R. Deformities of the auricle. In Converse JM, ed. Reconstructive Plastic Surgery, 2nd ed. Philadelphia: WB Saunders, 1977.
20. Crikelair G. A method of partial ear reconstruction for avulsion of the upper portion of the ear. Plast Reconstr Surg 17:438-443, 1956.
21. Brent B. The acquired auricular deformity: a systematic approach to its analysis and reconstruction. Plast Reconstr Surg 59:475-485, 1977.
22. Orticochea M. Reconstruction of partial losses of the auricle. Plast Reconstr Surg 46:403-405, 1970.
23. Dessy LA, Figus A, Fioramonti P, et al. Reconstruction of anterior auricular conchal defect after malignancy excision: revolving-door flap versus full-thickness skin graft. J Plast Reconstr Aesthet Surg 63:746-752, 2010.
24. Talmi YP, Wolf M, Horowitz Z, et al. "Second look" at auricular reconstruction with a postauricular island flap: "flip-flop flap." Plast Reconstr Surg 109:713-715, 2002.
25. Larrabee WF, Sherris DA. Ear. In Larrabee WF, Sherris DA, eds. Principles of Facial Reconstruction. Philadelphia: Lippincott-Raven, 1995.
26. Yotsuyanagi T, Yamashita K, Sawada Y. Reconstruction of the congenital and acquired earlobe deformity. Clin Plast Surg 29:249-255, 2002.
27. Pardue A. Repair of torn earlobe with preservation of the perforation for an earring. Plast Reconstr Surg 51:472-473, 1973.
28. Lin PY, Chiang YC, Hsieh CH, et al. Microsurgical replantation and salvage procedures in traumatic ear amputation. 69:E15-E19, 2010.
29. Mladick RA, Horton CE, Adamson JE, et al. The pocket principle: a new technique for the reattachment of a severed ear part. Plast Reconstr Surg 48:219-223, 1971.
30. Baudet J. A propos d'un procede original de reimplantation d'un pavilion de l'oreille totalement separe. Ann Chir Plast 17:67-72, 1972.
31. Zhou G, Teng L, Chang HM, et al. Free prepared composite forearm flap transfer for ear reconstruction: three case reports. Microsurgery 15:660-662, 1994.
32. Chiang YC. Combined tissue expansion and prelamination of forearm flap in major ear reconstruction. Plast Reconstr Surg 117:1292-1295, 2006.

# 39. Lip Reconstruction

James B. Collins, Raman C. Mahabir, Scott W. Mosser

## ETIOLOGIC FACTORS

- Trauma
- Cancer
  - Squamous cell carcinoma most common overall
  - Basal cell carcinoma most common on the upper lip

## LIP ANATOMY

- **Layers**
  - Skin
  - Subcutaneous fat
  - Muscle (e.g., orbicularis oris, mentalis)
  - Mucosa
- **External landmarks** (Fig. 39-1)
  - Commissure
  - Cupid's bow
  - Philtral columns: Ridges formed by decussation of orbicularis oris
  - Tubercle
  - White roll: Ridge formed by orbicularis oris
  - Red line: Wet-dry vermilion line
- **Aesthetic units of the lips**[1] (Fig. 39-2)
  - Upper lip
    - Lateral
    - Medial/philtral
  - Lower lip (one unit)

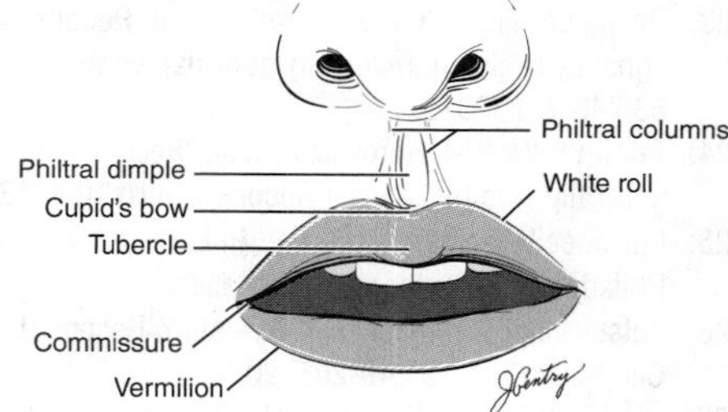


**Fig. 39-1** External anatomy of the lips.

> **TIP:** Many reconstructive techniques of the lip rely on the separation of aesthetic subunits.[2]

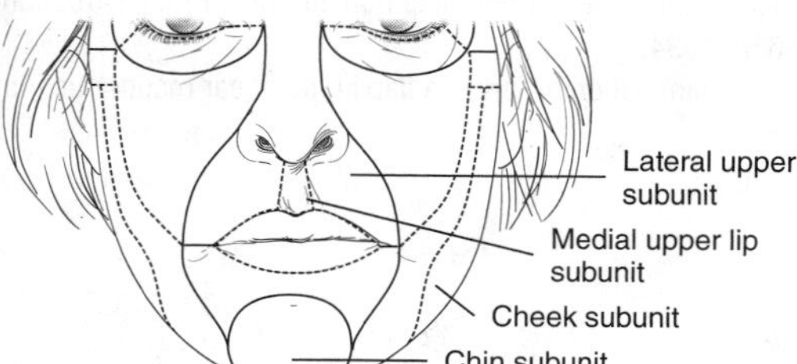


**Fig. 39-2** Aesthetic subunits of the face and lips.

- **Muscles of facial expression**[3,4] (Fig. 39-3) (Table 39-1)
  - Reconstructive techniques may damage innervation to these muscles.
  - **Modiolus:** Attachment site lateral to the commissure for multiple muscles

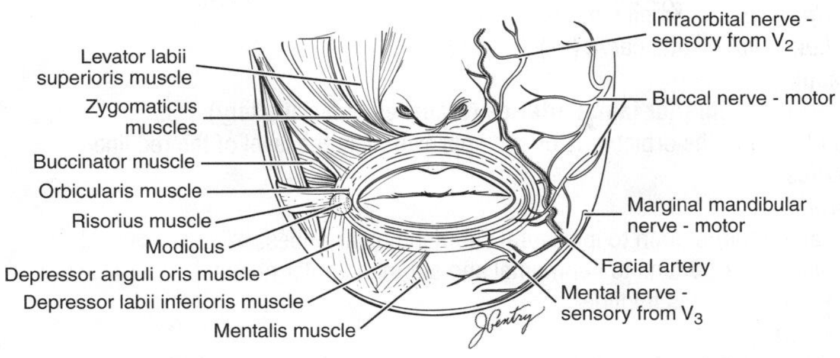


**Fig. 39-3** Internal anatomy of the lips.

**Table 39-1** *Origins, Insertions, and Actions of Muscles of the Lips*

| Muscle | Origin | Insertion | Innervation | Action |
|---|---|---|---|---|
| Buccinator | Alveolar process of maxilla and mandible, and along pterygomandibular raphe | Orbicularis oris | Buccal branch | Compresses cheeks |
| Depressor anguli oris | Lateral aspect of mental tubercle of mandible | Modiolus | Mandibular branch | Lowers angle of mouth |
| Depressor labii inferioris | Between mandibular symphysis and mental foramen, along oblique line of mandible | Skin of lower lip | Mandibular branch | Draws lip downward and laterally |
| Levator anguli oris | Maxilla, inferior to infraorbital foramen | Modiolus | Buccal branch | Elevates angle of mouth |
| Levator labii superioris | Maxilla, medial half of infraorbital margin | Modiolus and orbicularis oris of upper lip | Buccal branch | Elevates upper lip |
| Levator labii superioris alaeque nasi | Frontal process of maxilla | Upper lip orbicularis oris, nasal cartilages | Buccal branch | Elevates upper lip, flares nostrils |
| Mentalis | Incisive fossa of mandible | Skin of chin | Mandibular branch | Elevates and protrudes lower lip |
| Orbicularis oris | Alveolar border of maxilla, mandible | Circumferentially around mouth, interdigitates with other muscles | Buccal branch | Sphincter of lips, assists in lip protrusion |
| Platysma | Skin over deltopectoral region | Mandible and skin of lower face, including lip | Cervical branches | Lowers lower lip |
| Risorius | Parotid fascia | Modiolus | Buccal branch | Draws angle of mouth laterally |
| Zygomaticus major | Zygoma, anterior to temporal-zygomatic suture | Modiolus | Buccal branch | Draws angle of mouth superolaterally |
| Zygomaticus minor | Zygoma, posterior to zygomaticomaxillary suture | Skin of upper lip | Buccal branch | Elevates upper lip |

**TIP:** Reconstruction of orbicularis oris is important to maintain sphincteric activity of the lip.

- **Sensory innervation**
  - Trigeminal nerve
    - *Upper lip:* Infraorbital nerve ($V_2$)
    - *Lower lip:* Mental nerve ($V_3$)
- **Blood supply**
  - **Superior** and **inferior labial arteries** (branches of facial artery)
  - Found deep to the orbicularis oris at approximately the level of the red line
- **Lymphatics**[5]
  - *Lower lip*
    - Lateral thirds drain to ipsilateral submandibular nodes.
    - Medial third drains to submental and submandibular nodes.
      - It may cross midline.
  - *Upper lip*
    - Primarily drains to ipsilateral submandibular nodes
    - Occasionally drains to ipsilateral preauricular, infraauricular parotid, or submental nodes

## DESCRIPTION OF THE DEFECT

- **Size**
  - Absolute length
  - Percent of the total lip
- **Depth**
  - Partial or full thickness
- **Commissure involvement**

## GOALS OF LIP RECONSTRUCTION

- **Oral competence**
  - Muscular integrity
  - Oral aperture preservation
    - Reduction to $<$50% of the preoperative stoma produces significant dysfunction.

**TIP:** Patients with dentures require special consideration to maintain an adequate oral aperture.

- **Sensation**
- **Speech**
- **Cosmesis**
  - Aesthetic proportions and symmetry

**TIP:** A vermilion mismatch of >1 mm during repair can be noticed readily at a conversational distance.[6]

## REPAIR OF VERMILION DEFECTS[7,8]

- **Isolated volume deficiency**
  - V-Y advancement
    - Useful for a notch or vermilion defect
  - Lip switch
    - Useful for larger defects
    - Replaces wet and/or dry vermilion with identical tissue

**TIP:** Using wet vermilion to replace dry vermilion will result in chronically dry lips.

  - Fat grafting
    - Useful to replace volume
- **Subtotal vermilion deficiency** (<50%)
  - Axial myovermilion advancement flap[9] (Fig. 39-4)
  - Myomucosal V-Y advancement flap (Fig. 39-5)

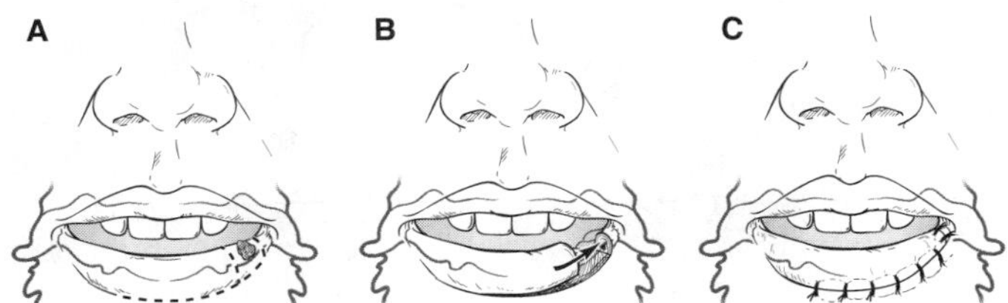


**Fig. 39-4** Axial myovermilion advancement flap. **A,** The flap is elevated deep to the labial artery. The position of the labial artery can be identified at the time of the resection of the lesion. **B** and **C,** Forward advancement of the flap allows primary closure of the defect.

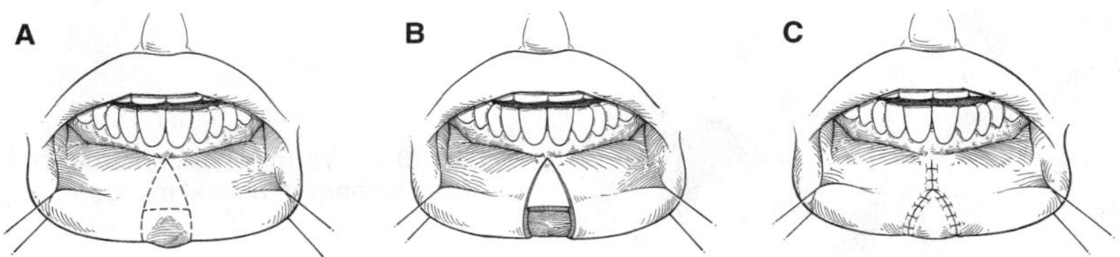


**Fig. 39-5** Myomucosal V-Y advancement flap. **A,** Focal lower lip vermilion deficiency. **B,** V design of the myomucosal advancement flap. **C,** Local volume increase following V-Y advancement flap.

- Vermilion lip switch flap[9] (Fig. 39-6)
- **Larger vermilion defects** (>50%)
  - Tongue flap
    - Two-stage procedure
    - Transfers ventral tongue tissue to lip defect
    - Suboptimal appearance compared with vermilion or oral mucosa reconstruction
- **Total vermilion deficiency**
  - Buccal mucosal advancement[9] (Fig. 39-7)
    - Wet buccal mucosa replaces deficient vermilion.
    - Resultant lip has good color.
    - It is prone to become dry and scaly.

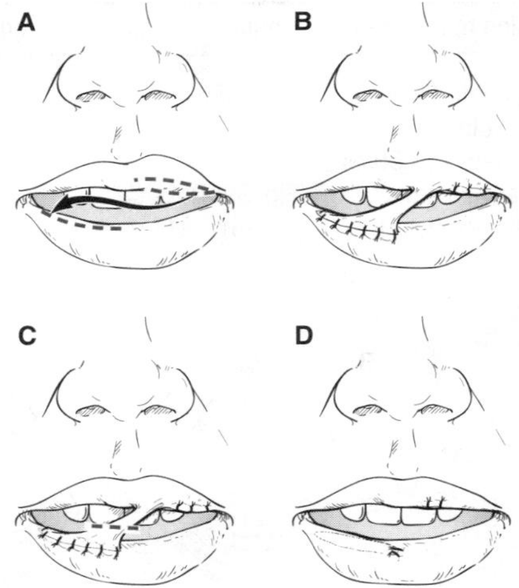


**Fig. 39-6** Vermilion lip switch flap. **A,** Left upper and lower lip volume deficiency. **B,** A right upper lip random vermilion pedicle flap is elevated. The transverse incision in the deficient left lower vermilion prepares the recipient bed. **C,** The pedicle is divided at 14 days. **D,** The flap adds volume to the left lower lip vermilion, and the donor site is closed primarily.

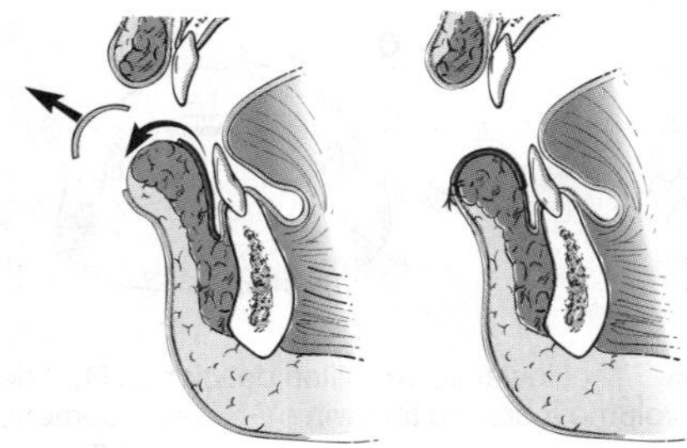

**Fig. 39-7** Vermilion reconstruction by advancement of buccal mucosa.

## FULL-THICKNESS LIP RECONSTRUCTION[10-13]

- **Rule of thirds**[9] (Fig. 39-8)
  - Standard method to determine options for lip reconstruction

Defect Size
A
Up to one third of the lip
Central defect
Perialar crescentic excision
Vermilion intact
Nasolabial flap
Lateral defect
Primary closure
One third to two thirds of the lip
Central defect
Abbé flap with perialar crescentic excisions or Karapandzic flap
Lateral defect
No commissure or philtrum involvement
Abbé flap
Commissure involved
Estlander flap
Commissure and philtrum involved
Estlander flap with contralateral perialar crescentic excision
Greater than two thirds of the lip
Sufficient cheek tissue
Central defect
Bernard-Burow
Lateral defect
Ipsilateral Bernard-Burow with contralateral perialar crescentic excisions
Insufficient cheek tissue
Distant/free flap
Defect Size
B
Up to one third of the lip
Close primarily
One third to two thirds of the lip
Sufficient lip tissue
Commissure involved
Karapandzic (first choice)
Estlander (second choice)
Commissure not involved
Abbé
Karapandzic
Insufficient lip tissue
Bernard-Burow
More than two thirds of the lip
Sufficient adjacent cheek tissue
Karapandzic for up to 80% defect or Bernard-Burow
Insufficient adjacent cheek tissue
Distant/free flap

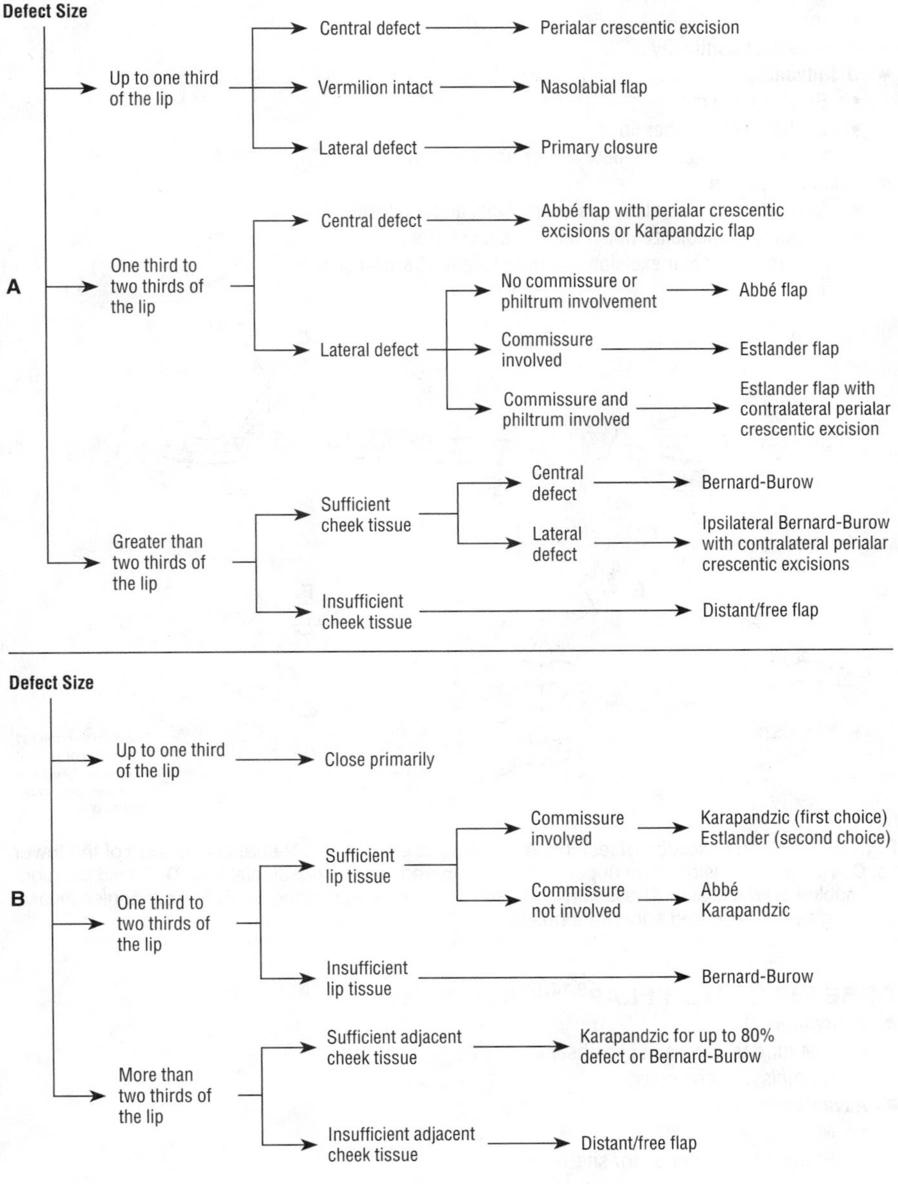

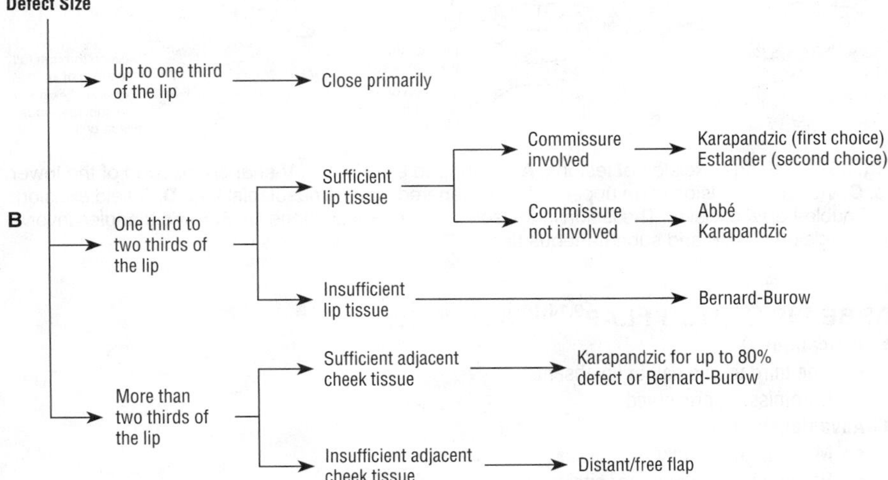

**Fig. 39-8** **A,** Algorithm for **upper lip** reconstruction. **B,** Algorithm for **lower lip** reconstruction.

## PRIMARY CLOSURE[9] (Fig. 39-9)

- **Indication**
  - Less than one third of lip absent
- **Advantages**
  - Single-stage procedure
  - Innervated
  - Muscular continuity
- **Disadvantages**
  - Small lip defects
  - Limited use in upper lip
    - Obliterates Cupid's bow and/or philtral elements
- **Technical pearls**
  - Accurate approximation of skin, muscle, and mucosa
  - Possible to medialize upper lateral lip elements
    - Crescentic alar excision useful to hide the vertical scar

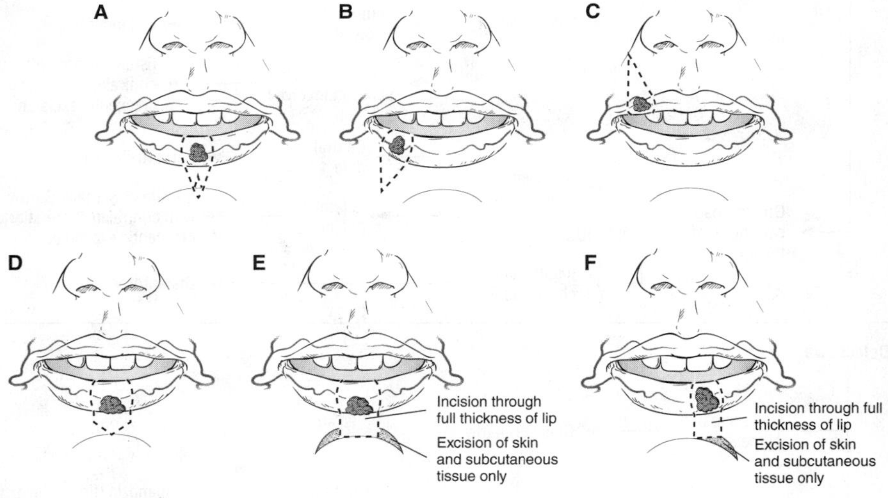


**Fig. 39-9** Wedge excision of lesions. **A,** W-shaped excision. **B,** V-shaped excision of the lower lip. **C,** V-shaped excision of an upper lip lesion, tapered into the nasolabial fold. **D,** Shield excision. **E,** Double-barrel excision. The lesion is excised in full thickness of the lip. Burow's triangles involve only excision of skin and subcutaneous tissue. **F,** Single-barrel excision.

## ABBÉ LIP SWITCH FLAP[9,14,15] (Fig. 39-10)

- **Indication**
  - One third to one half of lip absent
  - Commissure preserved
- **Advantages**
  - Muscular continuity
  - Primary closure of donor site

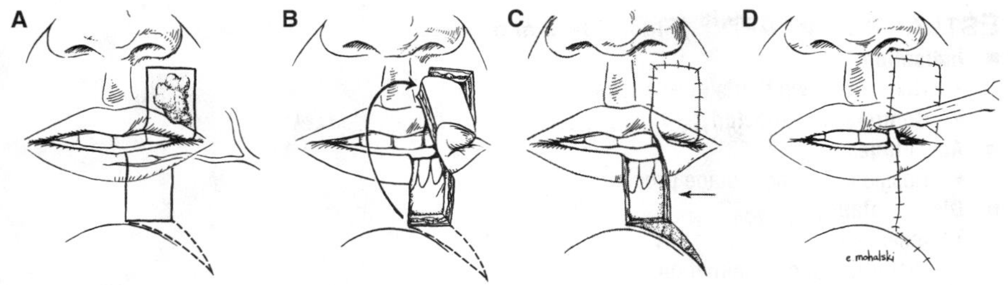


**Fig. 39-10** Abbé flap. **A,** Example of a rectangular design of a lip switch flap that fills an upper lip defect. The continuity of the labial artery is maintained in the pivoting portion of the flap. **B,** The flap is elevated in full thickness of the lip tissue and rotated into the upper lip defect. **C,** Excision of a Burow's triangle at the base of the donor site allows medial advancement of the lower lateral lip flap and primary closure of the donor site similar to the single-barrel excision. **D,** The pedicle is divided and inset at 14-21 days.

- **Disadvantages**
  - Two-stage procedure
    - Requires patient compliance
  - Insensate
- **Technical pearls**[8] (Fig. 39-11)
  - Flap design
    - Half the width of the defect
    - Full thickness
    - Rotation point should allow adequate mouth opening between first and second stages.
    - Leave a small cuff of muscle around the vascular pedicle.
  - Blood supply
    - Ipsilateral labial artery of opposite lip
  - Second-stage timing
    - 2 to 3 weeks
    - Test flap viability before flap take down.
    - Wedge resection may improve lip advancement.

**TIP:** An Abbé flap is preferred to a sliding reconstruction (e.g., Karapandzic, Estlander, or Bernard-Burow) in the upper lip, because it can preserve the Cupid's bow, oral commissure, and modiolus.

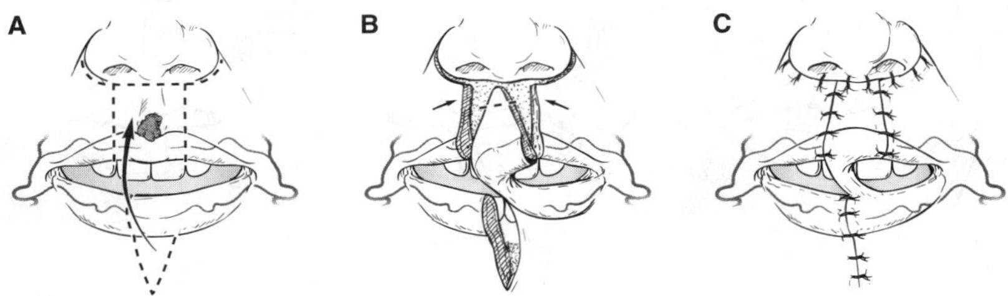


**Fig. 39-11** Combination of perialar crescentic excision and central Abbé flap. **A,** Flap elevation and perialar crescentic excisions. **B** and **C,** The flap pedicle is divided and inset at about 14 days.

## Estlander Flap[9,16] (Figs. 39-12 and 39-13)

- **Indication**
  - One half to two thirds of lip absent
  - **Commissure affected**
- **Advantage**
  - Possible for single-stage procedure
- **Disadvantages**
  - Insensate
  - Distortion of oral animation
    - ▸ Modiolus altered
    - ▸ May require secondary commissuroplasty
  - Tenuous vascular supply
- **Technical pearls**
  - Flap design
    - ▸ One third to one half the size of the defect
    - ▸ Full thickness
    - ▸ Leave a small cuff of muscle around the vascular pedicle.
  - Blood supply
    - ▸ Contralateral labial artery of opposite lip

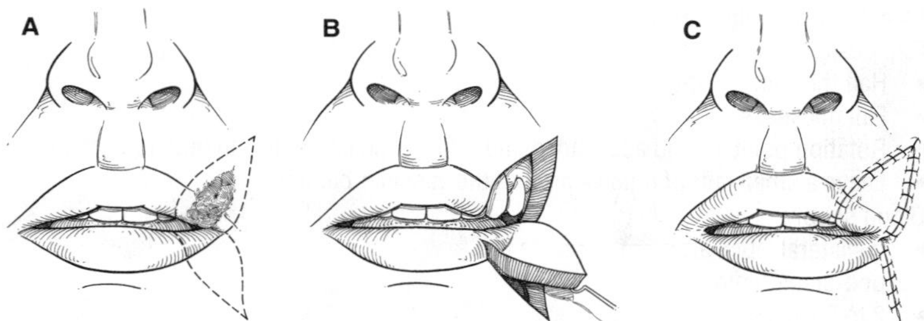


**Fig. 39-12** Estlander flap for upper lip reconstruction. **A,** The lower lip flap is designed to be no more than half the size of the upper lip defect. **B,** The flap is rotated about the vermilion, which harbors its blood supply from the contralateral labial artery. **C,** Three-layer closure of the inset flap and donor site.

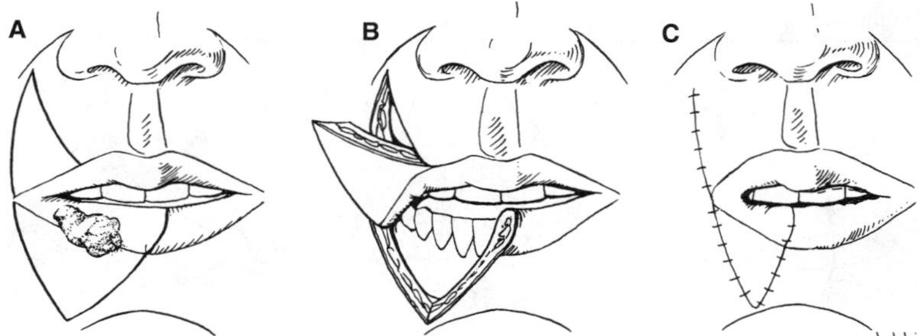


**Fig. 39-13** Estlander flap for lower lip reconstruction. **A,** The flap is designed to be one third to one half the size of the defect. The commissure must be involved. **B,** A full-thickness upper lateral lip flap is rotated into the lower lip defect. Blood supply to the flap is at the pivot point from the contralateral upper labial artery. **C,** The flap is inset, and the donor site is closed primarily.

## Karapandzic Flap[9,17,18] (Figs. 39-14 and 39-15)

- **Indication**
  - One third to two thirds of the lip absent
  - Central defect
- **Advantages**
  - Single-stage procedure
  - Sensate
  - Muscular continuity
    - Oral sphincter competence
  - Preserves the philtrum and modiolus
- **Disadvantages**
  - Microstomia in large defects (greater than two thirds of lip)
  - Upper lip may appear tight.
- **Technical pearls**
  - Flap design
    - Rotational, circumoral flaps
    - Intramuscular dissection to preserve vascular pedicle
  - Blood supply
    - Bilateral labial arteries
  - Technically, a modification of the Gillies fan flap that preserves neurovascular structures

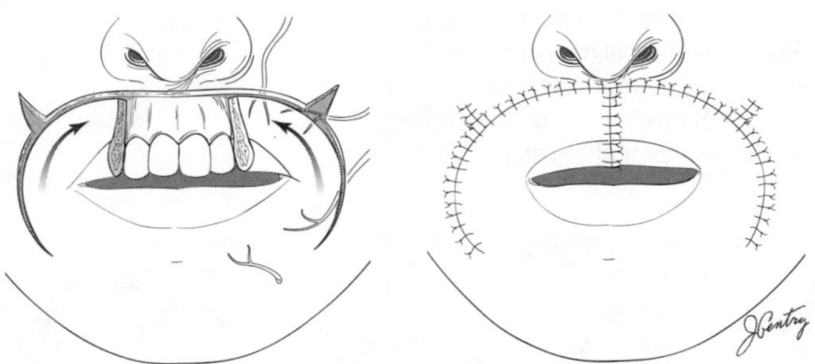

**Fig. 39-14** Upper lip Karapandzic flap with Burow's triangles.

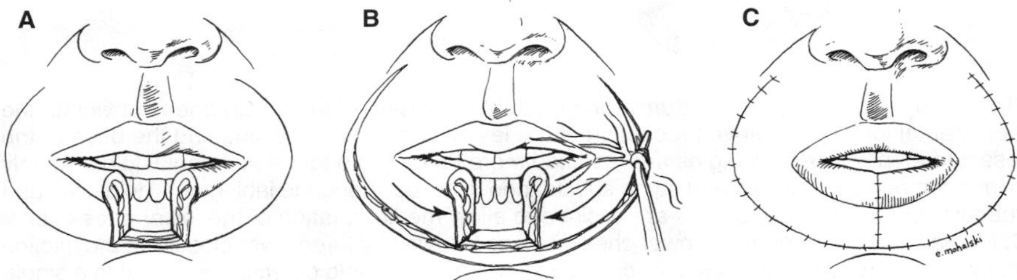


**Fig. 39-15** Lower lip Karapandzic flap. **A,** The width of the circumoral incision must be equal to the height of the defect at all points of the flap. **B,** The labial arteries and buccal nerve branches are identified and preserved bilaterally. **C,** Three-layer closure following medial advancement of the flaps.

## Bernard-Burow Cheiloplasty[19,20]

- **Indication**
  - Greater than two thirds of the lip absent
  - Central defect
- **Advantages**
  - Single-stage procedure
  - Local tissue flap reconstruction
- **Disadvantages**
  - Little or no muscle function
  - Oral sphincter incompetence
  - Insensate
  - Microstomia
- **Technical pearls**
  - Flap design
    - Burow's triangles allow medial advancement of lateral cheeks.
      - Designed after completing lip excision
      - Placed along anatomic subunit divisions (e.g., nasolabial fold and labiomental crease)
    - Buccal mucosal flaps can be used to reconstruct the vermilion.
  - Blood supply
    - Dermal plexus
  - Webster modification (Fig. 39-16)[12,21]
    - Excise skin and subcutaneous tissue only in Burow's triangles.
      - Preserves muscular innervation
    - Triangular excisions are located more laterally.
    - Paramental Burow's triangles are excised.
      - Advance inferior cheek skin.

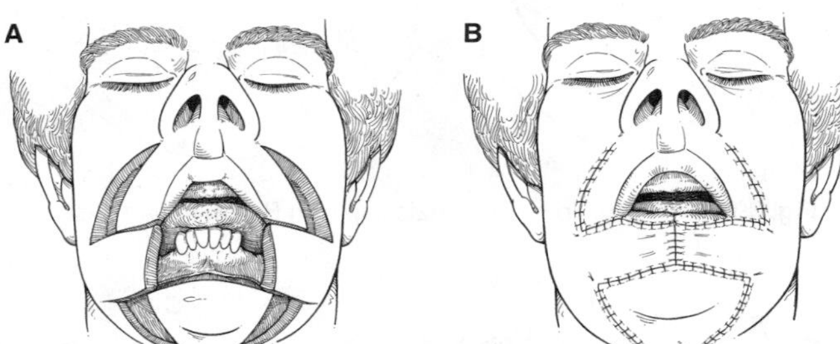


**Fig. 39-16** Modified Bernard-Burow procedure. **A,** Excision of the lesion does not violate the labiomental fold, but improved resection of the lesion is achieved by widening the base of the resected area. Burow's triangles are resected more laterally along the nasolabial fold and only involve the resection of skin and some subcutaneous tissue. Along the labiomental fold, skin and subcutaneous Burow's triangles are excised to allow medial rotation of the lower cheek flaps. **B,** Medial advancement of the lower cheek flaps is followed by three-layer closure at the midline and vermilion reconstruction with buccal mucosa. Nasolabial fold defects are closed in a single layer.

## Total Lip Reconstruction[22-25] (Fig. 39-17)

Total lip reconstruction can be performed with a radial forearm and palmaris longus composite free flap.[26,27]

- **Indication**
  - Total or near total loss of the lip
- **Advantages**
  - Well-vascularized coverage
  - Possible to include sensory innervation
- **Disadvantages**
  - No motor innervation
  - Poor color match
  - Difficult to reconstruct anatomic landmarks and vermilion
- **Technical pearls**
  - Flap design
    - ▸ Palmaris longus forms a sling to maintain lower lip height
  - Blood supply
    - ▸ Radial artery
  - Innervation
    - ▸ Lateral antebrachial cutaneous nerve
  - Excellent choice if local tissues have been irradiated

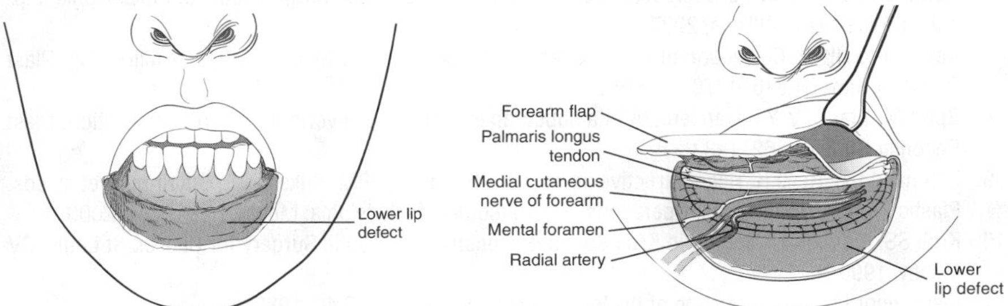


**Fig. 39-17** Total lip reconstruction with a free radial forearm fasciocutaneous flap and a palmaris longus tendon graft to the modiolus.

## POSTOPERATIVE CARE

- **Nutrition**
  - Proper-sized pieces or pureed/liquid diet
- **Oral hygiene**
  - Patients can swish and expectorate with oral solution if they have oral competence.
  - Gentle intraoral cleaning is performed with swab or soft bristled brush.

## Key Points

- ✓ Meticulous anatomic alignment of the vermilion border is essential.
- ✓ Anatomic landmarks should be preserved and/or reconstructed.
- ✓ Microstomia is a concern if the lip excision exceeds half.
- ✓ Up to one third of the lip can be closed primarily.
- ✓ An Abbé flap preserves the oral commissure.
- ✓ Estlander flaps are useful if the commissure is involved.
- ✓ Karapandzic flaps preserve innervation to the orbicularis oris.
- ✓ Bernard-Burow cheiloplasty compromises innervation of the orbicularis oris muscle.

## References

1. Burget GC, Menick FJ. Aesthetic restoration of one half the upper lip. Plast Reconstr Surg 78:583, 1986.
2. Harris L, Higgins K, Enepekides D. Local flap reconstruction of acquired lip defects. Curr Opin Otolaryngol Head Neck Surg 20:254, 2012.
3. Freilinger G, Gruber H, Happak W, et al. Surgical anatomy of the mimic muscle system and the facial nerve: importance for reconstructive and aesthetic surgery. Plast Reconstr Surg 80:686, 1987.
4. Gonzalez-Ulloa M. Restoration of the face covering by means of selected skin in regional aesthetic units. Br J Plast Surg 9:212, 1956.
5. Haagensen CD, Feind CR, Herter FP, et al. The Lymphatics in Cancer. Philadelphia: WB Saunders, 1972.
6. Boutros S, Thorne CH, Beasley RW, et al. Grabb & Smith's Plastic Surgery, 6th ed. Philadelphia: Lippincott Williams & Wilkins, 2007.
7. Kawamoto HK Jr. Correction of major defects of the vermilion with a cross-lip vermilion flap. Plast Reconstr Surg 64:315, 1979.
8. Spira M, Stal S. V-Y advancement of a subcutaneous pedicle in vermilion lip reconstruction. Plast Reconstr Surg 72:562, 1983.
9. Behmand RA, Rees R. Reconstructive lip surgery. In Achauer BM, Eriksson E, Guyuron B, et al, eds. Plastic Surgery: Indications, Operations, and Outcomes. Philadelphia: Mosby–Year Book, 2000.
10. Kroll SS. Lip reconstruction. In Kroll SS, ed. Reconstructive Plastic Surgery for Cancer. St Louis: CV Mosby, 1996.
11. MacGregor IA. Reconstruction of the lower lip. Br J Plast Surg 36:40, 1983.
12. Webster RC, Coffey RJ, Kelleher RE. Total and partial reconstruction of the lower lip with innervated muscle-bearing flaps. Plast Reconstr Surg 25:360, 1960.
13. Wilson JSP, Walker EP. Reconstruction of the lower lip. Head Neck Surg 4:29, 1981.
14. Abbé RA. A new plastic operation for the relief of deformity due to double harelip. Med Rec 53:477, 1898.
15. Cutting CB, Warren SM. Extended Abbé flap for secondary correction of the bilateral cleft lip. J Craniofac Surg 24:75, 2013.
16. Estlander JA. Eine methode aus der einen lippe substanzverluste der anderen zu ersetzen. Arch Kim Chir 14:622, 1872.
17. Jabaley ME, Clement RL, Orcutt TW. Myocutaneous flaps in lip reconstruction: applications of the Karapandzic principle. Plast Reconstr Surg 59:680, 1977.
18. Karapandzic M. Reconstruction of lip defects by local arterial flaps. Br J Plast Surg 27:93, 1974.
19. Freeman BS. Myoplastic modification of the Bernard cheiloplasty. Plast Reconstr Surg 21:453, 1958.

20. Madden JJ Jr, Erhardt WL Jr, Franklin JD, et al. Reconstruction of the upper and lower lip using a modified Bernard-Burow technique. Ann Plast Surg 5:100, 1980.
21. Seo HJ, Bae SH, Nam SB, et al. Lower lip reconstruction after wide excision of a malignancy with barrel-shaped excision or the Webster modification of the Bernard operation. Arch Plast Surg 40:36, 2013.
22. Freedman AM, Hidalgo DA. Full-thickness lip and cheek reconstruction with the radial forearm free flap. Ann Plast Surg 25:287, 1990.
23. Furuta S, Sakaguchi Y, Iwasawa M, et al. Reconstruction of the lips, oral commissure, and full-thickness cheek with a composite radial forearm palmaris longus free flap. Ann Plast Surg 33:544, 1994.
24. Sadove RC, Luce EA, McGrath PC. Reconstruction of the lower lip and chin with the composite radial forearm-palmaris longus free flap. Plast Reconstr Surg 88:209, 1991.
25. Godefroy WP, Klop WM, Smeele LE, et al. Free-flap reconstruction of large full-thickness lip and chin defects. Ann Otol Rhinol Laryngol 121:594, 2012.
26. Sasidaran R, Zain MA, Basiron NH. Lip and oral commissure reconstruction with the radial forearm flap. Natl J Maxillofac Surg 3:21, 2012.
27. Fernandes R, Clemow J. Outcomes of total or near-total lip reconstruction with microvascular tissue transfer. J Oral Maxillofac Surg 70:2899, 2012.

# 40. Mandibular Reconstruction

**Patrick B. Garvey, Jason K. Potter**

## GENERAL PRINCIPLES

- The type of reconstruction is primarily determined by the **location** and **size** of the mandibular defect.[1]
- Defects created as a result of trauma versus excision of benign or malignant tumors should be considered.
- Reconstructions for malignancy often will be subjected to postoperative radiotherapy and therefore are best reconstructed with vascularized bone flaps or soft tissue flaps.
- Donor site morbidity must be considered; however, to minimize donor site morbidity at the expense of the quality of the mandibular reconstruction is to confuse reconstructive priorities.[2]

## METHODS OF RECONSTRUCTION

### Collapse of Mandibular Defect Without Bone Reconstruction

- Acceptable for defects of the ascending ramus and lateral defects, particularly when the condylar head has been resected from the temporomandibular joint[1]
- **Advantages**
  - Speech and swallowing are typically good
  - Fast
- **Disadvantages**
  - Deviation of chin to affected side (crossbite)
  - Does not reestablish patient's bite/leaves patient with malocclusion

### Mandibular Reconstruction Plates (MRP) Alone

- Reconstruction plates are typically 1.5 to 2.4 mm thick
- Bone screws fixate plate to mandible
  - Traditional, "non-locking" screws simply hold plate against bone.
  - "Locking" screws have threaded screw heads that lock screws into reconstruction plate as well as threads that secure rigid screw-plate construct to the bone to create a more rigid and stable fixation.
- Some believe MRPs alone are appropriate for patients who are unable to tolerate longer procedures or who have a short life expectancy.
- **Advantages**
  - Fast
  - No donor site morbidity
- **Disadvantages**
  - **MRP fracture** will eventually occur if patient survives long enough, thus necessitating a flap reconstruction under far less advantageous conditions than those present at the time of initial tumor resection, particularly if the patient received postoperative radiotherapy.[3-6]
  - **Extrusion rate is high,** particularly when used in the anterior mandible or if the patient has postoperative radiotherapy.[7-10]

- Most MRP failures occur **within 18 months,** with a mean time to failure of **6-8 months.**[6]
- Patients reconstructed with MRP alone or MRP with soft tissue flaps lose significantly more days for secondary procedures compared with patients who have primary reconstruction with vascularized bone flaps.[6]

## Soft Tissue Flaps for Mandibular Reconstruction

- **Advantages**
  - Provide vascularized tissue bulk
  - Obliterate dead space
  - Provide coverage of neurovascular structures of neck
  - Prevent development of orocutaneous fistulas[1]
- **Disadvantages**
  - Do not reestablish occlusion
- **Common soft tissue flaps for mandible reconstruction**
  - **Pectoralis major**
    - Most commonly used flap for neck coverage
    - Pedicled flap that is reliable and easy to harvest
    - Vascular pedicle creates aesthetically displeasing bulge over ipsilateral clavicle unless a portion of the clavicle is resected.
  - **Anterolateral thigh (ALT) free flap**
    - Often used for posterior defects when temporomandibular joint (TMJ) has been resected or in patients with medical comorbidities.[1]
    - Based on the descending branch of the lateral circumflex femoral artery[11,12]
    - Minimal donor morbidity
    - Can be harvested at the same time that the tumor is being resected
  - **Vertical rectus abdominis myocutaneous (VRAM) free flap**
    - An alternative to the ALT flap with essentially the same indications
    - Based on the deep inferior epigastric artery (DIEA)
    - Donor site morbidity includes potential abdominal weakness, hernia, or bulging

**TIP:** Posterior mandibular defects in which the anterior mandible is spared do not necessarily require bone reconstruction, particularly when TMJ has been removed. Soft tissue flaps can produce similar aesthetic and functional results with shorter operative times and fewer complications.[1]

## Nonvascularized Bone Grafts

- **Indication**
  - Nonvascularized bone grafts are appropriate for traumatic or benign tumor defects <6 cm long that will not be subjected to postoperative radiotherapy.
  - >6 cm grafts: 83% success rate
  - >6 cm grafts: 25% success rate
- **Contraindications**
  - Radiotherapy: Extrusion, resorption, and infection in at least 50%-80% of cases[13]
  - Anterior mandibular defects
  - Cancer patients

**TIP:** Nonvascularized bone grafts are best performed in a delayed fashion.[14]

**Table 40-1** *Free Flap Donor Site Comparison for Mandible Reconstruction**

| | Tissue Characteristics | | Donor Site Characteristcs | | |
|---|---|---|---|---|---|
| **Donor Site** | **Bone** | **Skin** | **Pedicle** | **Location** | **Morbidity** |
| Fibula | A | C | B | A | A |
| Ilium | B | D | D | B | C |
| Scapula | C | B | C | D | B |
| Radius | D | A | A | C | D |

*Ranked in each category from best *(A)* to worst *(D).*

## VASCULARIZED BONE FREE FLAPS (Table 40-1)

- Compared with nonvascularized alloplastic bone grafts, vascularized bone free flaps provide 40% more strength, 56% more stiffness, higher complete arthrodesis rates, and superior functional outcomes.[15]
- **Indications**
  - Treatment of choice for **irradiated defects** or **bone defects >6 cm**[16]
- **Contraindications**
  - Posterior defects in patients with medical comorbidities, particularly when the condylar head has been resected from the TMJ

> **TIP:** Use of vascularized bone free flaps for mandibular reconstruction has been associated with lower failure rates than reconstructions with MRPs alone.

- **Common vascularized bone flaps for mandibular reconstruction** (Fig. 40-1)
  - **Free fibula osteocutaneous flap**[17]
    - Workhorse flap for mandibular reconstruction
    - **Blood supply:** Peroneal artery (branch of tibioperoneal trunk)[18,19]
    - **Pedicle length:** 6-10 cm
    - **Average useable bone length:** 24.4 cm (men), 22.6 cm (women)[20]
    - **Average maximum bone width:** 1.8 cm (men), 13.1 cm (women)[20]
    - **Suitability for implants:** Very good
    - **Soft tissue availability:** Very good
    - **Donor site disability:** Weight bearing in 2-5 days
    - **Advantages:**
      - Simultaneous harvest with two-team approach
      - Excellent bone length
      - Only choice for long defects
      - Can include overlying skin island(s) for floor of mouth and/or external skin resurfacing
      - Minimal long-term donor site morbidity
      - Bone suitable for endosteal implants to anchor dentures as part of dental rehabilitation
    - **Disadvantages:**
      - Lack of vertical height in reconstructed mandible
      - Skin island can be thick for endosteal implant emergence

## Outcomes

- Skin island was originally thought to be unreliable,[18] but with better understanding of anatomy and harvest techniques, skin island survival now approaches 100%.[19,21]
- Complication rates are increased with more osteotomies, particularly if bone segments are shorter than 2-3 cm.

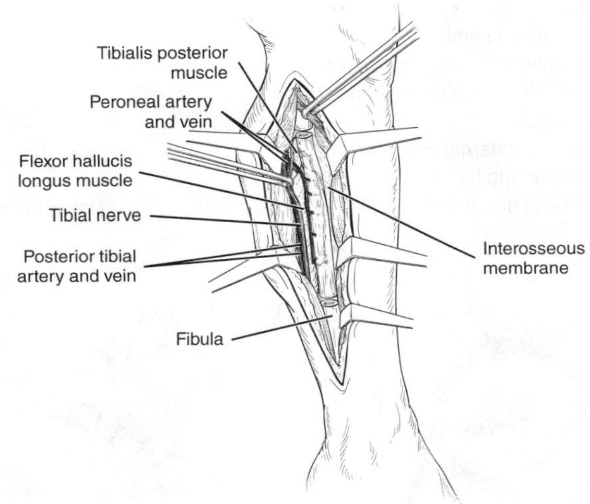


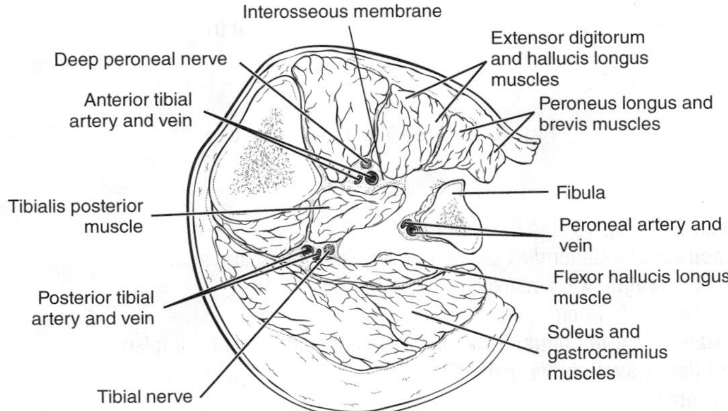


**Top:** Dissection of vascular bundle and completion of harvest
**Bottom:** Cross-section

**Fig. 40-1** Free fibula flap.

- **Free iliac crest bone flap** (Fig. 40-2)
  - **Blood supply:** Deep circumflex iliac artery (DCIA)
  - **Pedicle length:** 5-7 cm
  - **Usable bone length:** 14-16 cm
  - **Suitability for implants:** Excellent
  - **Soft tissue availability:** Internal oblique muscle can cover intraoral bone; external skin can be bulky
  - **Advantages:**
    - Excellent bone height
    - Internal oblique for intraoral cover
    - Bone suitable for endosteal implants
  - **Disadvantages:**
    - Poor skin for external coverage
    - Time-consuming harvest
    - Considerable donor defect that is prone to lateral abdominal wall hernias

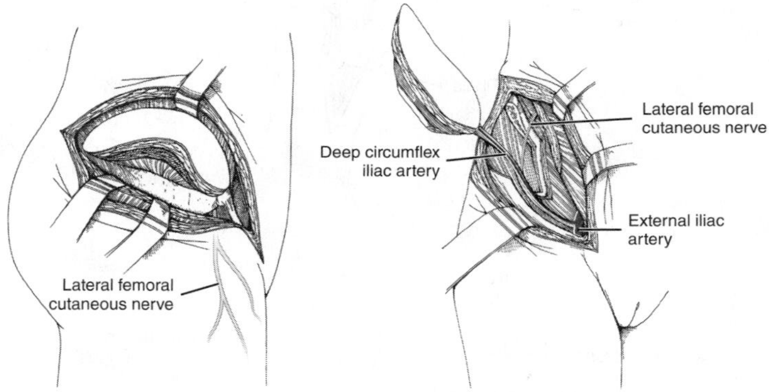


**Fig. 40-2** Free iliac crest bone flap.

- **Scapular flap** (Fig. 40-3, *A* through *C*)
  - **Blood supply:** Circumflex scapular artery from subscapular artery
  - **Pedicle length:** 4-6 cm, axillary artery to bone
  - **Bone size:** 10-14 cm
  - **Suitability for implants:** 60%-70% have adequate bone for implants.
  - **Soft tissue availability:** Extensive
  - **Advantages:**
    - Very large soft tissue
  - **Disadvantages:**
    - Harvest typically cannot begin until after tumor resection because of patient positioning.
    - Bone is thin.
    - Bone cannot tolerate multiple osteotomies, because it does not have a segmental blood supply.

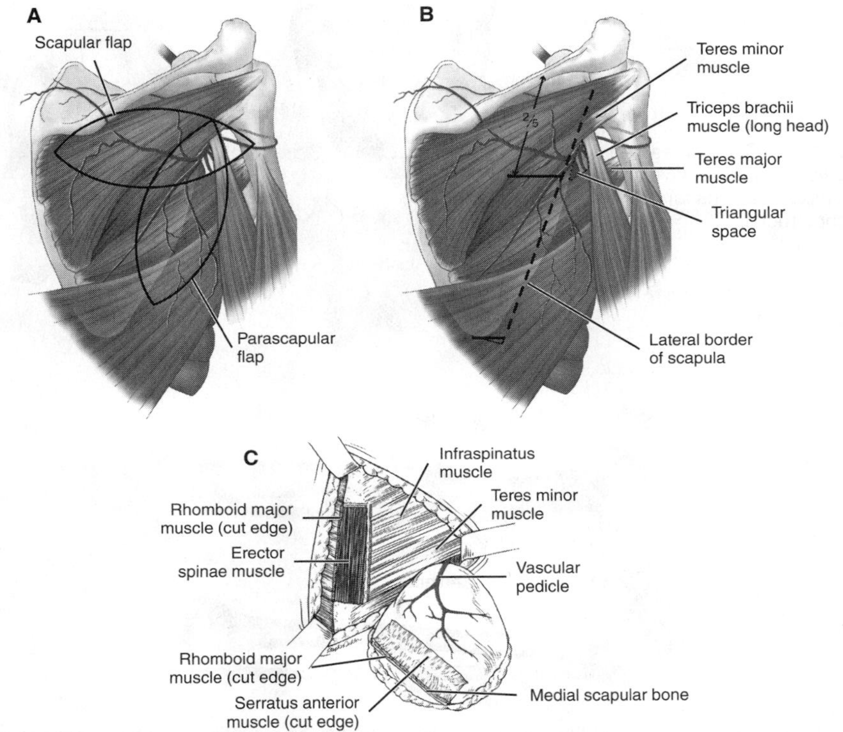


**Fig. 40-3 A,** The scapular and parascapular flaps are based on the transverse branch of the circumflex scapular artery and descending branch of the circumflex artery, respectively. **B,** The triangular space can usually be identified by palpation approximately two fifths the distance from the midportion of the spine of the scapula to its inferior border. **C,** The scapular osteocutaneous flap is isolated on its vascular pedicle and is observed for continuous perfusion.

- **Osteocutaneous radial forearm flap**
  - Radius provides inadequate bone stock for reliable mandibular reconstruction.

## COMPUTER-AIDED DESIGN (CAD) FOR VIRTUAL MANDIBULAR RECONSTRUCTION PLANNING

- Computer-aided design allows preoperative creation of optimized designs for mandibular reconstruction (Fig. 40-4).
- Three-dimensional computer images of the mandible and fibula are generated.
- Virtual mandibular defect is created.
- Virtual osteotomies in fibula model are made to optimally reconstruct contour of mandible.
- Patient-specific cutting guides (cutting jigs) for the mandible and fibula are manufactured preoperatively (Fig. 40-5).
- An MRP is prebent to the virtual mandibular reconstruction model.

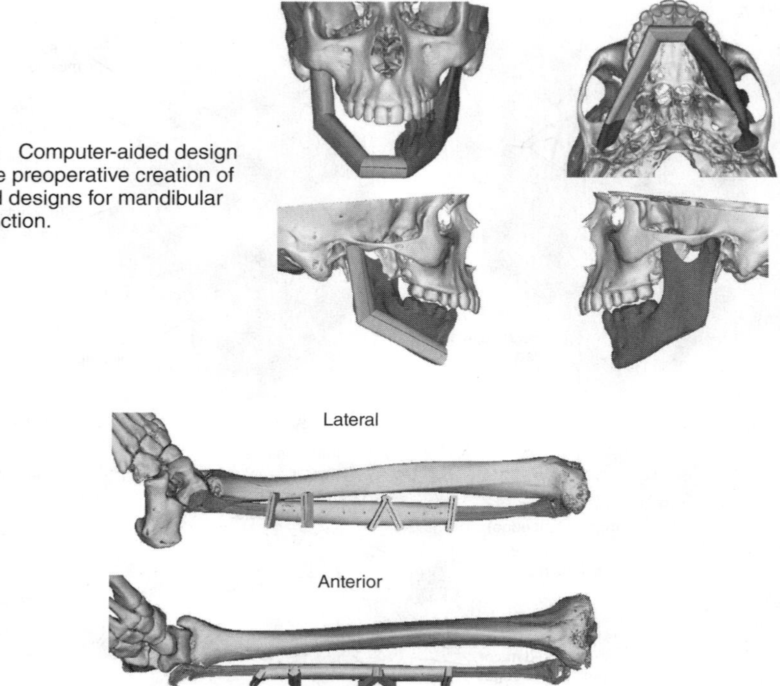


**Fig. 40-4** Computer-aided design allows the preoperative creation of optimized designs for mandibular reconstruction.

**Fig. 40-5** Patient-specific cutting guides (cutting jigs) for the mandible and fibula are manufactured preoperatively.

- Intraoperatively the mandible and fibula are cut according to the guides and affixed to the prefabricated MRP.
- **Advantages:**
  - Saves time in the OR
  - Improves accuracy of reconstruction
- **Disadvantages:**
  - Costly
  - Requires extra time for preoperative planning

## Key Points

✓ Reconstructive decisions are based on size and location of the mandibular defect.

✓ Defects ≥6 cm should be reconstructed with vascularized bone.

✓ Defects involving the anterior mandible should be reconstructed immediately with vascularized bone flaps.

✓ The free fibula osteocutaneous flap is the flap of choice for mandibular reconstruction.

✓ Preoperative mandible CAD modeling can save time and improve accuracy of the reconstruction.

## REFERENCES


1. Hanasono MM, Zevallos JP, Skoracki RJ, et al. A prospective analysis of bony versus soft-tissue reconstruction for posterior mandibular defects. Plast Reconstr Surg 125:1413-1421, 2010.
2. Momoh AO, Yu P, Skoracki RJ, et al. A prospective cohort of fibula free flap donor-site morbidity in 157 consecutive patients. Plast Reconstr Surg 128:714-720, 2011.
3. Kellman PM, Gullane PJ. Use of the AO mandibular reconstruction plate for bridging of mandibular defects. Otolaryngol Clin North Am 20:519-533, 1987.
4. Blackwell KE, Buchbinder D, Urken ML. Lateral mandibular reconstruction using soft-tissue free flaps and plates. Arch Otolaryngol Head Neck Surg 122:672-678, 1996.
5. Ueyama Y, Naitoh R, Yamagata A, et al. Analysis of reconstruction of mandibular defects using single stainless steel AO reconstruction plates. J Oral Maxillofac Surg 54:858-862, 1996.
6. Boyd JB, Mulholland RS, Davidson J, et al. The free flap and plate in oromandibular reconstruction: long-term review and indications. Plast Reconstr Surg 95:1018-1028, 1995.
7. Schusterman MA, Reece GP, Kroll SS, et al. Use of the AO plate for immediate mandibular reconstruction in cancer patients. Plast Reconstr Surg 88:588-593, 1991.
8. Kim MR, Donoff RB. Critical analysis of mandibular reconstruction using AO reconstruction plates. J Oral Maxillofac Surg 50:1152-1157, 1992.
9. Papazian MR, Castillo MH, Campbell JH, et al. Analysis of reconstruction for anterior mandibular defects using AO plates. J Oral Maxillofac Surg 49:1055-1059, 1991.
10. Cordeiro PG, Hidalgo DA. Soft tissue coverage of mandibular reconstruction plates. Head Neck 16:112-115, 1994.
11. Yu P. Characteristics of the anterolateral thigh flap in a western population and its application in head and neck reconstruction. Head Neck 26:759-769, 2004.
12. Garvey PB, Selber JC, Madewell JE, et al. A prospective study of preoperative computed tomographic angiography for head and neck reconstruction with anterolateral thigh flaps. Plast Reconstr Surg 127:1505-1515, 2011.
13. Adamo AK, Szai RL. Timing, results, and complications of mandibular reconstructive surgery: report of 32 cases. J Oral Surg 37:755-763, 1979.
14. Pogrel MA, Podlesh S, Anthony JP. A comparison of vascularized and nonvascularized bone grafts for reconstruction of mandibular continuity defects. J Oral Maxillofac Surg 55:1200-1206, 1997.
15. Goldberg VM, Shaffer JW, Field G, et al. Biology of vascularized bone grafts. Orthop Clin North Am 18:197-205, 1987.
16. Foster RD, Anthony JP, Sharma A, et al. Vascuarlized bone flaps versus nonvascularized bone flaps for mandibular reconstruction: an outcome analysis of primary bony union and endosseous implant success. Head Neck 21:66-71, 1999.
17. Cordeiro PG, Disa J, Hidalgo DA, et al. Reconstruction of the mandible with osseous free flaps: a 10-year experience with 150 consecutive patients. Plast Reconstr Surg 104:1314-1320, 1999.
18. Hidalgo DA. Fibula free flap: a new method of mandible reconstruction. Plast Reconstr Surg 84:71-80, 1989.
19. Garvey PB, Chang EI, Selber JC, et al. A prospective study of preoperative computed tomographic angiographic mapping of free fibula osteocutaneous flaps for head and neck reconstruction. Plast Reconstr Surg 130:542e-552e, 2012.
20. Chang EI, Clemens MW, Garvey PB, et al. Cephalometric analysis for microvascular head and neck reconstruction. Head Neck 34:1607-1614, 2012.
21. Yu P, Chang EI, Hanasono MM. Design of a reliable skin paddle for the fibula osteocutaneous flap: perforator anatomy revisited. Plast Reconstr Surg 128:440-447, 2011.

# 41. Pharyngeal Reconstruction

Phillip D. Khan, Raman C. Mahabir

## PHARYNGEAL ANATOMY[1-13] (Fig. 41-1)

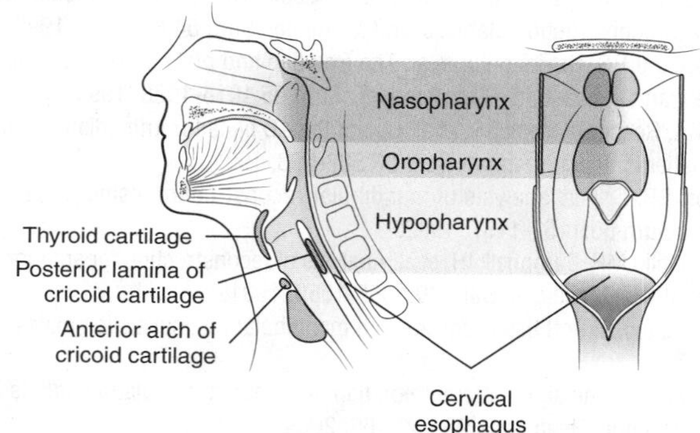


**Fig. 41-1** Subdivisions of the pharynx.

### NASOPHARYNX

Narrow space posterior to the nasal cavity (choanae) and above the soft palate, located immediately caudal to the central skull base

- **Boundaries**
  - Superior boundary: Sphenoid sinus and upper skull base (clivus)
  - Posterior boundary: Lower skull base (clivus) and first cervical vertebra
  - Inferior boundary: Soft palate
  - Anterior boundary: Choanae
- **Arterial blood supply**
  - Ascending pharyngeal artery (lateral walls)
  - Ascending palatine artery (pharyngotympanic tube region and soft palate)
  - Greater palatine artery
  - Artery to the pterygoid canal
- **Sensory**
  - Predominantly visceral through the pharyngeal plexus, mainly from CN IX.
  - Small area of anterior medial roof supplied by somatic sensory branches of maxillary nerve ($V_2$).

### OROPHARYNX

From the hard/soft palate junction to the aryepiglottic folds

- **Boundaries**
  - Superior boundary: Soft palate

- Inferior boundary: Hyoid bone and valleculae
- Ventral boundary: Base of tongue (ending at the circumvallate papillae)
- Lateral boundary: Tonsillar fossae
- Dorsal boundary: Dorsal pharyngeal wall

■ **Subsites**
- Soft palate
- Tonsils and tonsillar fossae
- Base of tongue
- Oropharyngeal walls

■ **Arterial blood supply**
- Soft palate: Palatine arteries
- Tonsil and tonsillar fossa: Posterior branches of the lingual artery, ascending pharyngeal artery, branches of facial artery, and palatine branches of the internal maxillary artery
- Base of tongue: Lingual arteries

■ **Sensory**
- Soft palate: Lesser palatine branch of maxillary nerve ($V_2$)
- Tonsil and tonsillar fossa: Middle and posterior palatine branches of maxillary nerve ($V_2$)
- Base of tongue: Lingual branch of CN IX
- Oropharyngeal wall: Pharyngeal plexus contributions (CN IX and X)

**TIP:** The tonsils, soft palate, and palatoglossal/palatopharyngeal folds are located in the oropharynx, not in the oral cavity. Just as the tongue base and oral tongue have different origins, innervation, function, and tumor behavior, so do the oral cavity and oropharynx.

## HYPOPHARYNX

From oropharynx (aryepiglottic folds) to esophageal inlet

■ **Boundaries**
- Superior boundary: Hyoid bone or level of pharyngoepiglottic folds
- Inferior boundary: Esophageal inlet at the level of cricopharyngeal muscle
- Anterior boundary: Larynx
- Posterior boundary: Retropharyngeal space

■ **Subsites**
- Anterior wall: Postcricoid
- Posterior wall: Separated from vertebral and paravertebral structures by potential retropharyngeal space
- Piriform sinus (one on each side)

■ **Arterial blood supply**
- Superior thyroid arteries with contributions from the lingual and ascending pharyngeal arteries

■ Sensory input assists with a **coordinated mechanism in swallowing.**
- CN IX and CN X to the nucleus solitarius in the brainstem; connected to nearby cranial motor neurons to assist in deglutination

**TIP:** Sensory fibers synapse in the jugular ganglion in the jugular foramen, along with Arnold's nerve from the external auditory canal. This accounts for referred otalgia.

### Cervical Esophagus

Area of esophagus situated superior to the sternum

- Squamous epithelial layer, submucosa rich in lymphatics, a muscular layer, and adventitial layer
- Inner circular and outer longitudinal layer of muscle
- Other pertinent anatomy in the area include the thoracic duct, carotid sheath, and lateral lobes of the thyroid.
- **Arterial blood supply**
  - Inferior thyroid artery
- **Sensory**
  - Sympathetic and parasympathetic contributions
  - CN IX, X, XI

> **TIP:** The esophagus has no serosa, making it different from the rest of the gastrointestinal tract.

## TUMOR BIOLOGY[4,5,7-11,13-16]

### Nasopharyngeal Cancer

- A large range of benign and malignant pathologies occurs at the confluence of the nasopharynx.
  - Most common **benign** tumor is **juvenile angiofibroma.**
  - Most common **malignant** tumor is **nasopharyngeal carcinoma.**
- Nasopharyngeal carcinoma has a strong correlation with ethnicity, diet, and Epstein-Barr virus.
- **Epidemiology**
  - Highest incidence is in southeast Asia.
    - Guangdong province: Age-adjusted incidence >30 per 100,000
    - Other ethnic groups include Eskimos, Polynesians, and indigenous Mediterranean population
  - Not common in U.S.
    - 1 in 100,000 in U.S. and European Caucasians
    - Highest incidence in first-generation ethnic Chinese immigrants
    - Decreasing incidence after first generation
  - Most commonly presents in males 30-50 years of age
- **Causes**
  - Genetic
  - Environmental
  - Diet high in preservatives and nitrosamines
  - Chemical fumes and wood dust
  - Smoking is NOT an associated risk factor
  - Epstein-Barr virus
- **Subtypes** (World Health Organization)[4,9]
  - Keratinizing (type I): Squamous cell carcinoma
  - Nonkeratinizing differentiated (type II): Transitional carcinoma
  - Nonkeratinizing undifferentiated (type III): Lymphoepithelial carcinoma
  - Basaloid squamous cell carcinoma
- **Clinical presentation**
  - More than 50% of cases present with **nodal metastasis.**
  - Common presenting symptoms
    - Neck lump
    - Blood in saliva

  - Deafness
  - Epistaxis
  - Nasal obstruction
  - Tinnitus
  - Cranial nerve palsy
- Concern for nasopharyngeal carcinoma should arise for any patient presenting with
  - Unilateral otitis media
  - Bilateral level V nodes
  - Skull base symptoms

> **TIP:** In workup of an unknown primary, random biopsies in bilateral fossae of Rosenmüller are recommended to rule out nasopharyngeal primary.

## OROPHARYNGEAL CANCER

- **Epidemiology and cause**
  - Incidence of 1-3/100,000 per year in the United States and Europe
  - Represents 10%-12% of all head and neck malignancies
  - Typically men, over the age of 50, with a long history of exposure to tobacco, alcohol, or both
  - Predominantly **squamous cell carcinoma** (90%) and associated with
    - Tobacco and alcohol consumption
      - Synergistic effect
      - Linked to 75% of cases in the Western world
    - HPV 16 and 18
      - Affects patients 10 years earlier with distinctly favorable prognosis
  - Other tumors include salivary gland, hematolymphoid tissue, mucosal malignant melanoma, tissue of lymphoepithelial origin
- **Clinical presentation** varies by region.
  - **Soft palate**
    - Generally easily detectable
    - 48% present with clinical evidence of neck disease.
  - **Tonsillar fossa**
    - Foreign body, otalgia, dysphagia impeding jaw mobility
    - **Most frequent location of tumors**
  - **Base of tongue**
    - Presents at advanced stages
    - **Difficult to detect**
      - Area nearly without pain fibers
    - Occult disease can present as a level II node (as in occult tonsillar disease)
    - Higher frequency of bilateral nodal disease
    - Ipsilateral nodal involvement in 70% of cases
  - **Oropharyngeal wall**
    - Generally presents late
    - Pain, dysphagia, bleeding
    - Frequent bilateral lymphatic spread

> **TIP:** Bilateral nodal metastasis increases with lesions closer to the midline.

## Hypopharyngeal Cancer

- **In general have the worst oncologic outcome of the head and neck cancers**
- **Epidemiology and cause**
  - 95% are **squamous cell carcinoma.**
  - Others include adenocarcinoma, lymphoma, and other pathologies.
  - **Tendency toward significant submucosal extent.**
  - Similar risk factors to other aerodigestive cancers.
  - Postcricoid cancer has a much higher incidence with Plummer-Vinson syndrome (iron-deficiency anemia, glossitis, splenomegaly, esophageal stenosis), especially in women.
- **Clinical presentation**
  - Most (over 75%) have advanced presentation (stages III and IV) and a high incidence of distant metastasis.
  - **Early-stage disease (I and II)**
    - 37% are asymptomatic at presentation.
    - Most common findings are gastroesophageal reflux disease (GERD) and sore throat
    - 25% with referred otalgia
  - **Advanced stage (III/IV)**
    - Over 90% present with a neck mass.
    - Shortness of breath, dysphagia, referred otalgia
- Incidence of a second neoplasm of the aerodigestive tract, either synchronous or metachronous to a tumor of the hypopharynx, has been reported to be 16% to 18%.

> **TIP:** Cross-innervation throughout the pharyngeal plexus leads to "cortical confusion." Connection through Arnold's nerve (CN X) can lead to **otalgia.** Be suspicious of patients who presents with ear pain, particularly if there are no abnormalities. They need a full workup, including nasopharyngoscopy.

# GENERAL RECONSTRUCTIVE PRINCIPLES

## Pharyngeal Function

- **Transit:** Passage of food and air, including air to the middle ear
- **Swallowing:** Coordinated act that propels a bolus and protects the airway
- **Speech:** Palate, tongue, and lips shape sound generated in larynx to create speech.

## Swallowing: Four Phases

- **Voluntary**
  - **Phase 1: Oral preparatory**
    - Lips, labial/buccal musculature, muscles of mastication
    - Rotatory jaw motion for chewing
    - **Tongue positioning of food, particularly the lateral rolling motion**
    - Bulging forward of the soft palate to seal the oral cavity posteriorly and widen the nasal airway
  - **Phase 2: Oral**
    - **Moves food from the front of the oral cavity to the pharynx,** where the pharyngeal stage of swallowing is initiated
    - **Tongue is the most critical part**
      - Shapes, lifts, and pushes food bolus upward and backward along the hard palate until food reaches the pharynx
    - Pharyngeal swallow usually triggered by CN IX

- **Programmed**
  - **Phase 3: Pharyngeal**
    - **Airway protection occurs during this stage**
    - Coordination between the medullary input of swallow and respiration
    - Respiration ceases for a fraction of a second during swallow
    - Some cortical input from tongue motion
    - Triggering of this phase programs five activities:
      - Velopharyngeal closure to prevent food reflux
      - Tongue base retraction, which propels the food bolus into the pharynx
      - Pharyngeal contraction to clear pharyngeal residue
      - **Elevation and closure of the larynx**
      - Cricopharyngeal and upper esophageal sphincter opening to allow food to pass
  - **Phase 4: Esophageal**
    - Begins when the bolus has passed through the upper esophageal sphincter
    - Greater variability in duration
    - Upper third consists of mixture of involuntary and voluntary muscle.
    - Lower two thirds is entirely involuntary muscle.

**TIP:** The pharyngeal stage is the most important, involving the transit of food into the esophagus and providing airway protection.

## Diagnostic Imaging and Evaluation of Swallowing

- **Bedside evaluation**
  - Assesses facial, lip, tongue, pharyngeal, laryngeal, and respiratory control
  - Sipping on a colored liquid allows detection of possible fistula.
- **Videofluoroscopy**
  - **Only procedure that allows observation of the upper aerodigestive tract during all four stages**
    - Cineradiography (high-resolution images/low frame rate) for mucosal detail
    - Video capture (low-resolution images/high frame rate) gives more dynamic evaluation with less radiation.
  - **Barium swallow**
    - Examines the anatomy and motility of the **esophagus**
    - For accurate evaluation of peristalsis without the effect of gravity, patient viewed in a supine position and in the AP plane
    - Evaluates esophagus for mass
  - **Modified barium swallow**
    - Examines the **oral cavity and pharynx**
    - Evaluates the dynamic coordination of the swallow reflex; can show subtle abnormalities
    - Differs from a barium swallow in that it evaluates laryngotracheal aspiration
    - Uses barium-rich substances of different consistencies
    - Guides clinical recommendations regarding eating strategies
  - **Contrast agents**
    - **Barium** may not be appropriate if perforations are suspected because of extravasation potential (causes inflammation and is not resorbed).
    - **Water-soluble contrast**
      - Less sensitive to small leaks; not as dense as barium
      - Often used first and followed by a barium swallow
      - May lead to chemical pneumonitis or pulmonary edema if aspirated

- **Functional endoscopic evaluation of swallowing with sensory testing (FEEST)**
  - Trained observer watches swallowing though an endoscope.
  - Can actively test sensation with puffs of air

**TIP:** Tracheostomy can paradoxically increase the risk of aspiration while providing increased pulmonary toilet (better suctioning), because it tethers the larynx and prevents normal elevation (early step in swallowing).

## TREATMENT AND RECONSTRUCTIVE PRINCIPLES BY SUBSITE[17-24]

**TIP:** The main criteria for successful treatment are locoregional control of the primary tumor, quality of life, and survival. When determining treatment modality and reconstruction, posttherapeutic function and the patient's quality of life must be considered.

### Overall Considerations[19,23,25-27]

- **Surgical approach**
  - **Transoral**
    - Lacks external incisions but can make visualization difficult
    - Access to anterior tongue, palate, and nasopharynx
    - Suitable for most small and medium-sized lesions and some large lesions of the upper aerodigestive tract
  - **Lateral and transhyoid pharyngotomy**
    - Used for resections too inferior for adequate transoral visualization
    - Lateral approach delivers tumor through an interval between the carotid sheath and larynx.
    - Careful planning of pharyngotomy to prevent cutting into tumor
    - Pharyngotomy can increase the risk of postoperative fistula.
    - Access to epiglottis, base of tongue, and deep posterior pharynx

**NOTE: Visualization of areas between the uvula and epiglottis is challenging through either transoral or pharyngotomy approaches. Wider field of vision may be needed with more invasive dissection. This comes at the expense of added morbidity.**

- **Mandibular swing**
  - Creates a wide field of view at the expense of disrupting structures nearby.
  - Incision is performed through the midline lip, down to the mental fold, around the mentum, and to the neck incision submentally.
  - Soft tissue incised and **mandibulotomy** performed
    - Leads to **significant postoperative morbidity and functional compromise**
  - Important to leave enough floor of mouth tissue laterally, if possible, for sufficient soft tissue closure
- **Minimally invasive approaches** (those not using transmandibular or translabial approaches)
  - Pull-through
    - Combination of transoral approach and lateral pharyngotomy
    - Avoids morbidity of mandibulotomy
  - **As discussed by Selber,[28,29] the future of pharyngeal reconstruction may lie in robotic surgery for ease of access without splitting the mandible.**

- **Allows locoregional control in the form of tumor resection, as well as a means of reconstruction** in confined areas.
- Superior visualization, access, and precision in areas difficult to manipulate even in normal conditions
  - Tumor resection
  - Flap inset
    - Local flaps such as the facial artery myocutaneous flap or random-pattern buccopharyngeal flaps
    - Free flaps

- **Neck Dissection**
  - Clinically positive neck typically treated with neck dissection
  - Clinically negative neck treated with either elective neck dissection or radiation
- **Complications**[30]
  - **Surgical:** Fistula, trismus, aspiration, muscular dysfunction (e.g., shoulder instability), chronic pain, dysarthria, flap loss, failure of reconstruction
  - **Radiotherapy**
    - Acute: Mucositis, dysphagia, xerostomia, loss of taste, dental issues, pain, skin changes, hair loss, loss of sebaceous gland function
    - Late: Osteoradionecrosis and decreased wound-healing ability
    - Modern changes to radiotherapy, such as intensity-modulated radiotherapy and improved technique, have decreased some complications.
- **Reconstruction**
  - Organized systematic approach
  - Multidisciplinary approach
  - Patient-related factors
    - Posttherapeutic function, quality of life, comorbid status
  - Provider-related factors
    - Surgeon experience, hospital resources, ancillary provider services available

## NASOPHARYNX

- **Treatment**
  - Almost always **nonsurgical**
    - Radiotherapy
    - Concurrent chemotherapy/radiotherapy
    - Neoadjuvant therapy followed by chemoradiation
  - Surgery is reserved for salvage with recurrent local and regional disease.
    - Various approaches include endoscopic, transnasal, transmaxillary, midfacial degloving, and transpalatal.
    - Open approaches have their own set of morbidities, which must be considered.
      - Scarring, trismus, dental malocclusion, cranial nerve injury, palatal defects, dysphagia, internal carotid injury
- **Reconstruction**
  - Generally two separate goals depending on clinical presentation
    - **Provide lining**
      - Skin/mucosal grafts
      - Free fasciocutaneous flaps such as radial forearm (FRFF)
      - Pedicled mucoperiosteal flap
    - **Obliterate dead space**
      - Flaps that provide more bulk

## Oropharynx

- Treatment decision depends on the location of the primary and the ability to control the primary and regional node involvement.
- Early stages can be managed surgically with or without postoperative chemoradiation therapy.
- Inoperable cases treated with chemoradiation therapy

**NOTE: Treatment options in this area have evolved with time.**[28,29]

- Traditionally they were addressed through transmandibular access, leading to increased morbidity and functional compromise.
- A shift away from ablative surgery and toward chemoradiation therapy has occurred to preserve physical structures.
- Side effects of chemoradiation such as persistent swallowing difficulties and velopharyngeal compromise have shifted focus back toward ablative surgery with soft tissue reconstruction.
- Minimally invasive techniques, as described by Selber,[28,29] give options for tumor resection and reconstruction in an attempt to maximize postoperative patient function.
  - This access provides treatment options for early and later stages of disease.

- **Soft palate** is the key structure in velopharyngeal competence.
  - Resection of >50% leads to velopharyngeal insufficiency.
  - **Treatment**
    - Early disease: Surgery alone or radiation alone
    - Advanced disease: Surgery and adjuvant radiotherapy with or without chemotherapy
  - **Reconstruction**
    - **Goals:** Functional velum and closure of oronasal communication
    - **Prosthesis**
      - Method of choice for hard palate defects and good for combined palatal defects
      - Some believe that rehabilitation is easier using this method.
      - Inferior for isolated soft palate defects because of lack of dynamic capability
    - **Primary closure and healing by secondary intention**
      - Good for marginal resection if the muscular raphe is not violated
    - **Local flaps**
      - When less than 50% of the soft palate has been resected
      - Uvulopalatal flap, buccinator myomucosal flap, superior constrictor advancement-rotation flap
    - **Free tissue transfer**[31,32]
      - Thin fasciocutaneous: FRFF, anterolateral thigh, lateral arm flap
      - Lacks dynamic capability
      - Dynamic reconstruction can be provided when a free flap is used in combination with a local pharyngeal flap
        - Improves speech, especially for those with >50% of soft palate resected
- **Base of tongue**
  - The tongue base is critical for **airway protection** and **swallowing.**
    - Consider laryngectomy when much of the tongue base is sacrificed to decrease the risk of aspiration.
    - Candidates for laryngeal preservation must have a good pulmonary reserve.
  - **Treatment**
    - Early: Surgery and/or radiotherapy
      - Transoral laser techniques
    - Advanced: Surgery with adjuvant radiotherapy ± concomitant chemotherapy

- **Reconstruction**
  - **Goals:** Maintenance of **airway, swallowing, articulation**
    - It is critical to use options that decrease tethering of components responsible for these processes.
  - Swallowing and speech require pliable tissue ideally with dynamic capability.
  - Reinnervation potential
    - Pharyngeal sensation to decrease aspiration risk
    - Motor function to enhance tongue and laryngeal elevation, creating a more physiologic swallow
  - Skin grafts and local flaps are not recommended in isolation because of deformation and tethering of the tongue.
  - **Regional flaps**
    - Pectoralis major muscle with skin graft or myocutaneous flap
    - Platysma myocutaneous[33]
      - Based on the submental branch of the facial artery
      - Advantage of simplicity and proximity to the defect, leading to tension-free closure
      - Lack of flap bulk and no sensory potential
      - Flap-related complications reported as high as 40%[10]
  - **Free tissue transfer** (reinnervation potential important)
    - Fasciocutaneous flaps may be harvested and folded in ways to increase **bulk** while providing options for sensory reinnervation (FRFF, ALT, lateral arm).
    - Myocutaneous flaps are bulkier and have motor potential.
    - Total or subtotal glossectomy defects are particularly challenging.[34,35]
      - Must provide **bulk** and **sensory innervation** if possible
        - Benefit of motor reinnervation is debatable, given that postoperative radiation may lead to fibrosis before muscle reinnervation.
        - Functional muscle transfer has varying results and often sacrifices the option for sensory reinnervation.[34]
          - Yu and Robb[34] did not seem to show substantial advantage for functional muscle transfer in these situations, especially in patients scheduled for postoperative radiotherapy.
      - Free fasciocutaneous flaps (ALT) suspended from the skull base/hyoid to form a sling

- **Pharyngeal wall**
  - **Treatment**
    - Early: Surgery and/or radiation
    - Advanced: Surgical resection, bilateral neck dissection, postoperative radiotherapy ± chemotherapy
  - **Reconstruction**
    - **Goal:** Thin, pliable tissue
    - Secondary intention and primary closure
      - Can be used for small defects of the posterior and lateral pharyngeal wall that do not have much effect on velopharyngeal function
      - Used with caution in previously irradiated patients
    - Skin grafting
    - Local flaps
      - Facial artery myomucosal flap (FAMM)
    - Regional flap
      - Pectoralis major

        - Platysma myocutaneous
        - Sternocleidomastoid flap
        - Temporoparietal flap
    - Free tissue transfer: FRFF, ALT, lateral arm

## Hypopharynx and Cervical Esophagus[20,36-47]

- The 5-year survival for patients with locally invasive cancer is **less than 35%.**
- Primary function of the hypopharynx is **deglutination.** It can be restored as a passive conduit, because the tongue is the most significant contributor to the propagation of the food bolus in combination with gravity.
- Reconstruction is designed to increase quality of life by addressing speech difficulties and swallowing issues.
- Defects are associated with the highest surgical complication rates in the head and neck.
- In addition to malignancy extirpation, reconstruction is also required for congenital problems, and corrosive and radiation injuries.
- **Treatment**
    - Early: Surgery and/or radiation/chemoradiation
        - Organ preserving therapy
            - Nonsurgical with radiation or induction chemotherapy and radiation
            - Surgical options such as transoral laser microsurgery and supracricoid hemilaryngopharyngectomy
    - Advanced: Surgical resection with radical neck dissection and postoperative radiation.
- **Reconstruction**
    - Goals: Protect the **airway,** restore pharyngeal **conduit, voice rehabilitation**
    - Disa et al[48] created a classification for defects requiring microvascular reconstruction:
        - Type I: Involves <50% of the circumference
        - Type II: Circumferential or involves >50% of the circumference
        - Type III: Extensive, noncircumferential deficiencies involving multiple anatomic levels
    - **Adequate mucosa**
        - Primary closure
            - Provided that there would be no compromise in the lumen, which would lead to dysphagia/stricture
            - Generally can be used when the pharyngeal lumen measures 28 to 32 French
            - In previously irradiated fields, there is a role for vascularized soft tissue coverage.
    - **Inadequate mucosa**
        - **Noncircumferential defect**
            - Skin grafts for smaller posterior defects
            - Mucosal or dermal grafts
            - Local rotation flaps
            - Regional flaps
                - Platysma, deltopectoral, internal mammary artery perforator (IMAP) flap
                - Pectoralis major muscle or myocutaneous flap[49]
                    - Advantage: Reliability and ease of harvest
                    - Disadvantage: Bulky, which can lead to postoperative stenosis, fistula problems, dysphagia
                - Pectoralis and deltopectoral flap used as salvage or primary repair
                - In general there is a higher fistula rate than with other forms of reconstruction if tubing is required.
            - Free fasciocutaneous flap (FRFF, ALT)

- **Circumferential defect**
  - Regional flap
    - Tubed pectoralis major flap (salvage)
  - Free fasciocutaneous flap[20]
    - Reported fistula (1%-27%) and stricture rates (2%-20%)[20]
    - Pharyngeal bypass tube helps to decrease this incidence.
    - FRFF
      - Also used for reconstruction of persistent fistula and hypopharyngeal stenosis
      - Functional advantage is speech quality after laryngopharyngectomy reconstruction
      - Successful oral intake in >75% of patients
      - Disadvantages: Donor scar, higher fistula rate, size limitations
    - ALT
      - Useful in thin patients
      - Can result in good functional results in terms of speech and swallowing
      - Versatile flap with low donor site morbidity
        - May be used as patch or tube
        - Can be designed as a two-skin-paddle flap for complex defects
      - Disadvantages: Anatomic variations, body habitus may preclude its use
    - Lateral arm flap and scapular flap

**TIP:** Free tissue transfer may require either an implantable monitor or incorporation of a segment of the flap in the closure for monitoring.

- Free enteric transplantation
  - Free jejunum
    - Moist, mucosal-lined tube with good size match
    - Segment of up to 20 cm can be harvested
    - Regains function (orient isoperistaltic)
    - Lower rate of fistula and stricture
    - Intrinsic mucus production may aid in swallowing
    - A sentinel loop of bowel is often left outside of the neck or skin paddle to monitor the flap
    - Disadvantages: High metabolic rate decreases ischemic tolerance, does not tolerate radiation as well as fasciocutaneous flaps, friable veins, abdominal incision
      - Postoperative dysphagia because peristalsis is not coordinated with the pharyngeal swallow
      - The mucus production can impair speech intelligibility.
      - Gives a coarse voice in patients using a tracheoesophageal puncture and voice prosthesis

**TIP:** The devascularized segment elongates after revascularization; therefore inset is performed under moderate tension to avoid kinking.

  - Free colon
    - Generally for wide defects that extend up into the oropharynx
    - Some using free ileocolon for voice restoration

  - Gastroomental flap
    - ❖ From greater curvature of the stomach
    - ❖ Omentum provides coverage of the vessels and suture lines.
    - ❖ Patients often are maintained on medication to reduce the production of stomach acid.

> **TIP:** In patients with poor pulmonary function, flaps that go through the thorax or mediastinum should be avoided (i.e., a subcutaneous plane, not retrosternal, should be used).

- **Voice, speech, and swallowing**
  - ▸ **Voice rehabilitation**
    - ♦ Nonsurgical management
      - – Electrolarynx
      - – Pneumatic artificial larynx
      - – Esophageal speech
    - ♦ Surgical management
      - – Neoglottis
        - ❖ Creation of a fistula between the trachea and esophagus
        - ❖ High rate of food regurgitation and high rate of fistula closure
      - – Tracheoesophageal puncture and prosthesis
        - ❖ Fistula created between the posterior trachea and anterior esophagus
        - ❖ Prosthetic device with one-way valve inserted
        - ❖ Air diverted into esophagus where the air **vibrates the walls** to create sound
        - ❖ Concerns of obstruction, infection, dislodgement, stenosis, esophageal perforation, and valve failure with regurgitation
      - – Other methods
        - ❖ Free jejunum or ileocolon for reconstruction of esophagus with a voice tube
        - ❖ Laryngeal transplantation
    - ♦ Tracheoesphageal voice (the benchmark); generated by artificial larynx and esophageal voice
  - ▸ **Factors affecting swallowing:**
    - ♦ Caliber of pharyngeal lumen, propulsive force of base of tongue, lubrication of the reconstructed segment, closure of the velopharynx
    - ♦ Stricture, flap redundancy, loss of normal anatomy such as the base of the tongue
  - ▸ **Factors affecting speech:**
    - ♦ Poor vibratory segment, cricopharyngeal spasm, accumulated secretions that give the voice a wet quality
- **Management of postsurgical complications**
  - ▸ Salivary bypass tubes reduce the incidence and severity of postoperative fistula.
  - ▸ Stenosis/stricture
    - ♦ Must rule out tumor recurrence
    - ♦ Dilation
    - ♦ Patch repair with skin or myocutaneous flap
  - ▸ Fistula
    - ♦ Assess the relationship to great vessels in the neck
    - ♦ Conservative drainage, washout, dressing, and antibiotics
    - ♦ May require coverage of vessels with vascularized soft tissue

## Key Points

- ✓ The pharynx is a shared conduit for speech, air transit, and swallowing.
- ✓ The main criteria for successful treatment are locoregional control of the primary tumor, quality of life, and survival.
- ✓ When determining treatment modality and reconstruction, posttherapeutic function and the patient's quality of life must be considered.
- ✓ Reconstruction of the pharynx generally entails restoring lining, reestablishing a conduit, or obliterating dead space to maintain and protect the airway, swallowing, and speech/articulation.
- ✓ Minimally invasive techniques such as robot assistance provide options for tumor resection and reconstruction to decrease morbidity and maximize postoperative function.

## References


1. Chen MY, Hua YJ, Wan XB, et al. A posteriorly pedicled middle turbinate mucoperiosteal flap resurfacing nasopharynx after endoscopic nasopharyngectomy for recurrent nasopharyngeal carcinoma. Otolaryngol Head Neck Surg 146:409, 2012.
2. Chepeha DB. Reconstruction of the hypopharynx and esophagus. In Flint PW, Haughey BH, Lund VJ, et al, eds. Cummings Otolaryngology: Head & Neck Surgery, 5th ed. Philadelphia: Elsevier, 2010.
3. Gherardini G, Evans RD. Reconstruction of the oral cavity, pharynx, and esophagus. In Thorne CH, Beasley RW, Aston SJ, et al, eds. Grabb and Smith's Plastic Surgery, 6th ed. Philadelphia: Lippincott Williams & Wilkins, 2007.
4. Glastonbury CM, Salzman KL. Pitfalls in the staging of cancer of nasopharyngeal carcinoma. Neuroimaging Clin N Am 23:9, 2013.
5. Harreus U. Malignant neoplasms of the oropharynx. In Flint PW, Haughey BH, Lund VJ, et al, eds. Cummings Otolaryngology: Head & Neck Surgery, 5th ed. Philadelphia: Elsevier, 2010.
6. Ong YK, Solares CA, Lee S, et al. Endoscopic nasopharyngectomy and its role in managing locally recurrent nasopharyngeal carcinoma. Otolaryngol Clin N Am 44:1141, 2011.
7. Saadeh PB, Delacure MD. Head and neck cancer and salivary gland tumors. In Thorne CH, Beasley RW, Aston SJ, et al, eds. Grabb and Smith's Plastic Surgery, 6th ed. Philadelphia: Lippincott Williams & Wilkins, 2007.
8. Schecter GL, Wadsworth TT. Hypopharyngeal cancer. In Bailey BJ, ed. Head & Neck Surgery: Otolaryngology, 2nd ed. Philadelphia: Lippincott Williams & Wilkins, 1998.
9. Tan L, Loh T. Benign and malignant tumors of the nasopharynx. In Flint PW, Haughey BH, Lund VJ, et al, eds. Cummings Otolaryngology: Head & Neck Surgery, 5th ed. Philadelphia: Elsevier, 2010.
10. Taylor MT, Haughey BH. Reconstruction of the oropharynx. In Flint PW, Haughey BH, Lund VJ, et al, eds. Cummings Otolaryngology: Head & Neck Surgery, 5th ed. Philadelphia: Elsevier, 2010.
11. Uppaluri R, Sunwoo JB. Neoplasms of the hypopharynx and cervical esophagus. In Flint PW, Haughey BH, Lund VJ, et al, eds. Cummings Otolaryngology: Head & Neck Surgery, 5th ed. Philadelphia: Elsevier, 2010.
12. Woodson GE. Laryngeal and pharyngeal function. In Flint PW, Haughey BH, Lund VJ, et al, eds. Cummings Otolaryngology: Head & Neck Surgery, 5th ed. Philadelphia: Elsevier, 2010.
13. Edge SB, Byrd DR, Compton CC, et al. AJCC Cancer Staging Manual, 7th ed. New York: Springer, 2002.
14. Lefebvre JL, Adenis A. Radiotherapy and chemotherapy of squamous cell carcinomas of the hypopharynx and esophagus. In Flint PW, Haughey BH, Lund VJ, et al, eds. Cummings Otolaryngology: Head & Neck Surgery, 5th ed. Philadelphia: Elsevier, 2010.

15. Witte MC, Neel HB III. Nasopharyngeal cancer. In Bailey BJ, ed. Head & Neck Surgery: Otolaryngology, 2nd ed. Philadelphia: Lippincott Williams & Wilkins, 1998.
16. Seikaly H, Rassekh CH. Oropharyngeal cancer. In Bailey BJ, ed. Head & Neck Surgery: Otolaryngology, 2nd ed. Philadelphia: Lippincott Williams & Wilkins, 1998.
17. Ariyan S. The pectoralis major myocutaneous flap. Plast Reconstr Surg 63:73, 1979.
18. Chepeha DB, Teknos TN. Microvascular free flaps in head and neck reconstruction. In Bailey BJ, ed. Head & Neck Surgery: Otolaryngology, 3rd ed. Philadelphia: Lippincott Williams & Wilkins, 2001.
19. Chim H, Salgado CJ, Seselgyte R, et al. Principles of head and neck reconstruction: an algorithm to guide flap selection. Semin Plast Surg 24:148, 2010.
20. Evans KF, Mardini S, Salgado CJ, et al. Esophageal and hypopharyngeal reconstruction. Semin Plast Surg 24:219, 2010.
21. Gurtner GC, Evans GR. Advances in head and neck reconstruction. Plast Reconstr Surg 106:672, 2000.
22. Hurvitz KA, Kobayashi M, Evans GR. Current options in head and neck reconstruction. Plast Reconstr Surg 118:112e, 2006.
23. Schusterman MA, Miller JA, Reece GP, et al. A single center's experience with 308 free flaps for repair for head and neck cancer defects. Plast Reconstr Surg 93:472, 1993.
24. Squaquara R, Evans KF, Spilimbergo SS, et al. Intraoral reconstruction using local and regional flaps. Semin Plast Surg 24:198, 2010.
25. Salgado CJ, Chim H, Schoenoff S, et al. Postoperative care and monitoring of the reconstructed head and neck patient. Semin Plast Surg 24:281, 2010.
26. Urken LM, Weinberg H, Buchbinder D, et al. Microvascular free flaps in head and neck reconstruction. Report of 200 cases and review of complications. Arch Otolaryngol Head Neck Surg 120:633, 1994.
27. Varkey P, Liu YT, Tan NC. Multidisciplinary treatment of head and neck cancer. Semin Plast Surg 24:331, 2010.
28. Selber JC. Transoral robotic reconstruction of oropharyngeal defects: a case series. Plast Reconstr Surg 126:1978, 2010.
29. Selber JC, Serletti JM, Weinstein G, et al. Transoral robotic free flap reconstruction of oropharyngeal defects: a preclinical investigation. Plast Reconstr Surg 125:896, 2010.
30. Tan BK, Por YC, Chen HC. Complications of head and neck reconstruction and their treatment. Semin Plast Surg 24:289, 2010.
31. Brown JS, Zuydam AC, Jones DC, et al. Functional outcome in soft palate reconstruction using a radial forearm free flap in conjunction with a superiorly based pharyngeal flap. Head Neck 19:524, 1997.
32. Kimata Y, Uchiyama K, Sakuraba M, et al. Velopharyngeal function after microsurgical reconstruction of lateral and superior oropharyngeal defects. Laryngoscope 112:1037, 2002.
33. Koch WM. The platysma myocutaneous flap: underused alternative for head and neck reconstruction. Laryngoscope 112:1204, 2002.
34. Yu P, Robb GL. Reconstruction for total and near-total glossectomy defects. Clin Plastic Surg 32:411, 2005.
35. Chana JS, Odili J. Perforator flaps in head and neck reconstruction. Semin Plast Surg 24:237, 2010.
36. Mardini S, Salgado CJ, Evans KF, et al. Reconstruction of the esophagus and voice. Plast Reconstr Surg 126:471, 2010.
37. Murray DJ, Novak CB, Neligan PC. Fasciocutaneous free flaps in pharyngolaryngo-oesophageal reconstruction: a critical review of the literature. J Plast Reconstr Aesthet Surg 61:1148, 2008.
38. Nakatsuka T, Harii K, Asato H, et al. Comparative evaluation in pharyngoesophageal reconstruction: radial forearm flap compared with jejunal flap. A 10-year experience. Scand J Plast Reconstr Surg Hand Surg 32:307, 1998.

39. Reece GP, Schusterman MA, Miller MJ, et al. Morbidity and functional outcome of free jejunal transfer reconstruction for circumferential defects of the pharynx and cervical esophagus. Plast Reconstr Surg 96:1307, 1995.
40. Robb GK, Lewin JS, Deschler DG, et al. Speech and swallowing outcomes in reconstructions of the pharynx and cervical esophagus. Head and Neck 25:232, 2003.
41. Schusterman MA, Shestak K, deVries EJ, et al. Reconstruction of the cervical esophagus: free jejunal transfer versus gastric pull-up. Plast Reconstr Surg 85:16, 1990.
42. Seidenberg B, Rosznak SS, Hurwitt ES, et al. Immediate reconstruction of the cervical esophagus by a revascularized isolated jejunal segment. Ann Surg 149:162, 1959.
43. Spyropoulou GC, Lin PY, Chien CY, et al. Reconstruction of the hypopharynx with the anterolateral thigh flap: defect classification, method, tips, and outcomes. Plast Reconstr Surg 127:161, 2011.
44. Triboulet JP, Mariette C, Chevalier D, et al. Surgical management of carcinoma of the hypopharynx and cervical esophagus: analysis of 209 cases. Arch Surg 136:1164, 2001.
45. Withers EH, Franklin JD, Madden JJ, et al. Immediate reconstruction of the pharynx and cervical esophagus with the pectoralis major myocutaneous flap following laryngopharyngectomy. Plast Reconstr Surg 68:898, 1981.
46. Yu P, Robb GL. Pharyngoesophageal reconstruction with the anterolateral thigh flap: A clinical and functional outcomes study. Plast Reconstr Surg 21:137, 1994.
47. Yu P, Hanasano MM, Skoracki RJ. Pharyngoesophageal reconstruction with the anterolateral thigh flap after total laryngopharyngectomy. Cancer 116:1718-1724, 2010.
48. Disa JJ, Pusic AL, Hidalgo DA, et al. Microvascular reconstruction of the hypopharynx: defect classification, treatment algorithm, and functional outcome based on 165 consecutive cases. Plast Reconstr Surg 111:652, 2003.
49. Bakamjian VY. A two-stage method for pharyngoesophageal reconstruction with a primary pectoral skin flap. Plast Reconstr Surg 36:1732, 1965.

# 42. Facial Reanimation

Daniel S. Wu, Raman C. Mahabir, Jason E. Leedy

## FACIAL NERVE ANATOMY

### FACIAL NERVE SUBDIVISIONS[1]

- **Branchial motor:** Voluntary control of muscles of facial expression, stylohyoid, stapedius, posterior belly of digastric
- **Visceral motor:** Parasympathetic innervation of lacrimal, submandibular, and sublingual glands and nasal mucosa
- **General sensory:** Sensation of the auricular concha, external auditory canal, and tympanic membrane
- **Special sensory:** Taste in anterior two thirds of the tongue

### THREE SEGMENTS

1. **Intracranial**
   - Primary somatomotor cortex of facial nerve is located in the precentral gyrus.
   - Facial nucleus is located in the dorsolateral pons.
   - Facial nucleus cell bodies that give rise to the **temporal branch** receive **bilateral** cortical input.
   - All other facial nucleus cell bodies receive **contralateral** cortical input.

> **TIP:** Ipsilateral supranuclear lesions give contralateral facial paralysis but maintain frontalis function.

2. **Intratemporal**
   - Facial nerve enters the internal auditory canal and travels with the acoustic and vestibular nerves for approximately 8-10 mm.
   - Facial nerve then enters the **fallopian canal** by itself, where it travels for 30 mm.
   - Meatal foramen is the narrowest portion of the fallopian canal, measuring 0.68 mm in diameter.
   - Fallopian canal has **three segments** (Fig. 42-1).
   1. **Labyrinthine segment**
      - 5-6 mm long, from entrance of the fallopian canal to the geniculate ganglion
      - Geniculate ganglion contains the nerve cell bodies of taste and sensation.
      - Narrowest segment: 1.42 mm diameter on average, nerve occupies 83% of available space
      - Greater petrosal nerve: First branch off geniculate ganglion, supplies parasympathetic nerves for lacrimal gland and sensory taste fibers from the palate
      - Junction of labyrinthine and tympanic segments formed by an acute angle: *Shearing occurs commonly*
   2. **Tympanic segment**
      - 8-11 mm long, from geniculate ganglion to bend at lateral semicircular canal

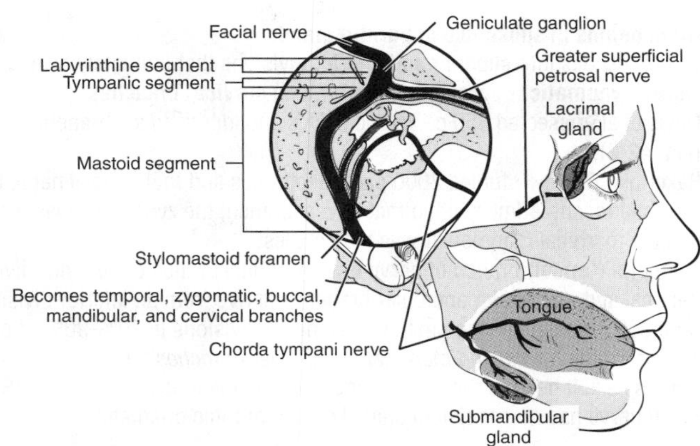


**Fig. 42-1** Facial nerve main divisions.

3. **Mastoid segment**
   - 9-12 mm long, from bend at lateral semicircular canal to stylomastoid foramen
   - Widest cross-sectional area
   - **Three nerve branches**
     - **Nerve to stapedius:** Motor function for stapedius muscle, allows dampening of loud sounds; cell bodies of this motor nerve not located in facial nucleus, therefore not affected by Möbius' syndrome
     - **Sensory branch to external auditory canal:** *Hitselberger's sign:* Hypesthesia of external auditory canal
     - **Chorda tympani:** Final intratemporal branch, joins lingual nerve to provide parasympathetic innervation to submandibular and sublingual glands; special sensory afferents from anterior two thirds of tongue

**TIP:** In children, the ratio of facial nerve diameter to fallopian canal diameter is less than in adults, which decreases the likelihood of facial nerve entrapment.

The facial nerve in the fallopian canal lacks sufficient identifiable topographic orientation to be clinically useful in selective fascicular nerve grafting.

3. **Extratemporal**
   - Starts where facial nerve exits **stylomastoid foramen;** nerve is protected by mastoid tip, tympanic ring, and mandibular ramus
   - **Nerve is superficial in children less than 2 years old.**
   - Travels along a course anterior to the posterior belly of the digastric muscle and along the styloid process to the posterior edge of the parotid gland
   - Facial nerve trunk 1 cm deep, just inferior and medial to the tragal pointer

- **Arborization begins in substance of parotid gland.**
  - Nerve first divides into superior and inferior divisions that ultimately give rise to **temporal, zygomatic, buccal, mandibular,** and **cervical branches.**
    - Davis et al[2] dissected 350 cadaveric halves and identified six branching patterns (Fig. 42-2).
    - Baker and Conley[3] studied 2000 parotidectomies and found facial nerve trunk trifurcation, sometimes with direct buccal branch; the zygomatic was most robust, and the marginal mandibular was the smallest.
    - Temporal (frontal) branch of nerve is the terminal branch of superior division.
    - Cervical and marginal mandibular branches derive from an inferior division.
    - Connections exist between major facial nerve divisions in 70%-90% of patients, *except for the frontal and marginal mandibular branches.*
    - Nerves lie just deep to the subcutaneous musculoaponeurotic system (SMAS) layer.
    - Facial nerve has no consistent spatial or topographic orientation.

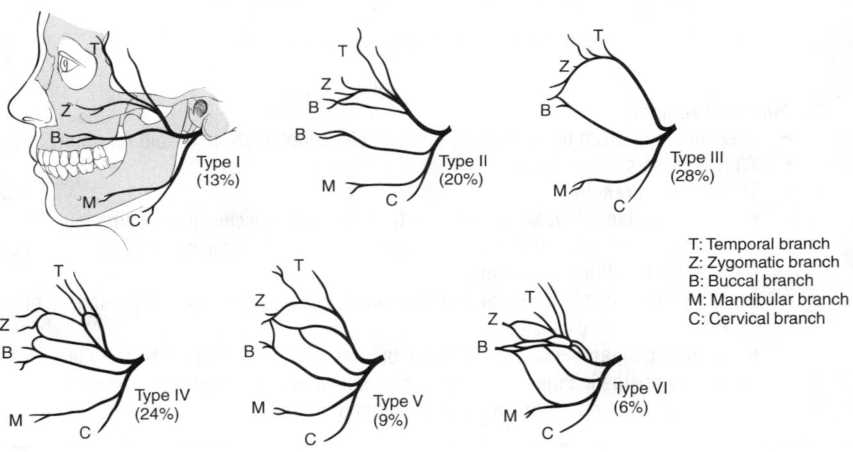


**Fig. 42-2** Facial nerve branching patterns.

## Temporal (Frontal) Branch Anatomy[4-9]

- Course is consistent from 0.5 cm below tragus to 1.5 cm above the lateral brow (Pitanguy's line).[10]
- It lies within temporoparietal fascia[11]
- Temporal nerve and superficial temporal artery reside in deep aspects of temporoparietal fascia. The most posterior rami of temporal branch may be either anterior or posterior to superficial temporal artery.[8]
- Temporal branch arborizes into one to five rami at zygomatic arch with frequent interconnections above zygomatic arch but not to other branches of facial nerve (Fig. 42-3).

## Marginal Mandibular Nerve Anatomy (Fig. 42-4)

- The nerve is connected to other rami in only 15% of cases.[3]
- When posterior to facial artery, the nerve is located above the inferior border of the mandible in 81% of cases and below it in 19%. When anterior to the facial artery, the nerve is above the inferior border in 100% of cases.[12]
- The nerve lies superficial to facial artery and anterior facial vein.
- Injury results in **drooling.**

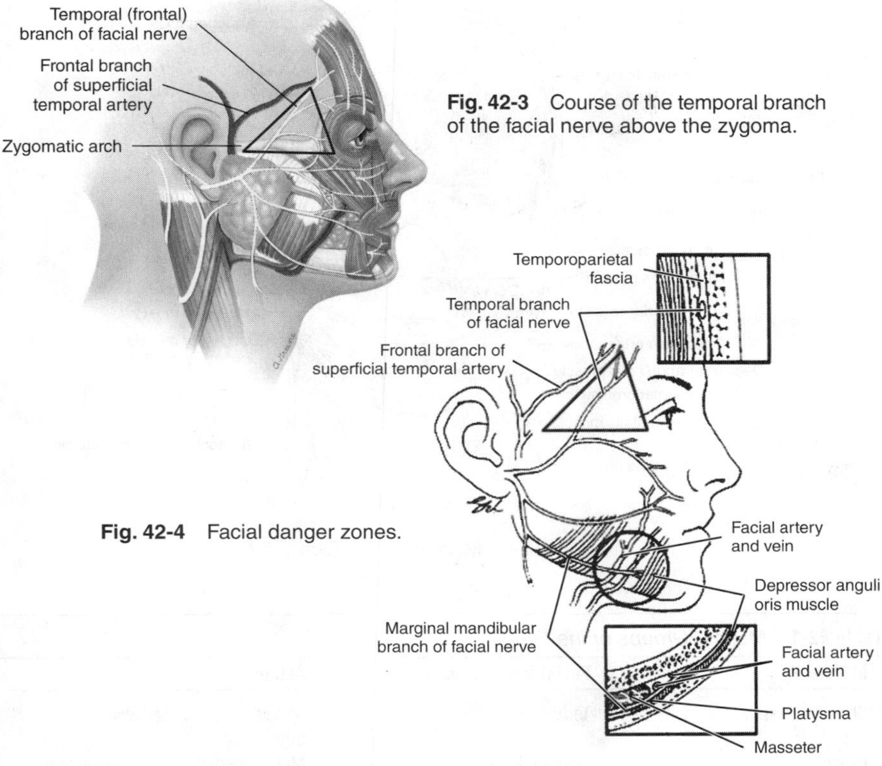


**Fig. 42-3** Course of the temporal branch of the facial nerve above the zygoma.

**Fig. 42-4** Facial danger zones.

## FACIAL MUSCULATURE (Fig. 42-5, Table 42-1)

- Orbicularis oris and 23 other paired muscles
- **Four layers**[13]
  - **Layer 1:** Depressor anguli oris, zygomaticus minor, orbicularis oculi
  - **Layer 2:** Depressor labii inferioris, risorius, platysma, zygomaticus major, levator labii superioris alaeque nasi
  - **Layer 3:** Orbicularis oris, levator labii superioris
  - **Layer 4:** Mentalis, levator anguli oris, buccinator

**TIP:** **Layer 4** muscles are innervated on their **superficial** surface; all other muscles receive innervation from their deep surfaces.

- Subtle movements of normal expression require a delicate balance among all the muscles. However, a few muscles create clinically significant movements that are important when evaluating facial paralysis.
  - **Frontalis:** Raises eyebrows
  - **Orbicularis oculi:** Closes eyelids
  - **Zygomaticus major and minor:** Smiling and grimacing
  - **Orbicularis oris:** Purses the lips
  - **Lower lip depressor:** Keeps lip from riding up during chewing

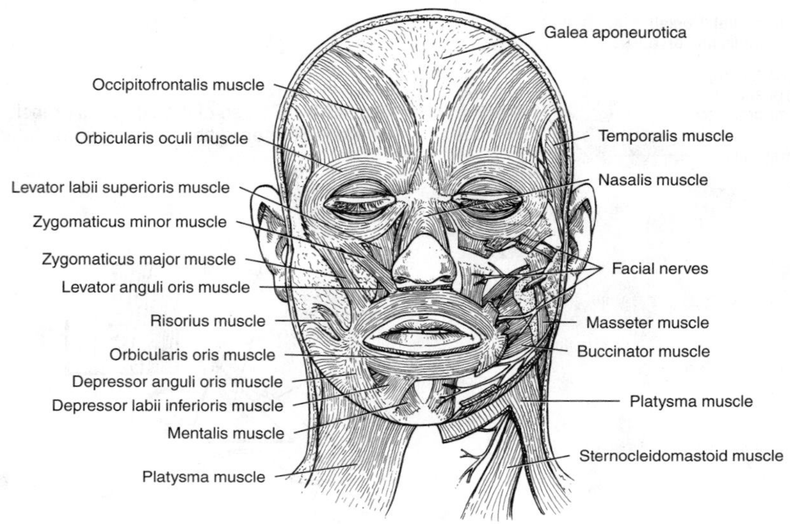


**Fig. 42-5** Muscles of the face.

**Table 42-1** *Muscle Groups of the Face*

| Muscle | Facial Nerve Branch | Action |
|---|---|---|
| Corrugator supercilii | Temporal | Moves eyebrow medially and downward |
| Procerus | Temporal | Moves medial eyebrow downward |
| Orbicularis oculi | Temporal and zygomatic | Closes eyelids and contracts skin around eye |
| Zygomaticus major | Zygomatic and buccal | Elevates corner of mouth |
| Zygomaticus minor | Buccal | Elevates upper lip |
| Levator labii superioris | Buccal | Elevates upper lip and midportion of nasolabial fold |
| Levator labii superioris alaeque nasi | Buccal | Elevates medial nasolabial fold and nasal ala |
| Risorius | Buccal | Aids smile with lateral pull |
| Buccinator | Buccal | Pulls corner of mouth backward and compresses cheek |
| Levator anguli oris | Buccal | Pulls angles of mouth upward and medially |
| Orbicularis oris | Buccal | Closes and compresses lips |
| Nasalis, dilator | Buccal | Flares nostrils |
| Nasalis, compressor | Buccal | Compresses nostrils |
| Depressor anguli oris | Buccal and marginal mandibular | Pulls corner of mouth downward |
| Depressor labii inferioris | Marginal mandibular | Pulls lower lip downward |
| Mentalis | Marginal mandibular | Pulls skin of chin upward |
| Platysma | Cervical | Pulls corner of mouth downward |

## DIFFERENTIAL DIAGNOSIS OF FACIAL PARALYSIS

### INTRACRANIAL

- Vascular abnormalities, aneurysms
- Central nervous system degenerative disorders
- Tumors of the intracranial cavity
- Trauma to the brain
- Congenital abnormalities and agenesis

### INTRATEMPORAL

- Bacterial and viral infections
- Cholesteatoma
- Trauma: Temporal bone fractures, penetrating trauma
- Bell's palsy
- Systemic conditions: Diabetes mellitus, HIV infection

### EXTRATEMPORAL

- Malignant parotid tumors
- Trauma: Particularly penetrating
- Primary tumors of the facial nerve
- Malignant tumors of ascending ramus of mandible, pterygoid, and skin

## UNILATERAL FACIAL PARALYSIS

### BELL'S PALSY[14]

- Idiopathic facial paralysis (Table 42-2)
- Accounts for 85% of all cases of facial paralysis
- **Most common** diagnosis in patients with facial paralysis: 15-40/100,000/year
- Associated with **pregnancy:** 17.4 of 100,000/year in women of child-bearing age versus 45 of 100,000/year in pregnant women
- **Diagnosis of exclusion** is used to avoid misdiagnosis and delay of treatment.

**Table 42-2** *Findings That Rule Out Bell's Palsy*

| Symptom/Finding | Diagnosis | Frequency Exclusive of Bell's Palsy |
|---|---|---|
| Simultaneous bilateral facial palsy | Guillain-Barré, sarcoidosis, pseudobulbar palsy, syphilis, leukemia, trauma, Wegener's granulomatosis | 100% |
| Unilateral facial weakness slowly progressing beyond 3 weeks | Facial nerve neuroma, metastatic cancer, adenoid cystic carcinoma | 100% |
| Slowly progressive unilateral facial weakness associated with facial hyperkinesis | Cholesteatoma, facial nerve neuroma | 100% |
| No return of facial nerve function within 6 months after abrupt onset of palsy | Facial nerve neuroma, adenoid cystic carcinoma, basal cell carcinoma | 100% |
| Ipsilateral lateral rectus palsy | Möbius' syndrome | 100% |
| Recurrent unilateral facial palsy | Facial nerve neuroma, adenoid cystic carcinoma, meningioma | 30% |

- **Proposed cause** is a viral-vascular insult to the facial nerve that causes edema of nerve within fallopian canal, which disrupts neural microcirculation, thereby impairing conduction of neural impulses or causing nerve degeneration.
- **Management**
  - No treatment
    - *All patients begin to recover function within 6 months of paralysis.*
    - All patients have improvement of paresis.
    - 71% of patients with total facial paralysis recover completely without sequelae.
    - Recovery begins within 3 weeks in 85% of patients but not until 3-6 months in 15% of patients.
    - Completeness of recovery decreases with age.
    - More damage to facial nerve results in more synkinesis and contracture.
  - Medical treatment (steroids)
    - Two studies document less denervation and significant improvement of facial grade at recovery if steroids are used within 24 hours.[15,16] The protocol involves prednisone 60 mg/day for 5 days, tapering to 5 mg/day by the tenth day of treatment.
    - Routine corticosteroids are NOT recommended in pediatric Bell's palsy.[17]
  - Surgical decompression
    - Labyrinthine segment, at a minimum, must be decompressed.

## TRAUMA

Trauma is the **second most common cause of facial paralysis,** usually caused by temporal bone fracture, penetrating wound, or birthing injury.

- **Temporal bone fractures**
  - These are classified as **longitudinal, transverse,** or **mixed** according to the long axis of the temporal bone.
  - Facial paralysis is more likely with **transverse** fractures.
  - Repair requires midcranial fossa or translabyrinthine approach with end-to-end coaptation of the transected nerve.
- **Penetrating wounds**
  - **In general, lacerations medial to the lateral canthus do not require repair because of nerve arborization.**
  - Repair should be performed **within 72 hours** to allow identification of distal branches by nerve stimulation.

> **TIP:** If soft tissue injury prohibits repair within first 72 hours, the nerve ends should be tagged to allow delayed repair.

  - Peripheral injuries to the temporal (frontal) and marginal mandibular branches that result in significant weakness should be repaired because of low likelihood of spontaneous recovery.

## TUMORS

- Paralysis can present variably: Sudden or slow progression, complete or incomplete, recurrent or single episode, possibly hyperkinesis (twitching)
- **High concern for neoplastic causes if:**
  - Unilateral facial weakness, slowly increasing for more than 3 weeks
  - Unilateral facial weakness, onset abrupt with no return of function in 6 months
  - Associated with hyperkinesis (twitching)

- **Types**
  - Primary facial nerve
  - Parotid
  - Acoustic neuroma (von Recklinghausen's disease)
  - Central nervous system
  - Cutaneous malignancy
  - Metastatic lesion
  - Cholesteatoma (benign)
  - Hemangiomas (benign)

### Viral Infection

- Can be caused by varicella-zoster (VZV), herpes simplex (HSV), or Epstein-Barr virus (EBV)
- **Ramsay Hunt syndrome:** Varicella-zoster virus infection with facial paralysis, ear pain, and varicelliform rash in external auditory canal; accounts for approximately 12% of all cases of facial paralysis.
  - Treatment involves prednisone (1 mg/kg/day divided twice per day) and acyclovir (800 mg 5 times/day) for 10 days.[18]

### Iatrogenic

- Postoperative facial paralysis after acoustic neuroma resection: Trauma, thermal injury, devascularization, edema, and reactivation of latent herpes virus infection

## BILATERAL FACIAL PARALYSIS

- 0.3%-2% of all cases of facial paralysis
- **Most commonly from Lyme disease** (36% in Teller and Murphy's review)[19]
  - Caused by the spirochete *Borrelia burgdorferi;* tick-borne disease
- **HIV infection** also a common cause

## RECURRENT FACIAL PARALYSIS

- **Melkersson-Rosenthal syndrome:** Recurrent facial nerve paralysis, noninflammatory facial edema, and congenital tongue fissures (lingua plicata)
  - Cause unknown, hereditary factor suspected
  - Can alternate sides
  - Treatment usually conservative, usually self-limited
  - Consider facial nerve decompression if significant increase in frequency, duration, and severity of facial paralysis or if disabling sequelae (synkinesis) and residual facial weakness
- **Bell's palsy** in approximately 10% of patients

## PEDIATRIC DIAGNOSES

### Etiologic Factors

- Congenital/developmental (Möbius syndrome, Chiari malformation, syringobulbia)
- Idiopathic (Bell's palsy)
- Traumatic (blunt, penetrating, iatrogenic, delivery)
- Infectious (Lyme disease, VZV, HSV, EBV, *Haemophilus influenzae*)
- Neoplastic (cholesteatoma, schwannoma, parotid tumor)

**NOTE: Facial nerve decompression is NOT recommended in the pediatric population for acute facial nerve paralysis.**[17]

### Möbius Syndrome

- Unilateral or bilateral loss of eye abduction
- Unilateral or bilateral, complete or incomplete, facial paralysis
- Facial paralysis may be accompanied by other cranial nerve palsies or congenital defects (extremity anomalies, defective brachial and thoracic musculature, micrognathia, mild mental retardation).
- Primary developmental defect of central nervous system
- Treatment: Free microvascular neuromuscular muscle transfer

### Hemifacial Microsomia

- Disorder of morphogenesis of the first and second branchial arches
- Facial paralysis in small percentage of patients

### Congenital Unilateral Lower Lip Palsy (CULLP)

- "Asymmetrical crying facies"
- Caused by intrauterine insult during fifth week of gestation
- Normal resting tone of facial muscles but have marginal mandibular nerve dysfunction when crying
- Other major congenital anomalies in 75% of affected children (cardiovascular, genitourinary, musculoskeletal, respiratory)

## FACIAL DYSKINESIAS

- *Dyskinesia* is a unilateral or bilateral, involuntary, uncontrollable contraction of facial muscles.

### Hemifacial Spasm

- Occurs in the middle-aged and elderly
- Spasms start in orbicularis oculi and can progress inferiorly to involve other facial muscles.
- Tonus phenomenon: Sustained contraction of facial musculature
- Cause: Vascular compression of facial nerve at brainstem
- Treatment: Microvascular decompression by mobilization of vessel and placement of nonabsorbable sponge between vessel and brainstem

### Essential Blepharospasm

- Occurs in older women
- Involuntary, spastic eyelid closure
- **Meige's syndrome:** Blepharospasm, grimacing mouth movements, tongue protrusion
- Treatment: Selective neurectomy, excision of periorbital muscles, botulinum toxin injection

### Facial Myokymia

- Continuous, undulating, writhing, wormlike contractions of facial muscles
- EMG characteristics: Recurrent, regular nerve discharges with short bursts of rapid-firing motor unit potentials
- Causes: Multiple sclerosis, polyradiculoneuropathy, radiation, peripheral nerve injury

## PATIENT EVALUATION

- History of weakness: Onset, duration, progression
- Physical examination[20,21]
  - Compensatory contralateral hypertonicity
    - Hypercontraction of nonparalyzed face that occurs in unilateral paralysis
    - Subconscious effort to correct position of paralyzed side
    - **S-shaped deformity** (Fig. 42-6). Hypercontraction of the contralateral, normal musculature of facial expression results in forehead wrinkling from frontalis contraction, brow elevation and palpebral opening, nasal alar elevation and prominence of the nasolabial fold with bowing of the dorsal nasal lines toward paralyzed side, and elevation of the lip with resultant pull of the midline of the lip (Cupid's bow) toward the normal side.
    - A line connecting the medial border of forehead wrinkling, nasal radix, nasal tip, midpoint of Cupid's bow, and midline of the chin results in an S shape that faces away from the paralyzed side (see Fig. 42-6).
  - Evaluate eyelid laxity, eyelid retraction, ectropion, lagophthalmos, corneal exposure, ptosis, excess skin, epiphora.
  - Bell's phenomenon: Reflex rotation of globe superiorly and temporally on eye closure
  - Corneal sensation: If no sensation, needs ophthalmology consult
  - Corneal light reflex
  - Visual acuity
  - Schirmer's test
  - Rate of eyelid closure and extent of eyelid excursion
  - Position of forehead skin and eyebrow
  - Evaluate for maxillary hypoplasia (congenital or traumatic)
    - "Negative vector": Anteriormost projection of globe lies anterior to lower lid and malar eminence.
    - *Increased risk of lid malposition and dry eye*
  - Evaluate nasal obstruction caused by nasal valve collapse (from paralysis of nasalis muscle).
  - Evaluate speech deficits, drooling, oral incompetence (from paralysis of orbicularis oris).

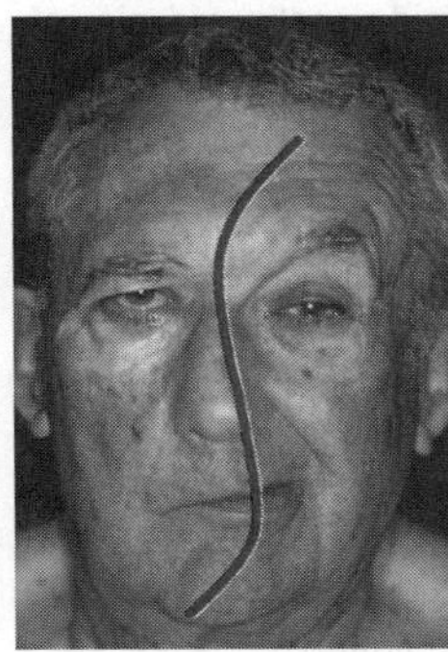

**Fig. 42-6** A line connecting the medial border of forehead wrinkling, nasal radix, nasal tip, midpoint of Cupid's bow, and midline of the chin results in an S shape that faces away from the paralyzed side.

- Grading facial nerve function
  - **House-Brackmann scale**[22]: Gross scale, most commonly used for reporting (Table 42-3)
  - **Burres-Fisch system,**[23] **Sunnybrook scale**[24]: Objective scales, used to limit subjectivity of evaluation
  - **Other scales**[25]: Botman and Jongkees, May, Stennert, Pietersen, Janssen, and Yanagihara

**Table 42-3** *House-Brackmann Scale*

| Grade | Description | Characteristics |
|---|---|---|
| I | Normal | Normal facial function |
| II | Mild dysfunction | Gross: Slight weakness on close inspection, normal at rest<br>Motion: *Forehead,* slight to moderate; *eye,* complete closure with effort; *mouth,* slightly weak with maximum effort |
| III | Moderate dysfunction | Gross: Obvious but not disfiguring, normal asymmetry and tone at rest<br>Motion: *Forehead,* slight to moderate; *eye,* complete closure with effort; *mouth,* slightly weak with maximum effort |
| IV | Moderately severe | Gross: Obvious weakness with disfiguring asymmetry at rest<br>Motion: *Forehead,* none; *eye,* incomplete closure; *mouth,* asymmetrical with maximum effort |
| V | Severe dysfunction | Gross: Only barely perceptible motion, asymmetry at rest<br>Motion: *Forehead,* none; *eye,* incomplete closure; *mouth,* slight movement |
| VI | Total paralysis | No movement |

## DIAGNOSTIC STUDIES

Most cases of facial paralysis are caused by Bell's palsy; therefore a **3-week period of observation** is acceptable before undergoing an extensive diagnostic workup.

### Tests for Etiologic Factors

Establish the cause of facial paralysis.

- **Serologic tests:** Syphilis, diabetes, viral titers
- **Radiographs:** Evaluate destructive lesions, opacification of mastoid air cells, widening of internal auditory canal.
- **CT scan:** Good for evaluating tumors and bony detail of the fallopian canal
- **MRI:** Good for evaluating pathologic and nonpathologic conditions of the nerve

### Prognostic Tests[14]

- **Nerve excitability test (NET)**
  - Subjective
  - Measures minimum stimulus to produce twitch of facial musculature
  - Difference of 3.0 milliamps or more between sides is abnormal.
- **Maximal stimulation test (MST)**
  - Subjective
  - Assesses facial movement with stimulus level that creates discomfort.
  - Any difference in facial movement between sides of the face is abnormal.
  - Becomes positive before NET does in lesions of facial nerve
  - 30% false-positive, 10% false-negative

- **Electroneurography (ENoG)**
  - Apply current to stylomastoid foramen region and record maximal muscle action potentials at nasolabial fold.
  - **Most accurate and reproducible test to determine prognosis**
  - When ENoG reveals 75%-95% degeneration within 2 weeks of onset, facial nerve decompression surgery may preserve the remaining axons.[18]
- **Electromyography (EMG):**
  - Measures muscle activity
  - Does not become positive until 14-21 days after onset of paralysis
  - Useful for late prognosis in complete nerve paralysis
  - Fibrillations are pathognomonic of denervation. In theory, muscles are still alive and can be reinnervated.

### Topographic Tests

Attempt to localize the intratemporal site or extent of involvement.

- **Schirmer's test:** Assesses lacrimation
- **Stapedial reflex:** Assesses function of nerve to stapedius muscle
- **Taste testing:** Assesses chorda tympani function

## GOALS OF SURGICAL TREATMENT

- Corneal protection
- Restoration of oral, nasal, and ocular sphincter control
- Normal appearance at rest
- Symmetry with voluntary motion
- Symmetrical, dynamic smile
- Symmetry with involuntary motion and controlled balance when expressing emotion
- No loss of other significant functions

## TREATMENT PLANNING

- **Analysis of the problem**
  - History
    - Was the nerve transected or anatomically intact?
    - Complete or incomplete paralysis
    - Duration of paralysis
    - Age and underlying comorbidities
    - Status of the eye
    - Patient expectation
  - Determine the greatest concern to the patient, functional or aesthetic.
  - Determine what can be reconstructed.
- Aim for realistic expectations of functional facial movement after intrinsic muscle reinnervation.
- Typically after **3 years,** facial muscles that have undergone denervation atrophy are no longer useful for further reconstruction.[17] However, presence of **fibrillations on EMG** is considered evidence of facial muscle viability and therefore indicates potential for useful function after reinnervation.

## TREATMENT TYPES (Table 42-4)

### REINNERVATION[26,27]

- Requires: Presence of viable facial muscle fibers, functional motor endplates, and unfibrosed facial nerve conduits for axonal regeneration
- Primary nerve repair (intracranial, intratemporal, extratemporal)
  - Must be tension free
  - More proximal the repair, expect more synkinesis
- Interpositional nerve graft
  - Nerve graft essential if any tension prevents primary repair
  - Axons grow **1 mm/day**
  - Donor nerves: Sural nerve, great auricular nerve, lateral or medial antebrachial cutaneous nerves
- Cross-facial nerve graft
- Hypoglossal-facial nerve transfer
- Hypoglossal-facial jump graft

**Table 42-4** *Algorithm for Management of Facial Paralysis*

| **Facial Paralysis: Temporal Branch** | |
|---|---|
| **Deformity** | **Treatment** |
| Brow ptosis | Brow lift |
| Dermatochalasis | Upper blepharoplasty |
| Lagophthalmos | Gold or platinum weight eyelid spring |
| Lower lid ectropion | Canthoplasty or lid shortening |
| **Facial Paralysis: Zygomatic, Buccal, and Marginal Mandibular Branches** | |
| **Time From Injury** | **Treatment** |
| <12 months | Nerve repair<br>Ipsilateral nerve graft<br>Cross-face nerve graft |
| 12-24 months | Nerve repair<br>Ipsilateral nerve graft<br>Hypoglossal-facial transfer<br>Hypoglossal-facial jump graft |
| >24 months | Static reconstruction<br>Cross-face nerve graft and delayed free-functional muscle transfer<br>Free-functional muscle transfer with CN XII or V neurotization |

### CROSS-FACE NERVE GRAFTING (Fig. 42-7)

- Technique is indicated when proximal ipsilateral facial nerve stump is unavailable for grafting, a distal stump is present, and facial muscles are capable of useful function after reinnervation.
- Use branches of contralateral functioning facial nerve to innervate paralyzed muscles.
- Sural nerve grafts are used to connect healthy peripheral nerve branches to corresponding branches of specific muscle groups on paralyzed side.
  - Some recommend using branch that produces maximum zygomaticus major activity for coaptation to cross-facial nerve graft; others recommend using distal buccal branches.
  - **One-stage:** Repair both ends at the same time.[28]

- **Two-stages:** Repair healthy end, then resect neuroma to verify graft success. Once nerve fascicles grow through graft, repair paralyzed side; perform second stage 9-12 months later, after positive Tinel's sign at distal end.

■ **"Babysitter" procedure** (if denervation time >6 months): Use partial hypoglossal-to-facial nerve graft to prevent atrophy and loss of motor endplates while axonal growth occurs through cross-face nerve graft.

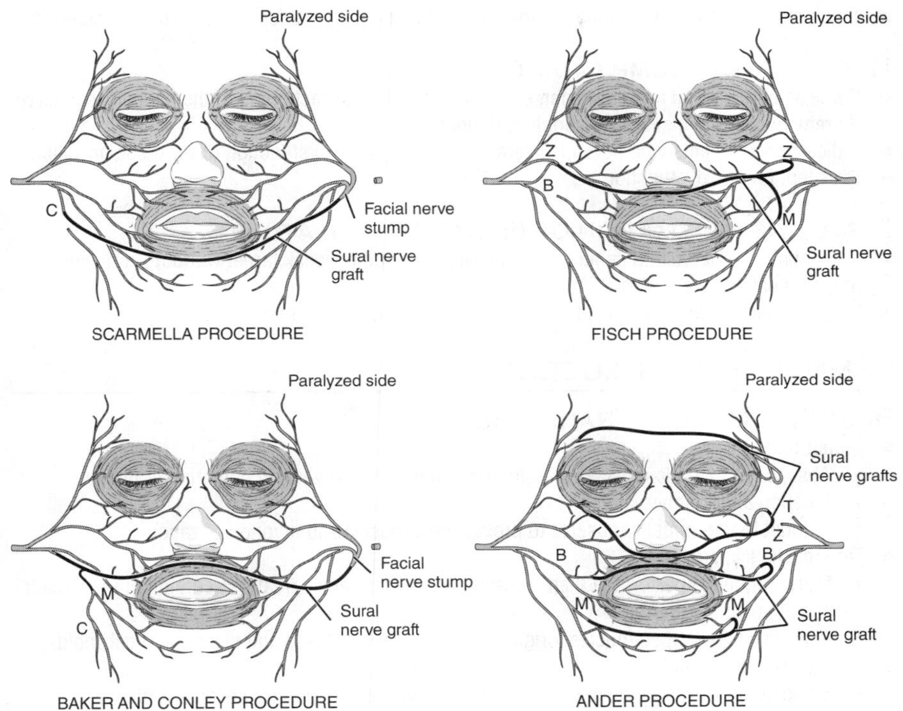


**Fig. 42-7** Techniques of cross-face nerve grafting. (*B,* Buccal branch; *C,* cervical branch; *M,* mandibular branch; *T,* temporal branch; *Z,* zygomatic branch.)

## Nerve Crossover

- Indicated when proximal ipsilateral facial nerve stump is unavailable for grafting, a distal stump is present, and facial muscles are capable of useful function after reinnervation
- Facial nerve stump coapted to hypoglossal (XII), masseteric (V), glossopharyngeal (IX), spinal accessory (XI), phrenic nerves, C7 nerve root, cervical plexus motor nerves (C4), recurrent laryngeal (VII)
  - Requires only a single suture line: A powerful source of reinnervation
  - Sacrifices donor nerve function and often results in difficulty coordinating facial movement, mass movement, and grimacing

### Hypoglossal Nerve Transfer

- Most common
- Best for immediate reconstruction of proximal facial nerve during tumor extirpation
- Provides excellent tone and normal appearance at rest
- Protects eye and allows intentional movement of face, no spontaneous facial expression
- Paralysis and atrophy of the ipsilateral tongue, usually well tolerated unless ipsilateral low cranial nerve dysfunction (CNs IX, X, XI) is present
- Involuntary grimacing with tongue movements, no spontaneous facial expression, synkinesis

### Hypoglossal-Jump Graft

- Same as hypoglossal nerve transfer, except involves partial sectioning of the hypoglossal nerve, thereby preserving ipsilateral hypoglossal function
- Indicated for patients who have ipsilateral low cranial nerve dysfunction or for those unwilling to accept tongue dysfunction

### Direct Neurotization of Facial Musculature[27]

- Implantation of nerve into denervated muscle to strengthen weak target without sacrificing muscle's native innervation
- Used to augment blink, smile, lower lip depressor, tongue movement

## DYNAMIC RECONSTRUCTION

### Regional Muscle Transfers[29]

- **Indications**
  - Absence of mimetic muscles after long-standing atrophy with no potential for useful function after reinnervation
  - Adjunct to the mimetic muscles to provide new muscle and myoneurotization
- **Temporalis transfer**
  - More frequently performed than masseter transfer because greater excursion of movement and adaptability to orbit
  - Anatomy: Fan-shaped muscle, originates from temporal fossa and inserts into coronoid process of mandible
  - Blood supply: Anterior deep temporal artery, posterior deep temporal artery, medial temporal artery
  - Innervation: Mandibular branch of trigeminal nerve
  - Can transfer and suture muscle with its fascial extensions to eyelids, ala of nose, oral commissure, and upper and lower lips
  - Can perform temporalis tendon transfer, where muscle is disinserted from coronoid and reinserted at oral commissure modiolus and dermis; prevents hollowing
- **Masseter transfer**
  - Technique to give motion to the lower half of face
  - Three muscle slips sutured to dermis of the lower lip, oral commissure, and upper lip.
  - During radical parotidectomy, masseter transposed with interdigitation into freshly denervated mimetic muscle to provide maximum myoneurotization
- **Digastric muscle transfer**
  - Used for injury to marginal mandibular nerve
  - Anterior digastric tendon mobilized and inserted into orbicularis oris at inferior vermilion border, medial to oral commissure

## Free-Functional Muscle Transfer[30,31]

- Indicated when facial muscles will not provide useful function after reinnervation
- Microneurovascular muscle transfer combined with cross-face nerve graft, ipsilateral nerve graft (facial nerve of motor nerve to masseter)
- Provides new, vascularized muscle that can pull in various directions
- **Ideal donor muscle characteristics**
  - Excursion is equal to that of normal side of face.
  - Reliable vascular and nerve pattern whose size is similar to that of recipient.
  - Removal of muscle leaves no functional deficit.
  - Location is distant enough from face to allow two operating teams to work simultaneously.
- **Gracilis muscle most commonly used**
- Other potential muscles: Pectoralis minor, serratus anterior, partial latissimus dorsi, partial rectus abdominis, extensor digitorum brevis, abductor hallucis, rectus femoris, and platysma
- Classically, two-stage operation: (1) Cross-facial nerve transfer followed by (2) functional free muscle transfer
- One-stage reconstruction if ipsilateral facial nerve is intact, or use of masseteric or spinal accessory nerve

## Static Reconstruction[21,32-35]

- **Indications:** Facial reanimation is neither possible nor indicated.
  - Elderly patients with poor prognosis or multiple medical comorbidities
  - Massive facial defects from trauma or cancer resection
  - Failed reanimation surgery
  - Atrophy of facial muscles
- **Goals**
  - Protect cornea
  - Restore facial symmetry at rest
  - Correct functional disability (drooling, obstructed airway, poor speech)

# TECHNIQUES

## Brow

- **Indications:** Brow ptosis (ipsilateral) and contralateral compensatory hypertonicity
- **Treatment:**
  - Brow lift
  - Direct (coronal, midforehead, brow incisions) or endoscopic
    - Coronal:
      - Incision: 4-6 cm posterior to anterior hairline
      - Elevation in subgaleal plane and superficial to superficial layer of deep temporal fascia forehead myotomies to release brow
      - Excise 1-2 cm of scalp
    - Midforehead (indirect brow lift):
      - Incision: In a deep brow rhytid
      - Dissection in subcutaneous plane to orbital rim
      - Suspend orbicularis oculi and skin to frontal periosteum
    - Superciliary
      - Incision: Superior brow hairline at junction of forehead and brow subunits
      - Pexy of orbicularis oculi to frontal periosteum

- Endoscopic:
  - Pexy of orbicularis to periosteum only, no skin excision
  - Smaller scars, visualization of supraorbital and supratrochlear nerves, less alopecia, faster recovery
- Considerations: Age of patient, hairline, scar location and prominence, incisional alopecia
- Adjunctive procedures: Younger patients tend to have more contralateral hyperfunctioning of facial nerve and may require temporary chemodenervation with brow elevation.

## Upper Eyelid

- **Supportive therapy:**
  - Lubrication of cornea
  - Use of tape or moisture chamber to prevent exposure and evaporation
  - Use of external weights for eye closure
  - Consider botulinum toxin A for chemodenervation of levator palpebrae and Müller's muscle in nonpermanent facial paralysis
- **Static surgical treatment:**
  - Lid loading: Placement of rigid weight under skin of upper lid to correct paralytic lagophthalmos
    - Can use gold plates or platinum chains
  - Tarsorrhaphy
    - Should not be primary treatment
    - Cosmetically disfiguring and decreases visual field
- **Dynamic surgical treatment:**
  - Lid (palpebral) spring
  - Temporalis muscle transfer (sling)
  - Adjunctive procedures: Blepharoplasty, brow lift, Müllerectomy, levator transection, lower lid repositioning

## Lower Eyelid

- **Lateral paralytic ectropion:** Caused by malposition and stretching of lateral canthal tendon
  - Lateral tarsal strip
  - Lateral transorbital canthopexy
- **Medial paralytic ectropion**
  - Precaruncular medial canthopexy
  - Transcaruncular medial canthopexy
- **Cicatricial ectropion**
  - Anterior lamellae: Full-thickness skin graft
  - Middle/posterior lamellae: "Spacer" graft with hard palate mucosa or acellular dermal matrix
  - Postoperative lower lid support needed
    - Frost stitch
    - Lower lid splint

## Midfacial Ptosis

- Suture suspension: Extended minimal access cranial suspension, multivectored suture suspension, suborbicularis oculi fat (SOOF) elevation

## Nasal Valve Stenosis

- Multivectored suture suspension
- Fascial slings
- Functional rhinoplasty

### Oral Commissure

- **Fascial slings**
  - Sling measured to reach from preauricular zygomatic arch to corner of mouth and extend to midline of upper and lower lip
  - Inferior portion of sling split for insertion into upper and lower lips
  - Subcutaneous tunnel from zygoma to oral commissure
  - Subcutaneous tunnel from oral commissure to upper and lower lips
  - Sutures to secure sling to orbicularis oris at nasolabial fold and oral commissure
  - Sutures to secure lip extensions at midline to orbicularis oris
- **Multivector suture technique**
  - Stab incisions made at lateral orbital rim and nasolabial fold at the nasal ala, midfold, and oral commissure
  - Suture passed subcutaneously from lateral orbital rim to three points of nasolabial fold using Keith needle
  - Polytetrafluoroethylene (PTFE) pledget is used and Keith needle passed back to orbital rim
  - Correct tension applied and sutures tied

## COMPLICATIONS

### Synkinesis[36]

- **Definition:** Unintentional motion in one area of the face produced during intentional movement in another area of the face
- **Pathophysiology:** Aberrant regeneration after injury with resultant innervation of nonnative muscle groups
- **Treatment:**
  - Physical therapy/biofeedback: Facial neuromuscular retraining
  - Botulinum toxin A

### Key Points

- ✓ Bell's palsy is the most common cause of facial nerve palsy and is a diagnosis of exclusion.
- ✓ Successful reanimation involves a thorough assessment with history and physical examination, in conjunction with causal and prognostic testing (i.e., EMG), and requires a discussion with the patient regarding goals of therapy. A combination of static and dynamic procedures may be necessary to achieve optimal outcomes.
- ✓ Corneal protection is essential to prevent exposure keratitis.
- ✓ Static procedures are useful for restoring facial symmetry in repose, but they do not address dynamic function.
- ✓ Free-functional muscle transfers are the best option to restore dynamic function.
- ✓ Successful free-functional muscle transfer involves postoperative physiotherapy.

### References

1. Chu EA, Byrne PJ. Treatment considerations in facial paralysis. Facial Plast Surg 24:164-169, 2008.
2. Davis RA, Anson BJ, Budinger JM, et al. Surgical anatomy of the facial nerve and parotid gland based upon a study of 350 cervicofacial halves. Surg Gynecol Obstet 102:385-412, 1956.
3. Baker DC, Conley J. Avoiding facial nerve injuries in rhytidectomy. Anatomical variations and pitfalls. Plast Reconstr Surg 64:781-795, 1979.

4. Ammirati M, Spallone A, Ma J, et al. An anatomicosurgical study of the temporal branch of the facial nerve. Neurosurg 33:1038-1044, 1993.
5. Babakurban ST, Cakmak O, Kendir S, et al. Temporal branch of the facial nerve and its relationship to fascial layers. Arch Facial Plast Sur 12:16-23, 2010.
6. Gagnon NB, Molina-Negro P. Facial reinnervation after facial paralysis: is it ever too late? Arch Otorhinolaryngol 246:303-307, 1989.
7. Gosain AK. Surgical anatomy of the facial nerve. Clin Plast Surg 22:241-251, 1995.
8. Gosain AK, Sewall SR, Yousif NJ. The temporal branch of the facial nerve: how reliably can we predict its path? Plast Reconstr Surg 99:1224-1233, 1997.
9. Zani R, Fadul R, DaRocha MA, et al. Facial nerve in rhytidoplasty: anatomic study of its trajectory in the overlying skin and the most common sites of injury. Ann Plast Surg 51:236-242, 2003.
10. Pitanguy I, Ramos AS. The frontal branch of the facial nerve: the importance of its variations in face lifting. Plast Reconstr Surg 38:352-356, 1966.
11. Stuzin JM, Wagstrom L, Kawamoto HK, et al. Anatomy of the frontal branch of the facial nerve: the significance of the temporal fat pad. Plast Reconstr Surg 83:256-271, 1989.
12. Dingman RO, Grabb WC. Surgical anatomy of the mandibular ramus of the facial nerve based on the dissection of 100 facial halves. Plast Reconstr Surg 29:266-272, 1962.
13. Freilinger G, Gruber H, Happak W, et al. Surgical anatomy of the mimetic muscle system and the facial nerve: importance for reconstructive and aesthetic surgery. Plast Reconstr Surg 80:686-690, 1987.
14. Anderson RG. Facial nerve disorders and surgery. Sel Read Plast Surg 9(20), 2001.
15. Austin JR, Peskind SP, Austin SG, et al. Idiopathic facial nerve paralysis: a randomized double blind controlled study of placebo versus prednisone. Laryngoscope 103:1326-1333, 1993.
16. Shafshak TS, Essa AY, Bakey FA. The possible contributing factors for the success of steroid therapy in Bell's palsy: a clinical and electrophysiological study. J Laryngol Otol 108:940-943, 1994.
17. Barr JS, Katz KA, Hazen A. Surgical management of facial nerve paralysis in the pediatric population. J Pediatr Surg 46:2168-2176, 2011.
18. Adour KK. Medical management of idiopathic (Bell's) palsy. Otolaryngol Clin North Am 24:663-673, 1991.
19. Teller DC, Murphy TP. Bilateral facial paralysis: a case presentation and literature review. J Otolaryngol 21:44-47, 1992.
20. Chan JY, Byrne PJ. Management of facial paralysis in the 21st century. Facial Plast Surg 27:346-357, 2011.
21. Meltzer NE, Byrne PJ. Management of the brow in facial paralysis. Facial Plast Surg 24:216-219, 2008.
22. House JW, Brackmann DE. Facial nerve grading system. Otolaryngol Head Neck Surg 93:146-147, 1985.
23. Burres S, Fisch U. The comparison of facial grading systems. Arch Otolaryngol Head Neck Surg 112:755-758, 1986.
24. Ross BG, Fradet G, Nedzelski JM. Development of a sensitive clinical facial grading system. Otolaryngol Head Neck Surg 114:380-386, 1996.
25. Brenner MJ, Neely JG. Approaches to grading facial nerve function. Semin Plast Surg 18:13-21, 2004.
26. Humphrey CD, Kriet JD. Nerve repair and cable grafting for facial paralysis. Facial Plast Surg 24:170-176, 2008.
27. Terzis JK, Konofaos P. Nerve transfers in facial palsy. Facial Plast Surg 24:177-193, 2008.
28. Smith JW. A new technique for facial reanimation. In Hueston JT, ed. Transactions of the Fifth International Congress of Plastic and Reconstructive Surgery. Melbourne: Butterworths, 1971.
29. Boahene KD. Dynamic muscle transfer in facial reanimation. Facial Plast Surg 24:204-210, 2008.

30. O'Brien MB, Pederson WC, Khazanchi RK, et al. Results of management of facial palsy with microvascular free-muscle transfer. Plast Reconstr Surg 86:12-22, 1990.
31. Sassoon EM, Poole MD, Rushworth G. Reanimation for facial palsy using gracilis muscle grafts. Br J Plast Surg 44:195-200, 1991.
32. Bergeron CM, Moe KS. The evaluation and treatment of lower eyelid paralysis. Facial Plast Surg 24:231-241, 2008.
33. Liu YM, Sherris DA. Static procedures for the management of the midface and lower face. Facial Plast Surg 24:211-215, 2008.
34. Seeley BM, To WC, Papy FA. A multivectored bone-anchored system for facial resuspension in patients with facial paralysis. Plast Reconstr Surg 108:1686-1691, 2001.
35. Seiff SR, Chang J. Management of ophthalmic complications of facial nerve palsy. Otolaryngol Clin North Am 25:669-690, 1992.
36. Husseman J, Mehta RP. Management of synkinesis. Facial Plast Surg 24:242-249, 2008.

# 43. Face Transplantation

Tae Chong

## INDICATIONS

- Facial defects in adults with functional deficits that cannot be reconstructed using conventional techniques
  - Nonreconstructible injury to the central face: eyes, nose, and mouth
    - Responsible for facial expression, communication, airway, eating, and control of oral secretions
      - Divided into three anatomic classifications: upper face, lower face, entire face
  - >25% of the facial area with or without loss of a central facial feature
  - Cleveland Clinic FACES score (Table 43-1)
    - Scoring system to identify ideal candidates for face transplantation based on the following factors:
      - Functional status
      - Aesthetic deficit
      - Comorbid conditions
      - Exposed tissue
      - Surgical history
    - Designed to facilitate patient selection and communication between centers, but has not been validated

**Table 43-1** *The Cleveland Clinic FACES Scoring System for Face Transplant Candidate Evaluation*

| Category | Point System | Totals |
|---|---|---|
| Functional status (SBSSS + KPS) | **Straus-Bacon Social Stability Score (SBSSS)** | 0-4 |
| | Steady job for last 3 years = 1 pt | |
| | Same residence for past 2 years = 1 pt | |
| | Married and lives with spouse/partner = 1 pt | |
| | Does not live alone = 1 pt | |
| | **Karnovsky Performance Score (KPS)** | 2-9 |
| | Capable of normal activity, minor symptoms = 9 pts | |
| | Normal activity with effort = 8 pts | |
| | Cares for self, unable to carry on normal activity/work = 7 pts | |
| | Requires occasional assistance, can take care of most tasks = 6 pts | |
| | Requires considerable assistance, needs frequent medical care = 5 pts | |
| | Disabled, requires special care and assistance = 4 pts | |
| | Severely disabled, hospital admission indicated = 3 pts | |
| | Very ill, urgently requiring admission = 2 pts | |

*FACES,* Functional status, *A*esthetic deficits, *C*omorbidities, *E*xposed tissue, *S*urgical history.

| Category | Point System | Totals |
|---|---|---|
| Aesthetic deficit (i.e., aesthetic units) | **Lateral**<br>Forehead (single side) = 1 pt<br>Brow (single side) = 1 pt<br>Perioral (single side) = 1 pt<br>Cheek (single side) = 1 pt<br>Ear (single side) = 1 pt<br>**Central**<br>Nose = 2 pts<br>Upper lip (upper perioral area) = 2 pts<br>Lower lip (lower perioral area) = 2 pts<br>Chin = 2 pts | 1-18 |
| Comorbidities | Cardiovascular status WNL = 1 pt<br>Hematologic status WNL = 1 pt<br>Hepatic status WNL = 1 pt<br>Nervous system status WNL = 1 pt<br>Pulmonary status WNL = 1 pt<br>Renal status WNL = 1 pt | 0-6 |
| Exposed tissue (i.e., depth) | Subcutaneous tissue = 5 pts<br>Muscle = 10 pts<br>Bone = 15 pts | 5-15 |
| Surgical history (SH)/recipient vessel patency (RVP) | Extensive SH (>10 surgeries)/below-average RVP = 2 pts<br>Moderate SH (5-10 surgeries)/average RVP = 4 pts<br>Minimal SH (<5 surgeries)/above-average RVP = 8 pts | 2-8 |

*WNL,* Within normal limits.

## CONTRAINDICATIONS

- **Psychiatric**
  - Active psychiatric disorder
  - Substance abuse
  - Cognitive and perceptual inability to understand risks of procedure
- **Medical**
  - Cancer: Active cancer diagnosis or high risk of cancer recurrence
  - Active infectious disease: HIV, hepatitis
  - Hematologic and immunologic conditions: Hypercoagulable disorders, systemic lupus erythematosus (SLE), scleroderma
- **Psychosocial**
  - History of medical noncompliance
  - Inadequate support network
  - Pregnancy
  - Congenital malformations: Difference with hand allotransplantation, based on a patient with neurofibromatosis who has undergone transplant

# RISKS

## Side Effects of Long-Term Immunosuppression

- Opportunistic infections: Bacterial, cytomegalovirus, fungal (oropharynx)
- Malignancy: Skin cancers, virally associated (Epstein-Barr virus [EBV]), Kaposi's sarcoma
- Metabolic: Hypertension, diabetes, renal insufficiency/failure, and gastrointestinal intolerance
  - Most are transient and reversible with change in medications or decrease in dosage.
- Complications of immunosuppression resulting in discontinuation of medications and subsequent allograft rejection

## Loss of Face Transplant

- Vascular compromise
  - Acute setting: <4%
- Irreversible allograft rejection
  - Acute
  - Chronic
- Challenges associated with transplant rescue operations
  - Technically difficult because many patients had >10 operations before transplant and exhausted many of their reconstructive flap options

## Death

- Chinese bear-mauling victim died after medical noncompliance.
- French burn victim with bilateral hand and face transplant had cerebral anoxia during reoperation.

# BENEFITS

## Functional Recovery

- Oral competence and mastication: Allow patient to eat and control secretions
- Ocular protection
- Social communication: Facial expression and improved speech
- Return of sensation
- Social reintegration

# ANATOMY AND SURGICAL PLANNING (Fig. 43-1)

- Facial allograft design based on missing functional and aesthetic units
- Functional components
  - Bony architecture: Osteotomies correspond to the missing structures
    - Midface
      - LeFort osteotomy lines
    - Mandible
      - Custom fit for small defects
      - Bilateral sagittal split osteotomies for larger defects
    - Presurgical modeling based on CT guidance
  - Facial mimetic muscles
  - Skin and mucosa
    - Lips
    - Buccal mucosa
    - Nose
    - Nasal mucosa

- Vascular perfusion
  - The entire facial vascularized composite allograft (VCA)
  - Including oral mucosa and bony skeleton; can be based on perfusion from one side because of robust collateral circulation
  - External carotid and external/internal jugular system
- Nerve reconstruction
  - Facial nerve
    - Coaptation of nerves as close to donor muscle as possible to avoid synkinesis
    - Based on length of recipient facial nerve; donor nerve may have to include the entire facial nerve trunk ± parotid gland
  - Trigeminal nerve branches for sensation
    - May require ostetomies to achieve greater length on the donor nerves
    - Recipient's sensory nerves may not be present because of injury.

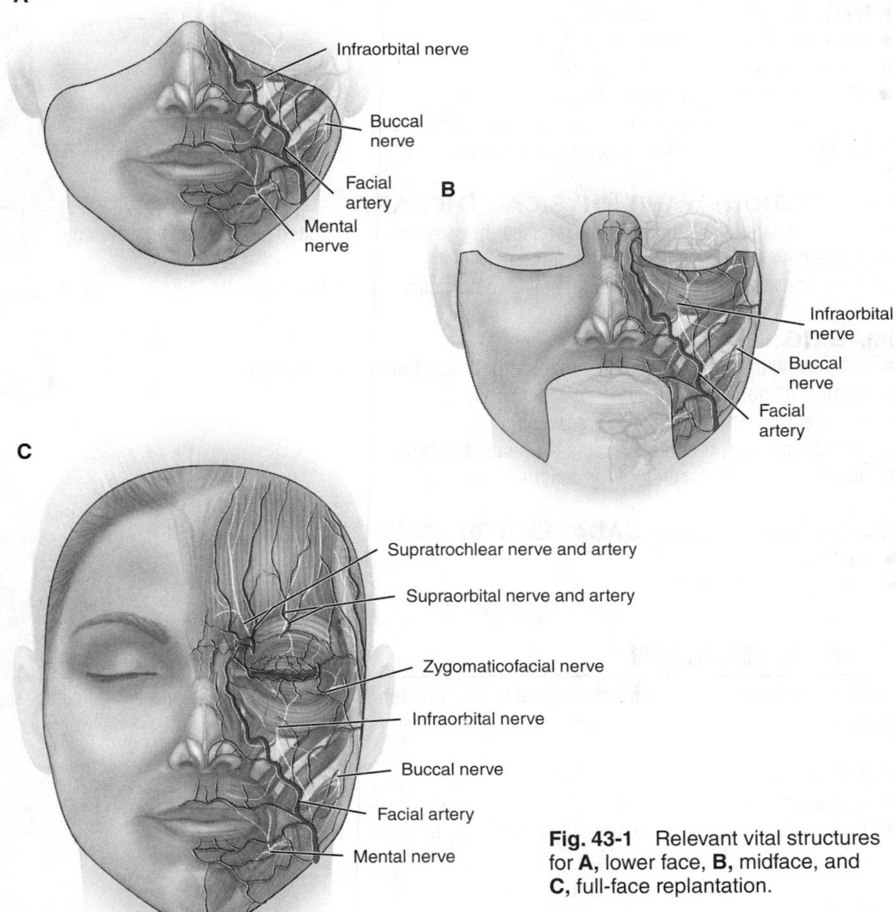


**Fig. 43-1** Relevant vital structures for **A,** lower face, **B,** midface, and **C,** full-face replantation.

## PREOPERATIVE EVALUATION

### Transplant Medical Clearance: Adults

- Physical health screening
- General well-being
  - Ability to tolerate immunosuppression and operation
- Infectious disease screening
  - Risk of opportunistic infections based on prior exposures and colonization
- Immunologic
  - ABO blood typing and HLA typing
  - Panel reactive antibodies
    - Reflect sensitization to potential donor antigen
    - Predictive of hyperacute rejection
    - May preclude transplant candidacy

### Psychiatric Clearance

- Rule out active psychiatric disorders.
- Assess patient for medical compliance.
- Confirm cognitive understanding and realistic expectations.
- Evaluate for postoperative regression and degree of coping skills.
- Assess and optimize the structure of home support.

### Occupational and Physical Therapy

- Evaluate candidacy and initiate exercises for postoperative speech and swallowing therapy.
- Assess need for physical therapy postoperatively.
- Evaluate level of engagement and ability to participate in postoperative therapy.

### Imaging

- CT scan with three-dimensional reconstruction, CT angiography, MRI
- Critical diagnosis of the defect
  - Identify components that are missing.
  - Identify components available for reconstruction.
- Identification of vasculature for anastomosis

### Multiple-Staged Cadaver Trials and Dissections

- For donor procurement
- For transplantation

## TRANSPLANTATION

Facial transplantation requires two surgical teams: one for donor dissection and one for recipient dissection.

### Donor

- Tracheostomy
- VCA procurement halted if any donor instability to allow solid organ procurement

- Transplant classification
  - Partial face
  - Midface
  - Full face
- Silicone prosthetic placed after procurement

### Recipient

- Tracheostomy
- Re-creation of the defect with removal of all prior reconstructions
- Identification of recipient vessels: External carotid and its branches and jugular drainage system

### Transplant Progression

- Vascular anastomosis
- Bony inset
- Intraoral/mucosal repair
- Neurorrhaphy
- Skin and all other soft tissue

## IMMUNOSUPPRESSION

### Induction

- Immunosuppression initiated before transplantation to prevent acute rejection of the transplant
- Depleting agent: Decreases lymphocytes
  - Antithymocyte globulin: Polyclonal antibody
  - Campath (alemtuzumab): Monoclonal antibody directed against cd52 (cell surface marker present on mature lymphocytes)
- Anti-IL-2 monoclonal antibody: Does not deplete the lymphocyte count but prevents T-cell activation via the IL-2–dependent pathway
- Calcineurin inhibitor: Prevents IL-2–dependent activation of lymphocytes
- Antiproliferative agent: Mycophenolate mofetil
- Steroid: General immunosuppressant with antiinflammatory properties

### Maintenance

- Most patients are on three-drug therapy with corticosteroids, tacrolimus, and mycophenolate mofetil.

## OUTCOMES

### Functional Recovery

- Sensory recovery within the first 6-8 months after surgery
- Motor recovery slower than sensory, but most patients able to control secretions, eat, and manage airway
- Social reintegration with improved speech and communication

## COMPLICATIONS

- **Infectious complications:** CMV, herpes virus, and fungal infections
  - Managed with appropriate antivirals and antifungals
    - Antivirals: Ganciclovir, acyclovir
    - Antifungals: Fluconazole,voriconazole, itraconazole
- **Metabolic:** Hyperglycemia, increased serum creatinine, and hyperlipidemia
- **Rejection episodes**
  - All transplant recipients thus far have had at least one episode of rejection.
  - *Skin is considered the most antigenic of all the components of a composite allograft.* (It is the earliest affected and appears to be the most severely injured.)
  - Symptoms of rejection most often manifest as cutaneous changes.
    - Diffuse edema
    - Erythema
    - Cutaneous rash
    - Mucosal lesions: Intraoral and intranasal
  - **Banff classification for VCA rejection:** 4 mm punch with H&E and PAS staining
    - **Grade 0:** No rejection
    - **Grade I:** Mild rejection—mild perivascular infiltrate (lymphocytic)
    - **Grade II:** Moderate rejection—moderate to dense perivascular inflammation, can include mild epidermal and adnexal involvement
    - **Grade III:** Severe rejection—dense inflammation with epidermal involvement, epithelial apoptosis/necrosis
    - **Grade IV:** Necrotizing rejection—necrosis of epidermis and/or other skin elements
  - Outcomes
    - All rejection episodes have been managed with modifications in the immunosuppressive protocol.
    - Treatment regimen includes:
      - Therapeutic dosage of calcineurin inhibitors (if levels low)
      - Topical steroids or tacrolimus
      - Pulse-dose steroids
      - Thymoglobulin or Campath for refractory episodes
- **Death (2):** Medically noncompliant patient and bilateral hand and face transplant recipient

## CONTROVERSIES

- Blind recipient
- Issues with transference of donor appearance
  - Largely refuted in soft tissue transplant, because the overall appearance is determined by the bony architecture
  - Complex ballistic injuries involve loss of both soft tissue and bony structure and have potential for appearance transfer.
- Multiorgan transplantation: Face and hand transplant
- Tolerogenic protocols vs. accepted standard immunosuppression
- Facial allotransplantation as first-line therapy after disfiguring injury
- Technique of transplantation: Preservation of native tissue as a lifeboat vs. removal of native tissue along facial subunits to optimize aesthetic result

## Key Points

- ✓ Face transplantation is indicated in adult patients with nonreconstructible defects of the central face and/or defects of >25% of the facial area with significant functional limitations.
- ✓ Face transplantation is contraindicated in patients with medical contraindications to chronic immunosuppression, lack of psychosocial support, history of medical noncompliance, and inability to understand the implications of face transplantation.
- ✓ Risks related to immunosuppression include opportunistic infections, malignancy, and metabolic complications, and the consequences of the loss of the face transplant
- ✓ Functional outcomes include return of sensation, motor recovery, and social reintegration.

## References

1. Siemionow M, Ozturk C. Face transplantation: outcomes, concerns, controversies, and future directions. J Craniofac Surg 23:254-259, 2012.
2. Siemionow M, Ozturk C. An update on facial transplantation cases performed between 2005 and 2010. Plast Reconstr Surg 128:707e-720e, 2011.
3. Siemionow M, Gharb BB, Rampazzo A. Pathways of sensory recovery after face transplantation. Plast Reconstr Surg 127:1875-1889, 2011.
4. Gordon CR, Avery RK, Abouhassan W, et al. Cytomegalovirus and other infectious issues related to face transplantation: specific considerations, lessons learned, and future recommendations. Plast Reconstr Surg 127:1515-1523, 2011.
5. Gordon CR, Siemionow M, Coffman K, et al. The Cleveland Clinic FACES Score: a preliminary assessment tool for identifying the optimal face transplant candidate. J Craniofac Surg 20:1969-1974, 2009.
6. Siemionow MZ, Papay F, Djohan R, Bernard S, Gordon CR, Alam D, Hendrickson M, Lohman R, Eghtesad B, Fung J. First U.S. near-total human face transplantation: a paradigm shift for massive complex injuries. Plast Reconstr Surg 125:111-122, 2010.
7. Siemionow M, Papay F, Alam D, et al. Near-total human face transplantation for a severely disfigured patient in the USA. Lancet 374:203-209, 2009.
8. Petruzzo P, Testelin S, Kanitakis J, et al. First human face transplantation: 5 years outcomes. Transplantation 93:236-240, 2012.
9. Petruzzo P, Kanitakis J, Badet L, et al. Long-term follow-up in composite tissue allotransplantation: in-depth study of five (hand and face) recipients. Am J Transplant 11:808-816, 2011.
10. Dubernard JM, Lengelé B, Morelon E, et al. Outcomes 18 months after the first human partial face transplantation. N Engl J Med 357:2451-2460, 2007.
11. Devauchelle B, Badet L, Lengelé B, et al. First human face allograft: early report. Lancet 368:203-209, 2006.
12. Guo S, Han Y, Zhang X, Lu B, et al. Human facial allotransplantation: a 2-year follow-up study. Lancet 372(9639):631-638, 2008.
13. Pomahac B, Pribaz J, Eriksson E, et al. Restoration of facial form and function after severe disfigurement from burn injury by a composite facial allograft. Am J Transplant 11:386-393, 2011.
14. Singhal D, Pribaz JJ, Pomahac B. The Brigham and Women's Hospital face transplant program: a look back. Plast Reconstr Surg 129:81e-88e, 2012.
15. Pomahac B, Pribaz J, Eriksson E, et al. Three patients with full facial transplantation. N Engl J Med 366:715-722, 2012.
16. Barret JP, Gavaldà J, Bueno J, et al. Full face transplant: the first case report. Ann Surg 254:252-256, 2011.
17. Cavadas PC, Ibáñez J, Thione A. Surgical aspects of a lower face, mandible, and tongue allotransplantation. J Reconstr Microsurg 28:43-47, 2012.

# Part IV

# Breast

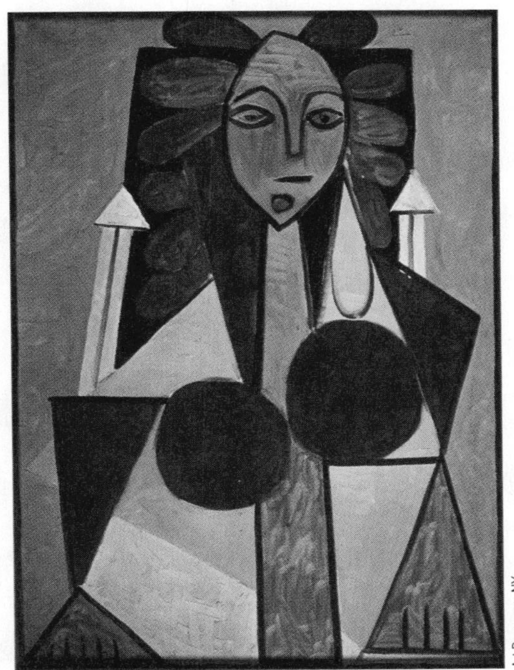

# 44. Breast Anatomy and Embryology

Melissa A. Crosby, Raman C. Mahabir

## EMBRYOLOGY AND DEVELOPMENT[1]

### EMBRYOLOGY

- Breast derives from ectoderm and develops during fourth week of gestation.
- Most tissue normally involutes except for a small thoracic portion that penetrates into the underlying mesenchyme.
- Mammary (milk) ridge develops at the sixth week, and extends from axilla to groin.
- From the eighth to tenth week of embryologic development, breast growth begins with differentiation of cutaneous epithelium of the pectoral region.
- Primary bud gives rise to secondary bud, which in turn gives rise to lactiferous ducts (modified sweat glands).
- Areolae develop by the fifth month.
- Toward the end of fetal development, acini develop around tips of lactiferous ducts creating mammary pit
- Supernumerary breasts *(polymastia)* and nipples *(polythelia)* can occur anywhere along the milk ridge.
  - The most common location for polymastia and polythelia is the **left chest wall,** below the inframammary crease.
  - **Polythelia** is the most common congenital breast anomaly, occurring in 2% of the population.

### DEVELOPMENT

- Puberty begins at age 10-12 years as a result of hypothalamic gonadotropin-releasing hormones secreted into the hypothalamic-pituitary portal venous system.
- The anterior pituitary secretes follicle-stimulating hormone (FSH) and luteinizing hormone (LH).
- FSH causes ovarian follicles to mature and secrete estrogens.
- Estrogens stimulate longitudinal growth of breast ductal epithelium.
- As ovarian follicles become mature and ovulate, the corpus luteum releases progesterone, which, in conjunction with estrogen, leads to complete mammary development.
  - Occurs between the superficial and deep layers of the superficial fascia. (Cooper's ligaments connect the two layers to each other and to the underlying musculature.)
- **Stages of breast development described by Tanner**[2]
  - **Stage 1:** Preadolescent elevation of nipple but no palpable glandular tissue or areolar pigmentation
  - **Stage 2:** Glandular tissue in the subareolar region; nipple and breast project as single mound
  - **Stage 3:** Further increase in glandular tissue with enlargement of breast and nipple but continued contour of nipple and breast in single plane
  - **Stage 4:** Enlargement of areola and increased areolar pigmentation with secondary mound formed by nipple and areola above level of breast
  - **Stage 5:** Final adolescent development of smooth contour with no projection of areola and nipple

## Menstrual Cycle

- **Follicular phase:** Days 4-14, mitosis and proliferation of breast epithelial cells
- **Luteal phase:** Days 14-28, progesterone levels rise, mammary ductal dilation and differentiation of alveolar epithelial cells into secretory cells, estrogens increase blood flow to breast
- **Premenstrual:** Estrogen peak, breast engorgement, breast sensitivity
- **Menstruation:** Breast involution and decrease in circulating hormones

## Pregnancy and Lactation

- Marked ductular, lobular, and alveolar growth occurs under the influence of estrogen, progesterone, placental lactogen, prolactin, and chorionic gonadotropin.
- **First trimester:** Estrogen influences ductular sprouting and lobular formation, early to late breast enlargement ensues, and dilation of superficial veins and increased pigmentation of NAC occurs.
- **Second trimester:** Lobular events predominate under the influence of progestins, and colostrum collects within lobular alveoli.
- **Third trimester:** By parturition, breast size triples because of vascular engorgement, epithelial proliferation, and colostrum accumulation.
- **Delivery:** Withdrawal of placental lactogen and sex hormones results in breast being predominantly influenced by prolactin.
- **Anterior** pituitary secretion of **prolactin** influences **milk production and secretion.**
- **Posterior** pituitary secretion of **oxytocin** leads to breast **myoepithelial contraction** and **milk ejection.**
- Tactile stimulation of nipples by nursing infant results in prolactin and oxytocin secretion.
- Postlactational involution occurs during the 3 months after nursing ceases; regression of extralobular stroma is a primary feature.

## Menopause

- Involves loss of glandular tissue and replacement with fat

# ANATOMY

## Vascular Supply[3] (Fig. 44-1)

- Arterial supply
  - **Skin** receives blood supply from subdermal plexus, which communicates through perforators with underlying deeper vessels supplying breast parenchyma
  - **Parenchyma** supplied by:
    - Perforating branches of internal mammary artery
    - Lateral thoracic artery
    - Thoracodorsal artery
    - Intercostal perforators
    - Thoracoacromial artery
  - **NAC** receives both parenchymal and subdermal blood supply.
  - **Venous drainage** mirrors the arterial supply and predominantly drains to the axilla.

**TIP:** In a normal breast, arterial collateralization is sufficient for survival on only a fraction of the arterial input.

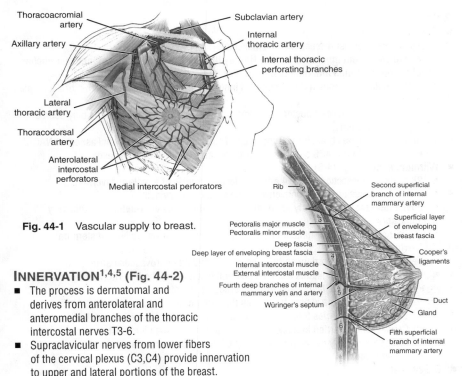

**Fig. 44-1** Vascular supply to breast.



## INNERVATION[1,4,5] (Fig. 44-2)

- The process is dermatomal and derives from anterolateral and anteromedial branches of the thoracic intercostal nerves T3-6.
- Supraclavicular nerves from lower fibers of the cervical plexus (C3,C4) provide innervation to upper and lateral portions of the breast.
- NAC sensation derives from the anteromedial and anterolateral **T4** intercostal nerve that travels along the pectoral fascia to innervate the NAC from the deep surface.
- Intercostobrachial nerve travels across axilla to supply upper medial arm.

> **TIP:** The intercostobrachial nerve is often injured during axillary dissection, resulting in anesthesia and paresthesias of the upper inner arm.

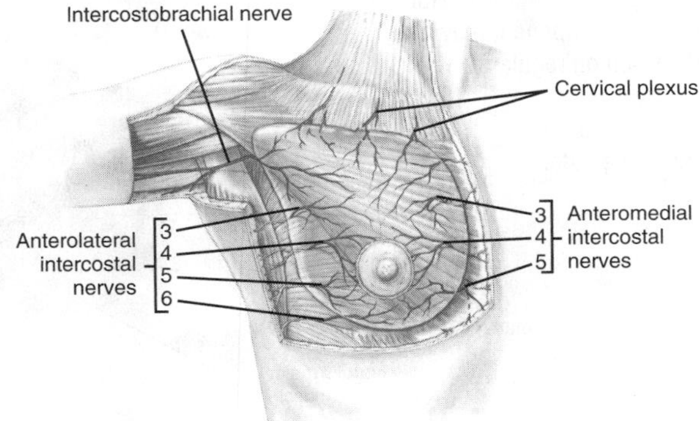


**Fig. 44-2** Innervation to breast.

## Anatomic Studies

- **Schlenz et al**[6]
  - 28 unilateral breast dissections in female cadavers
  - **Found consistent innervation of the NAC by the anterior and lateral cutaneous branches of the third through fifth intercostals nerves**
  - Lateral cutaneous branch (LCB) supplied innervation via posterior innervation of the nipple in 93%.
    - Fourth LCB provided posterior innervation in 93% of cases and was the only source 79% of the time.
  - Anterior cutaneous branch (ACB) had superficial course to supply medial aspect of NAC.
    - Third and fourth ACB combined to provide innervation in 57% of cases.
- **Würinger et al**[7,8] (Fig. 44-3)
  - 28 anatomic dissections and 14 arterial injection studies of female cadavers
  - Defined a "brassiere-like" connective tissue suspensory system
  - **Found neurovascular supply to the nipple runs along this well-defined suspensory apparatus**
    - Vertical ligaments originating from the pectoralis minor (laterally) and sternum (medially)
  - Define parenchymal borders and carries corresponding neurovascular structures
  - Horizontal septum originates from the pectoral fascia along the fifth rib; **Würinger's septum**
    - It merges with the lateral and medial vertical ligaments.
    - Breast parenchyma is bipartitioned as the septum runs anteriorly to the NAC.
    - Cranial aspect carries thoracoacromial and lateral thoracic arterial branches.
    - Caudal aspect carried branches of the fourth through sixth intercostals arteries.
    - Main contributory nerve to the nipple (LCB of fourth intercostals) was always found within septum.
- **O'Dey et al**[9]
  - Injection study of seven female cadavers with arterial distribution patterns mapped for 14 breasts
  - **Outlined four distinct arterial zones**
  - Largest territory supplied by branches of the internal mammary (zone 1) and lateral thoracic (zone 2)
  - Evaluated safety of eight different pedicles based on vascular reliability and regularity to the NAC
  - Concluded that pedicles with a lateral or medially based component may be safer strictly based on regularity of arterial anatomy
  - Study does not account for added safety with greater width.

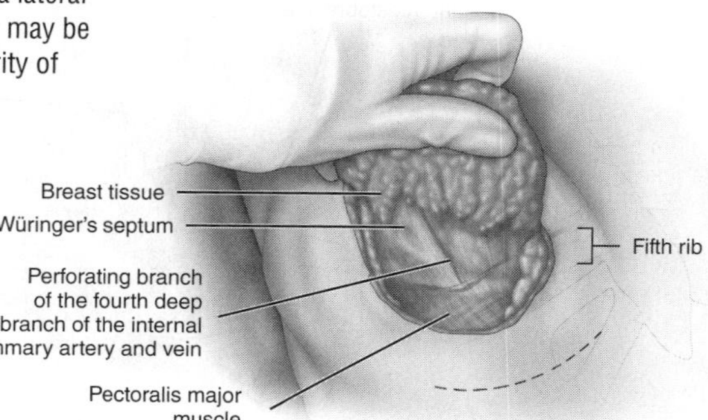


**Fig. 44-3** Würinger's septum.

## SKIN AND PARENCHYMA

- The adult breast extends from the second to the seventh rib in the midclavicular line, and medially from the sternocostal junction to the midaxillary line laterally.
- The inframammary fold (IMF) is the lower border of the breast and is a distinct anatomic structure that should be preserved whenever possible. **It represents fusion of the deep and superficial fascia with the dermis.** Distinct fibers crisscross, holding the skin in place (similar to the gluteal fold).[10]
- The adult breast also extends into the axilla, giving it a teardrop shape *(axillary tail of Spence).*
- The adult mammary gland is composed of multiple lobules that are connected and drained by 16 to 24 main lactiferous ducts.
- A **lobule** is the functional unit of the breast.
  - Lobules are situated in radial distribution (Fig. 44-4).
- Each lobule is composed of hundreds of **acini.**
  - Each acinus has secretory potential and is connected to lactiferous ducts by its own interlobular ducts.
- Each main lactiferous duct dilates as it approaches the nipple, forming a sinus *(lactiferous sinus* or *central collecting duct)* that functions as a reservoir for milk storage.
- Nipple contains orifices to drain each lactiferous duct; these may act as conduits for bacteria.
- **Morgagni's tubercles** are located near the periphery of the areola, which has elevations formed by openings of ducts of **Montgomery's glands.**
- **Montgomery's glands** are large sebaceous glands capable of secreting milk. They represent an intermediate stage between sweat and mammary glands and also act to lubricate the areola during lactation.
- Fat content varies but is responsible for most of the bulk, contour, softness, consistency, and shape of the breast.
- Fat content increases as glandular component subsides (e.g., after lactation or during menopause).
- The breast is supported by layers of **superficial fascia.**
  - **A layer of superficial fascia** is located near the dermis; it is difficult to distinguish unless patient is thin.
  - **A deep layer of superficial fascia** is present on the deep surface of the breast; a loose areolar plane exists between this layer and the deep fascial layer that overlies underlying musculature.
- **Cooper's ligaments** penetrate deep layer of superficial fascia into parenchyma breast to dermis; ptosis results from attenuation of these attachments.

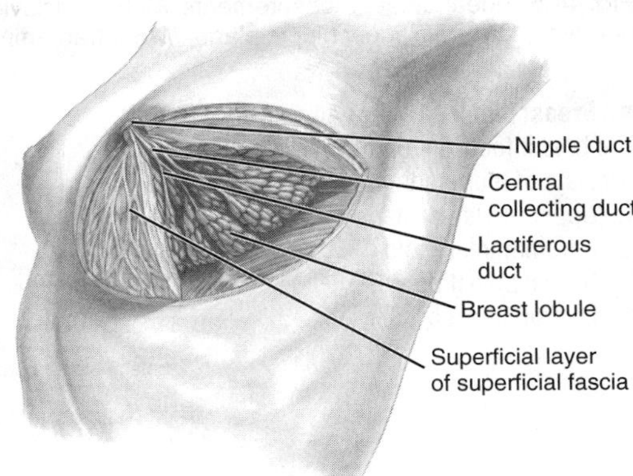


**Fig. 44-4** Lobules are situated in a radial distribution.

## BREAST SHAPE AND AESTHETICS[11] (Fig. 44-5)

- Less full above areola (upper pole) and fuller below (lower pole)
- Ideally in harmony with proportions of the chest, torso, and buttocks
- NAC: 19-21 cm from the sternal notch, 9-11 cm from midline, and 7-8 cm from IMF
- Medial cleavage: Function of medial origin of the pectoralis major and the medialmost extent of the breast parenchyma
- Ideally symmetrical in size, shape, volume, and ptosis
- Ptosis: Nipple position relative to IMF and breast parenchyma (see Chapter 46).

> **TIP:** Perfect symmetry is rare and should be noted and documented preoperatively.
>
> Women desiring full medial cleavage without bra support are often disappointed with aesthetic and reconstructive efforts. Preoperative counseling is helpful.

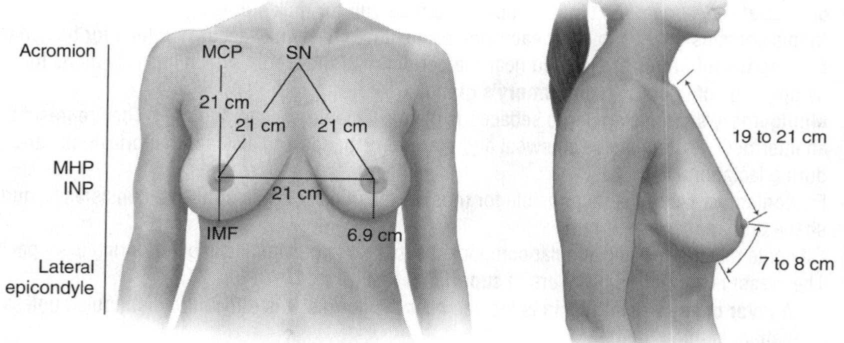


**Fig. 44-5** Ideal breast measurements. *MCP,* midclavicular point; *SN,* sternal notch; *MHP,* midhumeral plane; *INP,* ideal nipple plane; *IMF,* inframammary fold.

- **Breast footprint**[3] **(Fig. 44-6)**

The breast footprint on the chest wall consists of four landmarks

1. Upper breast border
2. Inframammary fold
3. Medial breast border
4. Lateral breast border

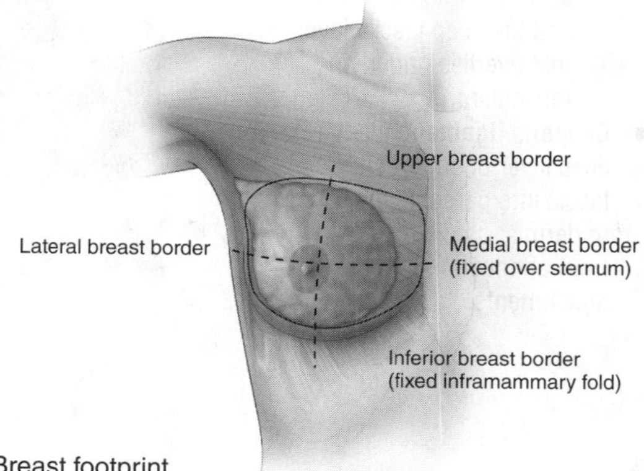


**Fig. 44-6** Breast footprint.

## UNDERLYING MUSCULATURE[11,12] (Fig. 44-7)

### Pectoralis Major

- **Origin:** Medial clavicle, sternum, anterior ribs (second to sixth), external oblique, rectus abdominis fascia
- **Insertion:** Upper humerus, 10 cm from humeral head on lateral side of intertubercular sulcus
- **Function:** Adduction and medial rotation of arm
- **Blood supply:** Internal mammary perforators, thoracoacromial artery, intercostal perforators, lateral thoracic artery
- **Innervation:** Medial (sternal portion) and lateral (clavicular portion) pectoral nerves *(named for origin in brachial plexus cord)*
- Upper medial portion of breast located over pectoralis major

**TIP:** Absence of sternal head of pectoralis major is seen in Poland's syndrome.

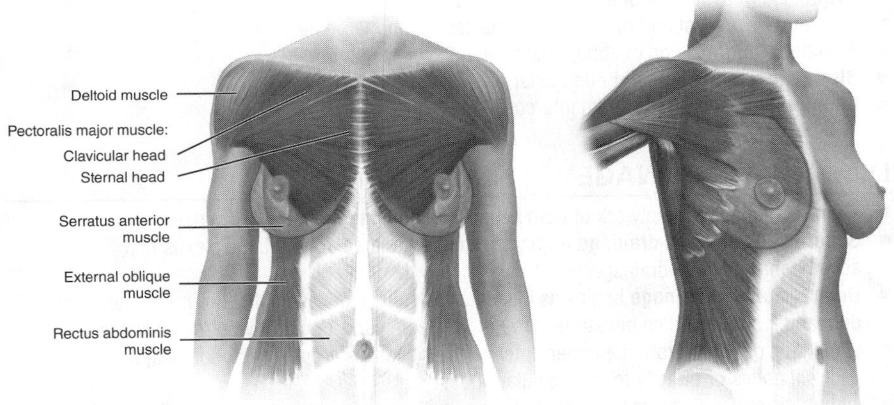


**Fig. 44-7** Underlying musculature.

### Pectoralis Minor

- **Origin:** Anterolateral surfaces of third to sixth ribs
- **Insertion:** Coracoid process of scapula
- **Function:** Draws scapula down and forward
- **Blood supply:** Pectoral branch of thoracoacromial artery, lateral thoracic artery, direct branch of axillary artery
- **Innervation:** Medial pectoral nerve

**TIP:** The pectoralis minor serves as a landmark during axillary dissection, because the lateral margin divides the superficial from the deep axillary nodes.

### Serratus Anterior

- **Origin:** Anterolateral aspects of upper eight ribs
- **Insertion:** Anterior surface of medial aspect of scapula
- **Function:** Stabilizes scapula against chest wall during abduction and elevation of arm in horizontal direction; also pulls scapula forward and laterally
- **Blood supply:** Lateral thoracic artery, branches of thoracodorsal artery
- **Innervation:** Long thoracic nerve

### Rectus Abdominis

- **Origin:** Pubic line
- **Insertion:** Third to seventh costal cartilages
- **Function:** Flexes the vertebral column and tenses abdominal wall
- **Blood supply:** Superior and inferior epigastric artery and vein, subcostal and intercostal perforators
- **Innervation:** Segmental motor nerves from seventh to twelfth intercostal nerves

### External Oblique

- **Origin:** External surface of lower anterior and lateral ribs
- **Insertion:** Iliac crest and medial abdominal fascial aponeurosis
- **Function:** Compression of abdominal contents
- **Blood supply:** Inferior eight intercostal arteries
- **Innervation:** Seventh to twelfth intercostal nerves

## LYMPHATIC DRAINAGE[13]

- There is an extensive network of both **superficial** and **deep** lymphatic drainage.
- **Superficial lymphatic drainage** originates from a periareolar lymphatic plexus that accompanies venous drainage.
- **Deep lymphatic drainage** begins as individual lymphatic channels that drain each lactiferous duct and lobule and then penetrate through the deep fascia of underlying musculature.
- Lymphatic drainage from the upper outer quadrant passes around pectoralis major to deep pectoral nodes or directly to subscapular nodes.
- Lymphatic efferent of breast travels to central axillary nodes, then to apical axillary nodes and to supraclavicular nodes.
- Medial lymphatic channels follow internal mammary perforating vessels and drain to parasternal nodes.
- **Most of breast drains into axillary nodes, with three levels identified.**
  - **Level I:** Lateral to lateral border of pectoralis minor
  - **Level II:** Behind pectoralis minor and below axillary vein
  - **Level III:** Medial to medial border of pectoralis minor
- **Rotter's nodes** are between pectoralis major and minor.

## Key Points

- ✓ The NAC is innervated by the anterolateral branch of the fourth intercostal nerve.
- ✓ Supernumerary nipples and breasts can occur anywhere along the milk line from the axilla to the groin.
- ✓ Attenuation of Cooper's ligaments leads to ptosis and increased breast mobility.
- ✓ The IMF is an important structure to preserve. Violation can be difficult to correct.
- ✓ Injury to the intercostobrachial nerve results in paresthesias or anesthesia of the upper medial arm.
- ✓ Perfect symmetry is rare.
- ✓ Medial cleavage is difficult to create if it does not exist in the native breast.
- ✓ Three levels of axillary lymph nodes exist.
- ✓ Poland's syndrome results in the absence of sternal head of pectoralis major.

## References

1. Bostwick J III. Anatomy and physiology. In Bostwick J III, ed. Plastic and Reconstructive Breast Surgery, vol 1, 3rd ed. St Louis: Quality Medical Publishing, 2010.
2. Tanner JM, ed. Growth at Adolescence, 2nd ed. Oxford: Blackwell Scientific, 1978.
3. Hall-Findlay EJ, ed. Aesthetic Breast Surgery: Concepts & Techniques. St Louis: Quality Medical Publishing, 2011.
4. Hanna MK, Nahai F. Applied anatomy of the breast. In Nahai F, ed. Art of Aesthetic Surgery: Principles and Techniques, vol 3, 2nd ed. St Louis: Quality Medical Publishing, 2011.
5. August DA, Sondak VK. Breast. In Greenfield LJ, Mulholland MW, Oldham KT, et al, eds. Surgery: Scientific Principles and Practice, 2nd ed. Philadelphia: Lippincott-Raven, 1997.
6. Schlenz I, Kuzbari R, Gruber H, et al. The sensitivity of the nipple-areola complex: an anatomic study. Plast Reconstr Surg 105:905-909, 2000.
7. Würinger E, Mader N, Posch E, et al. Nerve and vessel supplying ligamentous suspension of the mammary gland. Plast Reconstr Surg 101:1486-1493, 1998.
8. Wueringer E, Tschabitscher M. New aspects of the topographical anatomy of the mammary gland regarding its neurovascular supply along a regular ligamentous suspension. Eur J Morphol 40:181-189, 2002.
9. O'Dey DM, Prescher A, Pallua N. Vascular reliability of nipple-areola complex-bearing pedicles: an anatomical microdissection study. Plast Reconstr Surg 119:1167-1177, 2007.
10. Muntan CD, Sundine MJ, Rink RD, et al. Inframammary fold: a histologic reappraisal. Plast Reconstr Surg 105:549-556; discussion 557, 2000.
11. Jones G, ed. Bostwick's Plastic and Reconstructive Breast Surgery, 3rd ed. St Louis: Quality Medical Publishing, 2010.
12. Mathes SJ, Nahai F, eds. Reconstructive Surgery: Principles, Anatomy, & Technique, vols 1 and 2. St Louis: Quality Medical Publishing, 1997.
13. Haagensen CD, ed. Diseases of the Breast, 3rd ed. Philadelphia: WB Saunders, 1986.

# 45. Breast Augmentation

Jacob G. Unger, Thornwell Hay Parker III, Michael E. Decherd

## BACKGROUND/HISTORY

- Breast augmentation is the second most common cosmetic surgery (after liposuction), with nearly 300,000 performed in 2010.[1]
- Czerny[2] performed the first breast augmentation in 1895 with a lipoma.
- Through the early 1900s multiple injectables were used for augmentation, often with disastrous results.[3-5]
- Cronin and Gerow created the first silicone implant in 1961 with the Dow Corning Corporation.
  - Introduced in 1964 as a silicone envelope with a thick liquid silicone within and a Dacron patch
  - Considered the **first generation** silicone implant[6]
- Saline implants were introduced in the 1970s as an alternative to silicone.
- In 1992 the U.S. Food and Drug Administration (FDA) placed a moratorium on silicone implants for primary augmentation because of concerns about autoimmune and connective tissue disease.
  - In 1999 the **NIH Institute of Medicine and the National Academy of Sciences reviewed 17 epidemiologic studies and were unable to detect any link between silicone and systemic, autoimmune, or prenatal disease.**
  - Studies found silicone in local macrophages, lymph nodes, and breast tissue.
  - Studies did **not** demonstrate elevated systemic levels (normal liver, lung, and spleen).[7]
- Silicone implants have evolved through different generations.[8]
  - **First:** Thick shell and thick filler
  - **Second:** Thin shell and thin filler—less palpable, but higher rupture rate
  - **Third:** Thick reinforced shells, thick gel
  - **Fourth:** Refined, thinner shells and higher-quality gels (currently used)
  - **Fifth:** Cohesive gel form-stable devices
- U.S. FDA lifted moratorium on silicone implants for general use (aesthetic augmentation) in 2006 based on multiple meta-analyses.[9-11]
- Silicone implants are currently approved in the United States for:
  - Breast reconstruction
  - Breast augmentation in patients over 22 years of age[8] (Table 45-1)

**Table 45-1** *Generations of Silicone Gel–Filled Breast Implants*

| Implant Generation | Production Period | Characteristics |
|---|---|---|
| First | 1960s | Thick shell (0.25 mm average)<br>Thick viscous gel<br>Dacron patch |
| Second | 1970s | Thin shell (0.13 mm average)<br>Less viscous gel<br>No patch |
| Third | 1980s | Thick, silica-reinforced barrier coats shells |
| Fourth | 1992-present | Stricter manufacturing standards<br>Refined third-generation devices |
| Fifth | 1993-present | Cohesive silicone gel–filled devices<br>Form-stable devices |

## INDICATIONS[12]

- Enhance breast shape and volume
- Improve body image, symmetry, and balance
- Help clothes fit better
- Provide the appearance of a breast lift and increased cleavage
- Rejuvenation after postpartum deflation

## CONTRAINDICATIONS

- Body dysmorphic disorder
- Psychological instability
- Responding to peer, spousal, or parental pressure
- Attempting to salvage marriage or relationship, or to find husband
- Patient <18 years old
- Significant breast disease (severe fibrocystic disease, ductal hyperplasia, high-risk breast cancer)
- Collagen vascular disease

## PATIENT EVALUATION

### MEDICAL HISTORY

- Personal history of breast disease or cancer
- Family history of breast disease or cancer
- Pregnancy history: Breast size before, during, and after; plans for future children
- Mammography
  - Screening mammogram by age 35 years, if planning to operate on breast
- Current breast size
- Desired breast size

### PHYSICAL EXAMINATION

- **Cancer screening:** Masses, dimpling, discharge, and lymph nodes
- **Skin quality**
  - Tone
  - Elasticity
  - Striae

- **Asymmetries:** Chest wall, scoliosis, and breast
  - Difference in breast volume
  - Difference in inframammary fold (IMF) height
  - Difference in nipple-areola complex (NAC) height
- **Ptosis** (see Chapter 46)
  - Mild ptosis is improved by augmentation.
  - Moderate to severe ptosis may require mastopexy.
- **Measurements** (patient sitting up straight)
  - Height, weight, body frame (small to large)
  - Sternal notch to nipple distance (SN-N)
  - Nipple to IMF distance (N-IMF) during stretch
  - Base width (width of breast base)
  - Parenchymal coverage (pinch test)
    - Superior pole
    - Lower pole
  - Anterior pull skin stretch (centimeters of stretch from resting to maximal projection with pull at edge of areola)
  - Parenchymal fill (percentage of skin envelope filled by parenchyma)[13]

## IMPLANT CHOICE

### VOLUME

- **Patient preference**
  - Sizers placed in bra to establish desired volume (not recommended)
  - Photos of other women may help to establish shape and contour desires and unify the surgeon's and patient's expectations.
  - Digital imaging: Three-dimensional imaging is gaining popularity as ease of use and surgeon familiarity increase. This may be the best tool to align expectations of surgeon and patient.[14]

**CAUTION: The above-mentioned criteria do not guarantee postoperative results. This should be explicitly stated and documented.**

- **Surgeon's experience**
  - 125-150 ml to increase by one cup size
  - Larger body frames require larger implant volumes to increase cup size
- **Breast analysis**
  - **High five system**[13]
    - Objective measures to determine optimal implant and volume
    - Volume based on breast base width
    - Add or subtract volume based on skin stretch, breast envelope fill, and N-IMF.
    - Proven system with excellent reported results and low complication and reoperation rate
- **Intraoperative breast sizers**
- **Pitfalls of large implant volume**
  - Using an implant that is too large for the breast envelope will cause irreversible damage to the surrounding parenchyma.
  - Atrophy and thinning of both parenchyma and skin will occur.
  - Increased palpability may result.
  - Traction rippling occurs over time, especially laterally and inferiorly.

**TIP:** To create a long-lasting result, harmony between patient desires and what the tissue characteristics and envelope will allow is essential.

## Filler Types

- **Saline**
  - **Advantages**
    - Adjusts quickly to body core temperature
    - Leaks are safely absorbed by body
    - Easier to adjust for size and correct breast asymmetry
  - **Disadvantages**
    - Wrinkling
    - Leaks lead to complete deflation
    - Less natural feel
- **Silicone**
  - **Advantage**
    - More natural feel than saline
  - **Disadvantages**
    - Slow to adjust to body core temperature (e.g., implants remain cold after swimming)
    - Rupture may cause local inflammation and granulomas
  - **Construction**
    - Silicone shell with silicone filler
    - Silicone: Polymer of dimethylsiloxane; longer chains lead to increased viscosity

## Surface

- **Textured**
  - **Advantages**
    - Lower contracture rates in a subglandular plane (surface disorients collagen deposition)[15-17]
    - Less migration and implant rotation
    - Submuscular pocket placement likely equilibrates contracture risk between smooth and textured[16]
  - **Disadvantages**
    - Thicker shells
    - More palpable
    - Traction rippling
  - **Technique**
    - Intraoperative positioning of implant is critical, because textured surface resists migration or movement in pocket; base must be properly oriented along IMF.
- **Smooth**
  - **Advantages**
    - Thinner capsule formed
    - Less palpable: Preferable for patients with thin coverage
  - **Disadvantage**
    - Slightly higher contracture rates (especially in subglandular pocket)[17]

- **Polyurethane (PU)-covered (no longer available)**
  - **Advantage**
    - Dramatically low contracture rates (<1% over 10 years)
  - **Disadvantage**
    - Pulled from U.S. market because PU breaks down as a carcinogenic compound (although levels likely insignificant)
  - **Construction**
    - PU coating separates over weeks to months and becomes incorporated into the capsule, helping to disperse contractile forces.

**NOTE: Textured implants were developed to mimic the effect of PU on the capsule.**

### DIMENSION/SHAPE

- **Round (circular implant): Most commonly used in United States**
  - Low-profile
  - Moderate-profile
  - Moderate-plus-profile
  - High-profile
    - Increased projection for given base width at each level of projection
    - Increased volume for given base width
- **Anatomic (implant height different from width)**
  - Designed to give more natural breast shape
  - Increased implant height and projection for a given base width
  - Upper pole tapered; fuller lower pole, reducing upper pole collapse and filling lower pole of breast
  - Disadvantage: Must be oriented properly and symmetrically
  - Most textured to maintain position

**NOTE: Anatomic implants have regained national interest with the advent of commercially available "form-stable" implants that maintain their shape once placed with a breast pocket. Form-stable implants offer the advantage over cohesive gel of not drastically changing shape when the patient stands. Upper pole fill is maintained regardless of gravity or compressive forces. Gel implants augment and conform to the existing soft tissue envelope, whereas form-stable, shaped implants force the soft tissue envelope to conform around the implant's shape.**

## INCISION CHOICE[18] (Table 45-2)

### INFRAMAMMARY FOLD

- **Advantages**
  - Well hidden with mild ptosis or well-defined IMF
  - Best control of pocket development
  - Can avoid contact with breast ducts, which are colonized by bacteria, theoretically reducing the risk of biofilm formation and capsular contracture
- **Disadvantage**
  - Visible scar on breast (if not planned properly)
- **Technique**
  - Place incision at planned new IMF location, which may be lower than the preoperative IMF.
  - The new, postoperative IMF is best determined using the high five system.[13]
  - Keep most of the incision lateral to nipple, because it is more visible when placed medially.

**TIP:** This incision is commonly 5 cm in length for placement of silicone implants. By creating a line along the breast meridian the surgeon can place the incision along the IMF, drawn from 1 cm medial to the meridian, to 4 cm lateral. This is a safe way to place the incision in the appropriate location.

**Table 45-2** *Incision Options for Breast Augmentation*

| Factor | Axillary | Periareolar | Inframammary | Transumbilical* |
|---|---|---|---|---|
| **Implant Plane** | | | | |
| Submuscular | + | + | + | – |
| Subglandular | – | + | + | + |
| **Implant Type** | | | | |
| Saline, round | + | + | + | + |
| Saline, shaped | – | + | + | – |
| Silicone, round or shaped | – | + | + | – |
| **Preoperative Breast Volume** | | | | |
| High (>200 g) | + | + | + | + |
| Low (<200 g) | + | + | – | + |
| **Preoperative Breast Base Position** | | | | |
| High | + | + | + | + |
| Low | – | + | + | + |
| **Breast Shape** | | | | |
| Tubular | – | + | – | – |
| Glandular ptosis | + | + | + | + |
| Ptosis (grades I and II) | – | + | – | – |
| **Areolar Characteristics** | | | | |
| Small diameter | + | – | + | + |
| Light or indistinct | + | – | + | + |
| **Inframammary Fold** | | | | |
| None | + | + | – | + |
| High | + | + | – | + |
| Low | + | + | + | + |
| **Secondary Procedure** | – | + | + | – |

*Included for completeness, but generally not recommended.
+, Applicable; –, not generally recommended.

## PERIAREOLAR

- **Advantages**
  - Well hidden at interface of NAC and skin
  - Good access if diameter of areola >3.5 cm
  - No decreased nipple sensation compared with IMF technique[19]
- **Disadvantages**
  - May traverse and scar a cancer-prone organ
  - White or hypopigmented scar when placed within areola
  - Potential for visible scarring, especially risky if patient prone to hypertrophic scarring
  - Contamination theory suggests possible increased rate of capsular contracture from ductal bacteria.[20-22]
- **Technique**
  - Place around the lower half of the areola within areolar fade or at the junction of the areola and breast skin.
    - **Create a stair-step dissection**
      - Cut through skin and dissect inferiorly, following the subcutaneous plane to the inferior edge of the breast mound, then create a pocket.
      - This technique is preferred, because less parenchyma is disrupted and layered closure allows a discontinuous tract from the skin to the implant.

## TRANSAXILLARY

- **Advantages**
  - No breast scar
- **Disadvantages**
  - Potential scar visibility when sleeveless and raising arms
  - Difficult to insert silicone implants
- **Technique**
  - Although a blind procedure in the early 70s, now significantly advanced by endoscopic technique[23,24]
  - Make 2-3 cm horizontal incision at highest point of axilla, 1 cm behind border of pectoralis. Dissect medially in superficial subcutaneous plane, and continue to posterolateral border of pectoralis, incising vertically to enter subpectoral or subglandular plane.

> **TIP:** Avoid deep dissection in axilla; intercostobrachial and median brachial cutaneous nerves are vulnerable.

## TRANSUMBILICAL

- **Advantages**
  - Scar hidden and distant from breast
- **Disadvantages**
  - Difficult, blind dissection
  - High or asymmetrical placement
  - Difficult to make adjustments or corrections
  - Can only use saline implants
- **Technique**
  - **Blind dissection** from superior umbilical incision through inferomedial breast; expander or implant sizer inflated to create pocket, then replaced with permanent implant

## POCKET PLANE AND DISSECTION (Fig. 45-1)

### SUBGLANDULAR

- **Advantages**
  - Good projection and shape
  - Prevents distortion in muscular or active patients
- **Disadvantages**
  - Higher contracture rate[16,17]
  - Implant edges may be palpable
  - Interference with mammography[25]
- **Contraindication:** Thin parenchymal coverage (upper pole pinch test <2 cm)
- **Technique**
  - Dissection on top of pectoralis major, below gland

### SUBPECTORAL

- **Advantages**
  - Lower contracture rates[16,17]
  - Thick soft tissue coverage
  - Good preservation of nipple sensation
- **Disadvantages**
  - "Dancing breasts" during pectoralis contraction (animation deformity)
  - Lateral displacement of implant over time
  - Difficult to control upper pole fill
- **Relative contraindication**
  - Muscular or active patient
- **Technique**
  - Dissection below pectoralis major but above pectoralis minor
  - Does not disrupt inferior attachments of pectoralis if "total subpectoral" (rarely performed unless the patient has extremely thin lower pole coverage)

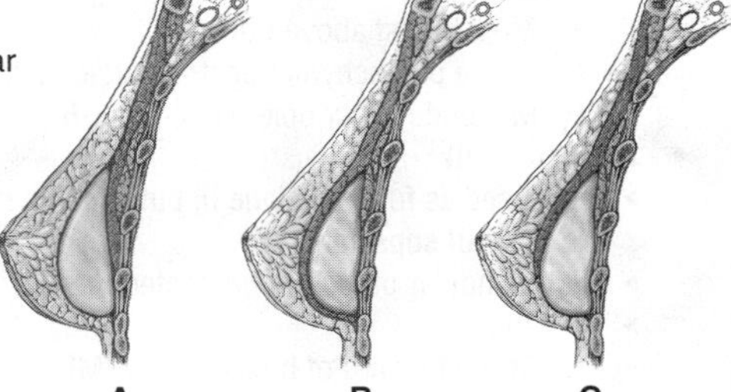


**Fig. 45-1** Implant location. **A,** Subglandular augmentation. **B,** Completely submuscular augmentation. **C,** Biplanar augmentation.

### BIPLANAR (DUAL PLANE)[26]

- **Advantages**
  - Subpectoral coverage of upper pole
    - Thick soft tissue coverage
    - Low contracture rate
  - Less implant displacement at rest and during pectoralis contraction
  - Allows implant to be positioned along IMF
  - Increases implant-parenchymal interface, which expands lower pole and prevents double-bubble deformity
  - Allows nipple to lie at the most projecting part of implant

- **Disadvantage**
  - Usually restricted to IMF incision when performing dual plane II and III
- **Contraindication**
  - IMF pinch test <0.4 cm: Requires complete retromuscular pocket placement
- **Rationale**
  - Complete muscle coverage restricts expansion of inferior pole, forcing implant superiorly and laterally.
  - Especially with ptotic and loose breast parenchyma, breast tissue may slide inferior to the axis of the implant while implant remains fixed higher on the chest wall, causing a type A double-bubble deformity **(Waterfall deformity).**
  - The inferior pectoralis attachments are released, and some superior pectoralis retraction occurs. This maximizes implant contact with lower pole breast parenchyma, with the advantage of upper pole coverage by the pectoralis. Further, releasing some attachments between the parenchyma and pectoralis allows the parenchyma to stretch and glide over the implant to be centered over the point of maximal projection.

> **TIP:** Do not release the sternal attachments of the pectoralis, because this will cause window-shading and decrease implant coverage.

- **Types** (Fig. 45-2)
  - **Dual plane I**[26]
    - Pectoralis released along IMF in addition to subpectoral dissection
    - Used for most typical breasts
    - Criteria
      - All breast above IMF (no ptosis)
      - Tight attachment of parenchyma to pectoralis
      - Minimally stretched lower pole (4-6 cm from NAC to IMF)
  - **Dual plane II**[26]
    - In addition to pectoralis release along IMF and subpectoral dissection, the pectoralis is separated from breast parenchyma **to level of inferior NAC.**
    - Criteria
      - Most breast above IMF
      - Loose parenchymal-pectoral attachments
      - Moderate lower pole stretch (5.5-6.5 cm from NAC to IMF)
  - **Dual plane III**[26]
    - Released as for dual plane II, but separation of pectoralis from parenchyma is continued **to level of superior NAC**
    - For glandular ptotic or constricted breasts
    - Criteria
      - At least a third of breast below IMF
      - Very loose parenchymal-pectoral attachments
      - Marked lower pole stretch (7-8 cm from NAC to IMF)
      - Can be used for grade 1 or mild grade 2 ptosis
      - Lower pole constricted
    - Constricted breast
      - Use radial and concentric scoring through breast parenchyma.

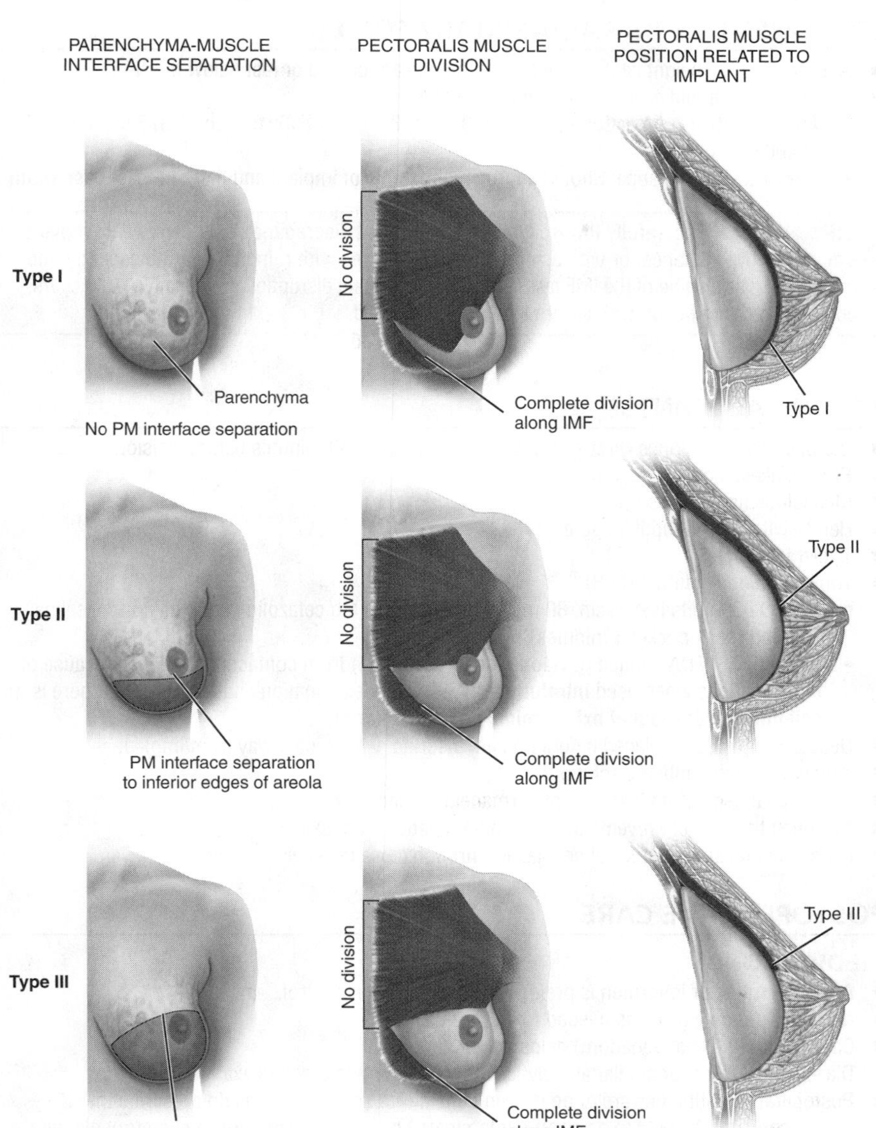


**Fig. 45-2** Dual plane augmentation techniques. The extent of dissection at the parenchyma-muscle interface *(left),* the position of the inferior edge of the divided pectoralis origins *(center),* and the pectoralis position relative to the implant *(right)* are shown. (*PM,* Parenchyma-muscle.)

## TREATMENT OF INFRAMAMMARY FOLD

- Appropriate IMF height centers the axis of the implant behind or just below the NAC.
- N-IMF length should correspond to implant volume.
  - Approximately 7 cm at 250 cc, 8 cm at 300 cc, 8.5 cm at 350 cc, 9 cm at 375 cc, 9.5 cm at 400 cc[13]
  - Areola-to-IMF distance: Should approximate radius of implant and half of breast base width

> **TIP:** IMF can be carefully lowered when a significant discrepancy exists between implant size and N-IMF distance, or with asymmetry. This is done with minimal sharp dissection and mostly blunt stretching of the IMF fascial planes. If complete disruption of the native IMF occurs, complete reconstruction with suture technique is needed.

## TECHNICAL POINTS[27]

- Perioperative antibiotics (first-generation cephalosporin 30 minutes before incision)
- Precise dissection
- Meticulous hemostasis
- Hand-switched monopolar cautery
- Talc-free gloves
- Triple antibiotic solution (TAB)[20]
  - Mix 50,000 units bacitracin, 80 mg gentamicin, and 1 g cefazolin in 500 cc normal saline solution (soak pocket 5 minutes).
  - In 2000 U.S. FDA banned povidone-iodine (Betadine) from contacting implants because of complications when used **intraluminally** (implant delamination and leakage), but there is **no scientific evidence that extraluminal contact is harmful.**
- Deep closing sutures placed before implant inserted, with knots away from implant
- Skin wiped with antibiotic solution
- Gloves changed before insertion of permanent implant
- No-touch technique: Prevents implant contamination from skin[28]
- For saline implants, sterile saline injected through closed system

## POSTOPERATIVE CARE

### Medications

- Acetaminophen or ibuprofen is preferred for routine pain control.
- Narcotics are only given as needed for severe pain.
- Carisoprodol (Soma, Vanadom) helps pectoralis relax.
- Diazepam (Valium) or similar anxiolytics are useful for pectoralis relaxation.
- Postoperative antibiotics are of no proven benefit, but some surgeons do prescribe them. (Some consider the field to be clean-contaminated by bacteria from breast secretory glands.)

### Brassiere and Dressing

- Steri-Strips, Dermabond, or Prineo System (Ethicon, Cincinnati, OH) for 2 weeks, or until it falls off
- Brassiere optional; no underwire or push-up bras for 6 weeks

### Activity

- Implant displacement exercises
  - Push implant medially and superiorly

- Begin postoperative day 3 or when not painful for patient
- Ten pushes, three times a day for 1 month, then once daily
- Aerobic exercise after 2 weeks
- Heavy lifting after 6 weeks

## COMPLICATIONS AND CONSENT

### CAPSULAR CONTRACTURE

The body naturally forms capsules around all implants. *Capsular contracture* is capsular tightening and compression that distort the implant.

- **Baker classification system**
  - I: **Normal,** soft, nonpalpable implant
  - II: **Palpable,** minimally firm to touch, not visible
  - III: **Visible,** easily palpated, and moderately firm
  - IV: **Painful,** hard, and breast distorted
- **Etiologic factors**
  - Subclinical infection[21,29-32]
    - Correlation well established, but causal relationship uncertain
    - *Staphylococcus epidermidis* most common, but many other types of bacteria implicated
  - Hypertrophic scar/inflammatory process hypothesis
    - Talc and operative towel fibers have been found within histologic studies of capsules.[33]
    - Foreign body reaction is thought to be a possible cause.[34]
- **Time course**
  - Most contractures occur within 1 year.
  - Late occurrence may be secondary to systemic bacterial seeding or capsular maturation.
- **Historical rates and risk factors BEFORE 1992 FDA ban**
  - **Pocket location**[34]
    - Subglandular: 32% contracture rate
    - Subpectoral: 12% contracture rate
  - **Filler**[35]
    - Silicone: 50% contracture rate
    - Saline: 16% contracture rate
  - **Implant surface**[15,36] (Fig. 45-3)
    - Smooth: 58% contracture rate
    - Textured: 11% contracture rate

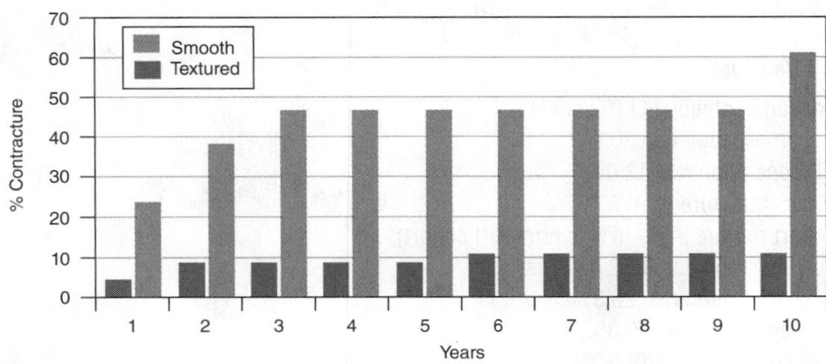


**Fig. 45-3** Ten-year development of subglandular capsular contracture in smooth versus textured implants.

- **Current data AFTER FDA reinstatement 2006[37] (Boxes 45-1 and 45-2)**
  - With significantly lower contracture rates, data have shown less correlation between implant texture, filler, or pocket choice.
  - Saline trial: 2001, Mentor Corporation (Santa Barbara, CA)[38]
    - 9% contracture rate with primary augmentation
    - 30% contracture rate with reconstruction
  - Saline trial: 2001, Inamed (Allergan) Corporation (Irvine, CA)[39]
    - 9% contracture rate with primary augmentation
    - 25% contracture rate with reconstruction
  - Silicone gel premarket approval trial: Mentor 2006, Allergan (previously Inamed) 2006, Sientra (Santa Barbara, CA) 2012[40]

**Box 45-1** *2006 Data by Manufacturer*

**Mentor (3-Year Data)**

- Primary augmentation (551 patients)
- Overall complication rate 36.6%
- Overall reoperation rate 15.4%
- Capsular contracture III/IV 8.1%
- MRI cohort rupture 0.5% (0% in non-MRI cohort)
- Revision augmentation (146 patients)
- Overall complication rate 50%
- Overall reoperation rate 28%
- Capsular contracture III/IV 18.9%
- MRI cohort rupture 7.7% (0% in non-MRI cohort)

**Allergan (4-Year Data)**

- Primary augmentation (455 patients)
- Overall complication rate 41.3%
- Overall reoperation rate 23.5%
- Capsular contracture III/IV 13.2%
- MRI cohort rupture 2.7% (0.4% in non-MRI cohort)
- Revision augmentation (147 patients)
- Overall complication rate 56.9%
- Overall reoperation rate 35.3%
- Capsular contracture III/IV 17.0%
- MRI cohort rupture 7.7% (0% in non-MRI cohort)

**Sientra (3-Year Data)**

- Primary augmentation (1115 patients)
- Overall complication rate 20.2%
- Overall reoperation rate 12.6%
- Capsular contracture III/IV 6.0%
- MRI cohort rupture 2.5% (0% in non-MRI cohort)
- Revision augmentation (362 patients)
- Overall complication rate 26.3%
- Overall reoperation rate 20.3%
- Capsular contracture III/IV 5.2%
- MRI cohort rupture 0% (0.4% in non-MRI cohort)

**Box 45-2** *FDA UPDATE 2011 DATA*

**Mentor Core Study (8-Year Data)**

- Large study (2007-2009) data (3-year follow-up)
- 41,900 patients silicone, 1030 saline
- Primary augmentation rupture rate 10.1%
- Revision augmentation rupture rate 6.3%
- Reoperation rate primary augmentation 10.8%
- Reoperation rate revision augmentation 14.6%
- Rupture rate primary augmentation 0.2%
- Rupture rate revision augmentation 1.0%
- Capsular contracture III/IV primary augmentation 5.3%
- Capsular contracture III/IV revision augmentation 11.8%

**Allergan Core Study (10-Year Data)**

- Large study (2007-2010) data (2-year follow-up)
- 41,342 patients silicone, 15,646 saline
- Primary augmentation rupture rate 13.6%
- Revision augmentation rupture rate 15.5%
- Reoperation: 6.5% silicone augmentation; 4.5% saline augmentation
- Rupture silicone 0.5%
- Saline deflation 2.5%
- Capsular contracture III/IV: 5.0% silicone; 2.8% saline

- **Treatment**
  - **Capsulectomy versus capsulotomy**
    - **Indications**[41]
      - Baker III or IV classification
      - Calcified or thick capsule
      - Ruptured silicone implant
      - Silicone granulomas
      - Infection around implant
      - Polyurethane implant
      - Previous implant needs to be replaced with larger-volume implant.
      - New plane needed (e.g., subglandular changes to subpectoral)
      - If primary plane was subpectoral, a **neosubpectoral pocket** may be used.[42,43]
        - This allows creation of a new pocket posterior to the muscle for control of pocket size and minimal trauma.
    - **Advantages**
      - Low contracture recurrence
      - Removal of potential contaminants
    - **Disadvantages**
      - Hemostasis more difficult
      - Anteriorly: Thins soft tissue coverage
      - Posteriorly: Risk of pneumothorax (if previous subpectoral implant)

- **Technique**
  - Subglandular plane: Complete capsulectomy is preferred in the subglandular plane, but caution is needed anteriorly with thin soft tissue coverage.
  - Subpectoral/dual plane: Anterior capsulectomy alone and posterior scoring or curettage; posterior capsule densely adherent to chest wall; risk of entering chest cavity

**CAUTION: Posterior capsulectomy in subpectoral or dual plane augmentations should be approached with extreme caution and only performed if required for calcifications or gross silicone contamination. Curettage of the posterior capsule creates a rough surface to facilitate adherence of the potential space and is often adequate.**

- **Open capsulotomy**
  - Controlled scoring through capsule, concentric and radial
  - 37%-89% recurrence
- **Closed capsulotomy**
  - Manual external compression in an attempt to break capsule
  - **Not recommended** because of risk of implant rupture and bleeding
  - 31%-80% recurrence
- **Breast massage and displacement exercises**
- **Exercise** (early, <2 weeks postoperatively)
  - This is a preventative measure that is commonly employed.
- **Pharmacotherapy**
  - Leukotriene inhibitors (e.g., montelukast [Singulair]): Some effect on prevention and improvement of contracture[44]

**CAUTION: Montelukast has been associated with rare liver toxicity.**

  - Papaverine hydrochloride (Pavabid)
  - Oral vitamin E
  - Intraluminal steroids: Reduced contracture but higher rate of implant rupture, skin erosion, atrophy, and ptosis; not recommended
  - Cyclosporine (Neoral, Sandimmune), mitomycin C (Mutamycin)

## Leakage or Rupture

- **Historical rupture rates**
  - Saline: 1% per year
  - Silicone[36]
    - 30% at 5 years
    - 50% at 10 years
    - 70% at 17 years
    - Current rupture rates as detailed above by newer studies
    - **Essentially both silicone and saline implants rupture at approximately 1% per year with fourth- and fifth-generation implants.**
- **Etiologic factors**
  - Fold flaw
  - Underfilling
  - Manufacturing flaws
  - Technical errors
  - Higher problem rates with thin-shell implants (second generation)

- **Diagnosis**
  - Examination
    - Asymmetry
    - Obvious deflation (less obvious with silicone)
  - Radiographs
    - Mammogram
      - Low sensitivity
      - Moderate specificity
      - Expense low
    - Ultrasound
      - Findings: Snowstorm, stepladder appearance
      - Moderate sensitivity
      - Moderate specificity
      - Expense moderate
    - MRI
      - Findings: **Linguine sign: sina qua non for intracapsular rupture**
      - High sensitivity
      - High specificity
      - Expense high
- **Treatment**
  - Treat as soon as possible to prevent further distortion of the deflated breast, contraction of the capsules, and local inflammation and granulomas from silicone leakage.
  - Remove implant and residual implant material.
  - Perform capsulotomy and capsulectomy as needed.
  - Implant may require replacement.

## Capsular Calcification[45]

- Related to implant age
- 0% occurrence for implants <10 years old
- 100% occurrence for implants >23 years old
- Remove by capsulectomy

## Nipple Sensation

- Permanent sensory change: 15% of patients

## Hematoma

- Rare: 0.5% of patients

## Clinical Infection of Implant

- Rare: <1% of patients
- Usually requires implant removal

## Asymmetry

- Almost universal
- Need to set levels of expectation with patient preoperatively

## Migration and Tissue Changes

- Bottoming out
  - Increased N-IMF distance, greater than half of base width
  - Related to poor tissue characteristics, large implant size, and overdissection of IMF
- Double-bubble deformity *type **A*** (waterfall deformity)
  - *Implant is **A**bove* breast mound.
  - Implant is held high on chest wall by total pectoral coverage or contracture, and loose parenchyma slides off pectoral muscles inferior to axis of the implant.
  - The dual plane approach helps to prevent this deformity.
- Double-bubble deformity *type **B***
  - *Implant is **B**elow* breast mound.
  - With significant overdissection of IMF, implant can slide caudal to the breast mound and create a second IMF below the native IMF and breast mound.
  - The native IMF will remain as a constricting band of soft tissue that compresses the implant and surrounding tissue to create the classic double bubble.

## Cancer Surveillance

- Implants cause interference with normal mammogram imaging.
- **Eklund mammogram views** displace breast and implant to increase parenchymal imaging after breast augmentation.
- **With appropriate imaging, no increased risk for cancer is found**; diagnosis not delayed; no difference in survival or recurrence.[25,46]

## Anaplastic Large Cell Lymphoma (ALCL)[47,48]

- There are 34 documented cases of ALCL in breast augmentation patients, and the FDA estimates possibly 60 cases in the world. This is a very small fraction of the millions of women with breast augmentation. Data are insufficient to show a clear link between ALCL and breast augmentation.
- The baseline risk of breast ALCL is 1 in 3 million; this may be increased to 1 in ~200,000 with breast implants.
- **Consider this diagnosis with late-presenting periimplant seromas.**
- Fluid should be submitted for cytologic evaluation with Wright-Giemsa–stained smears and cell block immunohistochemistry testing for cluster of differentiation (CD) and anaplastic lymphoma kinase (ALK) markers.
- No particular type of implant has been associated with ALCL.
- The FDA should be notified of any confirmed cases of ALCL.

## KEY POINTS

- ✓ Early mammograms are recommended for patients undergoing breast surgery (by age 30 to 35 years).
- ✓ **Eklund mammographic views** improve radiographic imaging of breast tissue after augmentation.
- ✓ It is important to note asymmetries during preoperative evaluations and discuss these with the patient. If there are asymmetries before surgery, there will be asymmetries afterward.
- ✓ Mild ptosis is improved with augmentation. However, when the N-IMF distance is >9.5 cm, the patient will likely need concomitant mastopexy.
- ✓ Subglandular augmentation is not recommended with thin upper pole coverage (superior pole pinch test is <2 cm).
- ✓ The dual plane technique takes advantage of extra upper pole pectoralis coverage while maximizing the implant-parenchymal interface in the lower pole. This can also help to prevent double-bubble deformity.
- ✓ Larger implants increase long-term detrimental effects on the breast.
- ✓ Textured implant surfaces are hypothesized to disorient collagen deposition, thereby potentially reducing contracture rates. The main indication for textured implants is to reduce mobility within the breast pocket.
- ✓ Bacterial contamination is likely one of the main etiologic factors for capsular contracture.
- ✓ Triple antibiotic irrigation and other techniques reduce contracture rates.
- ✓ MRI is the most sensitive and specific test for implant rupture or leakage.
- ✓ The risk for morbidity or mortality from breast cancer is no higher in breast implant patients.

## REFERENCES


1. American Society of Plastic Surgeons. Procedural statistics trends 1992-2012. Available at *www.plasticsurgery.org/public_education/Statistical-Trends.cfm.*
2. Czerny V. Plastischer ersatz der brusthuse durch ein lipoma. Zentralbl Chir 27:72, 1895.
3. Matton G, Anseeuw A, De Keyser F. The history of injectable biomaterials and the biology of collagen. Aesthetic Plast Surg 9:133-140, 1985.
4. Milojevic B. Complications after silicone injection therapy in aesthetic plastic surgery. Aesthetic Plast Surg 6:203-206, 1982.
5. Duffy DM. Injectable liquid silicone: new perspectives. In Klein AW, ed. Tissue Augmentation in Clinical Practice: Procedures and Techniques. New York: Marcel Dekker, 1998.
6. Cronin TD, Gerow FJ. Augmentation mammaplasty: a new "natural feel" prosthesis. In Transactions of the Third International Congress of Plastic Surgery. Washington, DC, Oct 1963.
7. Barnard JJ, Todd EL, Wilson WG, et al. Distribution of organosilicon polymers in augmentation mammaplasties at autopsy. Plast Reconstr Surg 100:197-203, 1997.
8. Adams WP Jr, Mallucci P. Breast augmentation. Plast Reconstr Surg 130:598e-612e, 2012.
9. Sánchez-Guerrero J, Colditz GA, Karlson EW, et al. Silicone breast implants and the risk of connective-tissue disease and symptoms. N Engl J Med 332:1666-1670, 1995.
10. Hennekens CH, Lee IM, Cook NR, et al. Self-reported breast implants and connective-tissue disease in female health professionals: a retrospective cohort study. JAMA 275:616-621, 1996.

11. Tugwell P, Wells G, Peterson J. Do silicone breast implants cause rhematologic disorders? A systematic review for a court-appointed national science panel. Arthritis Rheum 44:2477-2482, 2001.
12. Nahai F, ed. The Art of Aesthetic Surgery: Principles & Techniques, 2nd ed. St Louis: Quality Medical Publishing, 2011.
13. Tebbetts JB, Adams WP. Five critical decisions in breast augmentation using five measurements in 5 minutes. The high five decision support process. Plast Reconstr Surg 116:2005-2016, 2005.
14. Tepper OM, Small K, Unger JG, et al. 3D analysis of breast augmentation defines operative changes and their relationship to implant dimensions. Ann Plast Surg 62:570-575, 2009.
15. Collis N, Coleman D, Foo IT, et al. Ten-year review of a prospective randomized controlled trial of textured versus smooth subglandular silicone gel breast implants. Plast Reconstr Surg 106:786-791, 2000.
16. Wong CH, Samuel M, Tan BK, et al. Capsular contracture in subglandular breast augmentation with textured versus smooth breast implants: a systematic review. Plast Reconstr Surg 118:1224-1236, 2006.
17. Barnsley GP, Sigurdson LJ, Barnsley SE. Textured surface breast implants in the prevention of capsular contracture among breast augmentation patients: a meta-analysis of randomized controlled trials. Plast Reconstr Surg 117:2182-2190, 2006.
18. Hidalgo DA. Breast augmentation: choosing the optimal incision, implant, and pocket plane. Plast Reconstr Surg 105:2202-2206, 2000.
19. Mofid MM, Klatsky SA, Singh NK, et al. Nipple-areola complex sensitivity after primary breast augmentation: a comparison of periareolar and inframammary incision approaches. Plast Reconstr Surg 117:1694-1698, 2006.
20. Adams WP, Rios JI, Smith SJ. Enhancing patient outcomes in aesthetic and reconstructive breast surgery using triple antibiotic breast irrigation: six-year prospective clinical study. Plast Reconstr Surg 117:30-36, 2006.
21. Burkhardt BR, Dempsey PD, Schnur MD, et al. Capsular contracture: a prospective study of the effect of local antibacterial agents. Plast Reconstr Surg 77:919-932, 1986.
22. Bartsich S, Ascherman JA, Whittier S, et al. The breast: a clean-contaminated surgical site. Aesthet Surg J 31:802-806, 2011.
23. Price CI, Eaves FF, Nahai F, et al. Endoscopic transaxillary subpectoral breast augmentation. Plast Reconstr Surg 94:612-619, 1994.
24. Tebbetts JB. Axillary endoscopic breast augmentation: processes derived from a 28-year experience to optimize outcomes. Plast Reconstr Surg 118(7 Suppl):S53-S80, 2006.
25. Jakubietz M, Janis JE, Jakubietz RG, et al. Breast augmentation: cancer concerns and mammography—a literature review. Plast Reconstr Surg 113:117e-122e, 2004.
26. Tebbetts JB. Dual plane breast augmentation: optimizing implant-soft-tissue relationships in a wide range of breast types. Plast Reconstr Surg 107:1255-1272, 2001.
27. Rohrich RJ, Kenkel JM, Adams WP. Preventing capsular contracture in breast augmentation: in search of the Holy Grail. Plast Reconstr Surg 103:1759-1760, 1999.
28. Mladick RA. "No-touch" submuscular saline breast augmentation technique. Aesthetic Plast Surg 17:183-192, 1993.
29. Virden CP, Dobke MK, Stein P, et al. Subclinical infection of the silicone breast implant surface as a possible cause of capsular contracture. Aesthetic Plast Surg 16:173-179, 1992.
30. Dobke MK, Svahn JK, Vastine VL, et al. Characterization of microbial presence at the surface of silicone mammary implants. Ann Plast Surg 34:563-569, 1995.
31. Burkhardt BR. Effects of povidone iodine on silicone gel implants in vitro: implications for clinical practice. Plast Reconstr Surg 114:711-712, 2004.
32. Adams WP, Conner WC, Barton FE Jr, et al. Optimizing breast pocket irrigation: the post-betadine era. Plast Reconstr Surg 107:1596-1601, 2001.

33. Chandler PJ Jr. The deposition of talc in patients with silicone gel-filled breast implants. Plast Reconstr Surg 104:661-668, 1999.
34. Biggs TM, Yarish RS. Augmentation mammaplasty: a comparative analysis. Plast Reconstr Surg 85:368-372, 1990.
35. Gylbert L, Asplund O, Jurell G. Capsular contracture after breast reconstruction with silicone gel and saline-filled implants: a 6-year follow-up. Plast Reconstr Surg 85:373-377, 1990.
36. Marotta JS, Widenhouse CW, Habal MB, et al. Silicone gel breast implant failure and frequency of additional surgeries: analysis of 35 studies reporting examination of more than 8000 explants. J Biomed Mater Res 48:354-364, 1999.
37. U.S. Food and Drug Administration. Center for Devices and Radiological Health. FDA update on the safety of silicone gel-filled breast implants, June 2011. Available at *www.fda.gov/downloads/medicaldevices/productsandmedicalprocedures/implantsandprosthetics/breastimplants/ucm260090.pdf.*
38. Mentor Corporation. Saline implant premarket approval information, 2001. Available at *http://www.fda.gov/downloads/medicaldevices/productsandmedicalprocedures/implantsandprosthetics/breastimplants/ucm232436.pdf.*
39. Allergan Corporation. Saline implant premarket approval information, 2001. Available at *www.fda.gov//downloads/medicaldevices/productsandmedicalprocedures/implantsandprosthetics/breastimplants/ucm064457.pdf.*
40. Mentor, Allergan, and Sientra Corporations: silicone breast implant premarket approval information, 2003, 2005, 2012. Available at *www.fda.gov/medicaldevices/productsandmedicalprocedures/implantsandprosthetics/breastimplants/ucm063871.htm.*
41. Young VL. Guidelines and indications for breast implant capsulectomy. Plast Reconstr Surg 102:884-891, 1998.
42. Spear SL, Dayan JH, Bogue D, et al. The "neosubpectoral" pocket for the correction of symmastia. Plast Reconstr Surg 124:695-703, 2009.
43. Maxwell GP, Gabriel A. The neopectoral pocket in revisionary breast surgery. Aesthet Surg J 28:463-467, 2008.
44. Huang CK, Handel N. Effects of Singulair (montelukast) treatment for capsular contracture. Aesthet Surg J 30:404-408, 2010.
45. Peters W, Smith D. Calcification of breast implant capsules: incidence, diagnosis, and contributing factors. Ann Plast Surg 34:8-11, 1995.
46. Hoshaw SJ, Klein PJ, Clark BD, et al. Breast implants and cancer: causation, delayed detection, and survival. Plast Reconstr Surg 107:1393-1408, 2001.
47. U.S. Food and Drug Administration. Center for Devices and Radiological Health. Anaplastic large cell lymphoma (ALCL) in women with breast implants: preliminary FDA findings and analysis. Available at *www.fda.gov/medicaldevices/productsandmedicalprocedures/implantsandprosthetics/breastimplants/ucm239996.htm.*
48. de Jong D, Vasmel WL, de Boer JP, et al. Anaplastic large-cell lymphoma in women with breast implants. JAMA 300:2030-2035, 2008.

# 46. Mastopexy

Joshua A. Lemmon, José L. Rios, Kailash Narasimhan

## EPIDEMIOLOGY[1]

- The 2012 Plastic Surgery Statistics Report found that over 89,000 mastopexies were done in the United States.
- Compared to the year 2000, this is up 69%.
- 12,715 mastopexies performed in 2012 were on Massive Weight Loss Patients.
- Patients present typically between ages 40-54.

## TERMINOLOGY

### Ptosis

- *Ptosis* from Greek, meaning "falling"
- Describes descended breast parenchyma

### Mastopexy

- Surgical procedure designed to correct breast ptosis
- Often referred to as *breast lift*
- Indicated in women who desire improved breast contour without a volume change[1]

## HISTORICAL PERSPECTIVE AND REGIONAL DIFFERENCES[2]

- Historical perspective
  - History parallels that of breast reduction.
  - The procedures mostly involved elevation of the breast mound using suspension techniques.
  - Traditionally, mastopexy was performed using primarily skin excision techniques.
  - Since the mid-1990s, emphasis has been on internal shaping of the parenchymal tissue as well.
  - Classic skin excision patterns for mastopexy include:
    - Crescent
    - Periareolar
    - Circumvertical
    - Inverted-T designs
  - Internal shaping can be performed using various supportive materials or suturing of parenchymal pillars.
- Regional differences
  - North America
    - American surgeons use the **inferior pedicle** more frequently.
    - American surgeons use fascial sutures less often.
    - North American procedures usually do not incorporate autoaugmentation.
  - Latin America and Europe
    - Latin American and European surgeons prefer **superior pedicles.**

- Latin American and European surgeons use fascial sutures more often.
- Latin American surgeons use autoaugmentation more.

## ETIOLOGIC FACTORS, NATURAL CLINICAL HISTORY, AND CLASSIFICATION[3,4]

### Etiologic Factors

Ptosis results when the parenchymal volume decreases and the skin envelope and supporting structures do not retract.

- Young patients
  - May have thin skin or excessive breast size
- Middle-aged patients
  - Postpartum changes from lactation or engorgement
  - Subsequent gland atrophy and laxity of skin
  - Supporting Cooper's ligaments, dermal laxity, and ductal structures also stretched
- Postmenopausal patients
  - Factors such as atrophy, gravity, loss of skin elasticity from age, and weight gain all contribute.
  - The breast assumes a lower position on the chest wall; youthful breast contour is lost.

### Regnault Classification[1,5] (Fig. 46-1)

Ptosis is described by the relative positions of the nipple-areola complex (NAC) and inframammary fold.

- **Pseudoptosis or glandular ptosis**
  - The NAC is above or at the level of the inframammary fold, but most of the breast parenchyma has descended below the level of the fold.
  - Nipple-to-inframammary fold (N-IMF) distance has increased.
- **Grade I ptosis** (mild)
  - The NAC is at the level of the inframammary fold.
- **Grade II ptosis** (moderate)
  - The NAC is below the level of the inframammary fold, but above the most dependent part of the breast parenchyma.
- **Grade III ptosis** (severe)
  - The NAC is well below the inframammary fold, at the most dependent part of the breast parenchyma along the inferior contour of the breast.

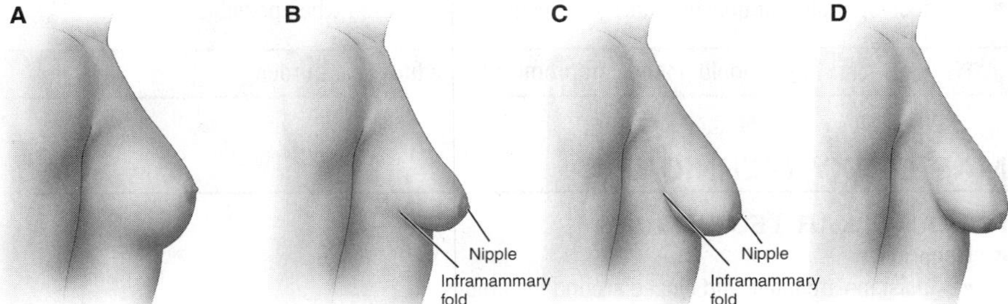


**Fig. 46-1** Regnault classification of breast ptosis. **A,** Pseudoptosis. **B,** Grade I ptosis. **C,** Grade II ptosis. **D,** Grade III ptosis.

## PREOPERATIVE EVALUATION[4,6]

### HISTORY

- Age
- Breast history: Lactation, pregnancy changes, size changes with weight loss or gain, tumors, previous procedures, family history of breast cancer, recent mammogram

### MEASUREMENTS

- Sternal notch-to-nipple distance: Allows detection of asymmetry in nipple position
- N-IMF distance: Measures redundancy of the lower pole skin envelope
- Classification of ptosis severity (see previous section)

### OTHER CONSIDERATIONS

- Skin quality: Presence of striae reflects inelastic quality of affected skin.
- Parenchymal quality: Fatty, fibrous, or glandular parenchyma
- Areolar shape and size: Areolae are often stretched, large, and asymmetrical.

### PHOTOGRAPHS

- Obtain AP, lateral, and oblique photographs.

### PATIENT EXPECTATIONS

- **Breast size**
  - Mastopexy techniques combine small amounts of parenchymal resection and redistribution with reduction of the skin envelope; this can result in reduced breast size.
  - Many patients seek restoration of upper pole fullness, which may necessitate simultaneous placement of an implant. (See Augmentation-Mastopexy, Chapter 47.)
- **Scar position**
  - Mastopexy procedures trade scars for improved contour.
  - Inform patients in detail, preoperatively, about scar placement and quality.
- **Other considerations**
  - Thorough patient education regarding procedural complications, use of drains, and recurrence of ptosis are essential components of preoperative preparation.

## GOALS OF MASTOPEXY SURGERY

- Reliable nipple-areolar transposition to an aesthetic position on the breast mound
- Obtain pleasing breast shape.
- Produce optimal scar quality: Short-scar techniques preferred when possible

**TIP:** Breast shape should not be compromised to reduce scar burden.

## MASTOPEXY TECHNIQUES

### PERIAREOLAR TECHNIQUES

- **General**
  - Incisions are made and closed around the areola.
  - Scars are therefore camouflaged at the areola-skin junction.

- **Patient selection**
  - Useful for mild and moderate ptosis.
  - Skin quality should be reasonable without striae, and parenchyma should be fibrous or glandular.
- **Techniques**
  - **Simple periareolar deepithelialization and closure**
    - Breast parenchyma is **not** repositioned, therefore this is only useful with mild ptosis.
    - This technique allows nipple repositioning.
    - Limited elliptical techniques can elevate the NAC approximately **1-2 cm.**[4]
  - **Benelli technique**[6,7] (Fig. 46-2)
    - This periareolar technique is used for patients with larger degrees of breast ptosis.
    - Technique allows parenchymal repositioning.
    - Areolar sizers are used to mark a new areolar diameter, and a wider ellipse is marked to reposition NAC and resect redundant skin envelope.
    - Undermining separates the breast gland from overlying skin.
    - Breast parenchyma is incised, leaving the NAC on a superior pedicle.
    - Medial and lateral parenchymal flaps are mobilized and crossed or invaginated at midline, narrowing breast width and coning the breast shape.
    - Periareolar incision is closed in purse-string fashion with permanent sutures.
  - **Other periareolar techniques**
    - Variations on the previous technique include use of mesh to support parenchyma[8] or use of breast implant to reduce amount of skin resection required.[5,9]
- **Advantages**
  - Short scar
  - Scar camouflaged at border of areola
- **Disadvantages**
  - Scar and areolar widening occur frequently.
  - Breast projection can be flattened.
  - Purse-string closure results in skin pleating that takes several months to resolve, and may be permanent.

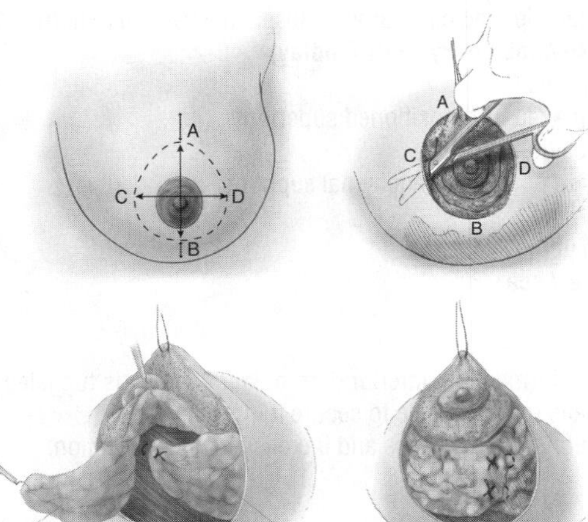


**Fig. 46-2** Benelli periareolar mastopexy. Markings, undermining, and parenchymal coning.

> **TIP:** If periareolar purse-string suture remains palpable, it can be removed with simple office-based procedure after 6 weeks.

## Vertical Scar Techniques

- **General**
  - Vertical mastopexy techniques are variations of vertical reduction mammaplasty techniques.
  - Incisions are closed around the areola and inferiorly toward the inframammary fold.
  - Techniques rely on parenchymal support inferiorly to narrow and cone the breast.
- **Patient selection**
  - Techniques can be applied to patients with all degrees of ptosis.
- **Techniques**
  - **Vertical mastopexy without undermining (Lassus)**[10] (Fig. 46-3)
    - Skin is incised as shown in Fig. 46-4.[11]
    - Inferior, ptotic skin, fat, and gland are resected en bloc, and the nipple is transposed superiorly without undermining.
    - Medial and lateral breast pillars are closed.
  - **Vertical mastopexy with undermining and liposuction (Lejour)**[12]
    - Skin is incised as shown in Fig. 46-4.[11]
    - Liposuction is performed in larger breasts to reduce parenchymal volume and mobilize superior dermal-parenchymal pedicle.
    - Inferior skin, fat, and gland are resected.
    - Wide undermining is performed, and medial and lateral breast pillars are closed inferiorly.
    - Skin is closed in a single vertical line; redundant skin remains as fine wrinkles between inferior sutures.
  - **Short-scar periareolar inferior-pedicle reduction (SPAIR) mammaplasty/mastopexy (Hammond)**[13]
    - Skin is incised as shown in Fig. 46-4.[11]
    - NAC is transposed to desired location based on an inferior pedicle.
    - Nipple is transposed and supported with parenchymal suspension sutures.
    - Inferior skin is tailor-tacked to create desired contour and closed in a vertical pattern.
  - **Medial pedicle vertical mammaplasty/mastopexy (Hall-Findlay)**[14]
    - Medial pedicle is designed to carry the NAC.
    - Lateral and inferior tissues are removed or repositioned superiorly.
    - Nipple is transposed to desired position.
    - Breast pillars are closed inferiorly to provide parenchymal support.
    - Skin is closed in vertical fashion.
    - Redundant skin is gathered along vertical closure.
    - Closure can also take the form of a **J scar.**[15]
- **Modifications**
  - Inferior chest wall–based flap[16]
    - Vertical mastopexy technique is performed, but inferior dermoglandular flap is tunneled superiorly under a sling of pectoralis major muscle to secure it in place.
    - Technique is designed to restore upper pole fullness and increase breast projection.

- **Advantages**
  - Limited vertical scar is achieved without horizontal inframammary fold incision.
  - Inferior parenchymal closure provides additional support to limit recurrent ptosis.
- **Disadvantages**
  - Immediate postoperative result often displays pronounced upper pole fullness that settles over time.
  - Inferior skin redundancy occasionally does not retract, requiring horizontal excision later.

**TIP:** To limit redundancy in inferior pole skin, the vertical closure is brought obliquely laterally (creating a J shape). This eliminates excessive inferior skin redundancy and prevents a medial horizontal scar.

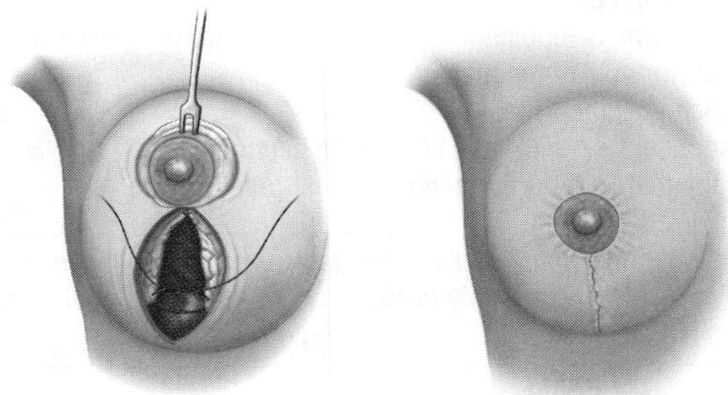

**Fig. 46-3** Vertical mastopexy without undermining. Inferior skin, fat, and gland are resected en bloc. The nipple is transposed to the desired position, followed by vertical closure of the medial and lateral breast pillars.

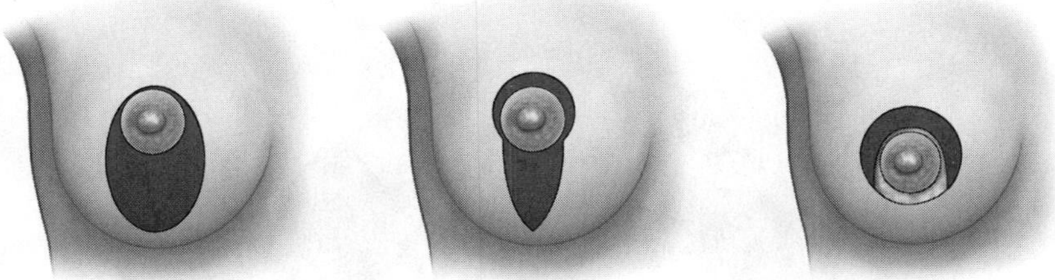

**Fig. 46-4** Vertical scar mastopexy techniques of Lassus *(left),* Lejour *(center),* and Hammond *(right).*

## Inverted-T Scar Techniques

- **General**
  - Incisions are closed around the areola, vertically to the vertical limbs, and horizontally to the inframammary fold.
- **Patient selection**
  - Inverted-T used for severe ptosis
  - Considered for mastopexy in patients with very poor skin quality and fatty parenchyma
- **Principles**
  - Frequently, Wise-pattern skin incision technique is used, because this breast reduction technique is popular.
  - Other skin excision patterns attempt to reduce the length of the horizontal scar[11] (Fig. 46-5).
  - Parenchymal resection is indicated for breast hypertrophy.
  - In most mastopexy patients, parenchymal support is obtained by inferior closure of the medial and lateral breast pillars.
  - The inferior parenchyma is repositioned superiorly to restore superior pole fullness or used to support the inferior pole of the breast.
    - Tunneled under a pectoralis sling[16]
    - Folded under superior pedicle and secured to pectoralis fascia[17]
    - Folded over to create supportive sling for lower pole[18]

> **TIP:** In traditional inverted-T mastopexy techniques, breast shape is maintained solely by the skin envelope. Modern variations rely heavily on parenchymal support to lend longevity to the result.

- **Advantages**
  - Surgeons are familiar with technique because of widespread use in reduction techniques.[19]
  - Results are predictable.
- **Disadvantages**
  - Scar burden
  - Recurrent ptosis probable if parenchymal support not used

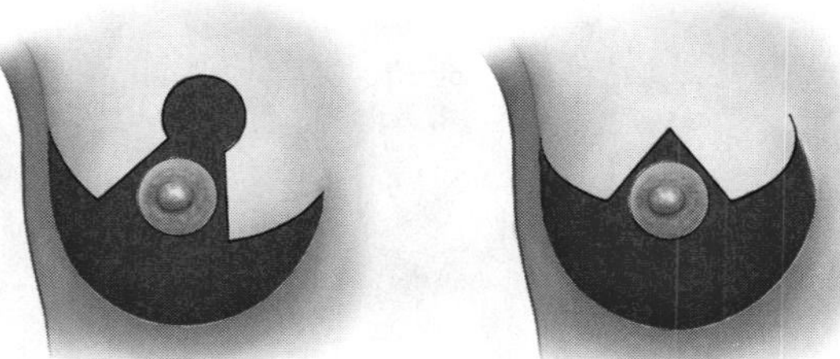

**Fig. 46-5** Skin incision patterns for inverted-T mastopexy techniques.

## POSTOPERATIVE CARE

- Drains, when used, are removed within the first 1-3 days postoperatively.
- Postoperative pain is treated with oral analgesics.
- A supportive brassiere is required for 6 weeks postoperatively to ensure full support during the healing process.
- Scar treatment begins 3 weeks postoperatively using the surgeon's preferred technique.
- Scar revisions, when necessary, are performed 1 year after initial surgery.

## COMPLICATIONS[4,6]

### HEMATOMA

- Relatively infrequent
- Patients should avoid using aspirin and antiplatelet medications for 10 days preoperatively.
- Tight hematomas require urgent reoperation for evacuation, hemostasis, and closure.

### INFECTION

- Uncommon problem
- Perioperative antibiotics used routinely to reduce risk of infection[20]

### WOUND HEALING PROBLEMS

- Mostly present in inverted-T procedures
- More common among smokers: Mastopexy not performed on active smokers for this reason[21,22]

### NIPPLE AND BREAST ASYMMETRY

- Inform patients preoperatively that perfect breast symmetry never will be achieved.
- Large asymmetries in nipple position, areolar size, and breast shape require revision surgery.

### SCAR DEFORMITIES

- Periareolar scar widening and medial horizontal inframammary fold scars are the source of frequent patient dissatisfaction.
- Scar revisions can be performed 1 year after initial surgery.

### RECURRENT PTOSIS

- Gravity and aging continue to affect the breast after mastopexy.
- Inferior parenchymal (not dermal) support is thought to decrease the likelihood of recurrent ptosis.
- Mastopexy is a temporary solution, and some deformity usually recurs in the long term.[4]

## SPECIAL CONSIDERATIONS

### AUGMENTATION-MASTOPEXY

- Loss of upper pole fullness with breast ptosis leads many surgeons to advocate placement of subglandular or subpectoral breast implants at the time of mastopexy.[4-6]
- Unfortunately, augmentation and mastopexy techniques work against each other.[23]
  - Mastopexy is designed to reposition the nipple, reshape the breast without tension to limit scarring, and reduce the size of the redundant skin envelope.
  - Augmentation increases the size of the skin envelope, the mass of the breast (subjecting it more to the force of gravity), and the tension of wound closure.
- Surgeons should consider staging augmentation and mastopexy in patients with moderate or severe ptosis.

## Mastopexy After Explantation

- Many patients with previously placed silicone gel implants seek explantation for various reasons, including rupture, fear of rupture, and capsular contracture.
- Often these patients benefit from simultaneous breast contouring procedures at the time of capsulectomy and implant exchange.[24]
  - Preexplantation ptosis is rarely corrected without formal mastopexy.
  - Good candidates are nonsmokers with mild to moderate ptosis, and adequate soft tissue coverage (>4 cm) over the implant.
  - In patients with sparse soft tissue coverage or severe ptosis, mastopexy should be staged 3 months after explantation.

**TIP:** Avoid mastopexy in all smokers.

- Choice of mastopexy technique depends on preoperative classification of ptosis[24] (Table 46-1).

**Table 46-1** *Breast Contouring at Time of Explantation and Choice of Technique*

| Ptosis Type | Characteristics | Technique |
|---|---|---|
| Pseudoptosis | • Adequate volume<br>• Good nipple position<br>• Nipple to inframammary fold: 6 cm | Inframammary fold wedge excision |
| Grade I | • Nipple repositioned <2 cm<br>• Areola: <50 mm diameter | Periareolar mastopexy<br>Vertical mastopexy |
| Grade II | • Nipple repositioned 2-4 cm | Wise-pattern mastopexy |
| Grade III | • Nipple repositioned >4 cm<br>• <4 cm breast thickness | Delayed mastopexy<br>(3 months, smoker) |

## Massive-Weight-Loss (MWL) Mastopexy

- The number of MWL surgeries is growing, leading to an increased number of mastopexies.
- Advantages of this procedure include elimination of axillary fat roll, autoaugmentation of breast using lateral fat roll tissue, control of skin envelope, and parenchymal shaping.
- However, scars are often long. To obtain proper shape, intraoperative tailoring is frequently necessary, which can lengthen operative time.
- Patients with deflated breasts who desire upper pole contour may require an implant in conjunction with mastopexy.
- **Breast characteristics of MWL patients**[25] (Fig. 46-6)
  - Poor shape, projection, and skin elasticity
  - Extreme ptosis and loss of volume
  - Flattening of breast against chest wall
  - Nipples distorted, ptotic, and often inferomedially translocated
- **Goals of reshaping surgery**
  - Use available breast tissue while maintaining ability to recruit additional volume.
  - Correct nipple position.
  - Reshape skin envelope without relying on it for support.
  - Eliminate lateral roll.
  - Create a defined lateral breast curvature.

- **Treatment principles**
  - MWL mastopexy can be tailored, based on breast shape, volume loss, and grade of ptosis.
  - Rubin has graded these deformities.[25]
    - **Severity grade 1** (ptosis grade I or II or severe macromastia)
      - Traditional mastopexy (preferably vertical technique) or
      - Standard breast reduction techniques or
      - Implant augmentation ± elevation of nipple through mastopexy scars
    - **Severity grade 2** (ptosis grade III, moderate volume loss, or constricted breast)
      - Traditional mastopexy (often requiring Wise pattern)
      - Consider implant augmentation to accompany mastopexy.
    - **Severity grade 3** (severe lateral roll and/or severe volume loss with loose skin)
      - Parenchymal reshaping techniques with dermal suspension
      - Consider autoaugmentation (see below).
      - Avoid implant augmentation if existing volume will create a reasonable result.
- **Dermal suspension autoaugmentation mastopexy**
  - For patients with sufficient parenchymal volume, severe ptosis, lateral skin fold
  - Surgical technique[25] (Figs. 46-7 through 46-9)
    1. Mark the patient with a Wise pattern, encompassing the lateral roll of tissue.
    2. Deepithelialize the entire Wise pattern area.
    3. Deglove the breast parenchyma.
    4. Elevate the medial and lateral parenchymal flaps.
    5. Suspend the dermal edge of flaps to rib periosteum.
    6. Plicate the dermis to shape the breast.
    7. Place sutures along the lateral edge of the breast to define its curvature.
    8. Redrape the skin.
    9. Release any dermis that is tethering the nipple.
    10. Close the skin.

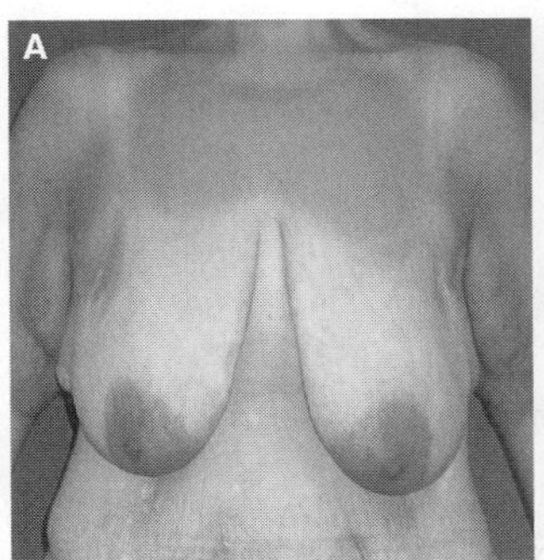

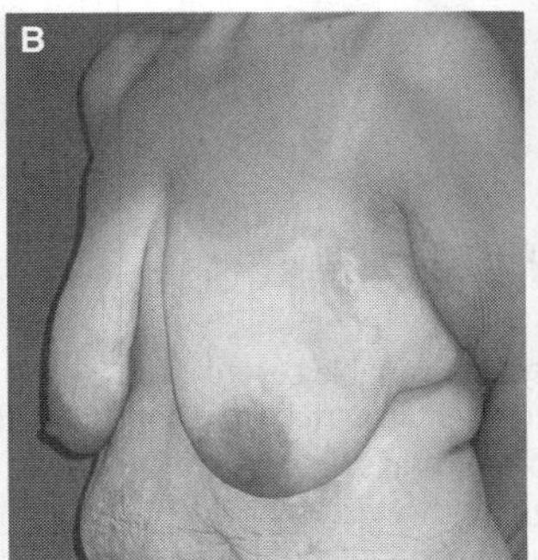

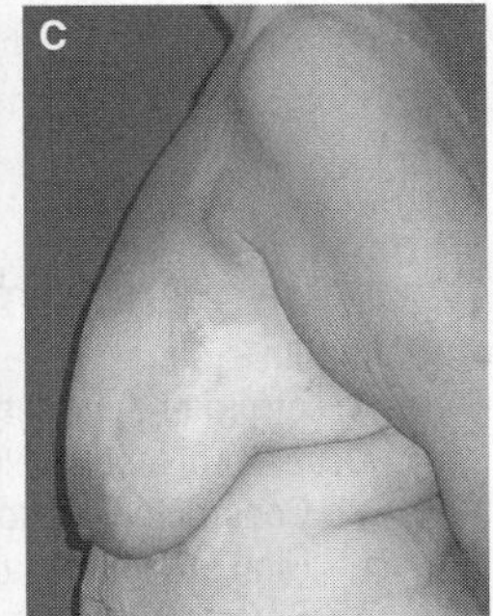


**Fig. 46-6 A-C,** Breast appearance after massive weight loss.

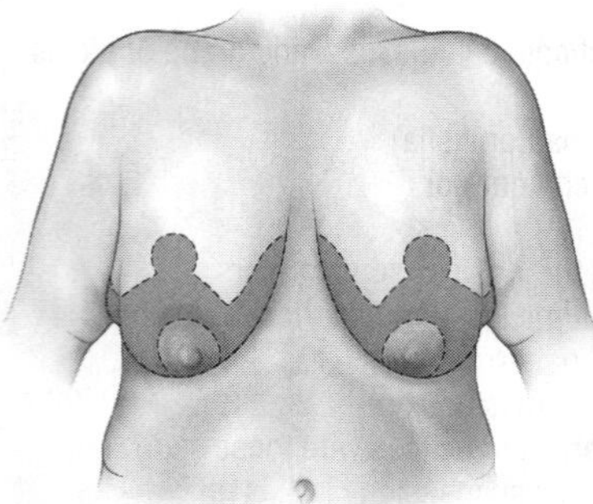

**Fig. 46-7** Wise pattern markings. *Shading* indicates areas to be deepithelialized.

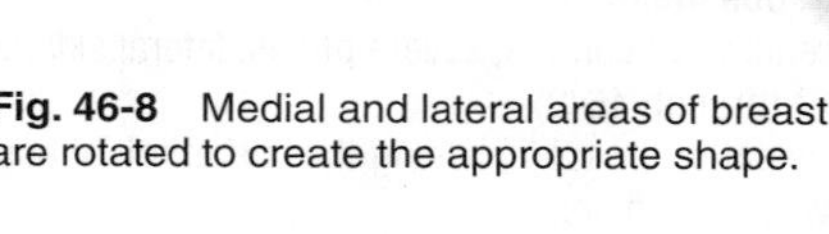

**Fig. 46-8** Medial and lateral areas of breast are rotated to create the appropriate shape.

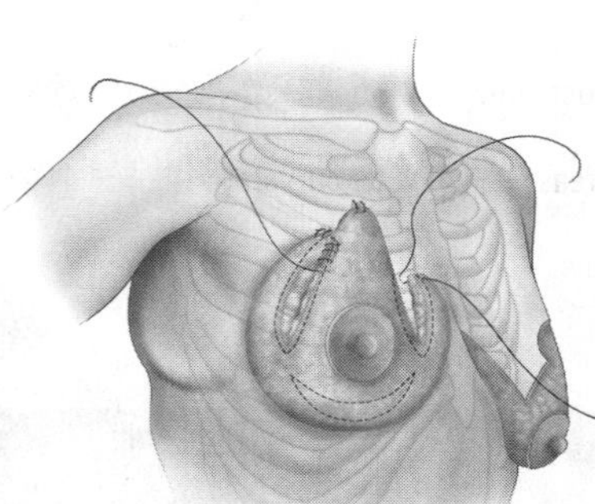

**Fig. 46-9** The breast is anchored to rib periosteum, and gland is reshaped.

## Tuberous Breast Deformity[26]

- **Definition**
  - Spectrum of deformity with variable severity[26]
  - Deficient breast development in vertical and horizontal dimensions
    - Constricted (narrowed) breast base
    - High inframammary fold
    - Breast parenchyma herniation into the areola resulting in disproportionately large areola
- **At consultation, these patients often seek mastopexy or augmentation.**

**TIP:** It is essential to identify and counsel these patients. They often are unaware of their anatomic abnormalities and that typical mastopexy techniques are not adequate.

- **Treatment goals**[26]
  - Expand breast circumference.
  - Expand skin envelope in the lower pole.
  - Release constriction at the breast-areola junction.
  - Lower the inframammary fold.
  - Increase breast volume (when appropriate).
  - Reduce areolar size and correct herniation.
  - Correct nipple location and breast ptosis.
- **Treatment options**[23]
  - Periareolar mastopexy techniques are used to reduce areolar size and reposition the NAC on the breast mound.
  - The breast parenchyma usually requires modification with inferior pole radial scoring, mobilization, or division.
  - Augmentation with permanent implants or expandable permanent implants usually is required to restore parenchymal volume.

**TIP:** Tissue expansion is necessary if there is severe inferior pole skin deficiency.

## OUTCOMES[2]

- **Long-term nipple position**
  - Ahmad and Lista[27] reviewed 1700 vertical scar procedures and evaluated measurements over time to determine position of the NAC.
    - Compared with preoperative markings, the NAC was 1.3 cm higher on postoperative day 5 and 1 cm higher at 4 years.
    - Distance from the IMF to the inferior border of the NAC did not lengthen over time, and pseudoptosis did not occur.
  - Swanson[2] reviewed 82 publications on mastopexy and reduction and various assessments on measurements such as breast projection, upper pole projection, nipple level, and breast convexity.
    - Techniques reviewed included inverted-T (with superior/medial, central, and inferior pedicles), vertical, periareolar, inframammary, and lateral.
    - Breast projection and upper pole projection were not increased significantly by any of the mastopexy or reduction procedures.
    - Nipple overelevation was common (41.9%), and teardrop areola deformity (53.8%) was significantly higher in patients with open nipple placement techniques.
    - Methods to increase upper pole fullness or projection, such as fascial sutures and autoaugmentation, generally did not maintain shape in the long term.[4]

## SURVEY COMPARISON OF VARIOUS TECHNIQUES

- Based on a survey of board-certified plastic surgeons, periareolar techniques had highest rate of surgeon dissatisfaction[28] and the highest rate of revision.
- Though most popular, the inverted-T group reported a significantly greater frequency of bottoming out ($p$ 0.043) and excess scarring along the inframammary fold ($p$ 0.001), compared with the short-scar and periareolar groups.

## KEY POINTS

- ✓ Classification of breast ptosis is determined by the nipple-areola position relative to the inframammary fold.
- ✓ Modern mastopexy techniques rely on inferior parenchymal support to elevate the gland on the chest wall and limit recurrent ptosis.
- ✓ Mild ptosis can be corrected with periareolar techniques alone.
- ✓ Moderate and severe ptosis require vertical, or vertical and horizontal, skin excision.
- ✓ Mastopexy and augmentation procedures have conflicting properties and should be combined cautiously.
- ✓ In MWL patients, longer scars may be needed to improve shape.
- ✓ It is important to identify patients with tuberous breast deformities, because specific techniques are required for treatment.

## REFERENCES


1. American Society of Plastic Surgeons. 2012 Plastic Surgery Statistic Report. Available at *http://www.plasticsurgery.org/documents/news-resources/statistics/2012-plastic-surgery-statistics/full-plastic-surgery-statistics-report.pdf.*
2. Swanson E. A retrospective photometric study of 82 published reports of mastopexy and breast reduction. Plast Reconstr Surg 128:1282-1301, 2011.
3. Hall-Findlay EJ. Mastopexy. In Hall-Findlay EJ, ed. Aesthetic Breast Surgery: Concepts & Techniques. St Louis: Quality Medical Publishing, 2011.
4. Jones GE. Mastopexy. In Jones GE, ed. Bostwick's Plastic & Reconstructive Breast Surgery, 3rd ed. St Louis: Quality Medical Publishing, 2010.
5. Kirwan L. Augmentation of the ptotic breast: simultaneous periareolar mastopexy/breast augmentation. Aesthet Surg J 19:34-39, 1999.
6. Grotting JC, Chen SM. Control and precision in mastopexy. In Nahai F, ed. The Art of Aesthetic Surgery: Principles & Techniques, 2nd ed. St Louis: Quality Medical Publishing, 2011.
7. Benelli L. A new periareolar mammaplasty: the "round block" technique. Aesthetic Plast Surg 14:93-100, 1990.
8. Goés JC. Periareolar mammaplasty: double skin technique with application of polyglactin or mixed mesh. Plast Reconstr Surg 97:959-968, 1996.
9. Spear S, Giese SY, Ducic I, et al. Concentric mastopexy revisited. Plast Reconstr Surg 107:1294-1299, 2001.
10. Lassus C. A 30-year experience with vertical mammaplasty. Plast Reconstr Surg 97:373-380, 1996.
11. Rohrich RJ, Thornton JF, Jakubietz RG, et al. The limited scar mastopexy: current concepts and approaches to correct breast ptosis. Plast Reconstr Surg 114:1622-1630, 2004.
12. Lejour M. Vertical mammaplasty and liposuction of the breast. Plast Reconstr Surg 94:100-114, 1994.
13. Hammond DC. Short scar periareolar inferior pedicle reduction (SPAIR) mammaplasty. Plast Reconstr Surg 103:890-901, 1999.
14. Hall-Findlay EJ. A simplified vertical reduction mammaplasty: shortening the learning curve. Plast Reconstr Surg 104:748-759, 1999.
15. Gasperoni C, Salgrello M, Gasperoni P. A personal technique: mammaplasty with J scar. Ann Plast Surg 48:124-130, 2002.

16. Graf R, Biggs TM, Steely RL. Breast shape: a technique for better upper pole fullness. Aesthetic Plast Surg 24:348-352, 2000.
17. Flowers RS, Smith EM Jr. "Flip-flap" mastopexy. Aesthetic Plast Surg 22:425-429, 1998.
18. Svedman P. Correction of breast ptosis utilizing a "fold over" deepithelialized lower thoracic fasciocutaneous flap. Aesthetic Plast Surg 15:43-47, 1991.
19. Rohrich RJ, Gosman AA, Brown SA, et al. Current preferences for breast reduction techniques: a survey of board-certified plastic surgeons in 2002. Plast Reconstr Surg 114:1724-1733, 2004.
20. Platt R, Zucker JR, Zalesnik DF, et al. Perioperative antibiotic prophylaxis and wound infection following breast surgery. J Antimicrob Chemother 31(Suppl B):43-48, 1993.
21. Gravante G, Araco A, Sorge R, et al. Wound infections in body contouring mastopexy with breast reduction after laparoscopic adjustable gastirc banding: the role of smoking. Obes Surg 18:721-727, 2008.
22. Hanemann MS Jr, Grotting JC. Evaluation of preoperative risk factors and complication rates in cosmetic breast surgery. Ann Plast Surg 64:537-540, 2010.
23. Spear S. Augmentation/mastopexy: "surgeon, beware." Plast Reconstr Surg 112:905-906, 2003.
24. Rohrich RJ, Beran SJ, Restifo RJ, et al. Aesthetic management of the breast following explantation: evaluation and mastopexy options. Plast Reconstr Surg 101:827-837, 1998.
25. Rubin JP, Toy J. Mastopexy and breast reduction in massive-weight-loss patients. In Nahai F, ed. The Art of Aesthetic Surgery: Principles & Techniques, 2nd ed. St Louis: Quality Medical Publishing, 2011.
26. Rees TD, Aston SJ. The tuberous breast. Clin Plast Surg 3:339-347, 1976.
27. Ahmad J, Lista F. Vertical scar reduction mammaplasty: the fate of nipple-areola complex position and inferior pole length. Plast Reconstr Surg 121:1084-1091, 2008.
28. Rohrich RJ, Gosman AA, Brown SA, et al. Mastopexy preferences: a survey of board-certified plastic surgeons. Plast Reconstr Surg 118:1631-1638, 2006.

# 47. Augmentation-Mastopexy

Purushottam A. Nagarkar

## GENERAL PRINCIPLES

- Augmentation-mastopexy is a technique used to simultaneously correct low volume and skin excess.
- **Augmentation** alone corrects relative **deficiency of volume.**
- **Mastopexy** alone corrects relative **excess of skin.**
- If volume deficiency and skin excess are significant enough that either procedure alone will result in a persistent relative mismatch, combined procedure is needed.
- **The revision rate is high (8%-20%).**[1-3]
- Gonzales-Ulloa[4] described the technique in 1960, followed by Regnault[5] in 1966.
- Surgical planning depends on relative locations of nipple and inframammary fold (IMF) (i.e., ptosis). Regnault described three categories[6,7] (Fig. 47-1):

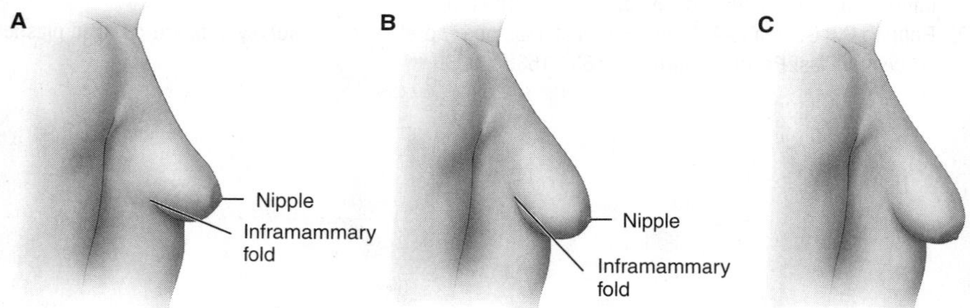


**Fig. 47-1** Regnault classification of breast ptosis. **A,** Grade I. **B,** Grade II. **C,** Grade III.

  - **Grade I:** Nipple at IMF
  - **Grade II:** Nipple below IMF
  - **Grade III:** Nipple at the lowest point on breast
- **Pseudoptosis:** Nipple at or above IMF but breast parenchyma below IMF[8] (Fig. 47-2, *A*)
- **Glandular ptosis:** Excess gland in the lower pole of the breast[8] (Fig. 47-2, *B*)

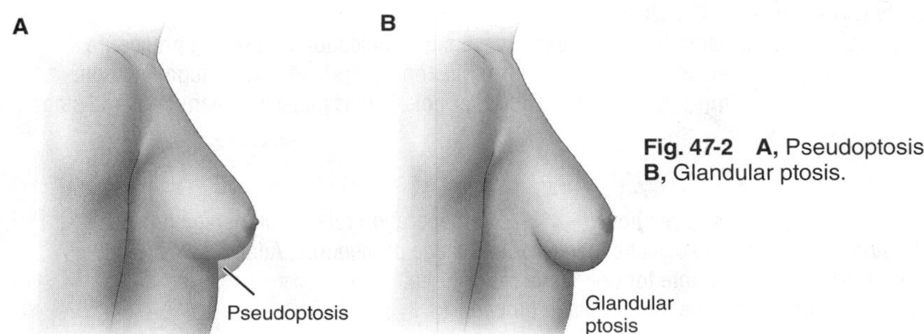


**Fig. 47-2** **A,** Pseudoptosis. **B,** Glandular ptosis.

## ALTERNATIVES

### Augmentation Alone

- Use if skin excess is minimal: i.e., minimal gland below IMF, minimal ptosis, AND
- Augmentation alone can provide appropriate projection and adequately correct ptosis by decreasing *relative* skin excess.

### Mastopexy Alone

- Use if volume deficiency is minimal, AND
- Skin resection alone will appropriately raise the nipple position and adequately correct projection by decreasing *relative* volume deficiency.

## INDICATIONS

- Ptosis (skin excess) combined with significant volume deficiency
- Periareolar mastopexy with augmentation requires[9]:
  - Nipple no more than 2 cm below the fold
  - Nipple-areola complex (NAC) at or above breast border, not pointing inferiorly
  - No more than 3 to 4 cm of associated breast ptosis
- More significant ptosis will require a vertical or Wise-pattern mastopexy.

## SINGLE-STAGE VERSUS TWO-STAGE PROCEDURE[10]

### Single-Stage Procedure

- Thought to be unpredictable, with higher revision rate than that of both procedures combined[11]
- **One of the most common causes for malpractice claims**[12]
- **Contraindications**[13,14]**:**
  - Constricted breast or skin deficiency
  - Unclear whether both procedures will be necessary
    - For example, no mastopexy required if patient has[13]:
      - No ptosis and no pseudoptosis (<2 cm of breast parenchyma below the IMF)
      - Alternatively, per Lee, Unger, and Adams,[15] skin stretch <4 cm and nipple-to-IMF (N-IMF) distance <10 cm
  - Significant asymmetry that is going to require an asymmetrical mastopexy for correction
  - Significant vertical skin excess that will require a large skin resection

## Two-Stage Procedure

- Per Lee, Unger, and Adams,[15] **vertical excess >6 cm** is indication for staging procedure.
  - If primary goal is ptosis correction, perform mastopexy first, and stage augmentation.
  - If primary goal is improved projection or upper pole fullness, place implant first, and stage the mastopexy.

## Outcomes (see Tables 47-1 and 47-2)

- Multiple large series have shown ~8%-20% reoperation rate for one-stage procedures.[1-3]
- Using his algorithm to select patients for two-stage procedures, Adams achieved:
  - 6.5% reoperation rate for one-stage procedures
  - 7% reoperation rate for two-stage procedures

# PREOPERATIVE EVALUATION

- Mammogram within the last year for selected patients: AMA and ACOG[16] guidelines
  - Age over 40 years, or
  - Age over 35 years with high risk for breast cancer, or
  - Personal history of breast cancer
- Detailed breast history, including previous breast surgery
- Understand goals. Does the patient want
  - Greater volume?
  - Greater projection?
  - A "lift" (i.e., nipple and glandular elevation)?
- **Set expectation that asymmetry is common at baseline;** therefore it is common at end point as well.
- Set expectation of reoperation rate of up to 20%.

# SURGICAL PLANNING AND TREATMENT

- Measurements (tissue-based planning)[15,17]
  - Pinch thickness in the superior pole of the breast: Results useful for choosing implant.
  - Skin stretch (SS): Nipple excursion on light traction; provides information on laxity in the anteroposterior dimension[15] (Fig. 47-3, *A* and *B*)
  - Nipple-to-IMF (N-IMF) distance on maximal stretch: Laxity in vertical dimension[15] (Fig. 47-3, *C*).
  - Vertical excess (VE): Anticipated excess skin/parenchyma to be resected
  - Base diameter (BD): Used to choose implant and define ideal N-IMF
- **Determine whether procedure needs to be staged**[15] (Fig. 47-4).
- **Choose appropriate implant material, shape, volume, location, approach.**
  - Material: Silicone versus saline; usually based on preference of patient and surgeon
  - Tissue-based planning to guide choice of implant volume and tissue plane
    - Higher risk of complications with subglandular implants in general
    - Risk increased when combined with mastopexy because of increased dissection, soft tissue disruption
  - Incision: Depends on choice of mastopexy incision
    - Inferior periareolar incision
    - IMF incision for vertical or Wise pattern mastopexy

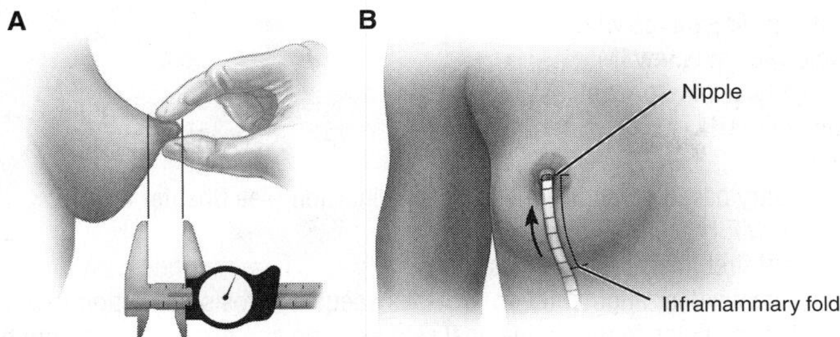


**Fig. 47-3** **A,** Skin stretch. **B,** Nipple-to-IMF stretch.

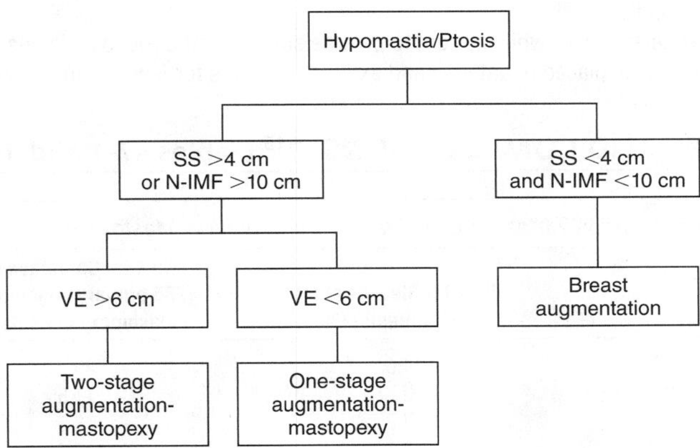


**Fig. 47-4** Algorithm for selecting mastopexy, one-stage augmentation-mastopexy, or two-stage mastopexy. (*N-IMF,* Nipple-to-IMF distance; *SS,* skin stretch; *VE,* vertical excess.)

- **Choose mastopexy incision**[9,18]
  - Periareolar for patients with:
    - Minimal ptosis: Nipple <2 cm below IMF, AND
    - NAC at or above breast border, not pointing inferiorly, AND
    - No more than 3-4 cm of associated breast ptosis
  - Vertical for patients with:
    - Nipple >2 cm below IMF, AND
    - Horizontal skin excess
    - Minimal vertical skin excess

- Wise pattern for patients with:
  - Nipple >2 cm below IMF
  - Both vertical and horizontal skin excess
- **Intraoperative details**
  - Markings
    - Details vary based on choice of mastopexy incision (see Chapter 46)
    - Midline, IMF, breast meridian
  - Place implant first, then perform mastopexy.
    - Determine whether augmentation provides adequate ptosis correction.
    - Tailor-tacking helps to determine final skin excision and prevents skin from being short.[19]

## POSTOPERATIVE CARE

- Consider covering incisions with semipermeable dressing (e.g., Tegaderm) or skin adhesive (e.g., Dermabond).
- Surgical brassiere is worn while upright to provide support and off-load incisions.
- No stress should be placed on internal and external incisions for 6 weeks to allow healing.

## OUTCOMES AND COMPLICATIONS[1,3,15] (Tables 47-1 and 47-2)

**Table 47-1** *Complication Rates for One-Stage Augmentation-Mastopexy*

| Complication | Rate for Stevens et al[1] (321 patients) (%) | Rate for Calobrace et al[3] (235 primary augmentation-mastopexy patients) (%) |
|---|---|---|
| Reoperation | 14.6 | 20 |
| Tissue related | 3.7 | 11.5 |
| Implant related | 10.9 | 8.5 |
| Implant rupture | 3.7 | 0.4 |
| Unattractive scarring | 2.5 | 2.1 |
| Recurrent ptosis or bottoming out | 2.2 | 3.0 |
| Nipple malposition or asymmetry | 2.2 | 3.0 |
| Capsular contracture | 1.9 | 3.8 |
| Breast asymmetry | 1.6 | 2.1 |
| Infection | 1.3 | 0.4 |
| Loss of nipple sensation | 1.2 | NA |
| Nipple loss or depigmentation | 0.6 | 2.6 |
| Implant malposition | 0.3 | 0.4 |
| Hematoma | 0.6 | 1.3 |
| Seroma | NA | 0.4 |

**Table 47-2** *Comparison of Complication Rates*

| Procedure | Number | Complication Rate (%) | Reoperation Rate (%) |
|---|---|---|---|
| One-stage augmentation-mastopexy | 91 | 10 | 6.5 |
| Two-stage augmentation-mastopexy | 14 | 7 | 7 |
| Mastopexy alone | 71 | 14 | 1.4 |

## Key Points

- ✓ The goal of augmentation-mastopexy is to correct ptosis while increasing volume.
- ✓ This can be a difficult and unpredictable technique, because two opposing breast characteristics and forces are treated simultaneously.
- ✓ Augmentation-mastopexy requires excellent patient selection and meticulous technique.
- ✓ Generally, if performing a single-stage procedure, place the implant first and then reassess to prevent being skin-short.

## References


1. Stevens WG, Freeman ME, Stoker DA, et al. One-stage mastopexy with breast augmentation: a review of 321 patients. Plast Reconstr Surg 120:1674-1679, 2007.
2. Spear SL, Boehmler JH IV, Clemens MW. Augmentation/mastopexy: a 3-year review of a single surgeon's practice. Plast Reconstr Surg 118(7 Suppl):S136-S147, 2006.
3. Calobrace MB, Herdt DR, Cothron KJ. Simultaneous augmentation/mastopexy: a retrospective 5-year review of 332 consecutive cases. Plast Reconstr Surg 131:145-156, 2013.
4. Gonzales-Ulloa M. Correction of hypotrophy of the breast by exogenous material. Plast Reconstr Surg Transplant Bull 25:15-26, 1960.
5. Regnault P. The hypoplastic and ptotic breast: a combined operation with prosthetic augmentation. Plast Reconstr Surg 37:31-37, 1966.
6. Regnault P. Breast ptosis: definition and treatment. Clin Plast Surg 3:193-203, 1976.
7. Kirwan L. Augmentation of the ptotic breast: simultaneous periareolar mastopexy/breast augmentation. Aesthet Surg J 19:34-39, 1999.
8. Hall-Findlay EJ, ed. Aesthetic Breast Surgery: Concepts & Techniques. St Louis: Quality Medical Publishing, 2011.
9. Davison SP, Spear SL. Simultaneous breast augmentation with periareolar mastopexy. Semin Plast Surg 18:189-201, 2004.
10. Nahai F, ed. The Art of Aesthetic Surgery: Principles & Techniques, 2nd ed. St Louis: Quality Medical Publishing, 2011.
11. Spear SL. Augmentation/mastopexy: "surgeon, beware." Plast Reconstr Surg 118(7 Suppl):S133-S134, 2006.
12. Gorney M. Ten years' experience in aesthetic surgery malpractice claims. Aesthet Surg J 21:569-571, 2001.
13. Spear SL, Giese SY. Simultaneous breast augmentation and mastopexy. Aesthet Surg J 20:155-164, 2000.
14. Spear SL, Dayan JH, Clemens MW. Augmentation mastopexy. Clin Plast Surg 36:105-115, 2009.
15. Lee MR, Unger JG, Adams WP. The tissue triad: a process approach to augmentation mastopexy. Plast Reconstr Surg (in press).
16. American College of Obstetricians-Gynecologists: Practice bulletin no. 122: breast cancer screening. Obstet Gynecol 118(2 Pt 1):372-382, 2011.
17. Tebbetts JB, Adams WP. Five critical decisions in breast augmentation using five measurements in 5 minutes: the high five decision support process. Plast Reconstr Surg 116:2005-2016, 2005.
18. Kirwan L. A classification and algorithm for treatment of breast ptosis. Aesthet Surg J 22:355-363, 2002.
19. Jones GE, ed. Bostwick's Plastic and Reconstructive Breast Surgery, 3rd ed. St Louis: Quality Medical Publishing, 2010.

# 48. Breast Reduction

**Daniel O. Beck, José L. Rios, Jason K. Potter**

## AESTHETICS[1] (Fig. 48-1)

### NAC

- Normal NAC: 38-45 mm diameter
- Placement at Pitanguy's point (transposition of IMF to anterior breast)

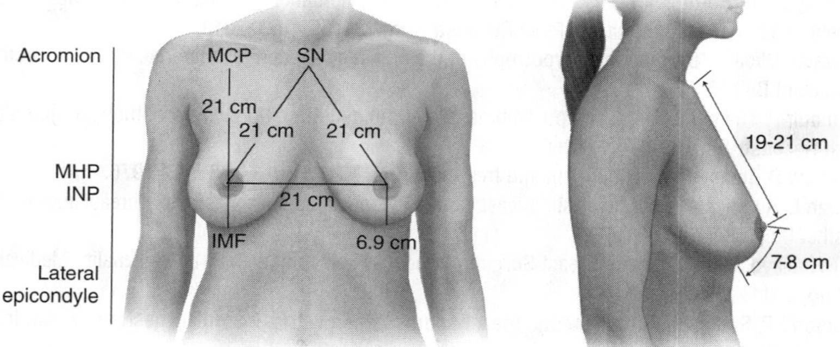


**Fig. 48-1** Ideal breast measurements. (*IMF,* Inframammary fold; *INP,* ideal nipple plane; *MCP,* midclavicular point; *MHP,* midhumeral plane; *SN,* sternal notch.)

### CLASSIC PENN NUMBERS[1]

- Notch-to-nipple distance: 21 cm
- Nipple-to-IMF distance: 6.9 cm

> **TIP:** Many patients need 22-24 cm (notch to nipple) or 10-12 cm (nipple to IMF) range for optimal shape.

## PATHOPHYSIOLOGY OF HYPERMASTIA

- Commonly, normal estrogen levels and number of receptors[2]
  - Suggests **abnormal excessive growth** in response to circulating estrogens
- Primarily an increase in fibrous tissue and fat, relatively smaller increase in glandular tissue

## INDICATIONS FOR SURGERY

### SYMPTOMS

- Back pain
- Neck pain
- Shoulder grooving
- Chronic headaches
- Numbness in upper extremities (ulnar distribution most common)
- Intertriginous infections, rashes, maceration
- Cervical or thoracic degenerative joint disease (DJD) in extreme cases
- Difficulty with wardrobe

### GIGANTOMASTIA (JUVENILE VIRGINAL HYPERTROPHY OF THE BREAST)

- Cause is unknown, and endocrine studies are usually normal.
- At least 1800 g is removed per breast.
- Condition mostly occurs in girls 11-14 years old.
  - Onset is with first menses.
- Regression is rare.
- Once growth ceases, early intervention may be warranted for severe symptoms.
- Surgical reduction is standard therapy.
- **Recurrence** is a recognized risk with pregnancy as circulating estrogens increase.
- Repeat reduction is standard treatment for recurrences.

### EVIDENCE

- **Netscher et al**[3]
  - Symptomatic hypermastia is better defined by symptom complex than volume of tissue removed.
  - There is no correlation between patient's weight and symptoms.
- **Kerrigan et al**[4,5]
  - Symptomatic hypermastia affects quality of life on par with other significant chronic medical conditions (e.g., kidney transplant).
  - Symptoms are more important than volume in determining health burden and surgical benefit.
  - Weight loss, special bras, and medical treatments are not successful.

## GOALS OF SURGERY

- Improve symptomatology.
- Decrease breast volume while creating a predictable and stable breast shape.
- Reposition the NAC in an anatomically correct position.
- Maintain vascularity and sensation to the NAC.
- Maintain parenchymal support for anatomic longevity.
- Resect skin adequately while ensuring tension-free closure.
- Minimize scars.

## SURGICAL OPTIONS

Many breast reduction pedicles and techniques have been described; only the more common are mentioned here.

### Suction Lipectomy

- **Indications and general points**
  - Used alone or with excisional techniques
  - Areolae in ideal location (may elevate slightly with decreased breast weight, but not reliable)
  - Older patients with heavy, predominantly fatty breasts and less concern for cosmesis
  - Patients must understand that breast shape not affected
    - Tendency toward flatter breast with residual ptosis
- **Benefits**
  - Smaller scars
  - Preserves NAC vascularity and innervation
  - Preserves lactation
  - Minimal disturbance of dermal and parenchymal support
- **Evidence**
  - **Courtiss**[6,7]
    - Up to 835 cc removed per breast
    - No calcifications on mammogram up to 2 years postoperatively
    - Pathologic examination of aspirate difficult
  - **Gray**[8]
    - Up to 2250 cc removed
    - Improvement of all grades of ptosis
    - No complications
- **Technique highlights**
  - Infiltrate with liposuction wetting solution (500-1000 ml).
  - Access tissue through medial and lateral IMF incisions.
  - Use 2.4-5 mm cannulas.
  - Postoperative garment is worn day and night for 6 weeks.
  - Postoperative edema and firmness may take months to resolve.

### Ultrasound-Assisted Lipectomy

- Indications are similar to those for suction-assisted lipectomy.
- Ultrasound energy may cause dermal and parenchymal retraction for mild ptosis correction.
- Extensive counseling and informed consent are required because of unknown effects of ultrasonic energy on breast tissue.

### Pedicle Designs

- **Inferior pedicle technique** (Fig. 48-2)
  - Safely remove up to 2500 g
  - Milk secreted postpartum by 72% of patients
  - Reliable technique for maintenance or improvement of pressure sensation to breast skin and NAC[9-12]
  - Pedicle width
    - 3:1 ratio recommended by Georgiade et al[13]
    - 6-8 cm adequate for most reductions; 8-10 cm in significantly large breasts

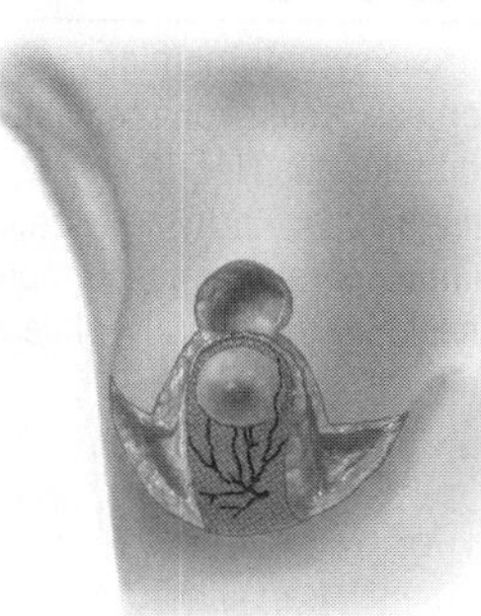

**Fig. 48-2** Inferior pedicle technique.

**TIP:** Nipple-to-IMF distances $>18$ cm may result in bulky pedicles, which may limit the extent of reduction.

- **Superior pedicle** (Fig. 48-3)
  - Perceived to result in less ptosis because of inferior tissue excision
  - Pedicle based on internal mammary perforator from the second intercostal space
    - Travels approximately 1 cm deep and enters just medial to the breast meridian
  - Must thin pedicle to allow inset
  - Tends to preserve breast projection
  - Technique recommended for NAC transpositions of $\leq 9$ cm and resections of $\leq 1200$ g.
  - Poor breast-feeding potential because NAC is based on dermal (not dermoglandular) pedicle
  - Demonstrated the greatest degree of breast skin[9] and NAC[7-9] sensory loss with 1-year follow-up

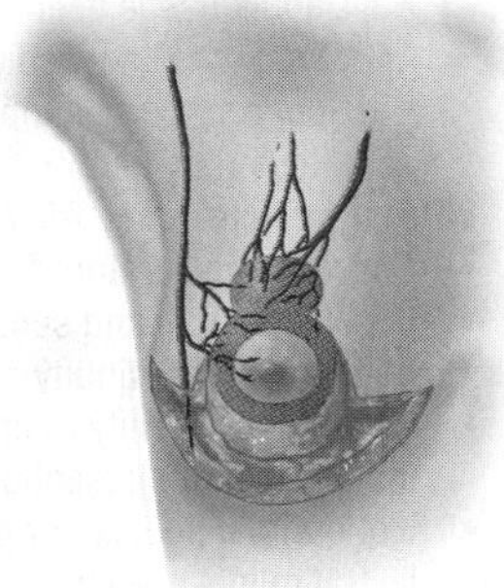

**Fig. 48-3** Superior pedicle.

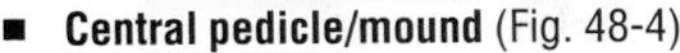

- **Central pedicle/mound** (Fig. 48-4)
  - Modification of inferior pedicle
  - Same blood supply as inferior pedicle but depends on arterial and venous flow through glandular component, not through dermal component
- **Medial pedicle** (Fig. 48-5)
  - Modified from horizontal bipedicle (Strombeck) techniques
  - Dermal or dermoglandular pedicle based on internal mammary perforators from third and potentially fourth intercostal space
  - Safe choice for small to moderate-sized reductions
    - Reliable preservation of NAC sensation shown in resections $>1200$ g[12]
- **Superomedial pedicle**[14] (Fig. 48-6)
  - Transition to a superomedial pedicle can increase safety in large-volume resections of up to 2000 g and NAC transpositions of up to 15 cm.

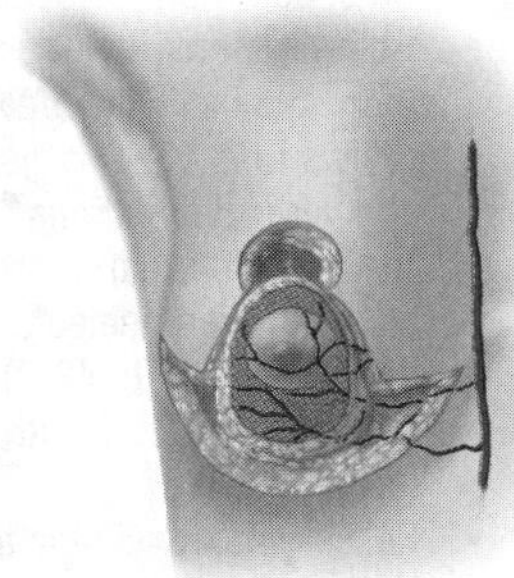

**Fig. 48-4** Central pedicle/mound.

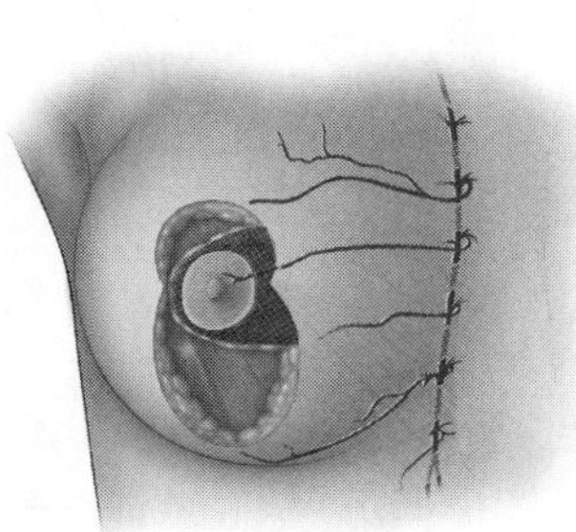

**Fig. 48-5** Medial pedicle.

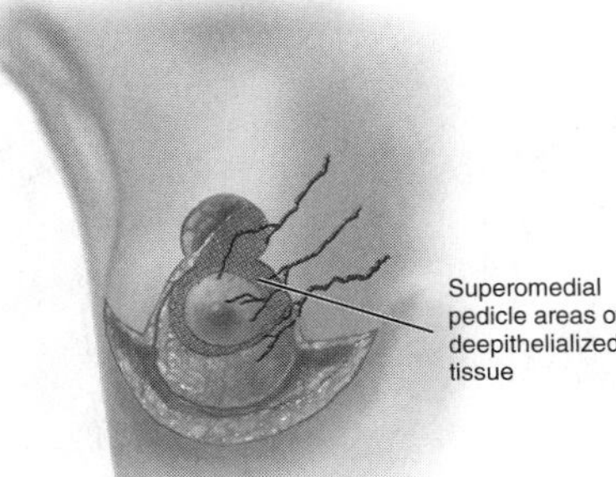


**Fig. 48-6** Superomedial pedicle.

- Base of medial pedicle is extended superiorly, slightly lateral to the breast meridian, to incorporate the descending artery from the second intercostal space.
- Extending the pedicle base may increase difficulty of inset.
  - Debulk tissue deep to the breast meridian to ease inset of stiff or bulky pedicle.
  - Superior blood supply is superficial and will not be affected by debulking.

▪ **Lateral pedicle**[14] (Fig. 48-7)
- Based on perforators from the lateral thoracic artery
- Vascularization and sensation to the NAC improved by maintaining continuity of Würinger's septum
- Advantages: Ability to create shorter pedicles and safety in large-volume resections.
- Not optimal pedicle for patients with excess axillary and lateral fullness where resection is limited

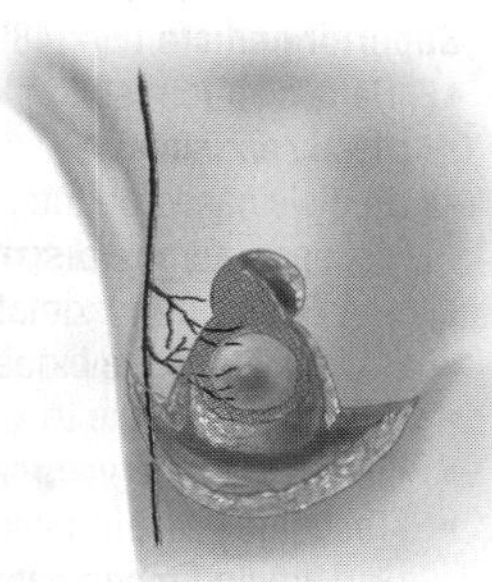

**Fig. 48-7** Lateral pedicle.

## Skin Resection Patterns

In general, patterns of skin resection are independent of pedicle design.

▪ **Inverted-T pattern** (Fig. 48-8)
- Most commonly associated with inferior pedicle
- Relies on integrity of skin to shape and hold breast parenchyma: "skin bra"
- Allows removal of large areas of skin in both horizontal and vertical directions
- Best suited for large breasts or poor quality skin that cannot be remodeled

▪ **Vertical pattern** (Fig. 48-9)
- Usually associated with superior or medial pedicle techniques
- Relies on parenchyma to shape skin
- Up to 1400-2000 g per reduction
- Eliminates horizontal scar
- Requires healthy skin (elasticity) for remodeling
- Dog-ear revision necessary in 10%-15% of patients

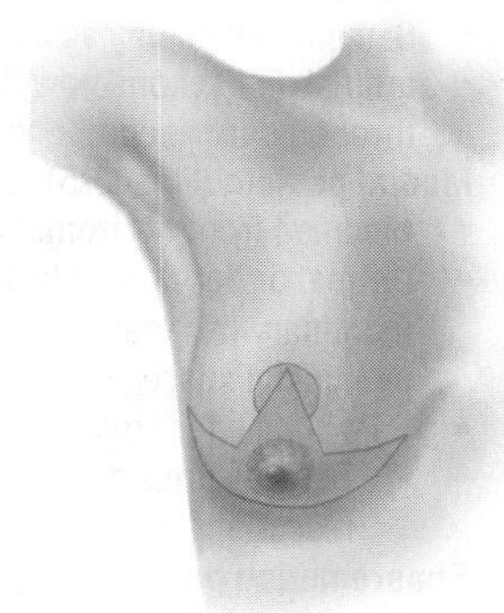

**Fig. 48-8** Inverted-T pattern.

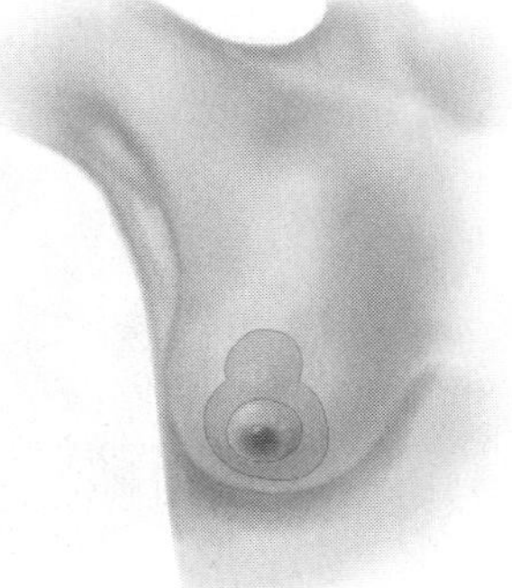

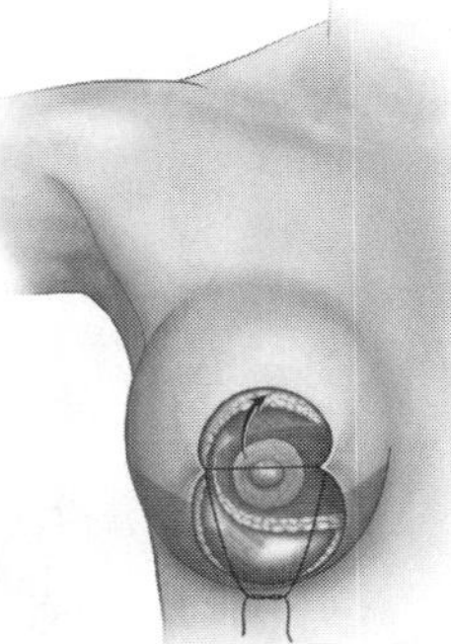

**Fig. 48-9** Vertical pattern.

- **Circumareolar pattern** (Fig. 48-10)
  - Not recommended for breast reduction or ptosis >2 cm
  - Tendency toward widening of NAC
- **No vertical scar pattern**[14-17] (Fig. 48-11)
  - Periareolar and inframammary scars only
  - Ideal candidate has significant ptosis (>5 cm between planned and existing NAC)
    - With <5 cm distance, breast may tend to be flattened or lack upper pole fullness
  - NAC based on a wide inferior pedicle
  - Most parenchymal resection occurs laterally
  - Superior breast skin advanced as an apron and secured along inframammary crease
  - Breast shaping (pillar sutures) often necessary
    - Can be converted to inverted-T pattern reduction if necessary

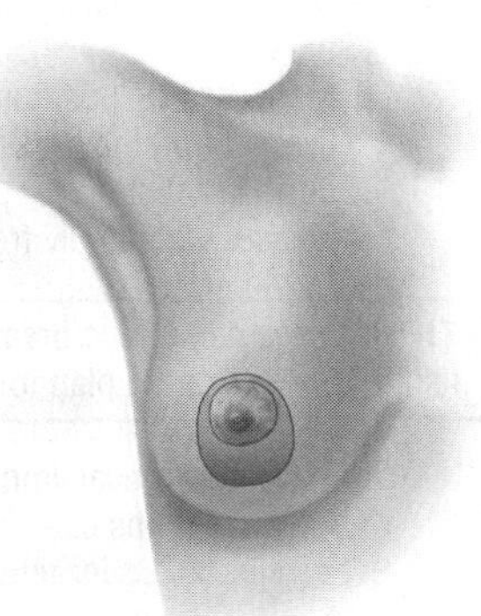

**Fig. 48-10** Circumareolar pattern.

**Fig. 48-11** No vertical scar pattern.

## Free-Nipple Grafting

- **Indications**
  - Patients with very long nipple-to-IMF distances (≥8 cm) seeking small postoperative breast size (B or small C cup)
  - Patients with significant systemic diseases that may impair blood flow
  - Patients with previous operations or chest wall radiation that may impair blood flow
  - Patients requiring short anesthesia times
- **Disadvantages**
  - Possible depigmentation in dark areolae
  - Loss of nipple sensation
  - Loss of lactation potential
  - Poor projection

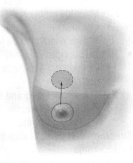

## Techniques[18]

- **Superior pedicle with inverted-T skin resection** (Fig. 48-12)
  - **Markings**
    1. Place patient in an upright position.
    2. Mark the midline.
    3. Mark the breast meridian to determine a new horizontal nipple position.

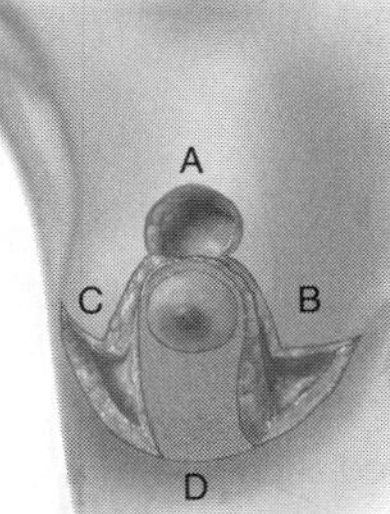


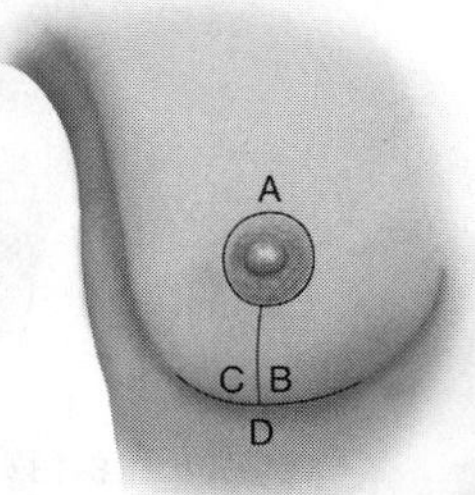


**Fig. 48-12** Superior pedicle with inverted-T skin resection.

4. Mark the vertical nipple location (Pitanguy's point) by transposition of IMF to front of breast.
5. Mark the IMF position, elevating mark a few millimeters onto the breast. This keeps the IMF scar on the breast and not on the chest, because the base of the breast is narrowed during reduction.
6. Measure bilaterally from notch to nipple and from midline to ensure symmetry.

> **TIP:** Large pendulous breasts demonstrate recoil of superior skin flap after elevation of the flap; it is important to plan for this when marking the new nipple location.

7. Mark the vertical limbs, which should measure approximately 7-8 cm under tension.
   - Long limbs can always be shortened on the operating table; short limbs may result in closure under tension, which may compromise shape and skin viability.
   - The angle of divergence determines amount of skin resection.
8. Connect vertical limbs to the medial and lateral aspects of the IMF marking following a lazy-S pattern.
9. Mark the pedicle approximately 10-12 cm from the midline.
10. Mark the areola at 42 mm; replace at 38 mm to minimize traction and distortion on the areola.
11. Mark any areas to be liposuctioned.

- **Technical Tips:**
  - Develop the pedicle before raising skin flaps. To avoid undercutting, bevel away from pedicle.
  - Sit the patient up and tailor-tack, as needed, to achieve desired shape.
  - Hidalgo[19] reviews the inverted-T pattern markings, along with modifications to improve aesthetic outcome.

- **Superomedial pedicle with vertical skin resection**[18] (Fig. 48-13)
  - **Markings**
    1. Place patient in an upright position.
    2. Mark the midline.
    3. Mark the upper breast border.
    4. Mark the position of the IMF.
    5. Transpose the level of the IMF to the breast and mark at the junction of the transposed IMF and breast meridian to determine the new nipple position.

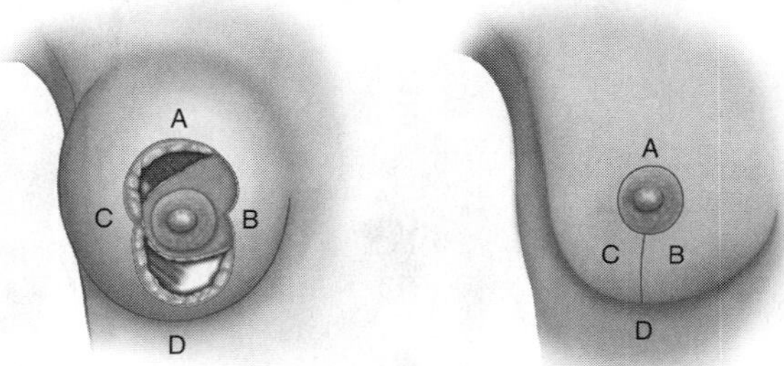


**Fig. 48-13** Superomedial pedicle with vertical skin resection.

6. Confirm that the new nipple position is 8-10 cm below the upper breast border at the intersection of the breast meridian.
7. Mark the top of the areolar opening 2 cm above the new nipple position.
8. Extend areolar markings to create 4 cm diameter opening upon closure.
9. Mark the vertical limbs by rotating the breast medially and laterally.
10. Join the vertical limbs at the meridian 2-4 cm above the IMF.
11. Design the pedicle with a 6-10 cm base; carry base slightly lateral to the meridian if a superomedial pedicle is desired.
12. Mark areas to be liposuctioned.

- **Technical Tips:**
  - **Creating a V pattern rather than a U when joining the vertical limbs above the IMF will prevent skin pucker on closure.**
  - After parenchyma is excised, approximate breast pillars, inset the NAC, and close the vertical incision in a gathering fashion, as needed.
  - Refer to Hall-Findlay[20] for an excellent review of this technique.

**TIP:** Symmetry in final breast shape and size is determined by what is left behind, not by what is removed.

## BREAST REDUCTION IN ADOLESCENTS

- 20 years of age or stabilization of breast size for 12-24 months preferred
- Surgery earlier only if severe physical or psychological symptoms
- **McMahan et al**[21]
  - Study included 48 women whose average age was 17.8 years at reduction.
  - 94% reported satisfaction (i.e., would recommend the surgery to a friend).
  - 60% complained of a prominent scar.
  - 35% reported changes in nipple sensation.
  - About 80% had relief of pain.
  - 72% had some regrowth of tissue; only one had reoperation for hypermastia.

## SECONDARY BREAST REDUCTION

- Causes include recurrence and inadequate primary reduction.
- Revision must be tailored to the presenting deformity, cause of deformity, previous surgical technique, and patient expectations.
- Use same pedicle as that used for first reduction, if known.
- Algorithm for the workup and treatment of recurrent mammary hypermastia (Fig. 48-14).[22]
  - Rule out malignancy as a possible cause.
  - With inadequate primary excision, surgical approach is dictated by the amount of tissue to be resected and knowledge of primary pedicle.

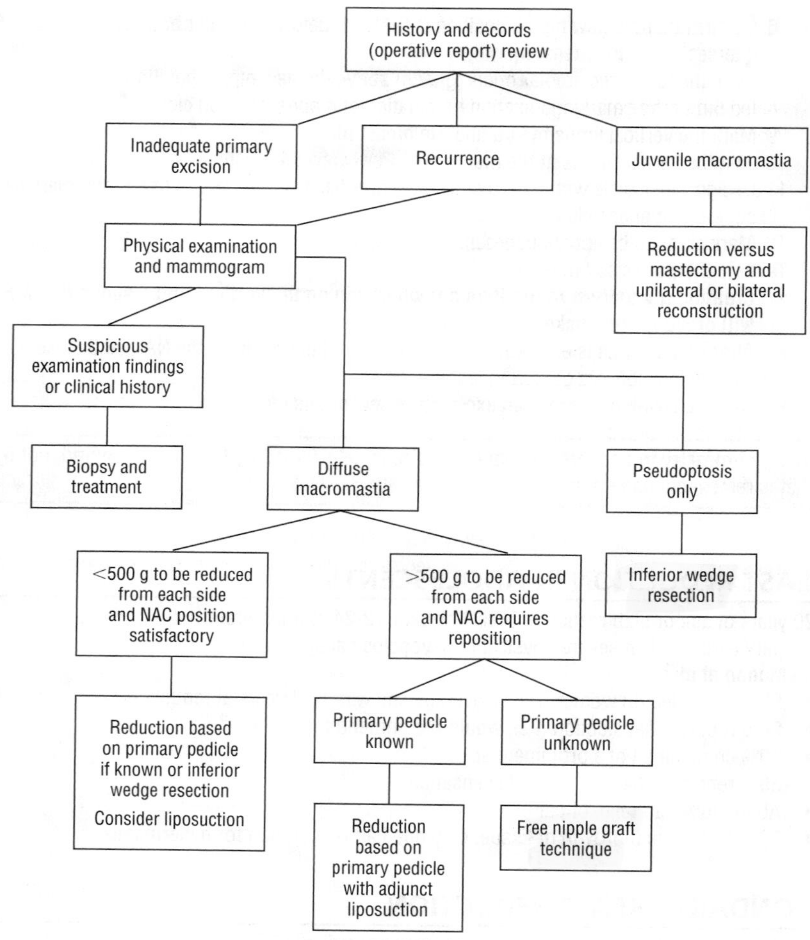


**Fig. 48-14** Algorithm for workup and treatment of recurrent mammary hypermastia.

- Data demonstrate mixed outcomes from use of transected pedicles.
  - **Hudson and Skoll**[23]
    - Two patients had previous pedicle transected; both developed NAC compromise.
    - One of five developed healing complications when pedicle was not transected.
    - Authors recommended free-nipple graft if primary pedicle is unknown.
  - **Losee et al**[24]
    - Two thirds of patients with transected pedicles had a complication that healed conservatively.
    - Authors concluded that it is safe to change pedicles.

## REDUCTION OF IRRADIATED BREASTS

- **Spear et al**[25]
  - No complications in three cases
  - Waited 6 months between cessation of radiation and surgery
  - Minimized pedicle length and flap undermining
- **Parrett et al**[26]
  - 12 patients had bilateral reduction; mean 86 months after lumpectomy and radiation
  - 42% complication rate in irradiated breasts
    - Seroma, fat necrosis, wound dehiscence, and cellulitis
  - 25% postoperative asymmetry
  - 4 of 12 had secondary surgery; 2 for complications and 2 for asymmetry

## BREAST INFILTRATION

- Infiltration with dilute epinephrine-containing solutions (e.g., liposuction wetting solution) reduces operative blood loss.
  - **Wilmink et al**[27]
    - 41 reductions performed after administration of infiltration solution versus 29 performed without
    - Infiltration solution: 0.25% prilocaine + 1:800,000 epinephrine
      - 40 ml to each breast; 20 ml injected to retroglandular space + 20 ml injected along incision markings
    - Reduction patterns; superomedial pedicle, inferior pedicle, or McKissock (bipedicle)
      - Average resection in each group approximately 1000 g
    - Blood loss significantly reduced in epinephrine-treated group as measured by
      - Total blood loss (ml)
      - Ratio of blood loss: tissue excised (g)
      - Postoperative drop in hematocrit/hemoglobin
    - Trend toward shorter hospital stay in treated group
    - No significance between groups in skin flap viability, postoperative drainage, or operation time
  - **Samdal et al**[28]
    - 12 bilateral reductions performed with administration of infiltration solution in one breast
      - No infiltration of contralateral breast
    - Infiltration solution: 1:1,000,000 epinephrine
      - 200 ml injected to retroglandular space + 40 ml injected along incision markings
    - Reduction patterns; superomedial pedicle or inferior pedicle
      - Mean resection: 685 g (infiltrated breast) and 669 g (noninfiltrated breast)
    - Epinephrine use significantly reduced mean intraoperative blood loss to <50% of the untreated contralateral control.
    - Epinephrine use significantly reduced operative time.
    - There was no significant difference in skin flap viability or postoperative drainage.

## POSTOPERATIVE DRAINS

- Studies do not demonstrate lower complication or hematoma rates attributable to drain use.
  - **Wrye et al**[29]
    - 49 consecutive patients with inferior pedicle reductions
    - One drained and undrained breast, per patient, chosen by randomization
    - No difference in complications or hematomas
  - **Corion et al**[30]
    - 107 patients with superomedial pedicle reductions
    - Prospective randomization to receive drains or not after bilateral reduction
    - No statistical difference in hematoma rate complications
    - Overall complication rate higher in patients with drains (40%-23%)
  - **Matarasso et al**[31]
    - Purpose: To determine rate of complications in reduction mammaplasty performed without drains
    - 50 patients; 84% superomedial pedicle, 14% inferior pedicle, 2% amputation-style reduction
      - Average total resection 953 g
    - Six total complications in 3/50 patients
      - Fat necrosis (4%), wound disruption (4%), hematoma (2%), partial nipple loss (2%)
    - No cases of infection or total nipple loss
    - No statistical difference in complication rate versus previously reported studies in patients with drains
    - Concluded that routine use of closed suction drainage after reduction mammaplasty is unnecessary
  - **Ngan et al**[32]
    - Retrospective review of reduction mammaplasty in 182 patients (333 breasts)
    - Age >50 years and resection weight >500 g associated with increased total drain output
    - Pedicle choice and BMI had no influence on drain output
    - Concluded that patients <50 years old with reductions <500 g may not need postoperative drains

## OUTCOME STUDIES

- **Miller et al**[33]
  - 93% of patients reported decrease in symptoms.
  - 62% of patients reported increase in activity.
- **Dabbah et al**[34]
  - 97% of patients reported symptom improvement (59% had complete elimination of symptoms).
- **Davis et al**[35]
  - Patients reported 87% overall satisfaction rate.
  - Main sources of dissatisfaction were breast size, shape, and scars.

## COMPLICATIONS

- **Nipple-areola compromise:** 4%-7% of patients
  - Monitoring options: Clinical examination, laser Doppler flowmeter
- **Altered nipple sensation:** 9%-25% of patients
  - Increased rates with increased amounts of resection
  - Improved sensation in patients with gigantomastia; likely from reduced traction on nerves to NAC
- **Unsatisfactory scarring:** 4% of patients
- **Wound-healing complications:** Up to 19% of patients
- **Breast-feeding**
  - **Aboudib et al**[36]
    - 91% of patients reported normal lactation postoperatively.
  - **Sandsmark et al**[37]
    - 65% of patients could breast-feed.
    - Supplemental feeding was needed in all cases.
  - **Brozowski et al**[38]
    - 69% of patients could breast-feed.
    - 18% needed supplemental feeding.
- **Other:** Fat necrosis, hypertrophic scarring, asymmetry, insufficient reduction, persistent pain, overreduction, infection, change in breast shape over time

## CANCER DETECTION

- Recommendations for preoperative mammography vary widely.
  - At a minimum, follow American Cancer Society guidelines.
  - Many surgeons recommend mammography for reduction patients >25 years of age.[39]
- Send all specimens to a pathologist.
  - Incidence of cancer in reductions is reported at 0.06%-1.8%.
- Obtain new baseline mammograms 6 months postoperatively.
  - Fat necrosis may trigger necrotic changes that are difficult to differentiate from breast carcinoma.
  - CT or MRI can be used when routine screening is unclear.

## WHAT TO DO IF THE NIPPLE TURNS BLUE OR DIES[40]

- **During flap elevation or pedicle formation:**
  1. Cease dissection.
  2. Ensure patient has adequate BP, urinary output, and temperature.
  3. Observe for 10-15 minutes for red bleeding from areola or pedicle borders.
  4. Convert to free-nipple graft if nonviable; be sure nonviable parenchyma underlying nipple is also resected.
- **During closure:**
  1. Open flaps and inspect.
  2. Evacuate hematoma if present.
  3. Check pedicle for kinking.

4. Ensure patient has adequate BP, urinary output, and temperature.
5. Resect more tissue to decrease pressure on pedicle with flap closure if needed.
6. If nipple returns to normal color, close.
7. Options are available if nipple is compromised with reclosure.
   - Convert to free-nipple graft.
   - Loosely approximate, allow 2-3 days for edema resolution, then attempt closure.

- **Postoperative:**
  1. If hematoma is obvious, release periareolar suture and return to operating room.
  2. If no hematoma is obvious, release periareolar suture(s).
     - If nipple returns to pink, leave wound open and close when edema resolves.
     - If nipple remains blue, return to operating room and use previous algorithms.

## Key Points

- ✓ The choice of procedure is based on needs and concerns of the patient. There is no single best procedure.
- ✓ Liposuction alone does not allow control of breast projection or nipple position.
- ✓ Inverted-T skin resection patterns are best suited for large breasts or those with significant skin excess.
- ✓ Vertical patterns use remodeled parenchyma to reshape skin.
- ✓ Accurate preoperative markings are essential to the success of all procedures.
- ✓ **With all techniques, patients must thoroughly understand the extent of breast scarring to ensure appropriate expectations.**

## References


1. Penn J. Breast reduction. Br J Plast Surg 7:357-371, 1955.
2. Jabs AD. Mammary hypertrophy is not associated with increased estrogen receptors. Plast Reconstr Surg 86:64-66, 1990.
3. Netscher DT, Meade RA, Goodman CM, et al. Physical and psychosocial symptoms among 88 volunteer subjects compared with patients seeking plastic surgery procedures to the breast. Plast Reconstr Surg 105:2366-2373, 2000.
4. Kerrigan CL, Collins ED, Kneeland TS, et al. Measuring health state preferences in women with breast hypertrophy. Plast Reconstr Surg 106:280-288, 2000.
5. Kerrigan CL, Collins ED, Striplin D, et al. The health burden of breast hypertrophy. Plast Reconstr Surg 108:1591-1599, 2001.
6. Courtiss EH, Goldwyn RM. Breast sensation before and after plastic surgery. Plast Reconstr Surg 58:1-13, 1976.
7. Courtiss EH. Reduction mammaplasty by suction alone. Plast Reconstr Surg 92:1276-1284, 1993.
8. Gray LN. Liposuction breast reduction. Aesthetic Plast Surg 22:159-162, 1998.
9. Schlenz I, Sandra R, Schemper M, et al. Alteration of nipple and areola sensitivity by reduction mammaplasty: a prospective comparison of five techniques. Plast Reconstr Surg 115:743-751, 2005.
10. Kuzbari R, Schlenz I. Reduction mammaplasty and sensitivity of the nipple-areola complex: sensuality versus sexuality? Ann Plast Surg 58:3-11, 2007.
11. Spear ME, Nanney LB, Phillips S, et al. The impact of reduction mammaplasty on breast sensation: an analysis of multiple surgical techniques. Ann Plast Surg 68:142-149, 2012.

12. Schrelber JE, Girotto JA, Mofid MM, et al. Comparison study of nipple-areolar sensation after reduction mammaplasty. Aesthet Surg J 24:320-323, 2004.
13. Georgiade NG, Serafin D, Morris R, et al. Reduction mammaplasty utilizing an inferior pedicle nipple-areolar flap. Ann Plast Surg 3:211-218, 1979.
14. Nahai F, ed. The Art of Aesthetic Surgery, 2nd ed. St Louis: Quality Medical Publishing, 2011.
15. Yousif NJ, Larson DL, Sanger JR. Elimination of the vertical scar in reduction mammoplasty. Plast Reconstr Surg 89:459-467, 1992.
16. Lalonde DH, Lalonde J, French R. The no vertical scar breast reduction: a minor variation that allows you to remove vertical scar portion of the inferior pedicle wise pattern T scar. Aesthetic Plast Surg 27:335-344, 2003.
17. Keskin M, Tosum Z, Savaci N. Seventeen years of experience with reduction mammaplasty avoiding vertical scar. Aesthetic Plast Surg 32:653-659, 2008.
18. Jones G, ed. Bostwick's Plastic and Reconstructive Breast Surgery, 3rd ed. St Louis: Quality Medical Publishing, 2010.
19. Hidalgo DA. Improving safety and aesthetic results in inverted T pattern breast reduction. Plast Reconstr Surg 103:874-886, 1999.
20. Hall-Findlay EJ. A simplified vertical reduction mammaplasty: shortening the learning curve. Plast Reconstr Surg 104:748-759, 1999.
21. McMahan JD, Wolfe JA, Cromer BA, et al. Lasting success in teenage reduction mammaplasty. Ann Plast Surg 35:227-231, 1995.
22. Rohrich RJ, Thornton JF, Sorokin ES. Recurrent mammary hyperplasia: current concepts. Plast Reconstr Surg 111:387-393, 2003.
23. Hudson DA, Skoll PJ. Repeat reduction mammaplasty. Plast Reconstr Surg 104:401-408, 1991.
24. Losee JE, Cladwell EH, Serletti JM. Secondary reduction mammaplasty: is using a different pedicle safe? Plast Reconstr Surg 106:1004-1008, 2000.
25. Spear SL, Burke JB, Forman D, et al. Experience with reduction mammaplasty following breast conservation surgery and radiation therapy. Plast Reconstr Surg 102:1913-1916, 1998.
26. Parrett BM, Schook C, Morris D. Breast reduction in the irradiated breast: evidence for the role of breast reduction at the time of lumpectomy. Breast J 16:498-502, 2010.
27. Wilmink H, Spauwen PH, Hartman EH, et al. Preoperative injection using a diluted anesthetic/adrenaline solution significantly reduces blood loss in reduction mammaplasty. Plast Reconstr Surg 102:373-376, 1998.
28. Samdal F, Serra M, Skolleborg KC. The effects of infiltration with adrenaline on blood loss during reduction mammaplasty: an early survey. Scand J Plast Reconstr Hand Surg 26:211-215, 1992.
29. Wrye SW, Banducci DR, Mackay D, et al. Routine drainage is not required in reduction mammaplasty. Plast Reconstr Surg 111:113-117, 2003.
30. Corion LU, Smeulders MJ, van Zuijlen PP, et al. Draining after breast reduction: a randomized controlled inter-patient study. J Plast Reconstr Aesthet Surg 62:865-868, 2009.
31. Matarasso A, Wallach SG, Rankin M. Reevaluating the need for routine drainage in reduction mammaplasty. Plast Reconstr Surg 102:1917-1921, 1998.
32. Ngan PG, Igbal HJ, Jayagopal S, et al. When to use drains in breast reduction surgery? Ann Plast Surg 63:135-137, 2009.
33. Miller AP, Zacher JB, Berggren RB, et al. Breast reduction for symptomatic macromastia: can objective predictors for operative success be identified? Plast Reconstr Surg 95:77-83, 1995.
34. Dabbah A, Lehman JA Jr, Parker MG, et al. Reduction mammaplasty: an outcome analysis. Ann Plast Surg 35:337-341, 1995.

35. Davis GM, Ringler SL, Short K, et al. Reduction mammaplasty: long-term efficacy, morbidity, and patient satisfaction. Plast Reconstr Surg 96:1106-1110, 1995.
36. Aboudib JH Jr, de Castro CC, Coelho RS, et al. Analysis of late results in postpregnancy mammoplasty. Ann Plast Surg 26:111-116, 1991.
37. Sandsmark M, Amland PF, Abyholm F, et al. Reduction mammaplasty: a comparative study of the Orlando and Robbins methods in 292 patients. Scand J Plast Reconstr Hand Surg 26:203-209, 1992.
38. Brozowski D, Niessen M, Evans HB, et al. Breast-feeding after inferior pedicle reduction mammoplasty. Plast Reconstr Surg 105:530-534, 2000.
39. Lemmon JA. Reduction mammaplasty and mastopexy. Sel Read Plast Surg 10(19), 2007.
40. Hall-Findlay EJ, ed. Aesthetic Breast Surgery: Concepts & Techniques. St Louis: Quality Medical Publishing, 2011.

# 49. Gynecomastia

Daniel O. Beck, José L. Rios

## DEFINITION

**Gynecomastia:** Benign proliferation of glandular tissue in the male breast
**Pseudogynecomastia** (lipomastia): Excessive development of the male breast from subareolar fat deposition without glandular proliferation

## DEMOGRAPHICS

- **It is the most common breast problem in men.**
- Most males experience some degree of gynecomastia during their lives, but definition and reporting are inconsistent.
- Overall incidence is 32%-36% (up to 40% in autopsy series).
- Up to 65% of adolescent boys are affected.
- Up to 75% of cases are **bilateral.**

## ETIOLOGIC FACTORS AND HISTOLOGY[1-3]

Primary causes are a relative or absolute excess of circulating estrogens, decreased circulating androgens, or enhanced sensitivity of breast tissue to circulating levels of estrogen.

### Clinical Classification

- **Idiopathic** *(most common)*
- **Physiologic**
  - **Neonatal:** Circulating maternal estrogens via placenta
  - **Pubertal:** Relative excess of plasma estradiol versus testosterone
  - **Elderly:** Decreased circulating testosterone, peripheral aromatization of testosterone to estrogen
- **Pathologic:** Box 49-1[3]
- **Pharmacologic:** Box 49-2[3]

### Histologic Classification[2]

- Degrees of stromal and ductal proliferation
  - **Florid:** Increased budding ducts and cellular stroma; seen in gynecomastia that is present for approximately 4 months
  - **Intermediate:** Overlapping florid and fibrous patterns
  - **Fibrous:** Extensive stromal fibrosis, minimal ductal proliferation; seen in gynecomastia that is present for >1 year

**Box 49-1** *PATHOLOGIC CLASSIFICATION OF GYNECOMASTIA*

**INCREASED SERUM ESTROGEN**

***Increased Endogenous Production***
Leydig or Sertoli cell tumors
Eutopic or ectopic human chorionic gonadotropin–secreting tumors
Adrenocortical tumors

***Higher Aromatization***
Aging
Obesity
Hyperthyroidism
Liver disease
Familial or sporadic aromatase excess syndrome
Klinefelter's syndrome
Testicular tumors
Adrenal tumors
Refeeding after starvation

***Exogenous Sources***
Topical estrogen creams
Oral estrogen ingestion

***Displacement of Estrogen From Sex Hormone–Binding Globulin***
Medications such as spironolactone and ketoconazole

***Decreased Estrogen Metabolism***
Cirrhosis

**DECREASED TESTOSTERONE SYNTHESIS**

***Primary Gonadal Failure***
Trauma
Radiation
Drugs
Klinefelter's syndrome
Congenital anorchia

***Secondary Hypogonadism***
Hypothalamic diseases
Pituitary failure
Kallmann's syndrome

***Decreased Androgen Action***
Androgen receptor defect
Antiandrogen drugs

**MISCELLANEOUS**

***Chronic Renal Failure***
***Liver Disease***
***HIV***
***Chronic Illness***
***Enhanced Breast Tissue Sensitivity***
***Environmental Agents***
Embalming agents
Lavender and tea tree oils
Phenothrin in delousing agents

**Box 49-2** *COMMON DRUGS ASSOCIATED WITH GYNECOMASTIA*

**Hormones**
Aromatizable androgens
hCG
Estrogens
Human growth hormone
Anabolic steroids
GnRH agonists/antagonists

**Antiandrogens**
Flutamide, bicalutamide
Finasteride, dutasteride
Spironolactone

**Antibiotics**
Isoniazid
Ketoconazole
Metronidazole

**Antiulcer Medications**
Cimetidine, ranitidine
Proton pump inhibitors

**Chemotherapeutic Medications**
Alkylating agents
Methotrexate
Vinca alkaloids

**Cardiovascular Medications**
Digoxin
Verapamil, diltiazem, nifedipine
Amiodarone
Captopril, enalapril

**Psychoactive Medications**
Diazepam
Antipsychotics
Antidepressants

**Drugs of Abuse**
Marijuana
Alcohol
Amphetamines
Heroin, methadone

**Others**
Metoclopramide
Phenytoin
HIV medications (protease inhibitors)
Stains
Theophylline

## RISK OF MALIGNANT TRANSFORMATION

- **No increased cancer risk for patients without Klinefelter's syndrome**
- **Klinefelter's syndrome:** Risk increases **60-fold** (1:1000 increases to 1:400)

## MALE BREAST CANCER

- Accounts for <1% of all breast cancer cases
- Mean age at detection: 65 years
- 75% ductal carcinoma, 20% lobular carcinoma, <5% inflammatory/Paget's disease, 1% other (medullary, mucinous, tubular, papillary)
- Increased risk
  - Family history of female breast cancer increases risk for male breast cancer
  - *BRCA-1* and *BRCA-2* mutations
  - Klinefelter's syndrome
  - Cryptorchidism
  - Orchitis
  - Radiation exposure
  - Exogenous estrogens
- Diagnostic mammography has 90% sensitivity and specificity to distinguish benign vs. malignant lesions.
  - Positive predictive value is approximately 55% because of low overall prevalence of male breast cancer.[3]

## PREOPERATIVE WORKUP

### HISTORY

- Age of onset
- Duration
- Symptoms
- Medications
- Recreational drug use
- Medical history

### PHYSICAL EXAMINATION

- Breast examination: Fat versus glandular predominance, laterality, ptosis, skin excess, masses
  - Differentiate true gynecomastia from pseudogynecomastia.
  - Rule out breast cancer.
- Testicular examination
- Thyroid, liver, or other abdominal masses
- Lack of male hair distribution
- Feminizing characteristics
- Additional diagnostic tests indicated by history and findings from physical examination
  - **General labs:** Blood testosterone, TSH/free thyroxine, luteinizing hormone (LH), human chorionic gonadotropin (hCG)
  - **Small, firm testes:** Karyotyping, because hallmark finding in cases of 47,XXY
  - **Abnormal testicular examination results or mass:** Testicular ultrasound, β-human chorionic gonadotropin (β-hCG), follicle-stimulating hormone (FSH), LH, serum testosterone, or estradiol

## CLASSIFICATION AND STAGING

### CLASSIFICATION

Webster[4]: Based on **tissue type**

- **Type I:** Glandular
- **Type II:** Fatty and glandular mix
- **Type III:** Simple fatty

Simon et al[5]: Based on **degree of tissue** and **skin excess**

- **Type I:** Minor breast enlargement without skin excess
- **Type II:** Moderate breast enlargement
  - IIa: Without skin excess
  - IIb: With minor skin redundancy
- **Type III:** Gross breast enlargement with skin excess creating a pendulous breast

### STAGING

Rohrich et al[6]

- **Grade I:** Minimal hypertrophy (<250 g) with no ptosis
  - Ia: Primarily glandular
  - Ib: Primarily fibrous
- **Grade II:** Moderate hypertrophy (250-500 g) with no ptosis
  - Ia: Primarily glandular
  - Ib: Primarily fibrous
- **Grade III:** Severe hypertrophy (>500 g) with grade I ptosis
- **Grade IV:** Severe hypertrophy with grade II or III ptosis

## MANAGEMENT

### IDIOPATHIC

- Observation
  - Gynecomastia often regresses after 3-18 months of enlargement.
  - Gynecomastia that is present for >12 months rarely regresses because of tissue fibrosis.
- Weight reduction if obese
- Surgery

### PHYSIOLOGIC

- Tamoxifen (Nolvadex) is particularly useful for "lump"-type gynecomastia.
- Clomiphene citrate is used with limited success.
- Aromatase inhibitors (letrozole, testolactone) show therapeutic potential in early trials but efficacy is not confirmed.
- Testosterone has limited ability to induce regression once gynecomastia is established.
  - Danazol, a synthetic testosterone derivative, has been used with some success in pubertal gynecomastia; however, side-effect potential is high.

### PATHOLOGIC

- Removal of testicular tumors
- Correction of underlying causes or disease

### Pharmacologic

- Removal of offending agent
- Change of medication

### Radiation[7]

- Prophylactic breast irradiation may have some benefit in reducing the incidence of gynecomastia in patients on long-term antiandrogen therapy (e.g., prostate cancer).
- Risk of malignancy with this type of exposure is not defined.
- There is no indication for use in cases of idiopathic gynecomastia.

## SURGICAL OPTIONS

### Techniques

- Periareolar or intraareolar incisions
  - Offer direct access for tissue resection
- Transaxillary incisions
  - For select cases; limited operative exposure
- All types of dermal and glandular pedicles for nipple relocation
- Free-nipple grafting
  - Allows en bloc resection of skin and breast tissue
- Traditional and ultrasound-assisted liposuction (UAL)
  - Basic tenets of UAL treatment
    - Superwet infiltration
    - Stab incisions at inferolateral aspects of intramuscular fat
    - Radial pattern across entire chest
    - Disruption of intramuscular fat
    - Avoid upper lateral pectoral region
  - Dressing: Two layers of Topifoam (3M Corporation, St. Paul, MN); compression vest for 4 weeks continuously, then 4 more weeks at night
- Arthroscopic shaver[8]
  - Allows precise resection of fibrous tissue after liposuction or en bloc resection

**TIP:** Tissue excision and liposuction may be performed as stand-alone procedures or combined in a two-stage approach. The choice of surgical technique(s) depends on the skin/tissue quality and the likelihood of skin redundancy after intervention.

## RESULTS AND COMPLICATIONS

### Excision (Courtiss)[9]

- Overresection in 18.7% of cases
- Poor scarring in 18.7% of cases
- Hematomas in 16% of cases
- Seromas in 9% of cases
- Underresection in 22% of cases

## UAL (Gingrass and Shermak)[10]

- No hematomas, skin necrosis, or other complications
- Results uniformly good to excellent at 4-year follow-up

## UAL (Rohrich et al)[6]

- 61 patients were treated for gynecomastia.
- UAL was more effective than suction-assisted liposuction (SAL) at treating the dense, fibrous tissue common in persistent (>12 months) gynecomastia.
- Overall, 87% of patients required only UAL.
- Staged skin excision was required by 33% of stage III and 57% of stage IV patients.
  - It was performed 6-9 months after UAL to allow maximal skin retraction.

## UAL With Excision (Hammond et al)[11]

- No nipple-areola complex (NAC) necrosis, hematoma, or infection
- One patient each with scar retraction, seroma, access port skin burn, epidermolysis, or decreased NAC sensation
- All patients pleased with results

## SAL With Excision (Babigian and Silverman)[12]

- Treated 20 patients who used anabolic steroids
- Resulted in two hematomas, two seromas, three recurrences

## Liposuction With Tissue Shaver (Petty et al)[8]

- 76 patients of 226 treated with combination procedure for gynecomastia
- Resulted in two seromas, one hematoma, one ultrasound burn, one skin buttonhole, four operations for recurrence
  - No significant difference in complication rate compared with patients undergoing single therapy (excision or liposuction)
- Objective conclusion of better patient satisfaction with liposuction plus shaver

## Key Points

- ✓ Gynecomastia is most commonly idiopathic.
- ✓ Most adolescent males (65%) experience transient gynecomastia.
- ✓ The risk of malignant transformation increases only in patients with Klinefelter's syndrome.
- ✓ A testicular examination is critical in patients with gynecomastia to rule out testicular tumors.
- ✓ Some medications and drug abuse are associated with the development of gynecomastia.
- ✓ UAL is the mainstay of initial treatment in most cases.

## REFERENCES

1. Wise GJ, Roorda AK, Kalter R. Male breast disease. J Am Coll Surg 200:255-269, 2005.
2. Banyan GA, Hajdu SI. Gynecomastia: clinicopathologic study of 351 cases. Am J Clin Pathol 57:431-437, 1972.
3. Deepinder F, Braunsein GD. Gynecomastia: incidence, causes and treatment. Expert Rev Endocrinol Metab 6:723-730, 2011.
4. Webster JP. Mastectomy for gynecomastia through a semicircular intra-areolar incision. Ann Surg 124:557-575, 1946.
5. Simon BE, Hoffman S, Kahn S. Classification and surgical correction of gynecomastia. Plast Reconstr Surg 51:48-52, 1973.
6. Rohrich RJ, Ha RY, Kenkel JM, et al. Classification and management of gynecomastia: defining the role of ultrasound-assisted liposuction. Plast Reconstr Surg 111:909-923, 2003.
7. Viani GA, Bernardes da Silva LG, Stefano EJ. Prevention of gynecomastia and breast pain caused by androgen deprivation therapy in prostate cancer: tamoxifen or radiotherapy? Int J Radiat Oncol Biol Phys 83:e519-e524, 2012.
8. Petty PM, Solomon M, Buchel EW, et al. Gynecomastia: evolving paradigm of management and comparison of techniques. Plast Reconstr Surg 125:1301-1308, 2010.
9. Courtiss EH. Gynecomastia: analysis of 159 patients and current recommendations for treatment. Plast Reconstr Surg 79:740-753, 1987.
10. Gingrass MK, Shermak MA. The treatment of gynecomastia with ultrasound-assisted lipoplasty. Perspect Plast Surg 12:101-106, 1999.
11. Hammond DC, Arnold JF, Simon AM, et al. Combined use of ultrasonic liposuction with the pull-through technique for the treatment of gynecomastia. Plast Reconstr Surg 112:891-895, 2003.
12. Babigian A, Silverman RT. Management of gynecomastia due to anabolic steroids in bodybuilders. Plast Reconstr Surg 107:240-242, 2001.

# 50. Breast Cancer and Reconstruction

Raman C. Mahabir, Janae L. Maher,
Michel Saint-Cyr, José L. Rios

## BREAST CANCER

### DEMOGRAPHICS/INCIDENCE[1]

- 2012 American Cancer Society statistics
  - There were 292,360 newly diagnosed patients with invasive or in situ breast cancer in 2012.
  - 2.5 million people in the United States are currently living with breast cancer.
- The lifetime risk for developing breast cancer is about 1 in 8 or **12%.**
- Breast cancer is the **second leading cause** of cancer deaths in women (lung cancer is the leading cause).
- Rates have been stable since 2004.
- Invasive ductal (65%) >ductal carcinoma in situ (DCIS) (10%-15%) >invasive lobular (10%) >phyllodes (<1%).

### CAUSE/PATHOPHYSIOLOGY[1,2]

- **Genetics**
  - 80% of cases are sporadic.
  - 15% are familial.
  - 5%-10% are from inherited mutations, including *BRCA1*/*BRCA2.*
  - 65% lifetime risk of developing breast cancer if *BRCA1* and/or *BRCA2* positive, and an 80%-95% risk reduction with prophylactic mastectomy
- **Risk factors**[3]
  - **Strong (RR >4.0):** Female; age (>65); biopsy-confirmed atypical hyperplasia; personal history of breast cancer; *BRCA1* and/or *BRCA2;* mammographically dense breasts
  - **Moderate (RR 2.1-4):** Two first-degree relatives with breast cancer; high dose radiation to chest; high endogenous estrogen or testosterone levels; high bone density (postmenopausal)
  - **Low (RR 1.1-2.0):** Alcohol consumption; Ashkenazi Jewish heritage; early menarche (<age 12); late menopause (>age 55); never breast-fed a child; nulliparity; late age at first full-term pregnancy (>age 30); hormone replacement therapy; personal history of endometrial, ovarian, or colon cancer; obesity; height (tall); high socioeconomic status
- **Pathology**
  - **Strong risk:** DCIS/lobular carcinoma in situ (LCIS)
  - **Moderate risk:** Atypical ductal/lobular hyperplasia
  - **Low risk:** Fibroadenoma with complex features, sclerosing adenosis, papilloma

## STAGING SYSTEMS[3]

- **TNM classification**
  - Primary tumor (T)
    - TX: Cannot be assessed T0: No evidence of tumor Tis: Carcinoma in situ
    - T1: <2 cm T2: >2 cm <5 cm T3 >5 cm
    - T4: Any size but invades chest wall or skin (includes inflammatory breast cancer)
  - Lymph nodes (N)
    - NX: Cannot be assessed N0: No evidence of spread N1: 1-3 axillary nodes
    - N2: 4-9 axillary nodes or enlarged internal mammary node
    - N3: 10 or more axillary + mammary nodes or supraclavicular nodes
  - Metastasis (M)
    - MX: Cannot be assessed M0: No distant disease
    - M1: Metastatic (most commonly bone, lung, brain, and liver)
- **Stage:** Assigned once TNM determined[4] (Table 50-1)
- **Surveillance, epidemiology, and end results (SEER) summary stage system**
  - Local: Cancer confined to the breast
  - Regional: Cancer spread to surrounding tissue or nearby lymph nodes
  - Distant: Cancer metastasized to distant organs
- **Molecular markers**
  - Estrogen receptor (ER) status: + or –
  - Progesterone receptor (PR) status: + or –
  - *HER2* expression: + or –
  - Cells without these receptors are called *triple negative.*

**Table 50-1** *Breast Cancer Staging*

| Anatomic Stage | Prognostic Groups | | |
|---|---|---|---|
| Stage 0 | Tis | N0 | M0 |
| Stage IA | T1* | N0 | M0 |
| Stage IB | T0 | N1mi | M0 |
| | T1* | N1mi | M0 |
| Stage IIA | T0 | N1† | M0 |
| | T1* | N1† | M0 |
| | T2 | N0 | M0 |
| Stage IIB | T2 | N1 | M0 |
| | T3 | N0 | M0 |
| Stage IIIA | T0 | N2 | M0 |
| | T1* | N2 | M0 |
| | T2 | N2 | M0 |
| | T3 | N1 | M0 |
| | T3 | N2 | M0 |
| Stage IIIB | T4 | N0 | M0 |
| | T4 | N1 | M0 |
| | T4 | N2 | M0 |
| Stage IIIC | Any T | N3 | M0 |
| Stage IV | Any T | Any N | M1 |

*T1 includes T1mi.
†T0 and T1 tumors with nodal micrometastases–only are excluded from stage IIA and are classified as stage IB.
*M,* Metastasis; *mi,* micrometastases; *N,* lymph nodes; *T,* primary tumor.

## TREATMENT

- **Breast conservation therapy** (BCT) (partial mastectomy/lumpectomy) removes a portion of the breast and typically requires postoperative radiotherapy.
  - 20-year follow-up studies demonstrate equivalent survival of patients treated by BCT and mastectomy. Local recurrence rates are higher for BCT but there was no effect on survival.[4]
  - Contraindications: Previous radiation, multifocal disease, serious connective tissue disorder, pregnancy, large tumors (>5 cm), inflammatory breast cancer, large cancer in a small breast
  - Oncoplastic surgery[5]
    - Defect can be corrected at the time of lumpectomy.
    - Often, using well-established breast reduction/mastopexy techniques
    - Several techniques described, typically relying on rotation/advancement of breast parenchyma
- **Mastectomy**
  - Nipple-sparing: Nipple-areola complex (NAC) preserved
  - Areola-sparing: Nipple removed but areola spared
  - Skin-sparing (SSM): NAC removed with the breast
  - Simple: NAC, skin, and breast removed but no axillary dissection
  - Modified radical: Simple + axillary lymph node dissection
  - Radical (rare): Simple + axillary lymph node dissection + removal of pectoralis major muscle
- **Sentinel lymph node biopsy:** Blue dye and radioactive tracer; 92% sensitivity and 100% specificity when done correctly
- **Survival (5-year):** Primarily influenced by initial cancer[3]
  - 0: 93% I: 88% IIA: 81% IIB: 74%
  - IIIA: 67% IIIB: 41% IIIC: 49% IV: 15%

## CHOOSING BREAST RECONSTRUCTION

- Substantial psychological benefit to reconstruction (immediate or delayed)[6]
- Why women choose breast reconstruction[7]
  - Eliminates need for external breast prosthesis
  - Prevents clothing limitations
  - Helps regain feelings of femininity and wholeness/improved "self-image"
- Why women decline breast reconstruction
  - Fear of complications
  - Belief they are too old
  - Fear it will interfere with cancer treatment and surveillance
- **Contraindications**
  - Absolute: Some form of reconstruction is almost always available to offer to a patient.
  - Relative/increased risk of complications: Advanced cancer stage, smoking, obesity, previous radiation, previous surgery in the area of the donor site (i.e., previous abdominoplasty in a patient requesting to use her abdominal tissue), medical comorbidities
- Patient education
  - Several states (CA, NM, NY, TX) have laws or are developing laws mandating that women receive written information on breast reconstruction before oncologic surgery to be able to make an informed decision regarding reconstruction.
  - Patients undergoing mastectomy must be offered a referral to a board-certified plastic surgeon to meet the standards set by the National Accreditation Program for Breast Centers (NAPBC).

## INSURANCE COVERAGE

- Women's Health and Cancer Rights Act of 1988
- Mandates coverage of breast reconstruction by **ALL** insurers *without specific time frame limitations*
- Includes contralateral breast-matching procedures

## PATIENT SELECTION

- Patient factors: Family support, home/work consideration, function, activities, recovery time
- Stage of breast cancer
- Comorbidities
- Anticipated skin defect (if immediate)
- Patient preference for size of final reconstruction
- Donor site availability
- Size and shape of contralateral breast (consider/offer prophylactic contralateral mastectomy)
- Need for adjuvant chemotherapy/radiotherapy
- Surgeon experience and preference

## TIMING

### IMMEDIATE RECONSTRUCTION

- **Advantages**
  - Typically the best cosmetic result because of preservation of anatomic landmarks and skin
  - Potential psychological benefit and immediate return of body image
  - Single-stage procedure with lower overall socioeconomic cost
  - Best for stage I and stage II breast cancer patients not expected to receive postoperative radiotherapy
- **Disadvantages**
  - Difficult to assess mastectomy flap viability
    - New technologies becoming available that may have a role in assisting with this[8]
  - Risk of postoperative radiotherapy requirements must be carefully evaluated to minimize the risk of future deformity.
  - Increased risk of postoperative complications
  - Postoperative complications can delay postoperative adjuvant chemotherapy or radiotherapy when required.

### DELAYED RECONSTRUCTION

- **Advantages**
  - No delay in postoperative chemotherapy/radiotherapy as a result of reconstructive complications
  - Allows careful monitoring of patients with advanced carcinomas (stages III and IV) over time before performing definitive reconstruction
  - Decreased risk of complications
  - Skin damage of mastectomy/radiation can be replaced at the time of reconstruction
  - Improved body image and increased vitality[9]
- **Disadvantages**
  - Loss of breast skin envelope and natural landmarks (e.g., the inframammary fold)
  - Recipient vessel dissection more tedious because of scarred/irradiated axilla or chest wall
  - Flap size requirement usually greater than with immediate reconstruction
  - Psychological morbidity of living with mastectomy defect

### Delayed-Immediate Reconstruction[10]

- Devised in response to inability to accurately predict nodal status and need for radiation
  - SSM with tissue expander placement
  - Performed when permanent pathology is available
    - If negative, proceed with reconstruction
    - If positive, consider deflation/removal of expander and delay reconstruction until after radiotherapy

## IMPLANTS AND TISSUE EXPANDERS

*Most common form of reconstruction in the United States*

- **Prerequisite:** Healthy mastectomy skin flaps to avoid prosthesis exposure
- Advantages
  - Lower initial cost compared with autologous reconstruction[11]
  - Technical ease (no specialized equipment required)
  - No additional scar or donor site morbidity
  - Shorter operative time and recovery compared with autologous tissue reconstruction
- Disadvantages
  - Early cost advantage of implant-based reconstruction over autologous tissue reconstruction disappears over time as a result of additional revision surgeries.[12]
  - Potential capsular contracture
  - Potential implant rupture or valve failure
  - Potential infection requiring implant removal
  - Increased probability of need for future surgery
  - Difficult to achieve symmetry in unilateral reconstruction

### One-Stage Immediate Reconstruction With Implants

- Obvious benefit of true immediate reconstruction with only one surgery
- Disadvantages: Limited size of reconstruction, less input into final size, insurance companies less likely to pay for later revisions/implant exchanges/changes, higher mastectomy flap necrosis, higher incidence of shape/volume asymmetry

### Two-Stage Immediate Reconstruction With Tissue Expander and Implant

- Minimizes tension and stress on skin flaps at time of mastectomy
- Increases flexibility in choosing final breast volume
- Offers a second surgery in which other revisions can be made as necessary

### Implant and Tissue Expander Size and Shape

- Consider base diameter of breast to be reconstructed (use contralateral breast in delayed cases).
- Consider projection, volume, and shape of preoperative or contralateral breast.
- Most reconstructions in the United States use silicone gel implants.

### Principles

- Ensure that placement of the tissue expander is submuscular (i.e., under pectoralis major muscle anteriorly and under slips of serratus anterior muscle laterally) or partially submuscular (i.e., upper pole of tissue expander is covered by the pectoralis muscle and lower pole is covered by subcutaneous tissue of lower mastectomy skin flap or acellular dermal matrix sling).

- Ensure that the inferior portion of the expander is placed precisely at the inframammary fold.
- Close lateral dead space by suturing skin flap to chest wall to prevent lateral migration of implant and tissue expander.
- Tissue expander may also be covered laterally with slips of serratus muscle to prevent lateralization.
- Tissue expander can be filled intraoperatively with 50-200 cc or more based on mastectomy skin flap quality and perfusion.
- Continue expansion 3 weeks postoperatively, injecting 25-100 cc weekly or biweekly as tolerated.
- Remove saline if there is blanching of the skin or patient discomfort.
- Overexpand 10%-15% beyond final breast volume to accommodate anticipated contracture and breast ptosis
- Maintain tissue expander in place at final volume for 1-3 months to allow capsule maturation before definitive implant placement.

> **TIP:** The expander itself has volume. The expanded volume is the volume of the fluid in the expander plus the volume of the expander. For example, a low-profile expander filled to 450 cc displaces ~540 cc (already 20% over expansion).[13]

## Outcomes and Long-Term Results[14,15]

- Preoperative radiation, smoking, and obesity increase the risk of postoperative complications.
- Diabetes and large breast size may increase the risk of postoperative complications.
- Chemotherapy and hormonal therapy do not have a clear risk of postoperative complications.
- Reconstruction does not appear to affect cancer surveillance or recurrence.
- 88% good to excellent aesthetic result at 3 years
- Satisfaction with reconstruction diminishes over time possibly from the incidence of reoperation/complications.
- Laterality of reconstruction (bilateral vs. unilateral) and radiation history are significant predictors of overall cosmesis.

## Variation for Large or Ptotic Breasts[16]

- Reduction pattern can be designed.
- Deepithelialize inferior skin that is normally discarded.
- Result is a skin flap–muscle pocket for the implant with double skin coverage at the point of the inverted T.
- High rate of complications

## Areas of Research/Development

- Many of these issues remain unresolved; hence preferences will be surgeon specific.
- Human acellular dermal matrix
  - Likely does not have a role in increasing rate of postoperative expansion or reducing pain[17]
  - Unresolved potential benefit to final shape/contour
  - Unresolved long-term potential benefit of reduced capsular contracture
- Use and duration of drains
- Use and duration of postoperative antibiotics

## PEDICLED FLAPS

### Latissimus Dorsi

- **Advantages**
  - Potential autologous reconstruction of small or medium-sized breasts[18]
  - Increases soft tissue coverage when used with tissue expander and implants
  - Reliable, large-diameter pedicle: Thoracodorsal artery and vein
  - Allows versatile skin paddle design that may be hidden by undergarments
  - Minimal long-term donor site morbidity
- **Disadvantages**
  - High seroma rate: Formation in up to 79% of patients; use of progressive tension sutures can significantly reduce seroma formation[19,20]
  - Often requires tissue expander and implant for increased breast projection and volume from atrophy/inadequate volume
- **Variations**
  - Extended latissimus dorsi myocutaneous flap[18]
  - Muscle-sparing latissimus dorsi flap[21]
  - Thoracodorsal artery perforator (TDAP) flap[22]

### Transverse Rectus Abdominis Muscle (TRAM) Flap[23]

- **Advantages**
  - Allows complete autologous reconstruction in many patients
  - Avoids disadvantages of implants
  - Good long-term result
  - Allows contouring of the abdominal area
- **Disadvantages**
  - Donor site morbidity: hernia/bulge, scarring, seroma, contour abnormality, weakness
  - Long recovery time
  - Reinforcement of rectus fascia often required (i.e., mesh or acellular dermal matrix)
  - Higher fat necrosis rate than free TRAM
- **Perfusion zones**[24] (Fig. 50-1)
  - **I:** Ipsilateral to pedicle, overlying the rectus muscle
  - **II:** Contralateral to pedicle, overlying contralateral rectus muscle
  - **III:** Ipsilateral to pedicle, lateral to the rectus muscle
  - **IV:** Contralateral to pedicle, lateral to contralateral rectus muscle
- **Reevaluation of perfusion zones**[25]
  - According to these authors, the ipsilateral TRAM flap side has an axial pattern of blood supply, and the contralateral side has a random blood supply
  - *Their conclusion: Hartrampf's zone III should be replaced by zone II and vice versa*
- **Surgical delay**
  - Optimal delay is 7-14 days
  - Division of the deep inferior epigastric artery and vein
  - Significantly increased perfusion pressure noted by end of 1 week[26]
  - No benefit by increasing delay past 3 weeks

**TIP:** Dissect deep inferior epigastric artery (DIEA) and vein (DIEV) as a lifeboat during pedicled TRAM flap harvest. If needed, enhance arterial inflow with DIEA or enhance venous outflow with DIEV once flap is transferred.

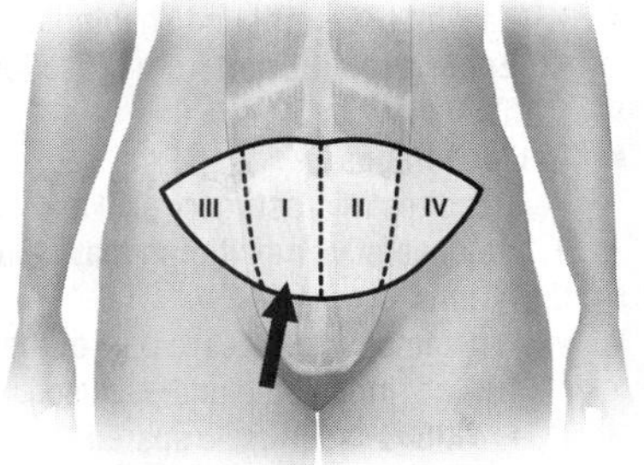


**Fig. 50-1** Classic perfusion zones.

- **Complications**[27-29]
  - Partial skin loss: 3%-25%
  - Fat necrosis: 4%-58.5%
  - Failure: 0%-8.5%
  - Fascial laxity: 4%-29.7%
  - Fascial defect: 0%-16%

# FREE FLAP BREAST RECONSTRUCTION

## RECIPIENT VESSEL OPTIONS[30]

- **Internal mammary (IM)**
  - **Advantages**
    - Easier access for microsurgery and better positioning for assistant surgeon
    - Typically good size match for vessels
    - Allows more medial placement of the flap compared with using thoracodorsal vessels; less lateral fullness
    - Avoids axillary dissection–related morbidity (lymphedema, shoulder stiffness, brachial plexus injury)
  - **Disadvantages**
    - Vessels can be thin walled and more fragile, especially veins.
    - The left IM vein tends to be smaller (or rarely absent) compared with the right IM vein.
    - Respiration changes the level of focus during microsurgery. (Patient vent settings can be changed to high volume low rate.)
    - Future use of IM artery for coronary artery bypass grafting may be compromised.
    - There is a small but potential risk for pneumothorax.
- **Thoracodorsal**
  - **Advantages**
    - Often exposed with the mastectomy/axillary node dissection
    - Consistent anatomy
  - **Disadvantages**
    - May be damaged by mastectomy/axillary node dissection
    - Lateral placement of the flap, increased axillary dissection and morbidity, difficult position for assistant surgeon
- **Alternate recipient vessels**
  - **Arteries:** Thoracoacromial, lateral thoracic, axillary, retrograde flow in IM artery
  - **Veins:** Thoracoacromial, lateral thoracic, axillary, retrograde flow in IM vein, cephalic turned up, external jugular turned down

## FREE TRAM FLAP

- **Advantages**
  - Robust blood supply, less fat necrosis and flap loss
  - Good vessel size match to either IM artery or thoracodorsal vessels
  - Less abdominal morbidity
  - No pedicle bulge from tunneling

- Ease of breast mound shaping/contouring
- **Zones are different** from those for a pedicled TRAM[24] (Fig. 50-2).

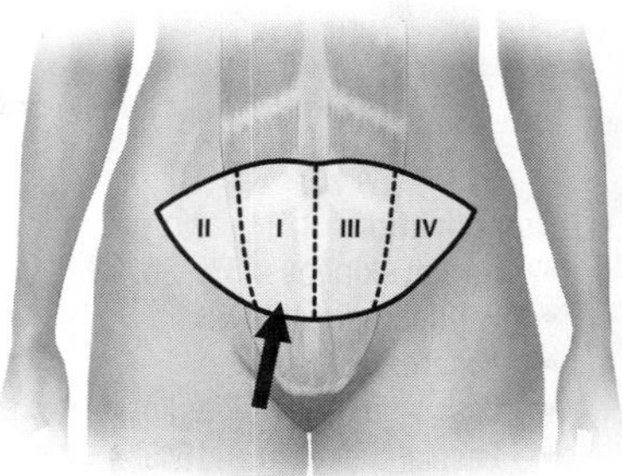


**Fig. 50-2** Free TRAM flap. Zones are different from those used for a pedicled TRAM flap. (*TRAM,* Transverse rectus abdominis myocutaneous.)

- **Disadvantages**
  - Requires microsurgery skill and equipment.
  - Postoperative monitoring may be more intensive.
- **Variations**[31]
  - **Muscle sparing:** Leave part of the muscle behind, innervated and perfused.
    - MS-0: No muscle spared
    - MS-1: Lateral muscle spared
    - MS-2: medial and lateral muscle spared
    - MS-3: All muscle spared[32]
  - **Fascia sparing:** No fascia is taken, or just a small cuff of fascia around the perforators.

**TIP:** Remember, the goal is breast reconstruction. Optimal perfusion to the flap is the key factor, followed by preservation of the muscle and fascia.[33] Improved abdominal closure methods may also help to minimize abdominal morbidity.[34]

- **Complications**[35-38]
  - Noninfectious wound complications may be as high as 28%-43%; however, most heal without intervention or long-term sequelae.
    - Fat necrosis: 3.3%-22.4%
    - Partial flap loss: 0%-7%
    - Abdominal hernia: 1.6%-6.3%
    - Total flap loss: 0%-4.7%
  - Increased in obese patients: Total flap loss, partial flap loss, mastectomy flap loss, hematoma, seroma, infection, hernia/bulge[35]

**TIP:** Dissect the superficial inferior epigastric vein (SIEV) as a lifeboat for additional venous outflow. The superficial venous system sometimes is dominant to the deep inferior epigastric system.

## Perforator Flaps

- **Options**
  - Deep inferior epigastric artery perforator (DIEP)
  - Periumbilical perforator (PUP)
  - Superior gluteal artery perforator (SGAP)
  - Inferior gluteal artery perforator (IGAP)
  - Posterior thigh (fasciocutaneous flap from descending branch of inferior gluteal artery)
  - Anterolateral thigh
  - Thoracodorsal artery perforator (TDAP)
- **Advantages**
  - Less donor site morbidity
  - Less functional deficit
- **Disadvantages**
  - Meticulous dissection with increased operating time
  - Decreased perfusion to flap with less perforators

## Alternate Flaps

- **Options**
  - Superficial inferior epigastric artery (SIEA)
  - Transverse upper gracilis myocutaneous (TUG)
  - Rubens (based on cutaneous perforators of the deep circumflex iliac artery [DCIA] and vein)
- **Advantages**
  - Minimal donor site morbidity (SIEA)
  - No functional deficit (SIEA/TUG)
  - Valuable alternatives for patients with small or medium-sized breasts with inadequate soft tissue bulk of the lower abdomen/gluteal region (TUG/DCIA)
- **Disadvantages**
  - Inconsistent anatomy (SIEA only present in 30%)
  - Vessel size mismatch (SIEA vessels can be small relative to recipient, may be better to use IM artery perforators)
  - Poor perfusion when trying to harvest extra tissue: Hemiabdomen only (SIEA) and limited in TUG
  - Potential contour deformity with high revision rate and risks lymphedema (TUG)

## ADJUVANT RADIATION[39]

- *Postmastectomy radiotherapy increases the rate of adverse events by 4.2-fold in breast reconstruction patients.*
- Postmastectomy radiotherapy with immediate reconstruction: Autologous tissue-based reconstruction had one fifth the risk of adverse events compared with implant-based reconstruction.
- Postmastectomy radiotherapy with delayed reconstruction: A similar pattern was seen.

## Prosthetic Reconstruction[40,41]

- Implant reconstruction in patients who receive radiotherapy is possible but associated with:
  - Increased overall complication rate >40% and a capsular contracture rate >40%
  - Decreased aesthetic results/patient satisfaction
  - 48% need autologous tissue in addition to or as replacement for implant reconstruction

## TRAM Flap Reconstruction

- **Pedicled TRAM**[42]
  - Total flap complications (infection, wound healing, hematoma/seroma, partial flap necrosis, flap loss, fat necrosis) were not significantly different between no-radiation and preoperative/postoperative radiation groups.
  - Aesthetic outcome, symmetry, and contracture were significantly better for no-radiation reconstruction group compared with preoperative/postoperative radiation group.
  - If radiotherapy is needed, delayed reconstruction after radiation is preferred (minimum 6 months), because it results in significantly less contracture and tends to provide better aesthetic outcomes.
- **Free TRAM Flap**[39,43]
  - No statistically significant difference in rates of major complications between autologous breast reconstruction patients who received preoperative radiotherapy and those who did not.
  - 88% vs. 9% complication rate for immediate reconstruction with postoperative radiotherapy versus delayed reconstruction (postoperative radiotherapy).
  - 28% of the immediate reconstruction group required second flap for correction of contour deformities.

**TIP:** If radiotherapy after mastectomy is probable (tumor size >5 cm or + lymph nodes), the best option may be delayed autogenous reconstruction.

## Key Points

✓ Immediate Breast Reconstruction
- Multidisciplinary planning and care are essential, as is the relationship with the oncologic surgeon.
- The importance of preserving IM artery perforators should be stressed (potential recipient vessels and blood supply to the mastectomy skin flaps).
- Ease of reconstruction is dictated by the quality of the mastectomy performed.
- A high-quality nipple-sparing/skin-sparing mastectomy that does not violate the breast's natural landmarks yields the best aesthetic results.

✓ Tissue Expanders
- If possible, tissue expanders should not be used in previously irradiated breasts. The complication rate and capsular contracture rate are higher in nonirradiated breasts.
- Partial submuscular coverage is the most common approach.
- The evidence for acellular dermal matrix use is unclear.
- The risk is significantly higher with previous radiation, smokers, obese patients, and patients with compromised mastectomy skin flaps; consider delayed reconstruction in these patients.

✓ Pedicled TRAM Flap
- The superior epigastric vessels can be very superficial in the rectus muscle; care must be taken to elevate the rectus fascia without injuring the underlying rectus muscle and pedicle.
- Surgeons should consider harvesting a portion of the deep inferior epigastric vessels with the pedicled TRAM flap to allow additional arterial inflow or venous outflow if needed.
- The subcutaneous tunnel needs to be wide enough to avoid compressing the TRAM pedicle.
- Bilateral pedicled TRAM flaps have significant abdominal donor site morbidity.
- Zone IV of the pedicled TRAM flap should be discarded and the viability in zone III carefully assessed, because this flap has a higher rate of fat necrosis.

✓ Free Flap Breast Reconstruction
- Surgeons should consider harvesting a portion of the SIEA and SIEV with a TRAM/DIEP flap for additional arterial and venous options.
- Zone IV of the free TRAM flap should be discarded when performing unilateral reconstructions, especially when a DIEP flap.
- When performing an SIEA flap, only the ipsilateral hemiabdomen should be used. (Tissue should not be used across the midline.)
- When using the thoracodorsal vessels as recipient vessels, the anastomosis should be performed proximal to the branch to the serratus from the thoracodorsal vessel. This preserves the latissimus dorsi flap for future reconstruction, if needed, via retrograde flow through the serratus branch.
- Most free TRAM flap failures can be linked to a technical error. (Kinking/twisting of the pedicle are the most common.)

## REFERENCES


1. American Cancer Society. Breast Cancer Facts & Figures 2011-2012. Atlanta, GA: American Cancer Society, Inc.
2. National Cancer Institute. BRCA1 and BRCA2: cancer risk and genetic testing. Available at *http://www.cancer.gov/cancertopics/factsheet/Risk/BRCA.*
3. Edge SB, Byrd DR, Compton CC, et al, eds. AJCC Cancer Staging Manual, 7th ed. New York: Springer, 2009.
4. Veronesi U, Carcinelli N, Mariani L, et al. Twenty-year follow-up of a randomized study comparing breast-conserving surgery with radical mastectomy for early breast cancer. N Engl J Med 347:1227, 2002.
5. Kronowitz SJ, Kuerer HM, Buchholz TA, et al. A management algorithm and practical oncoplastic surgical techniques for repairing partial mastectomy defects. Plast Reconstr Surg 122:1631, 2008.
6. Wellisch DK, Schain WE, Noone RB, et al. Psychosocial correlates of immediate versus delayed reconstruction of the breast. Plast Reconstr Surg 76:713, 1985.
7. Reaby LL. Reasons why women who have mastectomy decide to have or not to have breast reconstruction. Plast Reconstr Surg 101:1810, 1998.
8. Phillips BT, Lanier ST, Conkling N, et al. Intraoperative perfusion techniques can accurately predict mastectomy skin flap necrosis in breast reconstruction: results of a prospective trial. Plast Reconstr Surg 129:778e, 2012.
9. Wilkins EG, Cederna PS, Lowery JC, et al. Prospective analysis of psychosocial outcomes in breast reconstruction: one-year postoperative results from the Michigan Breast Reconstruction Outcome Study. Plast Reconstr Surg 106:1014-1025; discussion 1026, 2010.
10. Kronowitz SJ, Kuerer HM. Delayed immediate breast reconstruction. Plast Reconstr Surg 113:1617, 2004.
11. Spear SL, Mardini S, Ganz JC. Resource cost comparison of implant-based breast reconstruction versus TRAM flap breast reconstruction. Plast Reconstr Surg 112:101, 2003.
12. Kroll SS, Evans GR, Reece GP, et al. Comparison of resource costs between implant-based and TRAM flap breast reconstruction. Plast Reconstr Surg 97:364, 1996.
13. McCue JD, Lacey MS, Cunningham BL. Breast tissue expander device volume: should it be a factor? Plast Reconstr Surg 125:59, 2010.
14. ASPS evidence based clinical practice guideline for breast reconstruction with tissue expanders and implants (in press).
15. Cordeiro PG, McCarthy CM. A single surgeon's 12-year experience with tissue expander/implant breast reconstruction. II. An analysis of long-term complications, aesthetic outcomes, and patient satisfaction. Plast Reconstr Surg 118:832, 2006.
16. Hammond DC, Capraro PA, Ozolins EB, et al. Use of a skin-sparing reduction pattern to create a combination skin-muscle flap pocket in immediate breast reconstruction. Plast Reconstr Surg 110:206, 2002.
17. McCarthy CM, Lee CN, Halvorson EG, et al. The use of acellular dermal matrices in two-stage expander/implant reconstruction: a multicenter, blinded, randomized controlled trial. Plast Reconstr Surg 130 (5 Suppl 2):57S, 2012.
18. Heitmann C, Pelzer M, Kuentscher M, et al. The extended latissimus dorsi flap revisited. Plast Reconstr Surg 111:1697, 2003.
19. Delay E, Gounot N, Bouillot A, et al. Autologous latissimus breast reconstruction: a 3-year clinical experience with 100 patients. Plast Reconstr Surg 102:1461, 1998.
20. Rios JL, Pollock T, Adams WP. Progressive tension sutures to prevent seroma formation after latissimus dorsi harvest. Plast Reconstr Surg 112:1779, 2003.

21. Schwabegger A, Harpf C, Rainer C. Muscle-sparing latissimus dorsi myocutaneous flap with maintenance of muscle innervation, function, and aesthetic appearance of the donor site. Plast Reconstr Surg 111:1407, 2003.
22. Hamdi M, Van Landuyt K, Monstrey S, et al. Pedicled perforator flaps in breast reconstruction: a new concept. Br J Plast Surg 57:531, 2004.
23. Hartrampf CR, Scheflan M, Black PW. Breast reconstruction with a transverse abdominal island flap. Plast Reconstr Surg 69:216, 1982.
24. Zenn M, Jones G. Reconstructive Surgery: Anatomy, Technique, & Clinical Applications. St Louis: Quality Medical Publishing, 2012.
25. Holm C, Mayr M, Hofter E, et al. Perfusion zones of the DIEP flap revisited: a clinical study. Plast Reconstr Surg 117:37, 2006.
26. Codner MA, Bostwick J III, Nahai F. TRAM flap vascular delay for high-risk breast reconstruction. Plast Reconstr Surg 96:1615, 1995.
27. Garvey PB, Buchel EW, Pockaj BA, et al. DIEP and pedicled TRAM flaps: a comparison of outcomes. Plast Reconstr Surg 117:1711, 2006.
28. Hartrampf CR Jr. The transverse abdominal island flap for breast reconstruction. A 7-year experience. Clin Plast Surg 15:703, 1988.
29. Scheflan M, Dinner MI. The transverse abdominal island flap. I. Indications, contraindications, results, and complications. Ann Plast Surg 10:24, 1983.
30. Saint-Cyr M, Youssef A, Bae HW, et al. Changing trends in recipient vessel selection for microvascular autologous breast reconstruction: an analysis of 1483 cases. Plast Reconstr Surg 119:1993, 2007.
31. Nahabedian M, Tsangaris T, Momen B. Breast reconstruction with the DIEP flap or the muscle-sparing (MS-2) free TRAM flap: is there a difference? Plast Reconstr Surg 115:436, 2005.
32. Nahabedian MY, Dooley W, Singh N, et al. Contour abnormalities of the abdomen after breast reconstruction with abdominal flaps: the role of muscle preservation. Plast Reconstr Surg 109:91, 2002.
33. Garvey PB, Salavati S, Feng L, et al. Perfusion-related complications are similar for DIEP and muscle-sparing free TRAM flaps harvested on medial or lateral deep inferior epigastric artery branch perforators for breast reconstruction. Plast Reconstr Surg 128:581e, 2011.
34. Boehmler JH IV, Butler CE, Ensor J, et al. Outcomes of various techniques of abdominal fascia closure after TRAM flap breast reconstruction. Plast Reconstr Surg 123:773, 2009.
35. Chang DW, Wang BG, Robb GL. Effect of obesity on flap and donor site complications in free transverse rectus abdominis myocutaneous flap breast reconstruction. Plast Reconstr Surg 105:1640, 2000.
36. Schusterman MA. The free transverse rectus abdominis musculocutaneous flap for breast reconstruction: one center's experience with 211 consecutive cases. Ann Plast Surg 32:234, 1994.
37. Selber JC, Kurichi JE, Vega SJ, et al. Risk factors and complications in free TRAM flap breast reconstruction. Ann Plast Surg 56:492, 2006.
38. Sullivan SR, Fletcher DRD, Isom CD, et al. True incidence of all complications following immediate and delayed breast reconstruction. Plast Reconstr Surg 122:19, 2008.
39. Barry M, Kell MR. Radiotherapy and breast reconstruction: a meta-analysis. Breast Cancer Res Treat 127:15, 2011.
40. Kronowitz SJ, Robb GL. Radiation therapy and breast reconstruction: a critical review of the literature. Plast Reconstr Surg 124:395, 2009.
41. Spear SL, Onyewu C. Staged breast reconstruction with saline-filled implants in the irradiated breast: recent trends and therapeutic implications. Plast Reconstr Surg 105:930, 2000.
42. Spear SL, Ducic I, Low M, et al. The effect of radiation on pedicled TRAM flap breast reconstruction: outcomes and implications. Plast Reconstr Surg 115:84, 2005.
43. Tran NV, Chang DW, Gupta A. Comparison of immediate and delayed free TRAM flap breast reconstruction in patients receiving postmastectomy radiation therapy. Plast Reconstr Surg 108:78, 2001.

# 51. Nipple-Areolar Reconstruction

**Deniz Basci**

## INDICATIONS

- Reconstruction of the nipple-areola is usually the final stage of breast reconstruction. It visually transforms the breast mound into a natural-appearing breast.
- Studies have shown that all postmastectomy patients have severe alteration in body image with adverse psychological consequences after being diagnosed with breast cancer.[1]
- Retrospective analyses demonstrate that patient satisfaction with breast reconstruction highly correlates with the presence of a nipple and areola.[2]
- Nipple reconstruction plays an important role in acceptance of the reconstructed breast into the patient's own body image.
- Other conditions such as congenital abnormalities of the nipple, burn deformities, and complications after surgery, including breast reduction, may benefit from nipple reconstruction.

## PLANNING

- Timing of nipple reconstruction depends on the type of breast reconstruction and the need for adjuvant treatments.
- To ensure a stable underlying breast mound, ordinarily wait 3 months after autologous breast reconstruction or 3 months after the second stage of implant-based breast reconstruction to build the nipple.[3]
- Depending on the patient's level of sensation and anxiety, nipple reconstruction can be performed under intravenous sedation or with local anesthesia using 1% lidocaine without epinephrine.
  - Skin flaps after autologous breast reconstruction are often insensate.
  - Expander/implant-based breast reconstruction is associated with varying degrees of sensation.
- Nipple reconstruction is deferred until after completion of chemotherapy and radiotherapy.
- If nipple reconstruction is performed before completion of breast mound revisions, changes in breast shape may result in unpredictable, inappropriate positioning of the nipple, which can ruin an otherwise excellent result.
- There is essentially no downtime after nipple reconstruction; patients usually return to normal activities the following day.

## POSITIONING[4] (Fig. 51-1)

- Patients are marked in standing position with shoulders relaxed.

> **TIP:** Patient participation in determining optimal position helps improve satisfaction with the final result and can involve having the patient place a sticker of EKG lead on the desired position on the reconstructed breast.

- **Symmetry** is the ultimate goal (Fig. 51-2).
- Considerations to achieve proper nipple-areola complex (NAC) positioning:
  1. **Position of opposite nipple:** The reconstructed nipple should lie in the same transverse plane as the opposite nipple. The location is less critical with bilateral nipple reconstruction as long as the nipples appear to fall on the same transverse axis.
  2. **Position on breast mound:** The nipple should be centered on the breast and lie over the point of maximal convexity of the mound.
  3. **Projection:** Nipple height should equal that of the contralateral nipple.
  4. **Size and appearance of contralateral nipple**
     - Base width
     - Areolar size
     - Pigmentation

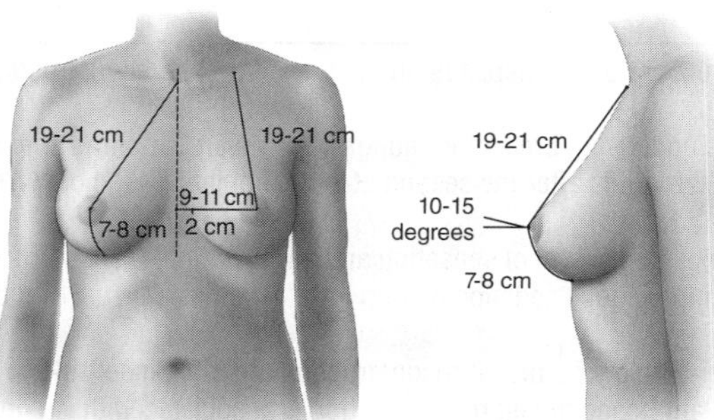


**Fig. 51-1** Positioning of the nipple-areola complex.

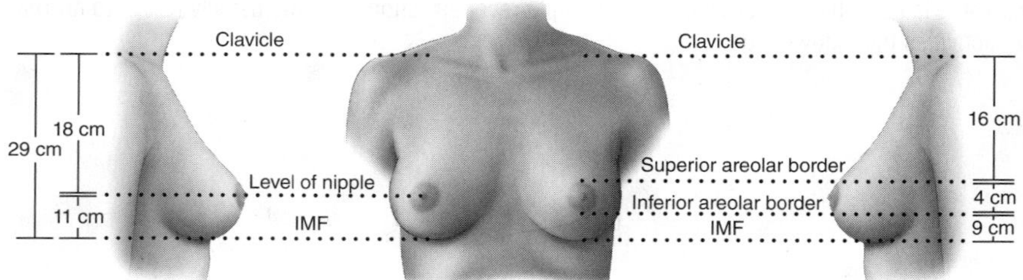


**Fig. 51-2** Symmetry of the NAC with the contralateral breast.

## SURGICAL TECHNIQUE

Methods for creating the NAC vary and include:

1. Local flaps
2. Nipple sharing
3. Reconstruction of areola

### LOCAL FLAPS: ADJACENT TISSUE REARRANGEMENT TO CREATE THE PAPULE

- Transfer of adjacent flaps of skin and subcutaneous fat are elevated to project beyond the breast mound.
- Flaps can be oriented in any direction on the breast and positioned along a scar **as long as blood supply enters away from the old scar.**
- Blood supply is based on subdermal plexus.
- The donor sites may be closed primarily or with skin graft.

**TIP:** The most important consideration when closing the donor site is to minimize tension that will almost certainly lead to a widened scar.

- Increased surface tension at the site of nipple reconstruction is associated with nipple projection loss and flattening of the breast silhouette where maximal convexity is desired.
- Skin grafts that fall within the pattern of the final areola are preferable to spread scars for overall outcome.
- No single technique is perfect, and the principle limitation of all techniques is **premature flattening** from scar contracture.

### COMMONLY USED LOCAL FLAPS FOR NIPPLE RECONSTRUCTION

- **Skate flap:** Predictable, versatile, best for matching a large opposite nipple[5] (Fig. 51-3)
  - A central dermal fat pedicle is elevated from the breast mound with lateral partial- or full-thickness "wings."
  - The wings are wrapped around the dermal fat pedicle.
  - Donor site defect is usually closed with small graft or primarily if tension is minimal.

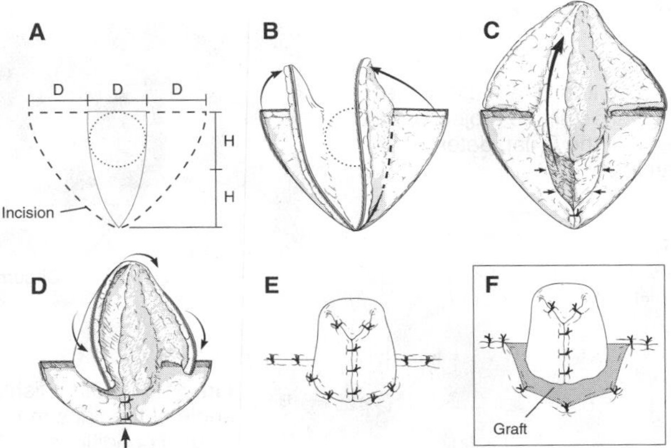


**Fig. 51-3 A-C,** Skate flap with primary closure of donor site. **D-F,** With skin graft.

- **Modified skate flap:** Without areolar grafting[4] (Fig. 51-4)
  - The circumference of the circular skin island is incised; the desired areola is marked on the larger skin island; the flap is designed leaving central vascularized pedicle intact; and the upper semicircle of extra skin is discarded.
  - After nipple flaps are positioned in the usual fashion, the two opposed semicircles are sutured together to re-create a circular areola, and the circumference of that areola is sutured to surrounding skin.
  - **Advantage:** Maintenance of the circular shape of the skin island that replaces the native NAC from skin-sparing mastectomy with autogenous tissue reconstruction
  - **Disadvantage:** More extensive procedure, requires incision and resuturing circumference of skin island

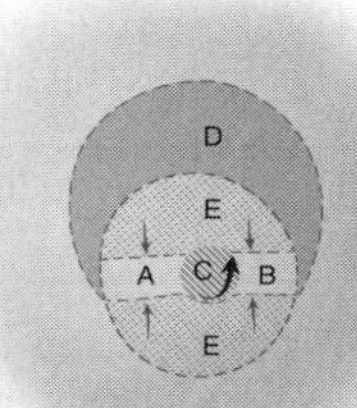


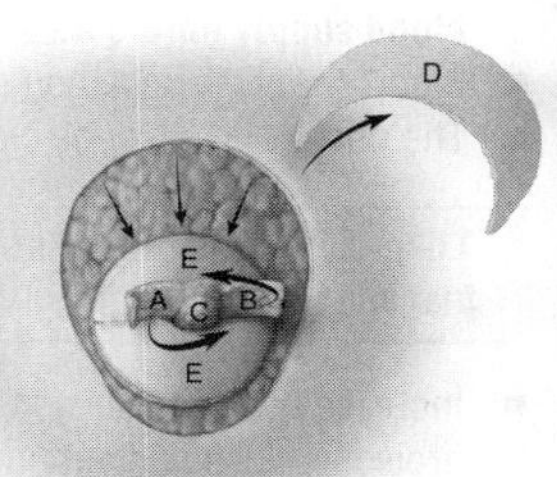


**Fig. 51-4** Modified skate flap without areolar grafting. (*A* and *B,* Modified C-V flaps; *C,* vascularized flap base; *D,* deepithelialized and resected; *E,* new areola.)

- **C-V flap:** Evolved from skate flap, uses two V flaps and a C flap to create the nipple[4,6] (Fig. 51-5)
  - Width of V flaps determines projection, and they are usually designed to be twice the desired projection.
  - Diameter of the C flap determines the diameter of the nipple.
  - **Advantage:** Donor site can be closed primarily.
  - **Disadvantage:** Use is limited in patients with thin skin, because they do not have subcutaneous bulk needed to create adequate projection.
- **Fishtail flap:** Modification of C-V flap[7,8] (Fig. 51-6)
  - V flaps are angulated to be <180 degrees from one another.

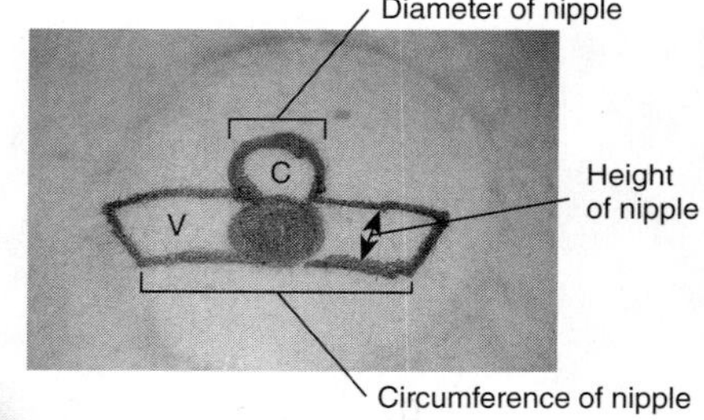


**Fig. 51-5** C-V flap. The width of the V flap determines nipple projection, and the diameter of the C flap determines nipple diameter.

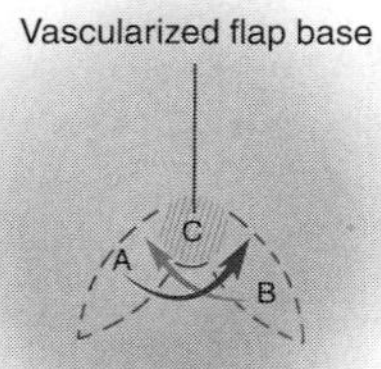


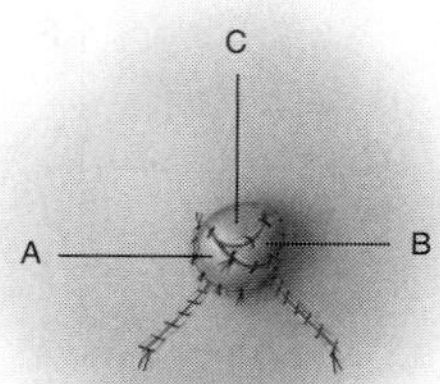


**Fig. 51-6** With a fishtail flap, the angle of the flaps may vary according to local conditions.

- **Star flap**[9]: Another derivative of the skate flap (Fig. 51-7)
  - Tapered arms wrap around a central composite flap to create the nipple papule.
  - Similar to C-V flap, the star has the advantage of primary closure over the skate flap, which usually requires skin graft.
  - **Advantages:** Straightforward design, easy to close
  - **Disadvantages:** Not much projection, three donor site scars

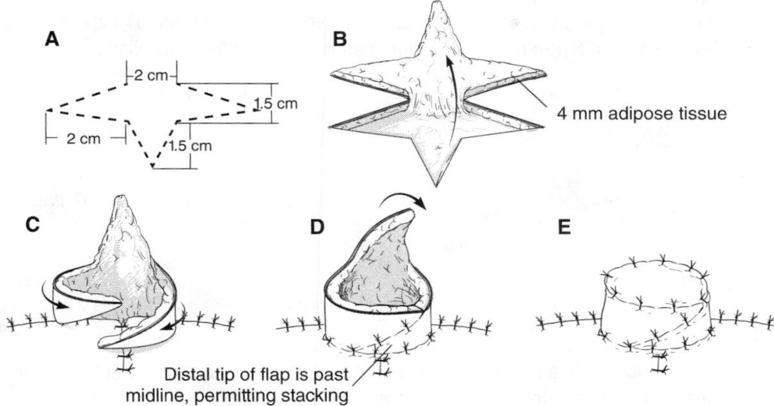


**Fig. 51-7** Star flap.

- **Bell flap**[10]: Useful for reconstruction of nipples with very little (<5 mm) projection (Fig. 51-8)
  - Pull-out flap that is folded over on itself; donor site closed primarily with periareolar purse-string suture
  - Maximal projection of the flap is half the flap length, because it is folded on itself.
  - Length/width ratio should not exceed 2:1.

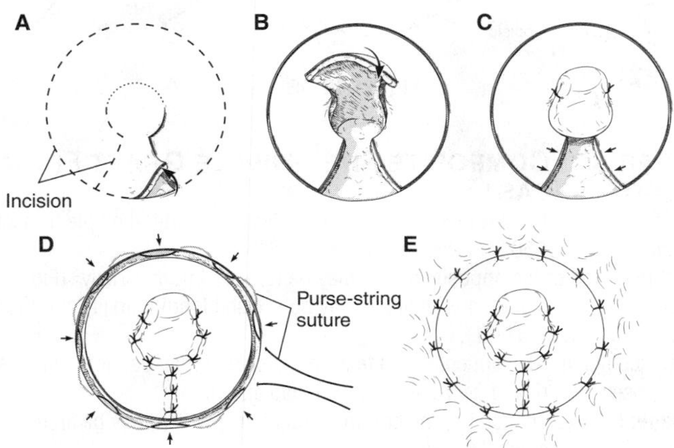


**Fig. 51-8** Bell flap.

- **Modified double-opposing tab (MDOT) flap**[5,11] (Fig. 51-9)
  - Long axis of the two flaps should be parallel to any preexisting scars to prevent interruption of blood supply.
  - Width of each flap should be at least 18 mm. Wider flaps will improve blood supply, but at the cost of creating an oval nipple.
  - Kroll et al[12] argued that this double flap has better blood supply for an equivalent amount of flap tissue than single flap techniques.
  - In a study of 155 nipples, projection was measured at 6 months. MDOT flap–reconstructed nipples maintained 5 mm more projection than those made from star flaps.[13]

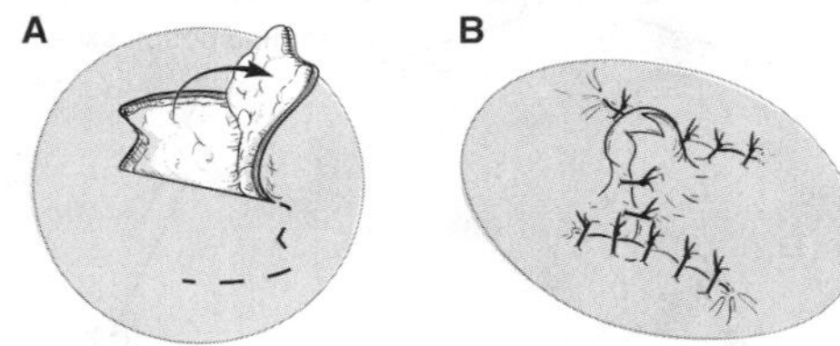


**Fig. 51-9** MDOT flap.

- **S flap**[5,14] (Fig. 51-10)
  - Excellent choice when a scar crosses the proposed location for reconstructed nipple
  - The length of each flap determines the projection of the nipple.
  - The width of each flap determines the width of the nipple.

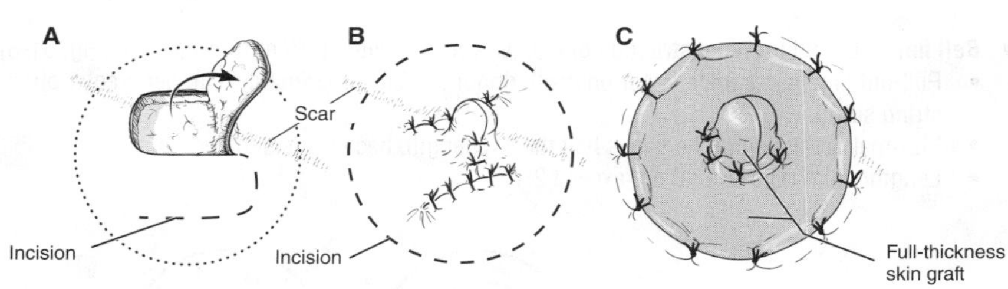


**Fig. 51-10** S flap.

## Nipple Sharing: Composite Free-Nipple Graft From the Opposite Breast

- This technique is considered for women with excessive contralateral nipple projection who are willing to sacrifice about 50% of their nipple height.[15,16]
- The distal three fifths of the opposite nipple may be removed transversely[5] (Fig. 51-11).
- Alternatively, half of the contralateral nipple may be excised longitudinally and the remaining nipple folded down[5] (Fig. 51-11).
- **Advantage:** Results in excellent color and texture match and may be more suitable for irradiated skin, which poses high risk of necrosis with local flap elevation[17]
- **Disadvantage:** Creates an insult to the contralateral nipple, which may be an unacceptable morbidity for many patients
- **Complication:** Pain, loss of sensation, cystic problems from blocked ducts, difficulty breast-feeding from donor nipple

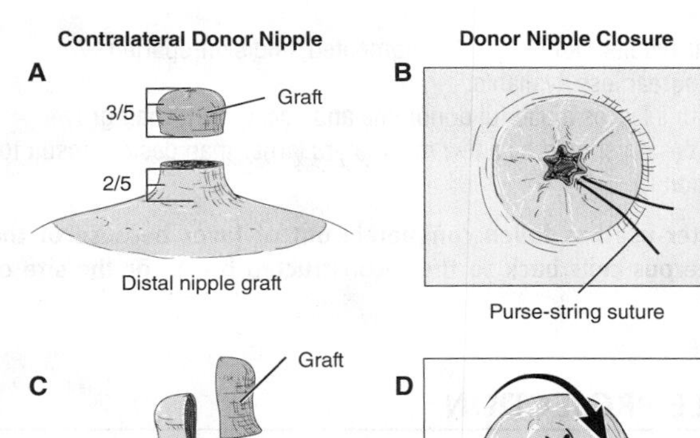


**Fig. 51-11** Techniques in nipple sharing.

## AREOLAR RECONSTRUCTION[4,8] (Fig. 51-12)

- **Tattooing:** Most popular technique, typically performed 3-4 months after nipple reconstruction, when most nipple shrinkage has occurred[18]
- Final color immediately after tattoo should be significantly darker than desired, because it fades within the first few weeks.
- Intradermal tattoos cannot hide spread scars from primary closure under tension, because scar tissue does not reliably accept pigments.
- Tattooing has been associated with decreased nipple projection.[19]
- **Skin grafts:** Full thickness can be taken from a number of locations.

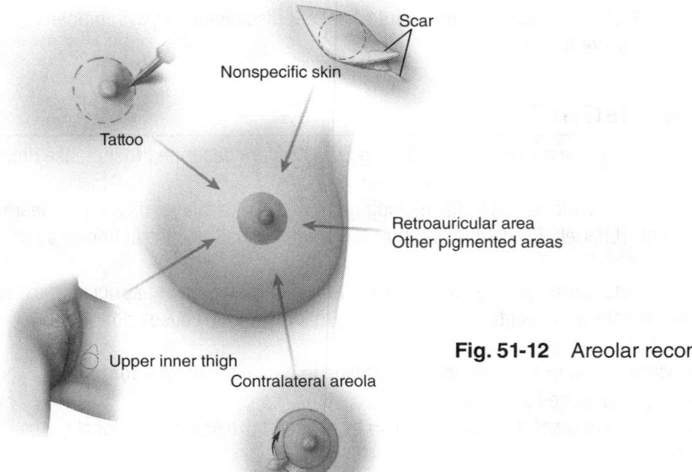


**Fig. 51-12** Areolar reconstruction.

- Lateral mastectomy scar dog-ear results, but skin is not pigmented, and skin-sparing mastectomy makes the lateral dog-ear less available.
  - Upper inner thigh; however, this leaves a painful donor site and occasionally hair grows
  - With skin grafts, the areolar design should be a few millimeters larger than desired result to accommodate graft contraction.

**NOTE: Banking the nipple for later use has fallen completely out of favor because of the known risks of transferring cancerous cells back to the reconstructed breast or the site of nipple banking.**

## RECONSTRUCTED NIPPLE PROJECTION

- Shestak et al[13] demonstrated that local flaps (star, skate, and bell) will flatten by 50%-70% in 2 years. (The bell flap lost significantly more projection than the other techniques.)
- Flattening of reconstructed nipples is thought to be related to:
  - Internal and external retraction forces of surrounding tissues
  - Shrinkage of the flap itself from inadequate subcutaneous fat
  - Poor flap design
  - Tissue memory
- **Most nipple projection loss occurs within the first 2 months postoperatively.**[13]
- Kroll[11] suggested that increasing flap width is the most important factor for obtaining long-term projection because of increased blood supply to reduce the risk of fat necrosis.

**NOTE: A common practice is to overbuild the nipple relative to the opposite nipple in anticipation of decreased long-term projection.**[20]

- It is easier to reduce the size of a reconstructed nipple during a secondary procedure than it is to increase it.

> **TIP:** The immediate postoperative nipple should be twice the desired final height.

- Jabor et al[21] showed that the principle determinant of patient dissatisfaction with nipple reconstruction is **excessive flattening.**

## IMPROVING PROJECTION

Because reconstructed nipples tend to shrink, multiple techniques are described to increase nipple projection.

- Nipple augmentation with various materials, including fat, dermis, cartilage, tissue-engineered cartilage, or AlloDerm (LifeCell, Branchburg, NJ) at the time of initial reconstruction or as a secondary procedure[22-25]
- Brent and Bostwick[26] and more recently Tanabe et al[27] reported on the use of auricular cartilage with local flaps to enhance and maintain projection, but this technique causes donor site morbidity.
- Cao et al[28] used experimental tissue-engineered cartilage to create an implant for nipple structure. Shape was maintained at 10 weeks.
- Nahabedian[29] described successful use of AlloDerm to augment projection with local tissue advancement flap.
  - Placement of a small piece of AlloDerm between apposing skin flaps
  - 38%-50% shrinkage of nipple at 6 months with this technique (less than historical controls)
  - Suggests AlloDerm may contribute to longevity and stability of reconstructed nipple projection

- Polyurethane implants and various other fillers have also been described to enhance projection with varied success; some reported difficulties in foreign-body implantation.[30]

> **TIP:** Avoid postoperative dressings that apply direct pressure on the nipple; this may contribute to fat necrosis and loss of nipple projection.

## COMPLICATIONS IN NAC RECONSTRUCTION

- Complications are uncommon but usually involve partial or total nipple necrosis.
- Wound-healing complications from ischemia of the reconstructed nipple result in increased wound contraction.
- Ischemic complications are unrelated to autologous vs. implant-based reconstruction.
- Incidence of tissue necrosis or delayed healing is higher with nipple reconstruction after radiotherapy than in nonirradiated patients.[31]
- Draper et al[31] demonstrated 22% wound-healing complication rate in patients with a history of radiotherapy.

## FLAT OR INVERTED NIPPLES

- Up to 10% of female population has flat or inverted nipples, either unilateral or bilateral.
- It is most commonly congenital, but nipple inversion can be secondary to mastitis, macromastia, breast reduction surgery, or carcinoma.[25]
- The condition presents cosmetic concerns and may interfere with ability to breast-feed.
- The anatomic defect is the **relative shortness of the lactiferous ducts,** which tethers the nipple and prevents projection, and the **paucity of normal dense collagenous tissue** surrounding the ducts.[32]
- Degree of severity is related to extent of retraction beneath the nipple and amount of dense connective tissue beneath the nipple to help with protrusion.
- In 1999 Han and Hong[33] described a grading scale of the inverted nipple.
  - Grade I: Nipple can be easily pulled out manually and maintains projection without traction.
    - Minimal or no fibrosis
    - No soft tissue deficiency
    - Normal lactiferous ducts
  - Grade II: Nipple can be pulled out manually but with less ease than grade I and tends to retract because of difficulty maintaining protrusion.
    - Fibrosis is moderate.
    - Lactiferous ducts retracted but do not need to be cut for release of fibrosis.
  - Grade III: Nipple is inverted, difficult to pull out manually, and promptly retracts.
    - Significant fibrosis, atrophic terminal duct lobular units
    - Short, retracted lactiferous ducts
    - Insufficient soft tissue bulk
- **Principles for treating this condition include**[25,34,35]**:**
  - Creation of tightness at the neck of the inverted nipple using a purse-string suture
  - Addition of bulk beneath the nipple (after sacrifice of the ductal system) using cartilage or adjacent dermal fat flaps
  - Release of the pathologic fibrous bands with or without disturbing the lactiferous ducts
  - Recurrence rates are variable but are lower when lactiferous ducts are released, although this precludes future lactation.[36]

## KEY POINTS

- ✓ Creation of an NAC is the final, essential step to reconstruction of a natural-looking breast.
- ✓ The benchmark for nipple reconstruction is not yet established.
- ✓ Patient participation in determining optimal position helps improve satisfaction with the final result.
- ✓ Numerous techniques of nipple reconstruction have been described, all of which are plagued with eventual loss of long-term projection of up to 50%-70%.
- ✓ The immediate postoperative reconstructed nipple should be twice the desired final height.
- ✓ Nipple reconstruction should be performed when there is reasonable symmetry between the two stable breast mounds and proper position can be more precisely determined.
- ✓ Composite graft of the contralateral nipple provides excellent texture and color match but comes at the cost of a reduced and scarred opposite nipple, which could lead to sensory deficits—an unacceptable morbidity for many women.
- ✓ The skate flap is the best for matching a large contralateral nipple.
- ✓ Closure of the donor site of a local flap under tension can result in stretched scar, which is unfavorable for tattooing, whereas well-healed, full-thickness skin graft is a far better recipient for tattoo.
- ✓ Prior radiotherapy creates a high risk of complications with nipple reconstruction.

## REFERENCES


1. Wilkins EG, Cederna PS, Lowery JC, et al. Prospective analysis of psychological outcomes in breast reconstruction: one year post-operative results from the Michigan Breast Reconstruction Outcome Study. Plast Reconstr Surg 106:1014-1025, 2000.
2. Wellisch DK, Schain WS, Noone RB, et al. The psychological contribution of nipple addition in breast reconstruction. Plast Reconstr Surg 80:699-704, 1987.
3. Nahabedian MY. Nipple reconstruction. Clin Plast Surg 34:131-137, 2007.
4. Bostwick J. Nipple areolar reconstruction. In Jones G, ed. Bostwick's Plastic & Reconstructive Breast Surgery, 3rd ed. St Louis: Quality Medical Publishing, 2010.
5. Spear SL, Little JW, Bogue DP. Nipple areola reconstruction. In Spear SL, ed. Surgery of the Breast: Principles and Art, 3rd ed. Philadelphia: Lippincott Williams & Wilkins, 2011.
6. Losken A, Mackay GJ, Bostwick J. Nipple reconstruction using the C-V flap technique: a long-term evaluation. Plast Reconstr Surg 108:361-369, 2001.
7. Strauch B, Vasconez LO, Hall-Findlay EJ, et al, eds. Grabb's Encyclopedia of Flaps. Philadelphia: Lippincott Williams & Wilkins, 2009.
8. Jones GE, ed. Bostwick's Plastic and Reconstructive Breast Surgery, 3rd ed. St Louis: Quality Medical Publishing, 2010.
9. Hartrampf CR, Culbertson JH. A dermal-fat flap for nipple reconstruction. Plast Reconstr Surg 73:982-986, 1984.
10. Eng JS. Bell flap nipple reconstruction—a new wrinkle. Ann Plast Surg 36:485-488, 1996.
11. Kroll S. Nipple reconstruction with the double opposing tab flap. Plast Reconstr Surg 104:511-514, 1999.
12. Kroll SS, Reece GP, Miller MI, et al. Comparison of nipple projection with the modified double apposing tab and star flaps. Plast Reconstr Surg 99:1602-1605, 1997.
13. Shestak KC, Gabriel A, Landecker A, et al. Assessment of long-term nipple projection: a comparison of three techniques. Plast Reconstr Surg 110:780-786, 2002.

14. Cronin E, Humphreys D, Ruiz-Razura A. Nipple reconstruction: the S flap. Plast Reconstr Surg 81:783-787, 1988.
15. Bhatty MA, Berry RB. Nipple-areola reconstruction by tattooing and nipple sharing. Br J Plast Surg 50:331-334, 1997.
16. Sakai S, Taneda H. New nipple-sparing technique that preserves the anatomic structure of the donor nipple for breastfeeding. Aesthetic Plast Surg 36:308-312, 2012.
17. Spear SL, Schaffner AD, Jesperson MR, et al. Donor-site morbidity and patient satisfaction using a composite nipple graft for unilateral nipple reconstruction in the radiated and nonradiated breast. Plast Reconstr Surg 127:1437-1446, 2011.
18. Spear SL, Aria J. Long-term experience with nipple-areola tattooing. Ann Plast Surg 35:232-236, 1995.
19. Beahin E. Decreased nipple projection following tattoo. Presented at the Twenty-fourth Annual Meeting of the American Society for Reconstructive Microsurgery, Beverly Hills, CA, Jan 2008.
20. Few JW, Markus JR, Casa LA, et al. Long-term predictable nipple projection following reconstruction. Plast Reconstr Surg 104:1321-1324, 1999.
21. Jabor MA, Shayni M, Collins DR, et al. Nipple-areolar reconstruction: satisfaction and clinical determinants. Plast Reconstr Surg 110:457-463, 2002.
22. Garramone CE, Lam B. Use of AlloDerm in primary nipple reconstruction to improve long-term nipple projection. Plast Reconstr Surg 119:1663-1668, 2007.
23. Bernard RW, Beran SJ. Autologous fat graft in nipple reconstruction. Plast Reconstr Surg 112:964-968, 2003.
24. Panettiere P, Marchetti I, Accorsi D. Filler injection enhances the projection of reconstructed nipple: an original easy technique. Aesthetic Plast Surg 29:287-294, 2005.
25. Evans KK, Rasko Y, Lenert J, et al. The use of calcium hydroxyapatite for nipple projection after failed nipple-areolar reconstruction: early results. Ann Plast Surg 55:25-29, 2005.
26. Brent B, Bostwick J. Nipple-areolar reconstruction with auricular tissues. Plast Reconstr Surg 60:353-361, 1977.
27. Tanabe HY, Tai Y, Kiyokawa K, et al. Nipple-areola reconstruction with a dermal fat flap and rolled auricular cartilage. Plast Reconstr Surg 100:431-438, 1997.
28. Cao YI, Lach F, Kim TH, et al. Tissue-engineered nipple reconstruction. Plast Reconstr Surg 102:2293-2298, 1998.
29. Nahabedian MY. Secondary nipple reconstruction with local flaps and AlloDerm. Plast Reconstr Surg 115:2056-2061, 2005.
30. Hallock GG. Polyurethane nipple prosthesis. Ann Plast Surg 24:80-85, 1990.
31. Draper LB, Bui DT, Chin ES, et al. Nipple-areola reconstruction following chest-wall irradiation for breast cancer: is it safe? Ann Plast Surg 55:12-15, 2005.
32. Schwager RG, Smith JW, Gray GF, et al. Inversion of the human female nipple, with a simple method of treatment. Plast Reconstr Surg 54:564-569, 1974.
33. Han S, Hong Y. The inverted nipple: its grading and surgical correction. Plast Reconstr Surg 104:389-395, 1999.
34. Pribaz JJ, Pousti T. Correction of recurrent nipple inversion with cartilage graft. Ann Plast Surg 40: 14-17, 1998.
35. Teimourian B, Adham MN. Simple technique for correction of inverted nipple. Plast Reconstr Surg 65:504-506, 1980.
36. Elsahy NI. An alternative operation for inverted nipple. Plast Reconstr Surg 57:438-491, 1976.

# Part V

## Trunk and Lower Extremity

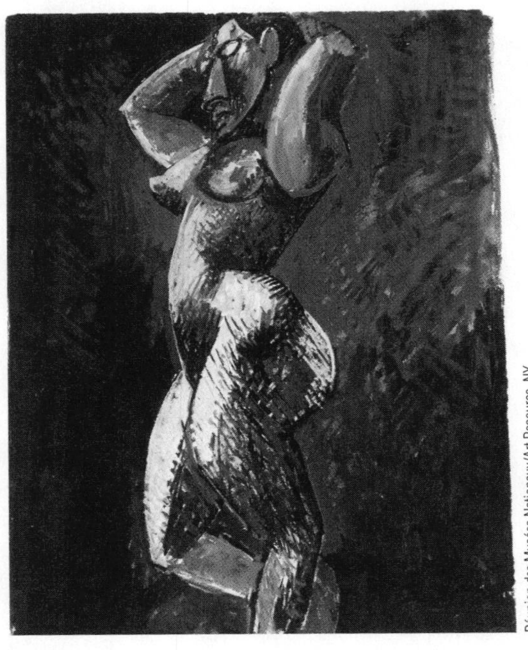

Part V opening art: Picasso, Pablo (1881-1973) © Artist Rights Society (ARS), NY. Nude With Raised Arms. Gouache on paper. Photo: JG Berizzi. Musée Picasso, Paris, France. Photo Credit: Réunion des Musées Nationaux/Art Resource, NY. © 2006 Estate of Pablo Picasso/ARS, New York.

# 52. Chest Wall Reconstruction

Jeffrey E. Janis, Adam H. Hamawy

## ANATOMY

### Pleural Cavity

- Visceral pleura
- Parietal pleura

**NOTE: Separate embryologic origins will result in anatomic differences between the visceral pleura and the parietal pleura, including arterial supplies, venous and lymphatic drainage patterns, and innervations.[1]**

### Thoracic Skeleton (Fig. 52-1)

- **Purposes**
  - Provides stable skeletal support
  - Protects vital organs (e.g., heart, lungs, great vessels, and some abdominal organs)
  - Contributes to respiratory function
  - Supports the upper extremities
- **Structures**
  - **12 paired ribs**
    - **True ribs,** or *vertebrosternal ribs (1-7, sometimes 8)*
      - Articulate directly with the sternum through costal cartilages
    - **False ribs,** or *vertebrochondral ribs (8-12)*
      - Connect with the costal cartilages superior to them rather than connecting directly to the sternum
    - **Floating ribs,** or *vertebral ribs (11 and 12)*
      - Do not communicate directly with either the sternum or the ribs superior to them
      - Articulate only with their own vertebral bodies
  - **Sternum**
    - Large, elongated, flat bone approximately 15-20 cm in length

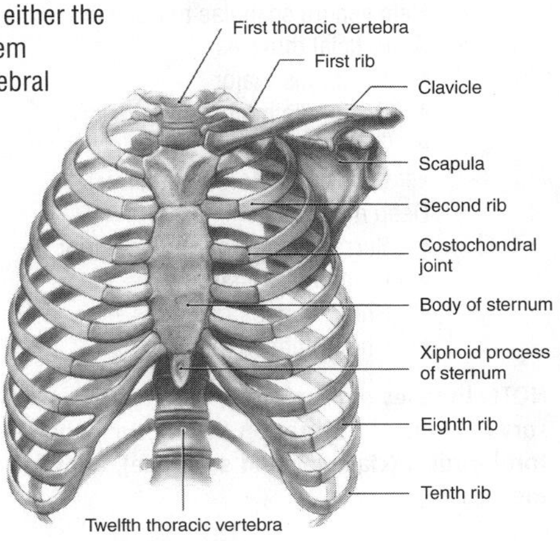

**Fig. 52-1** The bony thorax.

- ▸ **Divisions**
  - ♦ **Manubrium**
    - – Wider and thicker than the other two parts of the sternum
    - – Articulates with the clavicles and the first costal cartilage
    - – The *angle of Louis* represents the junction of the manubrium and body of the sternum—corresponds to the articulation with the second rib
  - ♦ **Body**
    - – Longest of the three parts
    - – Located anterior to T5 to T9
  - ♦ **Xiphoid**
    - – Smallest and most variable portion
    - – Usually ossifies and unites with the sternal body around age 40 years
- • **Clavicles**
- • **Thoracic vertebrae**

## THORACIC SOFT TISSUES[1] (Fig. 52-2)

- ■ Bony thorax is covered by muscle, subcutaneous tissue, and skin.
- ■ **Subdivisions of thoracic muscles**
  - • **Primary muscles of respiration**
    - ▸ Diaphragm
    - ▸ Intercostal muscles (external, internal, and innermost)
      - ♦ Neurovascular bundles run between the **internal** and **innermost** intercostals.
      - ♦ The bundles are positioned behind the costal groove inferior to the rib, with the vein positioned most superiorly, followed by the artery and the nerve in descending order **(VAN).**
      - ♦ All 11 intercostal spaces are wider anteriorly, and each intercostal bundle falls away from the rib posteriorly to become more central within each space.
  - • **Secondary muscles of respiration**
    - ▸ Sternocleidomastoid
    - ▸ Serratus posterior (superior and inferior heads)
    - ▸ Levatores costarum
  - • **Muscles that attach the upper extremities to the body**
    - ▸ Help secure scapulae to bony thorax
    - ▸ Superficial muscles
      - ♦ Pectoralis major
      - ♦ Pectoralis minor (anterior)
      - ♦ Trapezius
      - ♦ Latissimus dorsi (posterior)
    - ▸ Deep muscles
      - ♦ Serratus anterior and posterior
      - ♦ Levatores costarum
      - ♦ Rhomboideus major
      - ♦ Rhomboideus minor

**NOTE: In cases of respiratory distress, the pectoralis major and serratus anterior act as accessory muscles of respiration. This occurs when a person holds onto a table to fix his or her pectoral girdles (clavicles and scapulae), allowing these muscles to act on their attachments to the ribs.**

- **Internal mammary vessels**
  - Serve as important and useful recipient sites for microvascular tissue transfer, although rarely needed in chest wall reconstruction
  - **Anatomic studies**
    - According to Shaw,[2] when the mammary vessels are dissected at the fifth intercostal space, approximately 42% of the internal mammary veins are unsuitable for use.
    - Clark et al[3] discovered that the internal mammary veins gradually become smaller distally and often bifurcate, making them unsuitable for use as recipient vessels below the fourth intercostal space.
      - They concluded that the most consistent interval in which to find suitable recipient vessels was the **third intercostal space,** where 40% of the veins on the left and 70% of the veins on the right were ≥3 mm in diameter.
      - Furthermore, 90% of veins on the left and 40% of veins on the right bifurcated by the third rib.

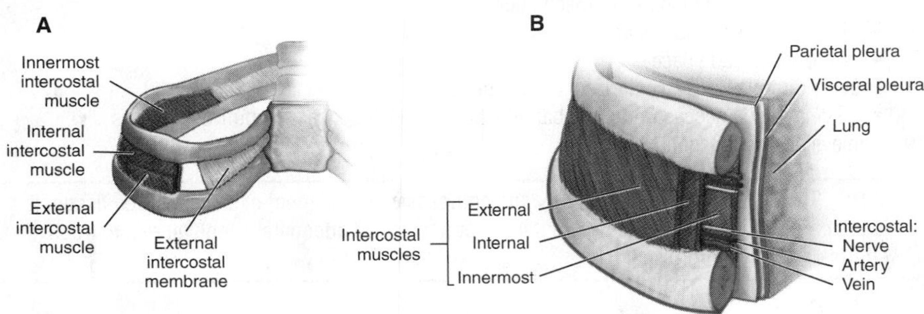


**Fig. 52-2 A,** The neurovascular bundle and **B,** the intercostal musculature.

## CHEST WOUNDS

### ETIOLOGIC FACTORS

- Trauma
- Tumor
- Infection
- Radiation
- Congenital

### PATIENT EVALUATION

- **History** (See Chapter 1 for general principles of managing complex wounds.)
  - Evaluate for underlying pulmonary disease.
    - Need preoperative pulmonary function tests (PFTs)
    - May help determine whether small defects require reconstruction
  - Obtain specific surgical history.
    - Previous thoracotomy may compromise latissimus dorsi and serratus muscles.
    - Previous subcostal incision may compromise rectus abdominis.
    - Previous axillary dissection may compromise thoracodorsal pedicle.
    - Previous coronary artery bypass graft may have used the internal mammary artery, thereby compromising the rectus abdominis or pectoralis major turnover.

> **TIP:** When in doubt, obtain radiologic imaging (e.g., CTA, MRA), and always read previous surgical reports.

- **Physical examination** (See Chapter 2 for general principles of managing complex wounds.)
  - Evaluate congenital disorders that may influence reconstructive options.
    - Poland's syndrome (pectoralis, latissimus dorsi)
    - Pectus excavatum (repair may have compromised vascular pedicles in the area)
    - Pectus carinatum (repair may have compromised vascular pedicles in the area)

### GOALS OF RECONSTRUCTION[4]

- Debride devitalized tissue and hardware, and obtain healthy wound bed.
- Restore skeletal stability and structure.
  - Reconstruct the skeleton if **more than four consecutive ribs are resected** or if the **defect is >5 cm.**
  - Restore normal respiratory mechanics.
  - Protect vital structures and organs.
  - Obliterate dead space.
- Provide durable well-vascularized soft tissue coverage.
  - Living tissue necessary to combat infection, fill dead space, and buttress repairs
- Achieve aesthetic results.

> **TIP:** There is no substitute for early and aggressive debridement of all devitalized tissue. It is the cornerstone of treatment, and if it is not performed adequately, then all reconstructive efforts will be compromised.

## RECONSTRUCTION OF PLEURAL CAVITY

- Defect usually results from complications of tumor resection (pulmonary or esophageal).
- Defect is usually present as bronchopleural or tracheoesophageal fistulas.
  - High morbidity and mortality rate

### GOALS OF RECONSTRUCTION

- Eradicate infection.
- Obtain airtight pleural cavity.

### TREATMENT

- Obliterate pleural space with local muscle flaps or omentum.
  - Latissimus dorsi
  - Serratus anterior
  - Pectoralis major
  - Rectus abdominis
  - Omentum
- Access muscle flaps or omentum through a previous thoracotomy incision, or create a second incision.
- To prevent ischemic failure it is imperative that the flap pedicle is not kinked or twisted.

## RECONSTRUCTION OF THORACIC SKELETON

### Defect Causes

- Usually caused by postoperative infection after cardiac surgery
- Can also occur after resection of chest wall tumors, trauma, or radiation
- **Sternotomy wound infections**[5] (Table 52-1)
  - **Incidence**[6]
    - Most common defect, likely after sternotomy wound infection/osteomyelitis
    - Occurs in up to **5%** of cardiac procedures
    - Can be life threatening
    - More common when internal mammary artery (IMA) is harvested
      - **0.3%** with **unilateral** IMA harvest, **2.4%** with **bilateral** IMA harvest
  - **Classification**
    - Pairolero and Arnold[7]
      - **Type 1:** Serosanguineous drainage within first 3 days, negative cultures, no cellulitis or osteomyelitis
        - Treatment: Reexplore, debride, reclose
      - **Type 2:** Purulent mediastinitis occurring within first 3 weeks, positive cultures, and cellulitis and/or osteomyelitis
        - Treatment: Reexplore, debride, flap
      - **Type 3:** Draining sinus tract from chronic osteomyelitis months to years after procedure
        - Treatment: Reexplore, debride, flap

**Table 52-1** *Starzynski Classification of Sternal Defects*

| Defect | Physiologic Deficit |
|---|---|
| Loss of upper sternal body and adjacent ribs | Minimal |
| Loss of entire sternal body and adjacent ribs | Moderate |
| Loss of manubrium and upper sternal body with adjacent ribs | Severe |

### Indications for Reconstruction

- **Defect affects more than four contiguous ribs or is >5 cm.**[8,9]
  - **Purpose:** Stabilize paradoxical motion and protect vital organs
  - May reconstruct smaller defect if underlying pulmonary disease (less tolerance for loss of respiratory mechanical efficiency)
  - May not reconstruct larger defects if previous radiotherapy
    - *Radiation stiffens chest wall through ischemic fibrosis, which leads to less paradoxical motion and loss of respiratory mechanical efficiency for a same-sized defect.*
- **If defect is located posteriorly and/or superiorly (shielded by the scapula), then a larger defect is tolerated.**

## Reconstructive Options

- **Alloplastic reconstruction**
  - **Mesh**[9-11]
    - **Polypropylene (Marlex)**
      - Semirigid
      - Reduces ventilator dependence and overall hospital stay
      - Can fragment or cause seroma formation
      - Can become infected
      - Forms fibrous capsule
    - **Expanded polytetrafluoroethylene (ePTFE) (Gore-Tex)**
      - Semirigid
      - Malleable and flexible
      - Does not become incorporated but forms a fibrous capsule
      - Prone to seroma formation
      - Expensive
  - **Methylmethacrylate**
    - Exothermic reaction
    - Rigid
    - Higher infection and extrusion rates
  - **Bone grafts**
  - **Acellular dermal matrix**[12]
    - Semirigid
    - Less prone to infection and becomes vascularized and incorporated
    - Prone to seroma formation
    - Expensive
  - **Titanium plate fixation**[13,14] (Fig. 52-3)
    - Applied transversely across the sternum and ribs to provide true fixation
    - Provides stable sternal repair for overlying tension-free pectoralis flap coverage
    - Results in earlier extubation (96% within first 24 hours)
    - Allows early return to mobility and activity
- **Autogenous tissue reconstruction**
  - **Locoregional flaps (most common)** (Table 52-2)
    - Pectoralis major
      - Advancement
      - Turnover
      - Composite myocutaneous
    - Latissimus dorsi
    - Rectus abdominis
    - Serratus anterior
    - Omentum
- **Vacuum-assisted closure**[15-18]
  - Provides bridge between debridement and definitive closure
  - Decreases wound size
  - Maintains stability
  - Can help splint chest, improve respiratory dynamics, and discontinue need for ventilator sooner
  - More comfortable
  - Acts as a "splint"
  - Improved survival from mediastinitis

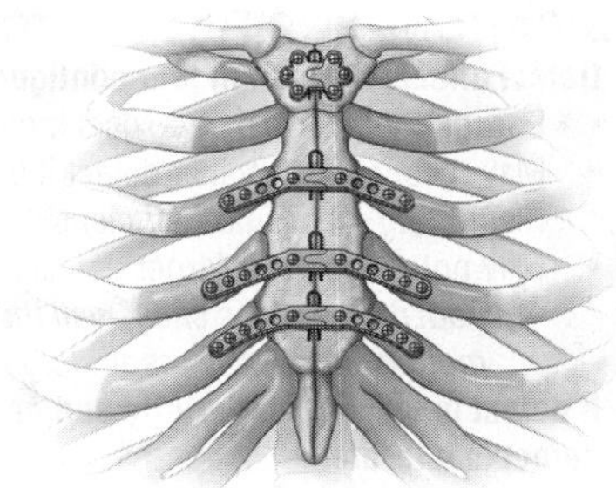

**Fig. 52-3** Transverse sternal plate fixation.

**Table 52-2** *Commonly Used Locoregional Flaps for Chest Wall Reconstruction*

| Flap | Mathes/ Nahai Flap | Origin | Insertion | Dominant Pedicle |
|---|---|---|---|---|
| Pectoralis major | V | Clavicle<br>Sternum<br>Upper seven ribs | Humerus | Pectoral branch of thoracoacromial artery |
| Latissimus dorsi | V | Spinous processes of lower six thoracic vertebrae<br>Thoracolumbar fascia<br>Iliac crest | Humerus | Thoracodorsal artery |
| Serratus anterior | III | Upper eight ribs | Scapula | Lateral thoracic artery and the serratus branch of the thoracodorsal artery |
| Rectus abdominis | III | Pubic symphysis and crest | Costal cartilages of ribs 5-7 | Superior and inferior epigastric artery |
| Omentum | III | Stomach<br>Duodenum<br>Gastrosplenic ligament | Transverse colon and gastrocolic ligament | Right and left gastroepiploic artery |

## RECONSTRUCTION OF THORACIC SOFT TISSUES[19]

### Partial-Thickness Defects

- Reconstruct with split-thickness skin grafts if wound bed is well perfused, or with local skin flaps.

### Full-Thickness Defects

- These are usually reconstructed with locoregional flaps.
- Larger defects may require free flap coverage from distant sites.

### Reconstructive Options

- **Anterior chest wall and mediastinum**
  - Pectoralis major
  - Latissmus dorsi
  - Omentum
  - Rectus abdominis
- **Anterolateral chest wall**
  - Latissmus dorsi
  - Omentum
  - Rectus abdominis
  - External oblique
  - Serratus anterior
  - Transverse thoracoabdominal flap
- **Diaphragmatic defects**
  - Direct suture repair
  - Acellular dermal matrix or mesh
  - Deepithelialized transverse rectus abdominis myocutaneous (TRAM)

- Latissmus dorsi
- Omentum

### Chronic Empyema and Bronchopleural Fistula

- **Eloesser flap**
  - Inferiorly based U-shaped flap from posterior chest wall turned into thoracic cavity
  - Allows passive drainage of empyema
  - Does not address bronchopleural fistula
- **Thoracoplasty**
  - Extraperiosteal removal of ribs to collapse chest wall
  - Treats both empyema and bronchopleural fistula in one surgery
  - Results in rib cage deformity
  - Interferes with scapulothoracic shoulder motion and function
  - Morbidity reduced by only resecting ribs in the upper chest
- **Muscle flap transfer into an intrathoracic position**
  - Omentum, rectus abdominis, or latissimus dorsi
  - Large deepithelialized fasciocutaneous paddle can be used to add bulk to fill defect.
  - Free tissue transfer may be used for larger defects or when local tissue is not available.

## CHEST WALL DEFORMITIES

There are various congenital chest wall abnormalities. Although most of them result in no noticeable physiologic impairment, some can be severe or even life threatening.

### Poland's Syndrome

- **Incidence**
  - Occurs in approximately 1:30,000 births[20]
  - No gender prevalence
  - Right side affected twice as often as left side
- **Current theory:** Syndrome caused by hypoplasia of subclavian artery secondary to kinking during week 6 of gestation
- **Components**[21-23]
  - Absence of sternal head of pectoralis major muscle
  - Absence of costal cartilages
  - Hypoplasia or aplasia of breast and subcutaneous tissue, including the nipple-areola complex
  - Deficiency of subcutaneous fat and axillary hair
  - Syndactyly or hypoplasia of ipsilateral extremity
- **Additional findings**
  - Absence or hypoplasia of pectoralis minor muscle
  - Shortening and hypoplasia of forearm
  - Variable deformities of the serratus, infraspinatus, supraspinatus, latissimus dorsi, and external oblique muscles
  - Total absence of anterolateral ribs with herniation of the lung
  - Symphalangism with syndactyly and hypoplasia or aplasia of middle phalanges
  - Occasionally associated with Möbius' syndrome (facial palsy and abducens oculi palsy) or childhood leukemia
- **Indications for treatment**
  - Patients with absent ribs
  - Female patients with breast asymmetry

- **Timing of surgery**
  - Delayed in females until after puberty to allow full development of the contralateral breast
- **Surgical techniques**
  - The ipsilateral latissimus dorsi is mobilized over a customized breast implant. The insertion of the latissimus dorsi is moved anteriorly on the humerus to establish an anterior axillary fold.[17]
  - Alloplastic meshes and custom-fabricated silicone moulages can also be used to correct the deformity.

## Depression Deformities (Pectus Excavatum)

- Also called *funnel chest*
- **Incidence**
  - **Most common chest wall deformity**
    - Occurs in 1:400 children
    - Approximately 10 times more common than pectus carinatum
  - Affects males more than females (4:1)
  - More than 30% have family history, although research has not proved genetic factors.[24]
  - Approximately 20% associated with other musculoskeletal abnormalities such as scoliosis (15%) and Marfan's syndrome
  - Congenital heart disease observed in 1.5%[25]
- **Pathophysiology**
  - Results from excessive growth of the lower costal cartilages, causing a posterior sternal depression
  - Sternum may rotate if depression deeper on right side than left side
  - Usually recognized within first year of life and progressively worsens as child grows older
  - Usually begins asymptomatically but eventually can result in significant pulmonary abnormalities
  - May result in a spectrum of severity, ranging from a mildly depressed sternum to sternal depression abutting the vertebral column
- **Indications for reconstruction**
  - Cosmesis
  - Psychosocial factors
  - Presence of respiratory or cardiovascular insufficiency
- **Timing of reconstruction**
  - Poor self-image is an important concern for many patients, particularly children and young adults or adolescents who are teased by peers. Because of these concerns, early repair is supported, with the best results reported in children 2 to 5 years of age.[26]
- **Surgical techniques**
  - Requires multiple osteotomies of the sternum and affected rib segments to help reposition the sternum and restore a normal contour
  - **Procedures**
    - Sternal osteotomy to reposition the sternum anteriorly
    - A modification that involves using a posterior strut (sternal strut) to support the repositioned sternum (Ravitch technique)[27]
    - The Nuss procedure is a minimally invasive modification that slips concave steel bars behind the sternum through two small incisions. The bar is flipped to a convex position to anteriorly displace the sternum and correct the deformity.

- The sternum is removed and repositioned in a front-to-back rotated position before stabilization (sternum turnover procedure).
- A silastic mold is created and implanted into the subcutaneous space to fill the defect without altering the thoracic cage.[28]

## PROTRUSION DEFORMITIES (PECTUS CARINATUM)

- Also called *pigeon chest*
- Defect characterized by an anterior protrusion deformity of the sternum and costal cartilages
- **Incidence**
  - Affects males more than females (4:1)
  - Family history (30%)
  - Associated with scoliosis (15%) and congenital heart disease (20%)[29]
- **Pathophysiology**
  - Defect typically not recognized until after first decade of life
  - Physiologic symptoms uncommon
  - **Types of defects**
    - *Chondrogladiolar protrusion*
      - Anterior displacement of the body of the sternum and symmetrical concavity of the costal cartilages
      - Most common of the three variants
    - *Lateral depression of the ribs on one or both sides of the sternum*
      - Poland's syndrome frequently associated with this type
    - *Pouter pigeon breast*
      - Upper or chondromanubrial prominence with protrusion of the manubrium and depression of the sternal body
      - Least common of the three variants
- **Surgical techniques**
  - Similar to pectus carinatum with resection of abnormal costal cartilages, repositioning of the sternum, and possible use of struts

## KEY POINTS

- ✓ A complete history and physical examination are critical before chest wall reconstruction, because the presence of significant comorbidities and previous surgeries can affect the outcome.
- ✓ Debridement of devitalized bone and cartilage is the cornerstone of treatment for infected sternal wounds.
- ✓ All foreign bodies need to be removed (e.g., sternal wires).
- ✓ Skeletal stability is reconstructed if the defect affects more than four contiguous ribs or is >5 cm in dimension, or if the defect causes significant pulmonary complications (e.g., flail chest with paradoxical movement).
- ✓ Restoration of skeletal stability is less likely in posteriorly located defects as a result of shielding by the scapula, and in patients with a history of radiotherapy, which stiffens the chest wall.
- ✓ Locoregional flaps, particularly muscle flaps, are the workhorses of reconstruction.
- ✓ It is rare for congenital deformities to significantly affect cardiorespiratory function. Indications for treatment are largely aesthetic.

## REFERENCES


1. Moore KL, Dalley AF, Agur AMR, eds. Clinically Oriented Anatomy, 7th ed. Philadelphia: Wolters Kluwer/Lippincott Williams & Wilkins, 2013.
2. Shaw WW. Breast reconstruction by superior gluteal microvascular free flaps without silicone implants. Plast Reconstr Surg 72:490-501, 1983.
3. Clark CP III, Rohrich RJ, Copit S, et al. An anatomic study of the internal mammary veins: clinical implications for free-tissue-transfer breast reconstruction. Plast Reconstr Surg 99:400-404, 1997.
4. Cohen M, Ramasastry SS. Reconstruction of complex chest wall defects. Am J Surg 172:35-40, 1996.
5. Starzynski TE, Snyderman RK, Beattie EJ Jr. Problems of major chest wall reconstruction. Plast Reconstr Surg 44:525-535, 1969.
6. Cosgrove DM, Lytle BW, Loop FD, et al. Does bilateral internal mammary artery grafting increase surgical risk? J Thorac Cardiovasc Surg 95:850-856, 1988.
7. Pairolero PC, Arnold PG. Management of infected median sternotomy wounds. Ann Thorac Surg 42:1-2, 1986.
8. Dingman RO, Argenta LC. Reconstruction of the chest wall. Ann Plast Surg 32:202-208, 1981.
9. McCormack PM. Use of prosthetic materials in chest wall reconstruction: assets and liabilities. Surg Clin North Am 69:965-976, 1989.
10. Hurwitz DJ, Ravitch M, Wolmark N. Laminated Marlex-methyl methacrylate prosthesis for massive chest wall resection. Ann Plast Surg 5:486-490, 1980.
11. Kroll SS, Walsh G, Ryan B, et al. Risks and benefits of using Marlex mesh in chest wall reconstruction. Ann Plast Surg 31:303-306, 1993.
12. Sodha NR, Azoury SC, Sciortino C, et al. The use of acellular dermal matrix in chest wall reconstruction. Plast Reconstr Surg 130(5 Suppl 2):S175-S182, 2012.
13. Cicilioni OJ, Stieg F III, Papanicolau G. Sternal wound reconstruction with transverse plate fixation. Plast Reconstr Surg 115:1297-1303, 2005.
14. Synthes. Titanium sternal plating system [brochure]. Available at http://www.synthes.com/MediaBin/US%20DATA/Product%20Support%20Materials/Brochures/CMF/MXBROSternalFixJ5756G.pdf.
15. Agarwal JP, Ogilvie M, Wu LC, et al. Vacuum-assisted closure for sternal wounds: a first-line therapeutic management approach. Plast Reconstr Surg 116:1035-1040, 2005.
16. Janis JE. Vacuum-assisted closure for sternal wounds: a first-line therapeutic management approach [discussion]. Plast Reconstr Surg 112:1041-1043, 2005.
17. Fuchs U, Zittermann A, Stuettgen B, et al. Clinical outcome of patients with deep sternal wound infection managed by vacuum-assisted closure compared to conventional therapy with open packing: a retrospective analysis. Ann Thorac Surg 79:526-531, 2005.
18. Sjogren J, Nilsson J, Gustafsson R, et al. The impact of vacuum-assisted closure on long-term survival after post-sternotomy mediastinitis. Ann Thorac Surg 80:1270-1275, 2005.
19. Netscher DT, Baumholtz MA. Chest reconstruction. I. Anterior and anterolateral chest wall and wounds affecting respiratory function. Plast Reconstr Surg 1124:240e-252e, 2009.
20. Freire-Maia N, Chautard EA, Opitz JM, et al. The Poland syndrome: clinical and genealogical data, dermatoglyphic analysis, and incidence. Hum Hered 23:97-104, 1973.
21. Hester TR Jr, Bostwick J III. Poland's syndrome: correction with latissimus muscle transposition. Plast Reconstr Surg 69:226-233, 1982.
22. Ohmori K, Takada H. Correction of Poland's pectoralis major muscle anomaly with latissimus dorsi musculocutaneous flaps. Plast Reconstr Surg 65:400-404, 1980.
23. Ravitch MM. Poland's syndrome: a study of an eponym. Plast Reconstr Surg 59:508-512, 1977.
24. Shamberger RC, Welch KJ. Surgical repair of pectus excavatum. J Pediatr Surg 23:615-622, 1988.

25. Shamberger RC, Welch KJ, Castaneda AR, et al. Anterior chest wall deformities and congenital heart disease. J Thorac Cardiovasc Surg 96:427-432, 1988.
26. Shamberger RC, Welch KJ. Chest wall deformities. In Ashcraft KW, Holder TM, eds. Pediatric Surgery, 2nd ed. Philadelphia: WB Saunders, 1993.
27. Ravitch MM. Congenital Deformities of the Chest Wall and Their Operative Correction, 5th ed. Philadelphia: Saunders-Elsevier, 2010.
28. Crump HW. Pectus excavatum. Am Fam Physician 46:173-179, 1992.
29. Shamberger RC, Welch KJ. Surgical correction of pectus carinatum. J Pediatr Surg 22:48-53, 1987.

# 53. Abdominal Wall Reconstruction

Georges N. Tabbal, Jeffrey E. Janis

## ANATOMY (Fig. 53-1)

- **Borders of the anterior/anterolateral abdominal wall include:**
  - **Superiorly:** Xiphoid process and costal cartilage of ribs 7 and 12
  - **Inferiorly:** Pubic tubercle and inguinal ligament
  - **Laterally:** Midaxillary line
- The abdominal wall is a layered construct with six components (listed below from superficial to deep.) These interact to perform two vital functions: *coverage* in the form of a skin envelope and myofascial *support.*
  1. **Skin and subcutaneous fat**
  2. **Superficial fascia**
     - Composed of two distinct layers: The *superficial fascial system* (historically referred to as *Scarpa's fascia*) is more fibrous in nature and has a faint yellow color, compared with the more superficially located Camper's fascia.
  3. **Myofascial anatomy**

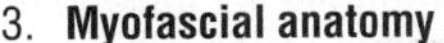

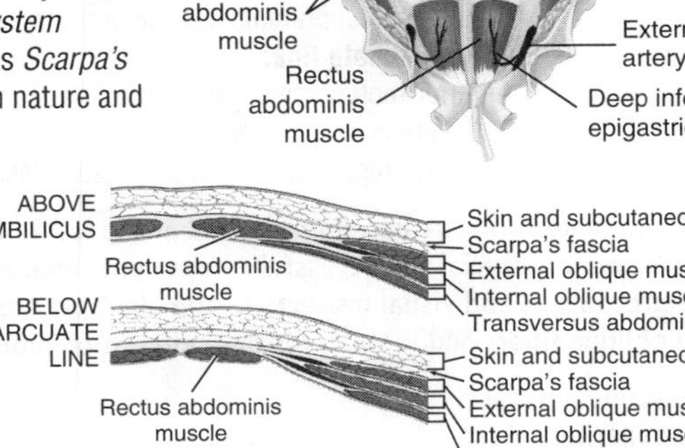

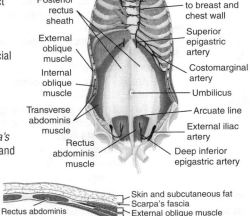


**Fig. 53-1** Anatomy.

- **Abdominal wall musculature**
- Consists of five paired muscles connected by a fascial lattice:
  - **Rectus abdominis**
    - Origin: Pubic ramus
    - Insertion: Xiphoid process and ribs 5-7

**NOTE: Three tendinous inscriptions traverse the muscle at the level of the umbilicus, xiphoid, and a point halfway between the two.**

  - **External oblique**
    - Origin: Lower eight ribs
    - Insertion: Linea alba through aponeurosis
    - Orientation: Muscle fibers run inferomedially

- **Internal oblique**
  - Origin: Thoracolumbar fascia, iliac crest, and inguinal ligament
  - Insertion: Costal margin and linea alba, through its aponeurosis
  - Orientation: Superomedially
- **Transversus abdominis**
  - Origin: Costal cartilages of ribs 6-12, thoracolumbar fascia, anterior iliac crest, and inguinal ligament
  - Insertion: Linea alba through aponeurosis
  - Orientation: Traverse horizontally toward the midline
- **Pyramidalis**
  - Functionally insignificant triangular muscle
  - Not present in everyone

- **Fascial interface**
  - **Linea alba**
    - Midline decussation of anterior rectus sheath
    - Course: Runs vertically from the xiphoid process to the pubis
  - **Linea semilunaris**
    - Fascial adherence that defines the lateral border of the rectus
- **Rectus sheath**
  - **Above the arcuate line:**
    - Anterior rectus sheath: Aponeurosis of the external oblique and anterior leaf of the internal oblique
    - Posterior rectus sheath: Posterior leaf of the internal oblique aponeurosis, transversus abdominis muscle, and transversalis fascia
  - **Below the arcuate line:**
    - Anterior rectus sheath: Aponeuroses of the external and internal obliques and transversus abdominis
    - Posterior rectus sheath: Transversalis fascia only

**NOTE: The arcuate (semicircular) line is found at the level of the anterior superior iliac spines. Its identification is crucial to successful component separation and is aided by digital palpation, electrocautery, and visual inspection, and electrocautery confirmation by tapping on the external oblique fibers and looking for the indentation along the semilunar line.**

4. **Transversalis fascia**
5. **Intraperitoneal fat**
6. **Parietal peritoneum**

- **Vasculature**
  - Vascular supply to the abdominal wall is robust with named vessels supplying each of the aforementioned muscles.
  - Abdominal skin and subcutaneous tissue receives rich collateralization from independent sources, allowing it to be raised as a random flap (e.g., during an abdominoplasty).
  - Best defined by *Huger zones*[3] (Fig. 53-2):
    - **Zone I:** Area that extends between the xiphoid and pubic symphysis, bordered by the lateral edges of the rectus muscles
      - Supplied by the superior epigastric (branch of the internal mammary) and deep inferior epigastric (medial branch of the external iliac) epigastrics, which collateralize within the middle third of the rectus, near the umbilicus
      - **Deep inferior epigastrics** are more dominant, providing rich number of perforators arranged in medial and lateral rows.
        - Most arise within 3 cm of the umbilicus.

**NOTE: The medial row is more dominant and can better perfuse a greater extent of the contralateral skin.**

- **Zone II:** Overlaps inferior aspect of zone I, bordered superiorly by a line connecting the right and left anterior superior iliac crests, and inferiorly by the pubic symphysis and paired groin creases.
  - Supplied by both DIEA perforators, as well as three arteries that all originate from the common femoral artery and travel in superficial plane (from lateral to medial):
    - Superficial circumflex femoral artery
    - Superficial inferior epigastric artery
    - External pudendal artery

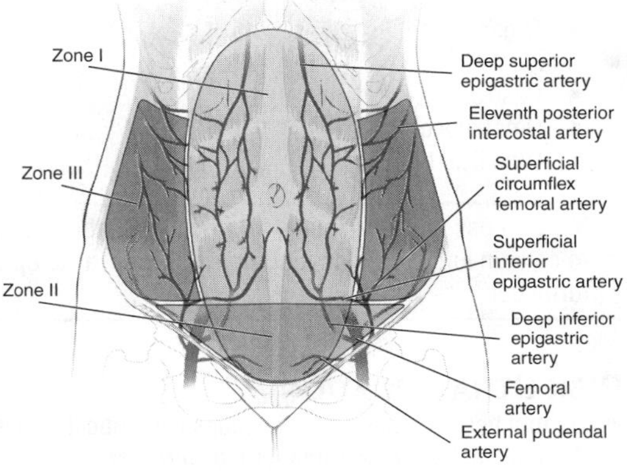

Fig. 53-2

- **Zone III:** Area superior to zone II and lateral to the lateral border of the rectus abdominis
  - Supplied by both thoracic intercostal perforators originating from T7-12, as well as the first lumbar neurovascular pedicle
  - Robust vascularity in this zone can adequately supply the entire abdominal wall if zone I and II blood supply should become compromised.

- **Innervation**
  - Ventral rami of T7 through L4 supply motor and cutaneous innervation to the abdominal wall.
    - Anterolateral abdominal wall supplied by thoracic perforators that travel below the internal oblique muscle
    - Rectus abdominis supplied by perforators that course more medially (in the same plane) before piercing the posterior rectus sheath
  - Iliohypogastric and ilioinguinal supply hypogastrium, branch between the oblique muscles *(where they are vulnerable to injury during component separation)*

# ETIOLOGIC AND RISK FACTORS

## MULTIFACTORIAL CAUSES

- Genetic factors include impairment of:
  - Collagen metabolism/expression
  - Tissue protease metabolism
- Iatrogenic
  - Failure of laparotomy incisions (in absence of other risk factors, incidence of primary failure rates of laparotomy incisions is 11%)[2,3]
  - Tumor resection
- Traumatic

- Infection
  - Superficial
  - Deep
  - Organ space
- Congenital
  - Gastroschisis
  - Omphalocele
  - Umbilical hernias

**TIP:** Loss of mechanical integrity within abdominal wall tissue and the resultant inability to contain and offset intraabdominal forces make up the fundamental mechanism for hernia formation.

## Risk Stratification

- Ventral hernia repair (VHR) includes two critical issues:
  1. Risk factors for **surgical site occurrences (SSOs) and infections**
     - Includes both *patient* and *wound factors* in addition to the *choice of repair material* used
     - Comorbidities associated with increased rates of wound infection include[4-6]:
       - Smoking
       - Diabetes
       - Chronic obstructive pulmonary disease
       - Coronary artery disease (CAD)
       - Nutritional status (preoperative serum albumin levels <2.0)
       - Obesity
       - Advanced age
       - Immunosuppression
       - Chronic corticosteroid use
  2. Risk factors for **hernia recurrence:**
     - Surgical technique
       - Critical principles of wound closure to prevent dehiscence[7]:
         - Wide tissue bites
         - Short stitch intervals
         - Nonstrangulating tension on the suture

**TIP:** Optimal wound closure should incorporate placement of fascial stitches from the fascial edge in 1 cm intervals.

     - Patient factors
       - Increased abdominal wall pressure
       - Compromised tissue integrity
     - Wound factors
       - Infection
         - Incidence of 4%-16%
         - Significantly increases rates of hernia recurrence (Recurrence rate when postoperative infection occurred was 80%, compared with 34% in those without infection.[8])

## PATIENT EVALUATION (see Chapter 1)

- **History**
  - Medical comorbidities
  - Surgical history (including dates, methods, and materials used during prior repairs)
  - Medications
  - Social history (including tobacco, alcohol, and illicit drug use)
  - Radiation
- **Physical examination**
  - Acute versus chronic defect
  - Anatomic tissues involved (i.e., partial versus full thickness)
  - Size and location of defect
    - Measured at the **superior, middle,** and **inferior** thirds of the abdomen
  - Wound contamination
  - Presence of ostomy
  - Presence of enterocutaneous fistula(s)
    - Must be adequately controlled before definitive reconstruction
    - Often associated with electrolyte imbalances and nutritional deficiencies
- Preoperative workup:
  - **Laboratory testing**
    - Albumin/prealbumin
    - Electrolytes (particularly if fistula or open wound is present)
- Imaging
  - CT
    - Aids in evaluation of the size and extent of the defect
    - Useful assessment tool of adjacent muscles, which may be required in reconstruction
  - Fistulogram

## CLASSIFICATION SYSTEMS

### GRADING OF HERNIA DEFECTS

- Efforts to improve risk stratification include a hernia grading system described by the Ventral Hernia Working Group (VHWG).
  - Grades were developed based on the risk of a surgical site complication, particularly infection.
  - They do *not* take into account hernia size, degree of complexity, proposed method of repair, or the risk of recurrence.
- **Four-tiered grading scheme**[9]:
  - **Grade 1** (low risk): Includes patients with no evidence of wound contamination or active infection and no comorbidities.
    - Low risk of complications
    - No history of wound infection
  - **Grade 2** (comorbid): Includes patients with comorbidities for increased risk of surgical site infections but without infection or evidence to support wound contamination
    - Smoking
    - Obesity
    - Diabetes
    - Immunosuppression
    - COPD

- **Grade 3** (potentially contaminated): Includes patients with evidence to support wound contamination
  - Previous wound infection
  - Presence of a stoma
  - Violation of the gastrointestinal tract
- **Grade 4** (infected): Actively infected patients
  - Infected mesh
  - Septic dehiscence

■ Validated three-tiered model (Rosen)

■ In an effort to challenge the strength and applicability of the VHWG grading scheme, Kanters et al[10] used a large cohort of patients to modify the classification scheme into a three-grade scheme (Fig. 53-3). This is the first *validated* grading system for hernia defects.
- The transition of the VHWG four-tiered grading scheme into a three-grade classification was done by restructuring grade 3 patients. In the new system:
  - Patients with a history of wound infection were classified in grade 2.
  - Patients with a stoma or a violation of their GI tract were placed in grade 3.
  - Grade 3 patients were then stratified based on their CDC wound contamination.

| Grade 1<br>Low Risk | Grade 2<br>Comorbid | Grade 3<br>Contaminated |
|---|---|---|
| Low risk of complications<br>No history of wound infection | Smoker<br>Obese<br>COPD<br>Diabetes mellitus<br>History of wound infection | A. Clean-contaminated<br>B. Contaminated<br>C. Dirty |
| Surgical site occurrence: 14% | Surgical site occurrence: 27% | Surgical site occurrence: 46% |

**Fig. 53-3** Modified hernia grading system.

# RECONSTRUCTION OF ABDOMINAL WALL DEFECTS

## PRINCIPLES OF REPAIR[9]

■ Patient optimization
- Nutritional status
- Blood sugar levels (<110 mg/dl)
- Smoking cessation (≥4 weeks preoperatively)
- Improved oxygenation in patients with chronic hypoxia
- Weight loss

■ Preparation of wound
- Reduce bioburden (if unable to manage successfully, a staged reconstruction is optimal, with serial debridement as necessary before definitive reconstruction)
- Lysis of adhesions, fistula takedown

■ Reapproximation and centralization of rectus muscles to the midline (to the extent possible) using component separation when appropriate

■ Appropriate use of reinforcement material

## Timing of Reconstruction

- **Immediate:** At tumor resection or hernia repair
- **Delayed:** Indications for staging or delayed repair include:
  - Patient instability
  - Injuries not yet fully declared
  - Active infection (grade 4 hernia) or inability to reduce bioburden in contaminated wounds (grade 3 hernia)

## Goals of Reconstruction[11]

- Prevent visceral eventration
- Tension-free skin reapproximation and provision of stable soft tissue coverage
- Restoration of physiologic tension of musculofascia
- Provide dynamic muscle support

# REPAIR MATERIALS

## Prosthetic (Alloplastic) Materials[12,13]

- Characteristics include:
  - Pore size: Affects fibrovascular ingrowth, tensile strength, and intensity of foreign body reaction while allowing serum drainage
    - Type I prosthetics: Macroporous materials
    - Type II: Uniformly microporous
    - Type III: Macroporous materials with multifilamenoutous or microporous components
    - Type IV: Biomaterials with submicronic pore size (i.e., Silastic sheeting)
  - Number and composition of fibers: Helps determine interstice size and material strength
- Polyglactin 910 (Vicryl) or polyglycolic acid (Dexon)
  - Absorbable meshed alloplastic material
  - Provides excellent temporary coverage and support
  - No need for removal, because it is absorbable
  - Will eventually result in hernia because of lack of permanence
- Polypropylene
  - Nonabsorbable meshed alloplastic material
  - Comes in microporous and macroporous
  - Comes in lightweight, midweight, and heavyweight
  - Durable and strong
  - Promotes fibrous ingrowth through its interstices
  - Can extrude, especially if thin soft tissue coverage
  - Can cause enterocutaneous fistulas, especially if not placed under mild tension (bowel erosion caused by folds)
  - Long-term disadvantages include stiffness with age that results in decreased abdominal wall pliability
- Expanded polytetrafluoroethylene (ePTFE) (Gore-Tex)
  - Nonabsorbable, nonmeshed alloplastic sheet
  - Allows no fibrous ingrowth (not meshed) and therefore does not incorporate (it encapsulates)
  - Easier removal
  - Soft and pliable
  - Causes fewer adhesions
  - Less adherent to bacteria
  - Does not allow egress of fluid

**CAUTION: Without fluid egress, problems can develop in open abdominal wounds; therefore Gore-Tex should be used with discretion.**

## Prosthetic (Alloplastic) Composite Materials

Newer composite prosthetics combine absorbable and nonabsorable materials or nonabsorable materials with tissue-separating barrier materials to help reduce complications and better duplicate the physiology of the native abdominal wall.

- Vypro I/II (Ethicon, Somerville, NJ)
  - Polypropylene with polyglactin-absorbable material used to improve handling and initial strength
- Ultrapro (Ethicon)
  - Polypropylene with poliglecaprone 25–absorbable material used to withstand increased abdominal pressures and improve handling while leaving less foreign body material
- Proceed (Ethicon)
  - Polypropylene composite with oxidized, regenerated cellulose for tissue separation
- Supramesh (Genzyme, Framingham, MA)
  - Macroporous polypropylene–coated with bioresorbable sodium hyaluronate and carboxymethylcellulose, which aids in improving tissue separation
- Bard Composix (Davol, a Bard Company, Warwick, RI)
  - Macroporous polyproylene bonded to ePFTE to allow fibrous ingrowth

**TIP:** When using prosthetic mesh as an underlay, omentum should be interposed between the bowel and the mesh. The mesh should be placed flat, tightly, and without wrinkles. Otherwise, an inlay technique is advised.

## Bioprosthetic Materials[14,15]

- Variety of porcine and bovine acellular dermal matrices of various sizes and thicknesses are now commonly employed.
- General consensus is that they are best used in contaminated wounds in which prosthetic mesh would be avoided.
- All undergo decellularization (reduces foreign body response).
  - Some are then *dehydrated:* Extends shelf-life, makes them easier to handle, reduces extensibility
  - A few varieties then undergo *chemical cross-linking:* Helps to control enzymatic degradation of the graft (beneficial in contaminated wounds)
- Proposed advantages
  - Host tissue remodeling: Incorporates into surrounding tissues by ingrowth of fibrocollagenous tissue and blood vessels while it degrades.
  - Resist infection: Thought to be better suited for use in contaminated wounds. Dermal exposure can be managed with local wound care (as opposed to removal).
  - Produce few visceral adhesions, compared with prosthetics, allowing their placement directly onto bowel.
- Main disadvantages include cost and lack of long-term data to support their use.
- In a systematic review published by Janis et al,[16] rates of hernia recurrence when using ADMs varied widely (from 0%-80%), with the highest rates occurring when ADM was used as a bridging technique.
- At present, no clear data exist to support the superiority of one material in VHR.

- Acellular human dermis (AlloDerm; LifeCell, Branchburg NJ)
  - Non-cross-linked, freeze-dried cadaveric dermis
  - Largest available size: 16 by 20 cm (prehydrated)
  - Original product requires a two-step rehydration process before use (10-40 minutes depending on thickness), although a newer, ready-to-use variant is now available.
  - Once hydrated, surface area expands 25%-40% to its normal physiologic surface area
- Acellular bovine dermis (SurgiMend; TEI Biosciences, Boston, MA)
  - Non-cross-linked fetal bovine dermal collagen (reported to have higher proportion of type III collagen)
  - Largest available size: 25 by 40 cm
  - Requires rehydration before use (~60 seconds in normal saline solution)
- Acellular porcine dermis (Strattice; LifeCell)
  - Non-cross-linked porcine dermis
  - Largest available size: 25 by 40 cm
  - Requires rehydration before use (~2 minutes in normal saline solution)
- Acellular porcine dermis (Permacol; Covidien, Mansfield, MA)
  - Undergoes chemical cross-linking, which inhibits degradation and reduces revascularization
  - Largest available size: 18 by 40 cm
  - Ready to use when opened
- Porcine small intestine mucosa (Surgisis Biodesign; Cook Surgical, Bloomington, IN)
  - Largest available size: 20 by 30 cm
  - Requires rehydration before use

## CHOICE OF REPAIR MATERIAL IN VHR

- Recommendations of the VHWG regarding the choice of repair material in the repair of incisional ventral hernias, based on hernia grade[9]:
  - **Grade 1:** Choice of repair material based on surgeon preference and patient factors
  - **Grade 2:** Increased risk of SSO suggests additive risk for use of synthetic repair materials and a potential advantage for appropriate biologic reinforcement
  - **Grade 3:** Permanent synthetic repair material generally not recommended; potential advantage for biologic repair material
  - **Grade 4:** Permanent repair material not recommended; biologic repair material should be considered

## SURGICAL TECHNIQUE

### Mesh Placement

- Material may be secured as:
  - *Underlay:* Deep to the primary repair or fascial edges (preferred method)
    - Retrorectus
    - Wide intraperitoneal underlay
  - *Overlay:* Superficial to the primary repair or fascial edges
  - *Interpositional:* Sutured as a bridge between the fascial edges of the hernia defect in one of three locations, edge-to-edge, anterior, or deep to the fascia (avoided because of high rates of recurrence)
  - *Doublelay "sandwich technique":* Repair is reinforced with biologic material both above and below the primary fascial repair.
- Minimum of 3-5 cm of overlap between material and fascia

## COMPONENT SEPARATION (Fig. 53-4)

- Young[17] published the original concept in 1961. This was popularized by Ramirez et al[18] in 1990.
- It described division of the external oblique aponeurosis, separation of the external oblique from the internal oblique, and the rectus muscle, from their posterior sheath, allowing medialization of a compound flap of rectus muscle with its attached internal oblique–transversus abdominis muscle complex.
- Medial advancement of each flap (distance doubled if bilateral release performed):
  - Epigastrium: 5 cm
  - Waist: 10 cm
  - Suprapubic area: 3 cm

**NOTE: Release of the rectus from its posterior sheath provides an additional 2 cm of advancement at all levels.**

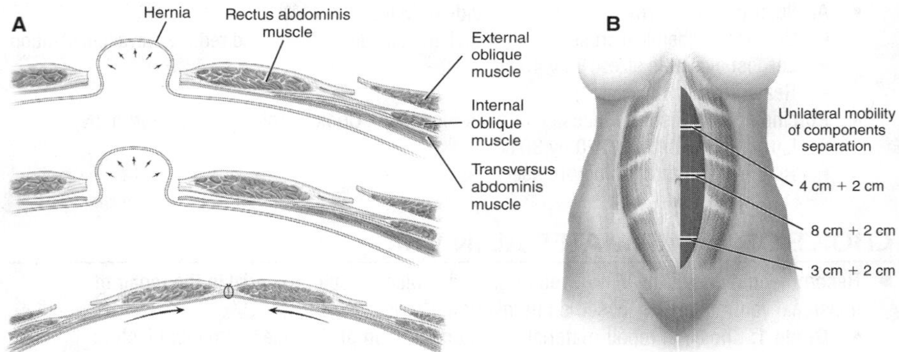


**Fig. 53-4 A,** Dissection of the abdominal wall musculature into components for medial advancement of separate muscle layers. **B,** Unilateral advancement distances for components separation.

## TECHNICAL MODIFICATIONS AND ADVANCEMENTS

- *Endoscopic-assisted* component separation was used to minimize dead space, limit exposure of the underlying myofascial tissue, and preserve blood supply to the overlying skin flap.
  - Lowe et al[19] made two small lateral incisions (one per side) and used a balloon device to develop subcutaenous pockets. The external oblique was released endoscopically.
  - Following a dissimilar order of operations, Maas et al[20] used balloon insufflation to develop a plane between the oblique muscles, *then* performed release endoscopically.
- *Perforator-sparing skin dissection* reduced incidence of wound complications (20% versus 2% compared with classical technique) and decreased rates of infection in clean-contaminated and contaminated cases.[21]
  - Sukkar et al[22] and Saulis and Dumanian[21] first described this method, which avoided lateral dissection at the level of the periumbilical perforators.
  - Instead they dissected subcutaneously above and below the level of the umbilicus to the linea semilunaris and accessed the external oblique. A lateral tunnel was made when these two pockets were connected.

- *Minimally invasive component separation with inlay bioprosthetic mesh* (MICSIB)
  - Described by Butler and Campbell,[23,24] this method preserves rectus abdominis perforators and the connections between subcutaneous tissue and anterior rectus sheeth, minimizing dead space and improving vascularity.[24]

## OTHER METHODS OF REPAIR

- *Retromuscular hernia* of the *Rives-Stoppa* repair uses the space between the rectus muscle fascia and the posterior rectus fascia.[25,26]
  - Limited by the lateral edge of the posterior rectus sheath
- *Transversus abdominis release* (TAR), an extension of the Rives-Stoppa method, uses a posterior component separation.[27,28]
  - Advantages include posterior rectus fascial advancement, perseveration of the neurovascular supply to the rectus abdominis muscle, creation of large space for sublay mesh, and wide lateral dissection.

**NOTE: TAR must *not be* combined with release of the external oblique (i.e., anterior abdominal component release).**

- *Tissue expansion* may include expansion of either skin/subcutaneous tissue and/or muscle fascia, depending on location of their placement.
  - Placement can be performed via an open approach through lateral incisions or endoscopically.
  - Case reports include successful closure of defects involving >50% of the abdominal area.
  - Disadvantages include the need for multiple procedures, prolonged recovery, and high complication rate.
- *Free tissue transfer* offers the potential for well vascularized, autologous soft tissue coverage of large defects.
  - Potential flaps include innervated tensor fascia lata, anterolateral thigh, and rectus abdominis.

## TREATMENT ALGORITHM

Proposed treatment guidelines from the VHWG include the following[9]:

- Assessment of patient risk factors for SSO is followed by hernia defect evaluation.
- Ultimate choice of repair material depends on the grade for risk of SSO.
- Special considerations include:
  - Grade 4 hernia defects should be repaired by open procedures.
  - Synthetic repair materials are most suitable for grade 1, some grade 2, and few grade 3 defects.
  - Conversely, biologic materials should be used in all grade 4 hernias, most grade 3 hernias, and some grade 2 defects.

## POSTOPERATIVE CARE

- Liberal use of progressive tension sutures[29]
- Abdominal binder to provide support, aid in tissue opposition/decreasing dead space; reminds patient to restrict activity during recovery period
- Early ambulation
- Epidural analgesia to increase patient comfort and decrease pulmonary complications
- Aggressive respiratory care
- Avoidance of strenuous activities or heavy lifting

## COMPLICATIONS

- Infection: Most common
- Seroma
- Cardiac, pulmonary, or other end-organ dysfunction
- Enterocutaneous fistula
- Abdominal compartment syndrome
- Recurrence: Associated with high BMI and infection, on average 20% rate of recurrence[30,31]

### KEY POINTS

✓ Preoperative patient optimization, wound bed preparation, and risk stratification maximize surgical outcomes.
✓ Primary fascial reapproximation with reinforcement is crucial to successful hernia repair.
✓ Delayed reconstruction is advised in the setting of gross contamination.
✓ Patients at risk for infection should undergo fascial reinforcement with biologic materials.
✓ Component separation and newer technical adjuncts/variants are highly useful to achieve primary facial closure.

## REFERENCES

1. Huger WE. The anatomic rationale for abdominal lipectomy. Am Surg 45:612-617, 1979.
2. Burger JW, Lange JF, Halm JA, et al. Incisional hernia: early complication of abdominal surgery. World J Surg 29:1608-1613, 2005.
3. Pollock AV, Evans M. Early prediction of late incisional hernias. Br J Surg 76:953-954, 1989.
4. Dunne JR, Malone DL, Tracy JK, et al. Abdominal wall hernias: risk factors for infection and resource utilization. J Surg Res 111:78-84, 2003.
5. Finan KR, Vick CC, Kiefe CI, et al. Predictors of wound infection in ventral hernia repair. Am J Surg 190:676-681, 2005.
6. Pessaux P, Lermite E, Blezel E, et al. Predictive risk score for infection after inguinal hernia repair. Am J Surg 192:165-171, 2006.
7. Carlson MA. Acute wound failure. Surg Clin North Am 77:607-636, 1997.
8. Luijendijk RW, Hop WC, van den Tol MP, et al. A comparison of suture repair with mesh repair for incisional hernia. New Engl J Med 343:392-398, 2000.
9. Breuing K, Butler CE, Ferzoco S, et al. Incisional ventral hernias: review of the literature and recommendations regarding the grading and technique of repair. Surgery 148:544-558, 2010.
10. Kanters AE, Krpata DM, Blatnik JA, et al. Modified hernia grading scale to stratify surgical site occurrence after open ventral hernia repairs. J Am Coll Surg 215:787-793, 2012.
11. DiBello JN, Moore JH. Sliding myofascial flap of the rectus abdominus muscles for the closure of recurrent ventral hernias. Plast Reconstr Surg 98:464-469, 1996.
12. Brown GL, Richardson JD, Malangoni MA, et al. Comparison of prosthetic materials for abdominal wall reconstruction in the presence of contamination and infection. Ann Surg 201:705-711, 1985.
13. Mathes SJ, Steinwald PM, Foster RD, et al. Complex abdominal wall reconstruction: a comparison of flap and mesh closure. Ann Surg 232:586-596, 2000.
14. Butler CE. The role of bioprosthetics in abdominal wall reconstruction. Clin Plast Surg 33:199-211, 2006.

15. Turza KC, Butler CE. Adhesions and meshes: synthetic versus bioprosthetic. Plast Reconstr Surg 130(5 Suppl 2):S206-S213, 2012.
16. Janis JE, O'Neill AC, Ahmad J, et al. Acellular dermal matrices in abdominal wall reconstruction: a systematic review of the current evidence. Plast Reconstr Surg 130(Suppl 2):183S-193S, 2012.
17. Young D. Repair of epigastric incisional hernia. Br J Surg 48:514-516, 1961.
18. Ramirez OM, Ruas E, Dellon AL. "Components separation" method for closure of abdominal-wall defects: an anatomic and clinical study. Plast Reconstr Surg 86:519-526, 1990.
19. Lowe JB, Garza JR, Bowman JL, et al. Endoscopically assisted "components separation" for closure of abdominal wall defects. Plast Reconstr Surg 105:720-729, 2000.
20. Maas SM, de Vries RS, van Goor H, et al. Endoscopically assisted "components separation technique" for the repair of complicated ventral hernias. J Am Coll Surg 194:388-390, 2002.
21. Saulis AS, Dumanian GA. Periumbilical rectus abdominis perforator preservation significantly reduces superficial wound complications in "separation of parts" hernia repairs. Plast Reconstr Surg 109:2275-2280; discussion 2281-2282, 2002.
22. Sukkar SM, Dumanian GA, Szczerba SM, et al. Challenging abdominal wall defects. Am J Surg 181:115-121, 2001.
23. Ghali S, Turza KC, Baumann DP, Butler CE. Minimally invasive component separation results in fewer wound-healing complications than open component separation for large ventral hernia repairs. J Am Coll Surg 214:981-989, 2012.
24. Butler CE, Campbell KT. Minimally invasive component separation with inlay bioprosthetic mesh (MICSIB) for complex abdominal wall reconstruction. Plast Reconstr Surg 128:698-709, 2011.
25. Rives J, Pire JC, Flament JB, et al. [Treatment of large eventrations. New therapeutic indications apropos of 322 cases] Chirurgie 111:215-225, 1985.
26. Stoppa RE. The treatment of complicated groin and incisional hernias. World J Surg 13:545-554, 1989.
27. Novitsky YW, Elliott HL, Orenstein SB, et al. Transversus abdominis muscle release: a novel approach to posterior component separation during complex abdominal wall reconstruction. Am J Surg 204:709-716, 2012.
28. Carbonell AM, Cobb WS, Chen SM. Posterior components separation during retromuscular hernia repair. Hernia 12:359-362, 2008.
29. Janis JE. Use of progressive tension sutures in components separation: merging cosmetic surgery techniques with reconstructive surgery outcomes. Plast Reconstr Surg 130:851-855, 2012.
30. Ko JH, Wang EC, Salvay DM, et al. Abdominal wall reconstruction: lessons learned from 200 "components separation" procedures. Arch Surg 144:1047-1055, 2009.
31. Souza JM, Dumanian GA. An evidence-based approach to abdominal wall reconstruction. Plast Reconstr Surg 130:116-124, 2012.

# 54. Genitourinary Reconstruction

Daniel R. Butz, Sam Fuller, Melissa A. Crosby

## EMBRYOLOGY

- **Germ layers:**
  - **Mesoderm:** Nephric system, gonads, wolffian ducts (mesonephric ducts), müllerian ducts (paramesonephric ducts)
  - **Endoderm:** Cloaca and membrane
  - **Ectoderm:** External genitalia
- Gonads start as genital ridges, which begin male or female differentiation at **6 weeks of embryologic life.** The testes precede differentiation of the ovaries by 1 week.
- Both mesonephric duct (i.e., primary duct of the male) and paramesonephric ducts (i.e., primary ducts of the female) are present in the developing fetus.
- **Differentiation of the ductal system:**
  - Regression of the **paramesonephric ducts (müllerian)**
    - Influenced by the **müllerian inhibiting substance**
    - Produced by **Sertoli cells**
    - Develop into the fallopian tubes, uterus, and upper portion of vagina in the absence of müllerian inhibiting substance
  - Masculine development of **mesonephric ducts (wolffian)**
    - Produced by the **interstitial cells of Leydig**
    - Influenced by the **testosterone analog**
    - Develops into the epididymis, vas deferens, and seminal vesicles
- **Female differentiation:**
  - The "default," occurring in the absence of müllerian inhibiting substance
  - Vaginal plate apoptosis by 22 weeks develops vaginal canal
  - Process complete by the fifth gestational month

**NOTE: The genital system is closely associated with the urinary system during development and should be evaluated if there are any developmental anomalies.**

## ANATOMY

### MALE

- **Penile layers:** Skin, dartos fascia (superficial), and Buck's fascia (deep)
- **Neurovascular bundle:** Deep dorsal vein, dorsal artery, and paired dorsal nerves of the penis/clitoris
- **Erectile tissue:** Paired corpora cavernosa and the corpora spongiosum

### FEMALE

- **Labia majora:** Skin, Camper's fascia, and Colles' fascia (continuous with abdominal Scarpa's fascia)

**NOTE: The labium majorum has an inferior attachment on the ischiopubic rami that prevents the spread of hematomas and infections.**

- **Labia minora:** Folds of skin without fat

**NOTE: The maximum distance from the base to the edge is >4 cm in terms of criteria for labioplasty.**

- **Clitoris:** Derived from undifferentiated phallus and has paired corpora, vestibular bulbs, and glans
- **Arterial supply:**
  - Internal pudenal artery
    - Perineal artery: Supplies perineum and scrotum/vulva
    - Common penile artery: Three branches (bulbourethral, dorsal, deep cavernosal)
  - Superficial and deep external pudenal artery
    - Branch off the medial side of the femoral artery
    - Supplies skin of lower abdomen and anastomoses with the internal pudenal artery to supply the genitalia
  - Testicular/ovarian arteries: Branch off aorta where gonads originate
- **Innervation:**
  - Pudenal nerve (S2-4)
    - Follows the course of the internal pudenal artery
    - Perineal nerve: Deep motor branch
    - Dorsal nerve of the penis/clitoris
    - Posterior scrotal/labial nerves
    - Inferior anal nerves
  - Ilioinguinal nerve (L1)
    - Anterior scrotal/labial nerve: Root of penis/mons and upper part of scrotum/labium majora

## CONGENITAL VAGINAL DEFECTS

### VAGINAL AGENESIS (MAYER-ROKITANSKY-KÜSTER-HAUSER SYNDROME)[1]

- Congenital absence of vagina: Occurs in **1:4,000-80,000 births**
- Caused by defect in paramesonephric duct development or fusion of urogenital sinus with paramesonephric duct
- Urinary abnormalities include ectopy, duplication, and agenesis; occur 25%-50% of the time
- **Clinical findings (two types)**
  - Genetic female with or without functioning uterus and absent vagina
  - Genetic female with or without functioning uterus, with absent vagina ± anomalies of skeletal, urinary (40%), or digestive system
- **Diagnosis**
  - Pelvic/rectal examination
  - Intravenous pyelogram (IVP) to rule out urinary abnormalities
  - Karyotype screening
  - Spinal radiographs to rule out associated vertebral abnormalities
- **Reconstruction**
  - **Nonoperative (Frank's/Ingram's technique):** Gradual dilation
    - 90% successful in motivated patient. Every patient should have a trial
  - **Málaga flap:** Vulvoperineal fasciocutaneous flaps
  - **Vecchietti procedure:** Laparoscopic technique that uses traction sutures to slowly pull a plastic bead internally 10-12 cm in 7-9 days[2]

- **McIndoe procedure:** Dissect tunnel in perineum above rectum and below bladder to peritoneal reflection; cavity lined with split- or full-thickness skin grafts
  - Patients wear stent for years, stenosis and fistulas common
- **Vascularized bowel segment:** Problems with mucus secretion and bleeding with intercourse
- **Other flaps:** Rectus abdominis flap, gracilis flap, pudendal thigh flap, ureter method, and inferior abdominal wall skin flap

## ACQUIRED VAGINAL/VULVAR DEFECTS[3]

### VAGINAL DEFECTS (Fig. 54-1)

- **Etiologic factors**
  - Cancer (colorectal, bladder), trauma
- Classification system and algorithm proposed by Cordeiro et al[3] based on anatomic location (Fig. 54-2)
- **Reconstruction flaps**
  - Modified Singapore fasciocutaneous flap
  - Vertical rectus flap
  - Bilateral gracilis flap
  - Colon transfer

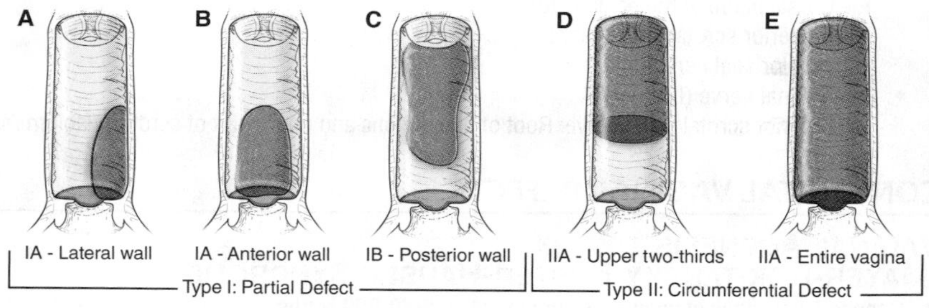


**Fig. 54-1** Acquired vaginal defects and correction.

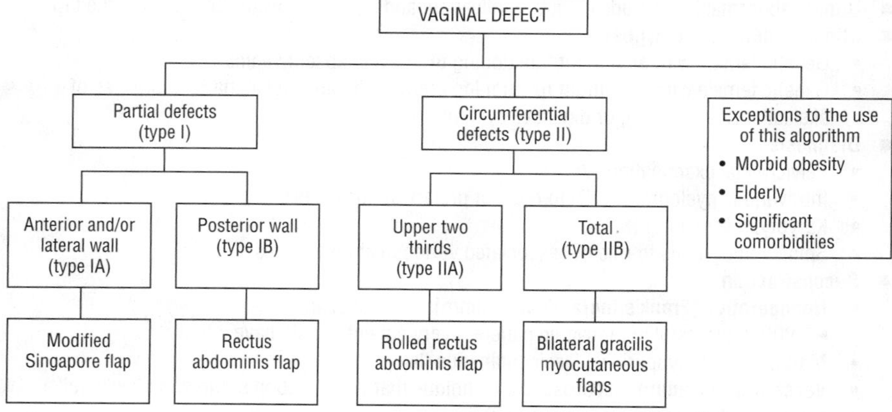


**Fig. 54-2** Classification system and algorithm proposed by Cordeiro based on anatomic location.

## Vulvar Defects

- **Etiologic factors**
  - Cancer, infection, trauma
- **Reconstruction**
  - Skin grafts
  - Fasciocutaneous medial thigh flaps
  - Gracilis myocutaneous V-Y advancement flaps
  - Pedicled ALT flaps

# CONGENITAL PENILE/SCROTAL DEFECTS

## Hypospadias[4] (Fig. 54-3)

The congenital development of the male urethra is incomplete. The meatus exits **ventrally** anywhere from the corona to the perineum.

- **Characteristics**
  - **The more proximal, the more severe the curvature and deformity**
  - Occurs in **1:150-300 males**[5]
  - Likely caused by genetic and environmental factors
  - Surgery performed between **6 and 9 months of age**
  - Ventral curvature of penis with prominent dorsal hood
  - **Meatus location**
    - **Distal third (50%):** Glanular, coronal, subcoronal
    - **Middle third (30%):** Distal penile, shaft, proximal penile
    - **Proximal third (20%):** Penoscrotal, scrotal, perineal
- **Reconstruction**
  - **Goals**
    - Release chordee
    - Create a new urethra
    - Advance urethral meatus to tip of penis
  - **Techniques**
    - **Glanular, coronal, and cases with minimal chordee**
    - **Meatal advancement and glanuloplasty (MAGPI)**
      - Vertical incision of the transverse mucosal bar distal to hypospadias meatus, which is closed transversely
      - Glanuloplasty achieved by midline approximation of lateral glanular wings, which are freed from corporal tunica
      - No urethral lengthening achieved

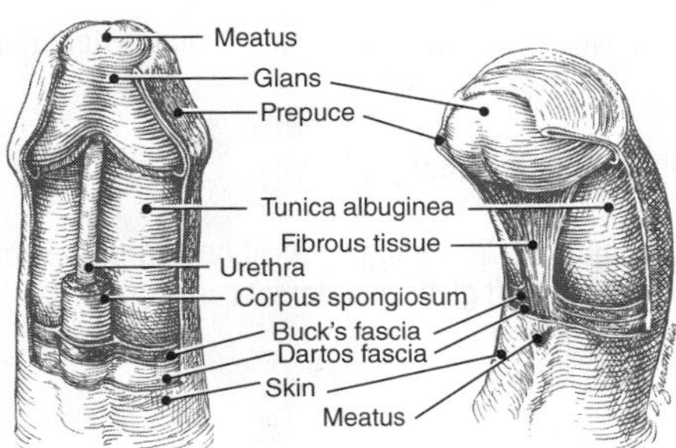


**Fig. 54-3** Hypospadias.

- ▸ **Urethral advancement**
  - ♦ Meatus and distal urethra freed from tunica albuginea of cavernous bodies and then from ventral skin for 1-2 cm
  - ♦ Distal urethra pulled through the tunneled glans and secured to tip of glans penis
  - ♦ Avoids urethral reconstruction, so fistula formation should not occur
- • **Distal defects**
  - ▸ **Tubularized incised plate (TIP) urethroplasty (i.e., Snodgrass)**
    - ♦ Most commonly used for **distal defects**
    - ♦ Longitudinal incision made through midline epithelium of urethral plate, extending from hypospadiac meatus to end of glans
    - ♦ Urethral plate tubularized on itself
    - ♦ Dorsal prepuce mobilized and rotated ventrally to cover urethroplasty
    - ♦ Glans wings closed over urethroplasty in midline
  - ▸ **Flip-flap technique**
    - ♦ Parallel incisions on each side of lateral plate to tip of glans form dorsal urethral wall
    - ♦ Meatal-based flip flap of ventral shaft skin makes up ventral wall
    - ♦ Lateral glans wings approximated over flip-flap urethroplasty after extension of meatus onto tip of glans
- • **Proximal defects**
  - ▸ **Full-thickness graft urethroplasty**
    - ♦ Ventral curvature corrected first by careful removal of chordee tissue
    - ♦ Skin graft harvested from inner surface of prepuce and rolled around catheter to form tube
    - ♦ Graft sutured in oblique fashion to normal urethra proximally and sutured to edges of triangular flap raised from the glans distally
    - ♦ Ventral defect may need coverage with prepuce flaps
  - ▸ **Preputial flap urethroplasty**
    - ♦ Island flap from skin of prepuce brought to ventral surface of penis, and its inner surface used for urethral reconstruction in form of a tube
    - ♦ Outer surface of flap used to cover ventral surface defect
- • **Complications**[6]
  - ▸ Complication rate approximately 10%, increases with age
    - ♦ **6% fistula**
    - ♦ **3% glans dehiscence**
    - ♦ **1% urethral stenosis**
    - ♦ Glans dehiscence, fistulas, and neourethral stricture

## EPISPADIAS

Epispadias is a severe congenital anomaly in which the urethral opening is on the **dorsal** aspect of the penis.

- ■ **Characteristics**
  - • Usually occurs in combination with **bladder exstrophy**
  - • Occurs in **1:30,000 males**
  - • Classified as **glanular, penile,** or **penopubic,** depending on location of urethral opening
  - • Penis short, wide, and stubby with flat and cleft glans and dorsal curvature
- ■ **Reconstruction**
  - • **Goals**
    - ▸ Penile lengthening
    - ▸ Correction of dorsal chordee

- Urethroplasty
- Penile skin coverage
- **Techniques**
  - **Young technique**
    - Penile skin used to construct longitudinal mucosal strip in shape of tube from neourethra
  - **Cantwell-Ransley technique**
    - Circumcising incision performed and shaft degloved down to base
    - Urethral plate outlined with lateral incisions and tubularized
  - **W-flap technique**
    - For secondary epispadias
    - W-shaped incision to produce bilateral, superiorly based groin flaps, with apex of each flap extending below penoscrotal junction
    - Dorsal chordee corrected and urethra reconstructed with full-thickness grafts
    - Dorsal defect covered with preputial skin flaps

## ACQUIRED PENILE/SCROTAL DEFECTS

### PEYRONIE'S DISEASE

This disorder of the penis involves connective tissue and affects 3%-9% of the male population 40-60 years old.

- **Characteristics**
  - Painful erections
  - Penile curvature during erection
  - Firm, palpable nodule or inelastic plaque on penile shaft
  - 10% also have Dupuytren's contracture of palmar fascia.
- **Surgical indications**[7]
  - Stable disease for 6 months
  - Inability to engage in coitus
  - Extensive plaque calcification
  - Failed conservative management
  - Patient desires most rapid and reliable results
- **Complications**
  - Persistence or recurrent curvature (6%-10%)
  - Shortening of penile length (more with plication)
  - Decreased rigidity (5%)
  - Decreased sexual sensation (20%)
- **Surgical techniques**
  - **Tunica plication procedure**
    - Males with minimal penile curvature (30-45 degrees) and relatively long erect penis
    - Circumcising incision with degloving of penile shaft
    - Tunica albuginea opposite area of maximum curvature identified and ellipse excised from each corporal body
    - Tunica defects closed primarily
    - Predicted loss of <20% of erect length
  - **Dermal graft procedure**
    - Curvature >45 degrees
    - Circumcising incision with complete degloving of penile shaft
    - Incisions made through Buck's fascia and mobilized off tunica albuginea

- Diseased tunica albuginea excised (plaque)
- Dermal graft used to cover corporal defects

## Penile Reconstruction[8]

- **Etiologic factors**
  - Trauma, female-male sex change, cancer
- **Reconstructive goals**
  - One-stage, reproducible operation with predictable results
  - Create competent neourethra that allows voiding while standing
  - Restore cosmetically acceptable penis with tactile and erogenous sensibility
  - Bring enough bulk to allow insertion of prosthesis if necessary
- **Reconstruction techniques** (most require penile implant)
  - Radial forearm flap (± unicortical radial bone): **Most popular technique**
  - Free sensate osteocutaneous fibula flap (obtain good sexual function without an implant)
  - Scapula flap, ± latissimus dorsi
  - Abdominal flaps (VRAM or DIEP flaps)
  - Less frequently used free flaps:
    - Gracilis flap
    - Ulnar forearm flap
    - Lateral arm flap
    - Dorsalis pedis flap
    - Groin flap
  - Urethral reconstruction with split- and full-thickness grafts taken from inner thigh, abdomen, or scrotum, and grafts of saphenous vein, appendix, ileum, or bladder

> **TIP:** Prosthesis placement should be delayed until the patient has protective sensation to minimize risk of prosthetic erosion and extrusion.

- **Subtotal defects**
  - Reconstruction technique depends on defect and missing components.
  - Total penile reconstruction is frequently required to achieve acceptable outcomes.
  - Reconstructive options include skin grafts and more complex repairs with free tissue transfer.
- **Traumatic amputation**
  - Attempt microvascular replantation.
  - Preservation: Rinse amputated part in saline, wrap in saline-soaked gauze, place in sterile bag, and place bag in ice slush.
  - Successful replantation has been reported after 16 hours cold ischemia and 6 hours of warm ischemia[9]

## Scrotal Reconstruction[10]

- **Etiologic factors**
  - Congenital anorchia, Fournier's gangrene, burn, traumatic loss, or tumor resection
  - **Partial lesions can frequently be closed primarily because of the elastic nature of the scrotal skin.**
  - **Goals**
    - One-stage operation with cosmetically acceptable result
    - Temperature regulation to preserve testicular function (approximately 32° C or 90° F)

- **Techniques**
  - Superomedial thigh flaps
  - Split-thickness or full-thickness skin graft
  - Pedicled ALT flap
  - Gracilis flap with split-thickness skin graft
  - Tissue expansion of perineal skin or remaining scrotal tissue

### FOURNIER'S GANGRENE[11]

- **Etiologic factors**
  - Perineal tissue necrosis caused by polymicrobial infection
  - Typically seen in **immunosuppressed** patients: diabetics, renal transplant recipients, cancer patients after chemotherapy or radiotherapy, and patients who have undergone medical or surgical perineal manipulation.
  - Organisms pass through Buck's fascia and spread along dartos fascia of the scrotum and penis to Colles' and Scarpa's fascia of the perineum and abdomen wall, respectfully.
  - Can be fatal if not recognized early and treated aggressively
- **Treatment**
  - **Urgent wide debridement to control infection**
  - Broad-spectrum antibiotics
  - Local wound care with topical antibiotics until wound controlled
  - Testes in thigh pouches (temporary) or sutured together to prevent retraction
- **Reconstruction**
  - Meshed/unmeshed split-thickness skin graft for penile shaft
  - See Scrotal Reconstruction above

## TRANSGENDER SURGERY

### TRANSSEXUALISM[12]

Transsexualism is characterized by a sense of discomfort and inappropriateness with one's anatomic sex; a desire to be rid of one's own genitals and live as a member of the opposite sex; a continuous disturbance for at least 2 years; and an absence of physical, psychological, intersex, or chromosomal abnormalities.

The Harry Benjamin International Gender Dysphoria Association has set standards of care and internationally accepted guidelines for treatment for transgender surgery.

- **Reconstruction**
  - **Goals**
    - Single stage
    - Aesthetically pleasing
    - Erogenous sensibility
    - Minimal morbidity
  - **Male to female**
    - Hormonal therapy and introduction into society as female for at least 2 years
    - Psychiatric clearance
    - Surgical interventions
      - Breast augmentation
      - Rhinoplasty
      - Male pattern hair removal

- Reduction of thyroid cartilage
- Feminizing genital surgeries (penectomy, penile inversion, skin grafts, and intestinal substitution)

- **Female to male**
  - Hormonal therapy and introduction into society as male for at least 2 years
  - Psychiatric clearance
  - Surgical interventions
    - Breast amputation or reduction
    - Hysterectomy and oophorectomy
    - Phallus construction (see above)
    - Neoscrotum (see above)

## Key Points

- ✓ Patients with Peyronie's disease may also have Dupuytren's contracture of the hands.
- ✓ The mesonephric duct develops into the epididymis, vas deferens, and seminal vesicles.
- ✓ The paramesonephric ducts develop into the fallopian tubes, uterus, and upper portion of the vagina.
- ✓ The goals for epispadias repair include penile lengthening, correction of dorsal chordee, urethroplasty, and penile skin coverage.
- ✓ The goals for hypospadias repair include release of chordee, creation of new urethra, and advancement of the urethral meatus to the tip of the penis.

## References

1. Eldor L, Friedman JD. Reconstruction of congenital defects of the vagina. Semin Plast Surg 25:142-147, 2011.
2. Miller RJ, Breech LL. Surgical correction of vaginal anomalies. Clin Obstet Gynecol 51:223-236, 2008.
3. Cordeiro PG, Pusic AL, Disa JJ. A classification system and reconstructive algorithm for acquired vaginal defects. Plast Reconstr Surg 110:1058-1065, 2002.
4. Horton CE, Devine CJ. Hypospadiea. In Converse JM, ed. Reconstructive Plastic Surgery, vol 7. Principles and Procedures in Correction Reconstruction and Transplantation, 2nd ed. Philadelphia: WB Saunders, 1977.
5. Macedo A Jr, Rondon A, Ortiz V. Hypospadias. Curr Opin Urol 22:447-452, 2012.
6. Yildiz T, Tahtali IN, Ates DC, et al. Age of patient is a risk factor for urethrocutaneous fistula in hypospadias surgery. J Pediatr Urol 2013 Jan 3. [Epub ahead of print]
7. Levine LA, Burnett AL. Standard operating procedures for Peyronie's disease. J Sex Med 10:230-244, 2012.
8. Babaei A, Safarinejad MR, Farrokhi F, et al. Penile reconstruction: evaluation of the most accepted techniques. Urol J 7:71-78, 2010.
9. Chou EK, Tai YT, Wu CI, et al. Penile replantation, complication management, and technique refinement. Microsurgery 28:153-156, 2008.
10. Chen SY, Fu JP, Chen TM, et al. Reconstruction of scrotal and perineal defects in Fournier's gangrene. Br J Plast Surg 64:528-534, 2011.
11. Ferreira PC, Reis JC, Amarante JM, et al. Fournier's gangrene: a review of 43 reconstructive cases. Plast Reconstr Surg 119:175-184, 2007.
12. Goldberg C, Bowman J. Care of the patient undergoing sex reassignment surgery (SRS), 2006. Available at *http://transhealth.vch.ca/resources/library/tcpdocs/guidelines-surgery.pdf.*

# 55. Pressure Sores

**Jeffrey E. Janis, Eamon B. O'Reilly**

## DEMOGRAPHICS[1]

### PREVALENCE[2-5]

- **General acute setting:** 10%-18% (average approximately 15%)
- **Long-term care facilities:** 2.3%-28% (average approximately 15%)
- **Home care setting:** 0%-29% (average approximately 15%)

### INCIDENCE[6-9]

- **General acute setting:** 0.4%-38%
- **Long-term care facilities:** 2.2%-23.9%
- **Home care setting:** 0%-17%
- **Highest incidences**
  - Elderly patients with femoral neck fractures (66%)
  - Quadriplegic patients (60%)
  - Neurologically impaired young (spinal cord injury [SCI] and veterans)
  - Chronic hospitalization and palliative care

### MORTALITY[1]

- Combined data support the conclusion that pressure sores are not directly the cause of increased mortality, but rather these patients succumb to their overall disease burden, which leads to severe malnutrition, immobility, and decreased tissue perfusion, which allow pressure sores to form.

### COSTS[10,11]

- National Pressure Ulcer Advisory Panel and the U.S. Department of Health and Human Services estimate a cost of **$20,900 to $151,700 per patient** to treat and heal ulcers acquired in hospitals. According to Medicare data, each diagnosis adds **$43,180** to a hospital stay.
- Total estimated cost for surgical and nonsurgical management is **$9.1 to $11.6 billion annually.**

### SUSCEPTIBLE AREAS[1]

- **Bony prominences**
  - Ischial tuberosity (28%)
  - Trochanter (19%)
  - Sacrum (17%)
  - Heel (9%)
  - Scalp

*The views expressed in this article are those of the authors and do not necessarily reflect the official policy or position of the Department of the Navy, Department of Defense, or the United States Government.*

# ETIOLOGIC FACTORS[12]

## EXTRINSIC FACTORS

- Mechanical forces on soft tissue
  - **Shear:** Mechanical stress **parallel** to plane
    - Stretches or compresses muscle perforators to the skin resulting in ischemic necrosis: ***superficial necrosis***
  - **Pressure:** Mechanical force per unit area **perpendicular** to plane[13] (Fig. 55-1)
    - Leads to tissue deformation, mechanical damage, blockage of vessels: ***deep necrosis***
    - Pressures of 2 times capillary arterial pressure for 2 hours produces irreversible ischemia in animal models
  - **Friction:** Resistance to movement between two surfaces
    - Outermost skin layer lost, resulting in increased water loss
    - Most often incurred during **patient transfers**
  - **Moisture**
    - Leads to skin maceration and breakdown
    - Most often the result of **incontinence**

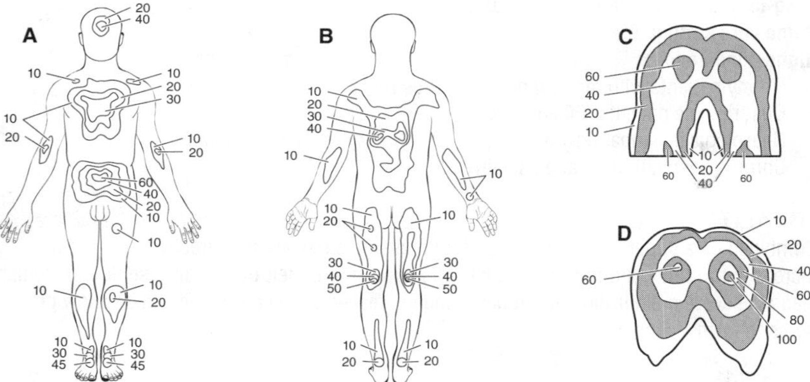


**Fig. 55-1** Pressure-distribution maps (in mm Hg) of a male figure. **A,** Supine. **B,** Prone. **C,** Sitting with feet hanging freely. **D,** Sitting with feet supported.

## INTRINSIC FACTORS

- Patient factors on soft tissue
  - **Ischemia/sepsis**
    - Causes decreased tissue perfusion and predisposes to necrosis
  - **Decreased autonomic control**
    - Can lead to excess perspiration, spasms, and lack of bowel or bladder control
  - **Infection**
    - *Staphylococcus aureus, Streptococcus* spp., *Corynebacterium* (skin), *Proteus mirabilis, Escherichia coli, Pseudomonas aeruginosa,* or *Enterococcus* spp.
  - **Increased age**
    - Decreased skin moisture, tensile strength
    - Increased friability
  - **Sensory loss**
    - Unable to experience discomfort from prolonged sitting or other position, leading to tissue ischemia

- **Vascular disease**
  - Diabetes, peripheral vascular disease, and smoking decrease tissue perfusion and predispose to necrosis.
- **Anemia**
  - Decreased wound healing capabilities
  - Weakness or fatigue that leads to prolonged immobilization
- **Malnutrition**
  - Diminished ability to heal wounds
  - Vitamin supplementation only effective if truly deficient
- **Altered level of consciousness**
  - Loss of protective reflexes or voluntary movements to off-load pressure

## RISK ASSESSMENT[14-17]

### BRADEN SCALE

- Most commonly used
- **Subscales**
  - Sensory perception
  - Skin moisture
  - Activity
  - Mobility
  - Friction and shear
  - Nutritional status
- **Minimum** value of **6**
- **Maximum** value of **23**
- **Subscales of sensory perception, mobility, moisture, and friction and shear most predictive**
- ***Lower scores indicate increased risk for developing pressure ulcers.***
- **Threshold scores for pressure sore development**
  - Tertiary care facilities: **16**
  - Veteran's hospitals: **19**
  - Skilled nursing care facilities: **18**

## CLASSIFICATION[18]

### NATIONAL PRESSURE ULCER ADVISORY PANEL STAGES[18] (Fig. 55-2)

- **Stage I:** Nonblanchable erythema of intact skin.
  - Can be seen within **30 minutes** and usually resolves after **1 hour**
  - Can be difficult to detect in dark-skinned patients
- **Stage II:** Partial-thickness skin loss that presents clinically as a blister, abrasion, or shallow open ulcer.
  - **2-6 hours** of pressure
  - Erythema lasts more than 36 hours.
- **Stage III:** Full-thickness tissue loss down to, but not through, fascia.
  - Subcutaneous fat *may* be exposed, the thickness of which varies by body site (i.e., bridge of nose vs. buttock).
  - Undermining and tunneling may be involved.
- **Stage IV:** Full-thickness tissue loss with involvement of underlying muscle, bone, tendon, ligament, cartilage, or joint capsule.

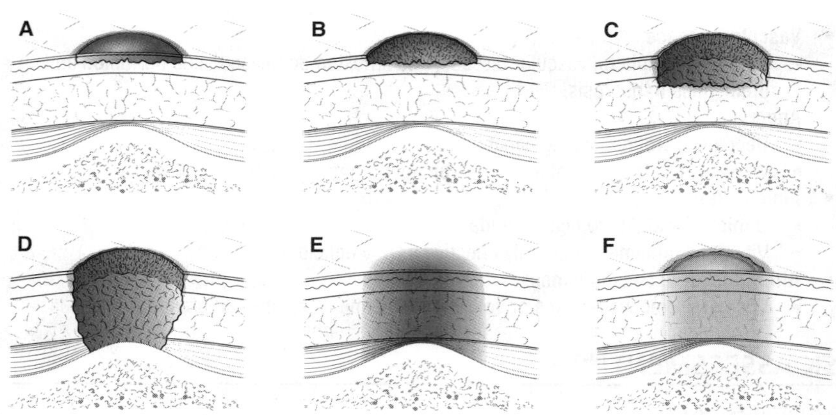


**Fig. 55-2** National Pressure Ulcer Advisory Panel stages. **A,** Stage I. **B,** Stage II. **C,** Stage III. **D,** Stage IV. **E,** Unstageable. **F,** Suspected deep tissue injury.

- **Unstageable:** Full-thickness skin or tissue loss, depth unknown
  - Depth of ulcers is obscured by slough (yellow to gray) and/or eschar.
  - Stable (dry) eschar on the heels acts as a biologic cover and should **not** be removed.
  - Ulcers are uniformly stage III or IV after surgical or biologic debridement.
- **Suspected deep tissue injury of unknown depth**
  - Purple area of intact skin or blood-filled blister may indicate deep tissue injury.
  - Wait for wound to evolve before staging.

## PREVENTION[19-24]

- Proper **skin care** to minimize moisture
- Care during **transfers**
- **Address spasticity**
  - Diazepam
  - Baclofen
  - Dantrolene sodium
- **Pressure dispersion**
  - Padding of pressure points (OR, ICU, hospital bed)
  - Pressure-relief behavior or alternate weight-bearing surfaces
    - **Kosiak's principle:** Tissue tolerates increased pressure if interspersed with pressure-free periods
      - Seated patients must be lifted for 10 seconds every 10 minutes.
      - Supine patients must be turned every 2 hours.
- **Support surfaces**
  - **Static pads**
    - At least **4 inches** of foam is required to provide modest protection.
    - Cochrane review found that specific intraoperative surgical padding is effective at preventing pressure ulcers.
    - Nonsurgical padding is less effective.

- **Alternating air cell mattresses**
  - Composed of air cells oriented perpendicularly to the patient
  - May facilitate dispersal of accumulated metabolites through the vascular and lymphatic channels
- **Low-air-loss mattresses**
  - Facilitate drying of the skin
  - Exert less than 25 mm Hg of pressure on any one point of the body
- **Air-fluidized beds**
  - Patient floats on ceramic beads while warm-regulated air is forced through, eliminating skin moisture.
  - Pressure is maintained at <20 mm Hg (capillary arterial pressure).
- ***No evidence via a Cochrane review that air-fluidized mattresses or low-air-loss mattresses are superior at preventing pressure ulcers vs. conventional support surfaces.***

■ **Minimize head-of-bed elevation** to reduce sacral shear and pressure (<45 degrees).
■ Pay attention to **incontinence** (urinary and fecal).
■ Ensure proper **nutrition.**
■ **Optimize** underlying medical comorbidities.

> **TIP:** Careful attention to preventive measures helps decrease the incidence and recurrence of pressure sores. It is critical to take a multidisciplinary approach to treat the whole patient, with significant input from an experienced physical medicine and rehabilitation physician.

## PATIENT EVALUATION

■ **History and physical examination**
- Determine etiologic factors for pressure sores.
- See Chapter 2.

■ **Pretreatment laboratory studies and imaging**
- Complete blood count
  - White blood cell count with differential
  - Hemoglobin/hematocrit
- Glucose/$HbA_1C$
- Erythrocyte sedimentation rate/C-reactive protein
- Albumin/prealbumin
- **Anemia, serum protein levels, and inflammatory markers have been shown to normalize *after* surgical management of pressure sores, indicating that factors such as low serum albumin are symptoms and not causes of the chronic process.**
- MRI[25]
  - Evaluates extent of osteomyelitis
    - **97% sensitive**
    - **89% specific**

> **TIP:** All medical comorbidities and both intrinsic and extrinsic factors should be documented and optimized before reconstruction to maximize success.

> **TIP:** If the extent of osteomyelitis is unknown or underappreciated, reconstruction is destined to fail.

## MEDICAL MANAGEMENT[1,26]

- **Relieve pressure**
  - Positional changes
  - Proper mattress, cushion, or wheelchair
- Control **infection**
- Control **extrinsic factors** (shear, moisture, friction)
- **Debridement:** Surgery vs. topical enzymatic agent
- **Dressings**
  - DuoDerm (ConvaTec, Princeton, NJ)
  - Wet-to-dry saline dressing changes
  - Dakin's solution if *Pseudomonas* spp. suspected

**TIP:** Dakin's solution (sodium hypochlorite and boric acid) is toxic to healthy tissue and should be used in dilute form (quarter strength) and only for a limited period (e.g., 3 days).

  - Silver sulfadiazine
  - Other topicals (e.g., hydrogels, absorbent foams)[27] (Fig. 55-3)

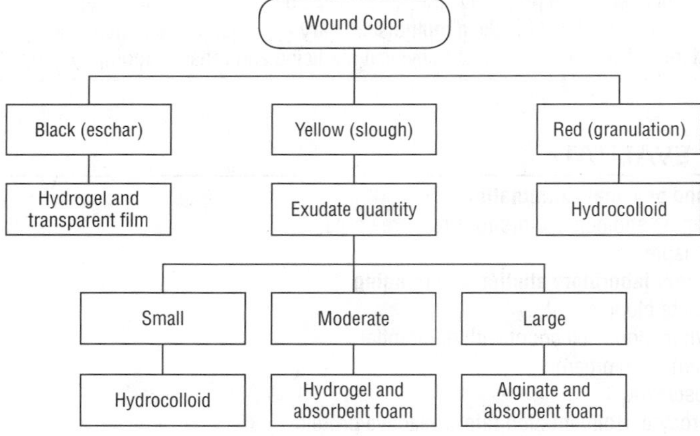


**Fig. 55-3** Simple algorithm for wound care in full-thickness, noninfected, chronic wounds.

- **Osteomyelitis** diagnosis critical to effective medical treatment
  - **Benchmark: bone biopsy**
  - MRI, CT, and plain film may be used in conjunction with physical examination for diagnosis.[28]
- **Negative-pressure wound therapy (NPWT)**
  - Effective for first-line treatment of stage III ulcers and some stage IV ulcers
  - May bridge stage IV ulcers to surgery
  - Effective for treatment of chronic wounds with 25% (average) faster healing rates

**TIP:** Vigilant management is crucial if NPWT is to be used as primary therapy. The device must be assessed at regular intervals for adequate seal and pressure points. The wound must be evaluated by a physician at least every 2 weeks for wound progression, otherwise surgery may be indicated.

## SURGICAL GUIDELINES[29]

- **Stage I** and **II** pressure ulcers usually can be managed **nonsurgically.**
- **Stage III** and **IV** pressure ulcers frequently require **surgical intervention.**
  - Consider the patient's **ambulatory status** to help with proper flap selection.
  - **Design flaps as large as possible** with suture lines away from area of direct pressure.
  - **Do not violate adjacent flap territories** for possible future flap coverage.
- **Staged operations:** Some evidence suggests one-stage debridement, ostectomy, and immediate reconstruction is as successful as staged debridement, negative-pressure therapy, and delayed reconstruction.[30]

### GOALS OF RECONSTRUCTION

- Debridement of all devitalized tissue
- Complete excision of pseudobursa
- Ostectomy of all devitalized or infected bone to clinically hard, healthy, bleeding bone
- Excellent hemostasis
- Obliteration of dead space with well-vascularized tissue
- Selection and creation of flaps that do not jeopardize future flap coverage
- Tension-free closure
- Pressure off-loading of reconstructed area

**TIP:** Infiltration of the peribursal area with wetting solution (1000 ml normal saline solution, plus 30 ml 1% plain lidocaine, plus 1 ampule epinephrine 1:1000) using a liposuction infiltration cannula can help decrease blood loss and hydrodissect the bursal tissues from the surrounding tissues.[31]

**TIP:** Coating the bursa with methylene blue dye before excision can help verify that all bursal tissue has been completely excised.

## RECONSTRUCTION BY ANATOMIC SITE

### SACRAL ULCERS

- **Common options**
  - **Lumbosacral flap (fasciocutaneous)**
    - Requires backgrafting at donor site
  - **Unilateral or bilateral gluteal fasciocutaneous flap versus myocutaneous rotation flap**
    - Segmental or full flap can be used depending on patient's ambulatory status.
    - Consider muscle flap if deep ulcer requires obliteration of dead space.
    - Flap can be rerotated in case of recurrence.
  - **Unilateral or bilateral gluteal myocutaneous V-Y advancement flap**
    - Flap can be readvanced in case of recurrence.

### ISCHIAL PRESSURE SORES

- **Common options**
  - **Gluteal fasciocutaneous flap versus myocutaneous rotation flap**
    - Segmental or full flap can be used depending on patient's ambulatory status.
  - **Posterior hamstring myocutaneous V-Y advancement flap**
  - Posterior thigh flap (fasciocutaneous)
  - Tensor fascia lata flap

### Trochanteric Pressure Sores

- **Common options**
  - **Tensor fascia lata**
  - Tensor fascia lata and **vastus lateralis**
  - **Girdlestone procedure** (proximal femurectomy and obliteration of dead space with vastus lateralis)

### Multiple Pressure Sores

- **Common options**
  - Treat with single stage if possible
  - If significant bony involvement, may require hip disarticulation, hemipelvectomy, or hemicorporectomy[32,33]
  - Total or subtotal thigh flaps

> **TIP:** Consider raising fasciocutaneous flaps with sharp scissors dissection instead of electrocautery to prevent thermal injury to the suprafascial vasculature.

> **TIP:** It is unnecessary to completely undermine all rotation flaps. Instead, check excursion constantly until a tension-free closure is possible. Further undermining jeopardizes blood supply.

## POSTOPERATIVE MANAGEMENT[34,35]

- **Pressure relief bed** for 3-6 weeks
- Culture-directed **antibiotics** with infectious disease consultation
- **Antispasmodics**
- **Bowel regimen** or ostomy care
- **Nutrition** optimization
- Active or passive range of motion of the uninvolved extremity
- Seat mapping
- Sitting protocol
- Education

## COMPLICATIONS[36]

- Hematoma
- Infection
- Wound dehiscence
- Recurrence
  - Overall recurrence rate **7%-82%**
  - Recent large meta-analysis (55 papers)[36]:
    - **Myocutaneous flaps:** Overall complication rate **18.6%,** recurrence rate **8.9%**
    - **Fasciocutaneous flaps:** Overall complication rate **11.7%,** recurrence rate **11.2%**
    - **Perforator flaps:** Overall complication rate **19.6%,** recurrence rate **5.6%**

## Key Points

- ✓ Proper and thorough evaluation of patients with pressure sores is critical. Surgery is the last thing to do. Identification of etiologic factors and appropriate treatment are key steps to a successful outcome.
- ✓ A multidisciplinary team consisting of a physical medicine and rehabilitation physician, infectious disease specialist, nutritionist, physical therapist, psychiatrist, and plastic surgeon can help optimize outcomes.
- ✓ Vitamin supplementation is not helpful for patients who do not have a true deficiency.
- ✓ Elderly patients with hip fractures, quadriplegics, and chronically hospitalized patients are at the highest risk for developing pressure sores.
- ✓ NPWT should be used as a management adjunct.
- ✓ Stage I and II pressure sores usually can be managed nonsurgically.
- ✓ Stage III and IV pressure sores frequently require flap surgery.
- ✓ Segmental muscle flaps or fasciocutaneous flaps should be used for ambulatory patients to decrease morbidity.
- ✓ Adhere to surgical principles when selecting flaps. Given the overall high rates of recurrence, choose rotation or advancement flaps that can be rerotated or readvanced.
- ✓ Be sure to seat map patients after reconstruction in case pressure dynamics have changed, especially after ostectomies.
- ✓ Prevention and education are critical.

## References


1. Janis JE, Kenkel JM. Pressure sores. Sel Read Plast Surg 9:1-42, 2003.
2. O'Brien SP, Wind S, Van Rijswijk L, et al. Sequential biannual prevalence studies of pressure ulcers at Allegheny-Hahnemann University Hospital. Ostomy Wound Manage 44(Suppl 3A):S78, 1998.
3. Langemo DK, Olson B, Hunter S, et al. Incidence and prediction of pressure ulcers in five patient care settings. Decubitus 4:25, 1991.
4. Baker J. Medicaid claims history of Florida long-term care facility residents hospitalized for pressure ulcers. J Wound Ostomy Continence Nurs 23:23, 1996.
5. Oot-Giromini BA. Pressure ulcer prevalence, incidence and associated risk factors in the community. Decubitus 6:24, 1993.
6. O'Sullivan KL, Engrav LH, Maier RV, et al. Pressure sores in the acute trauma patient: incidence and causes. J Trauma 42:276, 1997.
7. Lyder CH, Yu C, Stevenson D, et al. Validating the Braden scale for the prediction of pressure ulcer risk in blacks and Latino/Hispanic elders: a pilot study. Ostomy Wound Manage 44(Suppl 3A):S42, 1998.
8. Berlowitz DR, Bezerra HQ, Brandeis GH, et al. Are we improving the quality of nursing home care: the case of pressure ulcers. J Am Geriatr Soc 48:59, 2000.
9. Bergstrom N, Braden B, Kemp M, et al. Predicting pressure ulcer risk: a multisite study of the predictive validity of the Braden scale. Nurs Res 47:261, 1998.
10. Berlowitz D, VanDeusen Lukas C, Parker V, et al. Preventing pressure ulcers in hospitals: a toolkit for improving quality of care. Rockville, MD: Agency for Healthcare Research and Quality. Available at *http://www.ahrq.gov/research/ltc/pressureulcertoolkit/*.
11. Russo A, Steiner C, Spector W. Hospitalizations related to pressure ulcers among adults 18 years and older, 2006. Rockville, MD: Agency for Healthcare Research and Quality. Available at *http://www.hcup-us.ahrq.gov/reports/statbriefs/sb64.jsp*.
12. Enis J, Sarmiento A. The pathophysiology and management of pressure sores. Orthop Rev 2:26, 1973.
13. Lindan O, Greenway RM, Piazza JM. Pressure distribution on the surface of the human body. I. Evaluation in lying and sitting positions using a "bed of springs and nails." Arch Phys Med Rehabil 46:378, 1965.

14. Whitfield MD, Kaltenthaler EC, Akehurst RL, et al. How effective are prevention strategies in reducing the prevalence of pressure ulcers? J Wound Care 9:261, 2000.
15. Bergstrom N, Braden BJ, Laguzza A, et al. The Braden scale for predicting pressure sore risk. Nurs Res 36:205, 1987.
16. Braden NJ, Bergstrom N. Predictive validity of the Braden scale for pressure sore risk in a nursing home population. Res Nurs Health 17:459, 1994.
17. Cox J. Predictive power of the Braden scale for pressure sore risk in adult critical care patients: a comprehensive review. J Wound Ostomy Continence Nurs 39:613, 2012.
18. National Pressure Ulcer Advisory Panel (NPUAP). Pressure Ulcer Stages/Categories 2007. Available at *http://www.npuap.org/resources/educational-and-clinical-resources/npuap-pressure-ulcer-stagescategories/.*
19. Reuler JB, Cooney TG. The pressure sore: pathophysiology and principles of management. Ann Intern Med 94:661, 1981.
20. Krouskop TA. The role of mattress and beds in preventing pressure sores. In Lee BY, Ostrander LE, Cochran GV, et al, eds. The Spinal Cord Injured Patient: Comprehensive Management. New York: Demos Medical Publishing, 2002.
21. McLeod AG. Principles of alternating pressure surfaces. Adv Wound Care 10:30, 1997.
22. Goetz LL, Brown GS, Priebe MM. Interface pressure characteristics of alternating air cell mattresses in persons with spinal cord injury. J Spinal Cord Med 25:167, 2002.
23. McInnes E, Dumville JC, Jammali-Blasi A, et al. Support surfaces for treating pressure ulcers (Review). Cochrane Database Syst Rev 12:CD009490, 2011.
24. McInnes E, Jammali-Blasi A, Bell-Syer S, et al. Preventing pressure ulcers—Are pressure-redistributing support surfaces effective? A Cochrane systematic review and meta-analysis. Int J Nurs Stud 49:345, 2012.
25. Huang AB, Schweitzer ME, Hume E, et al. Osteomyelitis of the pelvis/hips in paralyzed patients: accuracy and clinical utility of MRI. J Comput Assist Tomogr 22:437, 1998.
26. Wooten MK. Management of chronic wounds in the elderly. Clin Fam Med 3:1, 2001.
27. Ladin DA. Understanding dressings. Clin Plast Surg 25:433, 1998.
28. Larson DL, Gilstrap J, Simonelic K, et al. Is there a simple, definitive, and cost-effective way to diagnose osteomyelitis in the pressure ulcer patient? Plast Reconstr Surg 127:670, 2011.
29. Conway H, Griffith BH. Plastic surgery for closure of decubitus ulcers in patients with paraplegia: based on experience with 1000 cases. Am J Surg 91:946, 1956.
30. Larson DL, Hudak KA, Waring WP, et al. Protocol management of late-stage pressure ulcers: a 5-year retrospective study of 101 consecutive patients with 179 ulcers. Plast Reconstr Surg 129:897, 2012.
31. Han H, Fen J, Fine NA. Use of the tumescent technique in pressure ulcer closure. Plast Reconstr Surg 110:711, 2002.
32. Barnett CC Jr, Ahmad J, Janis JE, et al. Hemicorporectomy: back to front. Am J Surg 196:1000, 2008.
33. Janis JE, Ahmad J, Lemmon JA, et al. A 25-year experience with hemicorporectomy for terminal pelvic osteomyelitis. Plast Reconstr Surg 124:1165, 2009.
34. Vasconez LD, Schneider WJ, Jurkiewicz MJ. Pressure sores. Curr Probl Surg 24:23, 1977.
35. Hentz VR. Management of pressure sores in a specialty center: a reappraisal. Plast Reconstr Surg 64:683, 1979.
36. Sameem M, Au M, Wood T, et al. A systematic review of complication and recurrence rates of musculocutaneous, fasciocutaneous, and perforator-based flaps for treatment of pressure sores. Plast Reconstr Surg 130:67e, 2012.

# 56. Lower Extremity Reconstruction

Jeffrey E. Janis, Eamon B. O'Reilly

## LOWER EXTREMITY WOUNDS[1]

### Etiologic Factors

- Trauma or open fractures
- Postsurgical dehiscence
- Compartment syndrome
- Tumor (e.g., sarcoma)
- Infection or osteomyelitis
- Radiation
- Vascular insufficiency
  - Arterial
  - Venous
- Diabetes

### Reconstruction Goals

- Debride devitalized tissue and obtain healthy wound bed
- Restore stability, structure, vascularity, and function
- Obliterate dead space
- Provide durable coverage of vital structures
- Aesthetic result

### Evaluation

- **ABCs:** Trauma evaluation is of paramount importance
- **Vascular** examination (e.g., palpable pulses, Doppler examination)
- **Neurologic** examination
- Assessment of size, depth, and exposure of vital structures
- Evaluation of radiographs

---

The views expressed in this article are those of the authors and do not necessarily reflect the official policy or position of the Department of the Navy, Department of Defense, or the United States Government.

# OPEN TIBIAL FRACTURES

## CLASSIFICATION[2,3] (Tables 56-1 and 56-2; Fig. 56-1)

- The **severity of soft tissue damage** is the foremost predictor of the clinical course and likelihood of healing.

**Table 56-1** *Gustilo Classification of Open Fracture*

| Type | Criteria |
|---|---|
| I | Open fracture with clean laceration <1 cm long |
| II | Open fracture with clean laceration >1 cm long without extensive soft tissue injury, flaps, or avulsions |
| III | Open fractures with extensive damage to soft tissue, including muscle, skin, and neurovascular structures |
| A | Adequate coverage available despite extensive damage |
| B | Extensive injury with periosteal stripping, bone exposure, and/or massive contamination |
| C | Open fracture with arterial injury requiring repair |

**Table 56-2** *Byrd Classification of Lower Extremity Trauma*

| Type | Criteria |
|---|---|
| I | Low-energy forces causing a spiral or oblique fracture pattern with skin lacerations <2 cm and a relatively clean wound |
| II | Moderate-energy forces causing a comminuted or displaced fracture pattern with skin laceration >2 cm and moderate adjacent skin and muscle contusion but *without* devitalized muscle |
| III | High-energy forces causing a significantly displaced fracture pattern with severe comminution, segmental fracture, or bone defect with extensive associated skin loss and devitalized muscle |
| IV | Fracture pattern as in type III but with extreme-energy forces as in high-velocity gunshot or shotgun wounds, a history of crush or degloving, or associated vascular injury requiring repair |

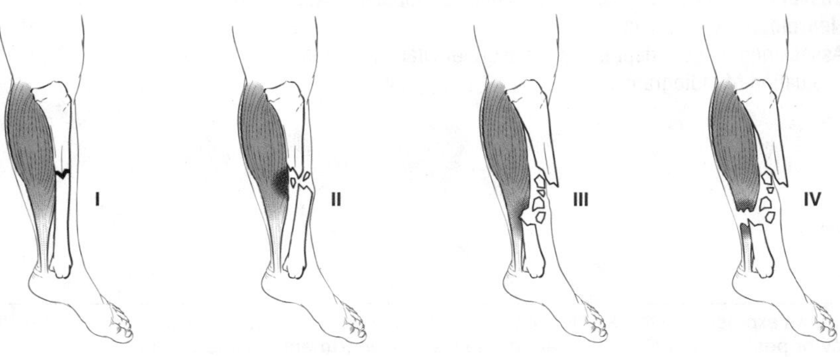


**Fig. 56-1** Byrd classification of lower extremity trauma.

## Prognostic Factors

- **Keller**[4]
  - Reviewed 10,000 tibial shaft fractures and found risk of systemic complications increased with presence of the following:
    - Comminution
    - Displacement
    - Bone loss
    - Distraction
    - Soft tissue injury
    - Infection
    - Polytrauma

**NOTE: Fracture location or configuration and concomitant fibular fracture have NO prognostic significance.**

## Order of Acute Treatment

1. **Reduction** and **stabilization** of fracture (usually external fixator)
2. Restoration of **vascular** inflow, if required
3. **Four compartment fasciotomies,** if required
4. Debridement and washout of wound
   - If vascular exposure, then immediate coverage
   - If no exposed vital structures, then repeat scheduled debridement

> **TIP:** The most important factor for the management of any open, lower extremity fracture is thorough debridement of devitalized tissue.

## Timing of Reconstruction

- **Byrd et al**[5] (Table 56-3)
  - Advocated radical bone and soft tissue debridement with flap coverage in the **first 5-6 days** after injury for type III and IV fractures
    - Muscle flap coverage during acute phase: Fewest complications and shortest hospitalization
  - Fractures not treated during the acute phase predictably entered a subacute, colonized, infected phase from **1 to 6 weeks** after injury
    - *Increased complication rate during subacute phase was attributed to difficulty in establishing adequate borders for bony debridement.*
  - Chronic phase (>6 weeks after injury) characterized by granulating wound, adherent soft tissue, and local areas of infection
    - Limits of bony debridement become well demarcated during chronic phase.
    - Devitalized and infected bone can be identified when cortical surfaces have nonadherent soft tissue and medullary bone is pale and fibrotic.
  - Incidence of infection for type III fracture: 5%
  - Incidence of infection for type IV fracture: 15%
  - Time to full-weight-bearing status: **Average 6 months** for types III and IV

**Table 56-3** *Biologic Phases of Open-Fracture Wounds*

| Category | Clinical Features | Time Since Injury |
|---|---|---|
| Acute | Contaminated but not infected<br>Hemorrhagic and edematous<br>Presence of ischemic and devitalized soft tissue and bone<br>Serosanguinous drainage | 1-5 days |
| Subacute | Colonized and infected wound<br>Seropurulent drainage<br>Erythema, increased swelling, cellulitis<br>Exudative wound surfaces late | 1-6 weeks |
| Chronic | Infection limited to scar and sequestra in fracture<br>Granulating, contracting wound<br>Soft tissues stuck to healthy bone outside of fracture | >6 weeks |

- **Yaremchuk et al**[6]
  - Reviewed patients with flap coverage at average of **17 days** after injury with infection rate at 14%
  - **Key difference:** *Complete removal of all bone fragments*
- **Godina**[7]
  - **Group I:** Free flap within 75 hours
    - Failure rate: 0.75%
    - Postoperative infection rate: **1.5%**
    - Time to union: 6-8 months
  - **Group II:** Flap between 3 days and 3 months
    - Failure rate: 12%
    - Postoperative infection rate: **17.5%**
    - Time to union: 12.3 months
  - **Group III:** Flap between 3 months and 12.6 years
    - Failure rate: 9.5%
    - Postoperative infection rate: **6%**
    - Time to union: 29 months
- Recent advances in both civilian and military experiences indicate that by using an **aggressive washout protocol,** in addition to **negative-pressure wound therapy (NPWT),** lower extremity injuries may undergo reconstruction in the subacute phase with excellent success rates.[8,9]

## Bony Reconstruction

- Performed to promote bone healing
- **Essential elements** for osseous healing of opposed fracture fragments: **blood supply** and **stabilization**
  - **Blood supply**[10-12] (Fig. 56-2)
    - **Nutrient artery**
      - Enters groove on posterior tibia and extends as a nutrient channel within the cortex (vulnerable to injury); then enters the medulla, where it divides into network of vessels supplying the cortex from the endosteal surface
      - **Endosteal circulation:** Supplies inner two thirds of the cortex
    - **Metaphyseal vessels**
    - **Periosteal vessels**
      - **Periosteal circulation:** Supplies outer third of the cortex, runs down long axis of the bone

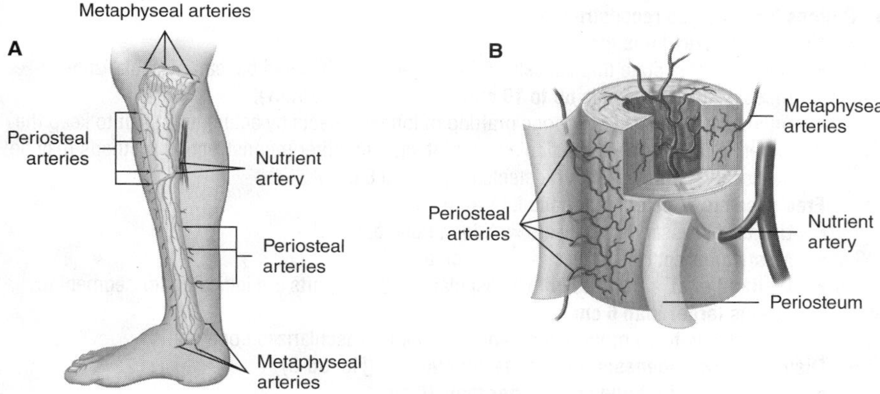


**Fig. 56-2** Blood supply to the tibia.

**NOTE: When a long bone is fractured, the nutrient vessels are disrupted, and the distal fragment is rendered avascular up to the point where the metaphyseal vessels enter the bone.** ***However, because periosteal vessels run transversely, the blood supply to the periosteum is maintained.***

- **Types of osseous callus**
  - **Periosteal**
    - Callus appears on **day 3.**
    - It provides ancillary external support to the fracture and always contains a zone of fibrocartilage.
    - Blood supply initially is from **surrounding soft tissues** and **periosteum.**
    - The periosteal callus is extremely important in the union of **displaced and comminuted fractures.**
  - **Medullary**
    - Callus is first noted on **day 4.**
    - Blood supply is solely from the **medulla.**
    - Stable, **nondisplaced** fractures heal with this type of callus, and **time to union is the shortest.**
  - **Intracortical**
    - Composed of woven bone
    - Blood supply intraosseous, extraosseous, or both
    - May be absent if bone fragments are too closely apposed for blood vessels to grow between them (e.g., compression plate fixation)
    - Fewer progenitor cells in adults than in children (so limited in amount of repair capability)
      - The periosteum is believed to be the origin of these cells.
      - Studies suggest that overlying soft tissues are important for osseous healing, because they provide an immediate source of blood supply to the fracture.
- **Options for stabilizing opposed fractures**
  - Plaster immobilization enclosing open wound (Trueta technique)
  - Internal fixation with plates, rods, and screws
  - External fixation

- **Options for bone gap reconstruction**
  - **Nonvascularized bone grafting**
    - Some authors state that cancellous bone grafts can be used beneath vascularized muscle flaps for defects **up to 10 cm.**[9]
    - An intact fibula facilitates bone grafting of longer defects by acting as a strut to keep the extremity at length. (If the fibula is not intact, then other reconstruction methods may be necessary, particularly with defects larger than 8 cm.)
  - **Free osseous or osteocutaneous flap transfer**
    - Usually necessary for patients with long bone gaps
    - **Most common:** Fibula, iliac crest, scapula
    - **Weiland et al[13]:** Concluded that vascularized bone grafts are indicated for segmental defects **larger than 6 cm**
    - May take up to 15 months for stable union after vascularized bone grafts
  - **Distraction osteogenesis (Ilizarov technique)**[14,15] (Fig. 56-3)
    - May be used for **bone gaps larger than 10 cm**
    - Involves radical debridement of the fractured bone ends and transection of the cortical bone outside the zone of injury, leaving the medullary bone and blood supply intact
    - Once corticotomy performed, insert Ilizarov pins near bone ends on either side of gap and apply distraction apparatus
    - Wait **7 days** before distraction
    - Distract at **1 mm/day** until defect spanned
    - Frame usually kept on for **1 year**
    - **Advantages**
      - The amount of bone generated is anatomically correct for the size of the defect.
      - Soft tissue defects can be closed by the docking method during the same process.
      - Blood transfusions are usually not required.
    - **Contraindications**
      - **Defects larger than 12 cm**
      - Compromised or deficient residual bone stock that cannot support two or three serial corticotomies
    - **Complications**
      - Pin-tract infection
      - Stiffness of adjacent joints
      - Severe pain

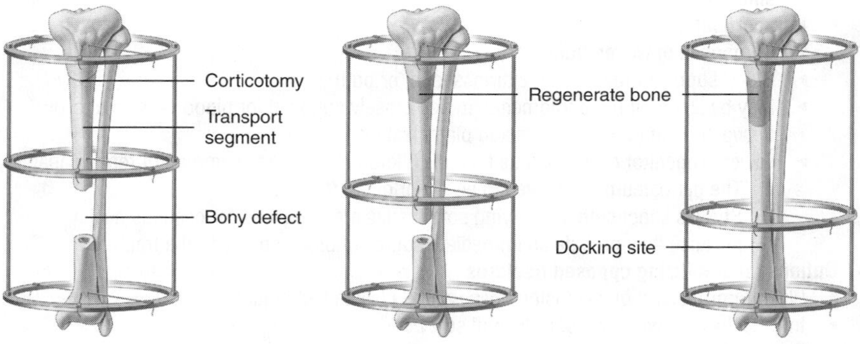


**Fig. 56-3** Bone transport.

## OPEN JOINT INJURIES

- In acute injury, obtain preoperative and intraoperative cultures, give broad-spectrum antibiotic agents, irrigate early and copiously, debride joint and injured soft tissues, and perform first-stage closure of wounds without drains.[16]
- The most common pathogens are *Pseudomonas* and *Klebsiella.*
- Soft tissue closure alone over chronically contaminated and open joints likely leads to **septic joint.**
- Studies of Trueta's closed plaster method have shown that joints allowed to remain open while patients ambulate heal without loss of the cartilaginous interface and without infection.[5]
- Second-stage muscle or soft tissue cover without water-seal closure can be performed.

## SOFT TISSUE RECONSTRUCTION

### GOALS

- Stable wound coverage
- Acceptable appearance
- Minimal donor site morbidity

### PRINCIPLES

- Adequate and thorough wound debridement
  - May require multiple serial debridements
- Control of any wound colonization or infection
  - Base antibiotic coverage on wound cultures
- Flap donor tissues should be harvested outside zone of injury

### LOCAL FLAPS

- **Thigh**
  - Extensive flap reconstruction not required because of large amounts of muscle tissue that can be advanced locally into wound and because of coverage with split-thickness skin graft, if necessary
  - Tensor fascia lata, gracilis, rectus femoris, vastus lateralis, biceps muscle flaps
- **Leg**
  - **Upper third** (in order of preference)
    - **Medial head of gastrocnemius**
      - Single, proximal neurovascular pedicle
      - Broad belly (larger than lateral head)
      - No functional deficit

> **TIP:** Score the fascia of the gastrocnemius to obtain greater muscular coverage of larger surface area defects.

    - **Lateral head of gastrocnemius**
      - Smaller
      - No functional deficit
    - **Proximally based soleus**
      - Can be reliably carried to a point approximately 5 cm above its tendinous insertion
      - Responsible for the venous pump
      - "Slow" muscle used for posture stabilization and slow gait
      - No functional deficit

- **Bipedicled tibialis anterior** (Fig. 56-4)
  - Extremely important for dorsiflexion of foot and should not be entirely sacrificed
  - Muscle function preserved when raised as a bipedicled flap
  - Transfer requires detaching dense anterior tibial connections while retaining segmental blood supply from anterior tibial artery.
  - Can use muscle-splitting approach and tibialis anterior for coverage of middle third
    - No functional deficit ensues
- **Middle third**
  - **Common options:**
    - **Proximally based soleus**
    - **Medial head of gastrocnemius**
    - **Lateral head of gastrocnemius**
    - **Flexor digitorum longus (FDL) for lower portion of middle third**
      - Can be transferred without significant functional loss
      - Used for small defects
      - Neurovascular pedicle usually enters at junction of proximal and middle third
    - **Extensor digitorum longus (EDL)**
      - Supplied by anterior tibial artery
      - Used for closure of small wounds (<5 cm)
      - Incision made 2 cm lateral to tibia
      - Located lateral to tibial artery
      - Preserve superficial peroneal nerve
      - If entire muscle used, then loss of toe extension is permanent
    - **Extensor digitorum hallucis (EDH) for lower portion of middle third**
      - Very narrow, so can only be used for small defects or to augment other flaps
      - To prevent great toe drop, distal tendon should be attached to EDL when dividing the muscle for transfer

A

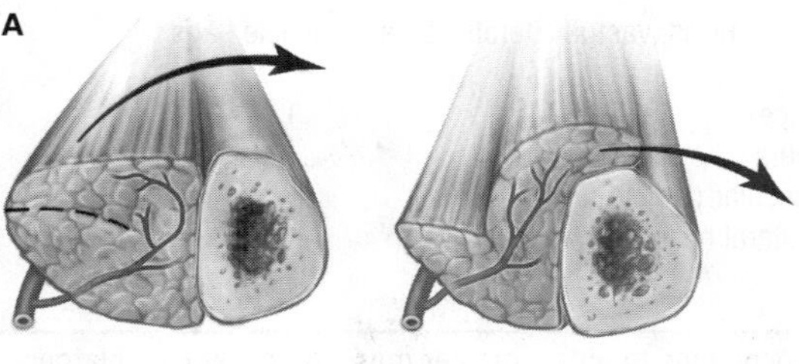

B

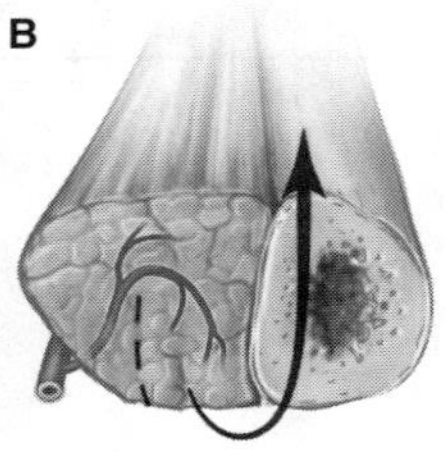

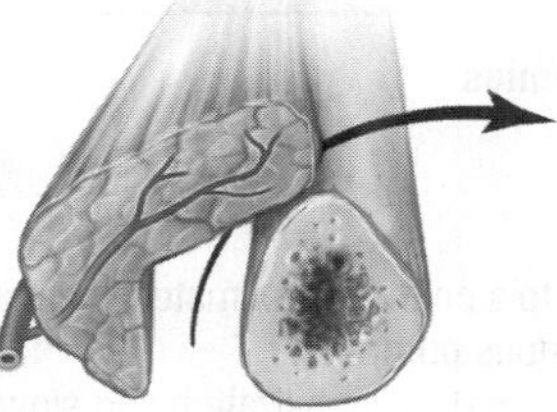

**Fig. 56-4** Technique of longitudinal splitting of the tibialis anterior muscle.

- **Flexor hallucis longus (FHL) for lower portion of middle third**
  - Primary function is to provide push-off for the great toe, so consider patient's occupation (e.g., athlete) before using
- **Tibialis anterior**

- **Lower third**
  - **Local flaps**
    - **Medial lower third:** Consider FHL, FDL, tibialis anterior, abductor hallucis, and extensor digitorum brevis muscle island flap
    - **Lateral lower third:** Peroneus brevis or tertius (very small; usually transferred with other flap) and lateral supramalleolar flap
  - **Distant flaps**
    - **Cross-leg flap**[17]
      - Can use if free flap is not an option
      - Local flap necrosis in **40%**
      - Infection in **28%**
      - Transferred as fasciocutaneous tissue units with length/width ratio 3:1 or 4:1
      - Can base on the axial blood supply of the posterior descending subfascial cutaneous branch of the popliteal artery
  - **Perforator flaps:** All fasciocutaneous flap skin perforators are either direct (source vessel to skin) or indirect (terminal branch of deeper tissue branch) perforator flaps (Fig. 56-5).
    - Perforator flap reconstruction particularly useful in the distal third, where the standard is otherwise free tissue transfer
    - **Sural artery flap**
      - Perforators from medial head of gastrocnemius more reliable
      - Most perforators found in distal half of the muscle near the midline raphe
      - Useful in upper-third and middle-third reconstruction, and in free tissue transfer
      - Venous drainage possibly unreliable
    - **Distally based (reverse) sural artery flap**[18,19]
      - *Neuro-skin* flap, because the sural nerve runs with median superficial sural artery
      - Arterial supply retrograde septocutaneous perforators connecting from the peroneal artery to the superficial sural
      - Small saphenous vein always included in the flap
      - Avoid compression of the pedicle.
      - Local flap necrosis in up to **21%**

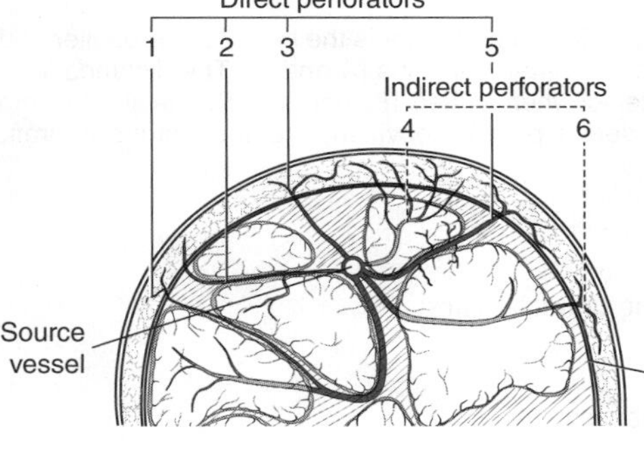


**Fig. 56-5** The distinct deep fascia perforators of Nakajima and colleagues can be considered more simply as either *direct* or *indirect* perforators.

- ♦ **Propeller flap**[20] (Fig. 56-6)
  - Described by Hyakusoku et al (90-degree rotation) and Hallock (180-degree rotation) as an alternative to free tissue transfer in the distal third[21,22]
  - Unequal length **island fasciocutaneous flap** based on a **single perforator** (e.g., peroneal artery perforators)
  - Pedicle occlusion prevented by maintaining pedicle length of at least **2 cm**
  - Partial flap loss in **11.3%** and venous congestion in **8.1%**[23]

> **TIP:** Numerous perforator flaps exist for the lower extremity, and especially the lower third of the leg. Judicious use of these flaps for reconstruction options must be weighed against relatively high complications rates such as partial flap loss and the inherent steep learning curves.[24]

- ■ **Foot**
  - **Split-thickness skin graft**
    - ▸ Can use even on calcaneus and first metatarsal head
      - ♦ Postoperative ink pad recordings have shown that patient's gait patterns change to enhance graft protection despite weight.[25]
  - Island instep fasciocutaneous or myocutaneous flap that preserves sensation
  - Toe fillet
  - Plantar digital web space island flap (for distal sole)

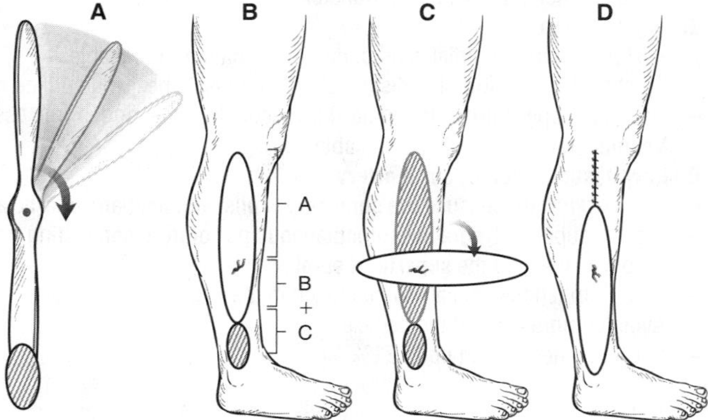


**Fig. 56-6 A,** The propeller flap concept. **B** and **C,** The perforator is the hub of the propeller and the pivot point of the flap and comprises two asymmetrical limbs (*A* and *B*). The distance from the longer limb *(A)* of the flap, which fills the defect when rotated 180 degrees. **D,** The shorter limb of the flap *(B)* is useful for closing the donor defect, possibly obviating the need for a skin graft.

## FREE TISSUE TRANSFER

- ■ Particularly useful for **lower-third** defects (classic)
- ■ **Use free flap when defect has the following characteristics:**
  - Large
  - Sacrifice of local tissue not desirable
  - Dead space after bony irrigation and debridement

- Local tissues or vessels damaged
- Local flap failure
- **Usual flaps**
  - Latissimus dorsi
  - Rectus abdominis
  - Serratus anterior
  - Gracilis
  - Scapular or parascapular
  - Radial forearm
  - Anterolateral thigh perforator flap
- Perform anastomosis outside of and **proximal** to the zone of injury
  - Can use vein grafts if necessary
  - Can perform end-to-end or end-to-side anastomoses
- Recent evidence suggests anastomosis may be performed distal to the zone of injury if necessary, with low complication rates.[26]
  - ***Must confirm flow is adequate across the zone of injury via either distal palpable pulses or angiography before embarking on distal anastomosis.***

**TIP:** Strongly consider performing end-to-side anastomoses to preserve blood flow to the distal lower extremity, especially when less than three-vessel runoff. Use either angiography or CTA liberally.

**NOTE: Integra (bilaminate neodermis) (Integra NeuroSciences, Plainsboro, NJ) can be used for any area of the lower extremity when there is a clean, vascular wound bed.**

## TISSUE EXPANSION IN THE LOWER EXTREMITY[27]

- Primary application for lower extremity is to resurface areas of unstable soft tissue or unsightly scar.
- Results are better in the thigh and buttocks.
- Complication rates are high if implant is placed below the knee.
  - **Infection rates:** 5%-30%

**TIP:** One of the most common causes of implant exposure is an inadequately dissected pocket.

## AMPUTATION

- Consider amputation if two or more of the following factors are present:
  - Three or more fascial compartments involved
  - Two or more tibial vessels injured
  - Failed vascular reconstruction
  - Cadaveric foot at initial examination
  - Severe muscle crush injury or muscle tissue loss
  - Age and functional status of the patient

## COMPARTMENT SYNDROMES

See Chapter 65 for more details.

- **Incidence** of compartment syndrome with tibial shaft fracture is **9.1%.**
- **An open tibial fracture does not allow adequate compartmental decompression (fasciotomies may still be required).**

### Signs and Symptoms

- **Pain** out of proportion to injury and with **passive** stretch
- **Pressure** from palpably swollen compartments
- **Paresthesia** of the involved compartment
  - Simple touch perception is diminished.
  - Loss of sensation over the saphenous nerve distribution should not be expected, because this nerve lies outside the compartments of the lower leg.
- **Paralysis** or decreased strength of involved compartment muscles
- **Pallor** of the involved compartment
- **Pulselessness** of the involved compartment

**NOTE: Distal pulses may or may not be palpable and/or this may be a late finding of compartment syndrome.**

## OSTEOMYELITIS

### Causes[28]

- Retained necrotic and infected bone
- Avascular or infected scar
- Dead space at the surgical site
- Inadequate skin cover
- Most common pathogen *Staphylococcus aureus*

### Incidence[29]

- Type III and IV open tibial fractures
  - **24%** infection rate without antibiotics
  - **4%** infection rate with prophylactic cephalosporin and aminoglycoside for 3 days

### Negative Pressure Wound Therapy

- Use of NPWT has allowed deescalation of the reconstructive ladder by managing preinfected wounds.[30]
- NPWT may temporize acute lower extremity injuries up to 7 days but does not obviate the need for definitive treatment.[31,32]
- Appropriately debrided wounds with osteomyelitis may be managed through an antibiotic course with NPWT.

### Treatment

- Aggressive debridement of all necrotic and infected bone and poorly vascularized and scarred soft tissues
- Dead space obliteration
- Stable, vascularized soft tissue coverage
- Often must balance opposing forces of internal fixation, wound coverage, and osteomyelitis

## CHRONIC WOUNDS OF THE LOWER EXTREMITY[33]

### Etiologic Factors

- Diabetic wounds
- Vascular insufficiency
- Venous stasis disease
- Lymphedema
- Osteomyelitis
- Cancer
- Radiation
- Vasculitis

### Patient Evaluation

- History
  - Comorbidities
    - Diabetes
    - Claudication
    - Rest pain
  - Onset, location, and drainage
  - Ambulatory status
  - Shoewear
  - Prior trauma
  - Prior ulcer
  - Prior treatment

### Physical Examination

- Size and depth
- Location
- Atrophic skin changes (hair or skin texture)
- Pulse examination
- Sensation
- Skin temperature
- Hemosiderin deposition
- Edema
- Ankle/brachial index

### Laboratory Studies

- Glucose or $A_1C$
- Radiographs (for osteomyelitis, calcification of vessels, etc.)
- Culture and sensitivities
- Biopsy

### Diagnosis and Treatment for Ulcer Types

- **General goals of treatment**
  - Complete healing of ulcer
  - Return to ambulatory status
  - Prevention of recurrence

- **Diabetic ulcers**
  - History of peripheral neuropathy
    - >40% incidence after 20 years of diabetes
  - Examination reveals decreased sensation
    - Protective sensation lost if patient cannot feel 5.07 Semmes-Weinstein filament (i.e., cannot appreciate 10 g of pressure)
- **Vascular insufficiency (arterial ulcers)**
  - History of claudication and/or rest pain
  - Abnormal pulses
  - Cool extremity with cyanosis and/or rubor and shiny hairless skin
  - Appear "punched out" and are painful
  - Check with transcutaneous $O_2$, duplex, MRA, or arteriogram
  - **Requires revascularization** by vascular surgeon
- **Venous stasis disease (venous ulcers)**
  - Chronic edema
  - Varicosities
  - Lipodermatosclerosis
  - History of deep venous thrombosis
  - Generally located in the "gaiter region," between the malleoli and gastrocnemius myotendinous junction ("bootstrap distribution")
  - Treat with **compression**
  - Can also attempt varicose vein stripping
- **Lymphedema**
  - Chronic edema with massively swollen leg and decreased skin blood flow
  - May have concomitant arterial disease
  - Treat with lymph-press pumps and leg wrapping techniques
  - Can surgically excise to fascia and skin graft (Charles procedure)
  - New techniques are promising for lymphovenous bypasses and lymph node transfers (see Chapter 58).
- **Osteomyelitis**
  - History of prior trauma
  - History of hardware placement
  - Chronic draining sinus tract that fails to close despite appropriate local wound care
  - MRI
  - Culture
  - Aggressive debridement of infected bone
  - Culture-directed antibiotics
  - Appropriate reconstruction (usually muscle-based flap)
- **Cancer**
  - Unusual ulcer appearance
  - History of coexisting malignancy
  - Biopsy
    - **Marjolin's ulcer:** Malignant SCC from transformation of chronic wounds (years)
  - Resection or amputation with margins
  - Reconstruction
- **Radiation**
  - History of prior radiation
  - Damaged vascularity to the affected area
  - Can pretreat with hyperbaric oxygen to stimulate angiogenesis at wound periphery

- Requires resection of irradiated tissue and free flap reconstruction
  - Local flaps are frequently ineffective because they are within the zone of radiation injury.

■ **Vasculitis**

- History of systemic inflammatory disease
  - Rheumatoid arthritis
  - Lupus
  - Scleroderma
- Disproportionate pain
- Confirmation by histopathology
- Treatment by calcium channel blockers, steroids, and antineoplastic drugs
- Should be overseen by a rheumatologist

## Key Points

✓ Radical debridement of all devitalized tissue (soft tissue and bone) is the key step to successful outcomes in posttraumatic situations.

✓ Obtain stable soft tissue coverage early to help decrease the incidence of complications.

✓ NPWT may help decrease edema, decrease bacterial counts, and stimulate blood flow to wounds before definitive coverage.

✓ The medial head of the gastrocnemius is the workhorse for upper-third lower extremity reconstruction.

✓ The soleus is the workhorse for middle-third lower extremity reconstruction.

✓ Free tissue transfer is the workhorse for lower-third lower extremity reconstruction.

✓ Integra can be used in any location as long as there is a clean, healthy wound bed (even if bone is exposed).

✓ Tissue expansion historically has not been reliably successful below the knee.

✓ Watch for compartment syndrome with lower extremity trauma.

✓ Amputation is an option in select cases and can result in an excellent functional outcome.

✓ Know the characteristics of the various chronic wounds of the lower extremity so that the proper diagnosis can be made and appropriate treatment selected.

## References

1. Hollenbeck ST, Toranto JD, Taylor BJ, et al. Perineal and lower extremity reconstruction. Plast Reconstr Surg 128:551e-563e, 2011.
2. Gustilo RB, Anderson JT. Prevention of infection in the treatment of one thousand and twenty-five open fractures of long bones. J Bone Joint Surg Am 58:453, 1976.
3. Gustilo RB, Mendoza RM, Williams DN. Problems in the management of type III (severe) open fractures: a new classification of type III open fractures. J Trauma 24:742, 1984.
4. Keller CS. The principles of the treatment of tibial shaft fractures. Orthopaedics 6:993, 1983.
5. Byrd HS, Spicer TE, Cierny G III. Management of open tibial fractures. Plast Reconstr Surg 76:719, 1985.
6. Yaremchuk MJ, Brumback RJ, Manson PN, et al. Acute and definitive management of traumatic osteocutaneous defects of the lower extremity. Plast Reconstr Surg 80:1, 1987.
7. Godina M. Early microsurgical reconstruction of complex trauma of the extremities. Clin Plast Surg 13:619, 1986.
8. Hou Z, Irgit K, Strohecker HA, et al. Delayed flap reconstruction with vacuum-assisted closure management of the open IIIB tibial fracture. J Trauma 71:1705, 2011.

9. Kumar AR, Grewal NS, Chung TL, et al. Lessons from operation Iraqi freedom: successful subacute reconstruction of complex lower extremity battle injuries. Plast Reconstr Surg 123:218, 2009.
10. Rhinelander FW. Tibial blood supply in relation to fracture healing. Clin Orthop Relat Res 105:34, 1974.
11. Macnab I, De Haas WG. The role of periosteal blood supply in the healing of fractures of the tibia. Clin Orthop Relat Res 105:27, 1974.
12. Christian EP, Bosse MJ, Robb G. Reconstruction of large diaphyseal defects without free fibular transfer in Grade IIIb tibial fractures. J Bone Joint Surg Am 71:994, 1989.
13. Weiland AJ, Moore JR, Daniel RK. Vascularized bone autografts: experience with 41 cases. Clin Orthop Relat Res 174:87, 1983.
14. Ilizarov GA, Devyatov AA, Kamerin VK. Plastic reconstruction of longitudinal bone defects by means of compression and subsequent distraction. Acta Chir Plast 22:32, 1980.
15. Cierny G III, Zorn KE, Nahai F. Bony reconstruction in the lower extremity. Clin Plast Surg 19:905, 1992.
16. Patzakis MJ, Dorr LD, Ivler D, et al. The early management of open joint injuries: a prospective study of one hundred and forty patients. J Bone Joint Surg Am 57:1065, 1975.
17. Dawson RL. Complications of cross-leg flap operation. Proc R Soc Med 65:2, 1972.
18. Almeida MF, da Costa PR, Okawa RY. Reverse-flow island sural flap. Plast Reconstr Surg 109:583, 2002.
19. Suga H, Oshima Y, Harii K, et al. Distally-based sural flap for reconstruction of the lower leg and foot. Scand J Plast Reconstr Surg 38:16, 2004.
20. Teo TC. The propeller flap concept. Clin Plast Surg 37:615, 2010.
21. Blondeel PN, Morris SF, Hallock GG, et al, eds. Perforator Flaps: Anatomy, Technique, & Clinical Applications, 2nd ed. St Louis: Quality Medical Publishing, 2013.
22. Hyakusoku H, Yamamoto T, Fumiiri M. The propeller flap method. Br J Plast Surg 44:53, 1991.
23. Gir P, Cheng A, Oni G, et al. Pedicled-perforator (propeller) flaps in lower extremity defects: a systematic review. J Reconstr Microsurg 28:595, 2012.
24. Hallock GG. The propeller flap version of the adductor muscle perforator flap for coverage of ischial or trochanteric pressure sores. Ann Plast Surg 56:540, 2006.
25. Woltering EA, Thorpe WP, Reed JK Jr, et al. Split thickness skin grafting of the plantar surface of the foot after wide excision of neoplasms of the skin. Surg Gynecol Obstet 149:229, 1979.
26. Spector JA, Levine S, Levine JP. Free tissue transfer to the lower extremity distal to the zone of injury: indications and outcomes over a 25-year experience. Plast Reconstr Surg 120:952, 2007.
27. Manders EK, Oaks TE, Au VK, et al. Soft tissue expansion in the lower extremities. Plast Reconstr Surg 81:208, 1988.
28. Ger R, Efron G. New operative approach in the treatment of chronic osteomyelitis of the tibial diaphysis. A preliminary report. Clin Orthop Relat Res 70:165, 1970.
29. Patzakis MJ, Wilkins J, Moore TM. Use of antibiotics in open tibial fractures. Clin Orthop Relat Res 178:31, 1983.
30. Liu DS, Sofiadellis F, Ashton M, et al. Early soft tissue coverage and negative pressure wound therapy optimises patient outcomes in lower limb trauma. Injury 43:772, 2012.
31. Hou Z, Irgit K, Strohecker KA, et al. Delayed flap reconstruction with vacuum-assisted closure management of the open IIIB tibial fracture. J Trauma 71:1705, 2011.
32. Stannard JP, Singanamala N, Volgas DA. Fix and flap in the era of vacuum suction devices: what do we know in terms of evidence based medicine? Injury 41:780, 2010.
33. Smith APS. Etiology of the problem wound. In Sheffield PJ, Smith APS, Fife CE, eds. Wound Care Practice, 2nd ed. Flagstaff, AZ: Best Publishing Company, 2007.

# 57. Foot Ulcers

Gangadasu Reddy

## TYPES OF FOOT ULCERS

- **Diabetic:** Neuropathic, neuroischemic, ischemic
- **Arterial/ischemic:** Nondiabetic
- **Venous or varicose**
- **Malignant:** Squamous cell carcinoma, basal cell carcinoma, malignant melanoma, Kaposi's sarcoma, Marjolin's ulcer
- **Infectious and others:** Tuberculosis, actinomycosis, burn, ulcerative colitis, etc.
- **Superficial:** Confined to the skin
- **Deep:** Tissue loss or infection deeper than the skin

## DIABETIC FOOT ULCERS

### EPIDEMIOLOGY

- Leading cause of foot ulcers and related complications like infections and amputations in the United States and Europe
- Incidence: 2.0%-6.8% per year[1-3]
- Usually the initial insult in the pathway to infection and amputation
- 25% of people with diabetes develop a foot ulcer during their lifetime.[4]
- 50% of ulcers get infected, and 20% of these require an amputation.[3]
- Lower extremity wound is a critical causal factor leading to 85% of amputations (major and minor).[5]
- Osteomyelitis in a diabetic without a preceding ulcer is uncommon.
- Hematogenous bone and soft tissue infections are very rare.
- Every case of osteomyelitis was preceded by ulceration.[6]
- Up to 60% of all nontraumatic amputations are in diabetics.

### CAUSES/RISK FACTORS

> **TIP:** The classic triad of risk factors for foot ulcers comprises peripheral neuropathy, foot deformity, and minor trauma.[7]

Causal pathways to foot ulceration are shown in Fig. 57-1.[8]

- **Neuropathy**

> **TIP:** Neuropathy is the most important risk factor for development of diabetic foot ulcers and amputations.[9]

- ***Sensory***
  - Loss of protective sensation
  - Impaired balance secondary to poor proprioception

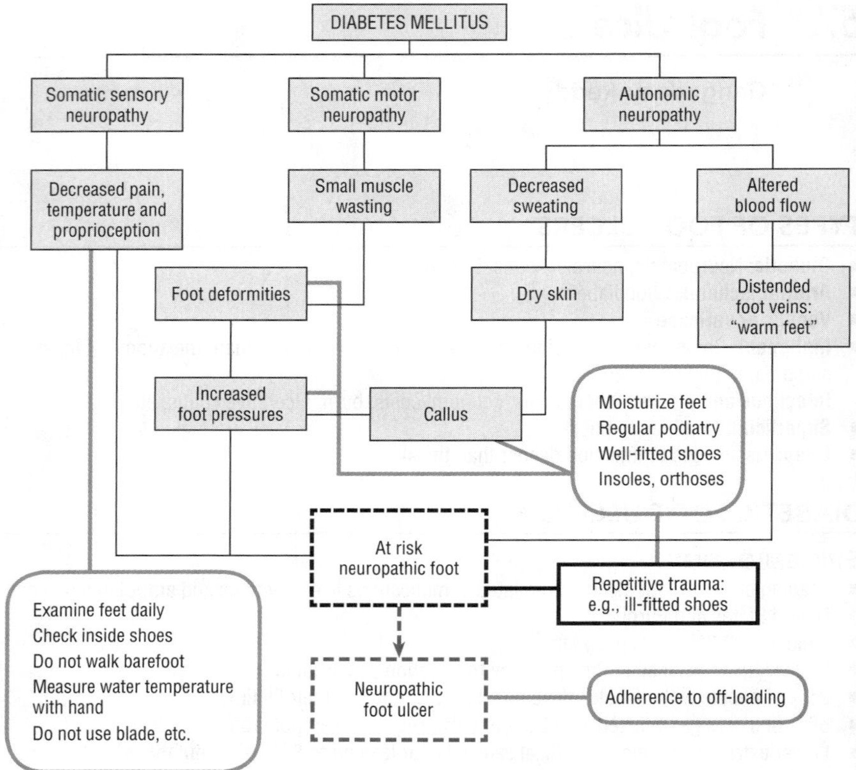


**Fig. 57-1** Causal pathways to foot ulceration emphasizing the key role of the patient in ulcer prevention.

> **TIP:** The only effective means of preserving sensory nerve function is by strict glucose control.[10]

- ***Motor***
  - Atrophy of intrinsic muscles of the foot
  - Overpowering of long flexors and extensors leading to foot deformities like claw toes, dislocated metatarsophalangeal joints
- ***Autonomic***
  - Decreased sweat and oil gland function leading to dry feet with cracks and fissures
  - Arteriovenous shunting[11]

> **TIP:** Surgical sympathectomy to improve blood flow to the foot is not beneficial in patients with longstanding diabetes because of the autosympathectomy effect caused by autonomic neuropathy.

- **Charcot's arthropathy or neuroarthropathy**
  - Characterized by abnormal sensory (loss of protective sensation, diminished or absent vibratory sensation) and motor (absent deep tendon reflexes) examination results, with normal vascular (bounding pedal pulses) examination results
  - Fracture and dislocation of the foot and ankle, mostly the **midfoot,** leads to Charcot's arthropathy.
  - Radiologic findings in Charcot's arthropathy **may mimic osteomyelitis.**
  - Patients with Charcot's arthropathy may be mistakenly treated for osteomyelitis even though they have never had a wound. Clinical findings of foot ulceration associated with positive bone scan (indium-111 WBC scan) or MRI suggests osteomyelitis.
- **Foot deformity**
  - Glycation of soft tissue leads to:
    - Joint stiffness
    - Decreased range of motion
    - Loss of footpad cushions
      - Limited joint mobility leads to uneven and increased distribution of pressure on the plantar aspect of the foot.[12]
  - Increased pressure and shear forces secondary to abnormal foot mechanics amplify the effects of neuropathy.
  - Structural deformities associated with plantar ulcers:
    - Ankle equinus
    - Hallux valgus
    - Hammertoe
    - Claw toes
    - Dislocated metatarsophalangeal joints
- **Trauma**
  - Bone deformities expose overlying skin to repetitive trauma.
  - Ill-fitting shoes and puncture wounds from sharp objects like nails can worsen the problem.
  - Injuries will go unnoticed because of loss of protective sensation, poor vision because of diabetic retinopathy, and lack of regular foot examination and care.
  - ***Edge effect***

Repetitive vertical stress and shear occur at the edge of an ulcer over a bony prominence.[13] At these pressure sites, maximal soft tissue damage occurs at the edge of the wound, and not at the center.

**TIP:** Ulcers persist because of pressure and repetitive trauma.[14]

- **Other risk factors**
  - Peripheral arterial disease (PAD)
  - Male gender
  - Increasing age >65 years
  - Obesity
  - Systemic risk factors like hypertension, hyperlipidemia, polycythemia
- **Vasculopathy**
  - Peripheral arterial disease contributes to foot ulceration in a third of all cases.
  - Arterial disease usually does not lead to development of an ulcer by itself, but it may impair healing of an already-developed ulcer.
  - In most diabetics, arterial insufficiency is from atherosclerosis of **large vessels,** and not because of small-vessel disease.
  - Lower extremity atherosclerosis is amenable to angioplasty and bypass, because the vessels above the knee and the vessels below the ankle are frequently spared.[15]

> **TIP:** A common misbelief regarding diabetic microangiopathy is that microcirculation in diabetics cannot be improved because of their underlying microangiopathy, even if they have palpable pedal pulses.

- Angiographic, physiologic, and histologic studies do not reveal the presence of a unique entity of "diabetic microangiopathy."[13]

■ **Sites of ulcers on the foot and their common causes**[16] (Fig. 57-2)

1. Heel ulcers: Gravitational (decubitus) pressure of the foot transmitted to the heel, and ischemia[7]
2. Great toe: Arthritis or limited motion of the first metatarsophalangeal joint
3. Tips of the toes: Clawing and constant pressure where the tip of the toe is bearing weight
4. Metatarsal heads (the ball of the foot): Site of high pressure and shear forces that are exposed to repetitive injury (normal walking)
5. Dorsum or sides of the foot: Ill-fitting shoes
6. Neuropathic ulcers occur on areas of elevated pressure like plantar aspect of foot.
7. Neuroischemic or ischemic ulcers develop on areas that are farthest away from the blood supply to that area like the tips of the toes or the lateral border of the foot.

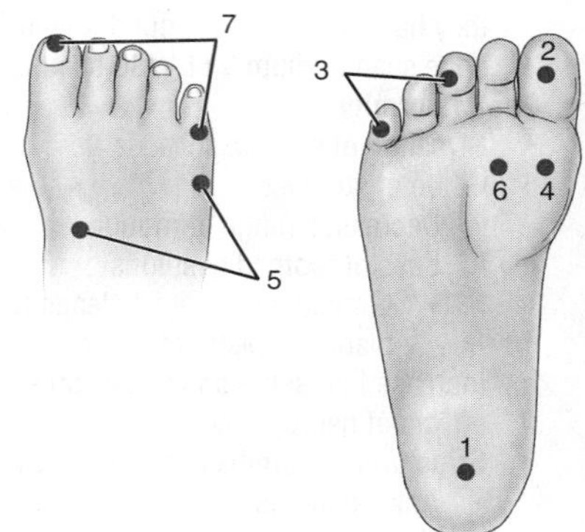


**Fig. 57-2** Ulcer sites in the foot and their causes.

> **TIP:** The most common location for a diabetic foot ulcer is under the hallux.

## Ulcer Evaluation

■ **History**

- Mechanism of injury: Puncture wounds, crush or shear injury, burn
- Duration: Acute or chronic
- Prior foot ulcers and their response to treatment
- Prior infections
- Prior amputations or revascularization procedures
- Claudication, rest pain
- Smoking
- Other risk factors (as outlined in the Causes/Risk Factors section)

■ **Physical examination**

- Systematic and thorough examination of both feet for calluses, corns, maceration between toes, nails
- Site and size
- Depth of ulcer: Superficial or deep
- Ulcer bed: Granulation or necrotic tissue, exposed vital structures
- Condition of surrounding tissue
- Amount of exudates
- Bone abnormalities: Claw toes, hammertoes, metatarsal heads pressing against the sole

- Infection: Erythema, tenderness, drainage, systemic signs of sepsis. Presence of crepitus suggests infection by gas-producing organisms and needs emergent treatment.
- Neurologic examination: Sensory and motor
- Vascular examination: Signs of ischemia like absent or diminished pulses, pallor with limb elevation or dependent rubor, delayed capillary refill, pale or cold foot, loss of hair
- Foot biomechanics: Range of motion, dorsiflexion and plantar flexion of toes and ankle
- Shoe wear: Assess for proper shoe fit, need for customized shoes, or other off-loading modalities.

## Classification of Diabetic Foot Ulcers/Wounds

- **Meggitt-Wagner System**[17,18]
  - Most commonly used classification system
  - ***Drawbacks***
    - Wound infection is included in grade 3 only.
    - Does not allow classification of superficial infected wounds
    - Does not address wounds of varying depths effected by PAD (except in grades 4 and 5)
  - ***Grade***
    - 0: Preulcerative/high-risk foot
    - 1: Superficial ulcer
    - 2: Deep to tendon, bone, or joint
    - 3: Deep with abscess/osteomyelitis
    - 4: Forefoot gangrene
    - 5: Whole foot gangrene
- **University of Texas Wound Classification System**[19] (Table 57-1)
  - Uses a 4 by 4 matrix
  - Consistently and systematically evaluated wounds taking into account wound depth, infection, and PAD

**Table 57-1** *University of Texas Wound Classification System*

| | | Wound Depth | | | |
|---|---|---|---|---|---|
| | | **0** | **1** | **2** | **3** |
| Comorbidities, infection, PAD | A | Preulcerative lesion or healed ulcer site | Superficial wound No tendon, capsule, or bone involvement | Wound extends to tendon or capsule | Wound extends to bone or into joint |
| | B | + Infection − PAD | + Infection − PAD | + Infection − PAD | + Infection − PAD |
| | C | − Infection + PAD | − Infection + PAD | − Infection + PAD | − Infection + PAD |
| | D | + Infection + PAD | + Infection + PAD | + Infection + PAD | + Infection + PAD |

*PAD,* Peripheral arterial disease.

**TIP:** Wound depth, infection, and PAD are the key factors predictive of healing, amputation, and final amputation level.

- **PEDIS System (International Working Group on the Diabetic Foot [IWGDF])**
  - **P**erfusion
  - **E**xtent/size
  - **D**epth/tissue loss
  - **I**nfection
  - **S**ensation
- **Infectious Disease Society of America (IDSA)/IWGDF**[20] (Table 57-2)
  - **Infection**
    - **Physical examination** is the best method to diagnose foot infection.
    - WBC count may be normal.
    - Chronic infections may have elevated ESR, C-reactive protein.
    - Radiologic manifestations may lag behind clinical manifestations by 2-3 weeks.
    - On radiographs, evaluate for fractures, dislocations, bone infection, foreign bodies, or subcutaneous gas.
    - ***Bacteriology***
      - Mild to moderate infections: *Staphylococcus aureus* and Streptococci species[10]
      - Severe infections: Mixed flora (Gram-positive cocci, Gram-negative aerobes and anaerobes)
      - Puncture wounds through footwear
      - High prevalence of *Pseudomonas* infections in nondiabetics[21]
      - *Staphylococcus* and *Streptococcus* species in diabetics[22]
    - ***Wound cultures***
      - Do not culture or treat ulcers with antibiotics if they are not infected.

**Table 57-2** *Classifications and Treatment of Diabetic Foot Ulcers/Wounds*

| Clinical Manifestations of Infection | PEDIS | IDSA | Treatment |
|---|---|---|---|
| No clinical features of infection | 1 | Uninfected | Not necessary |
| Local infection of skin and subcutaneous tissue (if erythema, >0.5 cm and <2 cm) | 2 | Mild | 1-2 weeks oral antibiotics (narrow-spectrum)<br>Outpatient treatment |
| Local infection involving tissues deeper to subcutaneous plane (abscess, bone, joints, fascia) | 3 | Moderate | 2-3 weeks IV/oral broad-spectrum antibiotics<br>Admit if associated complicating features like PAD, lack of home support |
| Local infection with systemic inflammatory response syndrome (SIRS) | 4 | Severe | 2-3 weeks IV broad-spectrum antibiotics for soft tissue<br>4-6 weeks for bone<br>Needs hospitalization |

Empiric MRSA treatment is recommended if infection is severe, there is a prior history of MRSA infection or colonization within last year, or local microbiology of the hospital suggests high MRSA prevalence. Empiric treatment for *Pseudomonas* is unnecessary except for patients with risk factors. *IDSA,* Infectious Disease Society of America; *IWGDF,* International Working Group on the Diabetic Foot; *PEDIS,* Perfusion, extent/size, depth/tissue loss, infection, sensation.

**TIP:** Obtain tissue culture specimens from the debrided base of the wound.

- *Osteomyelitis*
  - A positive **probe to bone test** may suggest bone infection, but a negative probe to bone test will most likely rule out osteomyelitis.[23]
  - **MRI** is the best noninvasive test to diagnose osteomyelitis.

**TIP:** Bone biopsy is the benchmark for diagnosing osteomyelitis.

- **Screening for neuropathy**
  - History of tingling, numbness, paresthesias, or "insects crawling on the feet"
  - Patients may complain that their feet are cold even though they have no ischemic signs.
  - Clinical examination and screening tests are not widely used and time consuming.
    - Semmes-Weinstein monofilament is the most commonly used method.
    - Vibration perception threshold

## Treatment of Diabetic Foot Ulcers

- **Multidisciplinary approach: diabetic foot team**

Providers are from podiatry, wound care, surgery, endocrinology, primary care, infectious diseases, dermatology, and rehabilitation medicine.

- **Six essentials of the ADA guidelines, treatment algorithm**
  1. Off-loading
  2. Debridement early and often
  3. Moist wound healing
  4. Treatment of infection
  5. Correction of ischemia (below-the-knee disease)
  6. Prevention of amputation
- **Other considerations**
  - Optimization of medical therapy
  - Foot baths can cause maceration of skin and are therefore contraindicated.
  - Topical antibiotics are not recommended for noninfected ulcers.
  - Data on use of silver-based dressings in infected wounds are not supportive.[24]
- **Off-loading**

**TIP:** Off-loading pressure is the most important aspect of neuropathic diabetic foot wound healing. The goal is to off-load the pressure at the ulcer while keeping the person ambulatory.[10,25]

- **Total contact casts**[26,27]

**TIP:** These are considered the benchmark of off-loading modalities.

  - *Advantages*
    - Entire plantar aspect of the foot and the lower leg remain in contact with the cast.
    - Pressure over the entire weight-bearing surface of the foot is **evenly distributed,** thereby permitting walking.
    - Foot ulcers should not be ischemic or infected before placement of this cast. Healing rates are 72%-100% over 5-7 weeks.
    - They must be applied by a skilled clinician.
    - Excellent patient compliance is ensured, because it is very hard for patients to remove them.

- ▸ ***Disadvantages***
  - ♦ Time consuming to place these casts
  - ♦ Need skilled, trained personnel for applying
  - ♦ Improperly placed casts can lead to ulcer formation.
  - ♦ Cannot be used on infected or ischemic wounds
- **Other off-loading methods**
  - ▸ Bed rest
  - ▸ Wheelchair
  - ▸ Crutches
  - ▸ Felted foam
  - ▸ "Half shoes"
  - ▸ Therapeutic shoes
  - ▸ Custom shoes
  - ▸ Custom splints

■ **Debridement**[28]

- ***Mechanical debridement***
  - ▸ Wet-to-dry dressings: Nonselective, painful, can lead to surface cooling, bacterial translocation possible, labor intensive
- ***Autolytic debridement***
  - ▸ Proteolytic enzymes in the wound break down the necrotic tissue when covered by an occlusive dressing.
- ***Enzymatic debridement***
  - ▸ Enzymatic preparations like collagenase are used to remove devitalized tissue.
- ***Maggot (larval) debridement***
  - ▸ Larvae of green blowfly *(Phaenicia sericata)* selectively consume devitalized tissue without affecting healthy granulation tissue.
  - ▸ Wounds are covered with a mesh dressing for 3 days.
  - ▸ Maggots are effective against methicillin-resistant *S. aureus* (MRSA) and vancomycin-resistant enterococcus (VRE)
  - ▸ Patient tolerance is poor because frequent clinic visits are needed for dressing changes, new batch of maggots is added each time, and treatment can be painful.
- ***Surgical debridement***
  - ▸ It is the most common and effective method.
  - ▸ Hydrosurgical debidement (Versajet; Smith & Nephew, Memphis, TN) allows precise depth of debridement using high-velocity stream of saline and centrally localized vacuum to debride necrotic tissue and biofilm (Venturi effect)
- **Timing of debridement**
  - ▸ For dry gangrene without cellulitis, the limb should first be revascularized.
  - ▸ With wet gangrene, the wound should be debrided and revascularized.

■ **Corrective surgery for the foot deformity**

- Considered in patients who failed appropriate off-loading methods or have recurrent ulceration despite proper preventive care
- **Ankle equinus**
  - ▸ Characterized by decreased ankle dorsiflexion
  - ▸ Surgical treatment
    - ♦ Achilles tendon lengthening: Endoscopic or open

- Risks of Achilles tendon lengthening
  - Infection
  - Rupture of the tendon
  - Charcot's neuroarthropathy
  - Overlengthening of the tendon
  - Transfer ulcer to the heel
- **Claw toes with toe ulcers**
  - Consider long flexor tenotomy if deformity is not reducible or persists despite off-loading and repeat debridements.
- **Hallux or first metatarsophalangeal ulcer**
  - Keller arthroplasty improves the motion and alignment of the first metatarsophalangeal joint by removing the proximal aspect of the proximal phalanx of the great toe.
- **Hammertoe and dorsal ulcer of PIP and DIP**
  - Manual reduction, resection arthroplasty, and joint arthroplasty
- **Plantarflexed metatarsal with metatarsal head ulcer**
  - Excision of sesamoid, surgical reduction of prominent condyle, isolated metatarsal head resection or panmetatarsal head resection

- **Wound closure**
  - ***Split-thickness skin graft***
    - Can be used to cover large granulation tissue defects
    - Outcomes are optimal when used on non-weight-bearing surfaces of the foot like the dorsum, medial and lateral aspects, or arch areas.
  - ***Tissue flaps***
    - Used to cover large soft tissue defects or when underlying critical structures are exposed.
    - Fasciocutaneous flaps:
      - Medial plantar artery flap can be rotated laterally to cover a subcuboid ulcer, or proximally to cover a plantar calcaneal defect.
      - Toe fillet flaps can cover submetatarsal head ulcers, but they require sacrificing that toe.
    - Muscle flaps
      - Small foot muscle flaps can be used to cover exposed bone.
      - Extensor digitorum brevis flap
      - Abductor hallucis (and digiti minimi) flap
  - ***Free flaps***
    - Used when adequate coverage of critical structures cannot be provided by local or regional tissues
- **Adjunctive treatments**
  - No compelling data favoring routine use of these expensive treatment modalities.
  - None of the adjunctive treatments have proven role in resolution of infection.
  - Can be considered in carefully selected diabetics who heal slowly or fail to respond to standard therapy.
  - ***Hyperbaric oxygen***
    - Data from controlled trials are conflicting regarding their efficacy in promoting diabetic foot-wound healing and their ability to decrease the rates of amputations.[27,29]
  - ***Negative-pressure wound therapy***[30,31]

Although earlier studies showed improved diabetic foot-ulcer healing, negative-pressure wound therapy cannot be used widely, especially in infected wounds, because of lack of sufficient high-level evidence.

- ***Ultrasound therapy***
  - Breaks biofilm
  - Decreases bioburden
  - Increases blood flow
  - Active cell stimulation
  - **Ennis et al**[32]
    - Wound-healing rate of recalcitrant diabetic foot ulcers in the treatment group (40 kHz noncontact ultrasound delivered by saline mist) was 40.7%. Healing rate in the control group (saline mist without ultrasound) was 14.3%.
- ***Growth factors***
  - Platelet-derived growth factor[33,34]: No improvement in wound healing despite initial studies showing some benefit
- ***Electrical stimulation***
  - Increases local perfusion and stimulates the release of growth factors
  - Double-blinded randomized controlled clinical study by Peters et al[35]
    - 65% of patients healed with active subsensory electrical stimulation compared with 35% of control patients over a 12-week period.
    - The response was more significant when patient compliance was taken into account and when electrical stimulation was used at least 3 days a week compared with patients who used it 0-2 days a week.
  - Lundeberg et al[36]
    - 64 diabetic patients with venous stasis ulceration
    - Wound reduction and proportion of wounds that healed were 61% and 31%, respectively, in the treatment group compared with 41% and 12.5% in the control group ($p < 0.05$).
- ***Radiant heat***
  - Wounds are hypothermic compared with core body temperature.
  - Radiant heat optimizes enzymatic processes involved in wound healing by creating a normothermic environment.
- ***Bioengineered tissue***
  - Apligraf (Organogenesis, Canton, MA) and Dermagraft (Advanced Tissue Sciences, La Jolla, CA) are used in shallow wounds without exposed deep structures.
  - **Apligraf** is a living dermal bilayer consisting of a dermis and epidermis.
  - **Dermagraft** is a cryopreserved single layer consisting of living fibroblasts on an absorbable mesh.
  - **GraftJacket** (Wright Medical Technology, Arlington, TN) is an acellular dermal matrix obtained from irradiated cadaveric skin.
    - It is used to cover exposed deep tissue, such as tendon and bone.

**TIP:** In general, skin grafts work well on non-pressure-bearing areas of the foot. Bioengineered tissue can be used on weight-bearing areas.

## RECURRENCE AND PREVENTION

- After an ulcer heals, the recurrence rate is very high, varying from 28% at 12 months to 100% at 40 months.
- Patients with a prior history of ulceration are **57 times more likely** to develop ulcer recurrence compared with those who had no ulcers.
- Toe ulcers have high rates of recurrence, because they have **underlying structural foot deformities.**
- **5 P's of prevention (Frykberg)**[37]
  - **P**odiatric care
  - **P**rotective shoes
  - **P**ressure reduction
  - **P**rophylactic surgery
  - **P**reventive education
  - Standard preventative foot care reduces the incidence of recurrent foot ulcers within the next year from nearly 60%-80% to 25%-33%.
- **Peripheral nerve decompression**
  - There are insufficient data supporting the efficacy of surgical nerve decompression at the sites of anatomic narrowing for treatment of diabetic neuropathy (American Academy of Neurology),[38] although there are conflicting studies on this, with some evidence to the contrary in the plastic surgery literature.
- **Fillers**
  - Fillers like silicone have been used to reduce pressure under bony prominences.[39]
- **Skin temperature monitoring**
  - In diabetics without protective sensation, the probable sites of foot ulceration can be identified very effectively by monitoring local skin temperature.
  - This home-monitoring method allows early detection of ongoing sites of inflammation that lead to ulceration.
  - Routine foot temperature monitoring reduces the incidence of diabetic foot ulceration by 73% (based on three randomized controlled trials).[40]
  - These thermometers need a prescription, are expensive, and are not reimbursed by insurance.

## ARTERIAL OR ISCHEMIC ULCER

- ***Assessment***
  - History of claudication, rest pain, gangrene
  - Clinical examination: Absent foot pulses, pallor with limb elevation or dependent rubor, atrophic integument, hair loss
  - Ankle-brachial index (ABI) $<0.9$ is suggestive of ischemia.
    - ABI may be unreliable in diabetics because of incompressible vessels from atherosclerosis.
  - Pulse volume recordings (plethysmography) assess physiologic status of foot perfusion either through straight-line flow from one- two- or three-vessel runoff, or through collateral circulation.
  - Skin perfusion pressure
  - Transcutaneous oxygen tension
  - Vascular duplex
  - CT angiography or MR angiography
  - Interventional angiography

- ***Management of arterial ulcers***
  - Diet modification
  - Exercise
  - Smoking cessation
  - Aspirin, clopidogrel, lipid-lowering medications like statins, cilostazo
  - Local wound care
  - Debridement
  - Amputations
  - Revascularization
    - Angioplasty, bypass
    - If clinical and/or noninvasive assessments suggest significant PAD

## VENOUS ULCER

- History of deep venous thrombosis (DVT), obesity, prolonged standing, pregnancy
- Physical examination
  - Swollen leg; ankle hyperpigmentation; varicosities; ulcers are usually located anywhere, extending from medial malleolus to lower part of the leg
- Clinically assess superficial and deep venous system and the competency of the valves or perforators.
- Venous duplex to rule out DVT and check the status of superficial veins, deep veins, and reflux at valve/perforator sites
- Treatment
  - Limb elevation, compressive dressings, local wound care, and control infection; surgical treatment for venous or valvular incompetencies

## MALIGNANT ULCER

- Cutaneous malignancies can manifest as nonhealing ulcers on the foot.
- Should have a high index of suspicion
- Obtain biopsy if ulcer looks suspicious or is not responding to optimal foot care.
- Marjolin's ulcer (SCC) develops at the site of chronically inflamed or scarred tissue like a prior burn or trauma.

## INFECTIOUS AND OTHER ULCERS (Table 57-3)

- History of travel or immunocompromised status
- Assess for other systemic manifestations of that disease.
- Obtain cultures and biopsies for tuberculosis, fungal, and atypical infections.
- Treat the underlying cause.

**Table 57-3** *Characteristics of Ulcers*

| | Venous | Arterial | Diabetic |
|---|---|---|---|
| Ulcer location | Medial malleolus<br>Trauma or infection may localize ulcers laterally or more proximally | Distal, over bony prominences<br>Trauma may localize ulcers proximally | Pressure points on feet (e.g., junction of great toe and plantar surface, metatarsal head, heel) |
| Ulcer appearance | Shallow, irregular borders<br>Base may be initially fibrinous but later develops granulation tissue | Round or punched-out, well-demarcated border<br>Fibrinous yellow base or true necrotic eschar<br>Bone and tendon exposure may be seen | Callus surrounding the wound and undermined edges are characteristic<br>Blister, hemorrhage, necrosis, and exposure of underlying structures are commonly seen |
| Physical examination | Varicose veins<br>Leg edema<br>Atrophie blanche<br>Dermatitis<br>Lipodermatosclerosis<br>Pigmentary changes<br>Purpura | Loss of hair<br>Shiny, atrophic skin<br>Dystrophic toenails<br>Cold feet<br>Femoral bruit<br>Absent or decreased pulses<br>Prolonged capillary refilling time | No sensation to monofilament<br>Bone resorption<br>Claw toes<br>Flatfoot<br>Charcot joints |
| Frequent symptoms | Pain, odor, and copious drainage from the wound<br>Pruritus | Claudication<br>Resting ischemic pain | Food numbness<br>Burning<br>Paresthesia |
| Ankle-to-brachial blood pressure ratio (ABI measured by Doppler ultrasonography) | >0.9 | ABI <0.7 suggests arterial disease<br>Calcification of vessels gives falsely high Doppler readings | Normal, unless associated with arterial component |
| Risk factors | Deep venous thrombosis<br>Significant leg injury<br>Obesity | Diabetes<br>Hypertension<br>Cigarette smoking<br>Hypercholesterolemia | Diabetes<br>Leprosy<br>Frostbite |
| Complications | Allergic contact dermatitis<br>Cellulitis | Gangrene | Underlying osteomyelitis |
| Treatment pearl | Compression therapy<br>Leg elevation | Pentoxifylline<br>Vascular surgery<br>Assessment if ABI <5 | Vigorous surgical debridement<br>Pressure avoidance |

*ABI,* Ankle-brachial index.

## Key Points

- ✓ Foot ulcers precede 85% of all lower extremity amputations.
- ✓ Neuropathy is the most important risk factor for development of diabetic foot ulcers.
- ✓ Only intensive glucose control has proved effective in preserving sensory nerve function.
- ✓ Bleeding below a callus or discoloration is a sign of preulcerative lesion.
- ✓ Because of autonomic neuropathy, there can be high arteriovenous shunting of blood. This can give the clinical picture of red and warm extremities despite severe underlying ischemia.
- ✓ Pressure is relieved by off-loading and debridement. This is fundamental to the treatment of diabetic neuropathic ulcers.
- ✓ Total contact casting is the benchmark of off-loading modalities.
- ✓ Skin temperature monitoring is a most effective means of identifying sites of impending ulceration.

## References


1. Armstrong DG, Lavery LA. Clinical Care of the Diabetic Foot, 2nd ed. Alexandria, VA: American Diabetes Association Press, 2010.
2. Lavery LA, Armstrong DG, Wunderlich RP, et al. Diabetic foot syndrome: evaluating the prevalence and incidence of foot pathology in Mexican Americans and non-Hispanic whites from a diabetes disease management cohort. Diabetes Care 26:1435-1438, 2003.
3. Pecoraro RE, Reiber GE, Burgess EM. Pathways to diabetic limb amputation: basis for prevention. Diabetes Care 13:513-521, 1990.
4. Singh N, Armstrong DG, Lipsky BA. Preventing foot ulcers in patients with diabetes. JAMA 293:217-228, 2005.
5. Lavery LA, Wunderlich RP, Tredwell J. Disease management for the diabetic foot: effectiveness of a diabetic foot prevention program to reduce amputations and hospitalizations. Diabetes Res Clin Pract 70:31-37, 2005.
6. Lavery LA, Armstrong DG, Wunderlich RP, et al. Risk factors for foot infections in individuals with diabetes. Diabetes Care 29:1288-1293, 2006.
7. Reiber GE, Vileikyte L, Boyko EJ, et al. Causal pathways for incident lower-extremity ulcers in patients with diabetes from two settings. Diabetes Care 22:157-162, 1999.
8. Vileikyte L, Boulton AJ. The diabetic foot: from art to science. The 18th Camillo Golgi lecture. Diabetologia 47:1343-1353, 2004.
9. Lavery LA, Armstrong DG, Vela SA, et al. Identifying high-risk patients for diabetic foot ulceration: practical criteria for screening. Arch Intern Med 158:157-162, 1998.
10. Reichard P, Nilsson BY, Rosenqvist U. The effect of long-term intensified insulin treatment on the development of microvascular complications of diabetes mellitus. N Engl J Med 329:304-309, 1993.
11. Calhoun JH, Overgaard KA, Stevens CM, et al. Diabetic foot ulcers and infections: current concepts. Adv Skin Wound Care 15:31-42, 2002.
12. Catanzariti AR, Haverstock BD, Grossman JP, et al. Off-loading techniques in the treatment of diabetic plantar neuropathic foot ulceration. Adv Wound Care 12:452-458, 1999.
13. Armstrong DG, Athanasiou KA. The edge effect: how and why wounds grow in size and depth. Clin Podiatr Med Surg 15:105-108, 1998.
14. Lavery LA, Armstrong DG, Wunderlich RP, et al. Predictive value of foot pressure assessment as part of a population-based diabetes disease management program. Diabetes Care 26:1069-1073, 2003.
15. LoGerfo FW, Coffman JD. Current concepts. Vascular and microvascular disease of the foot in diabetes. Implications for foot care. N Engl J Med 311:1615-1618, 1984.

16. Zenn MR, Jones G. Reconstructive Surgery: Anatomy, Technique, & Clinical Applications. St Louis: Quality Medical Publishing, 2012.
17. Wagner FW. The dysvascular foot: a system for diagnosis and treatment. Foot Ankle 2:64-122, 1981.
18. Meggitt B. Surgical management of the diabetic foot. Br J Hosp Med 227-332, 1976.
19. Armstrong DG, Lavery LA, Harkless LB. Validation of a diabetic wound classification system: the contribution of depth, infection and ischemia to risk of amputation. Diabetes Care 21:855-859, 1998.
20. Lipsky BA, Berendt AR, Cornia PB, et al; Infectious Diseases Society of America. 2012 Infectious Diseases Society of America clinical practice guideline for the diagnosis and treatment of diabetic foot infections. Clin Infect Dis 54:132-173, 2012.
21. Laughlin TJ, Armstrong DG, Caporusso J, et al. Soft tissue and bone infections from puncture wounds in children. West J Med 166:126-128, 1997.
22. Lavery LA, Walker SC, Felder-Johnson KL, et al. Infected puncture wounds in diabetic and non-diabetic adults. Diabetes Care 18:1588-1591, 1995.
23. Lavery LA, Armstrong DG, Peters EJG, et al. Probe to bone test for diagnosing osteomyelitis: reliable or relic? Diabetes Care 30:270-274, 2007.
24. Storm-Versloot MN, Vos CG, Ubbink DT, et al. Topical silver for preventing wound infection. Cochrane Database Syst Rev 3:CD006478, 2010.
25. Lavery LA, Vela S, Quebedeaux T, et al. Total contact casts: pressure reduction at ulcer sites and the effect on the contralateral foot. Arch Phys Med Rehabil 78:1268-1271, 1997.
26. Armstrong DG, Lavery LA, Bushman TR. Peak foot pressures influence the healing time of diabetic foot ulcers treated with total contact casts. J Rehabil Res Dev 35:1-5, 1998.
27. Sinacore DR, Mueller MJ, Diamond JE. Diabetic plantar ulcers treated by total contact casting. Phys Ther 67:1543-1547, 1987.
28. Attinger CE, Janis JE, Steinberg J, et al. Clinical approach to wounds: debridement and wound bed preparation including the use of dressings and wound-healing adjuvants. Plast Reconstr Surg 117(7 Suppl):S72-S109, 2006.
29. Wunderlich RP, Peters EJ, Lavery LA. Systemic hyperbaric oxygen therapy: lower-extremity wound healing and the diabetic foot. Diabetes Care 23:1551-1555, 2000.
30. Ubbink DT, Westerbos SJ, Evans D, et al. Topical negative pressure for treating chronic wounds. Cochrane Database Syst Rev 3:CD001898, 2008.
31. Gregor S, Maegele M, Sauerland S, et al. Negative pressure wound therapy: a vacuum of evidence? Arch Surg 143:189-196, 2008.
32. Ennis WJ, Foremann P, Mozen N, et al. Ultrasound therapy for recalcitrant diabetic foot ulcers: results of a randomized, double-blind, controlled, multicenter study. Ostomy Wound Manage 51:24-39, 2005.
33. Wieman TJ, Smiell JM, Su Y. Efficacy and safety of a topical gel formulation of recombinant human platelet-derived growth factor-BB (becaplermin) in patients with chronic neuropathic diabetic ulcers. A phase III randomized placebo-controlled double-blind study. Diabetes Care 21:822-827, 1998.
34. Steed DL. Clinical evaluation of recombinant human platelet-derived growth factor for the treatment of lower extremity ulcers. Plast Reconstr Surg 117:S143-S149; discussion S150-S151, 2006.
35. Peters EJ, Lavery LA, Armstrong DG, et al. Electric stimulation as an adjunct to heal diabetic foot ulcers: a randomized clinical trial. Arch Phys Med Rehabil 82:721-725, 2001.
36. Lundeberg TC, Eriksson SV, Malm M. Electrical nerve stimulation improves healing of diabetic ulcers. Ann Plast Surg 29:328-331, 1992.
37. Frykberg RG. The team approach in diabetic foot management. Adv Wound Care 11:71-77, 1998.
38. Chaudhry V, Stevens JC, Kincaid J, et al. Practice advisory: utility of surgical decompression for treatment of diabetic neuropathy: report of the Therapeutics and Technology Assessment Subcommittee of the American Academy of Neurology. Neurology 66:1805-1808, 2006.
39. Balkin SW, Kaplan L. Injectable silicone and the diabetic foot: a 25 year report. Foot 2:83-88, 1991.
40. Lavery LA, Armstrong DG. Temperature monitoring to assess, predict, and prevent diabetic foot complications. Curr Diab Rep 7:416-419, 2007.

# 58. Lymphedema

Benson J. Pulikkottil

## DEFINITION

*Lymphedema* is the buildup of proteinaceous fluid within the interstitial compartment secondary to abnormalities in the lymphatic transport system. It can result in soft and pitting edema that may progress to nonpitting edema and irreversible extremity enlargement,[1] leading to progressive fibrosis and obstruction of the lymphatics.[2]

## DEMOGRAPHICS

- Affects 200 million people worldwide
  - Most commonly affects[2]:
    - Lower extremity (90%)
    - Upper extremity (10%)
    - Genitalia (<1%)
- Incidence
  - After mastectomy: 24%-49%
  - After lumpectomy: 4%-28%[3]
  - After sentinel lymph node biopsy: 5%-7%[4]
- Can occur after treatment of other malignancies[1]:
  - Melanoma: 16%
  - Gynecologic malignancies: 20%
  - Genitourinary cancers: 10%
  - Head and neck cancers: 4%
  - Sarcomas: 30%

**TIP:** Cancer survivors with lymphedema have more than a $10,000/year increase in their treatment costs compared with those without lymphedema.[5]

## PHYSIOLOGY OF THE LYMPHATIC SYSTEM

- Clears the interstitial space of proteins and lipids and transports them to the vasculature based on differential pressures.[6]
- Superficial and deep systems.[6]
- Basic functional unit is the ***contractile lymphangion.***
- Blood vessels have a defined basement membrane, whereas lymphatics have several intercellular gaps that **allow movement of fat and proteins** into the lymphatics.
- Muscle does **not** contain lymphatics.
- Propulsion of lymph relies on **muscle contraction** to mobilize lymph from the higher pressures of the vascular system to the lower pressures of the lymphatic system.
- Lymphatic system can cycle half of the circulating albumin from the interstitium per day.[7]

## PATHOPHYSIOLOGY OF LYMPHEDEMA (Fig. 58-1)

- **Staging:** Four-stage system designated by the International Society of Lymphology[8]
  - **Stage 0:** Latent or subclinical condition. No edema is evident, but lymph transport is impaired.
    - Can occur months or years before overt edema.
  - **Stage I:** Early accumulation of proteinaceous fluid with edema that resolves with limb elevation. Pitting edema can occur.
  - **Stage II:** Pitting edema may or may not be present, but tissue fibrosis develops. Limb elevation as a sole therapy does not resolve tissue swelling.
  - **Stage III:** Lymphostatic elephantiasis with absent pitting. Acanthosis, fat deposits, warty growth, and other trophic skin changes develop.

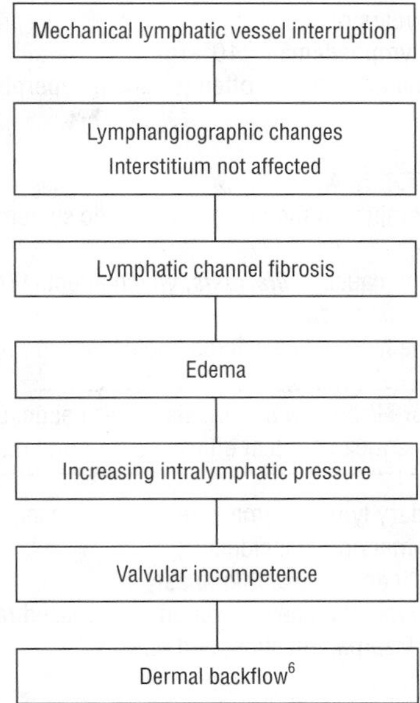


**Fig. 58-1** Pathophysiology of lymphedema.

## CLASSIFICATION

### PRIMARY LYMPHEDEMA

1. **Congenital lymphedema**
   - Also known as ***Milroy's disease***
     - Isolated and sporadic is the most common inheritance pattern
     - Occurs within first 2 years of life
     - Second most common type of primary lymphedema (10%-25%)
     - 3:1 lower extremity/upper extremity ratio
     - Commonly presents as bilateral lower extremity edema
     - 2:1 girl/boy ratio[6]
   - Autosomal dominant inherited inactivation mutation of VEGFR-3 tyrosine kinase (vascular endothelial growth factor receptor)[9,10]
   - Can be associated with intestinal lymphangiectasias and cholestasis[11]

2. **Familial lymphedema praecox**
   - Also known as ***Meige's disease***[12]
     - Presents during puberty
     - **Most common** form of primary lymphedema (65%-80%)
     - Incidence 1:100,000
     - 4:1 female/male ratio
     - Usually unilateral, affecting the foot and calf
     - Autosomal dominant inheritance
     - Associated with multiple anomalies: Vertebral, cerebrovascular malformations, hearing loss, and double row of eyelashes (distichiasis)[3]
3. **Lymphedema tarda**
   - Usually occurs after 35 years of age
   - Rarest form of primary lymphedema (<10%)[3]
   - Histologically, the lymphatic system is often tortuous, hyperplastic with an absence of competent valves.[2]

### SECONDARY LYMPHEDEMA

- Results from obstruction or injury of the normal lymphatic system by a defined disease process.[2]
- Worldwide the most common cause is ***filariasis,*** which affects 90 million people and is caused by the nematode *Wuchereria bancrofti.*
  - Adult worms obstruct the lymphatic systems and cause lymphedema.[13]

> **TIP:** The drug of choice for *W. bancrofti* filariasis is ivermectin. Circulating filarial antigen is pathognomonic and used as a means to test efficacy of treatment.

- In the United States, secondary lymphedema is related to consequences of treatment for malignancy (see previously mentioned incidences).[3]
- Can result from brachioplasty and medial thighplasty[14]
- Axillary node dissection and radiation have resulted in increased rates of lymphedema.[15,16]
- Notable risk factors include trauma, infection, and obesity.[3]

## NATURAL COURSE

- A significant latent period can occur before symptoms (1-5 years after surgery).[17]
- Initial mild soft edema of the involved extremity becomes fibrotic with time.
- **Potential consequences/complications:**
  - ***Erysipelas:*** Streptococcal dermal infection
  - ***Lymphangitis:*** Infection of the lymphatic vessels that starts distal to the channel
  - ***Lymphangiosarcoma:*** Rare malignant tumor associated with chronic lymphedema
    - Appears as bruising with multiple blue-red subcutaneous nodules in the affected extremity
    - Known as *Stewart-Treves syndrome* if it occurs after mastectomy
    - Mean survival ranges from 8-15 months.[6]
  - Negative psychological and social impact[18]
  - Massive local edema, also called *pseudosarcoma*[19]
    - In severely obese patients, folds of fat compress lymphatics and lead to edema, thickened epidermis, and dermal fibrosis.[20]
    - Most common location is the thigh.

## DIAGNOSIS

- **Differential diagnosis includes**[2,3]:
  - Cardiac failure
  - Renal failure
  - Proteinopathies
  - Lipedema
  - Deep venous thrombosis
  - Chronic venous insufficiency
  - Myxedema
  - Cyclical/idiopathic edema
  - Obesity
- **History**
  - Family history, recent surgery, infections, travel exposure, and prior episodes of symptoms[2]
- **Physical examination**
  - "Doughy" swelling of the extremity
  - Positive **Stemmer's sign**[21] (inability to grasp the skin of the dorsum of the second digit of the feet)
  - Peau d'orange skin changes caused by dermal fibrosis
  - Blunting of the involved digits
  - Circumferential limb measurements with a difference of **2 cm**[2,6]
- **Diagnostic studies**
  - **Contrast lymphography**
    - Direct injection of patent blue dye into the lymphatic channels
    - Rarely used because it is difficult and tedious, can worsen fibrosis, and is associated with adverse reactions[6]
  - ***Indirect lymphangiography***
    - Intradermal injection of water-soluble iodinated contrast material in conjunction with xeroradiography to evaluate lymphatics
  - **Isotopic lymphoscintigraphy**
    - *Most common diagnostic study to evaluate lymphedema*
    - Injection of nonionizing contrast agent (Tc 99m, Tc 99m-HAS, or Tc 99m dextran) into the interstitial space
    - Gamma camera follows the macromolecule and provides static and dynamic assessments of lymph flow.[6]
  - **MRI**
    - Provides details about lymphatic trunks and node
    - In chronic lymphedema the characteristic pattern of **"honeycombing"** in the epifascial compartment is noted.[6]
  - **CT**
    - Shows honeycombing and location of edema but is not as precise as MRI[6]
  - **Noninvasive techniques**
    - Bioelectric impedance analysis, tonometry, ultrasound, and perometry[3]

## TREATMENT

### CONSERVATIVE TREATMENT

- Benchmark is **complete decongestive therapy (CDT).**
  - Administered by a certified lymphedema therapist
  - Initial reductive phase, then a maintenance phase

- **Reductive phase** (3-8 weeks)
  - Manual lymph drainage
  - Multilayer short stretch compression bandaging
  - Therapeutic exercise
  - Skin care
  - Education in self-management
  - Elastic compression
- **Maintenance phase**[22]
  - Lifelong self-lymph drainage
  - Exercise
  - Skin care
  - Compression garments/bandages

- CDT has a 40%-60% mean reduction in excess volume in patients with pitting edema.[3]
- Preventative measures for lymphedema with strong scientific evidence (levels I and II) include:
  - Maintenance of normal body weight[23]
  - Avoidance of weight gain
  - Participation in supervised exercise programs

> **TIP:** Benefits from avoidance of venipuncture, limb constriction, limb elevation, heat and cold, air travel, and use of compression while flying have not been substantiated in the literature, and these measures may only provide a theoretical benefit to patients.[17]

## Surgical Treatment

- **Resection procedures**
  - First described by Charles in 1912[24]
    - Described radical circumferential excision of lymphedematous tissue deep to the fascial layer, with immediate coverage by a split-thickness skin graft from the excised skin[25]
  - The ***modified Charles procedure*** uses negative-pressure dressings after the initial debulking surgery, with skin grafting performed by day 5 or 7.[26]
  - More commonly, the ***Miller procedure*** is used for excision. It involves a longitudinal medial excision of skin and subcutaneous tissue with a layered closure and placement of closed-suction drains.[27]
- **Microsurgical approaches**
  - **General**
    - Supermicrosurgery (0.3-0.8 mm vessel diameter) allows lymph node transplantation, interposition lymph vessel transplantation, and lymphaticovenous anastomoses.
  - **Autologous lymph node transplantation**[28] (Fig. 58-2)
    - Recipient bed in the lymphedematous extremity is prepared through scar release until healthy tissue is found. A flap with superficial lymph nodes is harvested from the donor site with an artery and vein and microsurgically anastomosed to a recipient artery and vein.[1]
    - Benefits include:
      - Scar release
      - Recruitment of healthy, vascularized tissue
      - Addition of lymph nodes produces lymphangiogenetic VEGF-C (vascular endothelial growth factor C)
      - Immunologic system enhancement

- **Interposition lymph vessel transplantation**[29]
  - Baumeister et al[30] first reported lymph vessel transplantation in 1986.
  - Anatomic studies show 6-17 lymph vessels in the medial aspect of the thigh.[31]
  - *Technique:* Patent blue dye is subcutaneously injected into the first and second web spaces of the foot. Two or three ventromedial thigh lymph vessels are harvested. Depending on the location of the lymphatic obstruction, the interposition lymph grafts are positioned to bypass the obstruction and optimize lymph flow.[32]
  - Felmerer et al[32] noted enhanced lymphatic drainage in patients with secondary lymphedema in the upper and lower extremities, with complete symptomatic resolution in 3 of 14 patients and reasonable reduction of lymphedema in 9 of 14.
- **Lymphaticovenular bypass**[28] (Fig. 58-3)
  - Describes supermicrosurgical techniques to anastomose distal subdermal lymphatic vessels and adjacent venules <0.8 mm.[33]
  - *Technique:* 30-gauge needle used to inject 0.1-0.2 ml of isosulfan blue dye to identify lymph vessels. The subdermal region is dissected to identify and isolate a lymph vessel and its adjacent venule. A surgical bypass is performed using 11-0 or 12-0 nylon with a 50 μm needle.[33]
  - *Benefits:* Minimally invasive; minimal pain; usually discharged within 24 hours[33]
  - Chang[33] described lymphovenular bypass in 20 breast cancer patients and noted effective symptomatic improvement in 19 patients and quantitative lymphedema improvement in 13 patients using an average of 3.5 bypasses per patient.

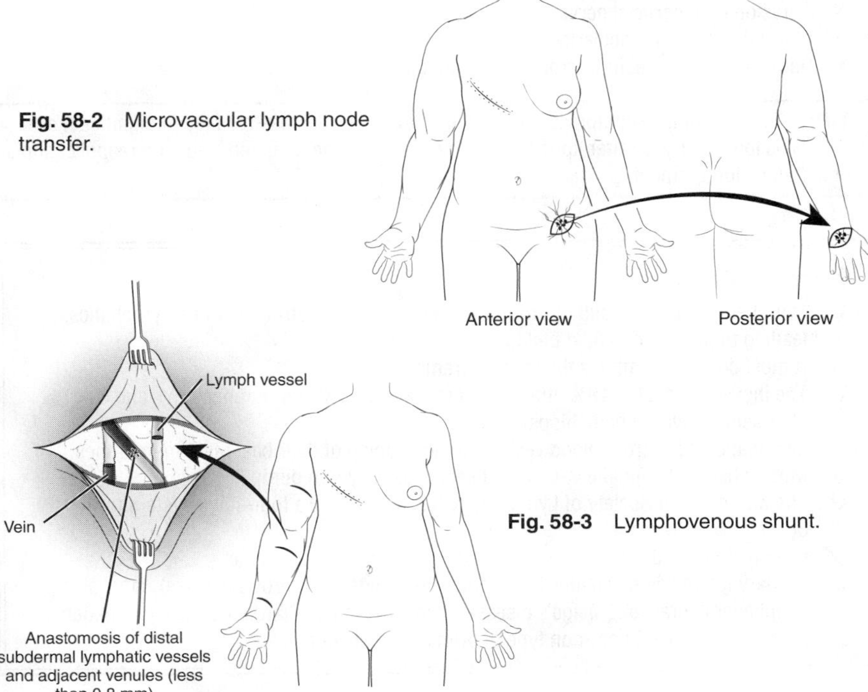


**Fig. 58-2** Microvascular lymph node transfer.

**Fig. 58-3** Lymphovenous shunt.

- **Suction-assisted lipectomy**
  - Liposuction of upper extremity lymphedema after breast cancer treatment reduced lymphedema volume by 104% after 1 year[34] and maintained results after 4 years with compression therapy.[35]
  - *Technique:* With general anesthesia and tourniquet control, circumferential liposuction is performed using special cutting cannulas through the lymphedematous tissue until required subcutaneous tissue is removed.
    - The postoperative incidence of cellulitis has been shown to be **four times** the preoperative incidence.[2]

## COMPLICATIONS[2]

- **Resection procedures**
  - Wound dehiscence
  - Lymphocele
  - Infection
  - Hematoma
- **Microsurgical techniques**
  - Lymphocele
  - Local infection and wound breakdown
  - Hematoma
  - Vascular thrombosis (2% risk)
- **Suction lipectomy**
  - Abrasion of superficial nerves
  - Disruption of skin vascularity
  - Damage to vital structures from sharp cannulas

**TIP:** Removal of arm compression garment for only a week has resulted in significant arm edema as long as 1 year after liposuction. However, arm edema is reduced with reapplication of compression garment.[6]

## KEY POINTS

- ✓ Lymphedema is the result of progressive fibrosis and obstruction of the lymphatics, leading to protein-rich fluid buildup in the interstitium.
- ✓ It most commonly affects the lower extremity.
- ✓ The incidence is 24%-49% after mastectomy, 4%-28% after lumpectomy, and 5%-7% after sentinel lymph node biopsy.
- ✓ Lymphatics differ from blood vessels in the gapping of their basement membranes.
- ✓ Muscle has no lymphatic vessels but serves as a "lymph pump."
- ✓ The International Society of Lymphology has designated a four-stage system to describe lymphedema.
- ✓ Lymphedema is divided into primary and secondary lymphedema.
- ✓ Primary lymphedema includes congenital lymphedema (Milroy's disease), familial lymphedema praecox (Meige's disease), and lymphedema tarda. Familial lymphedema praecox is the most common type of primary lymphedema.

- ✓ Filariasis is the most common cause for secondary lymphedema worldwide, whereas treatment after malignancy is the most common reason for this type of lymphedema in the United States.
- ✓ Chronic lymphedema can progress to lymphangiosarcoma (Stewart-Treves syndrome).
- ✓ Stemmer's sign is associated with lymphedema.
- ✓ Isotopic lymphoscintigraphy is the most common diagnostic study for identifying the condition. Honeycombing is a common pattern noted on MRI and CT, used for describing chronic lymphedema.
- ✓ CDT is the benchmark for conservative treatment.
- ✓ Patients with recalcitrant lymphedema may opt for surgical interventions, including resection, microsurgical approaches, and suction-assisted lipectomy.

## References


1. Becker C, Vasile JV, Levine JL, et al. Microlymphatic surgery for the treatment of iatrogenic lymphedema. Clin Plast Surg 39:385-398, 2012.
2. Raskin ER, Slavin SA, Borud LJ. Lymphedema. In Guyuron B, Eriksson E, Persing JA, et al, eds. Plastic Surgery: Indications and Practice. Philadelphia: Saunders Elsevier, 2009.
3. Warren AG, Brorson H, Borud LJ, et al. Lymphedema: a comprehensive review. Ann Plast Surg 59:464-472, 2007.
4. McLaughlin SA, Wright MJ, Morris KT, et al. Prevalence of lymphedema in women with breast cancer 5 years after sentinel lymph node biopsy or axillary dissection: patient perceptions and precautionary behaviors. J Clin Oncol 26:5220-5226, 2008.
5. Shih YC, Xu Y, Cormier JN, et al. Incidence, treatment costs, and complications of lymphedema after breast cancer among women of working age: a 2-year follow-up study. J Clin Oncol 27:2007-2014, 2009.
6. Beahm EK, Walton RL, Lohman RF. Vascular insufficiency of the lower extremity: lymphatic, venous, and arterial. In Mathes SJ, ed. Plastic Surgery, 2nd ed. Philadelphia: Saunders Elsevier, 2006.
7. Witte MH, Hanto D, Witte CL. Clinical and experimental techniques to study the lymphatic system. Vasc Surg 11:120-129, 1977.
8. International Society of Lymphology. The diagnosis and treatment of peripheral lymphedema. Consensus document of the International Society of Lymphology. Lymphology 36:84-91, 2003.
9. Karkkainen MJ, Ferrell RE, Lawrence EC, et al. Missense mutations interfere with VEGFR-3 signalling in primary lymphoedema. Nat Genet 25:153-159, 2000.
10. Irrthum A, Karkkainen MJ, Devriendt K, et al. Congenital hereditary lymphedema caused by a mutation that inactivates VEGFR3 tyrosine kinase. Am J Hum Genet 67:295-301, 2000.
11. Smeltzer DM, Stickler GB, Schirger A. Primary lymphedema in children and adolescents: a follow-up study and review. Pediatrics 76:206-218, 1985.
12. Wheeler ES, Chan V, Wassman R, et al. Familial lymphedema praecox: Meige's disease. Plast Reconstr Surg 67:362-364, 1981.
13. Szuba A, Shin WS, Strauss HW, et al. The third circulation: radionuclide lymphoscintigraphy in the evaluation of lymphedema. J Nucl Med 44:43-57, 2003.
14. Borud LJ, Cooper JS, Slavin SA. New management algorithm for lymphocele following medial thigh lift. Plast Reconstr Surg 121:1450-1455, 2008.
15. Coen JJ, Taghian AG, Kachnic LA, et al. Risk of lymphedema after regional nodal irradiation with breast conservation therapy. Int J Radiat Oncol Biol Phys 55:1209-1215, 2003.
16. Kissin MW, Querci della Rovere G, Easton D, et al. Risk of lymphoedema following the treatment of breast cancer. Br J Surg 73:580-584, 1986.

17. Cemal Y, Pusic A, Mehrara BJ. Preventative measures for lymphedema: separating fact from fiction. J Am Coll Surg 213:543-551, 2011.
18. Fu MR, Ridner SH, Hu SH, et al. Psychosocial impact of lymphedema: a systematic review of literature from 2004 to 2011. Psychooncology. 2012 Oct 9. [Epub ahead of print]
19. Farshid G, Weiss SW. Massive localized lymphedema in the morbidly obese: a histologically distinct reactive lesion simulating liposarcoma. Am J Surg Pathol 22:1277-1283, 1998.
20. Brewer MB, Singh DP. Massive localized lymphedema: review of an emerging problem and report of a complex case in the mons pubis. Ann Plast Surg 68:101-104, 2012.
21. Stemmer R. [A clinical symptom for the early and differential diagnosis of lymphedema] Vasa 5:261-262, 1976.
22. Cormier JN, Rourke L, Crosby M, et al. The surgical treatment of lymphedema: a systematic review of the contemporary literature (2004-2010). Ann Surg Oncol 19:642-651, 2012.
23. Ryan TJ. Lymphatics and adipose tissue. Clin Dermatol 13:493-498, 1995.
24. Karri V, Yang MC, Lee IJ, et al. Optimizing outcome of charles procedure for chronic lower extremity lymphoedema. Ann Plast Surg 66:393-402, 2011.
25. Charles RH. Elephantiasis scroti. In Latham AC, English TC, eds. A System of Treatment, vol 3. London: Churchill, 1912.
26. van der Walt JC, Perks TJ, Zeeman BJ, et al. Modified Charles procedure using negative pressure dressings for primary lymphedema: a functional assessment. Ann Plast Surg 62:669-675, 2009.
27. Miller TA, Wyatt LE, Rudkin GH. Staged skin and subcutaneous excision for lymphedema: a favorable report of long-term results. Plast Reconstr Surg 102:1486-1498, 1998.
28. Suami H, Chang DW. Overview of surgical treatments for breast cancer-related lymphedema. Plast Reconstr Surg 126:1853-1863, 2010.
29. O'Brien BM. Replantation and reconstructive microvascular surgery. Part I. Ann R Coll Surg Engl 58:87-103, 1976.
30. Baumeister RG, Siuda S, Bohmert H, et al. A microsurgical method for reconstruction of interrupted lymphatic pathways: autologous lymph-vessel transplantation for treatment of lymphedemas. Scand J Plast Reconstr Surg 20:141-146, 1986.
31. Kubik S. [Clinical anatomy of the lymphatic system] Verh Anat Ges 69:109-116, 1975.
32. Felmerer G, Sattler T, Lohrmann C, et al. Treatment of various secondary lymphedemas by microsurgical lymph vessel transplantation. Microsurgery 32:171-177, 2012.
33. Chang DW. Lymphaticovenular bypass for lymphedema management in breast cancer patients: a prospective study. Plast Reconstr Surg 126:752-758, 2010.
34. Brorson H, Svensson H, Norrgren K, et al. Liposuction reduces arm lymphedema without significantly altering the already impaired lymph transport. Lymphology 31:156-172, 1998.
35. Brorson H. Liposuction gives complete reduction of chronic large arm lymphedema after breast cancer. Acta Oncol 39:407-420, 2000.

# PART VI

# Hand, Wrist, and Upper Extremity

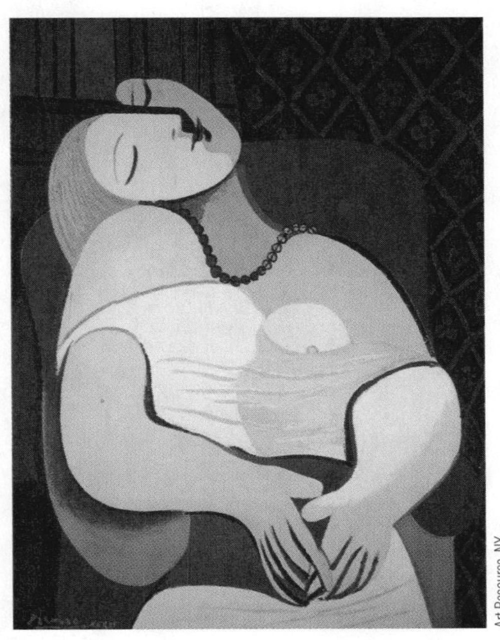

# 59. Hand Anatomy and Biomechanics

Douglas M. Sammer, David S. Chang

## ABBREVIATIONS

### Digits

- **IF:** Index finger
- **MF:** Middle finger
- **RF:** Ring finger
- **SF:** Small finger

### Joints

- **IP joint:** Interphalangeal joint
- **DIP joint:** Distal interphalangeal joint
- **PIP joint:** Proximal interphalangeal joint
- **MP joint:** Metacarpophalangeal joint
- **CMC joint:** Carpometacarpal joint
- **DRU joint:** Distal radioulnar joint

### Muscles

- **ADM:** Adductor digiti minimi
- **AdP:** Adductor pollicis
- **APL/APB:** Abductor pollicis longus/abductor pollicis brevis
- **ECRL/ECRB:** Extensor carpi radialis longus/extensor carpi radialis brevis
- **ECU:** Extensor carpi ulnaris
- **EDC:** Extensor digiti communis
- **EDM** or **EDQ:** Extensor digiti minimi or extensor digiti quinti
- **EIP:** Extensor indicis proprius
- **EPL/EPB:** Extensor pollicis longus/extensor pollicis brevis
- **FCR/FCU:** Flexor carpi radialis/flexor carpi ulnaris
- **FDM:** Flexor digiti minimi
- **FDP:** Flexor digitorum profundus
- **FDS:** Flexor digitorum superficialis
- **FPL/FPB:** Flexor pollicis longus/flexor pollicis brevis
- **ODM:** Opponens digiti minimi
- **OP:** Opponens pollicis
- **PL:** Palmaris longus
- **PQ:** Pronator quadratus
- **PT:** Pronator teres

# TERMINOLOGY

## Forearm and Hand

- **Radial** and **ulnar, dorsal** and **volar** (or **palmar**). *Avoid medial/lateral, anterior/posterior.*

## Digits

- Thumb
- Index finger
- Long or middle finger
- Ring finger
- Small or little finger

## Palm

- Thenar eminence
- Hypothenar eminence
- Midpalm: Area between thenar and hypothenar eminences

## Hand Motion

- **Thumb**
  - **Abduction:** Movement out of plane of palm (i.e., volar abduction) or in plane of palm (i.e., planar or radial abduction)
    - Abduction occurs at the CMC joint and refers to metacarpal motion.
  - **Flexion/extension:** Occurs at MP joint or IP joint of thumb—it is important to specify (i.e., IP joint extension)
  - **Opposition:** Combination of movements, including CMC joint rotation, resulting in the thumb pulp directly opposing the pulp of another finger
- **Fingers** (reference point is sagittal line through third ray)
  - **Abduction:** Movement is **away** from the long finger.
  - **Adduction:** Movement is **toward** the long finger.

# ANATOMY OF THE HAND

## Skin

- **Volar** skin is **thicker, less mobile,** and has **papillary ridges** for grasping.
- **Dorsal** skin is **thinner and more mobile,** and the subcutaneous tissue contains **veins** and **lymphatics.**

## Retinacular System

- **Volar fascia**
  - Anchors volar skin to bone for grasping, in contrast to loose skin on dorsum
  - **Superficial volar fascia:** Triangular-shaped fascia attached proximally to PL tendon; composed of longitudinal fibers, vertical fibers, transverse fibers, and natatory ligaments
- **Retaining ligaments of fingers**
  - Stabilize skin and extensor mechanism of digits and support neurovascular bundles
    - **Grayson's ligament:** Passes transversely from volar aspect of flexor tendon sheath to skin[1] (Fig. 59-1)
      - Prevents bowstringing of neurovascular bundle during finger flexion
    - **Cleland's ligament:** Passes from juncture of periosteum and flexor tendon sheath to skin laterally (see Fig. 59-1)
      - Lies dorsal to neurovascular bundle

- **Transverse retinacular ligament:** Lateral side of PIP joint, superficial to collateral ligament
  - Prevents dorsomedial displacement of lateral bands
- **Oblique retinacular ligament (ligament of Landsmeer):** Originates on volar aspect of middle phalanx and inserts on dorsal aspect of distal phalanx
  - Helps coordinate PIP joint and DIP joint motion

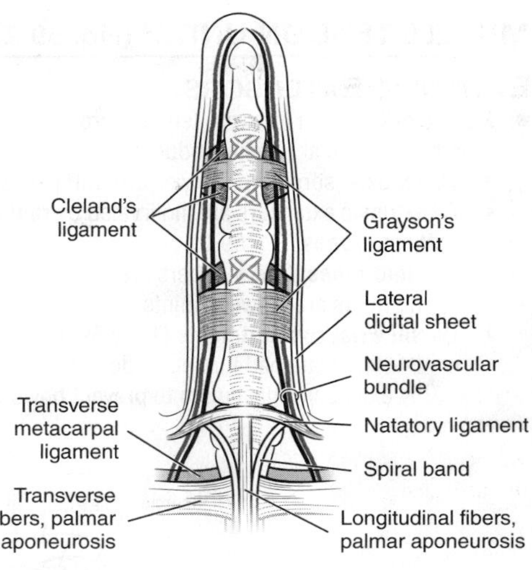


**Fig. 59-1** Distal volar and digital fascia.

## Deep Fascial Spaces

- **Potential spaces** that can be sites of infection
  - **Midvolar space**
    - **Boundaries**
      - **Dorsal:** Volar interossei and metacarpals
      - **Volar:** Volar aponeurosis and flexor tendons of ring, long, and small fingers
      - **Ulnar:** Hypothenar septum
      - **Radial:** Midvolar (oblique) septum
  - **Thenar space**
    - **Boundaries**
      - **Dorsal:** AdP
      - **Volar:** Index flexor tendon
      - **Ulnar:** Midvolar (oblique) septum
      - **Radial:** Adductor insertion and thenar muscle fascia
  - **Hypothenar space**
    - **Boundaries**
      - **Dorsal:** Hypothenar muscles
      - **Volar:** Small-finger flexor tendon
      - **Ulnar:** Hypothenar muscles
      - **Radial:** Hypothenar septum
  - **Interdigital web space**
    - Location of *collar button abscess*
    - **Boundaries**
      - **Dorsal:** Dorsal fascia and skin
      - **Volar:** Volar fascia
      - **Ulnar:** Extensor mechanism and MP joint capsule
      - **Radial:** Extensor mechanism and MP joint capsule
  - **Parona's space**
    - Infections can spread to this space from radial or ulnar bursa, or midvolar space.
    - **Boundaries**
      - **Dorsal:** Pronator quadratus
      - **Volar:** Digital flexors
      - **Ulnar:** FCU
      - **Radial:** Radial bursa (containing FPL)

## MUSCLE TENDON UNITS[2] (Fig. 59-2)

### Extrinsic Extensors

- Muscle bellies lie in forearm, tendons cross wrist to perform wrist and finger extension, and thumb extension and radial abduction.
  - Finger extensors primarily perform MP joint extension, and secondarily IP joint extension.
  - All extrinsic extensors are innervated by **radial nerve.**
  - **Extensor zones** (Fig. 59-3)
    - **Nine zones:** Odd numbers are over joints, starting with zone I over DIP joint; even numbers are between joints.
  - **Dorsal wrist compartments** (Table 59-1)
    - Six synovial-lined tunnels at dorsal wrist through which extensor tendons pass, covered by extensor retinaculum to prevent bowstringing

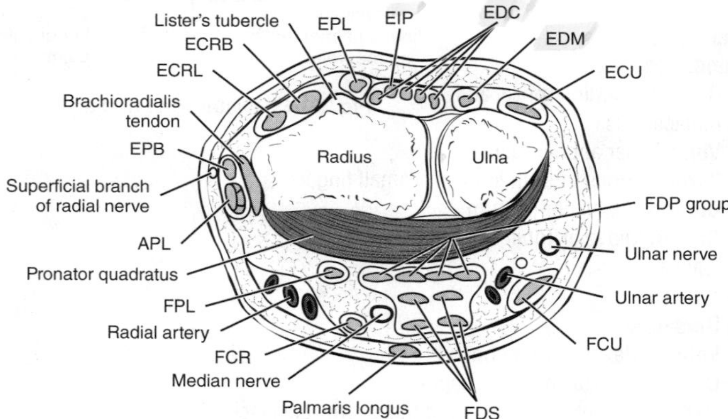


**Fig. 59-2** Cross-section of the wrist illustrating basic anatomic relations of major structures. Note the configuration of the flexor tendons (flexor digitorum superficialis *[FDS]* and flexor digitorum profundus *[FDP]* groups.) *APL,* Abductor pollicis longus; *ECRB,* extensor carpi radialis brevis; *ECRL,* extensor carpi radialis longus; *ECU,* extensor carpi ulnaris; *EDC,* extensor digitorum communis; *EDM,* extensor digiti minimi; *EIP,* extensor indicis proprius; *EPB,* extensor pollicis brevis; *EPL,* extensor pollicis longus; *FCR,* flexor carpi radialis; *FCU,* flexor carpi ulnaris; *FPL,* flexor pollicis longus.

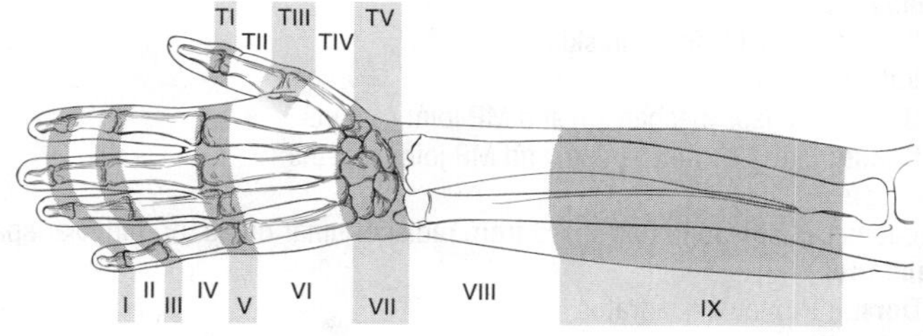


**Fig. 59-3** Extensor zones of the hand and forearm. The thumb has only two zones.

**Table 59-1** *Muscles of the Dorsal Wrist Compartments*

| Compartment | Muscle | Insertion | Action |
|---|---|---|---|
| First | APL | Base of first metacarpal | Extensor of first metacarpal and aids in abduction of thumb |
| | EPB | Base of proximal phalanx of thumb | Combines with EPL to extend thumb IP joint |
| Second | ECRL | Base of second metacarpal | Primarily radial deviation of wrist and secondarily wrist extension |
| | ECRB | Base of third metacarpal | Prime wrist extensor |
| Third | EPL | Passes around Lister's tubercle of radius and inserts on distal phalanx of thumb | Extends thumb IP joint |
| Fourth | EDC | No direct bony attachment to proximal phalanx (see Extensor mechanism below) | Extends MP joints and, with intrinsic muscles, extends IP joints<br>EDC to small finger absent in 50% of population |
| | EIP | Tendon lies ulnar to EDC tendon; functionally independent | Extends index finger while others are flexed |
| Fifth | EDM | Tendon lies ulnar to EDC tendon | Prime extensor of fifth MP joint, allows independent small finger extension<br>Abducts small finger |
| Sixth | ECU | Inserts on base of fifth metacarpal | Primarily ulnar deviation of wrist<br>Secondarily wrist extension |

- **ECRL, ECRB,** and **ECU** extend wrist.
- **EDC** has four tendons that extend index, long, ring, and small fingers.
- Index and small fingers have a **proprius tendon** (EIP and EDQ) in addition to EDC tendon.
  - *Proprius tendons (EIP and EDQ) lie* **ulnar** *to EDC tendon of respective digit.*
- **APL** radially abducts thumb metacarpal, **EPB** extends thumb MPJ, and **EPL** extends thumb IP joint.
- **Juncturae tendinum**
  - Tendinous interconnections between EDC tendons on dorsum of hand
  - Prevents independent action of extensors on single digit
  - Can also transmit MP joint extension to a finger even if its tendon is cut more proximally
- **Extensor mechanism** (Fig. 59-4)
  - Extensor mechanism on finger is *complex* and involves intermingling of extrinsic and intrinsic mechanisms.
  - EDC tendons insert onto extensor aponeurosis over the MP joint, and continue distally as **central slip.**

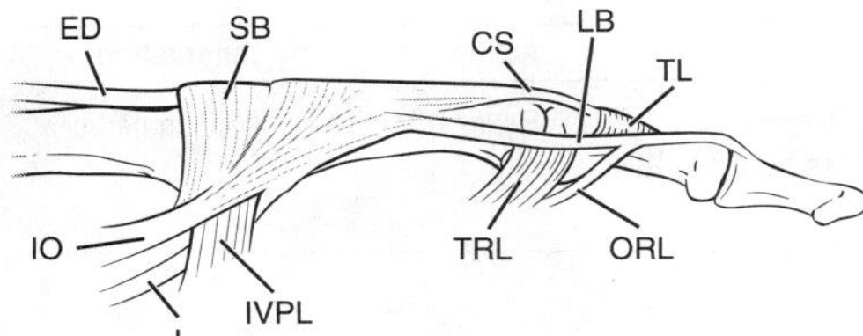


**Fig. 59-4** Extensor mechanism. *CS,* Central slip; *ED,* extensor digitorum; *IO,* interosseous; *IVPL,* intervolar plate ligament (deep transverse metacarpal ligament); *L,* lumbrical; *LB,* lateral band; *ORL,* oblique retinacular ligament of Landsmeer; *SB,* sagittal band; *TL,* triangular ligament; *TRL,* transverse retinacular ligament.

- Sagittal bands arise from volar plate and help stabilize the extensor tendon over the MP joint.
- Central slip inserts on the base of middle phalanx and contributes to PIP joint extension (along with the intrinsics).
- Two lateral slips arise from the central slip and join the intrinsics to become **conjoined lateral bands**, inserting on the base of distal phalanx as the **terminal tendon** and causing DIP joint extension.

## EXTRINSIC FLEXORS[3] (Tables 59-2 through 59-4)

- Muscle bellies lie in forearm, and tendons act to flex wrist, fingers, and thumb.
  - Innervated by **median and ulnar** nerves
    - **FDS** inserts on base of middle phalanx, causing PIP joint flexion, and is **median** nerve innervated.
    - **FDP** inserts on base of distal phalanx, causing DIP joint flexion. Index and long fingers are median nerve innervated, ring and small fingers are **ulnar** nerve innervated.
    - **FPL** inserts on base of thumb distal phalanx, causing thumb IP joint flexion, and is **median** nerve innervated.
    - **PL** inserts on superficial volar fascia **(unilateral absence in 15%, bilateral absence in 8%)**, and is **median** nerve innervated.
    - **FCR** inserts on index metacarpal, causing wrist flexion, and is **median** nerve innervated.
    - **FCU** inserts on small metacarpal, causing wrist flexion, and is **ulnar** nerve innervated.
- **Carpal tunnel** (see Fig. 59-2)
  - **Nine flexor tendons** (four FDS, four FDP, FPL) plus median nerve pass through carpal tunnel.
  - Long and ring finger FDS tendons stacked superficial to index and small finger FDS tendons within carpal tunnel
  - FDP and FPL tendons are deep to FDS tendons.

**Table 59-2** *Superficial Muscles of Forearm*

| Muscle | Insertion | Action | Innervation |
|---|---|---|---|
| PT | Midlateral radius | Pronates forearm, wrist, hand | Median nerve |
| FCR | Base of 2rd metacarpal (with a slip to 3rd) | Prime wrist flexor | Median nerve |
| PL | Attaches to volar aponeurosis | Ancillary wrist flexor<br>Absent in 10%-15%<br>Expendable as tendon graft | Median nerve |
| FCU | Pisiform and base of fifth metacarpal, and variably on fourth metacarpal and hook of hamate | Primarily ulnar deviator of wrist | Ulnar nerve |

**Table 59-3** *Intermediate Muscles of Forearm*

| Muscle | Insertion | Action | Innervation |
|---|---|---|---|
| FDS | Four tendons to index, long, ring, and small finger<br>Splits into radial and ulnar bands and passes dorsal to RDP tendon in finger, inserts on middle phalanx | Flexes PIP joint | Median nerve |

**Table 59-4** *Deep Muscles of Forearm*

| Muscle | Insertion | Action | Innervation |
|---|---|---|---|
| FDP | Distal phalanx after passing through Camper's chiasm (decussation of flexor digitorum superficialis) | Flexes DIP joints, fingers | Median nerve (radial half) Ulnar nerve (ulnar half) |
| FPL | Distal phalanx of thumb | Flexes DIP joints, thumb | Median nerve |

- **Flexor tendon zones**
  - Used to describe level of injury; determines treatment and prognosis[4] (Fig. 59-5)
    - **Zone I:** Distal to FDS insertion. Only the FDP is within the flexor tendon sheath.
    - **Zone II:** A1 pulley to FDS insertion. FDP and FDS are within the flexor tendon sheath (called *no-man's land* because of historically poor outcomes)
    - **Zone III:** Between carpal tunnel and A1 pulley
    - **Zone IV:** Within carpal tunnel
    - **Zone V:** Proximal to carpal tunnel

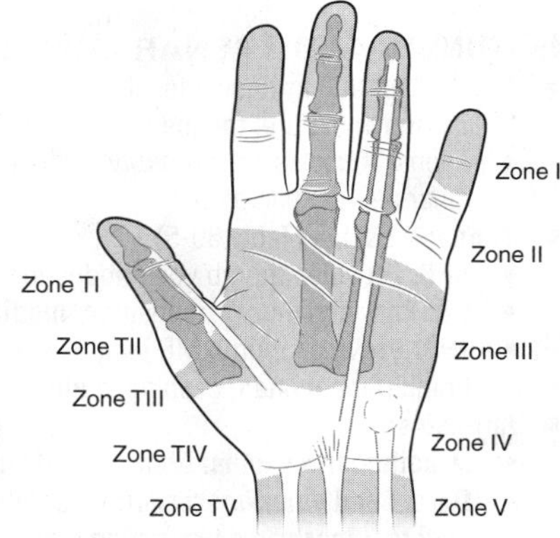


**Fig. 59-5** Flexor zones of the hand.

- **Camper's chiasm**
  - FDS tendon is superficial to the FDP in the forearm and palm.
  - FDS has a **longitudinal split** *(Camper's chiasm)* just proximal to its insertion on middle phalanx.
  - FDP passes through Camper's chiasm to become more superficial as it continues distally to its insertion on the distal phalanx.
- **Flexor tendon sheath**
  - From metacarpal heads to distal phalanges, flexor tendons lie within a tight fibroosseous sheath lined with synovium that functions as a pulley system[4] (Fig. 59-6).

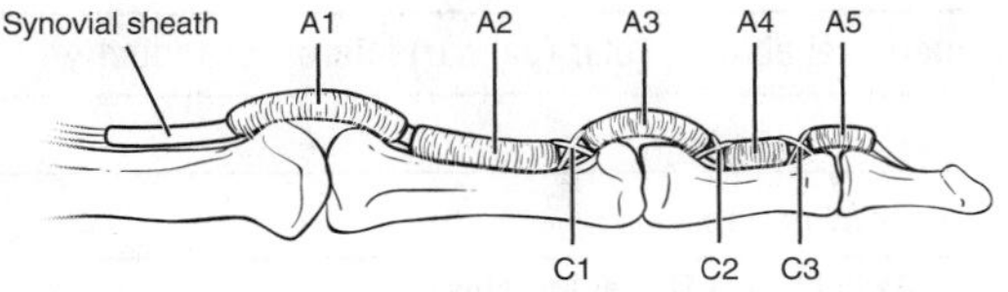


**Fig. 59-6** Flexor tendon sheath pulley system.

- **Pulleys**
  - Allow smooth excursion of tendons
  - Keep flexor tendons close to axis of rotation of joints (decreases moment arm)
  - Prevent bowstringing
  - Increase mechanical advantage of flexor tendons
- **Annular pulleys** (A1-A5)
  - Thickened regions of the flexor tendon sheath that function as strong pulleys
  - **Odd** numbers arise from **volar plates** of MP joint, PIP joint, and DIP joint.
  - **Even** numbers arise from **periosteum** of proximal and middle phalanges.
  - **A2** and **A4** pulleys are **most important** to prevent bowstringing

- **Cruciate pulleys** (C1-C3)
  - Thin portions of the flexor tendon sheath, with crisscrossing (cruciate) fibers
  - C1 lies between A2 and A3, C2 between A3 and A4, and C3 between A4 and A5.
  - Function like accordions and allow the flexor tendon sheath to compress and expand as the finger flexes and extends
- **Thumb**
  - A1 and A2 pulleys are over the MP joint and IP joint.
  - **Oblique pulley** lies between A1 and A2 pulleys and is **most important** to prevent bowstringing.

## Intrinsic and Thenar Muscles

- Both thenar and intrinsic muscles lie completely within the hand.
  - By nomenclature, the thenar muscles are considered separate from the intrinsic muscles.
  - Thenar muscles are *primarily* median nerve innervated, and intrinsic muscles are *primarily* ulnar nerve innervated.
- **Thenar muscles** (Table 59-5)
  - **APB:** Provides thumb volar abduction, **median** nerve innervated (recurrent motor branch)
  - **OP:** Provides thumb opposition, **median** nerve innervated (recurrent motor branch)
  - **FPB:** Provides thumb MP joint flexion, superficial head **median nerve** (recurrent motor branch) innervated; deep head **ulnar** innervated
- **Intrinsics**
  - **Hypothenar muscles:** Abduction of small finger, **ulnar** nerve innervated (Table 59-6)
  - **Dorsal and volar interossei:** Volar interossei adduct fingers, dorsal interossei abduct fingers, **ulnar** nerve innervated (Table 59-6)
  - **AdP:** Thumb metacarpal adduction, key pinch, **ulnar** nerve innervated
  - **Lumbricals:** Along with interossei, flex finger MP joints and extend finger IP joints. Arise from radial side of FDP. Ulnar two are **ulnar** nerve innervated, radial two are **median** nerve innervated.

**TIP:** The **median** nerve innervates the **"LOAF"** muscles: **l**ateral (radial) two lumbricals, **o**pponens pollicis, **a**bductor pollicis brevis, **f**lexor pollicis brevis (superficial head). All other intrinsic hand muscles are ulnar nerve innervated.

**TIP:** Think "**dab** with a **pad**": **d**orsal interossei **ab**duct, volar (**p**almar) interossei **ad**duct

**Table 59-5** *Radial and Ulnar Group Thenar Muscles*

| | Radial Group Thenar Muscles | | |
|---|---|---|---|
| **Muscle** | **Origin** | **Insertion** | **Action** |
| APB | Flexor retinaculum and tubercles of scaphoid and trapezium | Lateral side of base of proximal phalanx of thumb | Volar abductions, slight metacarpophalangeal flexion and interphalangeal extension |
| OP | Flexor retinaculum and tubercle of trapezium | Lateral side of first metacarpal bone | Rotates thumb pinch with index finger |
| FPB, superficial portion | Flexor retinaculum and tubercle trapezium | Medial side of base of proximal phalanx of thumb | Flexes and stabilizes MP joint |

| Muscle | Ulnar Group Thenar Muscles | | |
|---|---|---|---|
| | Origin | Insertion | Action |
| AP | Oblique head: Bases of second and third metacarpals, capitates, and adjacent carpal bones<br>Transverse head: Anterior surface of body of third metacarpal bone | Lateral side of base of proximal phalanx of thumb | Adducts thumb and flexes MP joint |
| FPB, deep portion | Flexor retinaculum and tubercle and trapezium | Medial side of base of proximal phalanx of thumb<br>Flexes MP joint | Flexes MP joint |

**Table 59-6** *Hypothenar Muscles*

| Muscle | Origin | Insertion | Action |
|---|---|---|---|
| ODM | Hook of hamate and flexor retinaculum | Medial border of fifth metacarpal | Rolls fifth metacarpal toward thumb<br>Flexes fourth and fifth metacarpal joints for better thumb opposition |
| FDM | Hook of hamate and flexor retinaculum | Medial side of base of proximal phalanx of small finger | Flexes MP joint |
| ADM | Pisiform bone | Medial side of base of proximal phalanx of small finger | Abducts small finger<br>Flexes fifth MP joint<br>Extends IP joints when MP joint is stabilized |
| PB | Flexor retinaculum and volar aponeurosis | Skin on medial side of palm | Pulls skin to help cup palm<br>Rudimentary muscle<br>Occasionally absent |

## VASCULATURE

### ARTERIAL (Fig. 59-7)

- **Radial artery**
  - Runs between brachioradialis and FCR tendons at wrist.
  - Splits into larger dorsal branch that courses through anatomic snuffbox to supply deep volar arch.
  - Smaller volar branch joins superficial volar arch.
- **Ulnar artery**
  - Lies radial to ulnar nerve at wrist and through Guyon's canal
  - Order of FCU tendon, ulnar nerve, and ulnar artery at the wrist in an ulnar to radial direction is tendon, nerve, artery.

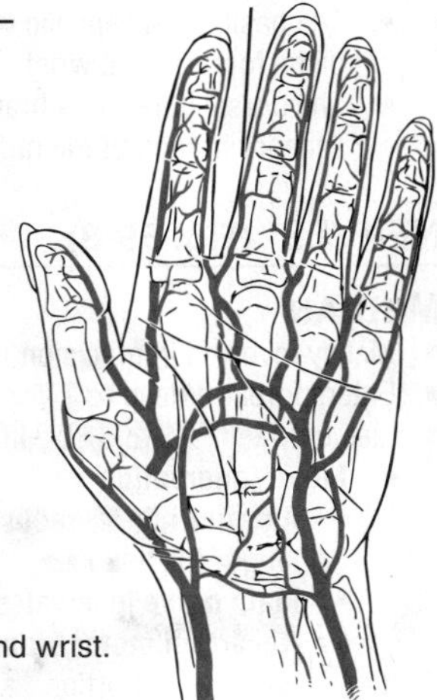


**Fig. 59-7** Arterial anatomy of the hand and wrist.

- Splits into larger volar branch that forms superficial volar arch.
- Smaller dorsal branch joins deep volar arch.

**TIP:** *Kaplan's cardinal line* is a line drawn across the palm from the apex of the first web space to the hook of hamate. It approximates the location of the superficial volar arch. The deep arch is 1 cm proximal to this line.

- **Superficial arch**
  - Gives rise to **common digital arteries** in interspaces
    - **Common digital arteries** lie **volar to common digital nerves in the palm**, then bifurcate at web space into radial and ulnar **proper digital arteries,** which lie **dorsal to the proper digital nerves in fingers.**
    - **Arteries are volar to nerves in palm, dorsal to nerves in fingers.**
    - Digital arteries arborize just distal to **DIP joint.**
    - At IP joints, digital arteries give off branches that pass under flexor tendons and anastomose with branch from other side to form vincular blood supply.
    - Primary blood supply to thumb is **princeps pollicis artery,** which arises from radial artery or deep volar arch.

**TIP:** Unlike the fingers, the thumb has a very robust dorsal blood supply and can survive reliably after loss of its primary volar blood supply.

### Veins and Lymphatics

- Venous and lymphatic drainage in the hand occurs in a volar to dorsal direction.

**NOTE: Because of this direction of drainage, and because of the looseness of dorsal skin, the dorsal hand swells easily.**

  - *Volar* infections can present with *dorsal* swelling.
- The basilic vein (ulnar side) and cephalic vein (radial side) are large, easily palpable vessels in the wrist and forearm.
  - The basilic and cephalic veins are surgical landmarks for important sensory nerves at the distal forearm and wrist.
  - The dorsal cutaneous branch of the ulnar nerve runs with the basilic vein, and the superficial sensory branch of the radial nerve runs with the cephalic vein.

## NERVES[2] (Fig. 59-8)

### Median

- Mainly involved in precision manipulation
- Enters forearm deep to PT or between two heads of PT
- Lies between FDS and FDP in forearm
  - **Motor innervation**
    - **Anterior interosseous branch** (arises in forearm) supplies FPL, index (and sometimes long) FDP, and PQ.
    - **Main nerve** innervates PT, FCR, FDS, PL.
    - **Recurrent motor branch** innervates intrinsic muscles of the thumb: APB, FPB (superficial portion), and OP.
    - **Small motor branches arising from common digital nerves** innervate lumbricals to index and long fingers.

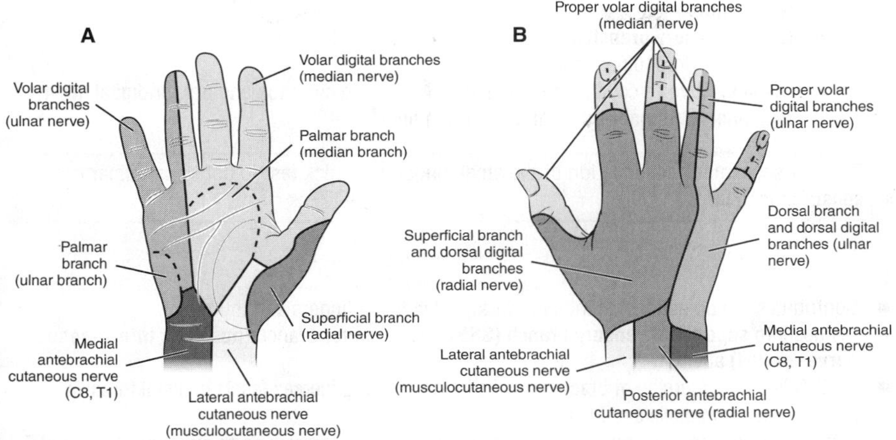


**Fig. 59-8** Sensory distribution. **A,** Volar. **B,** Dorsal.

**TIP:** Thumb opposition is a quick test to determine median nerve motor function (i.e., have the patient gesture "OK").

- **Sensory innervation**
  - **Volar cutaneous branch** arises **5 cm** proximal to wrist crease and innervates thenar eminence.
  - The main nerve divides into common and proper digital nerves, innervating the thumb and index, long, and ring (radial side) fingers.

**TIP:** Assessment of sensation at the volar tip of the index finger is a quick test to determine median nerve sensory function.

## ULNAR

- Essential for power grasp
- Passes through **cubital tunnel** at elbow, a common site for compression
- Enters forearm between two heads of FCU
- Lies under FCU in forearm and enters **Guyon's canal** (bounded by pisiform ulnarly, hook of hamate radially, volar carpal ligament volarly, and transverse carpal ligament dorsally) at the wrist
  - **Motor innervation**
    - **Forearm:** FCU and FDP to ring and small fingers
    - **Hand:** Deep motor branch, which arises within Guyon's canal, innervates hypothenar muscles (ADM, ODM, FDM), lumbricals to ring and small fingers, all interossei, deep head of FPB (superficial head is median innervated), and AdP.

**TIP:** Finger abduction and adduction and crossing of fingers are quick tests to determine ulnar nerve motor function.

- **Sensory innervation**
  - **Dorsal sensory branch** originates 5-7 cm proximal to ulnar styloid process and innervates dorsoulnar aspect of hand.
  - Distal to Guyon's canal, the main nerve divides into common and proper digital nerves that innervate small and ulnar side of ring finger.

> **TIP:** Assessment of sensation of the small finger is a quick test to determine ulnar nerve sensory function.

## Radial

- Contributes to supination, extends the wrist, extends the fingers and thumb
- Divides into **superficial sensory branch (SSBRN)** and motor branch **(posterior interosseous nerve, or PIN)** at elbow
- SSBRN lies on underside of brachioradialis in forearm and pierces fascia in distal forearm between brachioradialis and ECRL.
- PIN passes deep to or within the supinator in the proximal forearm and arborizes into a cauda equina.
  - **Motor innervation**
    - Main nerve innervates brachioradialis, ECRL, and ECRB before branching into SSBRN and PIN at elbow (some variability).
    - **PIN** innervates supinator and remaining extensors of wrist, finger, and thumb (ECU, EDC, EDM, APL, EPL, EPB, and EIP).

> **TIP:** Finger and thumb extension are quick tests to determine radial nerve motor function. When examining finger extension, only look at MP joint extension—the IP joints can be extended by the ulnar-innervated intrinsics. Make sure the wrist is in neutral position, because a flexed wrist position can cause MP joint extension by the tenodesis effect.

- **Sensory innervation**
  - **SSBRN** supplies sensibility to dorsoradial aspect of hand, and dorsum of thumb and index and long fingers to the IP joint.
  - **Lateral antebrachial cutaneous nerve** (continuation of myocutaneous nerve) has overlapping innervation with radial nerve at radial aspect of wrist.

> **TIP:** Assessment of first dorsal web space sensation is a quick test to determine radial nerve sensory function.

## Anomalous Interconnections

- **Martin-Gruber anastomosis**
  - Motor fiber connection from median to ulnar nerve in forearm
  - Affects 10%-25% of population
- **Riche-Cannieu anastomosis**
  - Motor fiber connection from ulnar to median nerve in the hand
  - Common[5]

**TIP:** A Martin-Gruber anastomosis can result in preserved ulnar nerve motor function in the hand after a high ulnar nerve injury. A Riche-Cannieu anastomosis can result in preserved thenar motor function after a more proximal median nerve injury.

## BONES AND JOINTS

### HAND

- **Bones**
  - Five metacarpals (Name them according to the corresponding digit [e.g., index metacarpal] rather than by number to prevent confusion.)
  - Three phalanges for each finger (proximal/P1, middle/P2, and distal/P3)
  - Thumb has two phalanges (proximal and distal).
- **MP joints**
  - Collateral ligaments pass obliquely in dorsal to volar direction, from metacarpal head to base of proximal phalanx.
  - Collateral ligaments are tightest and provide greatest stability when MP joints are flexed, and allow lateral movement with MP joint in extension.
  - **Volar plates:** Fibrocartilaginous part of joint capsule that provides additional stability and has strong distal attachment and loose proximal attachment, allowing MP joint hyperextension

**TIP:** When the hand is immobilized in a splint or cast, the MP joints should be flexed unless otherwise indicated. This stretches the collateral ligaments and prevents them from shortening and causing an extension contracture.

- **IP joints**
  - Collateral ligaments provide lateral stability throughout range of motion.
  - **Volar plates:** Unlike volar plate at MP joint, the **PIP joints** volar plates have strong proximal and distal attachments and prevent hyperextension.

### WRIST

- **Bones**
  - Organized into two rows: Proximal and distal carpal rows
  - **Proximal** row (scaphoid, lunate, triquetrum)
  - **Distal** (trapezium, trapezoid, capitate, and hamate)
  - *Pisiform is a sesamoid bone and lies within the substance of the FCU tendon.*
  - Scaphoid links proximal and distal rows and is ***the most commonly fractured carpal bone.***
- **Wrist joint**
  - Effectively composed of **radiocarpal** joint and **midcarpal** joint
    - Radius and ulna articulate with the proximal carpal row at radiocarpal joint.
    - Proximal and distal carpal rows articulate with each other at midcarpal joint.
  - Main movements are flexion-extension, radioulnar deviation, and circumduction, and are composed of radiocarpal and midcarpal motion.
- **CMC joints**
  - **Thumb CMC joint** is **saddle joint,** providing maximal mobility. It is stabilized by a complex of ligaments, including the critical volar beak ligament.
  - Index and long finger CMC joints have little mobility.
  - Ring and small-CMC joints have 20-30 degrees of flexion/extension, respectively.

**TIP:** Because the small finger CMC joint and thumb CMC joint have so much mobility, substantial fracture malunion is tolerated in these metacarpals with minimal loss of function.

- **Ligaments**
  - Organized into **extrinsic** and **intrinsic** ligaments
  - **Extrinsic** ligaments connect carpal bones to the radius and ulna, and **intrinsic** ligaments connect carpal bones to each other.
  - **Extrinsic** ligaments are divided into **dorsal** and **volar.**
    - **Volar extrinsic ligaments** are more important for wrist stability than the dorsal extrinsic ligaments.
  - **Intrinsic** wrist ligaments that connect bones of the same carpal row are called ***interosseous*** *ligaments.*

**TIP:** The scapholunate is the most commonly injured wrist ligament. This interosseous intrinsic ligament connects the scaphoid and lunate.

## DRU Joint

- Not a wrist joint, but a forearm joint
- Articulation of **ulnar head** with **sigmoid notch** of radius
- Allows the *radius to rotate around the fixed unit of the ulna*
- Allows forearm rotation (supination/pronation), along with sister joint at elbow (the proximal radioulnar joint, or PRU joint)
- **Triangular fibrocartilage complex (TFCC)** is primary stabilizer of DRU joint.
  - Consists of articular disc, distal radioulnar ligaments, ulnocarpal ligaments, and ECU tendon subsheath
  - Originates from radius, attaches to fovea and base of ulnar styloid, and transmits 20% of load across wrist
  - Central 80% of TFCC is avascular; poor healing potential in central portion

## Key Points

✓ The extrinsic finger extensors primarily extend the MP joints. IP joint extension is mainly performed by the intrinsics.

✓ An EDC laceration can be masked because of adjacent EDC pull through the juncturae tendinum.

✓ The FDS flexes the PIP joint. To test its function, hold the remaining fingers in extension and ask the patient to flex the affected finger.

✓ The FDP flexes the DIP joint. To test its function, hold the PIP joint of that finger in extension and ask the patient to flex the fingertip.

✓ Anastomoses between the median and ulnar nerves in the forearm and hand can mask ulnar or median nerve injuries.

## REFERENCES

1. Doyle JR, Botte MJ, eds. Surgical Anatomy of the Hand & Upper Extremity. Philadelphia: Lippincott Williams & Wilkins, 2003.
2. Beasley RW, ed. Beasley's Surgery of the Hand. New York: Thieme, 2003.
3. Lluch AL. Repair of the extensor tendon system. In Aston SJ, Beasley RW, Throne CH, eds. Grabb and Smith's Plastic Surgery, 5th ed. Philadelphia: Lippincott Williams & Wilkins, 1997.
4. Zidel P. Tendon healing and flexor tendon surgery. In Aston SJ, Beasley RW, Thorne CH, eds. Grabb and Smith's Plastic Surgery, 5th ed. Philadelphia: Lippincott Williams & Wilkins, 1997.
5. Harness D, Sekeles E. The double anastomotic innervation of thenar muscles. J Anat 109:461-466, 1971.

# 60. Basic Hand Examination

Jeffrey E. Janis

## HISTORY

### TRAUMA

- Determine age, occupation, and other pursuits.
- Determine whether the dominant hand is injured.
- Is there any history of previous trauma to the extremity?
- *When* did the injury occur?
- *Where* did the injury occur?
- *How* did the injury occur?
- *What* previous treatment has been administered?

### NONTRAUMA

- When did the pain, swelling, sensory change, or other symptoms begin?
- Is there a progression of symptoms, and in what order did they occur?
- How is function impaired?
- Are other joints or digits affected?
- What makes the pain (swelling, tingling) worse or better?
- Is it worse at some particular time (day or night)?

## PHYSICAL EXAMINATION[1,2]

- **Initial examination of the injured hand in the emergency room must establish the following:**
  - Is the injured hand or digit viable?
  - Is there a vascular injury?
  - Is there ischemic compartment syndrome?
  - Is there tendon damage?
  - Is there nerve injury?
  - Is the skeleton stable?
  - Is there actual or threatened skin loss?

### OVERVIEW

- **Skin**
  - Uncover the entire upper extremity.
  - Examine for swelling or edema.
  - Evaluate color.
  - Evaluate moisture and papillary ridges.
  - Examine, characterize, and document all wounds.
  - **Compare findings with the contralateral extremity.**
  - Note any atrophy (thenar or other muscle groups).

- **Motor function**
  - Determine active and passive range of motion (ROM).
  - Instruct patient, *"Make a fist."*
  - Instruct patient, *"Straighten out your fingers."*
  - Pain that is disproportionate to the injury or significant pain with passive motion may suggest serious underlying pathology such as ischemic compartment syndrome or suppurative flexor tenosynovitis.
  - Observe cascade of the fingers.
  - Determine whether patient can fully extend and flex each joint of the hand and wrist.
- **Sensation**
  - **Static two-point discrimination (2PD)** of digits should approach **6 mm.**
  - **Dynamic 2PD** should be approximately **3 mm.**
  - **Loss of sweating ability is** concomitant with the distribution of digital nerve interruption, as is **loss of papillary ridges.**
  - Glabrous skin will wrinkle after immersion in water for 5 minutes, *denervated skin will not.*
  - **Ten test** can be performed.
    - This is a simple, rapid, reliable, sensitive method to evaluate hand sensitivity.
    - Test has been validated in adults and children over 5 years old.[3,4]
    - Ask patient to rate sensation in affected area relative to a "10" baseline in unaffected area.
    - In adults, sensitivity is 87%, specificity is 52%.
- **Vascular**
  - Palpate radial and ulnar pulses.
  - Capillary refill should occur in <2 seconds.
  - **Allen's test** can be performed on the hand, as well as on individual digits.
  - Perform Doppler test when any question of vascular compromise remains.
- **Skeleton**
  - Swelling
  - Deformity
  - Abnormal ROM
  - Decreased ROM
  - Increased ROM (possible ligamentous injury)
  - Tenderness
- **Radiographs**
  - Carefully review all radiographs.
  - Take PA and lateral views at the least.
  - Reorder when inadequate, or add additional views as indicated.

**TIP:** Obtain comparison views of the contralateral side, particularly in children or when the wrist is involved.

  - Pay particular attention to insertion points of ligaments or tendons and to articular surfaces.

## ANATOMY (Figs. 60-1 through 60-3)

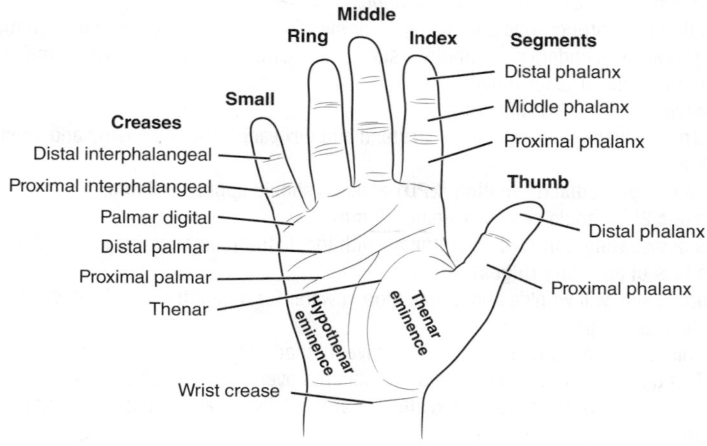


**Fig. 60-1** Surface anatomy of the hand.

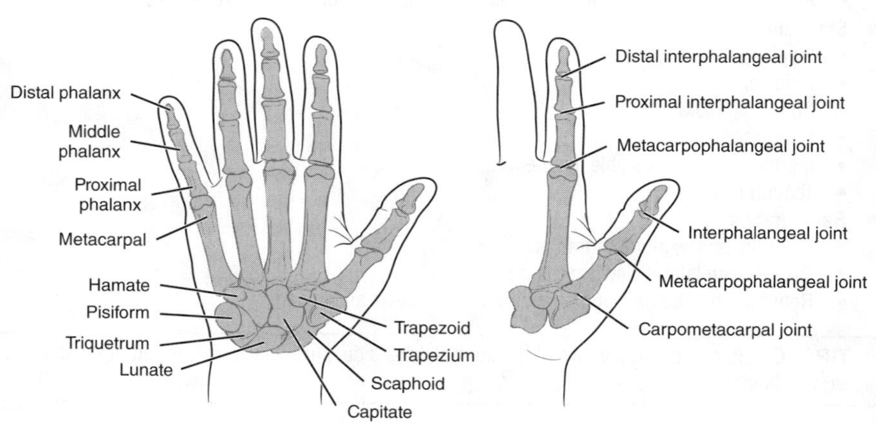


**Fig. 60-2** Skeleton of the hand and wrist.

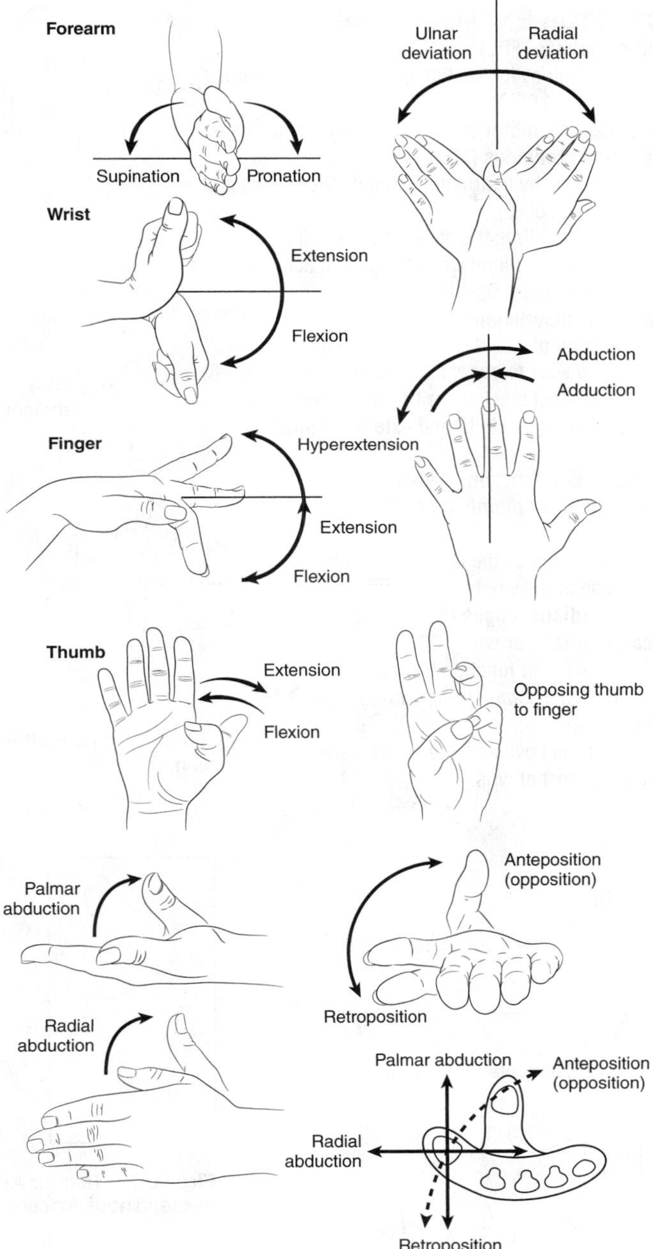


**Fig. 60-3** Terminology of the hand and digit motion.

## Specific Motor Examinations

- **Flexor pollicis longus (FPL)**
  - Test FPL function by instructing patient, *"Bend the tip of your thumb"* (Fig. 60-4).
  - Examiner can test motor strength by adding resistance.
- **Flexor digitorum profundus (FDP)**
  - Test FDP function by instructing patient, *"Bend the tip of your finger"* (Fig. 60-5).
  - The examiner stabilizes the patient's proximal interphalangeal (PIP) joint while the patient actively flexes distal interphalangeal (DIP) joint.
- **Flexor digitorum superficialis (FDS)**
  - Test the function of each FDS individually by instructing patient, *"Bend your finger at the middle joint"* (Fig. 60-6).
  - The examiner must block other fingers in extension.
- **Abductor pollicis longus (APL)** and **extensor pollicis brevis (EPB)**
  - Test APL and EPB function by instructing patient, *"Bring your thumb out to the side"* (Fig. 60-7).
  - The examiner palpates the taut tendons over the radial side of the wrist.
- **Extensor carpi radialis longus (ECRL)** and **extensor carpi radialis brevis (ECRB)**
  - Test ECRL and ECRB function by instructing patient, *"Make a fist and strongly bring your wrist back"* (Fig. 60-8).
  - The examiner then palpates the tendons over dorsoradial aspect of wrist.

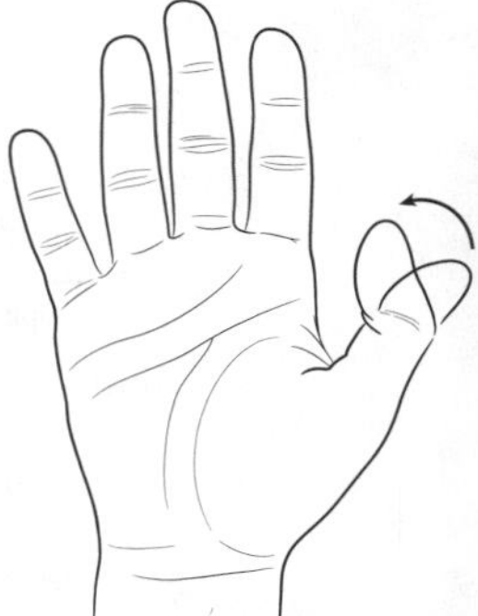

**Fig. 60-4** Test for FPL myotendinous function.

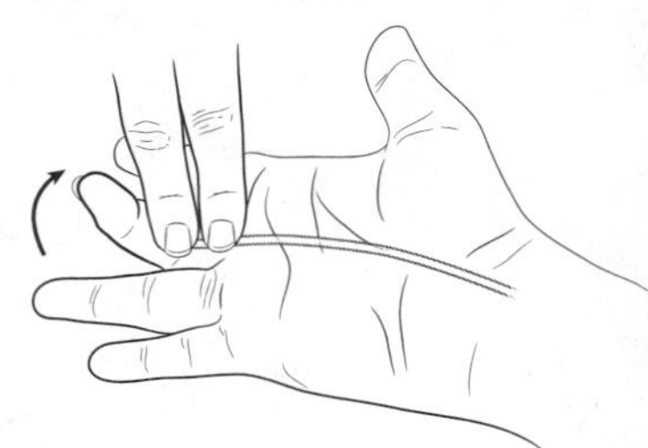

**Fig. 60-5** Test for FDP myotendinous function.

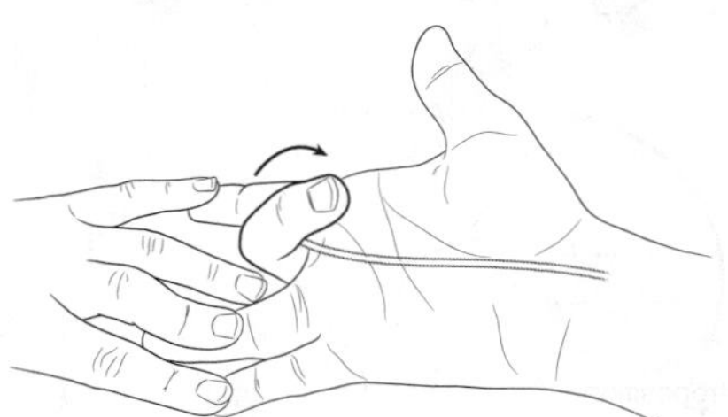

**Fig. 60-6** Test for FDS myotendinous function.

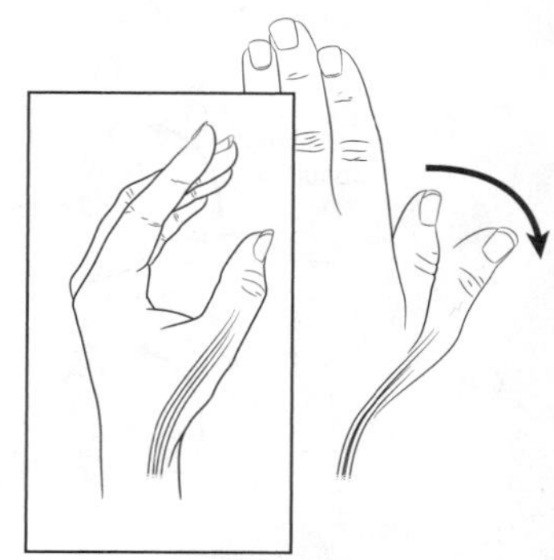

**Fig. 60-7** Test for APL and EPB myotendinous function.

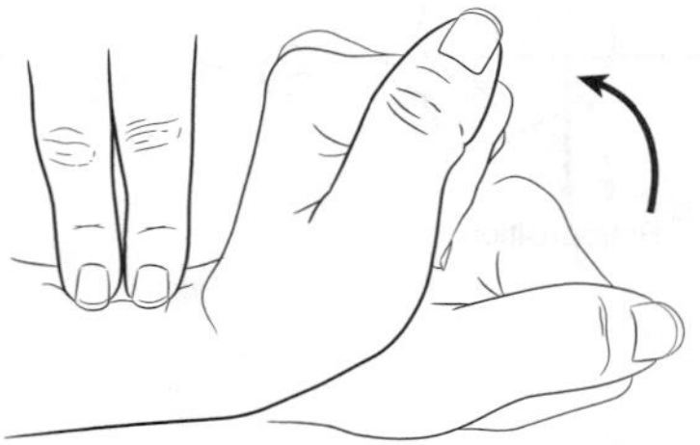

**Fig. 60-8** Test for ECRL and ECRB myotendinous function.

- **Extensor pollicis longus (EPL)**
  - Test EPL function by placing hand flat on the table and instructing patient, *"Lift only the thumb off the table"* (Fig. 60-9).
- **Extensor digitorum communis (EDC), extensor indicis proprius (EIP),** and **extensor digiti minimi** or **extensor digiti quinti (EDM or EDQ)** (Fig. 60-10).
  - Test EDC function by instructing patient, *"Straighten your fingers."*
  - Test EIP function by instructing patient, *"Stick out your index finger with the others in a fist."*
  - Test the function of EDM or EDQ by instructing patient, *"Stick out your small finger with the others in a fist."*
- **Extensor carpi ulnaris (ECU)**
  - Test ECU function by instructing patient, *"Pull your hand up and out to the side"* (Fig. 60-11).
  - The examiner palpates the tendon over the ulnar side of the wrist.
- **Thenar muscles**
  - The thenar muscles include the **abductor pollicis brevis (APB), opponens pollicis (OP),** and **flexor pollicis brevis (FPB).**
  - Test these muscles by instructing patient, *"Touch the thumb to the small finger"* (Fig. 60-12).

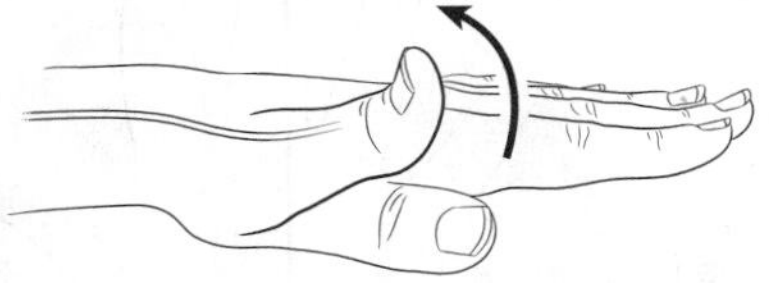

**Fig. 60-9** Test for EPL myotendinous function.

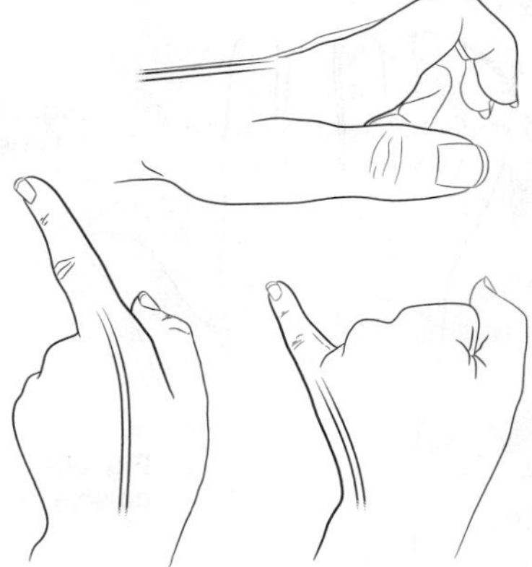

**Fig. 60-10** Test for EDC, EIP, and EDM (EDQ) myotendinous function.

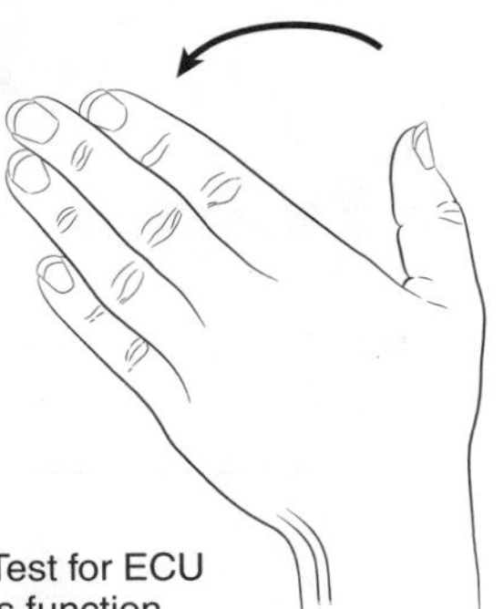

**Fig. 60-11** Test for ECU myotendinous function.

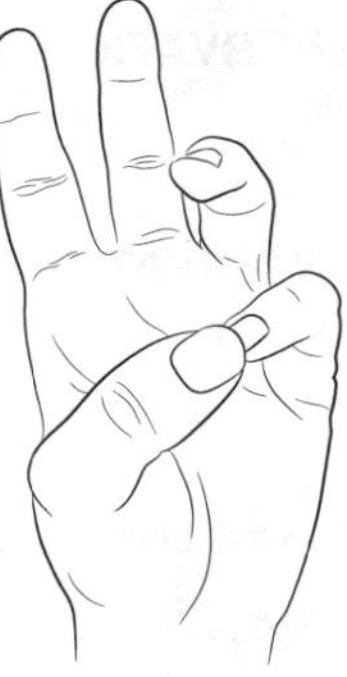

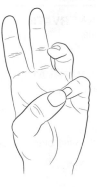

**Fig. 60-12** Test for thumb opposition.

- **Adductor pollicis (AdP)**
  - Test the function of adductor pollicis by having patient forcibly grasp a piece of paper between the thumb and radial side of the index P1 (Fig. 60-13).
  - This is *Froment's sign;* a positive response is shown in Fig. 60-13.
- **Interosseous muscles**
  - Test the interosseous muscle by applying resistance to the index and small finger and instructing patient, *"Spread your fingers apart"* (Fig. 60-14).
- **Hypothenar muscles**
  - The hypothenar muscles include the **abductor digiti minimi (ADM), flexor digiti minimi (FDM),** and **opponens digiti minimi (ODM).**
  - Test these muscles by instructing patient, *"Bring your little finger away from the others"* (Fig. 60-15).

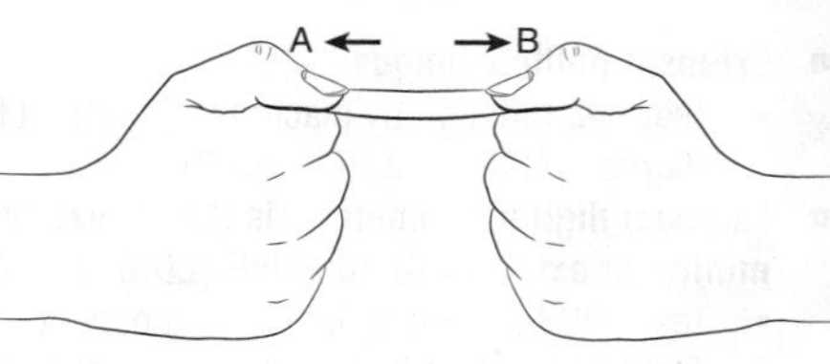


**Fig. 60-13** Froment's sign. Test is positive in *B* (compensatory flexion at IP joint.)

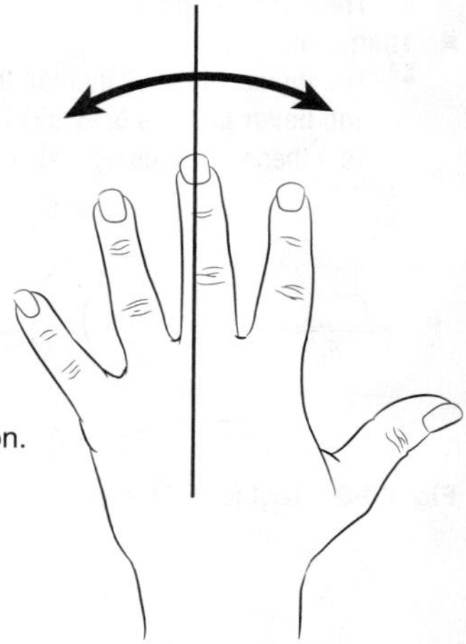

**Fig. 60-14** Test for interosseous muscle function.

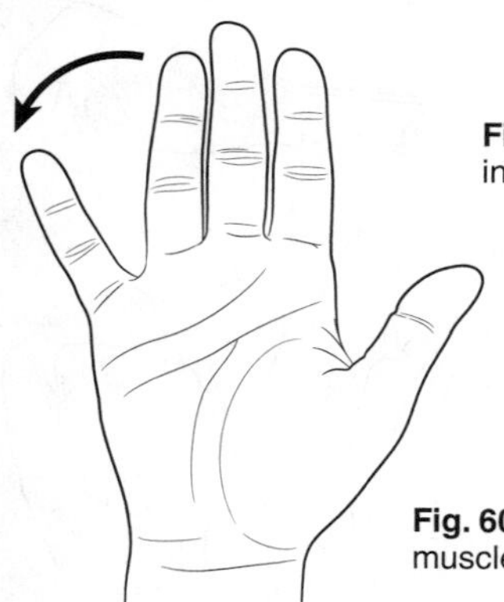

**Fig. 60-15** Test for hypothenar muscle function.

## SENSORY EXAMINATION

### Ulnar Nerve Innervation (Fig. 60-16)

- Ulnar half of ring finger
- All of small finger

### Median Nerve Innervation (Fig. 60-17)

- Volar surface of thumb
- Index finger
- Middle finger
- Radial side of ring finger
- Volar wrist capsule (terminal branch of **anterior** interosseous nerve)

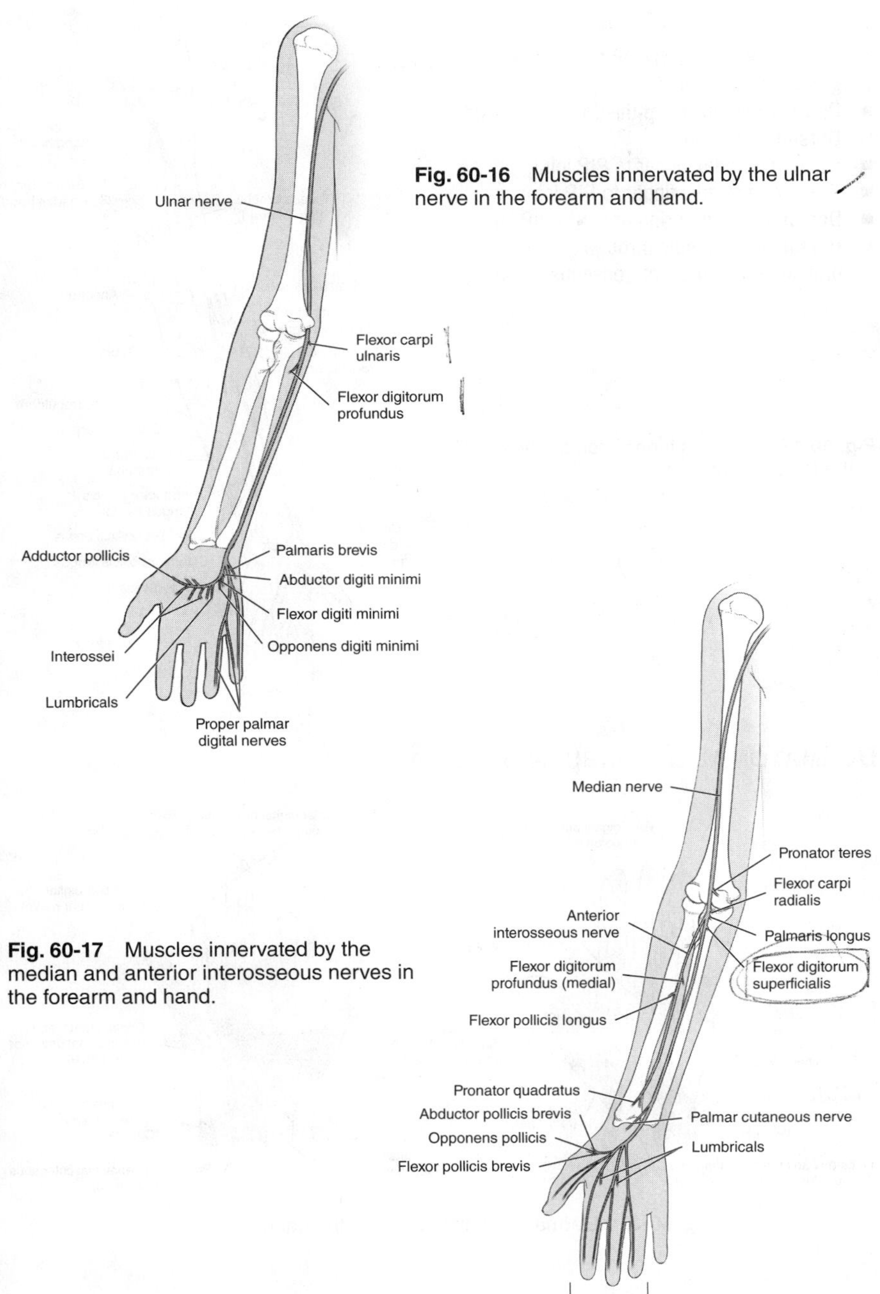


**Fig. 60-16** Muscles innervated by the ulnar nerve in the forearm and hand.

**Fig. 60-17** Muscles innervated by the median and anterior interosseous nerves in the forearm and hand.

## RADIAL NERVE INNERVATION (Fig. 60-18)

- Radial three fourths of the dorsum of hand
- Dorsum of thumb
- Dorsum of index finger to PIP joint
- Dorsum of middle finger to PIP joint
- Dorsoradial half of ring finger to PIP joint
- **Dorsal** wrist capsule through terminal branch of **posterior** interosseous nerve

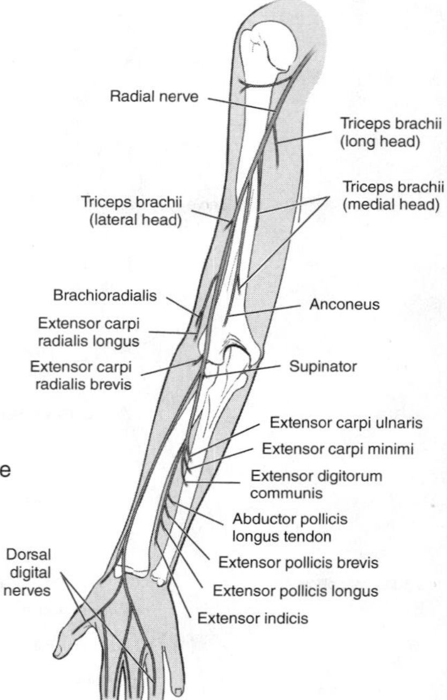


**Fig. 60-18** Muscles innervated by the radial nerve in the forearm and hand.

## DERMATOMAL DISTRIBUTION (Fig. 60-19)

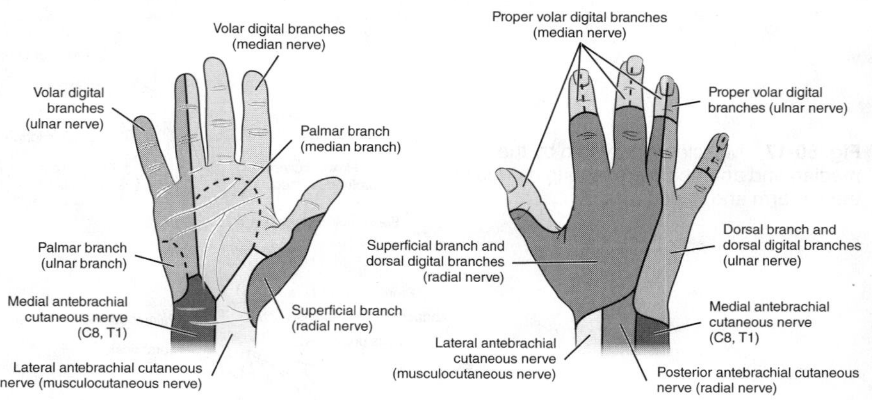


**Fig. 60-19** Dermatomal distribution of the hand and wrist.

## VASCULAR TESTS

### ALLEN'S TEST

- Determines **patency** of the ulnar and radial arteries (Fig. 60-20)
  1. Occlude both arteries.
  2. Exsanguinate the hand.
  3. Release the radial artery.
  4. Examine palm for pink color/capillary refill.
  5. Repeat for ulnar artery.

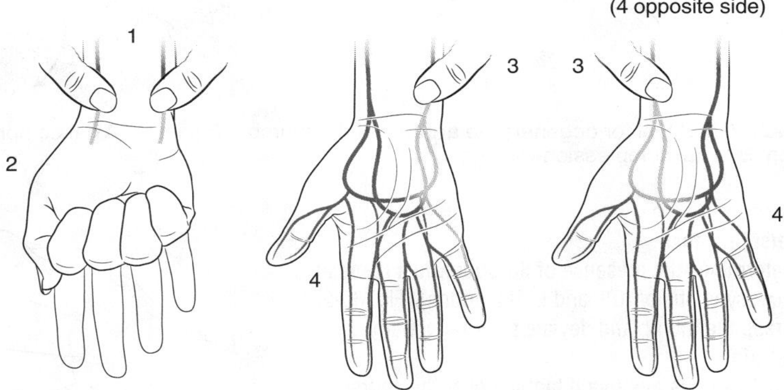


**Fig. 60-20** Allen's test for arterial patency.

**TIP:** This test also can be used on a single digit.

## CLINICAL SIGNS OF ACUTE PATHOLOGY

- **Tenderness in the snuffbox**
  - Tenderness during deep palpation of the anatomic snuffbox (between the EPL and EPB, just distal to the radial styloid) suggests a **possible scaphoid fracture** (Fig. 60-21).

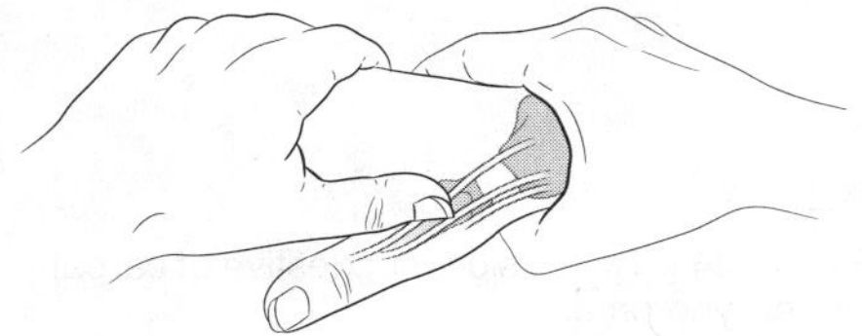

**Fig. 60-21** Fracture of the scaphoid with tenderness on deep palpation in the snuffbox area.

- **Grind test**
  - Test **degenerative arthritis** of the thumb metacarpophalangeal (MP) joint by compression and adduction (Fig. 60-22, *A*), or by compression and rotation (Fig. 60-22, *B*).

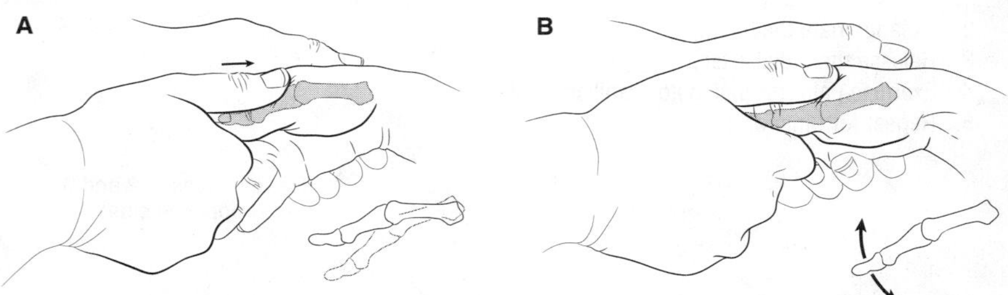


**Fig. 60-22** Grind test for degenerative arthritis of the thumb MP joint. **A,** Axial compression-adduction. **B,** Axial compression-rotation.

- **Finkelstein's test**
  - Determines the presence of **de Quervain's disease** (tenosynovitis of APL and EPB tendons) (Fig. 60-23)
  - Grasp the thumb and deviate the wrist ulnarly.
- **Tinel's sign**
  - Tinel's sign is **positive** if tapping over the course of the median nerve in the carpal tunnel creates paresthesias in the hand (Fig. 60-24). This suggests **carpal tunnel syndrome.**
  - Test the cubital and radial tunnels similarly.
- **Phalen's maneuver**
  - Perform by positioning the wrists in complete flexion for 1 minute (Fig. 60-25)
  - Paresthesias in the hand constitute a positive test and suggest **carpal tunnel syndrome.**
- **Durkan's compression test**
  - ▸ Perform by placing direct median nerve compression at the transverse carpal ligament for 30 seconds (Fig. 60-26).
  - Paresthesias in the hand constitute a positive test and suggest **carpal tunnel syndrome.**

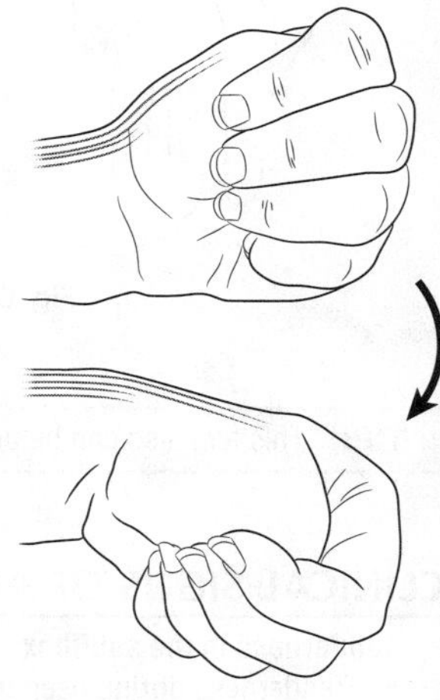

**Fig. 60-23** Finkelstein's test for de Quervain's disease.

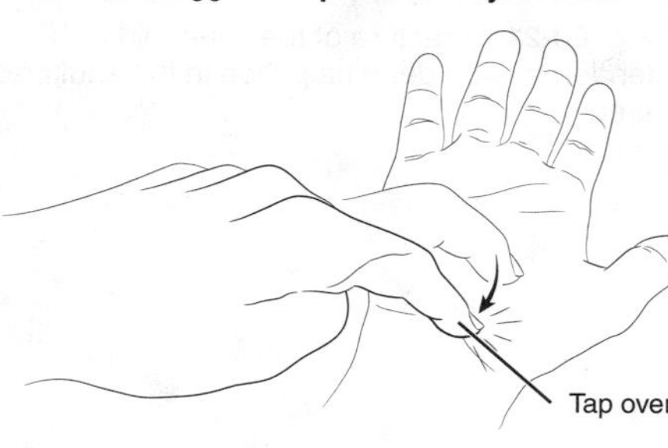


**Fig. 60-24** Tinel's sign, suggestive of carpal tunnel syndrome.

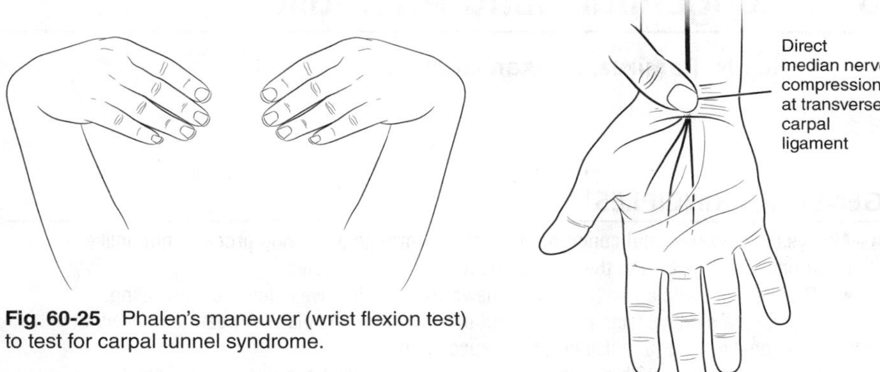


**Fig. 60-25** Phalen's maneuver (wrist flexion test) to test for carpal tunnel syndrome.

**Fig. 60-26** Durkan's compression test for carpal tunnel syndrome.

## Key Points

- ✓ Paresthesias in the hand constitute a positive test result and suggest **carpal tunnel syndrome.**
- ✓ It is imperative to obtain a thorough and proper history to design the most appropriate treatment.
- ✓ An organized approach to a physical examination will help to prevent inadvertent omissions.
- ✓ A static 2PD should be ≤6 mm, whereas the dynamic 2PD should be ≤3 mm.
- ✓ The immersion test helps to test innervation in children.
- ✓ Allen's test can be performed on digits and on the hand.
- ✓ Comparison of contralateral radiographs can be very helpful.
- ✓ Know key diagnostic maneuvers to test for abnormal pathology.

## References

1. American Society for Surgery of the Hand. The Hand: Examination and Diagnosis, 3rd ed. New York: Churchill Livingstone, 1990.
2. American Society for Surgery of the Hand. The Hand: Primary Care of Common Problems, 2nd ed. New York: Churchill Livingstone, 1990.
3. Strauch B, Lang A, Ferdar M, et al. The ten test. Plast Reconstr Surg 99:1074-1078, 1997.
4. Sun HH, Oswald TM, Sachanandani NS, et al. The 'Ten Test': application and limitations in assessing sensory function in the paediatric hand. J Plast Reconstr Aesthet Surg 63:1849-1852, 2010.

# 61. Congenital Hand Anomalies

Rey N. Ramirez, Ashkan Ghavami

## GENERAL PRINCIPLES[1-6]

- **Always address parental concerns.** Parents go through a grieving process, not unlike mourning, over the loss of the "perfect baby" that was expected.[2]
  - The first visit with a family and their newborn must involve extensive counseling.
  - Explain the medical facts known about the condition, the plan for treatment, need for additional testing (if indicated), and expectations.
    - Many children with congenital hand differences will have *near-normal ability to perform all activities.*
    - Knowledge of associated conditions is crucial, because some of these may be **more severe** than the limb anomaly. This can prevent unnecessary and distressing workups.
- Thorough history
  - Problems during pregnancy
  - Details of newborn period
  - Known medical comorbidities
  - Family history of congenital deformities
- Total body examination is always necessary. Look for a range of deformities from the craniofacial region to the toes.
- **Surgical timing is critical.**
  - Anesthesia risks are increased in children younger than 6 months.
  - Prioritize other medical and surgical problems.
  - Optimal hand size: Hand size doubles in the first 2-2½ years of life.
    - Important for any microsurgery
  - Consider child's maturity level (e.g., for rehabilitation and cooperation with splinting regimens).
  - Restoration of hand function at an early age may permit use of the hand during cognitive development.
    - Some surgeries (e.g., border syndactyly reconstruction) must be performed **before normal growth worsens the deformity.**
  - Time operation(s) before child starts school (largely to help social interaction).
- A meticulous dressing and a cast that cannot be removed are imperative. (An above-elbow full cast is almost always necessary.)

> **TIP:** Use toys and gadgets and assess primitive reflexes while visually observing the child's hand function.
>
> Do not assume that someone else has diagnosed other anomalies such as a sacral dimple, duplicate toes, an unusual facial appearance, or a known syndromic disorder that is associated with the hand anomaly.

## EMBRYOLOGY[7]

**Upper limbs develop from weeks 5 to 8.**

### Limb Outgrowth

- Upper limb bud emerges around week 4.
- Lateral plate mesoderm bulges out, covered by a thin layer of ectoderm.
- Development is triggered by T-box ***(TBX5),*** wingless-type MMTV ***(WNT),*** and fibroblast growth factor **(FGF).**
- Failure of limb induction is known as *tetramelia.*

### Apical Ectodermal Ridge (AER)

- Transient ectodermal thickening at leading edge of bud
- **FGF10** and **R-FNG** from the underlying mesoderm induce formation of AER.
- Induces underlying mesoderm to differentiate to a sub-AER population known as the *progress zone*
- Mesoderm produces morphogens (apical ectodermal ridge maintenance factor [**AERMF**]) that maintain the AER in feedback loop.

### Zone of Polarizing Activity (ZPA)

- Cluster of mesenchymal cells along postaxial (ulnar) border of limb bud
- Secretes sonic hedgehog **(SHH)** along an "ulnarizing" gradient
- Provides stimulus to AER in another reciprocal feedback loop

### Dorsal Ectoderm

- Produces **WNT7**
- Dorsalizes underlying mesoderm through the induction of Lim homeodomain transcription factor **LMX1B**

### Three Main Interactions Guide Formation

1. **Proximal to distal progression**
   - This is guided by the **AER.**
   - Reciprocal loop of **FGF** and **WNT** function maintains proximal-distal outgrowth.
   - Progressive loss of FGF function leads to loss of *radial structures* (e.g., thumb hypoplasia).
   - Removal of the AER causes a truncated limb.
2. **Dorsal to volar axis** (e.g., fingernails versus pulp; flexor versus extensor tendon)
   - This is guided by the **dorsal ectoderm.**
   - Disruptions cause abnormal dorsalization (e.g., nail-patella syndrome).
3. **Radial to ulnar axis cell differentiation** (or preaxial to postaxial, respectively)
   - This is guided by the **ZPA.**
   - ZPA expands limb width and *ulnarizes* the developing limb.
   - SHH induces ulnar formation and the four ulnar-sided digits in the hand.
   - Diminished ZPA function leads to reduction in limb outgrowth, volume, and width.
   - Loss of SHH function leads to *ulnar longitudinal deficiency.*

### Hand Plate Formation

- All hands begin as a hand plate (5 weeks' gestation) that develops into a hand by a combination of gradual recession of interdigit spaces and digital outgrowth.
- HOX transcription factors and SHH interact in a gradient to establish digit number and identity.

- SHH also induces an ulnar to radial **BMP gradient.**
  - BMPs induce apoptosis (programmed cell death) within interdigital spaces by repressing FGF.
    - *Syndactyly is thought to be failure of proper apoptosis between digits.*
- BMPs, SHH, and HOX induce formation of **phalanx-forming region** (PFR) for each digit, which regulates construction.
  - By **day 50,** individual digits and web spaces are well defined.

## CLASSIFICATION OF ANOMALIES[5]

**NOTE: Classification systems are less commonly used today, because there are many confounding variables.**

**International Federation of Societies for Surgery of the Hand Classification[5]**

I. **Failure of formation of parts**
   - Transverse arrest
   - Longitudinal arrest
   - **Examples:** Phocomelia, hypoplastic thumb; radial, central, or ulnar longitudinal deficiency

II. **Failure of differentiation of parts**
   - Soft tissue
   - Osseous
   - **Examples:** Synostosis, syndactyly, radial head dislocation, symphalangism, camptodactyly, clinodactyly, Kirner's deformity

III. **Duplication**
   - **Examples:** Polydactyly, mirror hand, duplicate thumb

IV. **Overgrowth**
   - **Examples:** Macrodactyly

V. **Undergrowth**

VI. **Constriction band syndrome**

VII. **Generalized anomalies and syndromes**
   - Certain disorders may fit into multiple classes or may **not** fit perfectly into a specific class.

## SYNDACTYLY[3,4,8]

- Congenital fusion of two digits

### ETIOLOGIC FACTORS

- Unknown failure of the process of recession at interdigit spaces

### INCIDENCE

- 1:2000 live births
- **Ten times** more common in whites than blacks
- **Twice** as common in males than females
- No difference between bilateral and unilateral
- **Long and ring finger** most commonly affected (57%)[1]
- Thumb-index finger most rare (3%)[6]

## Family History

- Reported in 15%-40% of cases[8]
- **Autosomal dominant inheritance with variable penetrance** when no other associated anomalies are present

## Associated Conditions

- **Familial** and **sporadic simple** syndactyly are generally **not associated** with systemic conditions.
- **Complicated** syndactyly may be associated with a syndrome.
  - **Poland's syndrome** (syndactyly, chest wall abnormalities) may be associated with symbrachydactyly (short fingers, syndactyly, hand hypoplasia).
  - **Apert syndrome** (craniosynostosis, complex syndactyly) is autosomal dominant and requires team-based approach, including craniofacial surgeons.

## Anatomy

- Cleland's and Grayson's ligaments thickened and coalesced
- Web space volar fascia extensive and thick
- Possibly stiff joints
- **Simple (cutaneous) form**
  - Ligaments usually normal
  - Duplicated sheaths, tendons, nerves, vessels
- **In complex and complicated forms**
  - Various fusion levels
  - Fingernail synechia
  - Abnormal tendons (especially in Apert syndrome)

## Clinical Presentation

- **Types**
  - **Simple:** No bony fusion
  - **Complex:** Presence of bony fusion
  - **Complicated:** In the presence of a syndrome
  - **Incomplete:** Web recessed to some degree
  - **Complete:** Syndactyly to fingertips
  - **Acrosyndactyly:** Associated with constriction bands
  - **Acrocephalosyndactyly** (Apert syndrome): Limb abnormalities with craniosynostosis

## Imaging

- **Radiographs are critical** for evaluating bony involvement and transverse bars (bony segments) or more complicated proximal joint and bony abnormalities.
- False-positive and false-negative results possible because of incomplete ossification
- **Arteriography** may be helpful in complex cases (e.g., Apert syndrome, multiple syndactyly) that will require multiple surgeries.

## Treatment

- **Timing**
  - Up to 40 different surgical techniques available
  - **Early** operative intervention at 4-6 months warranted for **border digits** (to prevent angular growth and deviation of the longer digit) or when **complex** (e.g., Apert syndrome with transverse bony components that will widen and worsen the deformity)
  - **Most commonly:** Assurance and waiting until hand is larger (6-12 months) best treatment choice

- **Simple syndactyly**
  - Most techniques use dorsal skin to lay into future proximal web space and limit skin grafting.
  - **Avoid scars and skin grafts in web space.**
    - Incisions in web space can lead to "web creep" postoperatively.
  - Use interdigitated ulnar and radial-based mirror image Z-flaps[9] (Fig. 61-1).
  - Make flaps large and simple.
  - Preserve paratenon.
  - Identify neurovascular bundles proximally and volarly first.
    - There may be a nonduplicated vascular supply.

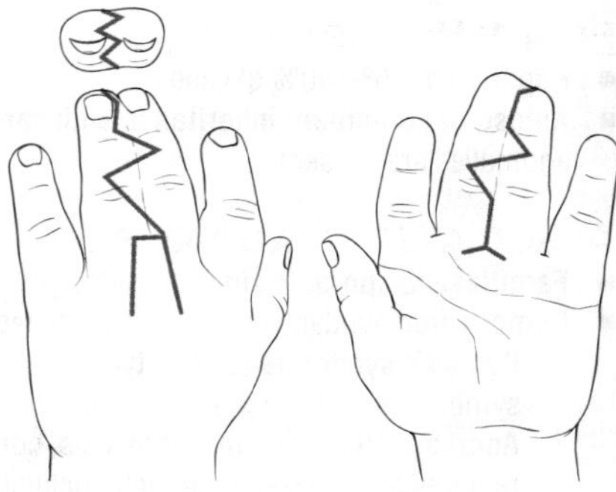

**Fig. 61-1** Incision markings for correction of syndactyly.

> **TIP:** Because vascular supply is uncertain, only operate on one side of a digit during a single surgery (e.g., syndactyly small/ring/long will require two surgeries to correct).

    - Digital artery bifurcation level is the **limit of proximal separation.**
    - Turn down tourniquet at least once to evaluate blood flow after separation of digits.
  - Controversy exists over the use of skin grafts.
    - **Skin graft technique**
      - Use full-thickness skin grafts with precisely templated designs.
      - Bolster skin grafts with nonadherent dressing and gauze.
      - Sutured bolsters are generally not required. If desired, consider Steri-Strips.
    - **No-graft technique**
      - Dorsal metacarpal artery flap to provide skin for commissure
      - Judicious debulking of the digit
      - Incomplete closure
  - Tip reconstruction
    - Hentz "pulp-plasty" with composite graft[2] (Fig. 61-2)
    - Buck-Gramcko "stiletto flap" to optimize tip fullness and contour[2]
  - **Long-arm cast** placement that *covers fingertips* prevents operative failure resulting from infection and early mobility.
- **Complex syndactyly**
  - Use technique similar to that described previously.
  - Divide bony elements while preserving joints when possible.
  - Preserve extensor and flexor tendon slips to each separated digit.
  - Plan on case-by-case basis, because presentation is quite variable.

**NOTE: The plan may change intraoperatively depending on findings.**

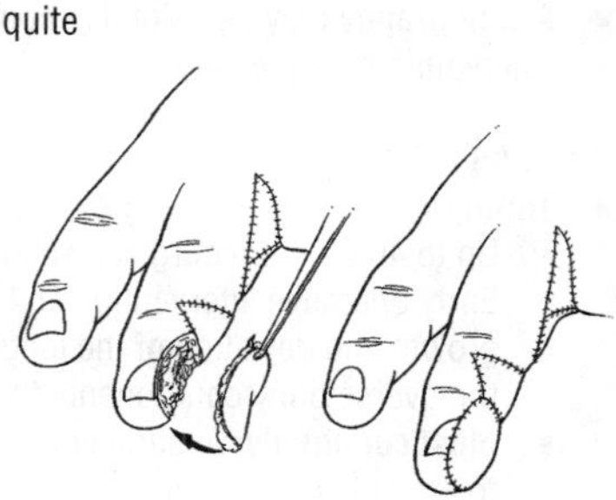

**Fig. 61-2** Hentz pulp-plasty. Composite grafts for radial or ulnar pulp defects after correction of syndactyly.

## CAMPTODACTYLY[3,10]

Congenital flexion contracture of the proximal interphalangeal (PIP) joint, **classically defined as involving the little finger.**

### Etiologic Factors

- Unclear
- **Common theories**
  - Abnormal lumbrical insertions and morphology
  - Extra or abnormal flexor digitorum superficialis slips
  - Abnormal extensor or PIP capsular structures
  - Bony abnormality of the PIP joint, especially when associated with stiffness

### Incidence

- Approximately 1% of population
  - Likely an underestimate because most cases do not seek medical attention
- Bilateral in two thirds of patients
- Up to 20% can present in adolescent females.

### Family History

- Usually sporadic
- Can be inherited as autosomal dominant trait with variable expressivity and incomplete penetrance

### Associated Conditions

- Generally an **isolated condition**
- Not considered camptodactyly when part of a syndrome

### Clinical Presentation

- **Type 1:** Apparent during infancy, usually isolated to small finger
- **Type 2:** Develops during preadolescence, more commonly in females; may progress rapidly during growth
- **Type 3:** Severe, involves multiple digits, and is part of a syndrome (most commonly arthrogryposis)
- Abnormal flexion posture of PIP joint (commonly little finger) that may be reducible versus irreducible; **painless without swelling**
- If actively reducible while stabilizing metacarpophalangeal (MP) joint, problem is MP joint instability
- Differentiate from arthrogryposis (multiple joint involvement, waxy skin, ulnar deviation), symphalangism (no active or passive motion, *absent skin creases*), boutonniere deformity (history of trauma, joint swelling, DIP hyperextension)
- Pain on extension (passive) may imply abnormal musculature (lumbrical).
- If associated brachydactyly and very stiff PIP joint without flexion-extension creases, then consider *symphalangism* (failure of joint formation)

> **TIP:** Always note the exact degrees of flexion contraction and passive/active correction that are possible.

## Imaging

- **True lateral radiograph of PIP joint is essential.**
  - Sometimes a bony synostosis is present.
- Dorsal ridge of proximal phalanx at PIP joint is often chiseled (flattened).
  - Flattened dorsal phalanx is often irreversible after correction.

## Treatment[2]

- ***Nonsurgical care is the mainstay.***
- Surgery very difficult with unpredictable outcome
- Complete correction never achieved
- **Nonoperative treatment**
  - When contracture is <30 degrees, activity is not inhibited and surgery rarely indicated
  - Splinting (dynamic versus static)
    - If correction achieved, repeat splinting may be necessary throughout growth during spurts
  - Stretching exercises
- **Operative treatment**
  - Surgery has **high failure rate** and is reserved for failure of conservative treatments.
  - Operation is usually required when **contracture is >60 to 90 degrees.**
  - Severe contraction (>90 degrees) may require early surgery because splint fitting is difficult.
  - **Technique**
    - Stepwise evaluation, including volar skin, tightness of FDS, and laxity of central slip
    - Surgical plan addressing each of these components
    - After release, soft tissue defect covered with either a midlateral, proximally based triangular rotation flap or a full-thickness skin graft
    - PIP joint maintained in position by K-wires

> **TIP:** Similar to an open capsular contracture release, perform a minimalist, stepwise release of tethering structures until satisfactory correction is achieved.

# CLINODACTYLY[2-5]

Curvature of the finger in radial/ulnar direction (<10 degrees may be considered a normal variant)

## Etiologic Factors

- Curvature usually results from abnormal middle phalanx.
- Physis may be "C-shaped" (bracketed) around one corner of phalangeal base.
- Phalanx may be triangular or trapezoidal in shape.
- *Delta phalanx* is the name for the triangular shape of the bony wedge (Fig. 61-3).
  - Bracket and abnormal shape prevent proper longitudinal growth.

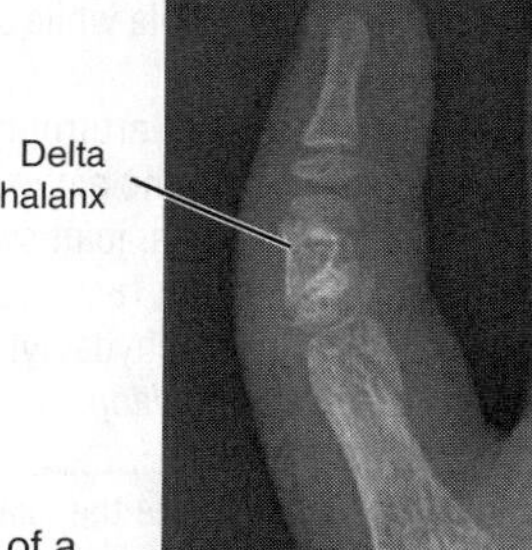


**Fig. 61-3** Radiograph of a delta phalanx.

## Incidence

- 1%-19.5%

## Family History

- Congenital ulnar angulation of small finger can be inherited in **autosomal dominant fashion with variable expression.**

### Associated Conditions

- In isolation, generally does not suggest syndromic conditions, especially familial clinodactyly

### Clinical Presentation

- Digit (commonly little finger) is abnormally angled in the radioulnar plane.
- Pain should not be a prevalent feature.
- Function is rarely limited.
- Most common site is **middle phalanx of small finger.**

### Imaging

- Plain radiographs in at least two views are necessary to evaluate growth plates and bony anomalies (e.g., presence of delta or bracketed phalanx).

### Treatment

- **Splinting is useless.**
- **Indications**
  - Most patients will present for aesthetic rather than functional reasons. *Avoid surgery in these patients, because scarring may limit function.*
  - Surgical correction is indicated for severe clinodactyly with shortening and angulation, particularly for radial digits where pinch is impaired.
  - Delta phalanx is present.
- Always use K-wires to hold corrections in place.
- **Physiolysis**
  - Bracket resection of longitudinal physis with preservation of growth plate and fat graft
  - Works well when true delta phalanx is resected
  - Can be performed when child is 3-4 years old
- **Osteotomy**
  - Closing, opening, or reverse wedge
  - Indicated when trapezoidal phalanx is present
  - May wait until skeletal maturity

> **TIP:** Any skin deficiencies after correction may require Z-plasty.

## POLYDACTYLY[3,4,11]

More than five digits on one hand

### Etiologic Factors

- Genetic disorder in *HOX* gene may be responsible
- Disruption of the AER or ZPA signaling pathways

### Incidence[4]

- **Very common deformity**
- True incidence skewed by "amputation" of extra digits in newborn nurseries
- Individuals of African descent: 1:300 (ulnar polydactyly)
- Whites: 1:3000

## Family History

- Usually sporadic
- May have strong inheritance pattern of dominant gene with variable penetrance, especially in those of African descent

## Ulnar-Sided Polydactyly (Postaxial)

Duplication of little finger

- More common in **those of African descent**
- **General classification** (used for ulnar-sided polydactyly)[5]
  - **Type A:** Supernumerary digit is well developed.
  - **Type B:** Digit is rudimentary and pedunculated.
- **Treatment**
  - Ligate when narrow stalk is present. This may be done in the nursery with clips or suture.
  - Allow autoamputation while cast is worn over several weeks.
  - Type A requires operative separation with transfer of important parts (ulnar collateral ligament, abductor digit quinti) to adjacent finger.

## Radial Polydactyly (Preaxial)

- More common in **whites**
- **Variations:** Soft tissue narrow stalk or bony elements with remnants or whole tendons, ligaments, and neurovascular tissue
- Surgical reconstruction more complicated (see below)

## Associated Conditions

- Type B postaxial polydactyly rarely has associated conditions.
- **Type A** postaxial polydactyly has up to **29% syndromic association,** which warrants workup.
- Postaxial polydactyly in whites is uncommon and may suggest underlying syndrome (e.g., chondroectodermal dysplasia or Ellis-van Creveld syndrome).
- Preaxial (thumb) duplication may be associated with systemic conditions and warrants workup.

## Imaging

- Radiographic evaluation probably not necessary in ulnar polydactyly but helpful and required in radial polydactyly
- Can be misleading because ossification not complete

## Wassel Classification of Thumb Duplication (Fig. 61-4)[9]

- **Type I is** least common: 2%.[1]
- **Type IV** is most common: 43%.[1]
- **Type VII** is most complex and requires at least one triphalangeal thumb.

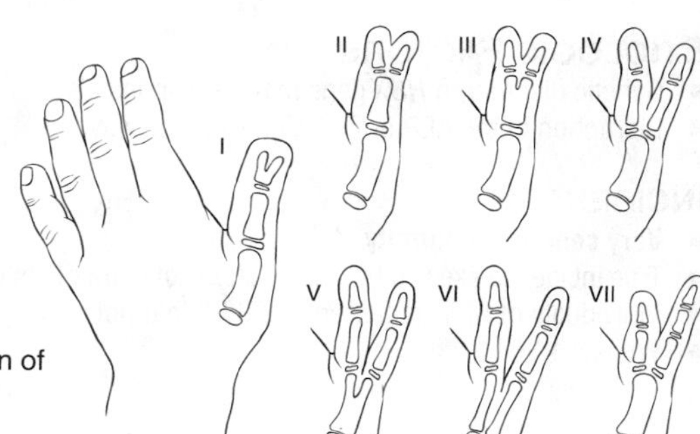


**Fig. 61-4** Wassel classification of thumb polydactyly.

- Zuidam classification[4] modifies the Wassel (which does not include more complex deformities).
  - **Type is still described by level of duplication, with modifier to describe the extra digit.**
    - **Type T: Triplication** in which three digits articulate with trapezium
    - **Type Tph: Triphalangism** in which one of the digits is triphalangeal
    - **Type H radial** or **Type IV H ulnar: Hypoplastic** extra digit radially or ulnarly, respectively
    - **Type D: Deviation** characterized by significant angulation at interphalangeal (IP) joint
  - **Type S: Symphalangism** or osseous union between two bones
  - Example: "Type IV H r" to describe a thumb with single metacarpal, ulnar thumb with two phalanges, radial thumb hypoplastic with a single phalanx

## TREATMENT

- **General guidelines**
  - Floating thumb with narrow stalk: Simple ligation
  - All others except floating thumb: Wait until 6-18 months of age
  - Preserve epiphyseal plates
  - In general, **ulnar thumb preserved to save the ulnar collateral ligament (UCL),** which provides MP joint stability for pinch
- **Wassel types I and II**
  - If each duplication is symmetrical and of equal size, **Bilhaut-Cloquet procedure** may be used with or without modifications[9] (Fig. 61-5).
    - This technique has largely fallen out of favor because of technical difficulty and poorer outcomes.
    - Nail ridging, stiffness, and joint arrest may be a problem with this technique. Consider modification by preserving most of one thumb (including physis, joint, and nail) and combining it with soft tissue of other thumb.
  - Close nail plate and repair as meticulously as possible.
  - Preserve pulp margins.

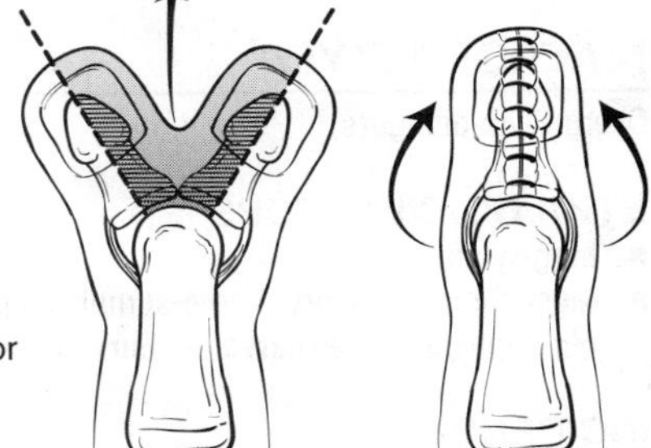

**Fig. 61-5** Bilhaut-Cloquet procedure for symmetrical distal polydactyly.

- **Wassel type III**
  - If duplication is bifid, Bilhaut-Cloquet procedure can be performed; otherwise, delete smaller thumb.
- **Wassel type IV**
  - Incise around base of sacrificed thumb with proximal and distal extensions (as Z's if necessary).
  - Shell out radial thumb (the one usually excised) sharply, preserving parts (tendon, ligament) as they are encountered and skin for closure.
  - Protect neurovascular bundle of retained thumb.

- Centralize digit on phalanx. Reduce metacarpal condyle if it is markedly wide[2] (Fig. 61-6).
- Pin from thumb tip through phalanges and metacarpal into the carpus with K-wire to maintain reduction.

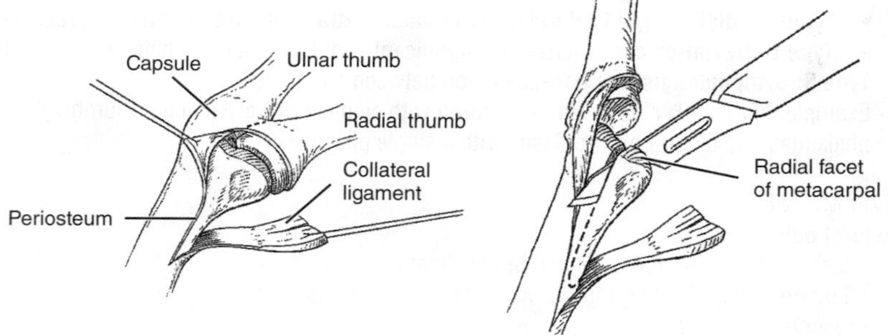


**Fig. 61-6** Correction of thumb polydactyly.

- Reconstruct collateral ligaments by preserving insertions or reattaching to remaining thumb.
- Reposition eccentric extensor and flexor tendons. Consider supplementing remaining thumb with tendons from sacrificed side.
- Identify and reattach/preserve abductor pollicis brevis.

■ **Wassel type V and VI**
- Reconstruct basal joint and metacarpals with osteotomy.

## MACRODACTYLY[4]

Overgrowth of digit(s)

### Etiologic Factors

- Largely unknown
- Most common theory: Nerve-stimulated pathology with abnormal neural control in distribution of peripheral nerve **(nerve territory–oriented macrodactyly)**

### Incidence

- Uncommon, <1% of all upper extremity anomalies

### Family History

- Usually sporadic

### Classification

- Four types described by Upton[12]
  - **Type I: Macrodactyly with lipofibromatosis of nerve**
    - Enlarged portion in specific nerve (median) distribution
    - Static subtype
      - Born with large digit(s); enlarge proportionately with age
    - **Progressive subtype**
      - Near-normal at birth; by age 3, enlarge disproportionately

- **Type II:** Associated with **neurofibromatosis** (von Recklinghausen's disease)
- **Type III: Macrodactyly with hyperostosis**—very rare
- **Type IV: Macrodactyly with hemihypertrophy**

## Associated Conditions

- Usually isolated
- Neurofibromatosis
- Klippel-Trénaunay-Weber syndrome (limb hypertrophy, hemangiomas, varicose veins)
- Limb hypertrophy
- Differential diagnosis includes tumor, vascular malformation, or lymphedema.

## Anatomy

- Skeleton is enlarged with advanced bone age, compared with normal digits.
- Soft tissue is diffusely enlarged.
- Osteoarthritic changes may present early.
- One of the digital arteries is often enlarged.
- Fatty infiltration of digital nerves is common, with significant enlargement.
- Thickened flexor sheath may cause triggering.

## Clinical Presentation

- Enlarged digits often have angular deformity, with radial deviation of radial digits and ulnar deviation of ulnar digits.
- Nerve hypertrophy may cause compression neuropathy.
- Though osseous growth ends at maturity, soft tissue enlargement may continue throughout adulthood.
- Approximately 10% are also associated with syndactyly.
  - **Type I**
    - Index then middle finger most commonly involved
    - Multiple digits usually involved
    - Predilection of median nerve distribution
    - 90% of cases unilateral
    - Hyperextension (volar growth >dorsal growth) and clinodactyly
  - **Type II**
    - **Usual signs of neurofibromatosis**
      - Six or more café-au-lait spots, multiple nodular peripheral nerve tumors
      - Autosomal dominant
      - Skeletal abnormalities may be present (30%): Scoliosis, bowing, tibial pseudarthrosis
      - Seizures, mental retardation possible
      - Often bilateral
  - **Type III**
    - Osteochondral periarticular masses that cause significant loss of motion and finger nodularity
    - Abnormal nerves not typically present
    - Incision scars prone to hypertrophy

- **Type IV**
  - Various forms
    - Segmental gigantism (only part of limb affected)
    - Hemihypertrophy (one side of body affected), associated with neurofibromatosis or Klippel-Trénaunay-Weber
    - Crossed gigantism (regions on both sides of the body affected)
  - Typically ulnar drift and flexion contraction of MP joints
  - Enlarged thenar and hypothenar eminences
    - Adduction contracture of thumb
  - May have renal, adrenal, and brain involvement

## IMAGING

- **Comparison of plain radiographs** is required to document growth variation.
- **Arteriogram** or **MRA** may be required to rule out vascular malformations.

## TREATMENT

> **TIP:** Psychological consequences can be disastrous and school-aged ridicule may be severe, because this deformity is difficult to conceal. Social counseling and thorough family discussions are imperative.

- Repeat surgery is often necessary.
- Surgery may be indicated for aesthetic or functional reasons.
- Involved digit is **never normal.**
- **Treatment goals:**
  - Control or reduce size.
  - Maintain sensibility
  - Maintain useful motion, especially of thumb joints
- **Common procedures:**
  - **Nerve decompression** if compression develops because of nerve enlargement
  - Limitation of growth
    - **Epiphysiodesis** (growth plate ablation) is effective to stop longitudinal growth. It is performed when digit is as long as the same digit in parent and can be combined with corrective osteotomy for deformity.
    - **Digital nerve stripping, digital artery ligation, compression bandaging** are less reliable methods.
  - **Skin and subcutaneous tissue resection** may decrease bulk.
  - **Wedge osteotomies** correct angular deformity.
  - Various bony shortening procedures exist, including multiple osteotomies, distal phalanx resection, and arthrodesis.
  - **Amputation**
    - Ray amputation for border digit
    - Transmetacarpal amputation of central digit with adjacent-digit transposition

> **TIP:** Amputation is a **very reasonable option** for many digits and should be discussed early with the family, especially for grotesque or functionally limiting cases. Most described procedures are unsatisfactory and continue to create deformities requiring additional surgery.

## RADIAL LONGITUDINAL DEFICIENCY[5,7,13-15]

Loss of the radial structures of the arm

### Background Factors

- Variously involves radial half of upper limb
- May be associated with a hypoplastic or absent radius, thumb hypoplasia
- **Essential to evaluation for other anomalies**
  - **Holt-Oram syndrome:** Autosomal dominant, septal defects, tetralogy of Fallot, mitral valve prolapse, PDA
  - **VACTERL: V**ertebral, **a**nal, **c**ardiac, **t**racheo**e**sophageal fistula, **r**enal, **r**adial, and **l**ower extremity abnormalities
  - **Blood dyscrasias**
    - **TAR: T**hrombocytopenia **a**bsent **r**adius syndrome
    - **Fanconi anemia:** Autosomal dominant, poor long-term prognosis. Early detection may allow life-saving bone marrow transplant.
- **Ulnar longitudinal deficiency** is much less common than radial deficiency.
  - Not associated with systemic conditions, does not require extensive workup
  - May include radial-sided hand abnormalities, including narrow web space or absent thumb
  - Based on ulna hypoplasia (may be difficult to distinguish from radial longitudinal deficiency)

> **TIP:** All patients with radial longitudinal deficiency should receive cardiac auscultation, echocardiography, renal ultrasound, CBC with differential, and a careful follow-up by the child's pediatrician.

### Etiologic Factors

- Disruption of axis formation or differentiation
- Mutations of FGF, SHH, or other signaling

### Classification[5]

- **Type N:** Thumb absence or hypoplasia
- **Type 0:** Thumb absence or hypoplasia, plus carpal absence, hypoplasia, or coalition, proximal radial synostosis or radial head dislocation
- **Type 1:** Type 0 plus radial shortening $>$2 mm shorter than ulna
- **Type 2:** Type 0 plus distal radius and proximal radius hypoplasia
- **Type 3:** Type 0 plus absent distal radial physis and proximal radius hypoplasia
- **Type 4:** Type 0 plus absent radius

### Anatomy

- Various small to absent intrinsic and extrinsic tendons/muscles, aberrant bony anatomy, joint instability or absence
- *Caveat:* Look for **pollex abductus,** which is an abnormal insertion of the flexor pollicis longus into the extensor mechanism.
  - Causes abduction on thumb flexion
  - May also be present in radial polydactyly

### Imaging

- Radiographs of the affected extremity, as well as additional testing for syndromic conditions

### TREATMENT

- Various, complex, and individualized depending on exact nature of deficiency (see Thumb Hypoplasia below)

## THUMB HYPOPLASIA[3,11]

A subset of radial longitudinal deficiency

### CLASSIFICATION

- Modified Blauth classification, by Manske and McCaroll[16]
  - **Type 1:** Diminution of thenar muscle bulk, smaller thumb elements
  - **Type 2:** Absence of thenar intrinsic muscles, plus lessened thumb-index web space, MP joint instability from UCL
  - **Type 3A:** Type 2 with extrinsic muscle abnormalities, even less bony (metacarpal) element; **stable** carpometacarpal (CMC) joint
  - **Type 3B:** Type 3A, with **unstable** CMC joint
  - **Type 4:** Floating thumb *(pouce flottant):* Small pedicle holding floating thumb
  - **Type 5:** Completely absent thumb

### IMAGING

- Multiview plain radiographs required to assess the joints (especially CMC and MP joints)

### TREATMENT

**TIP:** The decision to perform a pollicization is based on **CMC joint presence and integrity.**

- Thumb is reconstructed, addressing all components.
- **A normal-sized thumb with normal range of motion should never be expected or promised to the family.**
- More severe dysplasia or lack of elements will produce less pinch strength, thumb stability, and flexibility.
- Distinguishing type 3A from 3B can be difficult.
  - Routine use of thumb by the child during pinch and grasp signifies a stable 3A CMC joint.
  - A type 3B thumb will be ignored during use.
- **Type 1**
  - Often requires no treatment
  - Thumb augmentation/lengthening
- **Types 2-3A**
  - Thumb-index web space deepening with a four-flap Z-plasty (Fig. 61-7)[2,4,9]
  - Opponensplasty with ring-finger FDS

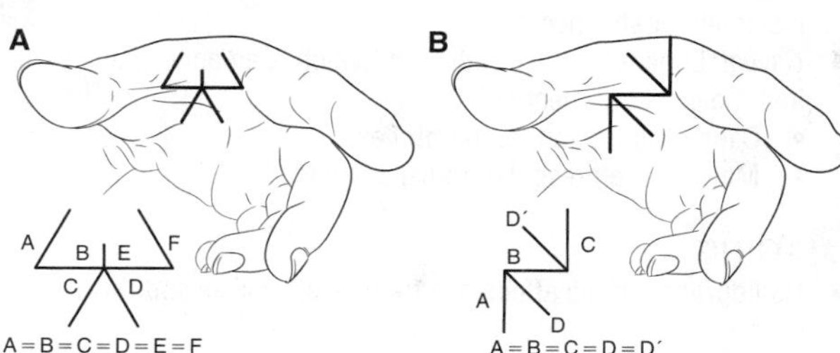


**Fig. 61-7** Thumb-index web space deepening with **A,** double opposing Z or **B,** four-flap reconstruction.

- UCL stabilization
- Use of abductor digiti quinti transfer (Huber) or EPL if FDS not available
- **Types 3B, 4, and 5**
  - Hypoplastic thumb is removed, followed by pollicization of index finger.
  - Mobility of index finger is assessed before decision to perform pollicization.
  - Microsurgical joint transfer to restore CMC has poorer results.

**TIP:** If the child does not bring the index finger into play or move it during the examination, he or she is not likely to move it as a new thumb after pollicization. However, it may still function as post for grasp.

## CENTRAL LONGITUDINAL DEFICIENCY (CLEFT HAND)[4,5,12,17]

*Functional triumph, but a social disaster.* – A. Flatt, MD

### Etiologic Factors

- Multifactorial, generally resulting in abnormalities of the AER

### Family History

- May be autosomal dominant and associated with a variety of syndromes

### Associated Conditions

- Split-hand, split-foot syndrome
- EEC (**e**ctodactyly, **e**ctodermal dysplasia, and **c**left lip/palate)
- Cornelia de Lange syndrome

### Anatomy

- Absent or deficient central digits
- Variable deficiency of the first web space
- Syndactyly of ring and small finger

### Clinical Presentation

- Patients rapidly develop adaptations for excellent function, even without corrective surgery.
- Characteristic deformity varies from generation to generation.
- It is often bilateral and associated with foot deformity.
- Phalanges may have bracketed epiphyses or double phalanges.
- Metacarpals may be absent, bifid, or duplicated.
- **Typical cleft hand:** Bilateral and familial. Syndactyly common. May be associated with cleft lip or palate
- **Atypical cleft hand:** Unilateral and spontaneous. Syndactyly rare. Associated with Poland's syndrome (chest wall abnormalities). Remaining digits may be markedly hypoplastic.
- Classification and treatment are largely based on the degree of first web space deficiency (Manske).[4]
  - **Type 1:** Normal first web space
  - **Type 2a:** Mildly narrowed web
  - **Type 2b:** Severely narrowed web
  - **Type 3:** Thumb/index syndactyly
  - **Type 4:** Index ray suppressed, thumb web space merged with cleft
  - **Type 5:** Thumb elements suppressed

### Imaging

- Radiographs are necessary to define osseous anatomy.

### Treatment

- Many patients will have excellent function despite aesthetic nature.
- Decisions for surgery require input from family.
- **Indications**
  - Progressive deformity (caused by deforming syndactyly or transverse bones)
  - Deficient first web space
  - Aesthetic appearance
  - Absent thumb
  - Involved feet perform well despite appearance and rarely require surgery.
- **Timing**
  - Early surgery may be indicated for transverse bones and syndactyly between digits of unequal length.
  - Remaining surgeries are performed at 1-2 years of age.
  - Syndactyly release
  - First web space deepening
  - Ulnar transposition of the index finger to the middle metacarpal
  - Closure of the commissure
  - Thumb realignment

## CONGENITAL BAND SYNDROME (STREETER'S SYNDROME)[4]

### Classification by Patterson[18]

- **Type I:** Simple constriction ring
- **Type II:** Constriction ring with deformity of distal part
- **Type III:** Constriction with variable fusion of distal parts (acrosyndactyly)
- **Type IV:** Complete intrauterine disruption

### Etiologic Factors

- **Two main theories**
  - **Internal (intrinsic) theory** (Streeter): Largely out of favor
    - Internal defect in embryo with possible genetic or sporadic etiologic factors
  - **Amniotic band (extrinsic) theory:**
    - Amniotic band may compress or encircle extremity or distal segment, causing local compression that heals and results in cleft.
    - Carter et al[2] theorized that swallowing of amniotic band may explain associated cleft lips, palates.
- **Clinical presentation**
  - **Check prenatal history**
    - Oligohydramnios, premature contractions, ruptures
    - Three-dimensional ultrasonography may improve intrauterine diagnosis.
  - Distal segment of extremity may present as **venous** and **edematous** (blue, purple, possibly weeping).
    - Initially observe most cases, even if edematous, as long as there is no vascular embarrassment distally. If necessary perform hemi–Z release (50% of constriction).
    - Early correction is often suboptimal, because Z-flaps are small and amount of correction is minimal with poor cosmetic result.

- Often confused with symbrachydactyly (distal "nubbins")
- May manifest as **acrosyndactyly**
  - Distal syndactyly with proximal separation or sinus
  - Reconstruction depends on available parts for transfer
  - May have fistulas and clefts or sinus tracts distal to web

### IMAGING

- Plain radiographs help evaluate any underlying bony abnormality and depth of soft tissue involved.

### TREATMENT

- Structures proximal to the constriction band will be **normal.**
- Impending amputations are rarely salvageable (dried necrotic segment in newborn).
- Release may improve neurologic compromise.
- Puffy digits that show no circulatory compromise can be watched.
- **Reconstruction**
  - Best to wait until extremity is larger (2-3 years) so that larger, more effective flaps can be used
  - Must excise full thickness of abnormal, scarred ring basin
    - Subcutaneous release in addition to skin is critical
  - **Upton and Tan method**[19]
    - Reverse (mirror) Z-flap of subcutaneous tissue from Z-flaps on skin layer and close as two layers
    - Not feasible for fingers
  - Staging not always necessary (may do circumferential)
  - **Procedures for acrosyndactyly**
    - Multiple surgeries may be necessary.
    - Early but minimal surgery to treat tethered border digits
    - Thumb web deepening (four-flap Z-plasty)
    - Release of skin bridges
    - Delayed, staged reconstruction of complete deformity

## TRIGGER THUMB[8,11]

### BACKGROUND

- ***Not a true congenital deformity; not in any classification scheme***
- Develops within first 2 years of life, **not present at birth**
- Bilateral in 25% of cases
- Thickening of FPL tendon *(Notta's node),* which catches on first annular pulley
- Congenital triggering of nonthumb fingers possibly caused by abnormal early FDS decussation

### CLINICAL PRESENTATION

- Thumb IP joint fixed in flexion and rest of thumb normal
- Occasionally presents as intermittent painful catching
- *Notta's node* palpable as moving with tendon at MP joint level
- Often discovered by parents when thumb fixed in flexion

### IMAGING

- Not necessary unless trauma suspected

### TREATMENT

- Conservative splinting and steroid injections are not very useful (different from adult trigger fingers).
- Approximately half of patients will resolve in 6 months with conservative treatment, including stretching.
- Easiest and most effective treatment is complete release of A1 pulley of thumb in controlled operating room environment.
    - Decision to go directly to surgery is controversial. Allow family to make informed decision.
    - Preserve as much pulley as possible after ranging tendon excursion in operating room.
- Congenital trigger finger may require release of abnormal tendon insertion in addition to A1 pulley.
- Cast with thumb tip exposed and in abduction-extension for minimal time, and allow early motion to prevent tendinous adhesions.

## KIRNER'S DEFORMITY[4]

Volar-radial curvature of the distal phalanx

### ETIOLOGIC FACTORS

- Abnormality of physis of the distal phalanx
- Tethering of the distal phalanx by abnormal FDP insertion

### INCIDENCE

- 0.15%, twice as common in females

### FAMILY HISTORY

- Often sporadic. Can be inherited as autosomal dominant trait with incomplete penetrance

### ASSOCIATED CONDITIONS

- Can be seen in Cornelia de Lange syndrome, Silver's syndrome, Turner's syndrome, and Down's syndrome
- Differential diagnosis includes physeal injury from trauma, burn, or frostbite

### ANATOMY

- Distal phalanx has curved shape.
- Dorsal physeal closure is delayed.

### CLINICAL PRESENTATION

- Progressive volar-radial curvature of the distal phalanx, usually the small finger
- Familial form usually present at birth and not progressive with growth
- Sporadic form develops in adolescence.
    - Initial swelling along dorsum of distal phalanx
    - Progressive deformity
- DIP motion preserved, minimal functional impairment

### IMAGING

- Radiographs are usually diagnostic, showing deformity and demonstrating epiphyseal abnormality with lengthening of the volar lip and metaphyseal sclerosis.

## TREATMENT

- Usually corrected for aesthetic reasons
  - Consider delaying surgery until patient old enough to participate in decision-making process.
- Splint during early swelling phase
- Early
  - Serial splinting
  - Partial release of abnormal flexor tendon
  - Dorsal hemiepiphysiodesis
- Late
  - Single or multiple osteotomies

### KEY POINTS

✓ Do not assume associated syndromes have been diagnosed. Order an appropriate workup and referrals.

✓ Timing of corrective surgery is critical and should be weighed against the anesthetic risk (greater risk if younger than 6 months), severity of deformity, and the goal of completing operative treatments by the time the child is of school age, which is when peer ridicule begins.

✓ Certain conditions have many operative descriptions associated with them. This may be a clue that an optimal treatment is not yet available (e.g., macrodactyly).

✓ Always consider basic hand surgery tenets, such as adequate blood supply, sensation, preservation of function, and basic goal of achieving a functional prehensile hand (sensate thumb opposition, pinch, and grip ability).

✓ Do not interfere with skeletal growth (be wary of growth plates).

✓ Social rehabilitation and support are as important as any other form of treatment.

✓ Many of these children do very well if they are appropriately managed, and go on to lead happy, successful, and independent lives.

## REFERENCES


1. Flatt AE, ed. Care of Congenital Hand Anomalies, 2nd ed. St Louis: Quality Medical Publishing, 1994.
2. Carter P, Ezaki M, Oishi S, et al. Disorders of the upper extremity. In Herring JA, ed. Tachdjian's Pediatric Orthopedics, vol 1, 4th ed. Philadelphia: Saunders Elsevier, 2007.
3. Goldfarb CA. Congenital hand differences. J Hand Surg Am 34:1351-1356, 2009.
4. Kay SP, McCombe DB, Kozin SH. Deformities of the hand and fingers. In Wolfe SW, Hotchkiss RN, Pederson WC, et al, eds. Green's Operative Hand Surgery, vol 2, 6th ed. Philadelphia: Elsevier, 2011.
5. Kozin SH. Upper-extremity congenital anomalies. J Bone Joint Surg Am 85:1564-1576, 2003.
6. McCarroll HR. Congenital anomalies: a 25-year overview. J Hand Surg Am 25:1007-1037, 2000.
7. Oberg KC, Feenstra JM, Manske PR, et al. Developmental biology and classification of congenital anomalies of the hand and upper extremity. J Hand Surg Am 35:2066-2076, 2010.
8. Lumenta DB, Kitzinger HB, Beck H, et al. Long-term outcomes of web creep, scar quality, and function after simple syndactyly surgical treatment. J Hand Surg Am 35:1323-1329, 2010.
9. Bentz ML, Bauer BS, Zuker RM, eds. Principles and Practice of Pediatric Plastic Surgery. St Louis: Quality Medical Publishing, 2008.
10. Kozin SH, Kay SP, Griffin JR, et al. Congenital contracture. In Wolfe SW, Hotchkiss RN, Pederson WC, et al, eds. Green's Operative Hand Surgery, vol 2, 6th ed. Philadelphia: Elsevier, 2011.

11. Kozin SH. Deformities of the thumb. In Wolfe SW, Hotchkiss RN, Pederson WC, et al, eds. Green's Operative Hand Surgery, vol 2, 6th ed. Philadelphia: Elsevier, 2011.
12. Upton J. Congenital anomalies of the hand and forearm. In McCarthy JG, ed. Plastic Surgery, vol 8, 2nd ed. Philadelphia: WB Saunders, 1990.
13. Al-Qattan MM, Al-Sahabi A, Al-Arfaj N. Ulnar ray deficiency: a review of the classification systems, the clinical features in 72 cases, and related developmental biology. J Hand Surg Eur Vol 5:699-707, 2010.
14. Goldfarb CA, Wall L, Manske PR. Radial longitudinal deficiency: the incidence of associated medical and musculoskeletal conditions. J Hand Surg Am 31:1176-1182, 2006.
15. James MA, Bedmar MS. Malformations and deformities of the wrist and forearm. In Wolfe SW, Hotchkiss RN, Pederson WC, et al, eds. Green's Operative Hand Surgery, vol 2, 6th ed. Philadelphia: Elsevier, 2011.
16. Manske PR, McCaroll HR Jr. Index finger pollicization for a congenitally absent or nonfunctioning thumb. J Hand Surg Am 10:606-613, 1985.
17. Upton J, Taghinia AH. Correction of the typical cleft hand. J Hand Surg Am 35:480-485, 2010.
18. Patterson TJ. Congenital ring-constrictions. Br J Plast Surg 14:1-31, 1961.
19. Upton J, Tan C. Correction of constriction rings. J Hand Surg Am 16:947-953, 1991.

# 62. Carpal Bone Fractures

**Joshua A. Lemmon, Timmothy R. Randell, Prosper Benhaim**

Carpal bone fractures are often significant wrist injuries that occur either in isolation or in association with more global carpal soft tissue injuries (see Chapter 53).[1]

## SCAPHOID

### FRACTURE INCIDENCE (Fig. 62-1)

- **Most frequently fractured carpal bone,** accounts for **70%** of all carpal bone fractures[2]
- Occurs most commonly in young men (age 15-30 years)
- Uncommon in children; carpus primarily cartilaginous and more resilient to injury
- Fractures often more distal in children than in adults

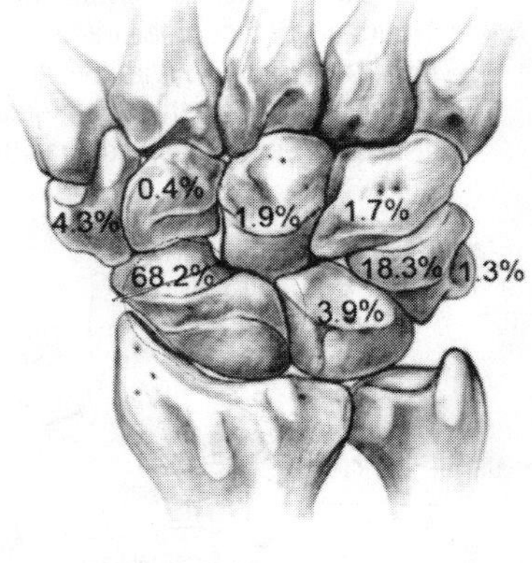

**Fig. 62-1** Relative incidence of carpal bone fractures.

### ANATOMY

- From Greek *skaphos*; has unique shape described as bean-shaped or peanut-shaped
- Surface **almost entirely articular** (80%) and covered with cartilage, *except for thin strip across dorsal waist.* Nutrient foramina are in this nonarticular region, allowing vascular supply.
- Dorsal ligamentous structures twice as strong as volar ligaments
- Only bone to bridge the proximal and distal rows of the carpus
- **Vascular supply**[3]
  - Two predominant vascular pedicles from the radial artery:
    - **Scaphoid tubercle:** Branch supplies the distal 20% of scaphoid.
    - **Dorsal ridge vessels:** Small perforating branches coming off radial artery penetrate through several foramina to supply proximal 80% of scaphoid.
  - No perforators supplying the scaphoid are found proximal to the waist, but a retrograde vascular supply is present.

> **TIP:** The unusual retrograde vascular supply limits healing of proximal scaphoid fractures and is the reason for the increased risk of avascular necrosis, delayed union, and nonunion.

## Kinematics

- Wrist kinematics are discussed in Chapter 63.
- Scaphoid and scapholunate interosseous ligament are important for coordination of proximal and distal carpal row motion.
- Unstable scaphoid fractures allow lunate and proximal scaphoid to extend while distal scaphoid continues to flex. This creates **dorsal intercalated segment instability (DISI).**
  - Creates an altered distribution of carpal loading and results in degenerative disease and progressive arthritic changes (**s**caphoid **n**onunion **a**dvanced **c**ollapse or SNAC wrist)

## Mechanisms of Injury (Fig. 62-2)

- **Two mechanisms**
  1. **Hyperextension:** With forced hyperextension to 95-100 degrees, the proximal half of the scaphoid is stabilized while the distal pole is unsupported. Load applied to the scaphoid is then concentrated at the waist (junction of supported and unsupported zones), and fracture occurs under tensile failure.[4]
  2. **Axial load (punch):** With the wrist in neutral position, an axial load is transmitted from the second metacarpal through the trapezium and trapezoid to impart volar shear force on the distal pole of the scaphoid. Fracture occurs most frequently at the waist.[5]

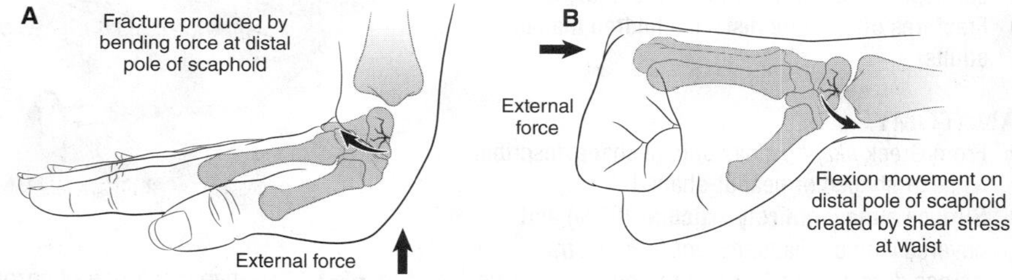


**Fig. 62-2** Mechanisms of scaphoid fracture. **A,** Hyperextension. **B,** Axial load.

## Evaluation

- **History**
  - Age
  - Sex
  - Handedness
  - Occupation
  - Mechanism of injury: Usually a fall on outstretched hand
  - Time since injury
- **Physical examination**
  - **Radial-sided wrist pain, edema, and ecchymosis:** Signs may be subtle
  - **Specific signs**
    - Tenderness in the anatomic snuffbox: Dorsal wrist between first and third dorsal compartments
    - Tenderness over the volar scaphoid tubercle and/or dorsal scaphoid with wrist in flexed position (proximal pole of scaphoid)
    - Tenderness with axial compression: Apply force axially through the first metacarpal

**TIP:** The clinical signs of scaphoid fracture are often inaccurate. Diagnosis relies mostly on high-quality radiography.

**TIP:** Isolated snuffbox tenderness is common. Most true scaphoid fractures will have either dorsal or volar tenderness as well.

## Radiographic Imaging

- **Five views of the wrist**[2]
  1. Posteroanterior (PA)
  2. Lateral
  3. Oblique
  4. Clinched fist PA: Extends scaphoid and accentuates waist fracture
  5. Scaphoid view: Fisted, semipronated, ulnar deviation

**TIP:** In a setting of high clinical suspicion, normal radiographs do not exclude a fracture. Place the hand in a thumb-spica splint, and repeat the examination and radiographic images after 14-21 days.[6]

- **Bone scan**
  - Performed when initial and repeated plain radiographs are normal, but the clinical suspicion for scaphoid fracture remains high
  - Increased Tc 99 activity seen in the fractured scaphoid
- **CT scan**
  - Obtain when plain radiographs demonstrate a nondisplaced fracture
  - Generally preferred over MRI in the nonacute setting to define bony alignment accurately (e.g., degree of displacement or angulation at fracture line)
  - Allows more detailed examination of scaphoid; reliably demonstrates when a fracture is displaced[7]
- **MRI**
  - Can detect presence or absence of acute fracture
  - Generally preferred over CT scan in acute setting, but expense often makes use impractical

## Treatment

- **Nondisplaced fractures**
  - **Nearly all nondisplaced scaphoid fractures heal well with immobilization.**
  - **Delayed treatment >4 weeks from injury increases fracture nonunion and complications.**[8]
  - Immobilize fractures in a long-arm thumb-spica cast for 6 weeks followed by 6 weeks in a short-arm thumb-spica cast.
    - ▸ Short-arm casts show a trend toward higher nonunion rates.[9]
  - Consider operative treatment with internal fixation (including percutaneous screw fixation) for high-demand patients who cannot tolerate 12 weeks of immobilization.
  - Internal fixation is also recommended for proximal pole fractures because of high rates of nonunion and avascular necrosis.[10]

- **Displaced fractures**
  - **All displaced scaphoid fractures require operative treatment.**
  - Multiple operative techniques are used and continue to evolve.
    - **Percutaneous screw fixation**[11]: Frequently used by modern surgeons
    - **Open reduction with screw fixation**
      - Solid (Herbert) or cannulated screws are placed across the fracture; these generally have a differential pitch and are designed to apply compression across the fracture site.
      - **Volar** approaches are often recommended for waist and distal fractures to preserve vascular supply to the scaphoid.
      - **Dorsal** approach allows better exposure of the proximal pole.

**TIP:** K-wires can be placed and used as "joysticks" to aid in reduction.

## COMPLICATIONS

- **Malunion**
  - **Improper reduction can lead to healing with inadequate alignment.**
  - A **humpback deformity** is the most common malunion.
    - *The distal pole of the scaphoid is flexed while the proximal pole is extended.*
    - Creates an angulated scaphoid on lateral radiographs and a foreshortened scaphoid on AP radiographs
    - Can lead to chronic pain, poor mobility, reduced grip strength, and degenerative arthritis
    - Treatment options (controversial)
      - Reoperate early.[12]
      - Perform correctional osteotomy with structural bone graft.[13]
      - Employ a conservative, nonoperative approach.[14]
- **Delayed union**
  - Occurs when symptoms persist, with no radiographic evidence of union after 4 months of adequate immobilization
  - Treatment controversial: Many treat with additional immobilization and observation, but open reduction and internal fixation (ORIF) increasingly used
- **Nonunion**
  - Trabeculation fails across the fracture site, and fracture lines become sclerotic.
  - Nonunions progress to degenerative arthritis and lead to **SNAC** wrist deformities (96% at 5 years).[15]
  - Early diagnosis and treatment of nonunions reduces development of degenerative wrist changes.[16]
  - Treatment options are controversial and vary according to anatomic location.
  - Goals are to restore alignment and promote healing.
    - Most surgeons suggest screw fixation and bone grafting of waist and distal pole nonunions, and vascularized bone grafting and screw fixation of proximal pole nonunions.[17]
    - **Vascularized graft options**
      - 1,2 Intercompartmental supraretinacular artery (1,2 ICSRA)
      - 2,3 ICSRA
      - Free medial femoral condyle vascularized graft
      - Pronator quadratus graft

## FRACTURES OF OTHER CARPAL BONES

### TRIQUETRUM[18]

- Second most commonly fractured carpal bone
- **Three fracture types:**
  1. **Dorsal cortical:** Avulsion fractures
     - Most common triquetrum fracture
     - Dorsal intercarpal ligament or lunotriquetral avulsions may pull small bony fragments off the dorsal rim.
     - Close inspection is required to detect wrist instability patterns or dislocations (see Chapter 63). Small avulsion fractures are easily missed on lateral radiographs and require careful evaluation.
     - Hyperextension and ulnar deviation can force impaction with the ulnar styloid, and a small ulnar-sided fracture of the dorsal rim occurs.
  2. **Body**
     - Isolated body fractures can occur from direct impact at the ulnar body of the hand, involving the medial tuberosity.
     - Other body fractures (sagittal, transverse, or comminuted) usually are secondary to crush injuries or part of a more complex global wrist injury.
  3. **Volar avulsion**
     - Avulsion of volar ulnar triquetral ligament and lunotriquetral interosseous ligament
- **Radiographic imaging**
  - AP
  - Lateral
  - 45-degree pronated oblique
    - The triquetrum is best viewed when the wrist is partially pronated.
  - CT scan to assess for occult fractures
- **Treatment**
  - Dorsal rim fractures usually heal with immobilization for 4 weeks in a short-arm cast or short-arm splint for minor chip avulsion fractures.
  - Displaced body fractures require ORIF, along with treatment of associated ligamentous injuries or dislocations.

### HAMATE

- **Two fracture types:**
  1. **Hamulus:** "Hook" of the hamate fractures
     - Fracture is caused most commonly by direct trauma to the hand while holding a racket, club, or bat (Fig. 62-3), also by falls on an outstretched hand.
     - Presentation includes pain and tenderness over the hamate and ulnar-sided hand edema.
     - Hook of the hamate pull test (HHPT): Wrist is supinated and ulnarly deviated. Force is then applied to the flexor tendons of the small and ring fingers, causing a displacing force on the hook of the hamate.[19]

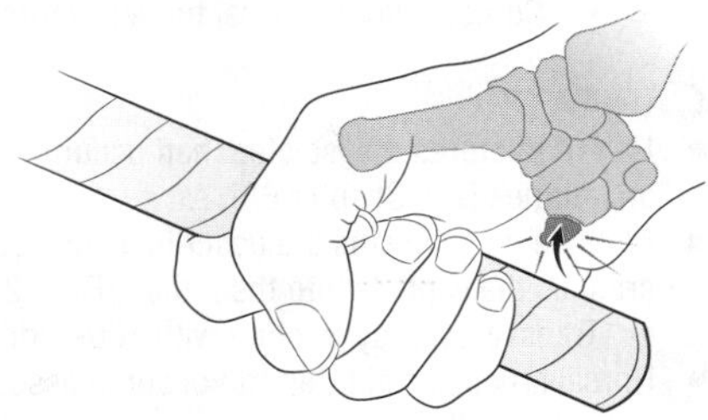

**Fig. 62-3** Typical mechanism of injury for hook of the hamate fractures.

    - A careful ulnar nerve examination is needed, especially of the deep (motor) branch, to exclude associated nerve injury.
    - Specialized radiographs (lateral, oblique, and carpal tunnel views) are needed to view the fracture.
    - CT scans are often required for adequate diagnosis.
    - Presentation of small-finger flexor tendon injuries can be delayed until pseudarthrosis and degenerative bony changes lead to attrition ruptures of the tendons.[20]
2. **Hamate body**
    - Usually represent a more complex wrist injury with axial fracture-dislocation patterns (see Chapter 63)
    - Most commonly result from a closed fist injury with axial force transmitted through fourth and fifth metacarpals
        - Hamate fractured in the coronal plane at fourth or fifth carpometacarpal (CMC) joint and dislocates dorsally

- **Treatment**
    - Nondisplaced hamulus fractures usually are treated with cast immobilization, but nonunion rate is high (>50%). Early surgical treatment yields best results.[21]
    - Treatment options for hamulus fractures include ORIF (no particular advantage) or excision of fragment (most common approach).
    - Nondisplaced hamate body fractures should be treated with cast immobilization.
    - Most hamate body fractures require ORIF because of other associated wrist injuries.

## TRAPEZIUM

- **Ridge fractures**
    - **Caused most commonly by avulsion of transverse carpal ligament**

> **TIP:** Carpal tunnel syndrome may occur in association with trapezium fractures and should be specifically excluded.

    - Fractures are thought to occur with hyperextension and abduction force to the thumb.
    - Treat with immobilization. Nonunions can result and should be treated with excision of bony fragment.
- **Body fractures**
    - Can occur when wrist is forced into extension and radial deviation, crushing the trapezium into the radial styloid
    - Also found in association with first metacarpal base fractures
    - Displaced body fractures treated with ORIF
        - Complications: Carpal tunnel syndrome, tendonitis, flexor carpi radialis rupture

## CAPITATE

- Half of fractures are isolated, half occur in association with other carpal injuries (e.g., greater arc injuries [see Chapter 63]).
- Multiple mechanisms are described, including **anvil mechanism,** whereby hyperextension crushes the capitate into the radius (Fig. 62-4).
    - Transverse body fracture with 180-degree rotation of the proximal fragment
- Dorsal articular fractures can occur in association with third metacarpal base fractures or third CMC dislocations.

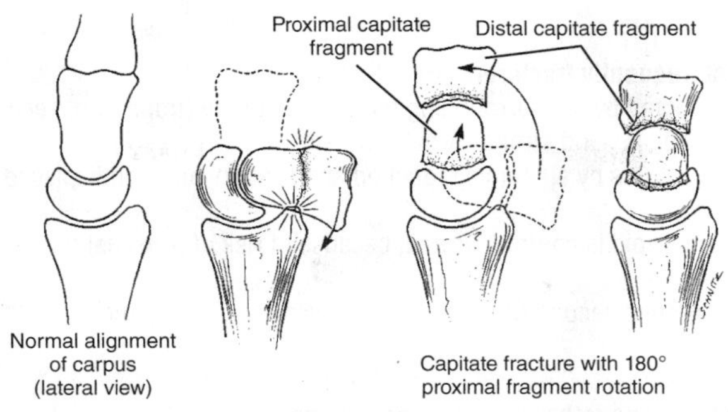


**Fig. 62-4** Anvil mechanism resulting in capitate body fracture.

- **Treatment**
  - Nondisplaced capitate fractures should be treated with cast immobilization, as long as ligamentous instability is excluded.
  - Displaced fractures can be treated with closed reduction and percutaneous pin fixation or open reduction, ligament repair, and internal fixation.

> **TIP:** Avascular necrosis of the proximal fragment is a recognized long-term sequela; therefore patients should be followed closely.

## LUNATE

- Rare fractures that usually occur in association with ligamentous injuries of the wrist
  - **Volar pole**
    - Often result from avulsion of the long and short radiolunate ligaments
    - Treat with anatomic reduction, giving attention to establishing normal ligamentous anatomy to support the midcarpal joint
  - **Dorsal pole**
    - Avulsion of the scapholunate or lunotriquetral ligaments can cause fractures, although these ligaments usually avulse off the neighboring bones rather than the lunate itself.
    - Caused by an axial load on a hyperextended and ulnarly deviated wrist.
    - Treatment should include repair of any associated ligamentous injuries.
  - **Body**
    - Fractures result from axial compression between capitate and lunate fossa on the radius.
    - CT scan is needed to assess displacement.
    - Displaced fractures require open reduction and fixation.
    - Prompt management is recommended because of risk of Kienböck's disease (avascular necrosis of lunate).
    - Nontraumatic fractures can be seen in Kienböck's disease.

**CAUTION: Lunate fractures have an increased risk of progression to Kienböck's disease.**

> **TIP:** A meticulous carpal ligamentous examination is needed when evaluating lunate fractures because of the high rate of associated injuries.

## Trapezoid

- This is the **least frequently fractured carpal bone.**
- Bone is **well-protected** by the surrounding osseous anatomy (trapezium, second metacarpal base, scaphoid, capitate, and strong carpal ligaments).
- Treat displaced fractures by anatomic reduction and fixation, and nondisplaced fractures by immobilization.[18]
- Excision of the trapezoid is contraindicated, because of risk of proximal migration of index metacarpal.
- Chronic injuries require second CMC joint arthrodesis.

## Pisiform

- This is a **sesamoid bone** rather than true carpal bone.
- It lies within the flexor carpi ulnaris tendon.
- Fractures occur as a result of direct trauma.
- Plain radiographs frequently do not demonstrate these injuries, and specific carpal tunnel view or CT scan may be necessary for diagnosis.
- **Ulnar nerve** is in close proximity; therefore *careful nerve examination is imperative.*
- **Treatment**
  - **Acute fractures** should be treated with **splint immobilization.**
  - **Chronic discomfort** and **nonunion** are best treated with **pisiform excision.**

## Key Points

✓ The scaphoid is the most commonly fractured carpal bone.
✓ The trapezoid is the least frequently fractured carpal bone.
✓ CT scans are necessary to accurately differentiate displaced and nondisplaced scaphoid fractures.
✓ Early operative treatment of nondisplaced scaphoid fractures can decrease the need for prolonged immobilization.
✓ Close follow-up is necessary for the treatment of scaphoid fractures to diagnose and treat delayed unions and nonunions.
✓ Whenever a carpal bone is fractured, median and ulnar nerve function should be carefully evaluated.
✓ Fractures of the triquetrum, hamate, lunate, and capitate often signal broader carpal injuries; precise imaging and a meticulous ligamentous examination are essential.

## References

1. Garcia-Elias M. Carpal bone fractures. In Watson HK, Weinzweig J, eds. The Wrist. Philadelphia: Lippincott Williams & Wilkins, 2001.
2. Wolfe SW. Fractures of the carpus: scaphoid fractures. In Berger RA, Weiss AP, eds. Hand Surgery. Philadelphia: Lippincott Williams & Wilkins, 2004.
3. Gelberman RH, Panagis JS, Taleisnik J, et al. The arterial anatomy of the human carpus. I. The extraosseous vascularity. J Hand Surg Am 8:367-376, 1983.
4. Weber ER, Chao EY. An experimental approach to the mechanism of scaphoid waist fractures. J Hand Surg Am 3:142-148, 1978.
5. Horii E, Nakamura R, Watanabe K, et al. Scaphoid fracture as a puncher's fracture. J Orthop Trauma 8:107-110, 1994.

6. Mittal RL, Dargan SK. Occult scaphoid fracture: a diagnostic enigma. J Orthop Trauma 3:306-308, 1989.
7. Nakamura R, Imaeda T, Horii E, et al. Analysis of scaphoid fracture displacement by three-dimensional computed tomography. J Hand Surg Am 16:485-492, 1991.
8. Langhoff O, Andersen JL. Consequences of late immobilization of scaphoid fractures. J Hand Surg Br 13:77-79, 1988.
9. Gellman H, Caputo RJ, Carter V, et al. Comparison of short and long thumb-spica casts for non-displaced fractures of the carpal scaphoid. J Bone Joint Surg Am 71:354-357, 1989.
10. Krimmer H. Management of acute fractures and non-unions of the proximal pole of the scaphoid. J Hand Surg Br 27:245-248, 2002.
11. Slade JF III, Jaskwhich D. Percutaneous fixation of scaphoid fractures. Hand Clin 17:553-574, 2001.
12. Nakamura P, Imaeda T, Miura T, et al. Scaphoid malunion. J Bone Joint Surg Br 73:134-137, 1991.
13. Lynch NM, Linscheid RL. Corrective osteotomy for scaphoid malunion: technique and long-term follow-up evaluation. J Hand Surgery 22:35-43, 1997.
14. Jiranek WA, Ruby LK, Millender LB, et al. Long-term results after Russe bone-grafting: the effect of mal-union of the scaphoid. J Bone Joint Surg Am 74:1217-1228, 1992.
15. Taleisnik J, Watson HK. Midcarpal instability caused by malunited fractures of the distal radius. J Hand Surg Am 20:57-62, 1995.
16. Reigstad O, Grimsgaard C, Thorkildsen R, et al. Scaphoid non-unions, where do they come from? The epidemiology and initial presentation of 270 scaphoid non-unions. Hand Surg 17:331-335, 2012.
17. Merrell GA, Wolfe SW, Slade JF III, et al. Treatment of scaphoid non-unions: quantitative meta-analysis of the literature. J Hand Surg Am 27:685-691, 2002.
18. Shah MA, Viegas SF. Fractures of the carpal bones excluding the scaphoid. J Am Soc Surg Hand 2:129-139, 2002.
19. Wright TW, Moser MW, Sahajpal DT. Hook of hamate pull test. J Hand Surg Am 35:1887-1889, 2010.
20. Neviaser RJ. Fractures of the hook of the hamate. J Hand Surg Am 11:207-210, 1986.
21. Scheufler O, Andresen R, Radmer S, et al. Hook of hamate fractures: critical evaluation of different therapeutic procedures. Plast Reconstr Surg 115:488-497, 2005.

# 63. Carpal Instability and Dislocations

Tarik M. Husain, Joshua A. Lemmon

## WRIST ANATOMY AND KINEMATICS[1]

The wrist is a complex joint that connects the distal forearm and the hand.

- Articulations exist between 14 bones and the pisiform.
- The pisiform is a sesamoid, providing a lever arm for the flexor carpi ulnaris tendon.
- The distal radius and ulna articulate with the two carpal rows (proximal and distal), and these articulate with the bases of the five metacarpal bones.
- The carpus is unique in that no muscles or tendons attach to any of the bones.
- *Carpal instability dissociative* (CID) is instability between bones within the same row[2] (Fig. 63-1).
- *Carpal instability nondissociative* (CIND) is instability of the entire proximal row relative to the radiocarpal or the midcarpal joint[2] (Fig. 63-2).

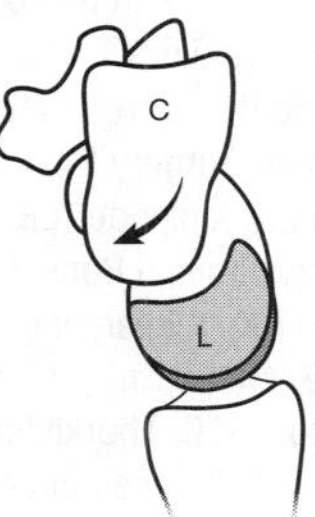


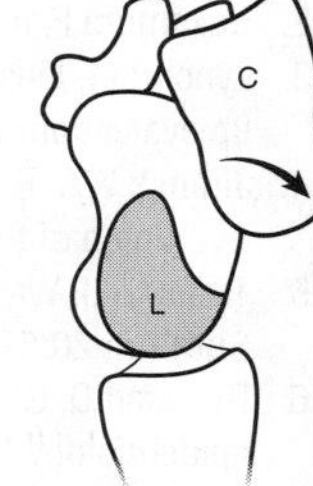


**Fig. 63-1** Carpal instability dissociative (CID).

### EIGHT CARPAL BONES[3] (Fig. 63-3)

- Arranged as a **distal** and a **proximal** carpal row
- **Proximal row**
  - Scaphoid (proximal pole)
  - Lunate
  - Triquetrum
- **Distal row**
  - Trapezium
  - Trapezoid
  - Capitate
  - Hamate
- **Pisiform**
  - **Sesamoid bone:** Lies within flexor carpi ulnaris tendon

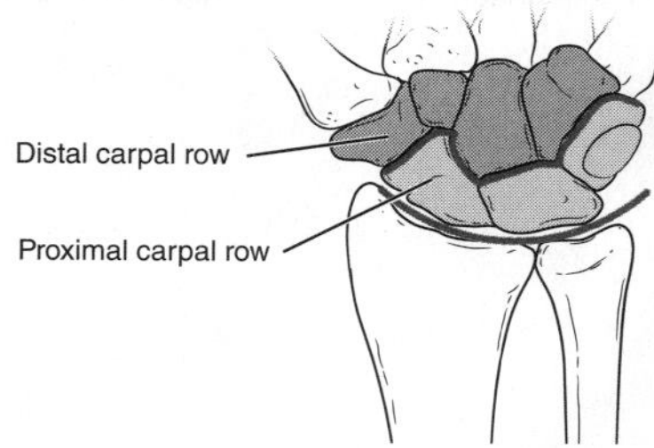


**Fig. 63-2** Carpal instability nondissociative (CIND) represents radiocarpal and/or midcarpal joint instability with **no** break between bones within either the proximal carpal or distal carpal row.

### COMPLEX LIGAMENTOUS SUPPORT SYSTEM[4] (see Fig. 63-3)

- **Extrinsic ligaments:** From radius and ulna to carpal bones
  - **Dorsal**
    - Dorsal radiocarpal (radiotriquetral) ligament
    - Radiolunate ligament
    - Dorsal radioscaphoid ligament

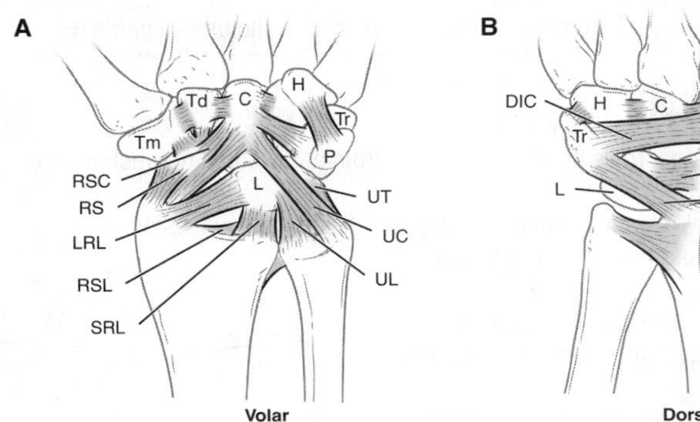


**Fig. 63-3** The ligamentous anatomy of the volar **(A)** and dorsal **(B)** wrist. (*C,* Capitate; *DIC,* dorsal intercarpal ligament; *DRL,* dorsal radiocarpal ligament; *DST,* dorsal scaphotriquetral ligament; *H,* hamate; *L,* lunate; *LRL,* long radiolunate ligament; *P,* pisiform; *RS,* radioscaphoid ligament; *RSC,* radioscaphocapitate ligament; *RSL,* radioscapholunate ligament, also known as ligament of Testut; *S,* scaphoid; *SRL,* short radiolunate ligament; *Td,* trapezoid; *Tm,* trapezium; *Tr,* triquetrum; *UC,* ulnocapitate ligament; *UL,* ulnolunate ligament; *UT,* ulnotriquetral ligament.)

- **Volar**
  - Radioscaphocapitate ligament
  - Long and short radiolunate ligaments
  - Radioscapholunate = *ligament of Testut*
  - Ulnolunate ligament
  - Ulnar collateral ligament
- **Intrinsic ligaments:** Interconnect carpal bones
  - Scapholunate interosseous ligament
  - Lunotriquetral ligament
  - Dorsal intercarpal ligament
- In general, **volar ligaments are stronger** than dorsal ligaments.

**NOTE: Berger[5] described a ligament-sparing approach to the dorsal wrist that in theory preserves wrist stability. This technique preserves the dorsal radiocarpal and dorsal intercarpal ligaments. No outcome-based studies have been conducted. The argument against it is that usually the wrist is immobilized postoperatively anyway; therefore the risk of instability is low (Fig. 63-4).**

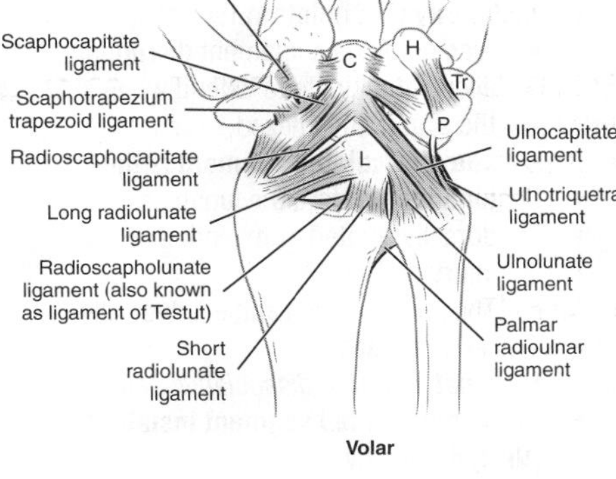


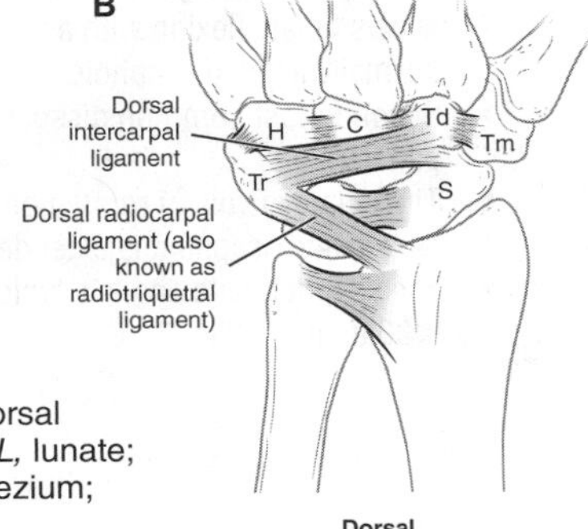


**Fig. 63-4** **A,** Volar ligaments of the wrist. **B,** Dorsal ligaments of the wrist. (*C,* Capitate; *H,* hamate; *L,* lunate; *P,* pisiform; *S,* scaphoid; *Td,* trapezoid; *Tm,* trapezium; *Tr,* triquetrum.)

**TIP:** The most frequently injured intercarpal ligament is the scapholunate ligament.

## Kinematics and Instability Patterns

- The proximal and distal carpal rows must move in a coordinated fashion to function as a stable joint.[6]
  - The proximal and distal rows move in synchrony with flexion and extension.
  - The movements are more complex during ulnar and radial deviation.
    - **Radial deviation:** The scaphoid flexes, and the lunate and triquetrum follow passively into flexion with it.
    - **Ulnar deviation:** The triquetrum is guided into extension by its articulation with the hamate, and the entire proximal row moves into extension with the triquetrum.
    - Coordinated carpal motion is possible because of the ligamentous support.
    - The normal scapholunate angle is between **30 and 60 degrees.**

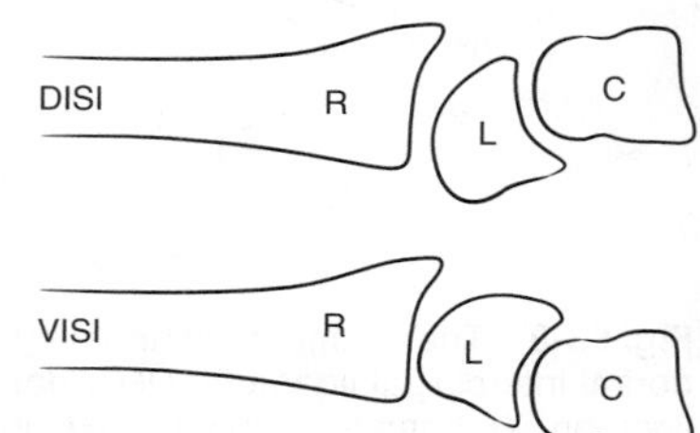


**Fig. 63-5** Dorsal intercalated segment instability *(DISI):* lunate tilts dorsally; and volar intercalated segment instability *(VISI):* lunate tilts volarly. (*C,* Capitate; *L,* lunate; *R,* radius.)

- When ligamentous support is absent, carpal motion is uncoordinated (Fig. 63-5).
  - **Dorsal intercalated segment instability (DISI) deformity**
    - A scapholunate ligament disruption allows the lunate to extend when the scaphoid is flexed.
    - **The intercalated segment is the lunate;** therefore the lunate is dorsally rotated or extended in this injury pattern.
    - The scapholunate angle is typically >60 degrees.
    - *Most common dissociative pattern*
  - **Volar intercalated segment instability (VISI) deformity**
    - A lunotriquetral ligament injury allows lunate flexion with a normally aligned scaphoid.
    - Second most common dissociative pattern
    - The lunate is volarly rotated or flexed, and scaphoid is extended.
    - The scapholunate angle is typically <30 degrees (Fig. 63-6).

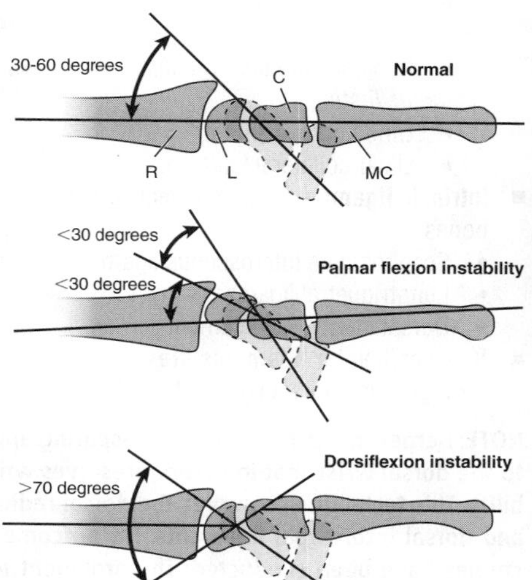


**Fig. 63-6** Scapholunate angle. (*C,* Capitate; *L,* lunate; *MC,* metacarpal; *R,* radius.)

## CARPAL INSTABILITY CLASSIFICATION (Table 63-1)

Carpal instability is characterized by loss of normal ligament and bony constraint.

- **Static versus dynamic versus predynamic**[7]
  - ***Static*** demonstrates radiographic malalignment of carpal bones.
  - ***Dynamic*** has normal radiographs, but malalignment is seen with stress as on clenched fist view.
  - ***Predynamic*** has normal radiographs and normal stress views, but scapholunate joint is mildly disrupted when the ligament is only stretched or partially ruptured. This is usually only seen arthroscopically.
- **CIND** (nondissociative): Tear of extrinsic ligament
- **CIC:** Combination of CID and CIND
- **CIA:** Carpal instability adaptive

**Table 63-1** *Analysis of Carpal Instability*

| Category I Chronicity | Category II Constancy* | Category III Etiologic Factors | Category IV Location | Category V Direction | Category VI Pattern |
|---|---|---|---|---|---|
| Acute <1 week (i.e., maximum primary healing potential) | Static† | Congenital | Radiocarpal | VISI | Carpal instability dissociative (CID) |
| Subacute 1-6 weeks (i.e., some primary healing potential) | Dynamic‡ | Traumatic | Intercarpal | DISI | Carpal instability nondissociative (CIND) |
| Chronic >6 weeks (i.e., little primary healing potential; surgical repair or reconstruction needed) | | Inflammatory | Midcarpal | Ulnar | Combinations (CIC) |
| | | Arthritis | Carpometacarpal | Radial | Carpal instability adaptive (CIA) |
| | | Neoplastic | Specific bone(s) | Ventral | |
| | | Iatrogenic | Specific ligament(s) | Dorsal | |
| | | Miscellaneous | | Proximal | |
| | | Combinations | | Distal | |
| | | | | Rotary | |
| | | | | Combinations | |

*This category also includes the concept of severity.
†Irreducible or reducible; ease of reducibility and degree of displacement may also be considered.
‡Degree of load required to cause displacement may also be considered.
*CIA,* Carpal instability adaptive; a carpal instability pattern that exists because the carpal bones have adapted to an extended deformity (e.g., a distal radius malunion); *CIC,* combination of CID and CIND (e.g., perilunate and axial injuries include both capsular [CIND] and intercarpal [CID] components.); *DISI,* dorsal intercalated segment instability; *VISI,* volar intercalated segment instability (volar flexion instability).

# LIGAMENTOUS INJURIES AND DISLOCATIONS

## Mechanism of Injury

- **Mayfield et al**[8] described the pathomechanics of progressive carpal injury.
  - Loading of the extended and ulnarly deviated wrist dissipates force through one of two arcs[3] (Fig. 63-7).
    - **Greater arc:** Injury progresses through **carpal bones.**
    - **Lesser arc:** Injury progresses only through **ligaments.**

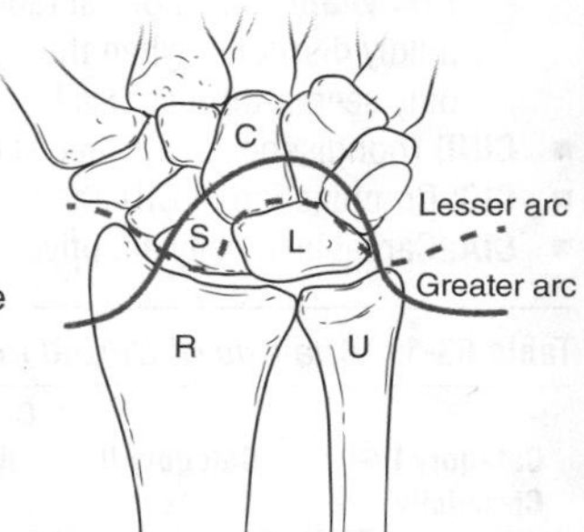


**Fig. 63-7** **Greater arc injuries** are fractures that involve the wrist's zone of vulnerability that includes the radial styloid, scaphoid, capitate, triquetrum, and the ulnar styloid. Lesser arc injuries sit within the greater arc, centered on the lunate; **lesser arc injuries** are pure ligamentous perilunate injuries. (*C,* Capitate; *L,* lunate; *R,* radius; *S,* scaphoid; *U,* ulna.)

> **TIP:** Carpal dislocations and injuries usually result from extreme hyperextension, ulnar deviation, and intercarpal supination; they can be caused by motor vehicle collisions or falls from a height.

- In this model, ligamentous injuries occur in a **stepwise progression.**
  - Scapholunate
  - Midcarpal capsule (radioscaphocapitate ligament)
  - Lunotriquetral ligament
  - Dorsal radiocarpal ligament (Fig. 63-8)

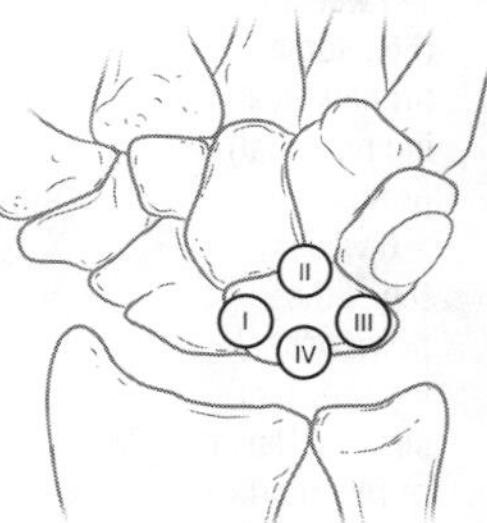


**Fig. 63-8** Stages of progressive perilunar instability. (*I,* Scapholunate failure; *II,* capitolunate failure; *III,* lunotriquetral failure; *IV,* dorsal radiocarpal ligament failure.)

## Ligamentous Injuries

- **Scapholunate (interosseous) ligament injuries**[9]
  - **Anatomy**
    - The scapholunate ligament is a C-shaped structure that connects the dorsal, proximal, and volar surfaces of the scaphoid and lunate (Fig. 63-9).
    - Several extrinsic volar ligaments lend additional support to the volar portion of this ligament.
  - **Mechanisms**
    - When an impact occurs to the hypothenar region, with the wrist in extension and ulnar deviation, the capitate is driven between the scaphoid and lunate. The lunate is pushed ulnarly and volarly; the scaphoid is pushed radially and dorsally.

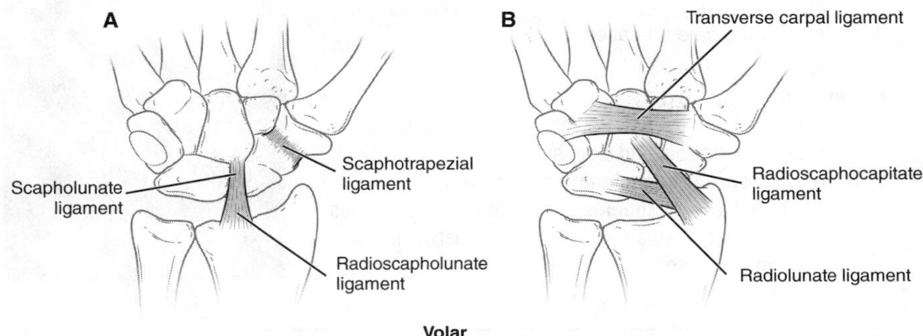


**Fig. 63-9** Intrinsic **(A)** and extrinsic **(B)** ligaments.

- The ligament will rupture given sufficient force, usually pulling away from the scaphoid and remaining attached to the lunate.
- Abnormalities also can be congenital (usually bilateral) or degenerative (e.g., arthritis).

- **History**
  - Patients have **radial-sided wrist pain and weakness,** especially with loading activities.
  - Patients usually have a history of a fall or sudden load on the wrist.
- **Physical examination**
  - Radial-sided wrist edema
  - **Tenderness in radial snuffbox** or over the scapholunate interval just distal to Lister's tubercle
  - Discomfort at extremes of wrist extension and radial deviation
  - **Positive ballottement test:** Dorsovolar stress of the scapholunate interval
  - **Positive Watson (scaphoid shift) test:** "Clunk" is felt during dynamic wrist loading. Scaphoid subluxates over dorsal rim of the radius when the wrist is moved from ulnar to radial deviation[10] (Fig. 63-10).
    - The examiner pushes on the distal pole of scaphoid in dorsal direction while ranging the wrist passively from ulnar deviation and slightly extended to radial deviation and slightly flexed.
    - In patients with an incompetent scapholunate ligament, the dorsal push on the scaphoid subluxates it out of the scaphoid fossa relative to the radius.
    - The "clunk" is the scaphoid reducing back into its anatomic position in the scaphoid fossa.

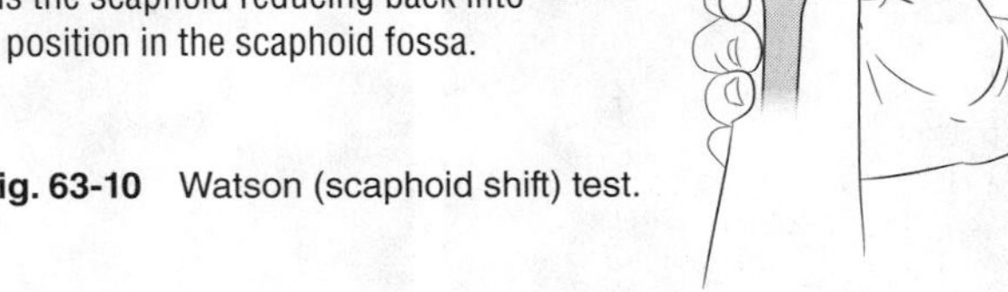

**Fig. 63-10** Watson (scaphoid shift) test.

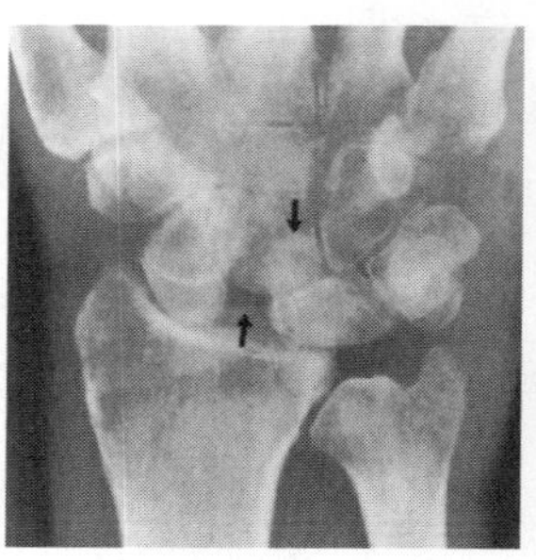

**Fig. 63-11** Scapholunate gap (Terry Thomas sign) *Arrows* indicate so-called geodes.

- **Imaging**
  - Six views of the wrist: PA, lateral, radial and ulnar deviation, flexion, and extension
    - **Increased scapholunate gap (3 mm):** Often called a **Terry Thomas sign,** referring to a famous English comedian with a large gap between his central incisors[10] (Fig. 63-11)

> **TIP:** The scapholunate gap should always be compared with the asymptomatic wrist, because up to 5 mm is considered to be within normal limits.

    - **Cortical ring sign:** Represents hyperflexed scaphoid wherein the distal pole is seen on end and appears as a cortical ring within 7 mm of the proximal pole[4] (Fig. 63-12)
    - Dorsiflexed lunate with a flexed scaphoid on lateral view: DISI deformity
    - Increased scapholunate angle

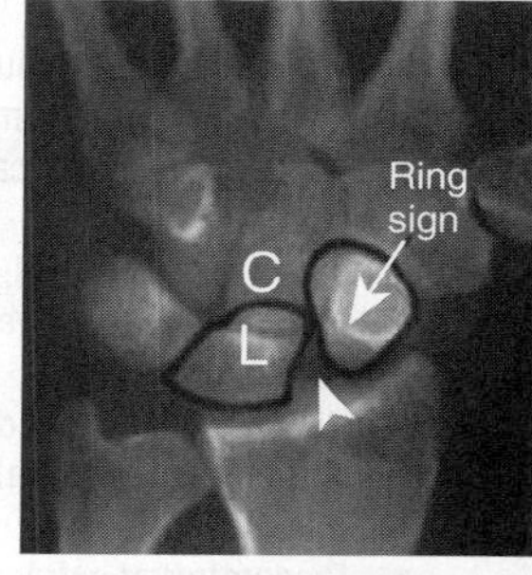


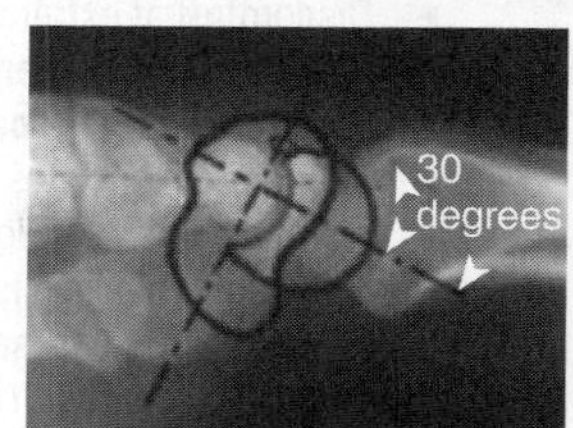


**Fig. 63-12** Cortical ring sign seen with DISI. The *arrowhead* points to an increased scapholunate gap. (*C,* Capitate; *L,* lunate.)

  - **Cineradiography or stress radiographs:** Allow detection of dynamic injuries that are thought to occur with injury to only dorsal portion of the ligament
    - Gapping of scapholunate junction seen with stress views
    - Clenched-fist view
    - Clenched-pencil view (Fig. 63-13)

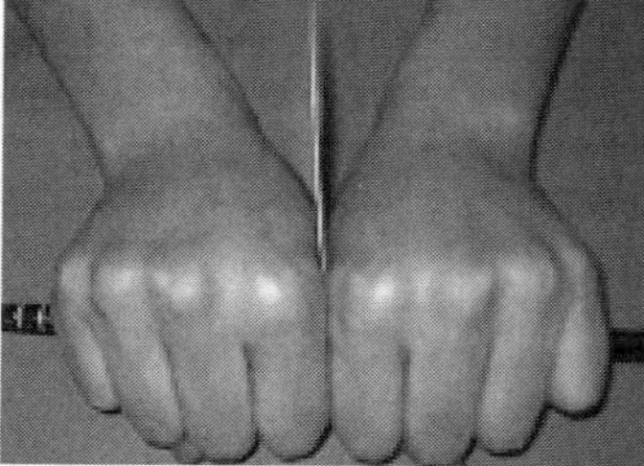

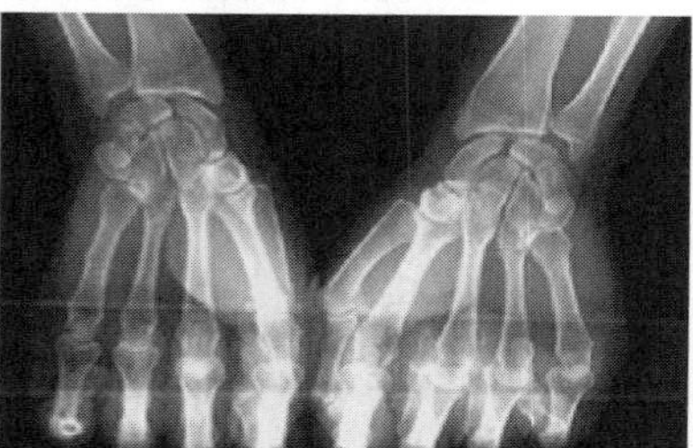

**Fig. 63-13** Clenched-pencil view.

- **Midcarpal or radiocarpal arthrography:** Used when standard radiographs are normal, which is common in subacute injuries
  - Contrast defines complete injuries, partial injuries, and other wrist pathologies.
  - Contrast passing from the radiocarpal joint to the midcarpal joint indicates a perforation in the ligament.
- **MRI**[4] (Fig. 63-14)
  - MRI with intraarticular contrast should be used to evaluate ligament tears.
- **Arthroscopy**[11] (Table 63-2)
  - **Benchmark for assessing the scapholunate ligament**
  - Aids staging the severity of the injury[11]

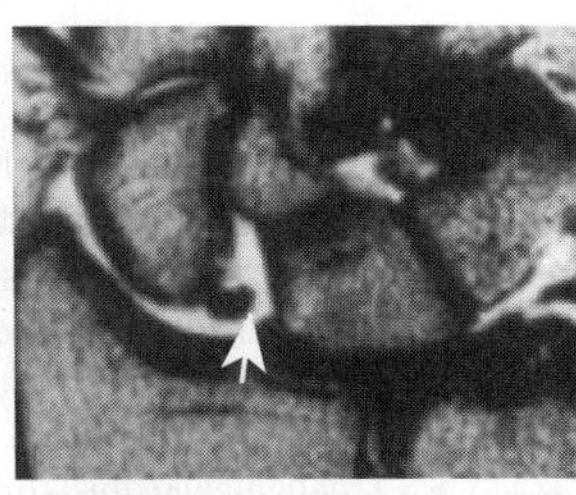

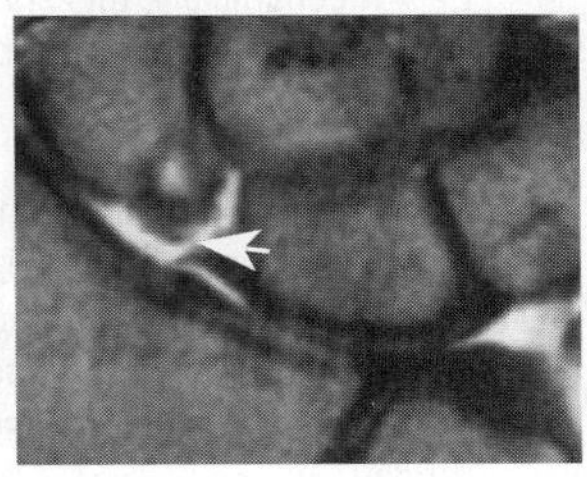

**Fig. 63-14** MRI of a scapholunate ligament tear. *Arrows* indicate the free edge of the ligament.

- **Treatment**
  - There is no consensus on the treatment of scapholunate ligament injuries.
  - Treatment options depend on the chronicity of the injury.
    - **Acute injuries:** Within **3 weeks** of injury
    - **Subacute injuries:** Within **3-6 weeks** of injury
    - **Chronic injuries:** >**6 weeks** from injury
  - Table 63-3 presents an algorithm for treatment.[9]

**Table 63-2** *Geissler Arthroscopic Grading System*

| Grade | Description |
|---|---|
| I | Attenuation/hemorrhage of SLIL (viewed from radiocarpal space)<br>No midcarpal malalignment |
| II | Attenuation/hemorrhage of SLIL (viewed from radiocarpal space) AND stepoff/incongruency of carpal alignment<br>Slight gap between carpals (<width of probe) |
| III | Stepoff/incongruency of carpal alignment (viewed from both radiocarpal and midcarpal space) AND scapholunate gap large enough to pass probe between carpals |
| IV | Stepoff/incongruency of carpal alignment (viewed from both radiocarpal and midcarpal space), gross instability, AND 2.7 mm arthroscope can pass through the gap between the scaphoid and lunate (positive drive-through sign) |

*SLIL,* Scapholunate interosseous ligament.

**Table 63-3** *Surgical Treatment of Scapholunate Injuries*

| Type | Radiographic Presentation | Treatment |
|---|---|---|
| Subacute | Dynamic deformity* | Conservative (splinting), arthroscopic pinning, capsulodesis |
| Acute | Static deformity | Open repair of SLIL |
| Late (chronic) | Static deformity | Open repair of SLIL and capsulodesis, capsulodesis alone, tenodesis alone, intercarpal fusion (STT or SC) |

*Dynamic deformity is present during stress (motion radiographs); positive clinical stress testing, positive arthroscopy, but negative arthrogram and normal static radiographs.
*SC,* Scaphocapitate; *SLIL,* scapholunate interosseous ligament; *STT,* scaphotrapezio-trapezoid.

## Surgical Options

- **Primary repair**
  - May be performed acutely, but usually combined with capsulodesis
- **Thermal (radiofrequency) shrinkage**
  - Described by Rosenwasser for predynamic instability and/or Geissler grade I and II injuries
    - Thermal energy causes collagen fibers to denature and shrink.
    - The temperature required to achieve the effect is about 70° to 80° C (<100° C to prevent tissue ablation).
    - Mechanically, this shrinkage tightens (shortens) the supporting ligaments, and this affects the relative motion between the scaphoid and lunate when examined clinically and with arthroscopy.
- **Percutaneous pinning**
  - Used as an adjunct to other surgical techniques to stabilize the lunate to the scaphoid as a form of internal immobilization
- **Capsulodesis (Blatt)**[2,12]
  - Uses **dorsal capsule** to act as a tether to prevent scaphoid flexion
  - The original technique used a pullout suture over a button, but suture anchor is usually used today.
- **Tenodesis**[4] (Fig. 63-15)
  - Technique described by Taleisnik and Linscheid[13] uses half of extensor carpi radialis longus (ECRL).
    - Leave attached distally, free proximally
    - Pass through scaphoid and triquetrum
    - Final attachment into capitate
  - Technique described by Brunelli and Brunelli[14] uses half of flexor carpi radialis (FCR).
    - Leave attached distally, free proximally
    - Pass volar to dorsal through scaphoid
    - Final attachment on distal radius
  - Van Den Abbeele et al[15] modification: Final attachment on lunate instead of DR
- Bone-ligament-bone
  - Tarsometatarsal joint autografts
  - Scapholunate interosseous ligament allograft
  - Bone retinaculum-bone autograft
  - Capitohamate joint
  - Third or second metacarpal-carpal bone
  - Long-term follow-up at 11.9 years demonstrated three failures in 14 patients.[16]

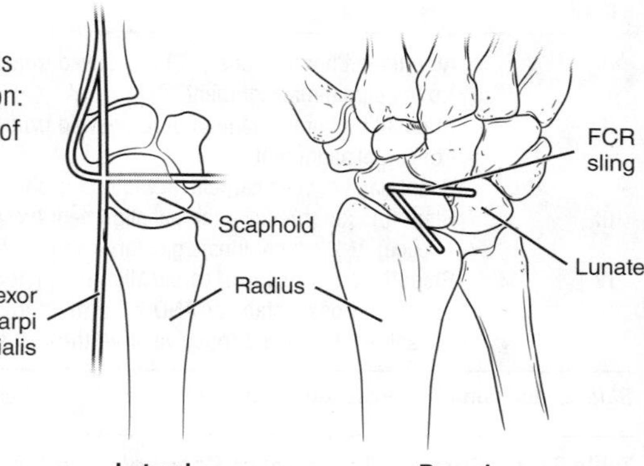


**Fig. 63-15** Tenodesis reconstruction of scapholunate joint. (*FCR,* Flexor carpi radialis.)

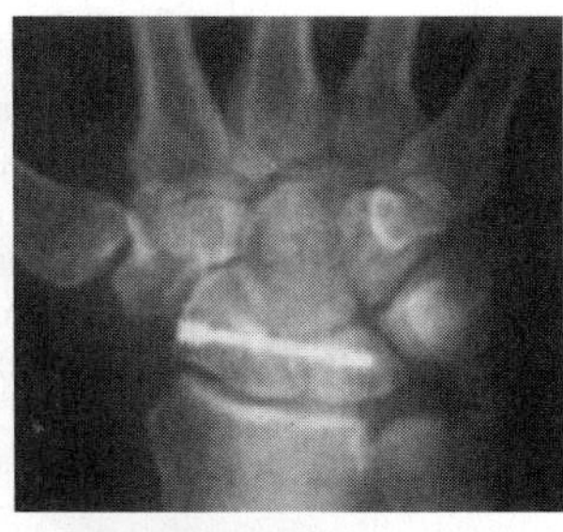

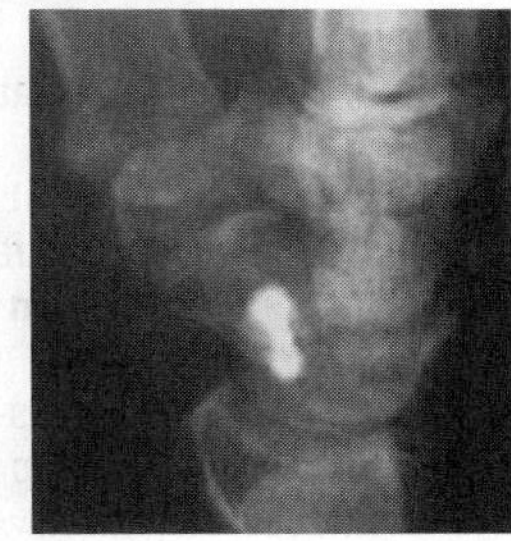

**Fig. 63-16** Reduction association scapholunate (RASL) procedure (pseudarthrosis of scapholunate joint).

- **Pseudarthrosis** (reduction association scapholunate [RASL])[9] (Fig. 63-16)
  - Described by Rosenwasser
  - Dorsal approach, followed by decortication of ulnar scaphoid and radial lunate
  - Uses a headless compression screw with differential pitch on either end, and a smooth shank
  - Usually prophylactic radial styloidectomy also performed, which assists with screw guidewire placement
- **Intercarpal fusion**
  - **Scapholunate fusion has been described but has low fusion rates, more commonly leading to pseudarthrosis, which was the basis for RASL.**
  - **Only 4 of 13 cases achieved fusion in one study.**[17]
- **Lunotriquetral ligament injuries**[3,18]
  - **Anatomy**
    - A C-shaped interosseous ligament spans the proximal, volar, and dorsal surfaces of the lunate and triquetrum, allowing coordinated motion between the triquetrum and lunate.
    - Ligament injury results in the lunate flexing with the scaphoid and proximal migration of the triquetrum during ulnar deviation, showing a **VISI** pattern of instability.
  - **Mechanism**
    - Injury often occurs as part of progressive perilunate instability, mentioned previously (see Fig. 63-9).
      - Occurs as the event just before complete lunate dislocation
      - Results from forceful hyperextension and ulnar deviation
    - Injury can also occur in isolation, showing a reverse perilunate instability pattern.[19]
      - Results from falling on outstretched hand in extension, with pronation and radial deviation
    - Chronic degenerative conditions can result in instability.[18]
      - Ulnar abutment syndrome
      - Inflammatory and crystalline arthropathies
  - **History**
    - Presentation is variable.
    - Patients usually recall a specific inciting event, usually a fall on an outstretched hand (FOOSH).
    - Symptoms may appear weeks to months after the injury.
    - Patients have **ulnar-sided wrist pain and weakness,** exacerbated by heavy use of the hand.
    - Patients may also describe a "clunk" or "clicking" when moving the wrist in radioulnar deviation.
  - **Physical examination**
    - Tenderness over lunotriquetral joint, immediately deep to the extensor digiti minimi tendon.

- **Provocative tests**
  - **Positive ballottement test:** Increased anteroposterior laxity, with pain, in lunotriquetral interval
  - **Positive shear test:** Dorsal force directed on triquetrum while stabilizing the lunate demonstrates increased laxity and elicits pain.
  - **Positive lateral compression test:** Pressure placed on medial tubercle of the triquetrum between the flexor carpi ulnaris and extensor carpi ulnaris tendons elicits pain.

**TIP:** Always compare positive results of provocative tests with those of the contralateral side.

- **Imaging**
  - For patients with isolated lunotriquetral injuries, the radiographic appearance is often normal.
  - **Obtain PA and lateral views of the wrist.**
    - May not demonstrate any findings if injury stable (or dynamic)
    - **Often a disruption in Gilula's arcs 1 and 2**[3] (Fig. 63-17)
  - The triquetrum moves proximally.
  - Lunotriquetral overlap also can be present.
    - Inspect lateral view for VISI deformity.
  - **Cineradiography or stress radiographs (clenched fist, ulnar or radial deviation)** help to detect dynamic injuries.

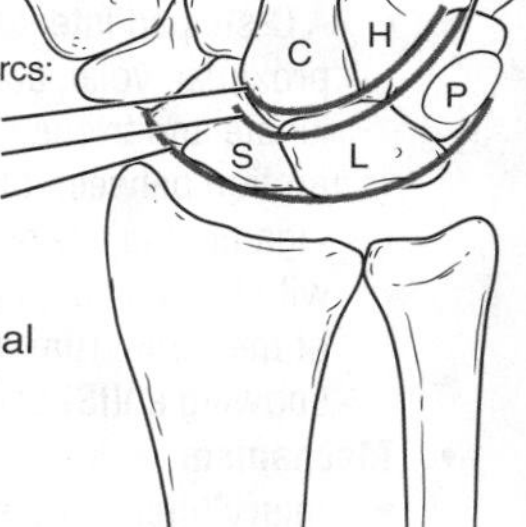


**Fig. 63-17** Gilula's arcs are smooth arcs that are formed by normal proximal *(1)* and distal *(2)* joint surfaces of the proximal carpal row and the normal proximal joint surface of the capitate and hamate *(3)*. (*C,* Capitate; *H,* hamate; *L,* lunate; *P,* pisiform; *S,* scaphoid; *Tr,* triquetrum.)

  - **Midcarpal or radiocarpal arthrography**
    - Rarely used
    - Mostly replaced by arthroscopy
  - **MRI**
    - Depends on multiple factors, including imaging protocol, radiologist's experience, and whether the tear is complete or incomplete
    - 89% sensitivity and 100% specificity reported[20]
  - **Arthroscopy**[21]
    - Benchmark **for assessing lunotriquetral joint**
    - Allows complete examination of wrist and triangular fibrocartilage complex
    - Additionally, arthroscopic treatment can be performed for various soft tissue injuries.
    - Geissler arthroscopic grading system of ligamentous injuries (see Table 63-2)
- **Treatment**

**There is no consensus on the treatment of lunotriquetral injuries.** Options depend on the **stability, chronicity,** and **severity** of the injury, as well as the demands of the patient.

  - **Nonsurgical management**
    - Indicated for stable or degenerative conditions
    - Immobilization using a molded cast with supporting pad under the pisiform or protective splint to prevent pronation
    - Nonsteroidal antiinflammatory drugs or corticosteroid injections
    - Consider arthroscopy if symptoms are not improved within 6 weeks.[3]

- **Surgical management**
  - **Arthroscopic debridement**
    - Usually performed at same time as diagnostic arthroscopy
    - Debridement of synovial hyperplasia in the fibrocartilaginous portion for symptomatic relief[22]
  - **Percutaneous pin fixation**
    - Only performed if no static VISI deformity
    - Arthroscopic guidance to examine lunotriquetral alignment
    - Immobilization postoperatively for 8 weeks before pin removal and rehabilitation
  - **Open repair**
    - Reserved for treatment of acute injuries
    - Dorsal or volar approaches
    - Ligament repaired directly with suture, bone tunnels, or suture anchors
    - Percutaneous pin fixation and immobilization also required
  - **Ligament reconstruction**
    - Performed when treating chronic and severe injuries with attenuated ligament remnants
    - Slip of extensor carpi ulnaris passed through drill holes and looped around the lunate and triquetrum to reconstruct ligament
    - Also, osteoligamentous autografts can be used (from dorsal capitohamate joint or tarsal joints).
  - **Lunotriquetral arthrodesis**
    - Consider for chronic dissociations
  - **Salvage procedures**
    - Indicated for patients with long-term static VISI deformities
    - Options: Proximal row carpectomy, four-corner arthrodesis, or total wrist arthrodesis

## PERILUNATE INJURIES AND PERILUNATE FRACTURE-DISLOCATIONS

- **Lesser arc injuries (dorsal perilunate or lunate dislocations)**[8,10,23]
  - **Anatomy**
    - The ligamentous anatomy of the wrist was reviewed earlier in this chapter.
    - **Space of Poirier**[24] (Fig. 63-18)
      - Area on the volar wrist capsule devoid of substantial ligamentous stability
      - **Site of capsular weakness that tears during perilunate injury**

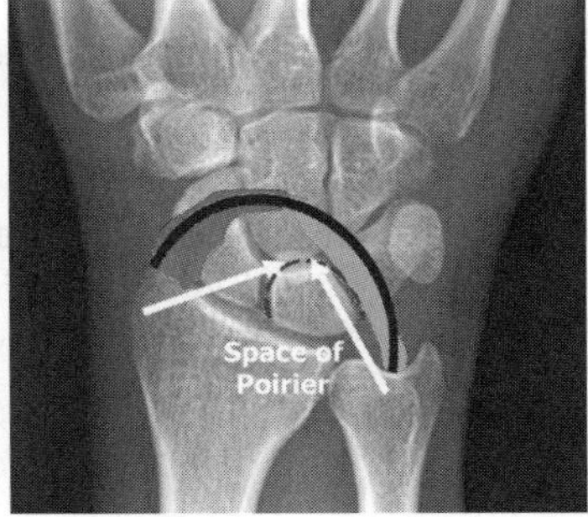


**Fig. 63-18** The space of Poirier *(white arrows)* is located between the lesser arc *(red dashed line)* and the greater arc *(black line).* The greater arc represents the zone of fractures and dislocations, the lesser arc represents the zone of dislocations, and the space of Poirier is the vulnerable zone between them. Fibers of the radioscaphocapitate ligament *(left)* and ulnocapitate ligament *(right)* interdigitate and form an arclike ligamentous structure called the *arcuate ligament* in the greater arc region. The lesser arc outlines the lunate. The scapholunate ligament and lunotriquetral ligament are part of the lesser arc, which does not extend to the distal radius and ulna.

- **Mechanism**
  - As with scapholunate ligament injuries, these injuries result from forceful wrist hyperextension, ulnar deviation, and intercarpal supination.
  - **A progressive perilunate instability pattern (four stages) ensues**[8] (see Fig. 63-8).
    - **Stage I: Scapholunate diastasis.** Scapholunate ligament disruption (DISI)
    - **Stage II: Dorsal dislocation of capitate.** Dorsal ligamentous attachments to the lunate are disrupted, space of Poirier is torn volarly, and the capitate dislocates dorsally relative to the lunate.
    - **Stage III: Lunotriquetral dissociation.** Lunotriquetral ligament disruption (VISI)
    - **Stage IV: Dislocation of lunate volarly.** External force pulls capitate proximally, which pushes lunate into volar dislocation after disruption of dorsal extrinsic ligamentous support.
  - Purely ligamentous injuries result from progressive injury along the **lesser arc.**
  - Perilunate fracture-dislocations result from progression along the **greater arc.**
- **History**
  - Patients present with a painful and swollen wrist after a high-energy hyperextension injury (usually a fall from a height or a motor vehicle collision).
- **Physical examination**
  - Wrist is acutely edematous.
  - Range of motion is very limited.
  - **Careful attention to sensation in the median nerve distribution is necessary.**

**CAUTION: As the lunate dislocates, the median nerve can be compressed acutely. Carefully elicit signs and symptoms to facilitate early carpal tunnel release, if necessary.**

- **Imaging**
  - Obtain PA and lateral views of the wrist.
    - **Gilula's arcs show multilevel disruption** with overlapping of bones across the midcarpal joint.
    - The lunate appears **triangular.**
    - The lateral view demonstrates the **spilled teapot sign** as the lunate tips volarly[24] (Fig. 63-19).
      - Dorsal dislocation of the capitate (perilunate dislocation) or complete volar dislocation of the lunate (lunate dislocation) is seen with severe injuries.
  - Traction views, CT scans, or repeat radiographs (after reduction) are required to accurately diagnose articular fractures obscured by a bony overlap.
- **Treatment**
  - **Closed reduction and immobilization**
    - *Closed reduction is the first step in all treatment methods.*

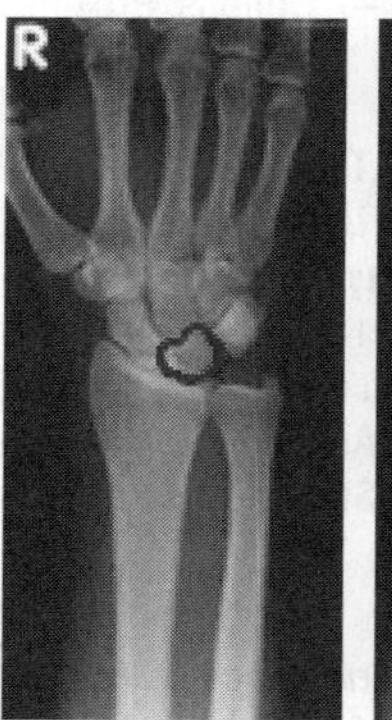

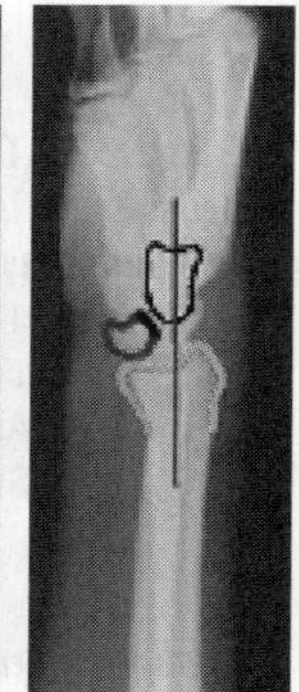

**Fig. 63-19** The spilled teapot sign indicates volar displacement of the lunate *(red)*. The capitate is outlined *(above)* and the distal radius *(below)*.

**TIP:** Closed reduction is performed most easily with a regional block and intravenous sedation; 10-15 minutes of uninterrupted traction should precede any attempt at reduction.

- **Tavernier's method** (Fig. 63-20)

♦ Most surgeon's advocate immobilization for 3 to 12 weeks.

▸ Careful follow-up with serial radiographs is necessary, because loss of reduction can occur.

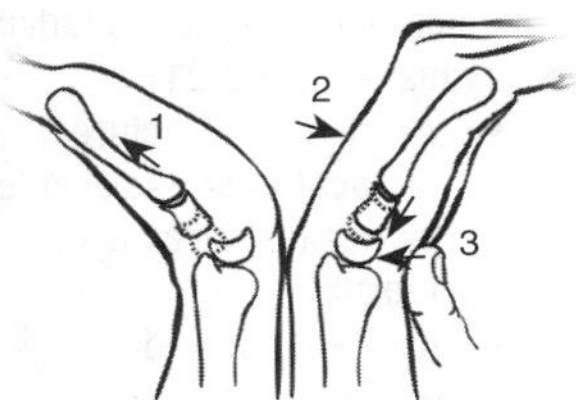


**Fig. 63-20** Tavernier's method for reduction of perilunate dislocations. *1,* Apply manual traction on the slightly extended wrist. *2,* Stabilize the lunate volarly with a thumb, and slowly flex the wrist without releasing traction until a snap occurs. This indicates that the proximal pole of the capitate has overcome the dorsal lip of the lunate. *3,* Release traction and bring the wrist back to neutral or slight flexion. Check reduction with a radiograph.

▸ **Closed reduction and percutaneous pin fixation**
  ♦ Careful reduction is performed, and slight adjustments to carpal alignment are made intraoperatively.
  ♦ Percutaneous pins are placed to hold reduction.
  ♦ Immobilize with cast (initially) and then use a splint for 12 weeks.

▸ **Open reduction, internal fixation, and ligament repair**
  ♦ **Most surgeons consider this method the treatment of choice.**
  ♦ Allows removal of intraarticular debris, more accurate reduction, and direct repair of ligamentous injuries (scapholunate ligament and volar capsule)
  ♦ Can use dorsal or dorsovolar combination approaches

**TIP:** Patients need to be counseled that loss of motion and diminished grip strength are common consequences despite appropriate treatment. Successful outcomes are dependent on timing of treatment, open versus closed injury, extent of chondral damage, residual instability, and fracture union.[25]

## CARPAL FRACTURE-DISLOCATIONS

### GREATER ARC INJURIES[10,22]

- If force travels along the greater arc, **bony fractures** rather than ligament injuries are generated.
- Injuries are named as perilunate dislocations along with associated fractures.
  - **Transscaphoid perilunate dislocation:** Fracture of scaphoid

**TIP:** Transscaphoid perilunate dislocation is the most common pattern of carpal dislocation.

  - **Transscaphoid, transcapitate perilunate dislocation:** Fracture of scaphoid and capitate

**TIP:** The proximal pole of the capitate fractures and rotates 90 to 180 degrees, making closed reduction nearly impossible.

- **Transscaphoid, transcapitate, transtriquetral perilunate dislocation:** Extremely rare
- **Transtriquetral perilunate dislocation:** Fracture of triquetrum
- Treatment options are identical to those for lesser arc injuries.
  - **Open reduction and internal fixation** is treatment of choice.

## Axial Fracture-Dislocations[26]

- These injuries usually result from a severe crush with dorsovolar compression.
- The carpus divides longitudinally, with one portion remaining aligned with the radius and the other displacing to the radial or ulnar side; the metacarpals follow their carpal attachments.
- **Types**[26] (Fig. 63-21)
  - **Axial-radial fracture-dislocations:** Radial column of carpus displaced distally and radially
    - Peritrapezoid
    - Peritrapezium
    - Transtrapezium
  - **Axial-ulnar fracture-dislocations:** Ulnar column displaced proximally and ulnarly
    - Transhamate peripisiform
    - Perihamate peripisiform
    - Perihamate transtriquetrum
- Associated soft tissue (vessel, nerve, and tendon) injuries are almost universal in these injury patterns.
- Dorsal approaches obtain fracture reduction and fixation.
- Volar approaches are necessary to repair associated soft tissue injuries.
- Outcomes are limited by associated tendon and nerve injuries.

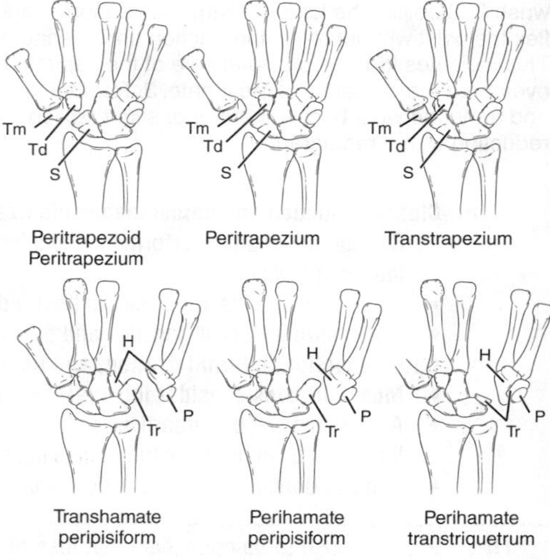


**Fig. 63-21** Axial fracture-dislocations of the carpus.

## ISOLATED CARPAL DISLOCATIONS[10]

- Isolated carpal bone dislocations, without the patterns described here, are extremely rare.
- They can occur when a localized force is concentrated over a single carpal bone.
- Treatment options include closed reduction, carpal bone excision, or open reduction and internal fixation.

## WRIST ARTHROSCOPY[27]

- First described by Chen[28] for diagnostic purposes
- Has advanced to many therapeutic applications
- Although arthroscopic examination is considered the benchmark for many intraarticular diagnoses, physical examination and imaging findings are still key adjuncts in interpreting findings as asymptomatic degenerative versus pathologic lesions.

## PATIENT PREPARATION (Fig. 63-22)

- Supine
- General anesthesia
- Arm abducted
- Padded tourniquet

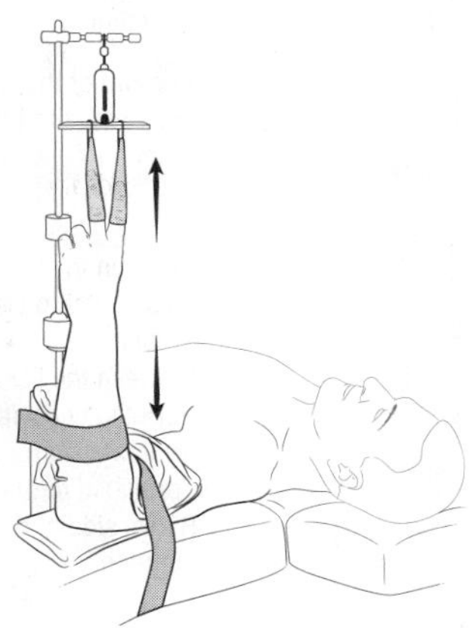

**Fig. 63-22** Wrist arthroscopy tower setup: wrist traction surface hand device is placed along the volar surface of the forearm so that the dorsal wrist can be accessed without interference from the traction device. The arms and forearm must both be strapped down to prevent countertraction to the weights that are applied through the fingers with the use of the Chinese finger traps. The space is opened up from traction across the wrist for clearer visualization through the arthroscope.

> **TIP:** Make sure that the tourniquet is placed ***proximally*** so that the arm can be secured within the sterile field. (This can make the entire case easier.)

- Fingers are suspended in traction, usually about 10 pounds.
- Arm is proximal to elbow and secured with either strap or Coban to a wrist tower.
- Surgeon usually faces dorsal side of wrist.
- Monitor is positioned so that the surgeon can easily view without turning head.
- Check equipment before starting case, including wrist tower with overhead traction device, finger traps, 2.7 mm 30-degree arthroscope, 3 mm hook-probe, thermal probe, mechanical shaver.
- Other specialized equipment may be used, including biters, graspers, and/or triangular fibrocartilaginous complex (TFCC) repair kit systems.

> **TIP:** Before making the incision, ensure that the camera and monitor are working and that pictures are being taken. White balance the camera on white gauze. Understand the function of all other buttons.

- Prime inflow so that it is ready to flow without air.
- Know how to adjust light intensity and field of view (making the circle larger or smaller).
- It is helpful to have a USB drive to save pictures.
- Remember that the scope is angled at 30 degrees. The viewing angle can be changed by rotating the scope for a full 360-degree view.

## PORTALS[2] (Table 63-4) (Figs. 63-23 and 63-24)

- Portals are named by two numbers that represent the interval between two extensor compartments.
- Usually two dorsal radiocarpal portals and two midcarpal portals are used.
- The most common radiocarpal portals are the 3-4, 4-5, and 6R portals.
- The most common midcarpal portals are the midcarpal radial (MCR) and midcarpal ulnar (MCU) portals.
- The midcarpal portals can be localized by advancing approximately 1 cm distal to the 3-4 and 4-5 portals.
- **The most common viewing portal is the 3-4 portal,** which is between the third and fourth extensor compartments (extensor pollicis longus and extensor digitorum communis) and usually is the first portal created.

**Table 63-4** *Wrist Arthroscopy Portals*

| Portal Name | Location | Purpose | Risks |
|---|---|---|---|
| 1-2 | Dorsum of the snuffbox, just radial to the EPL tendon | Not commonly used.<br>Inflow<br>Access to the radial styloid, scaphoid, lunate, and articular surface of the distal radius | Injury to the radial artery |
| 3-4 | Between the EPL and EDC, just distal to Lister's tubercle | Established first<br>Main radiocarpal arthroscopic viewing portal | Injury to EPL or EDC |
| 4-5 | Between the EDC and EDM in line with the ring metacarpal, slightly proximal to the 3-4 portal | Main radiocarpal instrumentation portal<br>Visualization of the TFCC | Injury to EDC or EDM |
| 6R | Radial side of the EDU tendon | Instrumentation portal<br>Visualize the triangular fibrocartilage and the ulnolunate, ulnotriquetral, and lunotriquetral ligaments | Injury to the dorsal sensory branch of ulnar nerve |
| 6U | Ulnar side of the ECU tendon | Dorsal rim of the TFCC or for instrumentation when debriding the volar LTIL | Injury to the dorsal sensory branch of the ulnar nerve |
| Radial midcarpal | Radial side of the third metacarpal axis proximal to the capitates, in a soft depression between the capitate and scaphoid | Visualization of the STT joint, scapholunate articulation, and distal pole of the scaphoid | Injury to the ECRB and EDC tendons |
| Ulnar midcarpal | 1 cm distal to the 4-5 portal, aligned with the fourth metacarpal, at the lunotriquetral-capitate-hamate joint | Visualization of distal lunate, lunotriquetral, and triquetrohamate articulation | Injury to the EDC and EDM tendons |
| Scaphotrapezio-trapezoid | Midshaft axis of the index metacarpal, just ulnar to the EPL at the level of the STT joint | Visualization of scaphotrapezial and scaphotrapezoid joints<br>Debridement of the STT joint | Injury to the small branches of the radial nerve<br>Injury to the radial artery |
| Triquetrohamate | Just ulnar to the ECU tendon at the level of the triquetrohamate joint | Inflow/outflow<br>Visualization, debridement of the TH joint | Injury to the dorsal cutaneous branch of the ulnar nerve |
| Volar radial | Just radial to the flexor carpi radialis tendon at the proximal wrist flexion crease | Visualization of the DRCL and the volar aspect of the SLIL<br>Visualization during DRU joint fracture reduction | Safe zone of 3 mm in all directions with respect to volar cutaneous branch of the median nerve (ulnarly) and radial artery (radially) |
| Volar ulnar | Interval between flexor tendons and flexor carpi ulnaris and the ulnar neurovascular bundle | Visualization of ulnar sling mechanism, dorsal radioulnar ligament, and volar aspect of the lunotriquetral ligament | Portal lies just radial to the ulnar artery |

*DRCL,* Dorsal radiocarpal ligament; *DRU joint,* distal radioulnar joint; *ECRB,* extensor carpi radialis brevis; *ECU,* extensor carpi ulnaris; *EDC,* extensor digitorum communis; *EDM,* extensor digiti minimi; *EDU,* extensor digiti ulnaris; *EPL,* extensor pollicis longus; *LTIL,* lunotriquetral interosseous ligament; *SLIL,* scapholunate interosseous ligament; *STT,* scaphotrapezio-trapezoid; *TFCC,* triangular fibrocartilage complex; *TH,* triquetrohamate.

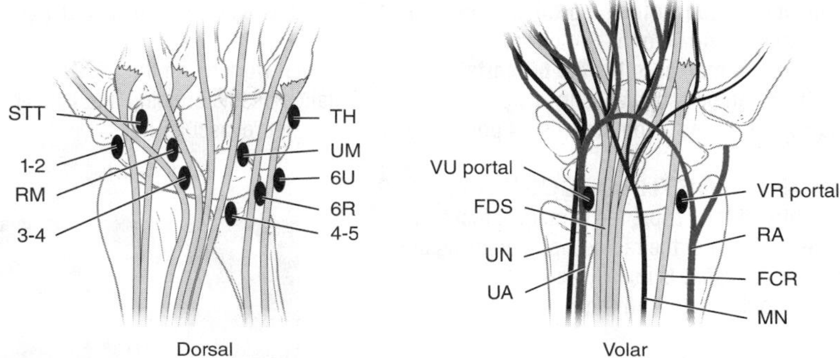


**Fig. 63-23** Portal anatomy. (*FCR,* Flexor carpi radialis; *FDS,* flexor digitorum superficialis; *MN,* median nerve; *RA,* radial artery; *RM,* radial midcarpal; *STT,* scaphotrapezio-trapezoid; *TH,* triquetrohamate; *UA,* ulnar artery; *UM,* ulnar midcarpal; *UN,* ulnar nerve; *VR,* volar radial; *VU,* volar ulnar.)

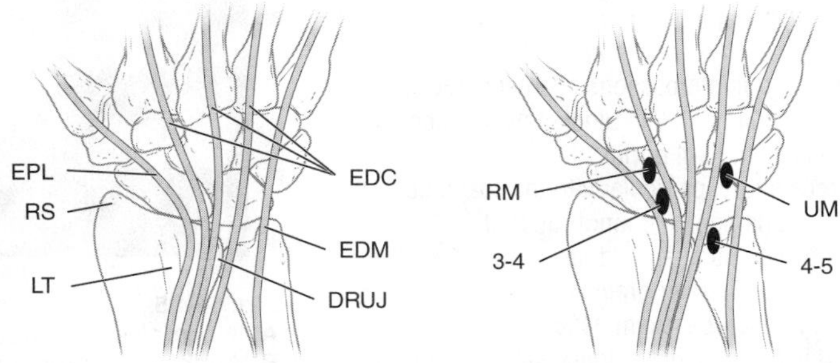


**Fig. 63-24** Portal anatomy with skin landmarks. (*DRUJ,* Distal radioulnar joint; *EDC,* extensor digitorum communis; *EDM,* extensor digiti minimi; *EPL,* extensor pollicis longus; *LT,* Lister's tubercle; *RM,* radial midcarpal; *RS,* radial styloid; *UM,* ulnar midcarpal.)

- Technique involves placing traction and then marking skin, including Lister's tubercle.
- Usually this portal is about 1 cm distal to Lister's tubercle and can be palpated in the concavity between the lunate and dorsal radius.
- A needle may be used to localize the joint. Approximately 5-10 ml of lidocaine 1% with epinephrine is injected for additional hemostatic control.
- The needle is directed approximately 10 degrees from dorsal distal to volar proximal to respect the natural volar tilt of the distal radius.
- A shallow skin incision is made with No. 15 blade, followed by blunt spread of mosquito forceps down to capsule.
- Dorsal veins are coagulated or retracted as necessary.
- The capsule is pierced in a controlled manner, using an index finger 2 cm from tip of mosquito forceps to act as a block to overpenetration.
- A blunt trocar is inserted into hole created by mosquito forceps in a controlled manner.
- Surgeon's preference determines whether wet or dry arthroscopy is performed. Usually, wet arthroscopy is preferred, in which case the inflow is switched ON.

- **The most common working portal is usually the 4-5 portal,** which is located about 1 cm ulnar and slightly proximal to the 3-4 portal.
- **The other common portal is the 6R portal,** particularly when working on the TFCC.
- An outflow can be established in any portal with an 18-gauge needle draining into a basin.
- Table 63-4 provides a complete list of portals and potential neurovascular risks.

## Diagnostic Arthroscopy (Fig. 63-25)

- Upon entry of the scope, the camera is focused.
- The vascular tuft of the radioscapholunate ligament *(ligament of Testut)* is usually seen.
- The scaphoid, lunate, and triquetrum are located superiorly.
- The distal radius articular surface, including the scaphoid and lunate fossa, is located inferiorly.
- The TFCC is located inferior and ulnar to the 3-4 portal and normally appears like a "trampoline."
- The membranous scapholunate ligament is just superior to the radioscapholunate ligament, between the scaphoid and lunate.
- The radioscaphocapitate ligament and long radiolunate ligament are radial to the portal.
- The lunotriquetral interosseous ligament, TFCC, ulnotriquetral ligament, and ulnolunate ligament are located ulnar to the 3-4 portal.
- Ligamentous injury, particularly to the scapholunate interosseous ligament and lunotriquetral interosseous ligament, should be classified according to the Geissler grading system.
- Systematic radiocarpal examination should be performed in a consistent manner, whether radial to ulnar or ulnar to radial. All ligaments and cartilage surfaces are assessed, and synovitic/inflamed areas and loose bodies are noted.
- Systematic midcarpal examination helps to evaluate ligaments from different view, evaluate chondral surfaces, and look for loose bodies.
- Chondral lesions are traditionally classified by the **Outerbridge system,**[29] which was originally designed for the knee:
  - **Grade I:** Softening and swelling of cartilage
  - **Grade II:** Fragmentation and fissuring, <0.5-inch diameter
  - **Grade III:** Fragmentation and fissuring, >0.5-inch diameter
  - **Grade IV:** Erosion of cartilage down to exposed subchondral bone
- **The ICRS (International Cartilage Restoration Society) system may be better suited to describe grade II and grade III lesions in the wrist as follows**[30]:
  - **Grade 0:** Normal
  - **Grade1:** Nearly normal (soft indentation and/or superficial fissures and cracks)
  - **Grade 2:** Abnormal (lesions extending down to <50% of cartilage depth)
  - **Grade 3:** Severely abnormal (cartilage defects >50% of cartilage depth)
  - **Grade 4:** Severely abnormal (through the subchondral bone)

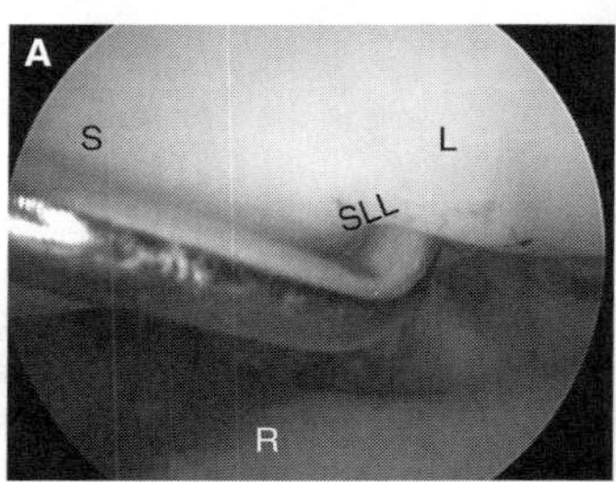


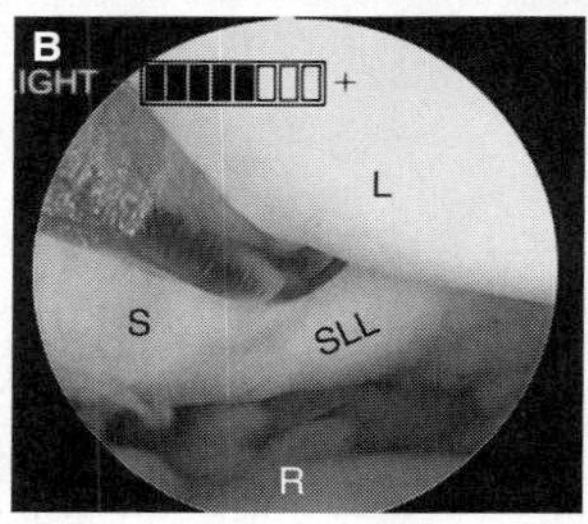


**Fig. 63-25** Arthroscopic images. **A,** Normal scapholunate joint. **B,** Abnormal scapholunate joint, Geissler stage 3 (width of probe). (*L,* Lunate, *R,* radius; *S,* scaphoid, *SLL,* scapholunate ligament.)

**Box 63-1** *PALMER CLASSIFICATION SYSTEM*

| **Class I: Traumatic (acute)** | **Class II: Degenerative (ulnar impaction syndrome)** |
|---|---|
| A. Central perforation | A. TFCC wear |
| B. Ulnar avulsion<br>With styloid fracture<br>Without styloid fracture | B. TFCC wear<br>+ Lunate and/or ulnar head chondromalacia |
| C. Distal avulsion (from carpus) | C. TFCC perforation<br>+ Lunate and/or ulnar head chondromalacia |
| D. Radial avulsion<br>With sigmoid notch fracture<br>Without sigmoid notch fracture | D. TFCC perforation<br>+ Lunate and/or ulnar head chondromalacia<br>+ Lunotriquetral ligament perforation |
| | E. TFCC perforation<br>+ Lunate and/or ulnar head chondromalacia<br>+ Lunotriquetral ligament perforation<br>+ Ulnocarpal arthritis |

*TFCC,* Triangular fibrocartilage complex.

- **TFCC**[31] (Box 63-1)
  - Palmer and Werner[31,32] used the term TFCC to describe the close anatomic and functional relationships of the soft tissue structures in the ulnar side of the wrist (Fig. 63-26).
  - Components of TFCC: Articular disc, dorsal and volar radioulnar ligaments, meniscus homolog, ulnar collateral ligament, and extensor carpi ulnaris sheath.
  - Palmer classified the abnormalities into type I (A-D) for acute traumatic injuries and type II (A-E) for chronic degenerative conditions that define the progressive spectrum of ulnocarpal impaction.

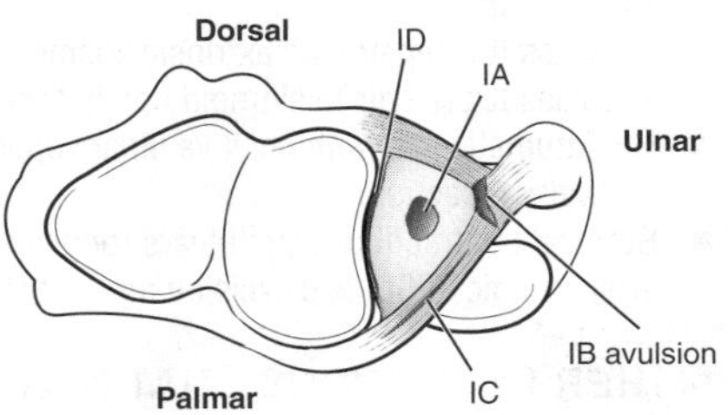


**Fig. 63-26** Anatomic depiction of Palmer's classification system.

## HISTORY

- Usually ulnar-sided wrist pain
- Pain with forearm rotation (pronation and supination)
- Typically from an acute traumatic injury or a chronic degenerative condition, usually ulnocarpal impaction
- Ask about mechanical symptoms such as popping, clicking, catching, or locking.
- Ask about instability symptoms such as giving way.

## PHYSICAL EXAMINATION

- Tenderness over the TFCC region: Palpate ulnar depression between distal ulna and carpus.
- TFCC compression test: Apply axial load during ulnar deviation.
- **Press test:** Provocative diagnostic maneuver. Seated patient is asked to push body weight off a chair using the affected wrist, creating an axial ulnar load. Positive test result is focal wrist pain.

- Test distal radioulnar joint (DRU joint) instability with the forearm in neutral, pronation, and supination by manually translating the ulnar head dorsal and volar to the distal radius. Compare result with the contralateral side.
- **Piano key sign:** The unstable distal ulna may be subluxated/dislocated dorsally or volarly. A push in the opposite direction may produce a palpable "clunk" similar to depressing a piano key.
- Look for a prominent ulna, which may indicate a dorsal distal ulnar dislocation (more common) or a volar dislocation.

## Imaging

- AP and lateral views of wrist are a minimum. Assess ulnar variance, which is relative length of ulna to the distal radius. Measure in either positive or negative millimeters. (*Ulnar positive* is an ulna longer or more distal than the distal radius at the level of the DRUJ).
- MRI is equipment sensitive.
- MRA (MRI with intraarticular contrast, not IV contrast) is most sensitive.

## Treatment

- Initial treatment is usually nonoperative if there is no DRU joint instability. Immobilize in a long arm cast for 4-6 weeks.
- Cortisone injections may be used for symptomatic relief but may inhibit healing of peripheral tears.
- Arthroscopy is indicated in patients with TFCC tears who have failed 3 months of nonoperative treatment.
- Early arthroscopic treatment may be considered for high-level athletes.
- Surgery is also indicated for acute DRU joint instability.
- Surgical treatment of type I tears:
  - Class IA (central tears): Debridement
  - Class IB: Repair
  - Class IC: Repair plus extrinsic ligament plication or open repair
  - Class ID: Repair to sigmoid notch if the DRU joint is unstable; debride if DRU joint is stable
  - Traumatic tear with positive ulnar variance may require concomitant ulnar shortening or wafer resection.
- Surgical treatment of type II tears (degenerative, ulnocarpal impaction) usually requires arthroscopic TFCC disc excision and wafer resection with ulnar shortening.

## Other Conditions That May Be Treated Arthroscopically

- Synovial biopsy
- Synovectomy
- Chondroplasty
- Loose body removal
- Ganglionectomy (dorsal or volar)
- Contracture release
- Scapholunate or lunotriquetral ligament tear, including thermal/radiofrequency shrinkage
- Reduction association of the scapholunate (RASL)
- Dorsal radiocarpal ligament repair
- Nondissociative midcarpal instability
- Bone resection, including proximal row carpectomy
- Radial styloidectomy
- Arthroscopic visualization for distal radius intraarticular fracture reduction
- Diagnostic for unexplained wrist pain that is unresponsive to nonoperative treatment and that is relieved with intraarticular anesthetic injection

## Key Points

- ✓ Carpal instability patterns are usually predictable.
- ✓ Lesser arc injuries are ligamentous, and greater arc injuries are bony.
- ✓ Scapholunate and lunotriquetral ligament injuries are best evaluated by wrist arthroscopy. Preoperative MRI is useful.
- ✓ Scapholunate ligament injuries are the most common ligamentous injury in the wrist. Look for signs of DISI deformity. There are multiple surgical options for this injury, but no consensus on optimal treatment.
- ✓ Perilunate dislocations and fracture-dislocations should be treated with early open reduction, internal fixation, and ligament repair, when possible.
- ✓ Know how to work up ulnar-sided wrist pain.
- ✓ Know the indications for wrist arthroscopy and how to grade ligamentous/cartilaginous injuries.
- ✓ Be aware of pertinent anatomy when creating wrist portals and performing wrist arthroscopic diagnostic examinations. This includes extensor compartment, volar wrist ligaments, and TFCC structures.

## References


1. Idler RS. Anatomy and biomechanics of the digital flexor tendons. Hand Clin 1:3-11, 1985.
2. Wolfe SW, Garcia-Elias M, Kitay A. Carpal instability nondissociative. J Am Acad Orthop Surg 20:575-585, 2012.
3. Butterfield WL, Joshi A, Lichtman D, et al. Lunotriquetral injuries. J Am Soc Surg Hand 2:195-203, 2002.
4. Walsh JJ, Berger RA, Cooney WP. Current status of scapholunate interosseous ligament injuries. J Am Acad Orthop Surg 10:32-42, 2002.
5. Berger RA. A method of defining palpable landmarks for the ligament-splitting dorsal wrist capsulotomy. J Hand Surg Am 32:1291-1295, 2007.
6. Horii E, Garcia-Elias M, An KN, et al. A kinematic study of the lunotriquetral dissociations. J Hand Surg Am 23:425-431, 1998.
7. Danoff JR, Karl JW, Birman MV, et al. The use of thermal shrinkage for scapholunate instability. Hand Clin 27:309-317, 2011.
8. Mayfield J, Johnson RP, Kilcoyne RK, et al. Carpal dislocation: pathomechanics and progressive perilunar instability. J Hand Surg Am 5:226-241, 1980.
9. Walsh JJ, Berger RA, Cooney WP, et al. Current status of scapholunate interosseous ligament injuries. J Am Acad Orthop Surg 10:32-42, 2002.
10. Garcia-Elias M, Geissler WB. Carpal instability. In Green DP, Hotchkiss RN, Pederson WC, et al, eds. Green's Operative Hand Surgery, 5th ed. Philadelphia: Churchill Livingstone, 2005.
11. Geissler WB, Freeland AE, Savoie FH, et al. Intracarpal soft-tissue lesions associated with an intra-articular fracture of the distal end of the radius. J Bone Joint Surg Am 78:357-365, 1996.
12. Blatt G. Capsulodesis in reconstructive hand surgery: dorsal capsulodesis for the unstable scaphoid and volar capsulodesis following excision of the distal ulna. Hand Clin 3:81-102, 1987.
13. Taleisnik J, Linscheid RL. Scapholunate instability. In Cooney WP, Linscheid RL, Dobyns JH, eds. The Wrist: Diagnosis and Operative Treatment, vol 1. St Louis: Mosby–Year Book, 1998.
14. Brunelli GA, Brunelli GR. A new technique to correct carpal instability with scaphoid rotary subluxation: a preliminary report. J Hand Surg Am 20(3 Pt 2):S82-S85, 1995.
15. Van Den Abbeele KL, Loh YC, Stanley JK, et al. Early results of a modified Brunelli procedure for scapholunate instability. J Hand Surg Br 23:258-261, 1998.

16. Soong M, Merrell GA, Ortmann F IV, et al. Long-term results of bone-retinaculum-bone autograft for scapholunate instability. J Hand Surg Am 38:504-508, 2013.
17. Zubairy AI, Jones WA. Scapholunate fusion in chronic symptomatic scapholunate instability. J Hand Surg Br 28:311-314, 2003.
18. Berger RA. Lunotriquetral joint. In Berger RA, Weiss AP, eds. Hand Surgery. Philadelphia: Lippincott Williams & Wilkins, 2004.
19. Reagan DS, Linscheid RL, Dobyns JH, et al. Lunotriquetral sprains. J Hand Surg Am 9:502-514, 1984.
20. Magee T. Comparison of 3-T MRI and arthroscopy of intrinsic wrist ligament and TFCC tears. AJR Am J Roentgenol 192:80-85, 2009.
21. Osterman AL, Seidman GD. The role of arthroscopy in the treatment of lunatotriquetral ligament injuries. Hand Clin 11:41-50, 1995.
22. Weiss AP, Sachar K, Glowack KA, et al. Arthroscopic debridement alone for intercarpal ligament tears. J Hand Surg Am 22:344-349, 1997.
23. Garcia-Elias M. Perilunar injuries including fracture dislocations. In Berger RA, Weiss AP, eds. Hand Surgery. Philadelphia: Lippincott Williams & Wilkins, 2004.
24. Taljanovic MS, Goldberg MR, Sheppard JE, et al. US of the intrinsic and extrinsic wrist ligaments and triangular fibrocartilage complex—normal anatomy and imaging technique. Radiographics 31:e44, 2011.
25. Sawardeker PJ, Kindt KE, Baratz ME. Fracture-dislocations of the carpus: perilunate injury. Orthop Clin North Am 44:93-106, 2013.
26. Yaghoubian R, Goebel F, Musgrave DS, et al. Diagnosis and management of acute fracture-dislocation of the carpus. Orthop Clin North Am 32:295-305, 2001.
27. Wolf JM, Dukas A, Pensak M. Advances in wrist arthroscopy. J Am Acad Orthop Surg 20:725-734, 2012.
28. Chen YC. Arthroscopy of the wrist and finger joints. Orthop Clin North Am 10:723-733, 1979.
29. Outerbridge RE. The etiology of chondromalacia patellae. J Bone Joint Surg Br 43:752-757, 1961.
30. Brittsberg M, Winalski CS. Evaluation of cartilage injuries and repair. J Bone Joint Surg Am 85:58-69, 2003.
31. Henry MH. Management of acute triangular fibrocartilage complex injury of the wrist. J Am Acad Orthop Surg 16:320-329, 2008.
32. Palmer AK, Werner FW. The triangular fibrocartilage complex of the wrist—anatomy and function. J Hand Surg Am 6:153-162, 1981.

# 64. Distal Radius Fractures

**Wendy L. Parker, Georges N. Tabbal, Zach J. Barnes**

## DEMOGRAPHICS AND PATHOPHYSIOLOGY

- Most common fracture presenting to emergency departments (one sixth of all fractures)
- 3% of all upper extremity injuries
  - Incidence: >640,000 annually
  - Women aged 60 to 70 most commonly affected
- Fall from standing height onto outstretched hand (FOOSH) most common mechanism
- **Bimodal distribution:**
  - Physiologically young, typically active males sustain high-energy injuries (usually sports related).
  - Physiologically older, most commonly inactive females have low-energy fragility fractures (usually osteoporotic fractures, 90% extraarticular).

## PATHOPHYSIOLOGY

### ANATOMY AND KINEMATICS[1] (Fig. 64-1)

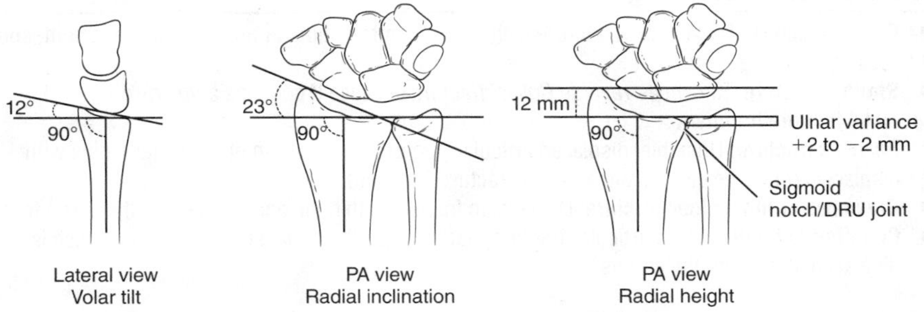


**Fig. 64-1** Normal anatomic parameters of the distal radius.

- **Extraarticular**
  - Metaphyseal flare begins 2 cm proximal to radiocarpal joint.
  - Dorsally concave, housing the dorsal extensor compartments
  - Dorsal cortex thin, easily comminuted
  - Volarly convex, thicker cortical bone
  - Distal margin both volarly and dorsally is insertion site of extrinsic ligaments.
  - The only tendon to insert onto the distal radius is the **brachioradialis.**
  - Distal radius described as having **three columns**[2]:

- **Intraarticular** (Fig. 64-2)[3]
  - Distally, made up of the triangular scaphoid and circular lunate facets, separated by an articular ridge often involved in fracture pattern
  - Sigmoid notch ulnarly, articulating with the ulnar head
  - TFCC acts as a stabilizer of the distal radioulnar joint (DRU joint).
  - Arises from ulnar aspect of lunate fossa and inserts at base of ulnar styloid (fovea)
  - Volar and dorsal extrinsic ligaments support carpus and regulate motion.
  - Volar ligaments are stouter and more defined than dorsal ligaments.
  - Radius bears 82% of the axial load when the wrist is in neutral ulnar variance.[4]

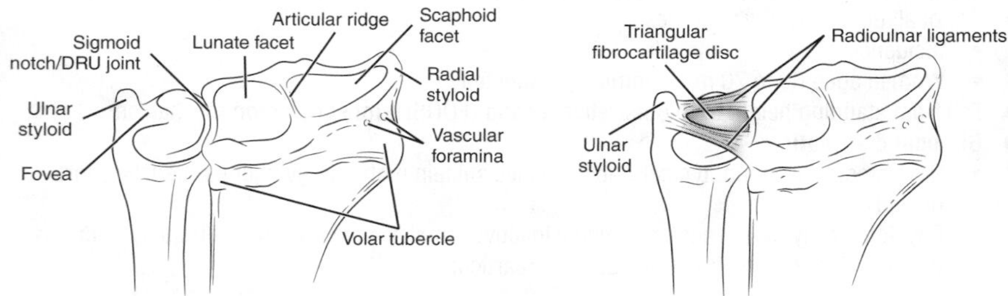


**Fig. 64-2** Intraarticular anatomy of distal radius and ulna.

## NOMENCLATURE (Fig. 64-3)

- **Colles' fracture:** Distal radius fracture with *dorsal* comminution, angulation, displacement, and radial shortening
- **Smith's fracture:** Known as *reverse Colles' fracture* because it contains a *volarly* displaced distal fracture fragment
- **Barton's fracture:** Unstable, displaced articular fracture–subluxation of the distal radius with displacement of the carpus and articular fracture fragment
- **Die punch or lunate load fracture:** Depression fracture within the dorsal aspect of the lunate fossa
- **Chauffeur's fracture:** Intraarticular fracture that includes the radial styloid process, which is displaced along with the carpus

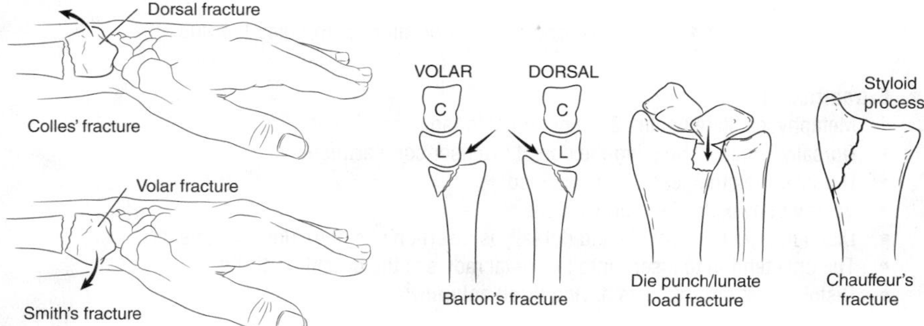


**Fig. 64-3** Types of fractures.

## CLASSIFICATIONS

- Numerous classification systems have been developed to aid in diagnosing and treating distal radius fractures (albeit with little success in achieving that goal).
- Interobserver agreement is *moderate* for Mayo[5] (Fig. 64-4) and *fair* for Frykman[6] (Fig. 64-5), Melone, and AO classifications.
- The Mayo classification is intuitive: it broadly groups fractures into extraarticular and intraarticular. From there the groups follow classic anatomic fracture patterns through the radiocarpal joint involving either the scaphoid fossa, the lunate fossa, or both.
- **Frykman:** Relies on radiocarpal and radioulnar joint involvement with the presence or absence of an ulnar styloid fracture to categorize injuries[7]

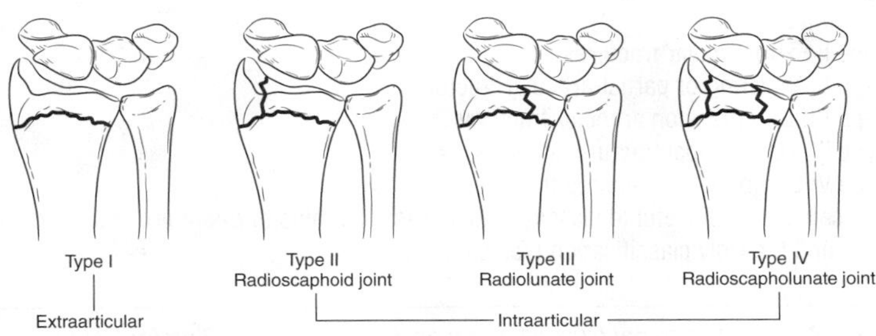


**Fig. 64-4** Mayo classification.

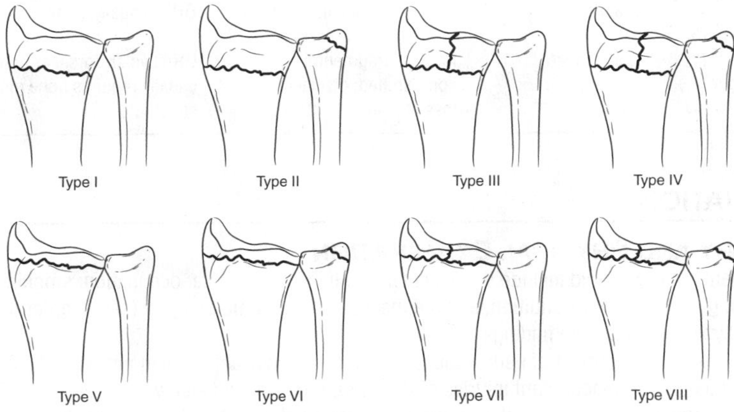


**Fig. 64-5** Frykman classification.

**Table 64-1** *Frykman Classification of Radius Fractures*

| Ulnar styloid fracture | No | Yes |
|---|---|---|
| Extraarticular | I | II |
| Intraarticular, involving radiocarpal joint | III | IV |
| Intraarticular, involving radioulnar joint | V | VI |
| Intraarticular, involving radiocarpal + radioulnar joints | VII | VIII |

- **Melone:** Categorizes distal radius fractures based on the involved parts (diaphyseal shaft, radial styloid, dorsal medial facet, and volar medial facet). The importance of the radiolunate articulation is emphasized, which by definition applies to only articular fractures. A fifth group represents severely comminuted fractures.[8]
- **AO (Association for the Study of Internal Fixation):** Fractures are organized into three groups (A, B, and C) based on fracture severity. Each group is subdivided into nine divisions based on the extent of articular involvement, metaphyseal fragmentation, and orientation of the articular fracture lines.[9]
  - Type A: Extraarticular fractures
  - Type B: Partial articular fractures
  - Type C: Complete articular fractures
- **Jupiter and Fernandez**[10]**:**
  - Type I: Extraarticular fractures
  - Type II: Shearing or partial-articular fractures
  - Type III: Compression articular fractures
  - Type IV: Radiocarpal fracture dislocations
  - Type V: Complex, high-energy fractures
- Often it can be more useful to classify logically as it pertains to treatment modality: The Good, the Bad, and the Ugly classification (Table 64-2).

**Table 64-2** *Simplified Clinical Classification and Management Plan for Distal Radius Fractures*

| | | | |
|---|---|---|---|
| Good | Extraarticular | Noncomminuted | CR and cast; CRRP; ORIF |
| Bad | Intraarticular | 2-4 part; little comminution; reducible | ORIF; usually volar |
| Ugly | Intraarticular | Multiple fragments; comminuted; displaced with loss of height | ORIF; volar/dorsal or both; usually requires bone graft or substitute |

# EVALUATION

## History and Physical Examination

- Pertinent history should include the patient's age, hand dominance, occupation, smoking status, general medical condition, and the mechanism and time of injury (see Chapter 60).
- Key physical examination findings:
  - Thorough assessment of neurovascular function (specifically median nerve)
  - Evaluation for concomitant injuries of the wrist, forearm, and elbow
  - Tenderness to palpation of the carpus or instability of the intercarpal ligaments
  - Evaluation of the DRU joint
    - Point tenderness over the ulnar styloid may suggest a fracture
    - A positive fovea sign is sensitive and specific for a TFCC injury
    - Instability of the DRU joint through the radius-ulna translation suggests DRU joint instability

## Commonly Associated Injuries

- Carpal tunnel syndrome: Reported incidence of 8%[11]
- Scapholunate ligament: Most common; occurs in 6.7% of extraarticular fractures, although incidence is 21.5% with intraarticular fractures[12]
- Compartment syndrome: Rare, reported incidence of 1%

- TFCC injury and DRU joint instability
  - Found in large percentage (40%-85%) of unstable distal radius fractures
  - When an ulnar styloid fracture is present, the reported incidence is as high as 50%, most commonly with fractures at the base of the styloid

## RADIOGRAPHIC IMAGING

### RADIOGRAPHY

- Main diagnostic test
- Standard films:
  - PA
  - Lateral
  - Modified lateral (10-30 degrees cephalic): Helps assess the articular surface and is particularly useful intraoperatively (i.e., to confirm that the joint space is free of hardware); obtained by taking a lateral view with the distal forearm elevated off of horizontal.
  - Traction view: Aids in assessing degree of fracture comminution and articular component of the fracture.
- Radiographs of joints above and below the injury site are obtained to rule out concomitant injuries.

**TIP:** The integrity of a lateral radiograph can be assessed by referencing the relative position of the pisiform to the distal pole of the scaphoid. In a "true" lateral, they will overlap 50%.

## RADIOGRAPHIC MEASUREMENTS AND PARAMETERS

- **Articular step-off:** *The most important determinant of outcome*
  - An articular step-off as minimal as 1 mm can lead to pain and stiffness,[13,14] although some refute the validity of this finding.

**NOTE: Radiographic degenerative joint disease (DJD) does not necessarily correlate with functional status.**

- **Radial height:** Measured on PA radiograph as the distance between a line drawn perpendicular to the shaft of the radius (passing through the sigmoid notch at the distal tip of the ulna articulation) and another line that intersects the tip of the radial styloid
  - Normal = 11 to 12 mm.
  - Loss of radial height results from comminution and impaction of fracture fragments into the metaphysis
  - Ulnar variance changes of ≥3 mm can lead to acquired positive ulnar variance, ulnar impaction syndrome, and joint instability.

**NOTE: Clinical interpretation of this measurement necessitates comparison with the noninjured wrist.**

- **Volar tilt:** Measured on lateral radiograph as the angle between the distal radial articular surface and a line drawn perpendicular to the shaft of the radius
  - Normal = 11 degrees (range 2-20 degrees).
  - Chronic cases can lead to ulnar midcarpal instability.

**TIP:** Generally, the goal of treatment is to place the wrist in at least "neutral" (i.e., zero degrees angulation) position or better.

- **Radial inclination:** Measured on PA radiograph as the angle between a line drawn from the tip of the radial styloid to the ulnar corner of the distal end of the radius and a line drawn perpendicular to the shaft of the radius
  - Normal = 19 to 29 degrees, with average of 24 degrees.
  - Loss of radial inclination will translate into increased load across the lunate.

**NOTE: With fracture reduction, acceptable inclination should be >10-15 degrees.**

- **Teardrop angle:** Measured on lateral radiograph as the angle between a line drawn parallel to the subchondral bone along the volar rim of the lunate facet to a line drawn parallel to the central axis of the radial shaft.
  - Normal = 70 degrees.
  - Often reduced in extraarticular, dorsally displaced fractures and articular fractures secondary to axial loads
  - Strong indicator of articular incongruity within the lunate facet
- **AP distance:** Measured on lateral radiograph as the distance between the apices of the dorsal and volar rims
  - Normal = 19.1 mm, slight gender disparity exists (men = 17.8 mm, women = 19.1 mm)[15]
  - Indicates discontinuity between the volar and dorsal rims when elevated

**TIP:** Rule of 11s. These radiographic findings can be remembered as factors of 11: Volar tilt 11 degrees, radial length 11 mm, radial inclination 22 degrees.

## TREATMENT (Fig. 64-6)

### NONOPERATIVE

- **Principles of Intervention: ARMS**
  - **A**rticular congruity: Reduce wear and degenerative changes
  - **R**adial alignment and length: Restore kinematics of carpus and radioulnar joint
  - **M**otion: Digits, wrist, and forearm to optimize functional return
  - **S**tability: Preserve length and alignment during healing
- **Closed reduction and casting**
  - All patients with closed, nondisplaced extraarticular fractures, regardless of age or activity level
  - At least one attempt at closed reduction should be made on all displaced extraarticular fractures.
  - Follow-up is required for subsequent displacement. Splint/cast changes will likely be needed.
  - Serial radiographs
  - Only in elderly, inactive patients can 20 degrees dorsal angulation and 5 mm of shortening be accepted.

**TIP:** Late attrition rupture of the extensor pollicis longus (EPL) can occur with this fracture.

  - Closed reduction technique
    - Carpal tunnel symptoms should be investigated, before **and** after reduction.
    - Anesthesia achieved with hematoma block by infiltrating 10 ml 1% lidocaine into the fracture plane.

**TIP:** Look for "flash back" of blood to confirm correct location. Then infiltrate using repetitive "serial" steps in which several milliliters of anesthetic are expelled, followed by gentle aspiration of the hematoma/lidocaine mix.

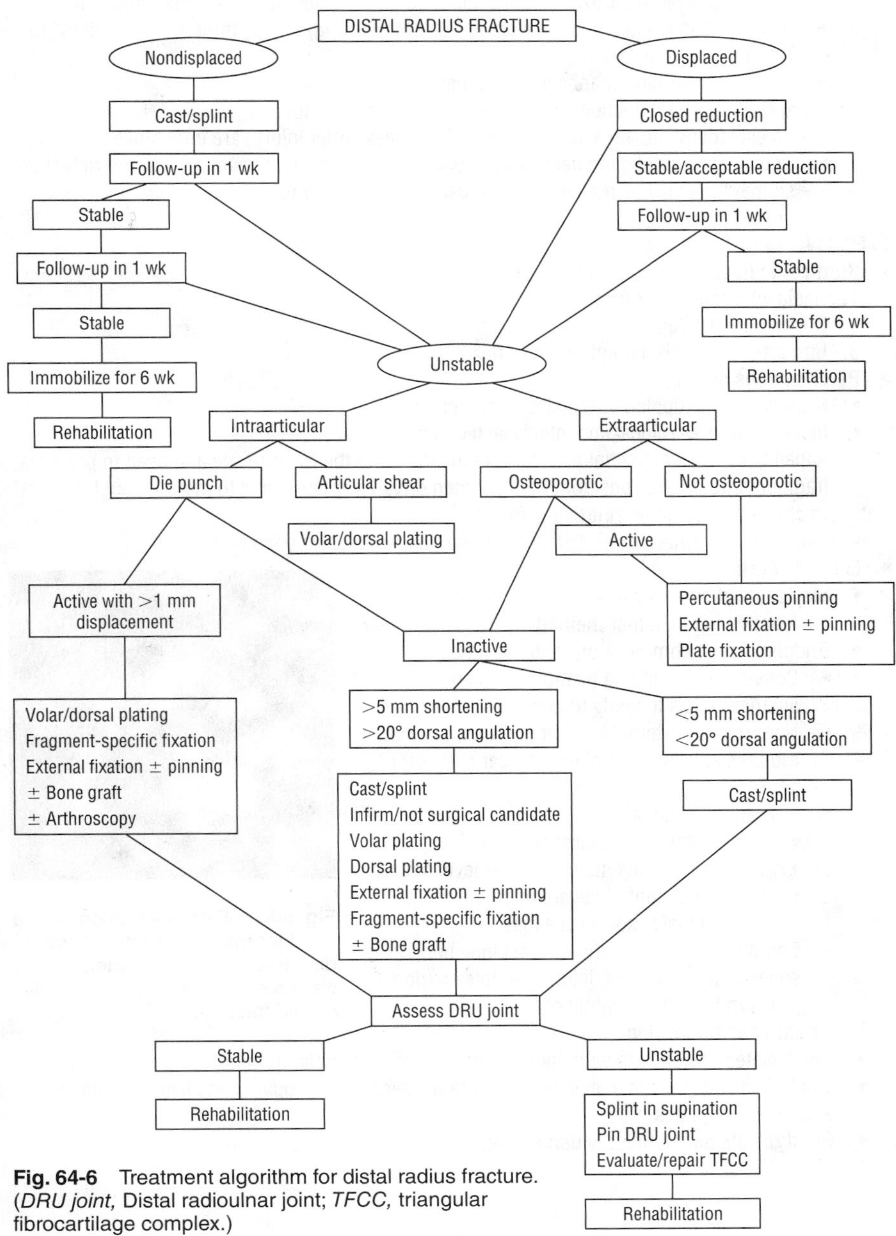


**Fig. 64-6** Treatment algorithm for distal radius fracture. (*DRU joint,* Distal radioulnar joint; *TFCC,* triangular fibrocartilage complex.)

- Extremity is placed under traction to distract soft tissues and unlock fracture fragments. Consider the use of finger traps (5-10 pounds for 10-15 minutes).
- With aid of assistant (who places countertraction above the elbow): The fracture is recreated by hyperextending the distal fracture fragment, which is immediately distracted distally to clear the proximal radial shaft, and then flexed to restore anatomic reduction.
- A sugar-tong plaster splint is placed (to allow swelling) using "three-point molding" to help maintain fracture reduction.
- Postreduction radiographs are essential.

- Adequate fracture reduction warrants a trial of closed therapy.
  - Weekly follow-up visits (during the initial 3 weeks after injury) are imperative.
  - Repeat radiographs are necessary to discover fractures that have fallen out of reduction so that they may be managed judiciously with operative fixation.

## Operative

- **Surgical indications**[16]
  1. Radial shortening >3 mm
  2. Dorsal tilt >10 degrees
  3. Intraarticular displacement or step-off >2 mm
- **Percutaneous pinning**
  - Best used as a supplement to closed reduction
  - Includes both extrafocal and interfocal techniques
  - Kapandji (interfocal) technique: Pins are inserted into the fracture site and used to pry distal fragment into optimal position. Pins are then driven from proximal to distal through the fracture site, providing **relative** stability.
  - Indicated for extraarticular distal radius fractures with good bone stock.
- **External fixation** (Fig. 64-7)
  - May be used alone, or more commonly in conjunction with another method
  - Bridging (most common) or nonbridging
    - Conventional bridging fixation relies on ligamentotaxis to apply traction.[17]
    - Nonbridging external fixation obviates this, but requires at least 1 cm of intact volar cortex for pin purchase.
    - Indications include[18]:
      - Temporizing polytrauma patients
      - Transferring patients to a higher level of care
      - Initial treatment of severe open fractures with extensive soft tissue loss
    - Complications common: Pin tract infection, superficial radial nerve injury (complex regional pain syndrome), unsightly scars

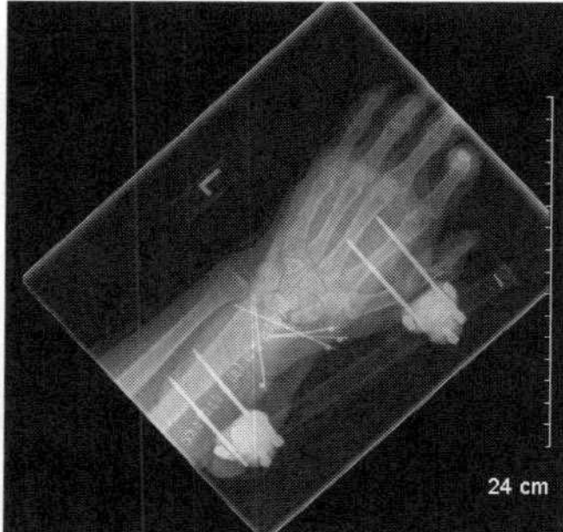


**Fig. 64-7** External fixation device used for management of distal radius fractures. Percutaneous pins were also used to stabilize a radial styloid fracture.

- **Fragment-specific fixation**
  - Small plates designed to withstand forces of immediate wrist motion
  - Limited use because of high incidence of radial sensory neuropathy and lengthy time to apply traction plates
  - Good results but technically demanding

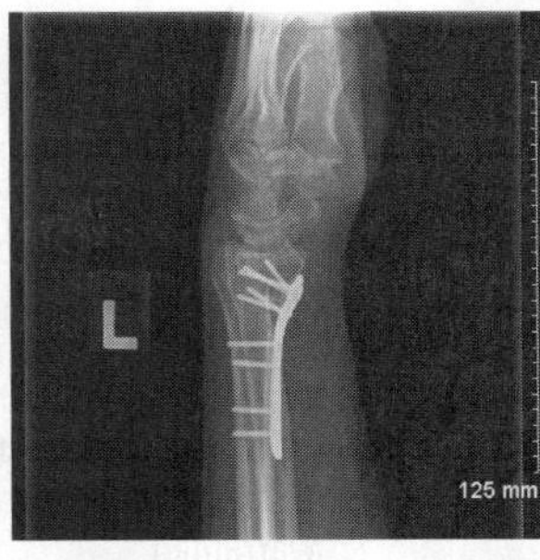


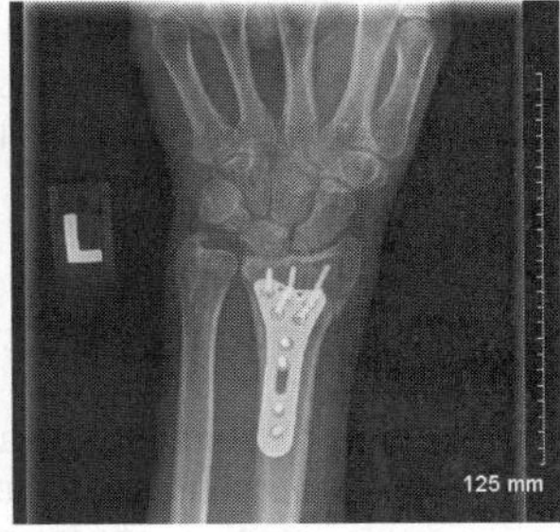


**Fig. 64-8** Fractures stabilized with volar plates in two patients.

- **Open reduction internal fixation (ORIF)**[19]
  - Unstable, displaced >1 mm
  - Original plating systems were dorsal. However, complications (extensor tendon irritation and rupture) led to lower-profile plates and the now-popular use of volar plating techniques. May also be assisted by arthroscopy.
  - *Articular congruity is paramount.*
  - Surgical approach: **Volar** approach and plating has become utilitarian in modern treatment (Fig. 64-8).
    - Allows improved early functional outcomes resulting from direct visualization of fracture, improved stability of fixation construct, reduced periods of postoperative immobilization, and faster returns of function.
  - Two general designs of plating mechanisms[20]:
    - **Buttress plates:** Designed to help reduce intraarticular fractures because of their antiglide effect
    - **Spanning plates:** Span metaphyseal comminution; rely on direct reduction of the fracture fragments, which they then can only help maintain. Two subdivisions:
      - **Conventional** plate design: Stability of the construct relies on screw purchase of the far cortex.
        - Disadvantages include potential collapse of the far cortex if already comminuted and reliance on anatomic contouring of the plate to the fracture.
      - **Locking** plate design: Achieves stability via transmission of axial forces to the screw/plate interface, sparing the need for screw purchase into the far cortex
        - Advantages include preserved periosteal blood supply of the proximal bony cortex.
  - Bone grafting or substitute
    - Filling of metaphyseal defects after reduction to length
    - Autologous still the benchmark; however, bone substitutes becoming more common because of ease and lack of further defect or secondary donor site
    - Most common: Demineralized bone matrix (DBX), cadaveric cancellous bone chips, hydroxyapatite (HA), and injectable bone cement
    - Some substitutes even confer strength to the repair, especially in osteoporotic bone.
- **Management of the TFCC:** After fixation, stability of DRU joint should be assessed with the **piano key test** intraoperatively, which is performed as follows:
  - The forearm is in neutral position while radioulnar joint undergoes dorsovolar shucking.
  - Alternatively, the radius or ulna can be manually displaced in both dorsal and volar directions while the other is stabilized.
  - Diagnosis of a complete peripheral tear of the TFCC has a sensitivity of 0.59, specificity of 0.96, and positive predictive value of 0.91.[21]
  - Stability on examination (negative test result): Treat with placement of a routine volar resting splint.[22]

- Instability of DRU joint on examination (positive test result) indicates disruption to the TFCC (Fig. 64-9).
  - If instability occurs in only certain positions of forearm rotation, treatment involves placement of a sugar-tong splint and/or radioulnar pinning with forearm in 60 degrees of supination for 6 weeks.
  - Management of gross instability elicited in all positions, however, is based on the presence of a large ulnar styloid fracture:
    - If absent, direct repair of the TFCC acutely is warranted.
    - If present, proceed with ORIF of the styloid fragment and reassess the DRU joint. Continued instability warrants direct repair of TFCC as above.

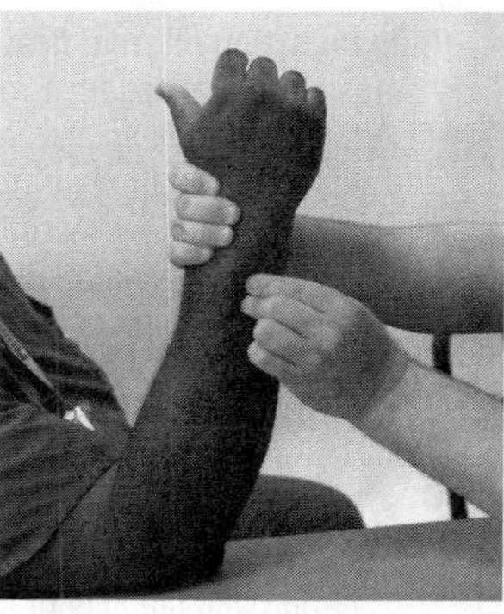

**Fig. 64-9** Clinical assessment of the DRU joint.

- Specific concerns[23]
  - **Pediatric fractures:** Management guidelines differ substantially, because fracture plating is highly avoided and fixation is dependent on pinning.
  - **Elderly patients:** Radiographic malunion has little effect on functional outcomes. Thus general consensus is for less aggressive treatment, because much higher degrees of displacement may be tolerated.

## ROUTINE POSTOPERATIVE CARE

- **Immediate**
  - Postoperative splint: Long-arm or sugar-tong to prevent forearm rotation
  - Digital ROM exercises
- **Early**
  - First follow-up: 7-14 days, evaluate incisions and sutures. Check reduction on radiograph.
  - Convert to removable splint if favorable fixation, reliable patient, and fracture pattern.
  - Begin forearm rotation and gentle, active wrist motion exercises.
  - If unfavorable (highly comminuted, microfragment fixation): Continue in short- or long-arm cast. Consider therapy at 4-6 weeks.
  - Evaluate with radiographs at 6 weeks.
- **Chronic**
  - OT may be beneficial formally for up to 3 months.
  - Therapy can progress ROM, strengthening for up to 1 year.
  - Least deforming tendon forces on fracture are thought to occur with forearm in supination.

## COMPLICATIONS

- **Early**
  - Overlooked associated injury
    - Ligamentous most common, ulnar styloid fracture, or carpal fractures
  - Loss of reduction, ± hardware failure
  - Infection or wound-healing problem
  - Iatrogenic injury to nerve, vessel, tendon

- Median/ulnar neuropathy, iatrogenic or postoperative carpal tunnel syndrome (CTS) (consider concomitant release in high-energy injuries or massive edema)
- Compartment syndrome (consider concomitant fasciotomies in high-energy injuries or massive edema)

■ **Late**
- Malunion or nonunion
- CTS
- Chronic regional pain syndrome: Less common than previously thought (<3% at 12 weeks)
- Hypertrophic scarring
- **Extensor pollicis longus** (EPL) or other tendon ruptures
- Joint stiffness, tendon adhesions
- Arthritis

## OUTCOMES

■ **Locking versus nonlocking volar plate fixation**
- Locking plates seem to provide benefits regarding surgical technique and comfort, improvement in implant anchorage (especially in osteoporotic bone), and reduced need for additional bone grafting.[24]

■ **Wrist pain after volar locking plates**
- Volar locking plates maintained reduction; however, incidence of wrist pain was significant. It was typically more often radial (45 versus 25). Logistic regression showed female sex and intraarticular fracture correlated significantly with radial-sided wrist pain.[25]

■ **Closed reduction and plaster cast fixation (CRPCF) versus external fixation (EF) in patients 65 and older**
- Fractures were AO type A or C, dorsally displaced without articular step-off or gap. Though not statistically significant, complications were more frequent in CRPCF group. All achieved union.[26]

### KEY POINTS

✓ Fractures of the distal radius are common with a bimodal distribution.
✓ High-quality radiographic assessment is instrumental both during the evaluation at the time of injury and at follow-up treatment.
✓ Thorough physical examination with specific attention to median nerve symptoms is paramount.
✓ Attempts at closed reduction/casting may obviate the need for operative intervention but warrant close follow-up.
✓ Advances in plate design, specifically volar plates with locking screws, allow maintenance of articular reduction while stabilizing comminution at the far cortex.

## REFERENCES

1. Smith DW, Brou KE, Henry MH. Early active rehabilitation for operatively stabilized distal radius fractures. J Hand Ther 17:43-49, 2004.
2. Rikli DA, Regazzoni P. Fractures of the distal end of the radius treated by internal fixation and early function. A preliminary report of 20 cases. J Bone Joint Surg Br 78:588-592, 1996.
3. Spinner EB. Kaplan's Functional and Surgical Anatomy of the Hand, 3rd ed. Philadelphia: Lippincott Williams & Wilkins, 1984.

4. Palmer AK, Werner FW. Biomechanics of the distal radioulnar joint. Clin Orthop Relat Res 187:26-35, 1984.
5. Berger RA, Weiss AP, eds. Hand Surgery. Philadelphia: Lippincott Williams & Wilkins, 2004.
6. Wolfe SW, Pederson WC, Hotchkiss RN, et al, eds. Green's Operative Hand Surgery, 6th ed. Philadelphia: Elsevier, 2011.
7. Frykman G. Fracture of the distal radius including sequelae—shoulder-hand-finger syndrome, disturbance in the distal radio-ulnar joint and impairment of nerve function. A clinical and experimental study. Acta Orthop Scand 108:103+, 1967.
8. Melone CP Jr. Distal radius fractures: patterns of articular fragmentation. Orthop Clin North Am 24:239-253, 1993.
9. Lichtenhahn P, Fernandez DL, Schatzker J. [Analysis of the "user friendliness" of the AO classification of fractures] Helv Chir Acta 58:919-924, 1992.
10. Jupiter JB, Fernandez DL. Comparative classification for fractures of the distal end of the radius. J Hand Surg Am 22:563-571, 1997.
11. Dresing K, Peterson T, Schmit-Neuerburg KP. Compartment pressure in the carpal tunnel in distal fractures of the radius. A prospective study. Arch Orthop Trauma Surg 113:285-289, 1994.
12. Richards RS, Bennett JD, Roth JH, et al. Arthroscopic diagnosis of intra-articular soft tissue injuries associated with distal radial fractures. J Hand Surg Am 22:772-776, 1997.
13. Trumble TE, Schmitt SR, Vedder NB. Internal fixation of pilon fractures of the distal radius. Yale J Biol Med 66:179-191, 1993.
14. Trumble TE, Schmitt SR, Vedder NB. Factors affecting functional outcome of displaced intra-articular distal radius fractures. J Hand Surg Am 19:325-340, 1994.
15. Medoff RJ. Essential radiographic evaluation for distal radius fractures. Hand Clin 21:279-288, 2005.
16. Garrett WE, Swiontkowski MF, Weinstein JN. The Treatment of Distal Radius Fractures. Guidelines and Evidence Report. Rosemont, IL: American Academy of Orthopaedic Surgeons, 2009.
17. Eichenbaum MD, Shin EK. Nonbridging external fixation of distal radius fractures. Hand Clin 26:381-390, 2010.
18. Bindra RR. Biomechanics and biology of external fixation of distal radius fractures. Hand Clin 21:363-373, 2005.
19. Trumble TE, Budoff JE, eds. Hand Surgery Update IV. Rosemont, IL: American Society for Surgery of the Hand, 2007.
20. Nana AD, Joshi A, Lichtman DM. Plating of the distal radius. J Am Acad Orthop Surg 13:159-171, 2005.
21. Lindau T, Adlercreutz C, Aspenberg P. Peripheral tears of the triangular fibrocartilage complex cause distal radioulnar joint instability after distal radial fractures. J Hand Surg 25:464-468, 2000.
22. Sammer DM, Chung KC. Management of the distal radioulnar joint and ulnar styloid fracture. Hand Clin 28:199-206, 2012.
23. Wysocki RW, Ruch DS. Ulnar styloid fracture with distal radius fracture. J Hand Surg 37:568-569, 2012.
24. Osti M, Mittler C, Zinnecker R, et al. Locking versus nonlocking palmar plate fixation of distal radius fractures. Orthopaedics 35:e1613-e1617, 2012.
25. Kurimoto S, Tatebe M, Shinohara T, et al. Residual wrist pain after volar locking plate fixation of distal radius fractures. Acta Orthop Belg 78:603-610, 2012.
26. Aktekin CN, Altay M, Gursoy Z, et al. Comparison between external fixation and cast treatment in the management of distal radius fractures in patients aged 65 years and older. J Hand Surg Am 35:736-742, 2010.

# 65. Metacarpal and Phalangeal Fractures

Tarik M. Husain, Danielle M. LeBlanc

## DEMOGRAPHICS[1]

- **Most common fractures of the upper extremity (10%)**
- **Outer rays** (thumb and fifth finger) are most commonly injured.
- 70% of all metacarpal and phalangeal fractures occur between ages 11 and 45.
- Operative fixation was first performed only 80 years ago.
- Degree of stabilization before or after closed reduction determines whether protective splints and/or early mobilization can be used.
- Operative fixation of hand fractures has increased for the following reasons:
  - Improved materials, implant designs, and instrumentation
  - Better understanding of biomechanical principles
  - More demanding public expectations
  - Better imaging: Radiographs, CT, MRI, fluoroscopy
  - Increased number of specialists in hand surgery
  - Improved anesthesia: Regional blocks, monitored anesthesia care (MAC)
  - Hand therapy

## ANATOMY

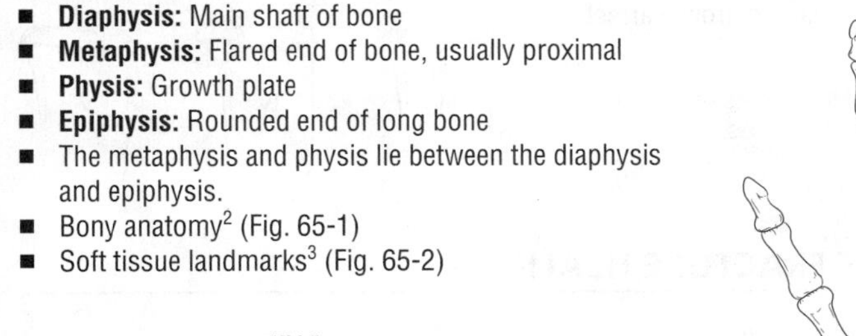

- **Diaphysis:** Main shaft of bone
- **Metaphysis:** Flared end of bone, usually proximal
- **Physis:** Growth plate
- **Epiphysis:** Rounded end of long bone
- The metaphysis and physis lie between the diaphysis and epiphysis.
- Bony anatomy[2] (Fig. 65-1)
- Soft tissue landmarks[3] (Fig. 65-2)

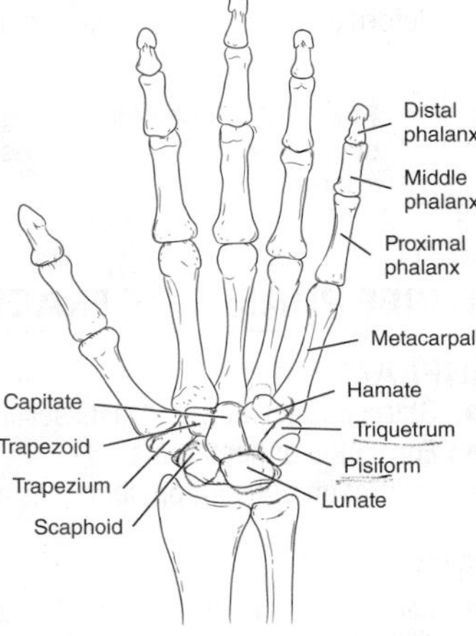


**Fig. 65-1** Bones of the hand and wrist.

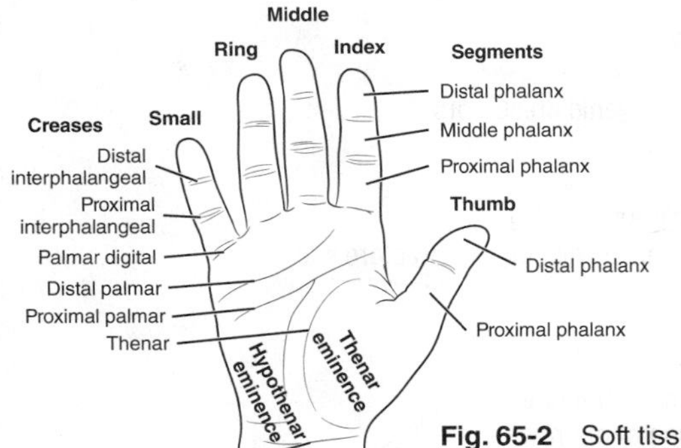


**Fig. 65-2** Soft tissue landmarks of the hand.

## FRACTURE TERMINOLOGY

- **Closed:** Intact skin over fracture and hematoma
- **Open:** Wound allows interaction between fracture and environment. (NOTE: "Compound fracture" is an outdated term and should not be used.)
- **Simple:** Two bone fragments
- **Comminuted:** More than two bone fragments
- **Transverse:** Fracture perpendicular to long axis of bone
- **Oblique:** Fracture tangential to long axis of bone
- **Spiral:** Fracture plane oblique and rotated
- **Impaction:** End-on stress force causing compression without displacement
- **Longitudinal:** Parallel to long axis of bone
- **Pathologic:** Fracture in tumor-laden or osteoporotic bone
- **Stress:** Fracture in normal bone caused by cyclic loading
- **Greenstick:** Incomplete fracture involving only one cortex
- **Avulsion:** Bone chip caused by distraction forces on tendon or ligament
- **Intraarticular:** Through articular surface

### Salter-Harris Fracture Classification: Pediatric Fractures[4] (Fig. 65-3)

- **Salter-Harris I:** Through growth plate only
- **Salter-Harris II:** Through metaphysis and growth plate
- **Salter-Harris III:** Through epiphysis and growth plate
- **Salter-Harris IV:** Through epiphysis, growth plate, and metaphysis
- **Salter-Harris V:** Crushed growth plate, may cause deformity in future secondary to growth arrest

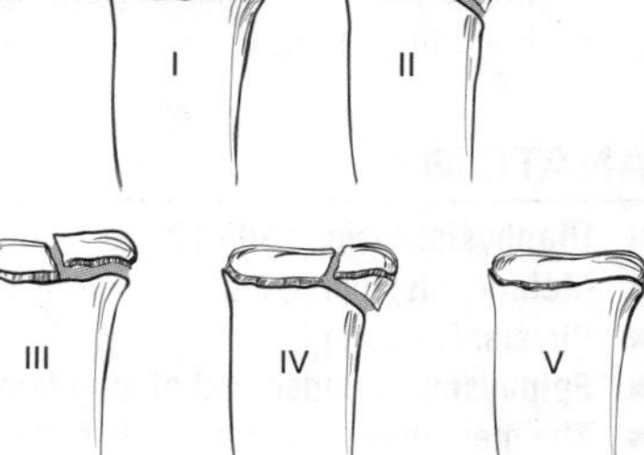


**Fig. 65-3** Salter-Harris classification system of pediatric fractures.

## THREE PHASES OF FRACTURE HEALING

### Inflammation

- Starts immediately and lasts several days
- Formation of hematoma
- Infiltration of hematopoietic cells and osteogenic precursors

### Repair

- Begins at <24 hours and peaks at 2-3 weeks
- Collagen deposition and cartilaginous callus formation over fracture site
- Endochondral ossification

### Remodeling

- Lasts months to years, depending on type of fracture
- Lamellar bone formation and repopulation of marrow
- Resorption of callus

**TIP:** External callus is not visible on plain radiographs until 3-6 weeks after formation. Clinical bony union averages 4-8 weeks; however, total bony healing time is approximately 5-7 months.[5]

**TIP:** In general, avoid NSAIDs in settings of acute fracture, because animal studies report adverse fracture healing and increased nonunion rates. There is some level IV evidence that a short-duration NSAID regimen may be safe. NSAIDs disrupt the inflammatory phase of fracture healing.[6]

## DIAGNOSIS

- History: Hand dominance and occupation, mechanism of injury
- Physical examination: Area(s) of tenderness, deformities, malrotation
- Neurovascular status: Needs to be checked and documented before anesthetization
- Soft tissue injury: Open or closed
- When documenting open wounds, use a grid system referencing the finger involved and soft tissue landmark (see Fig. 65-2).
  - Example: 2 cm transverse laceration over ring finger volar digital crease
  - It is also helpful to photograph the wound.
- Radiographs: AP/lateral at a minimum, often oblique and specialized views
- Plan is determined by considering the balance between early motion and adequate fracture stabilization.
  - Early motion may lead to fracture displacement or nonunion/malunion.
  - Long-term immobilization and/or surgical fixation may lead to stiffness.

## TREATMENT

**A treatment plan depends on many factors:**

- Patient age, occupation, health, and compliance
- Fracture location and geometry
- Clinical deformity
- Open or closed classification
- Associated soft tissue injury
- Stability

## COMPLICATIONS

### INFECTION

- Incidence 2%-11% in open fractures
- Usually results from contaminated wound or delay in treatment
- Antibiotics generally recommended for 24 hours for open fractures
- Management: Eradicate sepsis, obtain union of fracture, and regain function

### MALUNION

- **Malrotation:** Functional impairment caused by digital overlap on flexion
- **Angulation:** Lateral or volar angle deformity
- **Shortening:** Prevents balance of extensor or flexor excursion
- All types of malunion: Usually corrected with osteotomy, with or without bone graft

## Nonunion

*Nonunion occurs when fracture site fails to heal.*

- Usually results from unstable fracture reduction, contamination
- Atrophic: Lack of callus. Requires bone grafting.
- Hypertrophic: Callus has formed, but radiolucency persists and immobilization is insufficient. Requires more rigid fixation.
- Treatment: Corrective osteotomy and possible bone graft

## Loss of Motion

- Tendon adhesions
- Capsular contracture
- Immobilization for >4 weeks
- Associated joint injury
- Multiple fractures per finger
- Crush injury

# METACARPAL FRACTURES

## Metacarpal-Head Fractures

- Rare occurrence
- Result from axial loading, direct trauma, dislocation
- Usually intraarticular
- **Indications**[7]
  - **Nonoperative**
    - Closed fractures with articular congruency
    - Metacarpophalangeal (MP) joint stability by stress testing
    - <20% articular surface involvement
  - **Operative**[1]
    - >25% of the articular surface
    - >1 mm of articular step-off
    - Irreducible fracture
    - Malrotation: Difficult to determine on radiographs, must be assessed clinically; look for "scissoring" of fingers
    - Soft tissue injury such as tendon, nerve, or vessel laceration
    - Two-part fractures amenable to headless screws
    - Open fractures, particularly clenched fist injuries with presumed oral contamination
    - Comminuted fractures may need K-wires, spacers, or external fixation.
- **Treatment**[5]
  - Nonoperative options
    - Immobilize with wrist extended about 20-30 degrees, MP joints flexed 70-90 degrees, and interphalangeal (IP) joints in full extension (safe position) for 2-3 weeks, followed by ROM exercise (Fig. 65-4).
    - This maintains maximum stretch of collateral ligaments and decreases rate of stiffness.
  - **Surgical options**
    - Closed reduction/pinning
    - Open reduction internal fixation with pins/screws

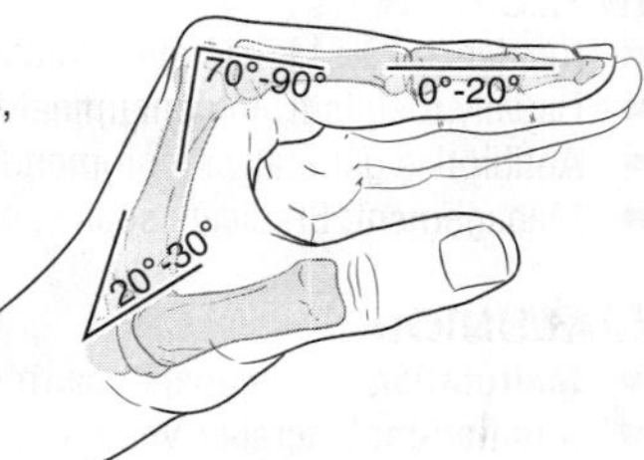

**Fig. 65-4** Safe position or intrinsic plus position of the hand.

- External fixation
- Prosthetic arthroplasty
- Arthrodesis

- **Simple fractures**
  - Surgically treated, open using dorsal approach with minicondylar plate or screws
  - K-wires also used, but may delay joint mobilization
  - May also use buried headless compression screws
- **Comminuted fractures**
  - K-wire fixation or cerclage wire is preferred, because risk of avascular necrosis is lower.
  - External fixator is required if proximal phalanx is also fractured or soft tissue loss is severe.
  - Fixation technique depends on fragment size and number.
- **Severe comminuted fractures**
  - May benefit from implant arthroplasty **except in index finger** (implant failure common because of shear stress), **extensive metacarpal bone loss,** or **extensive soft tissue loss**
  - MP arthrodesis only a salvage procedure

## METACARPAL NECK FRACTURES

- Common occurrence
- Occur when axial load applied to clenched fist
- **Apex dorsal angulation** because intrinsic muscles lie volar to axis of rotation of MP joint and maintain flexed head posture[5]
- Almost always heal and nonunion is rare; however, angular malunion is common
- *Boxer's fracture:* Small finger metacarpal neck fracture
  - Misnomer because professional boxers rarely get this type of fracture
  - True boxers more likely to have sagittal band ruptures at the MP joint, resulting in extensor tendon subluxation known as *boxer's knuckle*[1]
- **Indications for treatment**
  - **Angulation deformity**
    - Index and middle fingers: At least 10-15 degrees
    - Ring finger: At least 30-40 degrees
    - Small finger: At least 50-60 degrees
  - **Rotational deformity** or **scissoring:** Digital overlap in flexion
  - **Shortening:** >3 mm
  - **Extensor lag**

> **TIP:** Ring and small fingers can better compensate for fracture angulation, because carpometacarpal (CMC) joints have 20-30 degrees of mobility in sagittal plane, whereas index and middle fingers are less mobile at CMC joint.

- **Treatment**[5,7]
  - Most closed MC neck fractures are treated nonoperatively with dorsal block cast or ulnar gutter splint (intrinsic plus) for 3-4 weeks.
  - When performing closed treatment, counsel patient that the knuckle may appear depressed, but full function is usually expected.
  - If reduction cannot be maintained, then use K-wire fixation in crossed/transverse/intramedullary configuration.
  - Plate fixation should be last resort to avoid extensive dissection and MP stiffness.

- **Closed reduction is performed to treat malrotation or pseudoclawing.**
  - Perform this under local anesthetic or hematoma block.
  - **Jahss maneuver**[1] (Fig. 65-5): Flexing the MP joint to 90 degrees relaxes the intrinsic muscles and tightens collateral ligaments, allowing proximal phalanx to place upward pressure on metacarpal head while placing downward pressure on metacarpal shaft.
  - Stable reduction is held by molded splint with wrist extended 20-30 degrees, MP joint flexed 90 degrees, and proximal interphalangeal (PIP) joint in extension for 12-14 days. (Do not keep PIP joints flexed, because this may lead to long-term stiffness.)
  - Unstable reduction can be treated by crossed K-wires or transverse K-wires applied to intact adjacent metacarpal shaft.

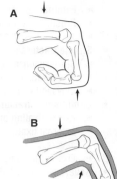

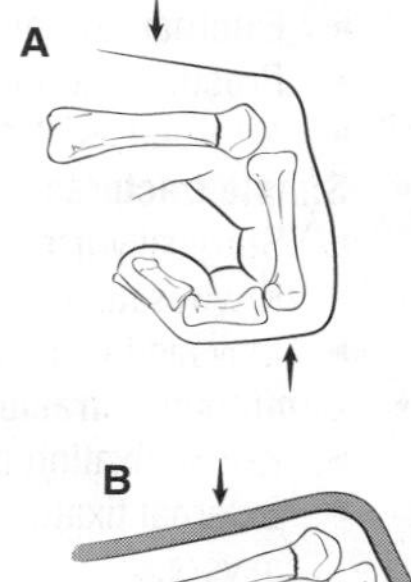


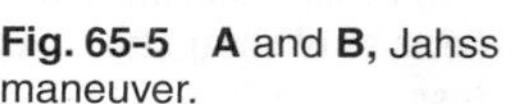


**Fig. 65-5** **A** and **B,** Jahss maneuver.

**TIP:** Closed reduction is difficult if fracture is more than 5-7 days old.[8]

- **Open reduction**
  - Dorsal approach is through a longitudinal incision adjacent to extensor tendon overlying fractured metacarpal; juncturae tendinum can be divided and repaired with permanent suture.
  - Use K-wires or minicondylar plate.
  - Immobilize patient for 10 days in molded splint; confirm alignment using radiography, then protect active ROM.

■ There are many controversial articles on the treatment of metacarpal neck fractures, and no clear consensus.
- Hansen and Hansen[9] reported better ROM and less pain with functional brace versus casting and elastic bandage treatments.
- Hunter and Cowen[10] reported that patients had no significant disability with up to 70 degrees of angulation.
  - According to their protocol, reduction was not attempted for angulation $<40$ degrees.
- Statius Muller et al[11] found no statistical difference between cast immobilization versus immediate mobilization in fractures with angulations $\leq 70$ degrees.
- Tavassoli et al[12] compared three different casting techniques and found no difference with regard to ROM, grip strength, or maintenance of reduction.

## Metacarpal Shaft Fractures

■ Classification based on radiographs: **Transverse, oblique** (or spiral), **comminuted**
- **Transverse**
  - Caused by axial load, apex dorsal angulation, interosseous muscles are deforming force
  - Reduce if angulation $>30$ degrees in small finger, $>20$ degrees in ring finger, and any angulation in index/middle finger

- **Oblique/spiral**
  - Caused by torsional forces
  - Can cause rotational malalignment; difficult to judge by radiographs and requires clinical assessment
  - Flex all fingers simultaneously and look for scissoring.
- **Comminuted**
  - Caused by direct impact, often associated with soft tissue injury, usually results in shortening

■ **Apex dorsal angulation:** Caused by interosseous muscles

■ **Indications for treatment:**

- **Dorsal angulation**
  - Index or middle fingers: At least 10 degrees
  - Ring finger: At least 20 degrees
  - Small finger: At least 30 degrees
- **Rotational deformity:** Digital overlap in flexion
- **Shortening in excess of 3 mm:** Alters length-tension relationship of intrinsic muscles, causing weakness

> **TIP:** 10 degrees of rotation equals 1.5 cm of digital overlap.[13]

■ **Treatment**

- Closed reduction and plaster/fiberglass immobilization
- Most metacarpal shaft fractures are stable.
  - Rettig et al[14] reported that 82% of metacarpal fractures were minimally displaced or nondisplaced.
  - Burkhalter cast: Advocated closed treatment if no rotational deformity, with short arm cast and dorsal hood in safe position[15] (see Fig. 65-4)
- **Operative reduction**
  - Indicated for **unstable reductions, multiple fractures, or open fractures**
  - Fixation method dependent on fracture pattern
  - Exposure through longitudinal dorsal incision adjacent to extensor tendon that overlies fractured metacarpal; juncturae tendinum divided and repaired with permanent suture; reduction held with bone clamps
- **Closed reduction and percutaneous pinning**
  - Antegrade or retrograde pinning
  - Pins may interfere with extensor tendon function if not buried
  - May also use transverse K-wires (usually two distal, one proximal)
- **Open reduction and internal fixation**
  - Melone[16] found that about 10% of phalangeal and metacarpal fractures were irreducible by closed means.
  - Indications:
    - Open fractures
    - Multiple fractures
    - Unstable fractures
    - Malalignment/malrotation

- **Open reduction options:**
  - **K-wires**
    - May be used for nearly any fracture pattern
    - Technically easy with minimal dissection
    - Universally available
    - Configuration may be crossed, transverse, longitudinal (intramedullary), or combination[1] (Fig. 65-6, *A*).
    - Not rigid
    - May loosen or migrate
    - Risk of pin tract infections
  - **Composite (tension band) wiring**[1] (Fig. 65-6, *B*)
    - Combination of K-wires (0.035 inch or 0.045 inch) with monofilament steel wire, usually 24- or 26-gauge
    - Principle: Tensile force converted to a compressive force
  - **Cerclage and interosseous wiring**
    - Cerclage wire is circumferential wiring for oblique and spiral metacarpal shaft fractures.
    - Excellent results have been reported but it is not popular method.
  - **Intramedullary fixation**[17] (Fig. 65-7)
    - Best indication: Transverse fracture
    - Easy to perform, allows early active motion
    - Commercially available systems (Small Bone Fixation System; Biomet, Warsaw, IN)
    - Disadvantages: Rotational instability (although a derotational pin may be used), pin migration, and fracture distraction.
  - **Interfragmentary compression screws (lag screws)**
    - Indicated for *long oblique fractures*
    - Stable enough for early active ROM
    - Fracture length should be twice bone diameter.
    - Use bone clamp to hold reduction.
    - Screws are usually 2.7, 2.4, or 2 mm.
    - Screw should be placed a minimum of two screw head diameters from fracture margin.
    - Trajectory of drill should be perpendicular to the fracture site.
    - Near drill hole should be same diameter as screw diameter.
    - Far drill hole should be smaller diameter than screw diameter.
    - Differential drill hole diameters allow the screw to compress across the fracture site.
  - **Plate fixation**
    - More stable than K-wires or interosseous wiring
    - Requires extensive dissection and periosteal stripping
    - Disadvantages: Tendon adhesions, plate loosening or breakage, stiffness, malunion/nonunion
    - Most implants are made of stainless steel or titanium.
    - Titanium is more expensive but has lower incidence of corrosion, easier to contour, and modulus of elasticity approaches that of bone.

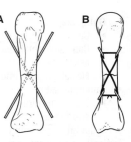

**Fig. 65-6** **A,** Crossed K-wires. **B,** Tension band wiring.

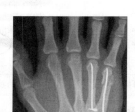

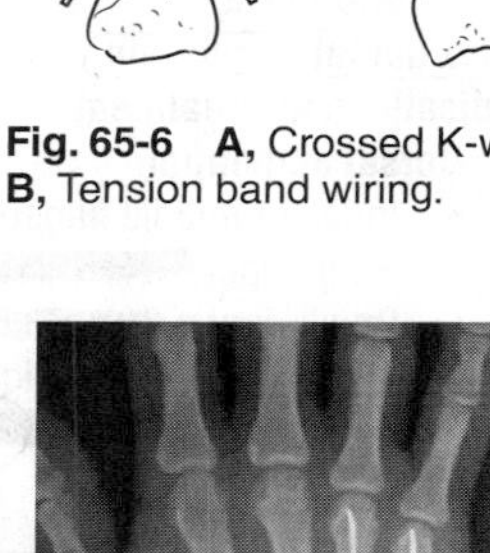

**Fig. 65-7** Intramedullary fixation.

- **External fixation**[1] (Fig. 65-8)
  - Respects bone biology
  - Fracture fragments not stripped of periosteal blood supply
  - Adjustable
  - If adequate stability, can initiate early ROM
  - Complications: Pin tract infections, osteomyelitis, fracture through pin holes, overdistraction/nonunion, impairment of tendon gliding
- **Bioabsorbable fixation**
  - Infrequently used in United States, but more common in Europe
  - Bioabsorbable plates reported to have torsional rigidity comparable with 2.3 mm titanium plating
  - Advantage: Removal unnecessary
  - First generation: Polyglycolic acid
  - Newer generation: Poly-L-lactide
  - High rates of inflammatory response (up to 25%)

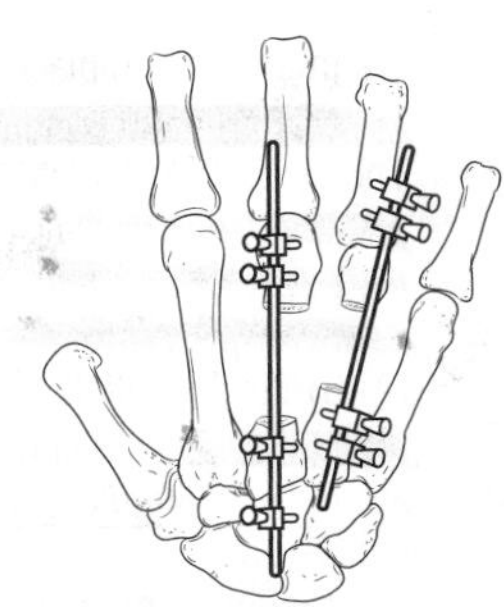

**Fig. 65-8** External fixation.

> **TIP:** Use lag screw technique for oblique or spiral fractures, when the ratio of length of fracture plane/width of bone is 2:1 to 3:1 at the fracture site.

## Segmental Loss of Metacarpal Shaft

**NOTE: Segmental loss almost always involves open injury with soft tissue loss; initial management requires debridement.**

- **Treatment**
  - Open injury requires thorough debridement and maintenance of length.
  - Freeland et al[18] believed the best time to restore osseous stability was within 10 days of injury, with bone graft and internal fixation.
  - Provisional stabilization maintains length.
    - Transfixation pins, external fixation, methylmethacrylate spacers, or combination can be used.
    - Most defects can be bridged with autogenous iliac crest corticocancellous graft[1] (Fig. 65-9).

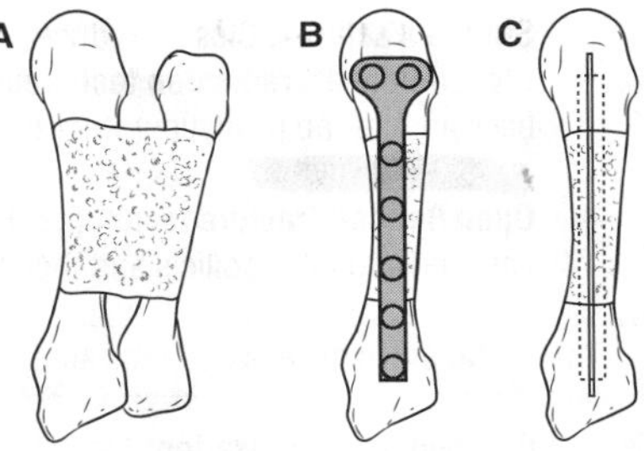


**Fig. 65-9** **A-C,** Corticocancellous bone graft.

## Metacarpal Base Fractures

- Rare occurrence
- Result from axial load on volar flexed wrist or partially flexed thumb
- Usually intraarticular
- **Bennett fracture:**
  - Single volar/ulnar fracture fragment of thumb base metacarpal
  - Unstable intraarticular thumb fracture of metacarpal base, two-part fracture

- Fragment held in place by anterior oblique or volar beak ligament
- The deforming forces: Abductor pollicis longus (APL) proximally and abductor pollicis brevis (APB)/flexor pollicis brevis (FPB) distally, causing apex dorsal angulation and subluxation
- The reduction maneuver: Longitudinal traction, pressure at the thumb MC base, and pronation[1] (Fig. 65-10)

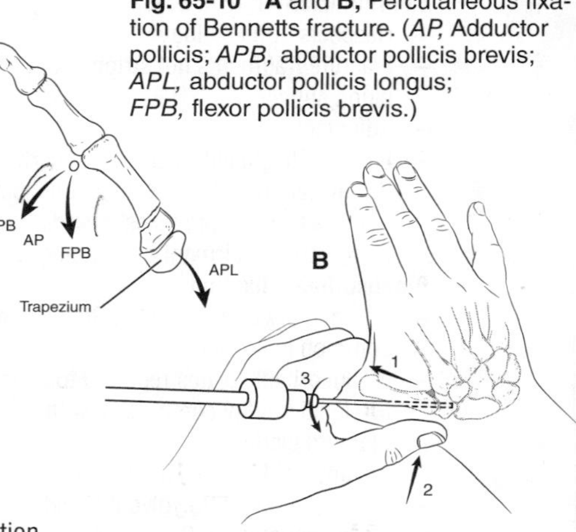


**Fig. 65-10** **A** and **B,** Percutaneous fixation of Bennetts fracture. (*AP,* Adductor pollicis; *APB,* abductor pollicis brevis; *APL,* abductor pollicis longus; *FPB,* flexor pollicis brevis.)

- **Reverse Bennett fracture:**
  - Unstable intraarticular fracture
  - Dislocation of fifth metacarpal base, causing proximal and dorsal subluxation of metacarpal
  - Displacement accentuated by flexor carpi ulnaris (FCU), extensor carpi ulnaris (ECU), and abductor digiti minimi (ADM)
- **Rolando fracture:** Any comminuted intraarticular fracture of thumb metacarpal base
- **Indications for treatment**
  - **Usually operative** because of unstable dislocation component
  - Open versus closed technique depends on fracture morphology

**TIP:** Open reduction is indicated in multiple CMC joint dislocations.

- **Treatment**
  - **Simple fractures:** Closed, reduced, and stabilized with K-wire fixation
  - **Closed Bennett reduction technique:** Longitudinal traction with pressure on metacarpal base and thumb pronation; K-wires placed through thumb metacarpal into trapezium and second metacarpal
  - **Open Bennett fracture technique:** Performed through radial border incision located between abductor pollicis and thenar muscles with screw or K-wire fixation

**TIP:** No pin is necessary in the actual Bennett fracture fragment.

- **Rolando fracture fixation:** Closed K-wire preferred because of comminuted fragments; if feasible, miniplate fixation on larger fragments
- **Severely comminuted fractures:** May require oblique traction pin or quadrilateral external fixator
- **Reverse Bennett fracture-dislocations:**
  - Inherently unstable
  - Difficult to follow radiographically to assess redislocation or resubluxation without proper views and/or C-arm fluoroscopy
  - Reduce by longitudinal traction and volar pressure at base of small finger metacarpal
  - Pin small finger to ring finger metacarpal and also small finger to hamate.
  - May also plate
  - If small finger/hamate joint arthritis develops, can perform arthrodesis

- **Open reverse Bennett reduction:** Performed through dorsal ulnar incision with protection of dorsal sensory branch of ulnar nerve; fixation held with multiple K-wires

- **Metacarpal fracture complications**
  - Malunion: Usually apex dorsal after transverse
  - Malrotation
    - Weckesser advocated osteotomy through base with 25 degrees of correction.
    - Transverse metacarpal ligament limits maximal rotation.
  - Intraarticular malunion: Rarely correctable
  - Osteomyelitis
    - Remove metallic implants, check radiographs, debride, external fixation, antibiotic spacer, IV antibiotics
    - Second stage: Bone graft and plate/screw fixation
  - Nonunion: Hypertrophic rare, atrophic common
  - Tendon adhesions

## PHALANGEAL FRACTURES

### DISTAL PHALANX FRACTURES

- Distal phalanx fractures are the **most common fractures of the hand.**
- **Thumb** and **middle finger** are most commonly injured.
- See Chapters 67 and 68 for discussion of fingertip and nail bed injuries.
- **Classification**
  - **Tuft fractures**
    - History
      - Doors are most common cause of trauma.
      - Smashing between two objects
      - Lacerations from yard or workshop tools
      - Thin/sharp object versus wide/dull object
    - Examination
      - Long finger is the most frequently injured.
      - Nail bed is usually injured distally.
      - Lacerations may be simple, stellate, crush, or avulsion.
    - Radiographs: 50% chance of bone injury with nail bed injury
    - Treatment
      - Closed fractures frequently present with subungual hematoma.
      - Decompress wound with a small drill bit, heated paper clip, or battery-powered electrocautery.
      - Can immobilize for 14 days
      - Comminuted fractures rarely require fixation.
      - Focus on approximating pulp and nail matrix.
      - Nail should be removed if nail matrix injury is suspected.
      - Fractures rarely unite, but they clinically heal with fibrous union.
      - If a closed fracture undergoes decompression or nail removal, it has been converted into an open fracture. Therefore oral antibiotics are indicated.
  - **Shaft fractures**
    - Transverse or longitudinal orientation
    - Treatment:
      - Nondisplaced fractures usually stabilized by soft tissues
      - Displaced fractures usually associated with nail matrix laceration and may require K-wire pinning

- **Intraarticular fractures**
  - Avulsion fracture of insertion of extensor tendon called ***mallet finger*** (bony or soft tissue only)
  - Dorsal base fracture with secondary mallet finger deformity caused by hyperextension of distal interphalangeal (DIP) joint
  - Epiphyseal separation from hyperflexion common in children; can result in foreshortened digit and decreased ROM at DIP joint
  - Volar base fracture from forceful flexion and profundus tendon avulsion

■ **Treatment**

- **Nondisplaced** fractures stabilized by surrounding tissue
- **Comminuted** fragments reduced by careful approximation of soft tissues
- **Displaced** fractures stabilized with longitudinal K-wires
- Immobilization with finger cast for $<$3 weeks, excluding PIP joint

**TIP:** Comminuted tuft fractures often fail to unite but are stabilized by fibrous union.[19]

- Symptomatic nonunion may be treated by crossed K-wires and bone graft using open volar midline approach.[20]
- **Mallet finger** treatment discussed in Chapter 70.
  - Extension splinting for 8 weeks.
  - May require pinning in noncompliant patient
  - Surgical indication
    - If more than a third to half of the articular surface is displaced
    - Volar subluxation of distal phalanx
    - Extension block pinning (Fig. 65-11)

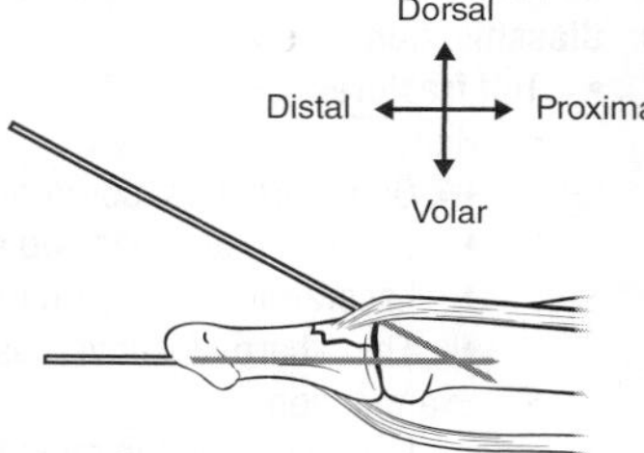


**Fig. 65-11** Extension block pinning.

- **Epiphyseal fractures** (Seymour injury)
  - In children, a transverse laceration of the nail matrix causes the avulsed nail plate to lie superficial to the nail fold.
  - Treatment
    - Irrigation and debridement
    - Fracture reduction
    - Repair of the lacerated nail matrix
    - Replacement of the nail plate beneath the nail fold to act as a stent to reduction
  - Failure to recognize fracture may result in osteomyelitis or septic arthritis (or both).

## Middle and Proximal Phalanx Fractures[21]

■ **Classification**[5,22]

- **Phalangeal head articular fractures (unicondylar versus bicondylar)**
  - Classified by Weiss and Hastings[23]
    - Type I: Stable fractures without displacement
    - Type II: Unicondylar, unstable fracture
    - Type III: Bicondylar, comminuted fractures
- **Neck fractures**
  - Subcapital fractures uncommon in adults but common in children

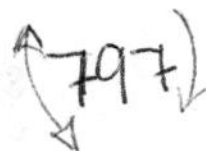

- **Shaft fractures**
  - Transverse, spiral, or oblique
  - Critical to evaluate rotational deformity
    - Flex/extend fingers while observing nail plates.
    - Compare results with those of contralateral hand.
    - Any overlapping of fingers is a surgical indication.
  - Nondisplaced fracture treatment: Buddy taping and/or splinting
  - Displaced fracture that reduces: Stabilize with intrinsic plus immobilization
  - Surgical treatment
    - K-wires
    - Interfragmentary screws
    - Wiring
    - Plate fixation
  - Requires extensive dissection and can result in stiffness with need for plate removal and subsequent tenolysis

TIP: Proximal phalanx shaft fractures anglulate apex volar because of flexion of the proximal fragment by the interossei. Middle phalanx shaft fractures can angulate apex volar or apex dorsal, depending on the location of the fracture in relation to the insertion of the flexor digitorum superficialis (FDS) tendon.[24]

- **Base fractures**
  - Typically involve impaction with **apex volar** angulation
  - Up to 25 degrees of angulation tolerated but may result in loss of motion
  - *Malunion:* "**Pseudoclawing**" possible when hyperextension of MP at fracture site and extensor lag at PIP joint
  - **Lateral volar base avulsions:** Result of detached collateral ligament
  - **Gamekeeper's thumb:** Proximal phalanx avulsion of ulnar collateral ligament at ulnar volar base
  - **Dorsal base avulsion fractures:** From detached central slip with PIP dislocation (see Chapter 66)
- **Pilon fractures**
  - Comminuted intraarticular fractures at base of middle phalanx
  - Caused by axial load

■ **Treatment**

- **Articular fractures (condylar head)**
  - Require stabilization with K-wires, miniplates or lag screws, depending on fracture morphology
  - Displaced fractures require open reduction using dorsal approach through central slip and lateral band.
- **Neck fractures**
  - **Nondisplaced fractures:** Can be treated with closed reduction and splinting
  - **Displaced fractures:** Head fragment often rotated 90 degrees, with articular surface facing dorsal and fracture surface volar
  - Open reduction from dorsal approach with displacement of interposed volar plate and stabilization with K-wires

- **Shaft fractures**
  - **Stable, nondisplaced fractures:** Require splinting in safe position to prevent collateral ligament and volar plate contracture (see Fig. 65-4)
  - **Unstable, displaced fractures:** May require closed fixation with K-wires, lag screws, interosseous wires, or miniplates
  - **Comminuted shaft fractures:** May require external fixator
- Base or **pilon fractures (including PIP joint fracture/dislocations)**
  - **Gamekeeper's thumb:** Requires fixation of fragment displacement that is at least 2 mm; also requires thumb spica immobilization
  - Displaced collateral ligament avulsion fractures of all other digits: Require open reduction and repair if joint laterally unstable
  - Usually require open reduction and fixation to preserve articular surface
    - K-wires
    - Screws
    - Dynamic external fixation[25] (Fig. 65-12)
    - Hook-plate[26] (Fig. 65-13)
    - Hemihamate arthroplasty[27]
  - Reduction or correction osteotomy: Required if **angular malunion is at least 25 degrees** to prevent loss of motion and pseudoclaw deformity (hyperextension of MP at fracture site with extensor lag)

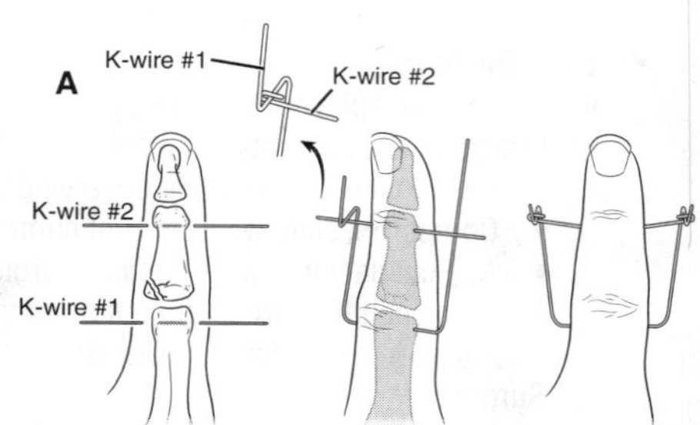


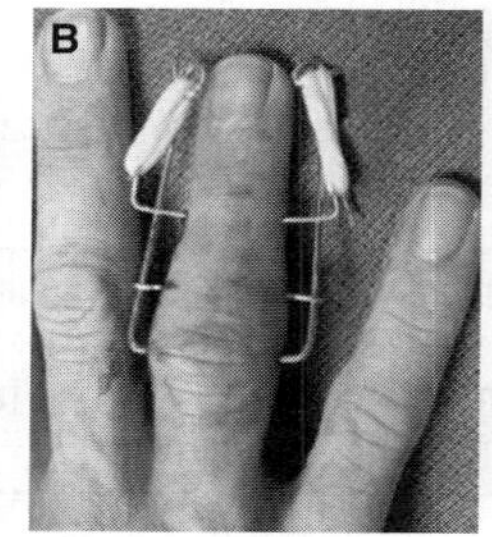


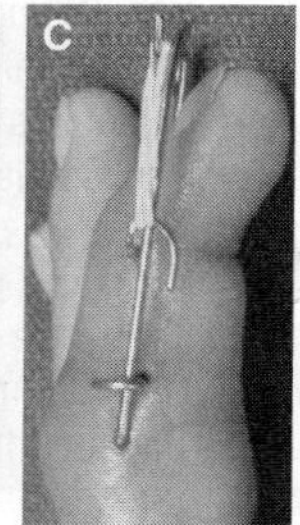


**Fig. 65-12 A-C,** Dynamic external fixation.

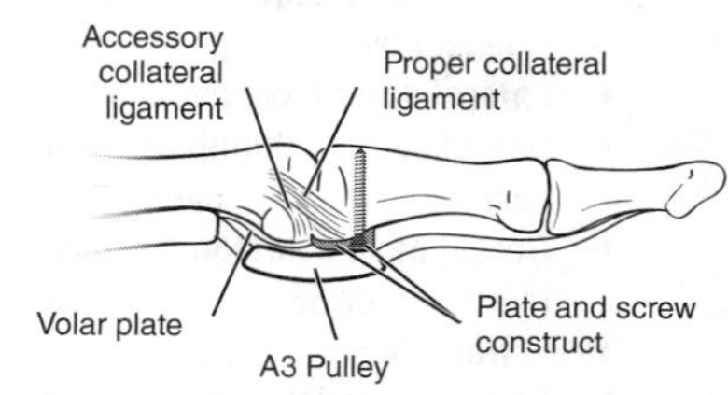


**Fig. 65-13** Hook-plate fixation.

**Box 65-1** *INDICATIONS FOR METACARPAL AND PHALANGEAL FRACTURE FIXATION*

- Irreducible fractures
- Malrotation (spiral and short oblique)
- Intraarticular fractures
- Subcapital fractures (phalangeal)
- Open fractures
- Segmental bone loss
- Polytrauma with hand fractures
- Multiple hand or wrist fractures
- Fractures with soft tissue injury (e.g., vessel, tendon, nerve, skin)
- Reconstruction (e.g., osteotomy)

## Key Points

- ✓ The Salter-Harris classification is used only with pediatric fractures.
- ✓ In general, metacarpal and phalangeal fractures are treated operatively if there is scissoring, rotation, or shortening.
- ✓ The Jahss maneuver may help with closed reduction of a fifth metacarpal neck fracture (boxer's fracture).
- ✓ Only a small amount of rotation is needed to produce a significant amount of digital overlap.
- ✓ Lag screws are ideal for long oblique fractures and should be placed perpendicular to the fracture and the long axis of the bone. Both should be at least two screw-head diameters away from the fracture.
- ✓ Avoid opening comminuted fractures, if possible.
- ✓ In general, avoid plating metacarpal and phalangeal fractures if they are amenable to K-wire or intramedullary fixation.
- ✓ In general, immobilize in the safe position (see Fig. 65-4).

## References


1. Day CS, Stern PJ. Fractures of the metacarpals and phalanges. In Wolfe SW, Hotchkiss RN, Pederson WC, et al, eds. Green's Operative Hand Surgery, 6th ed. Philadelphia: Churchill Livingstone, 2011.
2. Zenn MR, Jones G. Reconstructive Surgery: Anatomy, Technique, & Clinical Applications. St Louis: Quality Medical Publishing, 2012.
3. American Society for Surgery of the Hand. Hand Anatomy. Available at *http://www.assh.org/Public/HandAnatomy/Pages/default.aspx.*
4. PediatricEducation.org. What are the Salter-Harris Fracture Types? Available at *http://www.pediatric-education.org/2005/10/03/.*
5. Stern PJ. Fractures of the metacarpals and phalanges. In Green DP, Hotchkiss RN, Pederson WC, eds. Green's Operative Hand Surgery, 4th ed. Philadelphia: Churchill Livingstone, 1999.
6. Kurmis AP, Kurmis TP, O'Brien JX, et al. The effect of nonsteroidal anti-inflammatory drug administration on acute phase fracture-healing: a review. J Bone Joint Surg Am 94:815-823, 2012.
7. Weinstein LP, Hanel DP. Metacarpal fractures. J Hand Surg Am 2:168-180, 2002.
8. Opgrande JD, Westphal SA. Fractures of the hand. Orthop Clin North Am 14:779-792, 1983.
9. Hansen PB, Hansen TB. The treatment of fractures of the ring and little metacarpal necks. A prospective randomized study of three different types of treatment. J Hand Surg Br 23:245-247, 1998.
10. Hunter JM, Cowen NJ. Fifth metacarpal fractures in a compensation clinic population. A report on one hundred and thirty-three cases. J Bone Joint Surg Am 52:1159-1165, 1970.
11. Statius Muller MG, Poolman RW, van Hoogstraten MJ, et al. Immediate mobilization gives good results in boxer's fractures with volar angulation up to 70 degrees: a prospective randomized trial comparing immediate mobilization with cast immobilization. Arch Orthop Trauma Surg 123:534-537, 2003.
12. Tavassoli J, Ruland RT, Hogan CJ, et al. Three cast techniques for the treatment of extra-articular metacarpal fractures. Comparison of short-term outcomes and final fracture alignments. J Bone Joint Surg Am 87:2196-2201, 2005.
13. Freeland AE, Jabaley ME, Hughes JL. Stable Fixation of the Hand and Wrist. New York: Springer-Verlag, 1986.
14. Rettig AC, Ryan R, Shelbourne KD, et al. Metacarpal fractures in the athlete. Am J Sports Med 17:567-572, 1989.
15. Hamilton SW, Aboud H. Finite element analysis, mechanical assessment and material comparison of two volar slab constructs. Injury 40:397-399, 2009.

16. Melone CP Jr. Rigid fixation of phalangeal and metacarpal fractures. Orthop Clin North Am 17:421-435, 1986.
17. Hand Innovations. The first percutaneous locked flexible intramedullary nail system for hand fractures. Available at *http://www.biomet.com/traumaTransition/country/pr/products/files/SBFS%20Surgical%20Technique.pdf.*
18. Freeland AE, Jabaley ME, Burkhalter WE, et al. Delayed primary bone grafting in the hand and wrist after traumatic bone loss. J Hand Surg Am 9:22-28, 1984.
19. Schneider LH. Fractures of the distal phalanx. Hand Clin 4:537-547, 1988.
20. Itoh Y, Uchinishi K, Oka Y. Treatment of pseudarthrosis of the distal phalanx with the palmar midline approach. J Hand Surg Am 8:80-84, 1983.
21. Freeland AE, Sud V. Unicondylar and bicondylar proximal phalangeal fractures. J Hand Surg Am 1:14-24, 2001.
22. London PS. Sprains and fractures involving the interphalangeal joints. Hand 3:155-158, 1971.
23. Weiss AP, Hastings H II. Distal unicondylar fractures of the proximal phalanx. J Hand Surg Am 18:594-599, 1993.
24. McNealy RW, Lichtenstein ME. Fractures of the metacarpals and phalanges. West J Surg Obstet Gynecol 43:156-161, 1935.
25. Ruland RT, Hogan CJ, Cannon DL, et al. Use of dynamic distraction external fixation for unstable fracture-dislocations of the proximal interphalangeal joint. J Hand Surg Am 33:19-25, 2008.
26. Kang GC, Yam A, Phoon ES, et al. The hook plate technique for fixation of phalangeal avulsion fractures. J Bone Joint Surg Am 94:e72, 2012.
27. Yang DS, Lee SK, Kim KJ, et al. Modified hemihamate arthroplasty technique for treatment of acute proximal interphalangeal joint fracture-dislocations. Ann Plast Surg 2012 Dec 13. [Epub ahead of print]

# 66. Phalangeal Dislocations

Rohit K. Khosla, Douglas S. Fornfeist

## CLINICAL EVALUATION OF THE JOINT[1-3]

- Assess functional stability of the joint under digital or wrist block.
- **Active stability**
  - Evaluate active range of motion of the involved joint.
  - Full or near-complete range of motion indicates joint stability.
  - *Dislocation with motion indicates an unstable joint.*
- **Passive stability**
  - Lateral stress is applied to joint at full extension and at 30 degrees of flexion to assess integrity of collateral ligaments.
  - Dorsal stress and volar stress are applied to joint.
  - Compare joint laxity with an uninjured digit and contralateral digit to confirm injury from patient's normal joint laxity.
- Review routine plain radiographs, which must include at least three views of the affected area (AP, lateral, and oblique).
  - The joints proximal and distal to the area of concern should be visualized radiographically.
- Joint may dislocate in **dorsal, lateral,** or **volar** direction.

**NOTE: Dislocations are described according to the position of the distal bone relative to normal joint alignment.**

## GRADING OF COLLATERAL LIGAMENT SPRAIN

**Grade I:** Gross stability with microscopic tear
**Grade II:** A grossly intact ligament with some abnormal laxity when joint is stressed
**Grade III:** Complete tear of collateral ligament with gross instability

## FINGER METACARPOPHALANGEAL JOINT

### ANATOMY

- **Features of metacarpophalangeal (MP) joint ligament box complex that resist ligament injury and dislocation**
  - Protected position at base of finger
  - Intrinsic ligamentous structure
  - Surrounding support structures, which include flexor and extensor tendon systems, sagittal bands, and tendons of the intrinsic muscles

- **Volar plate**
  - Forms floor of joint
  - Supported laterally by deep transverse metacarpal (intervolar plate) ligament that links each ligament box complex to the adjacent joint[3] (Fig. 66-1)
- **Cam effect**
  - A cam is a construct that translates rotary motion into linear motion.
  - The rotary flexion of the MP joint places linear stretch on the collateral ligaments.
  - The metacarpal head has a nonspherical shape and is wider on the volar side. Therefore the collateral ligaments become stretched taut in flexion relative to extension.
  - There is broader, more stable articulation between the metacarpal head and proximal phalanx with more than 70 degrees of flexion. **This produces increased lateral stability when the MP joint is in flexion and allows some abduction-adduction when the joint is in extension.**

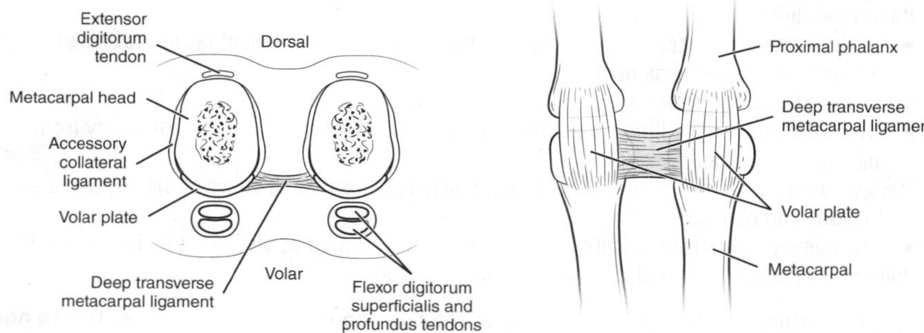


**Fig. 66-1** The intervolar plate ligaments span in a transverse direction and link the ligament box complex of each metacarpophalangeal joint. They provide increased stability to the volar plate.

## Dorsal MP Joint Dislocation

- Usual mechanism of injury is **forced hyperextension of digit** (e.g., from a fall on an outstretched hand).
- These injuries are rare and are primarily seen in the **index finger,** followed by the **small finger.**

**TIP:** Central digit MP dislocation is seen only with concomitant dislocation of a border digit.

## Classification of Dorsal MP Joint Dislocation

- **Simple MP subluxation**
  - **Incomplete dislocation:** Proximal phalanx is locked in 60-80 degrees of hyperextension.
  - It is reduced by flexing the wrist to relax flexor tendons. Initially increase deformity by hyperextension of the joint, and then apply dorsal pressure at the base of the proximal phalanx while gradually flexing the MP joint.
- **Complex MP subluxation**
  - **Complete and irreducible dislocation:** Metacarpal head protrudes volarly between the lumbrical and flexor tendons. Volar plate becomes impinged in the previous joint space.
  - Flexor tendon sheath remains attached to the volar plate and is held taut. Distal joints are held in flexion. This maintains a tight tendon-lumbrical encirclement and prevents reduction.

- **Requires open reduction and release of the A1 pulley:** This relaxes tension of the tendon-lumbrical mechanism.
- Immobilize the MP joint postoperatively in 30 degrees of flexion for 2 weeks. Then allow active range of motion with 10-degree dorsal blocking splint for 2 weeks.

### Volar MP Joint Dislocation

- These injuries are extremely rare.
- **Most are managed with closed reduction.** If unsuccessful, proceed with open reduction.

### Collateral Ligament Rupture of MP Joint

- Isolated ulnar collateral ligament (UCL) rupture is extremely rare.
- Isolated radial collateral ligament (RCL) rupture is more common.
  - They are typically seen in athletes after forced ulnar deviation of digit with MP joints flexed.
  - They typically occur in ulnar three digits.
  - They typically present late with persistent swelling and dysfunction of involved digit.
  - Presentation includes tenderness on radial aspect of joint, pain with passive MP flexion, and instability of joint with ulnar deviation of proximal phalanx.
- **Treatment of RCL rupture**
  - Immobilize joint in 30 degrees of flexion for 3 weeks.
  - Reevaluate joint laxity at 3 weeks. Buddy-tape it to adjacent digit for additional 2-3 weeks if joint instability persists.
  - Surgical repair is indicated if instability or pain persists after more than 6 weeks of nonoperative treatment.

## THUMB MP JOINT

### Anatomy

- Range of motion of the thumb MP joint is the most variable in the body.
- Primary arc of motion is flexion-extension. Minor arcs of motion are abduction-adduction and pronation-supination.
- **Collateral ligaments** provide lateral stability.
  - **Proper collateral ligaments** arise from condyles of the metacarpal head and insert on the volar proximal phalanx.
  - **Accessory collateral ligaments** originate on the volar metacarpal head and insert on the sesamoid bones and volar plate.
  - Additional lateral stability is provided by thenar muscle secondary insertions via adductor and abductor aponeuroses.
- Volar support of the joint is provided by the volar plate and thenar intrinsic muscle insertions to sesamoid bones.

### Acute UCL Injury (Skier's Thumb)[4]

- **UCL** injuries are *10 times more common* than **RCL** injuries in the thumb MP joint.
- They usually occur from forced radial deviation of the joint (e.g., falling on an outstretched hand with thumb abducted).

**TIP:** *Distal* tears of the UCL insertion are *five times more common* than proximal tears.

- **Avulsion fractures** of the proximal phalanx can occur with UCL tears.
  - Typically they are small fracture fragments that do not involve the articular surface and are managed with cast immobilization.
  - Large fracture fragments with more than 2 mm displacement require closed reduction percutaneous pinning (CRPP) or open reduction and internal fixation (ORIF).
- **Stener lesion**
  - These occur only with complete UCL rupture.
  - Adductor aponeurosis becomes interposed between the distal stump of the UCL and the insertion point at the base of the proximal phalanx.
  - **The UCL will not heal in this situation without surgical repair.**
- **Treatment of acute UCL ruptures**
  - **Partial UCL tears** are effectively treated with **cast immobilization** for 4 weeks followed by 2 weeks of splint immobilization with active range of motion exercises.
  - **Complete UCL** tears require **operative exploration and repair.**
    - Reattach ligament avulsions with a bone-anchoring technique.
    - Central ligament tears can be repaired with nonabsorbable braided sutures.
    - Immobilize thumb postoperatively in thumb spica cast for 4 weeks and follow with 2 weeks of splint immobilization and active range of motion exercises.

## Chronic UCL Injury (Gamekeeper's Thumb)

- This is seen in patients with untreated acute complete tear, unrecognized Stener lesion, or progressive attenuation of the UCL.
- Patients present with chronic pain, swelling, and weakness of the affected thumb.
  - *Chronic* is defined as symptoms **lasting longer than 6 weeks.**
- Osteoarthritis of the joint should be ruled out on plain radiographs before reconstruction.
- Surgical reconstruction of the ligament is best achieved with free tendon graft.
  - All scar and remnant of the UCL must be resected.
  - Options for tendon graft include palmaris longus (PL), strip of flexor carpi radialis (FCR), abductor pollicis longus (APL), plantaris, or toe extensor.
  - Immobilize thumb postoperatively in thumb spica cast for 6 weeks. Follow with 2 weeks of splint immobilization and active range of motion exercises.
  - Temporary pinning of the MP joint may be needed to correct the volar subluxation of the proximal phalanx on the metacarpal head.

## RCL Injury

- This occurs with forced adduction or torsion on a flexed MP joint.
- There is no equivalent Stener-type lesion, because the abductor aponeurosis is much broader than the adductor aponeurosis and prevents ligament interposition.
- Tear can occur on the proximal or distal end.
- Treatment of acute RCL ruptures
  - **Manage partial tears nonoperatively,** similar to partial UCL injury.
  - Isolated complete tears can be managed nonoperatively, similar to partial tear.
  - Operative repair is indicated for **complete tears associated with volar subluxation of the proximal phalanx.** Repair with free tendon graft is similar to complete UCL reconstruction.

## Dorsal Dislocation of Thumb MP Joint

- These are much more common than volar dislocations.
- They are seen with hyperextension injuries that cause complete rupture of volar plate with at least partial tear of collateral ligaments.

- Most are easily reducible.
  - Immobilize thumb in 20 degrees of MP joint flexion for 2 weeks. Follow with active flexion in 20-degree dorsal blocking splint.
  - Immobilize thumb for up to 4 weeks if there is a significant collateral ligament injury.

**TIP:** Irreducible dislocations are a result of entrapment of the volar plate, sesamoid bone, or flexor pollicis longus (FPL) and require open reduction.

## PROXIMAL INTERPHALANGEAL JOINT

Dislocation of the proximal interphalangeal (PIP) joint is the most common ligament injury in the hand.

### ANATOMY

- Normal 100- to 110-degree arc of rotation
- **Lateral collateral ligaments**
  - 2-3 mm thick
  - **Proper collateral ligament:** Inserts on volar base of middle phalanx
  - **Accessory collateral ligament:** Inserts on volar plate
  - Avulse proximally in 85% of injuries
- **Volar plate**
  - Forms floor of joint and is suspended laterally by collateral ligaments
  - Confluent with periosteum of proximal and middle phalanx
  - Prevents hyperextension and allows full flexion
  - Secondary stabilizer against lateral deviation of joint when collateral ligaments are incompetent or torn
- **Ligament box complex** (Fig. 66-2)
  - Provides stability to PIP joint and strength that resists joint displacement
  - ***Must be disrupted in at least two planes for dislocation to occur***

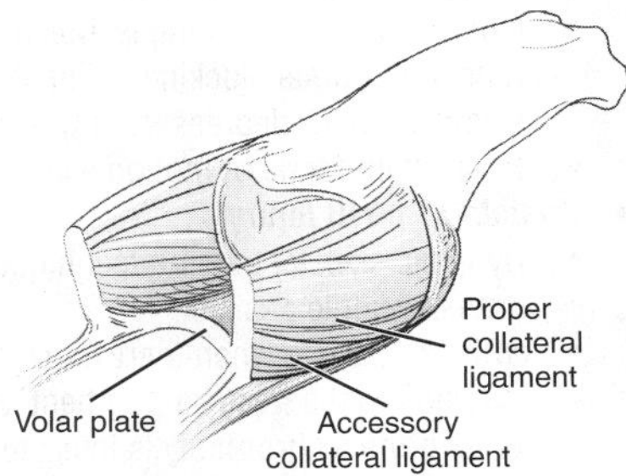


**Fig. 66-2** The ligament box complex provides joint stability.

### DORSAL DISLOCATION OF PIP JOINT[5]

- These injuries are frequently seen with PIP joint hyperextension that includes longitudinal compression of digit.
- Avulsion of volar plate occurs distally in 80% of injuries.
- Proximal volar plate avulsion can produce a trapped osteochondral fragment between proximal and middle phalanx. This is irreducible and requires open reduction.

### CLASSIFICATION OF DORSAL DISLOCATIONS

- **Type I (hyperextension):** Partial or complete avulsion of volar plate. The middle phalanx locks in 70-80 degrees of hyperextension. Partial articulation of joint remains intact.
- **Type II (dorsal dislocation):** Complete dorsal dislocation of middle phalanx. Avulsion of the volar plate is associated with a major split of the collateral ligaments. The base of the middle phalanx rests on the condyles of the proximal phalanx without apposition of the articular surface.

- **Type III (fracture-dislocation):** Avulsion fracture of volar middle phalanx with volar plate
  - **Stable fracture-dislocation**
    - Small triangular fragment **less than 40% of volar articular surface** of middle phalanx
    - Dorsal portions of the collateral ligaments intact, which makes complex stable after reduction
  - Unstable fracture-dislocation
    - **Disruption of more than 40% of volar articular surface** of middle phalanx
    - Most of collateral ligament–volar plate complex attached to fracture fragment
    - Difficult to maintain closed reduction

## Treatment of Acute PIP Dislocations[5,6]

- **Type I injury**
  - Treatment includes closed reduction and immobilization in 20-30 degrees of flexion for 1 week.
  - Avoid prolonged immobilization.
  - Edema and stiffness may persist for 6 months.
- **Type II injury**
  - Treatment includes closed reduction and immobilization in 20-30 degrees of flexion for 2-3 weeks.
- **Stable type III injury**
  - Treatment includes closed reduction and immobilization with dorsal blocking splint in 20-30 degrees of flexion for 3 weeks.
  - Extension block splinting is effective. Adequate reduction must be ensured before splinting. Start with dorsal blocking splint at degree of potential redisplacement. Reduce flexion of splint by 10-15 degrees each week.
  - Follow with range of motion exercises after 3 weeks.
- **Unstable type III injury**
  - Dynamic skeletal traction techniques are effective for comminuted fracture patterns through base of middle phalanx.
  - ORIF is effective when there is a large volar fracture fragment. Preserve the volar plate insertion to the fracture fragment. Stabilize repair using Kirschner wires or mini–lag screw.
  - **Volar plate arthroplasty** is indicated when fracture-dislocation is not amenable to ORIF. Immobilize PIP joint for 3 weeks. Then allow unrestricted PIP flexion with dorsal blocking splint for 1-3 weeks. Then proceed with unrestricted active extension of joint. Best results are achieved if repair is made within 6 weeks of injury. There is a significant risk of recurrent dislocation.
  - **Hemihamate arthroplasty** is another treatment option[7-9] (Fig. 66-3). This is indicated for comminuted, unstable PIP palmar lip fractures with dorsal dislocation of the joint, as well as ulnar condylar plateau fractures of the middle phalangeal base. It can also be used to salvage failed volar plate arthroplasty, ORIF, and external fixation.

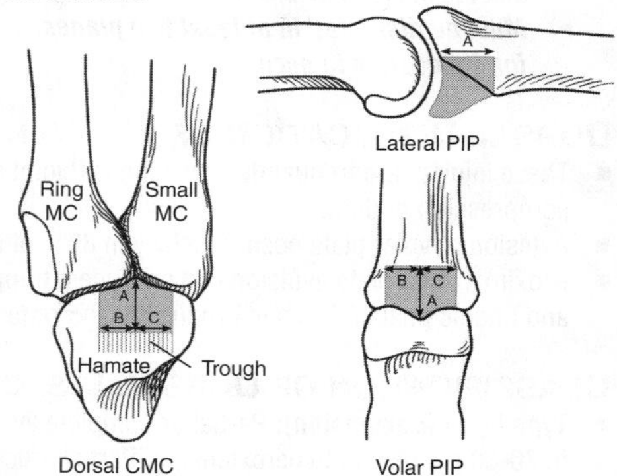


**Fig. 66-3** Hemihamate arthroplasty. (*CMC,* Carpometacarpal; *MC,* metacarpophalangeal; *PIP,* proximal interphalangeal.)

- The hemihamate procedure involves the harvest of an osteochondral graft from the dorsum of the hamate to include a small portion of the articular facet for the fifth metacarpal. This is then fashioned to fit into the bony defect at the base of the middle phalanx, restoring the volar lip of the middle phalangeal base. The graft is usually secured using small bone screws, and motion is initiated in the finger within 3-5 days. One recent series reported an average arc of motion of 87 degrees with good maintenance of the joint space up to 8 years after surgery. Union rates reported to this point are 100%. Though technically demanding, this procedure can serve as a viable alternative in patients with unstable type III injuries involving more than 50% of the articular surface.

## Chronic PIP Subluxation (Hyperextension)

- Results from **untreated type I injury** resulting in **swan neck deformity**
- Pain caused by lateral bands that snap across the condyles of the proximal phalanx
- Must distinguish **volar plate injury** from **extensor mechanism imbalance**
  - Stabilize PIP joint in full extension and have patient actively extend distal interphalangeal (DIP) joint. Volar plate is damaged if DIP joint extends normally.
- Repaired with flexor digitorum superficialis (FDS) tenodesis ("sublimis sling")
  - The radial slip of the FDS tendon is passed through the proximal phalanx from the ulnar to the radial side.
  - Anchor tendon to the periosteum to hold PIP joint in 5 degrees of flexion.
  - Apply dorsal blocking splint, and allow immediate active flexion.
  - Motion is unrestricted after 6 weeks.

## Lateral Dislocation of PIP Joint

- This is seen with **rupture of a collateral ligament** and at least **partial volar plate avulsion.**
- **Assess PIP stability after reduction of the joint.** More than 20 degrees of deformity on lateral stress testing indicates complete collateral ligament disruption with injury to secondary stabilizer.
- Reduce the joint and buddy-tape it to an adjacent uninjured digit.

**TIP:** Most lateral dislocations can be managed nonoperatively with early range of motion.

- Surgical repair is indicated for subacute or chronic injuries with persistent PIP instability and dysfunction.

## Volar Dislocations of PIP Joint

- Rare injuries
- **Types of volar dislocations**
  - **Volar dislocation without rotation:** Tear through the central slip of the extensor mechanism
  - **Volar rotatory subluxation:** Occurs when rotation occurs on one intact collateral ligament. The condyle of the proximal phalanx usually ruptures between the central slip of the extensor tendon and the ipsilateral lateral band as the middle phalanx displaces volarly.
  - Volar fracture-dislocation
- **Treatment**
  - Nonrotatory volar dislocations can be reduced easily. Splint in full extension for 4-6 weeks.

**TIP:** Most rotatory volar dislocations can be reduced and managed nonoperatively.

- ▸ Apply gentle traction with MP and PIP joints flexed to relax volarly displaced lateral band.
- ▸ Gentle rotatory motion disengages the intraarticular portion and allows reduction.
- ▸ Test active range of motion of PIP joint after reduction.
- ▸ Immobilize digit in full extension for 6 weeks if unable to actively extend fully at PIP joint after closed reduction.
- Volar fracture-dislocations should be managed with CRPP or ORIF with a mini–lag screw. This depends on the size of the dorsal fracture fragment.

### Collateral Ligament Fibrosis

- This condition is a late inevitable consequence of PIP joint dislocation.
- Fibrosis evolves over **10-12 months** after injury.
- Minimize fibrosis with consistent rehabilitation as soon as joint is stable.
- Low-dose prednisone taper after 4 weeks of injury can reduce edema and enhance recovery of movement.
- **Collateral ligament excision for PIP contracture release**
  - Operative intervention is indicated if range of motion is less than 60 degrees after compliant rehabilitation efforts and patient's quality of life is significantly impaired.
  - Both collateral ligaments usually must be excised. Lateral bands must be preserved.
  - Full passive range of motion must be achieved before testing active excursion.

## DISTAL INTERPHALANGEAL JOINT AND THUMB INTERPHALANGEAL JOINT

### Anatomy

- Ligamentous anatomy of DIP joint and thumb IP joint is analogous to that of PIP joint.

### Dislocations of DIP and Thumb IP Joints

- Much less frequent than PIP dislocations
- Enhanced stability of these joints provided by **adjacent insertions of flexor and extensor tendons**
- Usually dorsal or lateral
- **Can treat most with closed reduction;** joint immobilized with dorsal splint in slight flexion for 2-3 weeks
- Irreducible dislocations rare and usually caused by a trapped volar plate
  - Requires operative reduction

### Dorsal Fracture-Dislocations of DIP and Thumb IP Joints

- This condition is a volar fracture fragment of a distal phalanx.
- Stable closed reduction must be achieved if a volar fracture fragment is not avulsed with the FDP-FPL tendon.
- Operative intervention is required if FDP-FPL is avulsed.
- Volar plate arthroplasty is indicated if there is an unstable fracture-dislocation.

## Key Points

- ✓ Dislocations are described as the position of the distal bone relative to normal joint alignment.
- ✓ The **cam effect** describes the stretch of the digit MP joint collateral ligaments during flexion. This stabilizes the joint during flexion.
- ✓ Complete tears of the thumb MP ulnar collateral ligament are associated with **Stener lesions.** These require operative repair to prevent chronic joint instability.
- ✓ Dislocations of the PIP joint are the most common ligament injury in the hand.
- ✓ The ligament box complex must be disrupted in at least two planes for dislocation to occur.
- ✓ Unstable fracture-dislocations typically occur when more than 40% of the volar articular surface is disrupted.
- ✓ Unstable type III PIP fracture-dislocations are very difficult to treat. Options include dynamic external fixation, ORIF, volar plate arthroplasty, and hemihamate arthroplasty.
- ✓ Volar plate injury must be distinguished from extensor tendon imbalance in patients with posttraumatic swan neck deformities before repair.
- ✓ Collateral ligament fibrosis will develop after PIP dislocations and will disrupt the function of the digit.
- ✓ The severity of collateral ligament fibrosis is reduced with early rehabilitation as soon as the joint is stable after injury.

## References

1. Glickel SZ, Barron OA, Catalano LW. Dislocations and ligament injuries in the digits. In Green DP, Hotchkiss RN, Pederson WC, et al, eds. Green's Operative Hand Surgery, 5th ed. Philadelphia: Churchill Livingstone, 2005.
2. Jobe MT, Calandruccio JH. Fractures, dislocations and ligamentous injuries. In Canale ST, ed. Campbell's Operative Orthopaedics, 10th ed. New York: Elsevier, 2003.
3. Eaton RG, Littler JW. Joint injuries and their sequelae. Clin Plast Surg 3:85-98, 1976.
4. Stener B. Skeletal injuries associated with rupture of the ulnar collateral ligament of the metacarpophalangeal joint of the thumb: a clinical and anatomic study. Acta Chir Scand 125:583-586, 1963.
5. Deitch MA, Kiefhaber TR, Comisar BR, et al. Dorsal fracture-dislocation in the proximal interphalangeal joint: surgical complications and long-term results. J Hand Surg Am 24:914-923, 1994.
6. Eaton RG, Malerich MM. Volar plate arthroplasty of the proximal interphalangeal joint: a review of ten years' experience. J Hand Surg Am 5:260-268, 1980.
7. Williams RM, Hastings H II, Kiefhaber TR. PIP fracture/dislocation treatment technique: use of a hemi-hamate resurfacing arthroplasty. Tech Hand Up Extrem Surg 6:185-192, 2002.
8. Hastings H. Hemi-hamate resurfacing arthroplasty. In Strickland JW, Graham TJ, eds. Master Techniques in Orthopedic Surgery: The Hand, 2nd ed. Philadelphia: Lippincott Williams & Wilkins, 2005.
9. Calfee RP, Kiefhaber TR, Sommerkamp TG, et al. Hemi-hamate arthroplasty provides functional reconstruction of acute and chronic proximal interphalangeal fracture-dislocations. J Hand Surg 34:1232-1241, 2009.

# 67. Fingertip Injuries

Joshua A. Lemmon, Tarik M. Husain

## ANATOMY[1,2]

The **fingertip** is the portion of the digit **distal to the insertion of the profundus and extensor tendons** (Figs. 67-1 and 67-2).

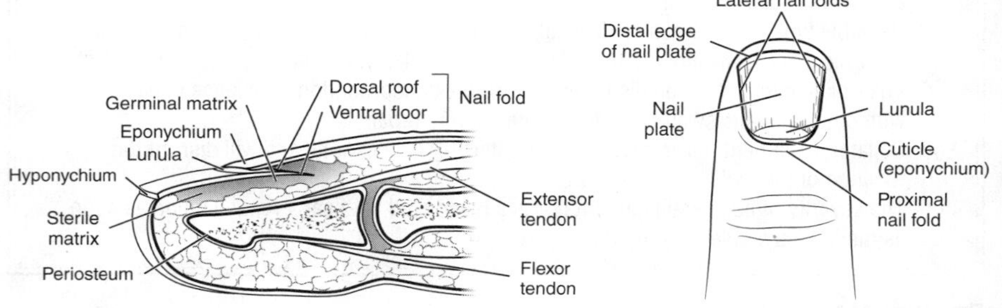


**Fig. 67-1** Lateral view of fingertip.

**Fig. 67-2** AP view of fingertip.

### PERIONYCHIUM

- Nail complex
- Constitutes dorsum of fingertip
- Begins approximately 1.2 mm distal to extensor tendon insertion
- See Chapter 57 for anatomic details.
- Fingertip injuries: May involve nail plate, nail bed, hyponychium, eponychium, and paronychium

### SKIN

- Glabrous
- Thick epidermis with deep papillary ridges that create fingerprints

### PULP

- Fibrofatty tissue
- Rich vasculature
- Stabilized by fibrous septa that extend from dermis to periosteum of distal phalanx
- Stabilized laterally to distal phalanx by extensions from Cleland's and Grayson's ligaments
- **Distal pulp:** Multipyramidal structure of fibroadipose tissue compartments
- **Proximal pulp:** Two layers of spherical tissue compartments
- Volar pulp: **56%** of fingertip volume[1]

### INNERVATION[3]

- Digital nerves carry mainly sensory fibers from C6, C7, and C8.
- Digital nerves arise from either the median or the ulnar nerve in the palm.

- Common digital nerves are initially deep to the arteries in the palm, but distally they are more superficial.
- At the level of the metacarpophalangeal (MP) joints, they have become proper digital nerves, located more superficial relative to their corresponding artery.
- Proper digital nerves split into **three branches (trifurcation)** just distal to the distal interphalangeal (DIP) joint (Fig. 67-3)
- One branch innervates the nail bed, one the distal fingertip, and one the volar pulp.

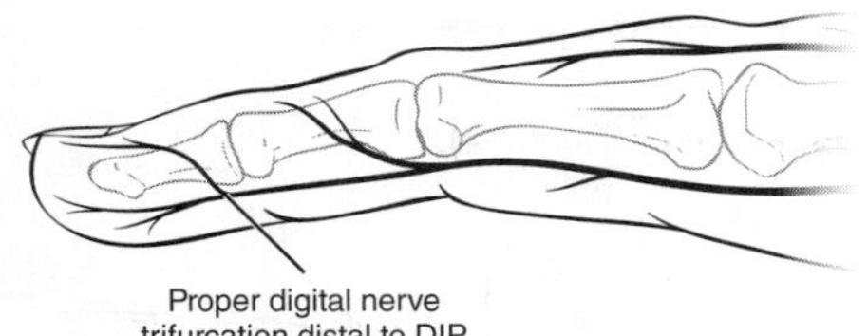


**Fig. 67-3** Lateral view of proper digital artery and nerve trifurcation.

### Vascular Supply

- Proper digital artery divides into **three branches (trifurcation)** (see Fig. 67-3).
- The three branches are interconnected distally by **two anastomotic arches.**
    - One arch is parallel to the lunula.
    - Second arch is parallel to the free edge of the nail.
- One branch continues laterally, and two dorsal branches arise from each artery.
    - One branch supplies nail fold.
    - The other branch arborizes at the level of the midnail and continues into volar pulp.
- Venous drainage[4]
    - Dorsal veins are dominant.
    - Veins around the lateral nail wall and distal pulp form an arch over the distal phalanx, surrounding the nail fold proximally.
    - Midline, longitudinal veins connect to a middle venous arch over the middle phalanx.
    - Valves are present even in the most distal veins.

## EVALUATION

### History

- **Age:** Children are treated differently from adults, and older patients have limited treatment options.
- **Gender:** Aesthetic outcome is often more important to female patients.
- **Hand dominance:** Dominant-hand injuries are treated more aggressively.
- **Occupation:** A manual laborer might be treated differently from a musician.
- **Determine mechanism of injury.**
- **Tobacco use:** Random-pattern flaps are discouraged in smokers.
- **Comorbid medical illnesses:** Patients with rheumatoid arthritis or Dupuytren's disease may not be candidates for some regional flaps because of contracture risk (e.g., thenar flap, cross-finger flap). Patients with diabetes mellitus are prone to infection and wound-healing difficulties.

### Physical Examination

- Perform complete hand examination; do not neglect the rest of the hand.
- Give special attention to the injured digit.
    - Assess the flexor and extensor tendons.

**TIP:** Associated mallet injury is common.

- Measure defect size (in cm$^2$).
- Determine the composition of the missing or nonviable tissue (e.g., nail plate, nail bed, skin, pulp, bone).

**TIP:** This information may best be obtained after digital block anesthesia and thorough irrigation.

- Note the presence of exposed bone.
- Evaluate the geometry of the injury to guide treatment[5] (Fig. 67-4).

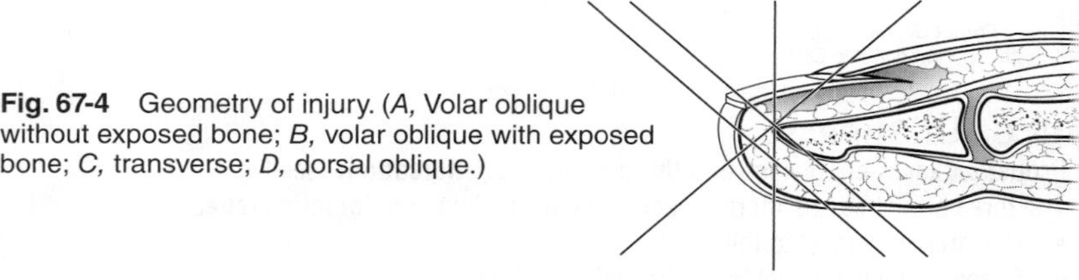


**Fig. 67-4** Geometry of injury. (*A,* Volar oblique without exposed bone; *B,* volar oblique with exposed bone; *C,* transverse; *D,* dorsal oblique.)

### Digit-Specific Radiographs

- Obtain AP and lateral films.
- Radiographs should include the amputated piece, if present.

## TREATMENT PLANNING[6]

The ideal treatment for a particular patient is either fingertip reconstruction or revision amputation. This decision should be made *along with the patient* by an experienced surgeon in a **patient-specific** and **digit-specific** fashion.

**TIP:** The size of the defect, the presence of exposed bone, and the geometry of the injury help guide reconstruction methods.

### Goals of Fingertip Reconstruction

- Provide durable coverage.
- Preserve length.
- Preserve sensation.
- Minimize pain, including prevention of neuroma.
- Minimize donor site morbidity.
- Maintain joint function.
- Provide an aesthetically acceptable result.

**TIP:** The primary goal is a painless fingertip with durable/sensate skin.

## Reconstructive Options: Reconstructive Ladder

- Healing by secondary intention
- Skin grafting
- Composite grafting
- Homodigital flaps
- Heterodigital flaps
- Regional flaps
- Microsurgical replantation or reconstruction

## SKIN GRAFTS

### Split-Thickness Skin Graft (STSG)

- 56% of patients considered their results good after STSG versus 90% treated by secondary intention.[7]
- Complications
  - Graft failure
  - Hypoesthesias
  - Cold sensitivity

### Full-Thickness Skin Graft (FTSG)

- Consider for soft tissue defect $>1\ cm^2$
- More durable, less contraction, and greater sensibility than STSG
- Harvest graft from the thenar eminence.
  - Excellent color match, hairless
  - May be as wide as 2 cm
- Close donor site primarily.

## HOMODIGITAL FLAPS

- The source of donor tissue is the **injured digit.**
- These flaps provide immediate, near-normal sensibility.
- Donor tissue must be from outside the zone of injury.
- *This method often requires a small amount of bone shortening to facilitate flap inset.*

### Volar V-Y Advancement Flap (Atasoy et al)[8]

- Useful for **dorsal oblique** and some **transverse** geometry injuries
- Uses tissue adjacent to wound
- Designed with wound edge as base of triangular flap
- Can only advance distal edge **1 cm** unless incision carried proximal to distal interphalangeal (DIP) flexion crease

- Can design flap more proximally to cross DIP flexion crease and include neurovascular pedicles for increased advancement[9] (Fig. 67-5)
- Contraindication: Volar oblique injury[5] (see Fig. 67-4)
- Conflicting outcome studies
- According to Atasoy et al,[8] 56 of 61 patients had normal sensibility and normal motion.
- Repeat studies by other investigators showed much higher rates of complications, including cold intolerance, difficulty with grasp, paresthesias, and poor sensibility.

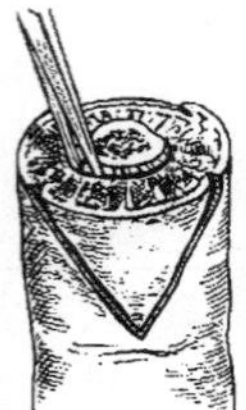
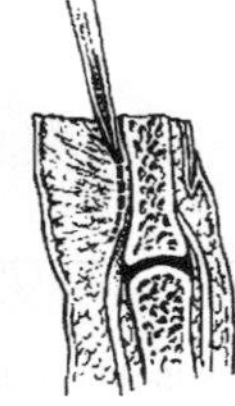
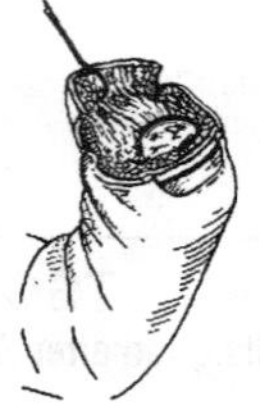
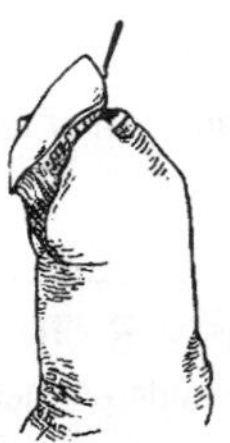
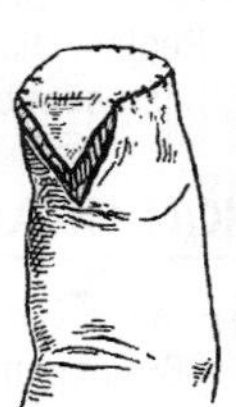

**Fig. 67-5** Volar V-Y advancement flap.

## Furlow's Modified Volar V-Y Advancement "Cup" Flap[10]

- Modification of classic V-Y volar advancement for volar oblique injuries
- Flap design extended across DIP and proximal interphalangeal (PIP) volar flexion creases
- Elevated just volar to flexor sheath, including neurovascular bundles laterally
- Flap advanced distally and lateral edges folded together and "cupped" over distal injury
- Use of digit possibly limited by postoperative fingertip and volar scars

## Volar Advancement Flaps (Moberg)[11]

- Technique is used mostly for the **thumb** because of unique dorsal and volar blood supply.
- Radial and ulnar midaxial incisions are made dorsal to the neurovascular bundles, which are **included in the flap.**
- Flap elevation is in plane just volar to the tendon sheath.
- Advancement is limited to **1.0 cm** without additional modifications.
- A transverse incision at base increases advancement to **1.5 cm.**
- **Dellon's modification** of flap design into the web space increases advancement to **3.0 cm**[12] (Fig. 67-6).

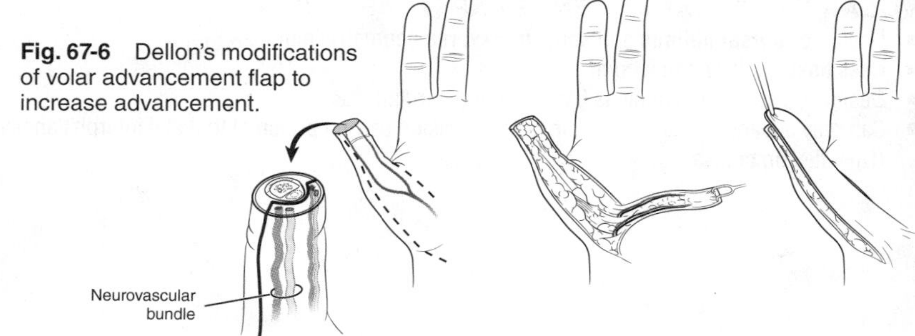


**Fig. 67-6** Dellon's modifications of volar advancement flap to increase advancement.

## Bilateral Triangular V-Y Advancement Flaps (Kutler)[13]

- Described for **transverse amputations,** but perhaps most useful for **lateral oblique** injuries
- Triangular flaps designed along lateral aspects of distal tip
- Advanced distally and centrally to cover injury

## Oblique Triangular Neurovascular Island Flap[14]

- Useful for **volar oblique** injuries up to 2 cm in size
- Unilateral triangular flap design
- Neurovascular pedicle dissection: Extend proximally to web space for increased advancement[9] (Fig. 67-7)

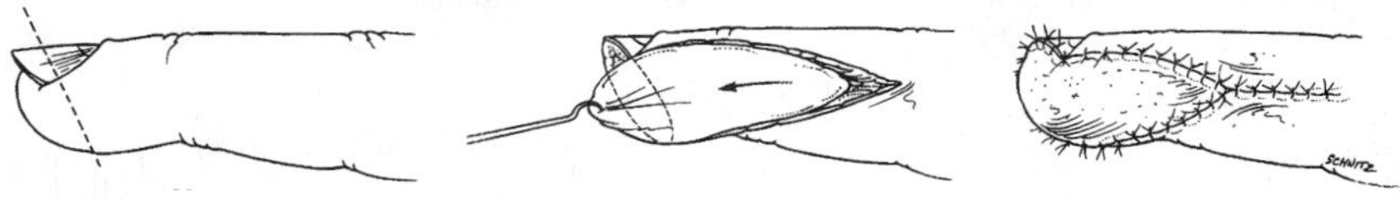

**Fig. 67-7** Oblique triangular island flap.

## Other Homodigital Flaps

- Surgeon's familiarity and preference determine more frequent use of these techniques.
- Hueston's flap[15]
- Souquet's flap[16]
- Step-advancement flap[17]
- Reverse digital artery flaps[18]

# HETERODIGITAL FLAPS

- Can cover **larger areas than homodigital flaps**
- Violates a normal digit
- Often requires cortical relearning
- **Sensibility not as good as with homodigital flaps;** for example, protective sensation was preserved with cross-finger flaps but not tactile gnosis (0% tactile gnosis in 54 patients).[19]

## Cross-Finger Flap[20] (Fig. 67-8)

- Useful for large **volar oblique** injuries
- Flap raised on dorsum of injured digit's adjacent middle phalanx and elevated just dorsal to paratenon
- Flap left pedicled to donor site along lateral margin adjacent to injured digit
- Injured finger flexed and flap inset over defect
- Flap division at 8 to 10 days
- Postoperative sensibility relatively poor (as previously described)

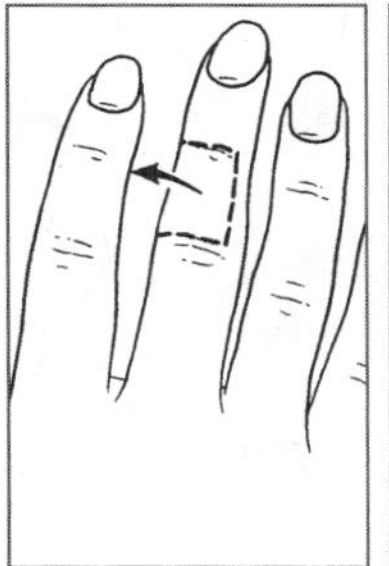

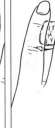

Flap design

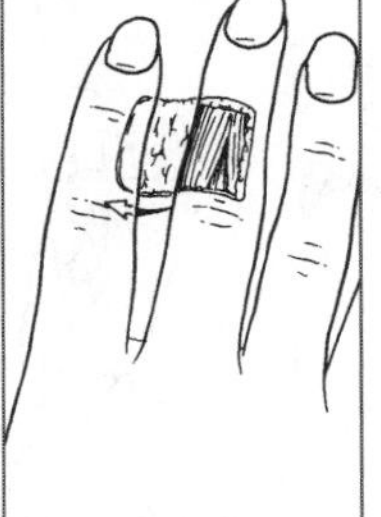

Arc to adjacent digit

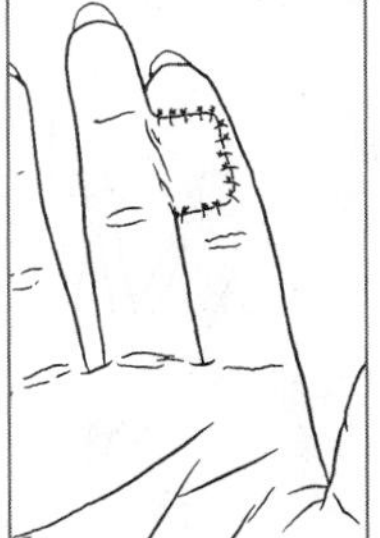

Flap inset

**Fig. 67-8** Cross-finger flap.

- Donor digit frequently bothered by cold intolerance and sensitivity
- Aesthetic deformity on dorsum of donor finger often troubling for women

## Heterodigital Neurovascular Pedicled Flaps (Fig. 67-9)[21,22]

- More commonly used for **ulnar thumb pulp defects**
- Can provide stable coverage for larger injuries compared with homodigital flaps
- Donor site reconstructed with skin grafting
- Requires cortical relearning, which occurs in only 40% of cases[23]
- Involves dissection of middle or ring finger proper digital artery and nerve proximally to bifurcation of common digital source
- Larger volar access incisions necessary to tunnel pedicle and inset flap in defect

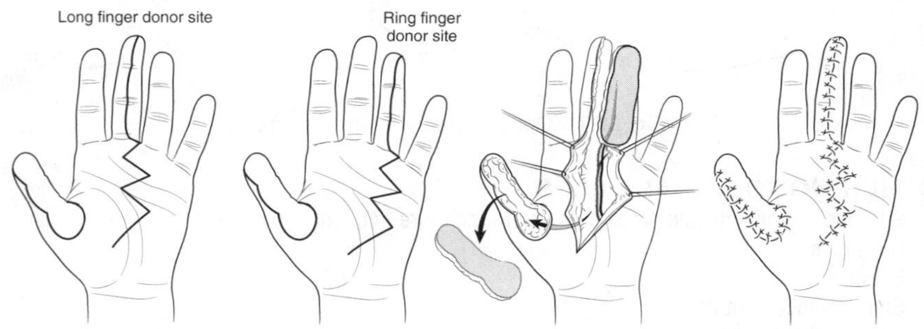


**Fig. 67-9** Neurovascular pedicled flap.

## First Dorsal Metacarpal Artery Flap[22,24] (Fig. 67-10)

- Additional option for reconstruction of volar thumb injuries
- Neurovascular pedicled flap based on dorsal first metacarpal artery
- Allows transfer of tissue from dorsum of index finger proximal phalanx
- Flap includes terminal branch of superficial radial nerve to provide **protective sensation**
- Like other neurovascular pedicled flaps, requires cortical relearning and skin grafting of donor site

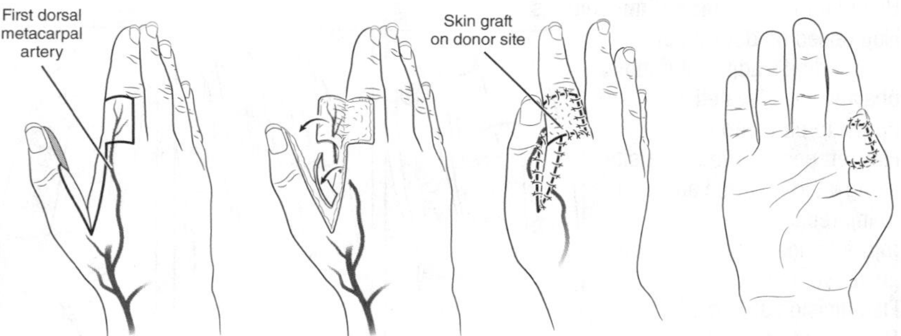


**Fig. 67-10** First dorsal metacarpal artery flap.

## First Dorsal Metacarpal Artery Perforator Flap (Quaba Flap)[25] (Fig. 67-11)

- Useful for coverage of the dorsum of the hand and fingers to the PIP joint, and the distal palm and web spaces
- When the reverse flap is used, coverage may be extended past the PIP joint.
- Based off perforators from the dorsal communicating branch of the common digital artery, also known as the *Quaba perforator*
- Perforators are primarily distal to the junctura tendinum in the distal third of the dorsum of the hand.
- Flow through this perforator can be antegrade through the dorsal metacarpal artery (DMA) or retrograde from the volar system or the dorsal digital arteries.

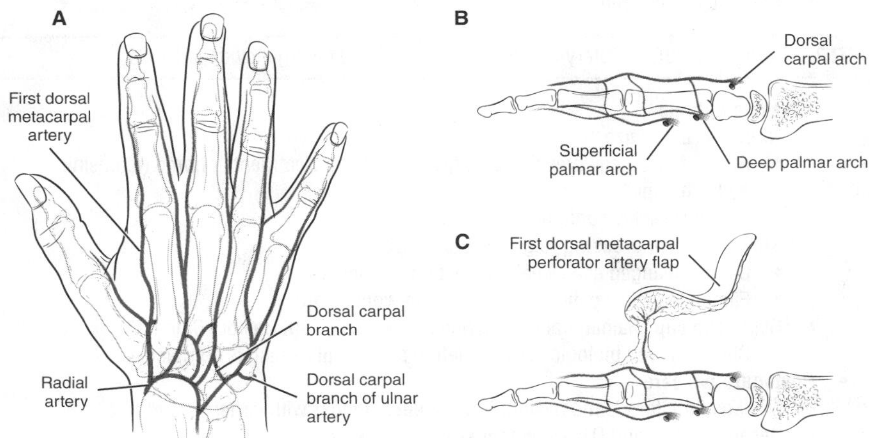


**Fig. 67-11** **A,** Vascular supply to the first dorsal metacarpal artery perforator (Quaba) flap. **B,** Sagittal view of the arterial anatomy of the hand; the dorsal metacarpals are joined, and on occasion replaced, by perforators from the deep volar arch and/or volar metacarpal arteries. **C,** Planning: The arterial basis of the flap is a direct branch from the dorsal metacarpal artery. The site of entry of this vessel into the dorsal skin is the axis of the flap. It is situated 0.5 to 1 cm proximal to the adjacent MP joint. A useful intraoperative guide to this point is the intertendinous connection.

# REGIONAL FLAPS

## Thenar Flap[26,27]

- Used for large **volar oblique** injuries of **index** and **middle** fingers
- Flap of skin and subcutaneous tissue elevated on thenar eminence
- Injured digit flexed, and flap inset over injury
- Flap division at 10-14 days
- Often discouraged in patients older than 40 years for fear of joint contractures, but some report good results in older adults[28]
- **Contraindicated** in patients with rheumatoid arthritis, Dupuytren's disease, or other illnesses that preclude prolonged finger flexion

## TREATMENT OF INJURY TYPES: AN ALGORITHMIC APPROACH

Treatment method selection follows focused injury evaluation with attention to **injury size** and **geometry**, as well as **patient-specific** and **digit-specific** factors.

### SOFT TISSUE LOSS WITHOUT EXPOSED BONE[5] (see Fig. 67-4, *A*)

- **Healing by secondary intention**
  - Digital tip injuries <**1.5 cm$^2$** heal with excellent results by secondary intention.[29]
  - **Procedure**
    - Local digital block with 1% lidocaine
    - Finger tourniquet not necessary, may hinder evaluation of viable tissue
    - Copious irrigation and cleansing with surgical scrub solution
    - Debridement of clearly nonviable tissue
    - Hemostasis ensured

> **TIP:** Battery-operated cautery devices are helpful in the emergency department.

  - **Dressing options**
    - **Nonadherent gauze**
      - Allows twice-daily dressing changes and wound treatment at home (e.g., sink hydrotherapy)
      - Best for heavily contaminated injuries
    - **Semiocclusive dressing** (e.g., Tegaderm, OpSite)
      - Can be changed each week by treating physician
      - Eliminates initial patient involvement in wound care
    - **Hyphecan cap** (Hainan Kangda Marine Biomedical Corp, Haikou, China)[30]
      - Chitin-derived biologic dressing left in place until healing is complete
  - **Postoperative care**
    - Average time for wound healing is **3-4 weeks** (longer with larger wounds).
    - Desensitization and OT begin after soft tissue heals.
- **Skin grafting**
  - Full-thickness and split-thickness grafts are harvested from the **hypothenar eminence** and allow coverage with glabrous skin.
  - Does **not** provide consistently good results[31]
    - Increased incidence of cold intolerance
    - Increased incidence of postoperative tenderness
    - Does not allow patients to return to work earlier
  - For these reasons, skin grafting should be used only if wound is too large to heal by secondary intention, and if other techniques for reconstruction are impractical or not feasible (e.g., large volar skin avulsion without exposed tendon or bone).

### SOFT TISSUE LOSS WITH EXPOSED BONE

- **Bone shortening**
  - In some circumstances, bone can be minimally shortened to convert an injury with exposed bone to one without exposed bone, allowing healing by secondary intention.
  - Procedure is performed only for small wounds (<1.5 cm$^2$) with minimal area of exposed bone.
  - Distal phalanx serves as support for nail bed; therefore **nail bed must be shortened 2 mm proximal to the distal extent of the distal phalanx** to prevent postoperative hook-nail deformity.[32]

> **TIP:** The bone should never be shortened beyond the insertion of the flexor or extensor tendons.

- **Dorsal oblique injury** (see Fig. 67-4, *D*)
  - Relative preservation of volar tip pulp and glabrous skin
  - Reconstruction with **volar V-Y advancement flap**[5]
  - **Procedure** (see Fig. 67-5)
    1. Digital block with 1% lidocaine
    2. Thorough irrigation and cleansing
    3. Debridement of nonviable tissue
    4. Finger exsanguination and digital tourniquet
    5. Sterile matrix removed 2 mm proximal to the end of distal phalanx
    6. Flap designed with wound edge as the base of a triangular flap
    7. Full-thickness elevation of volar flap under loupe magnification
    8. Fibrous septa that anchor pulp sharply released from distal phalanx
    9. Flap mobilized distally
    10. Limited bone shortening as needed to facilitate inset
    11. Inset into defect, secured to nail bed with 6-0 chromic gut suture
    12. Lateral edges contoured and secured with 5-0 nylon suture
    13. Donor site closed in V-Y fashion
    14. Bulky dressing or volar protective splint applied
    15. Desensitization and OT after soft tissue heals
- **Volar oblique injury**[5] (see Fig. 67-4, *B*)
  - Technique preserves nail complex, but leaves deficiencies in volar skin and pulp.
  - Technique should be **digit-specific** to preserve most important aspects of each digit.
  - **Thumb**
    - Maintaining sensation is important for precision.
    - Sensation is best with homodigital flaps.
    - The **classic thumb tip procedure is the Moberg volar advancement flap.**[11]
    - Modifications may be required to increase advancement, as described previously.
    - Heterodigital flaps are required for large injuries (e.g., Littler neurovascular island flap, cross-finger flap, or first dorsal metacarpal artery flap).
  - **Index finger**
    - Like the thumb, the index finger is involved with pinch grip and precision activity.
    - **Sensibility is of greatest importance.**
    - Use homodigital flap reconstruction when possible.
      - **Furlow's modified volar V-Y advancement** can be used for large injuries (up to 1.5 $cm^2$).
      - Larger injuries, up to 2 $cm^2$, can be reconstructed with **homodigital oblique triangular neurovascular island flap** (see Fig. 67-7).
    - **Thenar flaps** are preferred over cross-finger flaps for larger injuries, because postoperative sensibility is better; cross-finger flaps rarely achieve more than protective sensation.[19,33]

> **TIP:** The thenar flap is the best option for large injuries of the index finger tip.

- A Moberg volar advancement flap is feasible for the index finger, but unlike the thumb the index finger has no dedicated dorsal arterial supply.
  - Dorsal skin is supplied by perforating branches of the common digital arteries.
  - Dorsal skin necrosis can occur unless these branches are preserved.
  - To preserve these branches a vertical spreading technique, rather than sharp dissection, is used during flap elevation.
  - Excellent results are reported.
  - Advancement is limited to 1.5 cm.

**TIP:** This is a difficult technique to use on the index finger and should be done meticulously and only by an experienced surgeon.

- **Middle finger**
  - The middle or long finger is the central digit of the hand; its **length** is required for a normal aesthetic pattern of the hand.
  - **Sensibility is of secondary importance to length.**
  - Because most homodigital flaps require some bone shortening, the thenar flap should be used initially to limit shortening.
- **Ring and small fingers**
  - The main role of the ulnar two digits is **power grip.**
  - Durable coverage, length, minimal pain, and adequate joint mobility are the most important considerations.
  - Sensibility is of limited importance.
  - Homodigital flaps may sacrifice length, as previously indicated.
  - Additionally, homodigital flaps can result in volar scars that extend across the contact surface of these fingers during power grip.
  - **A heterodigital, cross-finger flap is an appropriate reconstructive method.**
    - Postoperative sensibility is limited, but length and durable coverage are preserved, volar scars are avoided, and MP and PIP joint mobility are maintained.
  - **Procedure (for ring finger)**
    1. Best performed in operating room with regional anesthesia
    2. Injury irrigated, cleaned, and debrided
    3. Upper extremity exsanguinated and tourniquet placed
    4. Flap designed on dorsum of middle finger over middle phalanx
    5. Flap elevated just dorsal to extensor paratenon; elevated from radial to ulnar direction
    6. FTSG harvested from forearm and secured to radial border of the injury on ring finger
    7. Ring finger flexed into position, flap inset over injury, and skin graft secured over donor site
    8. Volar protective splint applied
    9. Flap divided in 8-10 days
    10. Desensitization and OT started after soft tissue heals

- **Transverse injury**[5] (see Fig. 67-4, *C*)
  - This type of injury results in equal deficiencies in volar pulp and dorsal nail complex.
  - Use techniques described for dorsal oblique and volar oblique injuries.
    - **Volar V-Y advancement flaps** are useful for relatively distal injuries, but require prohibitive bone shortening if injury goes through proximal half of sterile matrix.
    - Other **homodigital, heterodigital,** or **regional flaps** are used, as described for volar oblique injuries.

- **Lateral oblique injury**
  - Use with injury in the sagittal plane and with radial or ulnar-sided tissue loss.
  - Previously mentioned homodigital flaps can be used.
  - Additionally, a **lateral pulp flap** may be used.[34]
    - The remaining volar pulp is sharply elevated off periosteum of the distal phalanx and advanced laterally into defect; a raw surface remains on lateral aspect.
    - The wound is allowed to reepithelialize with moist wound care.

### Composite Grafting

- Nonmicrosurgical replantation of amputated fingertip
- Typically recommended only for children younger than 2-6 years[35,36]
- **Not recommended for patients >6 years old**
- May use only a biologic dressing that allows underlying healing by secondary intention
- Attempts made to improve graft take by postoperative cooling and subcutaneous pocket placement
- Though traditionally composite grafting not recommended for adults, retrospective studies in adults show success of composite grafts, including those with bone[37]
- Graft survival rates up to 93% described in adults by refining surgical technique, including excision of bony segment, defatting, deepithelialization, tie-over suturing, and finger splinting to increase the graft survival[38]
- Discouraged in severe crush injuries

## REVISION AMPUTATION

### Indications

- Patient preference
  - Manual laborers may request well-performed termination rather than reconstruction to speed recovery and return to work.
- Heavy contamination and human bites should be staged, with initial debridement and delayed amputation.
- Injury **proximal to the lunula** is best treated with **nail ablation** and **revision amputation.**
- Perform if injury is proximal to the insertion of the flexor or extensor tendons

### Technical Considerations

- The remaining skeleton should be contoured to a smooth, tapered end.
- The distal phalanx should be completely removed, if injured.
- Digital nerves should be divided at least 1 cm proximal to the injury and placed away from contact surfaces.
- Digital arteries and dorsal veins should be ligated or cauterized to prevent hematomas.
- To prevent a **quadrigia effect,** the profundus tendon should **not** be advanced distally. The *quadrigia effect* is a restriction in flexion of adjacent digits, resulting from a common muscular origin of the profundus tendons.
- The profundus tendon can be secured to the A4 pulley to prevent a **lumbrical plus** deformity; extension at the PIP with attempted flexion results from retracting flexor digitorum profundus (FDP) tendon and lumbrical origin, increasing lumbrical pull.
- Completely ablate the nail bed, including the dorsal roof, to prevent problematic remnants.

## MICROSURGICAL REPLANTATION

- Microsurgical replantation techniques are practiced and reported mostly in Japan and other Asian countries, where cultural differences place greater importance on the presence of a normal fingertip.
- Replantation of fingertips is performed only at tertiary referral centers in the United States.
- Replantation should be considered in all children, young women, and musicians.

### KEY POINTS

- ✓ Injuries without exposed bone that are $<1.5$ cm$^2$ are best managed with healing by secondary intention.
- ✓ Skin grafting should rarely be used.
- ✓ Injury geometry dictates reconstructive options.
- ✓ Homodigital flaps provide better postoperative sensibility than heterodigital flaps and are preferred for the thumb and index fingers.
- ✓ Shortening should be avoided if at all possible when treating middle fingertip injuries.
- ✓ Composite grafting should be performed in children $<6$ years old. Composite grafting may be performed cautiously in adults using special techniques.
- ✓ Revision amputation is a preferred treatment for many patients and should be discussed with every patient before pursuing fingertip reconstruction.

## REFERENCES

1. Murai M, Lau HK, Pereira BP, et al. A cadaver study on volume and surface area of the fingertip. J Hand Surg Am 22:935-941, 1997.
2. Zook EG. Anatomy and physiology of the perionychium. Hand Clin 6:1-7, 1990.
3. Midha R, Zager EL, eds. Surgery of Peripheral Nerves: A Case-Based Approach. New York: Thieme, 2008.
4. Moss SH, Schwartz KS, von Drasek-Ascher G, et al. Digital venous anatomy. J Hand Surg Am 10:473-482, 1985.
5. Fassier PR. Fingertip injuries: evaluation and treatment. J Am Acad Orthop Surg 4:84-92, 1996.
6. Lemmon JA, Janis JE, Rohrich RJ. Soft-tissue injuries of the fingertip: methods of evaluation and treatment. An algorithmic approach. Plast Reconstr Surg 122:105e-117e, 2008.
7. Holm A, Zachariae L. Fingertip lesions: an evaluation of conservative treatment versus free skin grafting. Acta Orthop Scand 45:382-392, 1974.
8. Atasoy E, Ioakimidis E, Kasdan ML, et al. Reconstruction of the amputated finger tip with a triangular volar flap. A new surgical procedure. J Bone Joint Surg Am 52:921-926, 1970.
9. Chao JD, Huang JM, Wiedrich TA. Local hand flaps. J Am Soc Surg Hand 1:25-44, 2002.
10. Furlow LT Jr. V-Y "cup" flap for volar oblique amputation of fingers. J Hand Surg Br 9:253-256, 1984.
11. Moberg E. Aspects of sensation in reconstructive surgery of the upper extremity. J Bone Joint Surg Am 46:817-825, 1964.
12. Rohrich RJ, Antrobus SD. Volar advancement flaps. In Blair WF, ed. Techniques in Hand Surgery. Baltimore: Williams & Wilkins, 1996.
13. Kutler W. A new method for fingertip amputation. JAMA 133:29-30, 1947.
14. Venkataswami R, Subramanian N. Oblique triangular flap: a new method of repair for oblique amputations of the fingertip and thumb. Plast Reconstr Surg 66:296-300, 1980.
15. Hueston J. Local flap repair of fingertip injuries. Plast Reconstr Surg 37:349-350, 1966.
16. Souquet R. The asymmetric arterial advancement flap in distal pulp loss (modified Hueston's flap). Ann Chir Main 4:233-238, 1985.

17. Evans DM, Martin DL. Step-advancement flap for fingertip reconstruction. Br J Plast Surg 41:105-111, 1988.
18. Lai CS, Lin SD, Chou CK, et al. A versatile method for reconstruction of finger defects: reverse digital artery flap. Br J Plast Surg 45:443-453, 1992.
19. Nishikawa H, Smith PJ. The recovery of sensation and function after cross-finger flaps for fingertip injury. J Hand Surg Br 17:102-107, 1992.
20. Gurdin M, Pangman WJ. The repair of surface defects of fingers by trans-digital flaps. Plast Reconstr Surg 5:368-371, 1950.
21. Littler JW. The neurovascular pedicle method of digital transposition for reconstruction of the thumb. Plast Reconstr Surg 12:303-319, 1953.
22. Green DP, Hotchkiss RN, Pederson WC, eds. Green's Operative Hand Surgery, 6th ed. Philadelphia: Churchill Livingstone, 2011.
23. Oka Y. Sensory function of the neurovascular island flap in thumb reconstruction: comparison of original and modified procedures. J Hand Surg Am 25:637-643, 2000.
24. Holevich J. A new method of restoring sensibility to the thumb. J Bone Joint Surg Br 45:496-502, 1963.
25. Quaba AA, Davison P. The distally-based dorsal hand flap. Br J Plast Surg 43:28-39, 1990.
26. Gatewood MD. A plastic repair of finger defects without hospitalization. JAMA 87:1479, 1926.
27. Flatt AE. The thenar flap. J Bone Joint Surg Br 39:80-85, 1957.
28. Barbato BD, Guelmi K, Romano SJ, et al. Thenar flap rehabilitated: a review of 20 cases. Ann Plast Surg 37:135-139, 1996.
29. Mennen U, Weise A. Fingertip injuries management with semi-occlusive dressing. J Hand Surg Br 18:416-422, 1993.
30. Halim AS, Stone CA, Devaraj VS. The Hyphecan cap: a biological fingertip dressing. Injury 29:261-263, 1998.
31. Holm A, Zachariae L. Fingertip lesion: an evaluation of conservative treatment versus free skin grafting. Acta Orthop Scand 45:382-392, 1974.
32. Kumar VP, Satku K. Treatment and prevention of "hook nail" deformity with anatomic correlation. J Hand Surg Am 18:617-620, 1993.
33. Melone CP Jr, Beasley RW, Carstens JH Jr. The thenar flap: analysis of its use in 150 cases. J Hand Surg Am 7:291-297, 1982.
34. Elliot D, Jigjinni VS. The lateral pulp flap. J Hand Surg Br 18:423-426, 1993.
35. Elsahy NI. When to replant a fingertip after its complete amputation. Plast Reconstr Surg 60:14-21, 1977.
36. Moiemen NS, Elliot D. Composite graft replacement of digital tips. A study in children. J Hand Surg Br 22:346-352, 1997.
37. Lee KS, Lim YS, Choi J, et al. Composite graft including bone tissue: a case report of successful reattachment of multiple fingertip oblique amputation. J Plast Reconstr Aesthet Surg 66:e43-e46, 2012.
38. Chen SY, Wang CH, Fu JP, et al. Composite grafting for traumatic fingertip amputation in adults: technique reinforcement and experience in 31 digits. J Trauma 70:148-153, 2011.

# 68. Nail Bed Injuries

Joshua A. Lemmon, Bridget Harrison

## DEMOGRAPHICS

- The hand is the most frequently injured body part; the **fingertip** is the most commonly injured part of the hand.[1,2]
- Injuries are most common in males age 4-30 years.
- They account for two thirds of hand injuries in children.
- The **middle** finger is most commonly injured because of increased exposure distal to other digits.[3]
- Most injuries involve the **nail bed** and **soft tissue of the fingertip.**

## ANATOMY[4,5] (Fig. 68-1)

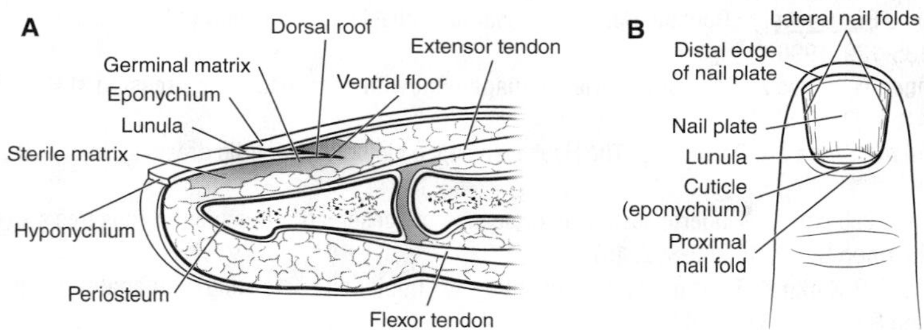


**Fig. 68-1** **A** and **B,** Anatomy of the fingertip and nail bed.

### Nail Plate

- Composed of hard, keratinized, squamous cells attached to nail bed
- Loosely attached to germinal matrix, but densely adherent to sterile matrix

### Perionychium

- Consists of nail folds, nail plate, nail bed, hyponychium

### Hyponychium

- Junction of sterile matrix and fingertip skin beneath distal nail margin
- Contains highest concentration of lymphatics of any dermal area in the body

### Paronychium

- Skin on each side of the nail

> **TIP:** The paronychium is the lateral nail fold. The perionychium includes the paronychium, nail plate, and nail matrix. A paronychia refers to a soft tissue infection around the fingernail.

### EPONYCHIUM
- Skin proximal to nail that covers nail fold

### NAIL FOLD
- Composed of the ventral floor and the dorsal roof
- **Ventral floor:** Site of the **germinal matrix**
- **Dorsal roof:** Hosts cells that impart **nail shine**

### LUNULA
- White arc just distal to the eponychium
- Caused by **persistence of nail cell nuclei** in the germinal matrix
- Distal to this location, nuclei absent and nail is clear

### GERMINAL MATRIX
- Lies on ventral floor **proximal** to distal border of lunula
- Immediately distal to the insertion of extensor tendon
- Responsible for **90%** of nail production
- Injury leads to nail absence

### STERILE MATRIX
- Nail bed **distal** to lunula
- Responsible for nail plate adherence
- Secondary site of nail production
- Injury leads to nail deformity

### INNERVATION
- Sensation to nail bed supplied by dorsal branches of digital nerves

### BLOOD SUPPLY
- Terminal branches of volar digital arteries and capillary loops

## PHYSIOLOGY AND FUNCTION[4-6]

### NAIL GROWTH OCCURS IN THREE LOCATIONS
1. **Germinal matrix**
   - Produces nail by **gradient parakeratosis**
     - Basilar cells, close to the distal phalanx periosteum, duplicate and enlarge (macrocytosis).
     - Newly formed cells are driven dorsally in a column toward the nail.
     - These cells flatten and elongate in response to the resistance of the nail, assimilate into the nail itself, and stream distally.
     - Cells initially retain nuclei. As cells become nonviable, they slowly lose nuclei.
     - When cells reach distal lunula, so few nuclei remain that nail becomes clear.
2. **Dorsal roof of nail fold**
   - Produces nail by same mechanism as germinal matrix, but these cells lose nuclei more rapidly
   - Imparts shine to nail plate

3. **Sterile matrix**
   - Amount of nail produced in this location varies by individual.
   - It adds squamous cells, contributing to **nail strength** and **thickness.**
   - Continued nail growth allows nail adherence; overlying nail plate is securely anchored by linear ridges in sterile matrix epithelium.

### Variable Nail Growth

- Nail growth rate generally **3-4 mm** per month
- **Growth more rapid in:**
  - Longer digits
  - Summer months
  - Young persons
    - Twice as rapid in persons <30 years, compared with those over 80
  - Nail biters

**TIP:** It takes about 100 days to grow a complete nail.

### Nail Function

- Fingernail serves as a counterforce to the fingertip pad, increasing its sensitivity.
  - **Two-point discrimination decreases when fingernail is absent.**
- Fingernail is used almost exclusively for picking up fine objects (e.g., pins, needles).

## ETIOLOGIC FACTORS/PATHOPHYSIOLOGY[6]

- Nail bed is positioned between two relatively unyielding structures: **distal phalanx** and **nail plate;** thus it is well protected.
- Required force must be great enough either to cause fracture of distal phalanx or to deform nail plate.
- Most injuries result from crushing force, compressing delicate nail bed between solid nail plate and solid bone.
- Other injuries result from penetration of nail plate by foreign objects such as machinery or tools.

## EVALUATION

### History

- Age
- Gender (aesthetic importance of nail greater in women)
- Handedness
- Occupation
- Mechanism of injury
- Time of injury

### Complete Hand Examination

- Special attention to injured digit
  - Extensor tendon function: Mallet deformity possible
  - Flexor tendon function
  - Tip sensation

## Digit-Specific Radiographs

- AP and true lateral views

> **TIP:** 50% of nail bed injuries are associated with distal phalangeal fractures, so make certain a radiograph is obtained.

## Digital Block[7] (Fig. 68-2)

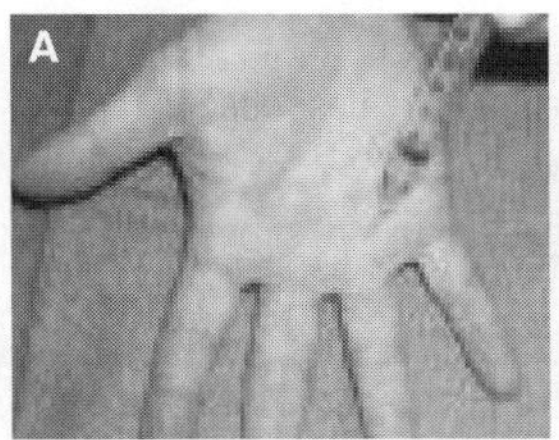

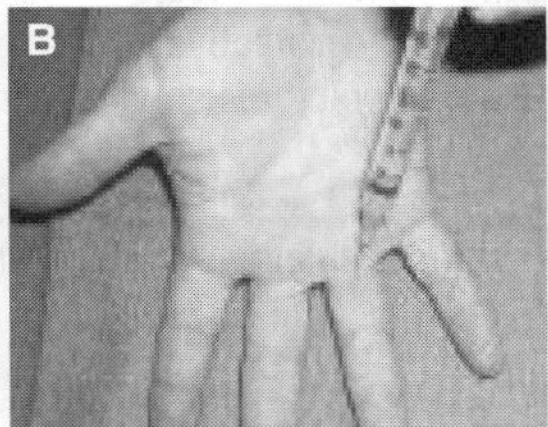

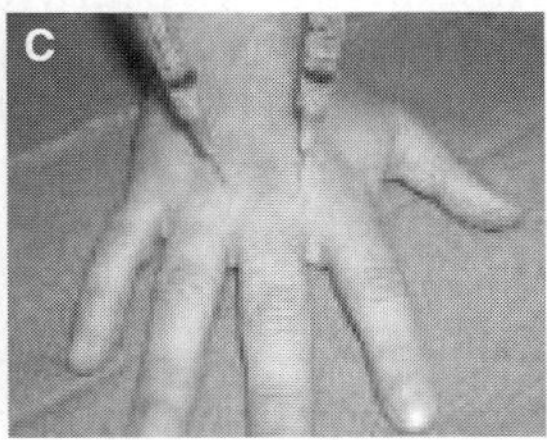


**Fig. 68-2** Digital block.

- Adequate cleaning of fingertip and complete assessment of injury are required.
- A distal wing block may be used for isolated nail surgery by injecting both lateral edges of the proximal nail fold, proceeding along the lateral nail fold into previously anesthetized skin[8] (Fig. 68-3).
  - Pain from this method of injection may require initial application of a topical anesthetic or cryogen spray.

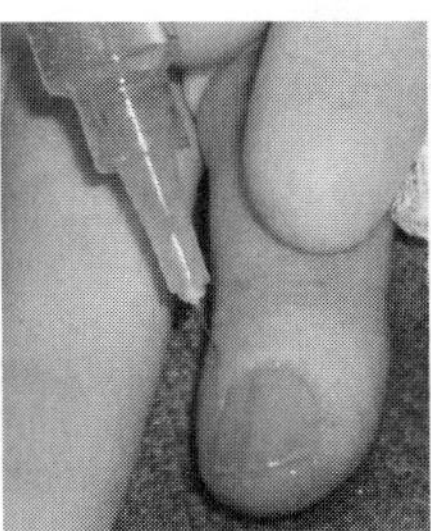

**Fig. 68-3** Distal wing block.

## Prognosis

- Determined by extent of injury
- Associated with poor aesthetic and functional outcomes
  - Comminuted distal phalanx fracture
  - Severe soft tissue loss
  - Nail bed fragmentation or avulsion lacerations

# CLASSIFICATION

- **Injury type**[9]
  - **Type I:** Small (25%) subungual hematoma
  - **Type II:** Larger (50%) subungual hematoma
  - **Type III:** Nail bed laceration associated with distal phalangeal fracture
  - **Type IV:** Nail bed fragmentation
  - **Type V:** Nail bed avulsion

- **Laceration type** (in order of increasing severity)
  - Simple lacerations
  - Stellate lacerations
  - Severe crush
  - Nail bed avulsion

## TREATMENT

### Underlying Phalangeal Fractures

- **Tuft fractures** are best managed with only **protective splinting.**
- More proximally significant or displaced fractures should be managed as described in Chapter 65.

> **TIP:** A ***Seymour fracture*** is an extraarticular transverse fracture of the distal phalanx with associated nail bed injury and is usually seen in children.

### Simple Subungual Hematoma (Type I, Type II Injuries)

Historically, nail removal and nail bed inspection and repair were recommended if hematoma stained more than 25% to 50% of nail bed. More recent data suggest that **trephination alone** gives equivalent good results with all hematoma sizes.[10,11]

- **Nail trephination for subungual hematoma** (Fig. 68-4)
  - **Indications**
    - Nail margin and nail plate intact
    - No associated displaced distal phalanx fracture
    - Patient complains of pain; otherwise, observation alone sufficient
  - **Technique**
    - Use a digital block with 1% lidocaine without epinephrine.
    - No digital tourniquet is necessary.
    - Prepare the finger with Betadine.
    - Ophthalmic battery-powered cautery or heated paper clip is used to penetrate nail plate and evacuate underlying hematoma.
    - Irrigate with isotonic saline solution.
    - Cover with nonadherent and sterile gauze.
    - Protective finger splint is worn for 1 week.
    - Prescribe antibiotics for a tuft fracture (now that it is converted to an open fracture).

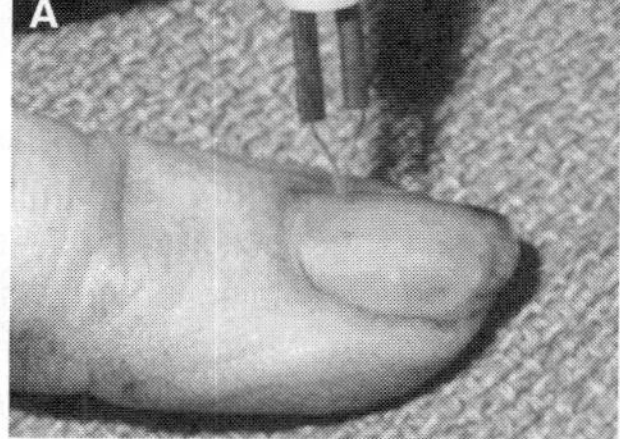


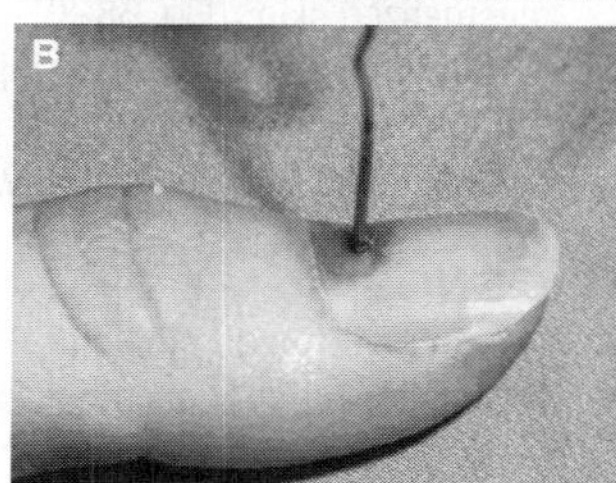


**Fig. 68-4** Trephination of the nail. Both the **A,** ophthalmic cautery method and **B,** heated paper clip method are effective.

> **TIP:** The underlying hematoma will cool the cautery tip and prevent injury to the underlying nail bed.

## Simple and Stellate Lacerations (Type III Injuries)[12]

- Nail plate is removed and nail bed is explored when nail margin or nail plate is disrupted and when associated with a displaced fracture of distal phalanx.
- **Nail bed laceration primary repair:**
  - **Indications**
    - Simple or stellate nail bed lacerations
  - **Technique**
    - Use a digital block with 1% lidocaine without epinephrine.
    - Exsanguinate finger and create a tourniquet at base of finger using half-inch Penrose drain or small sterile glove.
    - Prepare finger with Betadine.
    - Remove nail with Kutz or Freer elevator, tenotomy scissors, or curved iris scissors.
      - *Careful technique is essential to prevent iatrogenic nail bed injury.*
    - If laceration involves germinal matrix, incisions should be made perpendicular to nail fold margin to allow elevation of nail fold and improve exposure.
    - Examine laceration and perform minimal debridement; crushed and bruised nail beds often survive.
    - Running 6-0 or 7-0 chromic gut suture repairs simple lacerations.
    - Interrupted and running sutures are often necessary to accurately repair stellate lacerations.
    - If nail plate is available, replace it in the nail fold.
      - This splints the repair and prevents formation of nail fold adhesions (synechiae), which lead to ridging.
      - Drainage is through a hole made in nail plate.
    - When nail plate is not available or excessively damaged, secure silicone sheeting or sterile foil (from suture package or nonadherent gauze package) over repair and in nail fold.
    - Hold nail plate or other material in place with 5-0 chromic or nylon half-buried horizontal mattress or figure-of-eight suture, secured proximal to the nail fold. Suture can be removed at first postoperative visit to prevent formation of an epithelialized tract.
    - Place nonadherent, sterile gauze and a protective finger splint for dressing.
- Simple nail bed lacerations may be repaired with Dermabond (2-octylcyanoacrylate), which is faster than suture repair and provides similar cosmetic and functional results.[13,14]

**TIP:** Always use loupe magnification.

## Nail Bed Avulsions and Severe Crush Injuries (Type IV, Type V Injuries)[15-18]

- **Characteristics**
  - These are common in industrial workers, carpenters, and manual laborers who work with power machinery (e.g., saws, belts, drills, and presses)
  - Large areas of nail bed tissue are absent or irreparably damaged.
  - If left to heal by secondary intention, **misshapen and nonadherent nail plates are common.**
    - Spontaneous regeneration may occur if repair of available nail matrix is performed and nail splint is placed.[19]
  - Replace like tissue with like tissue; avulsed nail bed or nail bed grafting is used when possible.

> **TIP:** When nail bed grafting is not possible, split-thickness skin grafts can be placed over the defect, but nonadherent nail plates and poor aesthetic outcomes are common.

- **Nail bed avulsion repair with retained segment**
  - **Indications**
    - Injury too complex for primary repair
    - Large segment of nail bed tissue retained on avulsed portion of nail plate
  - **Technique**
    - Digital block and exposure as for type III injuries
    - Avulsed segment of nail bed carefully removed from back of nail plate and used as free graft
      - Removed segment placed directly on periosteum with good results
      - Secured with 7-0 chromic gut suture under loupe magnification
    - Dressing and nail plate replacement and postoperative treatment as for type III injuries
- **Nail bed avulsion repair with lateral bipedicled advancement**
  - **Indications**
    - Narrow ($<$2 mm) germinal matrix avulsions
    - Narrow ($<$2 mm) sterile matrix avulsions (less frequently described)
  - **Technique**
    - Digital block, finger tourniquet, and exposure as for type III injuries
    - Nail bed undermining performed lateral to defect on either side
      - Performed with Freer or Cottle periosteal elevator
      - Usually requires extensive undermining to lateral nail fold
    - Tissue advanced medially to cover defect
    - Sutured with 6-0 or 7-0 chromic gut suture
      - **Must be tension free** or suture will tear the tissue and create nail deformity
- **Nail bed avulsion repair with split-thickness nail bed graft**[16-18]
  - **Indications**
    - Large area of avulsed or irreparably damaged sterile matrix
    - Retained segment not available
  - **Technique**
    - Discuss potential donor sites (same digit, toe, etc.) with patient.
    - Technique is best performed in operating room.
    - Use digital or regional block with digital or upper extremity exsanguination and tourniquet.
    - Expose nail bed as described previously.
    - Template of defect is made using foil from suture package.
    - If defect is less than 50% of nail bed, a split-thickness nail bed graft can be harvested from the same digit using the foil template.
    - When defect is larger than 50% of nail bed, a split-thickness nail bed graft should be harvested from the great toe.[17]
    - Harvest split-thickness nail graft with No. 15 scalpel.
      - View blade through nail bed at all times to ensure proper thickness (0.007-0.010 inch).
      - Harvesting is best done using an operating microscope.
    - Sew graft in place with 7-0 chromic gut suture; proper longitudinal orientation is not necessary for injuries in the sterile matrix.
    - The nail plate makes the best dressing when available; otherwise, fine mesh gauze or silicone sheeting provide excellent results.
    - Dressings will be pushed forward and off by the new advancing nail.
    - Protective splinting is performed as previously described.

- **Nail bed avulsion repair with full-thickness nail bed graft**
  - **Indications**
    - Germinal matrix avulsion injuries too wide (0.2 mm) for repair with bipedicled advancement
  - **Technique**
    - Procedure begins as with split-thickness technique.
    - The lateral nail bed of the great toe is the best donor site.
    - Remove toenail, elevate the nail fold, and excise the lateral nail bed (full thickness) from distal margin to most proximal extent of germinal matrix.
    - Close donor site by advancement of lateral nail fold and primary closure.
    - Use template to design graft dimensions.
    - Secure graft to defect with 7-0 chromic gut suture.
      - **MUST** maintain proper longitudinal orientation
    - Use nail plate, fine mesh gauze, or silicone sheeting for dressing.
- **Nail bed avulsion repair with bilaminate neodermis**[20]
  - **Indications**
    - Avulsion injuries involving proximal half of nail bed
  - **Technique**
    - Artificial dermis is applied as a substitute for the missing part of the nail bed.
    - If necessary, scarred nail bed is excised.
    - Fixate dermis to surrounding tissue using 5-0 nylon.
    - Silicone membrane is removed 3-6 days after application and covered with polyethylene film.
    - Dressings are changed every 2-3 days until wound is completely healed.

## POSTOPERATIVE CARE

- Protective digital splint and bulky dressing suffice for adults unless associated injury requires greater immobilization.
- More bulky, usually plaster, immobilization is required to ensure compliance in children.
- Antibiotics are recommended if there is an associated distal phalanx fracture.
- Patients are seen in office, and dressings are removed after 5-7 days.
- Protective splinting is continued for 2 weeks.
- Inform patients that nail growth is usually stunted or absent for up to 21 days.[21]
- Desensitization protocols and occupational therapy should be started after soft tissue healing is adequate.
- Follow up monthly for 3 months and then at 6 months and 1 year.
- Three nail cycles (approximately 1 year) are required before final nail appearance can be assessed reliably.

## COMPLICATIONS

- **Hook-nail deformity** (Fig. 68-5)[22]
  - Also known as "parrot beak" deformity
  - Likely to occur with loss of bony support
  - Prevent by avoiding excessive tension from tight suturing and preserving bony and soft tissue support

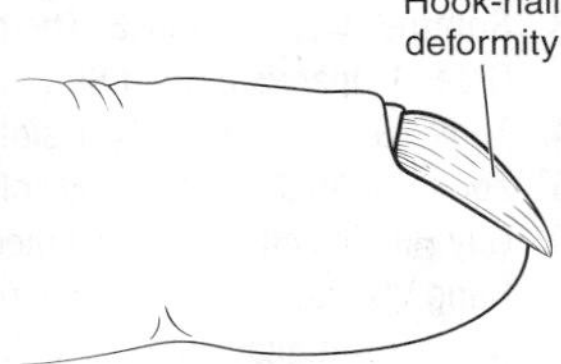


**Fig. 68-5** Hook-nail deformity.

- Prevent by shortening nail bed back to level of remaining distal phalanx
- Once established, repair accomplished by excision of the scarred tissue and replacement with a local flap, full-thickness skin graft, or bone grafting with local flap[23]

▪ **Nail ridges**
- Caused by scar beneath the nail bed

▪ **Split nail**
- Caused by ridge or longitudinal scar in germinal or sterile matrix
- Requires scar excision and nail bed repair or replacement

▪ **Nonadherence**
- Consequence of scar in sterile matrix

▪ **Nail absence**
- Usually caused by injury of germinal matrix
- Free microvascular transfer from toe most reliable treatment, but creates scars on foot, toe, and finger[24]

▪ **Dull nail**
- Cosmetic deformity from injury to dorsal roof, which is responsible for shiny surface of the nail

▪ **Short nail**
- Complex repair can be performed with osteoonychocutaneous free flap from toe.
- Bakhach flap deepithelializes proximal eponychium, which is then slid proximally through periungual incisions to lengthen the nail bed.[25]

## Key Points

✓ Nail production occurs primarily in the germinal matrix.
✓ It takes 100 days to grow a fingernail.
✓ Nail trephination is the best treatment for simple subungual hematomas.
✓ Loupe magnification is necessary for nail bed repairs.
✓ The nail plate makes the best dressing for the nail bed.
✓ Split-thickness nail bed grafting is best for sterile matrix avulsion injuries.
✓ Full-thickness nail bed grafting is best for germinal matrix avulsion injuries.

## References

1. Chau N, Gauchard GC, Siegfried C, et al. Relationships of job, age, and life condition with the causes and severity of occupational injuries in construction workers. Int Arch Occup Environ Health 77:60-66, 2004.
2. Sorock GS, Lombardi DA, Hauser RB, et al. Acute traumatic occupational hand injuries: type, location, and severity. J Occup Environ Med 44:345-351, 2002.
3. Sommer NZ, Brown RE. The perionychium. In Wolfe SW, Hotchkiss RN, Pederson WC, et al, eds. Green's Operative Hand Surgery, 6th ed. Philadelphia: Elsevier, 2011.
4. Zook EG. Anatomy and physiology of the perionychium. Hand Clin 18:553-559, 2002.
5. Zook EG. Anatomy and physiology of the perionychium. Hand Clin 6:1-7, 1990.
6. Guy RJ. The etiologies and mechanisms of nail bed injuries. Hand Clin 6:9-19, 1990.
7. Hung VS, Bodavula VKR, Dubin NH. Digital anaesthesia: comparison of the efficacy and pain associated with three digital nerve block techniques. J Hand Surg Br 30:581-584, 2005.
8. Jellinek NJ. Nail surgery: practical tips and treatment options. Dermatol Ther 20:68-74, 2007.

9. Van Beek AL, Kassan MA, Adson MH, et al. Management of acute fingernail injuries. Hand Clin 6:23-35, 1990.
10. Roser SE, Gellman H. Comparison of nail bed repair versus nail trephination for subungual hematomas in children. J Hand Surg Am 24:1166-1170, 1999.
11. Dean B, Becker G, Little C. The management of the acute traumatic subungual haematoma: a systematic review. Hand Surg 17:151-154, 2012.
12. Brown RE. Acute nail bed injuries. Hand Clin 18:561-575, 2002.
13. Strauss EJ, Weil WM, Jordan C, et al. A prospective, randomized, controlled trial of 2-octylcyanoacrylate versus suture repair for nail bed injuries. J Hand Surg Am 33:250-253, 2008.
14. Langlois J, Thevenin-Lemoine C, Rogier A, et al. The use of 2-octylcyanoacrylate for the treatment of nail bed injuries in children: results of a prospective series of 30 patients. J Child Orthop 4:61-65, 2010.
15. Shepard GH. Management of acute nail bed avulsions. Hand Clin 6:39-56, 1990.
16. Shepard GH. Perionychial grafts in trauma and reconstruction. Hand Clin 18:595-614, 2002.
17. Brown RE, Zook EG, Russell RC. Fingertip reconstruction with flaps and nail bed grafts. J Hand Surg Am 24:345-351, 1999.
18. Hsieh SC, Chen SL, Chen TM, et al. Thin split-thickness toenail bed grafts for avulsed nail bed defects. Ann Plast Surg 52:375-379, 2004.
19. Ogunro O, Ogunro S. Avulsion injuries of the nail bed do not need nail bed graft. Tech Hand Up Extrem Surg 11:135-138, 2007.
20. Sugamata A. Regeneration of nails with artificial dermis. J Plast Surg Hand Surg 46:191-194, 2012.
21. Gellman H. Fingertip-nail bed injuries in children: current concepts and controversies of treatment. J Craniofac Surg 20:1033-1035, 2009.
22. Strick MJ, Bremner-Smith AT, Tonkin MA. Antenna procedure for the correction of hook nail deformity. J Hand Surg Br 29:3-7, 2004.
23. Pandya AN, Giele HP. Prevention of the parrot beak deformity in fingertip injuries. Hand Surg 6:163-166, 2001.
24. Endo T, Nakayama Y. Microtransfers for nail and fingertip replacement. Hand Clin 18:615-622, 2002.
25. Adani R, Marcoccio I, Tarallo L. Nail lengthening and fingertip amputations. Plast Reconstr Surg 112: 1287-1294, 2003.

# 69. Flexor Tendon Injuries

Joshua A. Lemmon, Prosper Benhaim, Blake A. Morrison

## ANATOMY[1-6]

### Muscles and Tendons

- Flexion of the fingers and thumb is powered by **flexor digitorum profundus** (FDP), **flexor digitorum superficialis** (FDS), and **flexor pollicis longus** (FPL) **muscles.**
  - **FDS** tendons have a **common muscle belly** at the forearm level. Each **FDP** tendon has its own **individual muscle belly** at the forearm level.
  - Each FDS tendon divides into two equal halves at the level of the metacarpal head (Camper's chiasma).
    - Each half rotates laterally and dorsally around the FDP tendon.
    - FDS slips rejoin deep (dorsal) to the FDP tendon at the distal end of the proximal phalanx[1] (Fig. 69-1).
    - FDS then inserts on volar aspect of middle phalanx as two separate slips.
    - Small finger FDS tendon may be diminutive or completely absent.[7]

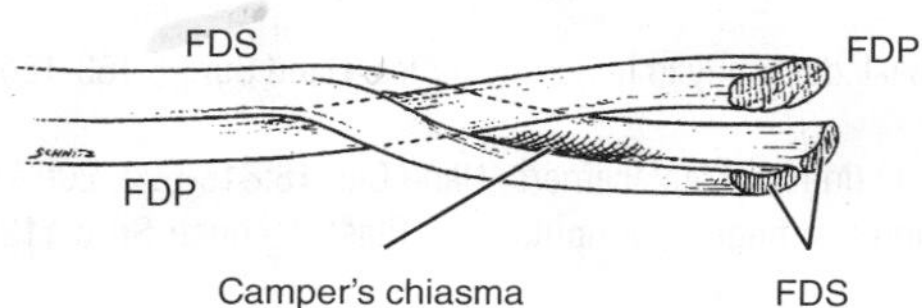


**Fig. 69-1** Arrangement of flexor digitorum profundus *(FDP)* and flexor digitorum superficialis *(FDS)* tendons within the flexor tendon sheath.

  - FDS tendons power flexion of the **proximal interphalangeal (PIP) joints.**
    - Origin: Medial epicondyle and coronoid process of ulna (humeroulnar head) and proximal shaft of radius (radial head)
    - Insertion: Middle phalanx
    - Innervation: Median nerve
    - Middle and ring finger FDS tendons are volar to the index and small finger FDS tendons at the distal forearm; useful for realignment when multiple tendon lacerations present (spaghetti wrist injury)
  - **FDP** tendons power flexion of the **distal interphalangeal (DIP) joints.**
    - Origin: Proximal ulna and interosseous membrane
    - Insertion: Volar base of distal phalanx
    - Innervation
      - Index and middle finger: Anterior interosseous branch of median nerve
      - Ring and small finger: Ulnar nerve
    - Origin of lumbrical muscles: Radial side of each FDP tendon at palm level (index and middle lumbricals are unipenniform, ring and small finger lumbricals are bipenniform)

- **FPL** powers flexion of the thumb interphalangeal (IP) joint.
  - Origin: Proximal radius and interosseous membrane (radial head) and medial epicondyle or coronoid process (accessory head)
  - Insertion: Volar base of thumb distal phalanx
  - Innervation: Anterior interosseous nerve branch of the median nerve
- Tendons of these muscles each lie within a tendon sheath.
  - The sheath is a synovial-lined channel that allows smooth tendon gliding.
  - The synovial fluid environment provides tendon nutrition.
  - Each sheath is reinforced with thickened areas known as ***pulleys.***

## Pulley System

- Pulleys hold the tendons close to the phalanges at all positions of extension and flexion, maximizing mechanical efficiency.
- There are **five annular (A)** and **three cruciate (C)** pulleys[1] (Fig. 69-2).
- Odd-numbered annular pulleys are at the joints levels: A1 at metacarpophalangeal (MP) joint, A3 at PIP joint, A5 at DIP joint.
- A2 pulley is at proximal portion of proximal phalanx; A4 pulley is at middle portion of middle phalanx.

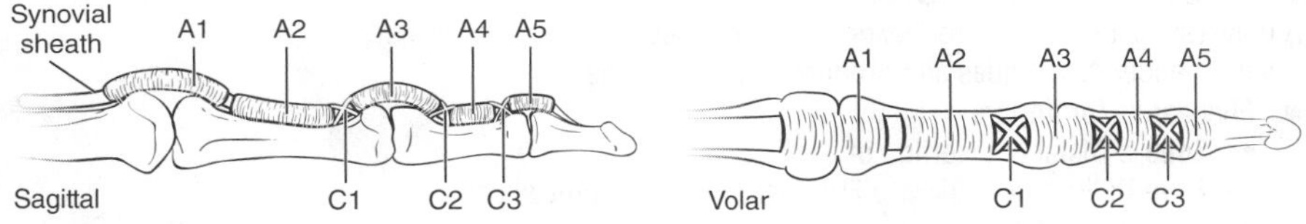


**Fig. 69-2** Components of the flexor tendon sheath. *A1-A5* are annular pulleys. *C1-C3* are cruciate pulleys.

> **TIP: Mnemonic:** *"proximal proximal" and "middle middle"*

- Transverse fibers of the **p**almar **a**poneurosis make up the **PA** pulley, also known as the ***A1 pulley.***

> **TIP:** The A2 and A4 pulleys are the most important components for proper flexor tendon function. Injury to these pulleys can lead to flexor tendon bowstringing.

- The **pulley system of the thumb** reflects its unique anatomy, with one less tendon and one less intercalated joint than the fingers. The thumb has only two annular pulleys (A1, A2) and an intervening oblique pulley.
- Injury to the oblique pulley in the thumb can lead to bowstringing of the FPL tendon.

## Tendon Nutrition

- **Direct vascular supply**
  - **Myotendinous junction:** Supplies short segment near proximal end of tendon
  - **Bony junction (Sharpey's fibers):** Supplies a short distal segment
  - **Vincula:** Fibrovascular structures (mesotenon folds) that directly supply the tendons within the tendon sheath[8] (Fig. 69-3)

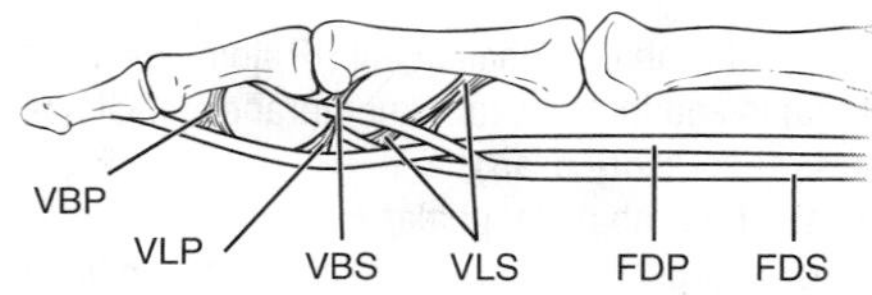


**Fig. 69-3** Vincula of the flexor tendons. (*FDP,* Flexor digitorum profundus; *FDS,* flexor digitorum superficialis; *VBP,* vinculum breve profundus; *VBS,* vinculum breve superficialis; *VLP,* vinculum longum profundus; *VLS,* vinculum longum superficialis.)

- **Vincula arise from transverse communicating branches of the digital arteries.**
  - Two vincula to the FDS tendon: Vinculum breve superficialis (distal), vinculum longum superficialis (proximal)
  - Two vincula to the FDP tendon: Vinculum breve profundus (distal), vinculum longum profundus (proximal)
- *Vincula enter the tendons dorsally. It is theoretically best to repair tendon with sutures placed volarly to minimize effect on blood supply.*

■ **Synovial diffusion:** Provides most of the tendon nutrition within the sheath

## Flexor Tendon Zones (Verdan)

A universal nomenclature for flexor tendon injuries has been established.
Recommended techniques and prognoses vary by zone.

■ **Five zones for fingers**[9] (Fig. 69-4)
- **Zone I:** Distal to insertion of the FDS
- **Zone II:** From A1 pulley to FDS insertion (within the sheath: "no man's land")
- **Zone III:** From distal end of the carpal tunnel to A1 pulley
- **Zone IV:** Within the carpal tunnel
- **Zone V:** Proximal to the carpal tunnel

■ **Five zones for thumb**
- **Zone T I:** Distal to interphalangeal (IP) joint
- **Zone T II:** From A1 pulley to IP joint
- **Zone T III:** Over thenar eminence
- **Zone T IV:** Within the carpal tunnel
- **Zone T V:** Proximal to the carpal tunnel

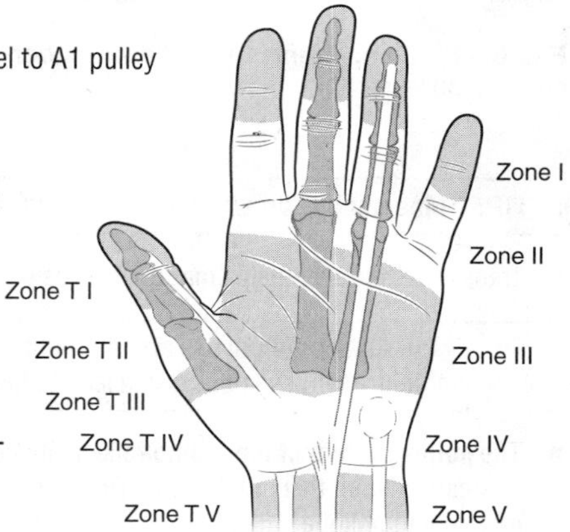

**Fig. 69-4** Flexor tendon zones of the digits.

# Histology[10]

## Tendon Composition

■ **Collagen:** Mostly type I
■ **Ground substance:** Elastin and various mucopolysaccharides
■ **Tenocytes:** Specialized fibroblasts

## Tendon Structure

■ **Endotenon:** Fascicular arrangement with bundles of tenocytes and collagen fibers held together by fine layer of connective tissue
■ **Epitenon:** Septa of endotenon joined together externally to form fibrous outer layer
■ **Paratenon:** Tendons covered by loose layer of adventitial tissue proximal to tendon sheath

## PATIENT EVALUATION

### HISTORY

- Age
- Handedness
- Occupation
- Mechanism of injury, including how hand was positioned during the injury
- Time of injury
- Previous treatment
- History of tobacco use
- Tetanus status

### PHYSICAL EXAMINATION

- Characterize and document open wounds.
- Evaluate arterial supply to the digit; handheld Doppler probes are useful.
- Examine the resting position of the hand (i.e., in obtunded adult or pediatric patients who may not be able to cooperate with examination).
- Evaluate for nerve injury.

> **TIP:** Sensation should be evaluated with static and moving two-point discrimination tests before using local anesthetic.

- Test individual tendon function.
  - Each FDS and FDP must be assessed while blocking movement of adjacent digits.
  - The FDP is examined by blocking PIP flexion in each digit (each FDP tendon has an independent muscle belly).
  - The FDS is examined by preventing flexion of the other digits (all FDS tendons share a common muscle belly).
- Recognize normal variants.
  - FDS tendon for small finger is absent in **15%** of population.
  - **Linburg's syndrome:** Adhesions between FPL tendon and index finger FDP tendon within the carpal tunnel cause the index finger to flex with flexion of the thumb IP. This occurs in **30%** of the population.

### HAND RADIOGRAPHS

- AP, lateral, and oblique views to rule out fractures or retained foreign bodies

## PREOPERATIVE CONSIDERATIONS, TIMING OF REPAIR, AND TREATMENT OPTIONS[11-16]

> **TIP:** Emergency flexor tendon repair is not required unless the digit is devascularized.

### PRIMARY REPAIR (<24 HOURS)

- Preferred option when feasible
- **Contraindications**
  - Gross contamination or human bites
  - Evidence of active infection (cellulitis, purulence)
  - Lack of stable soft tissue coverage

## Delayed Primary Repair (>24 Hours but <2 Weeks)

- Reasonable option for heavily contaminated wounds
- Functional results comparable to primary repair

## Secondary Repair

- **Early (2-5 weeks)**
  - Performed before significant muscle contraction
  - Functional results similar to delayed primary repair
  - Increased risk of infection and prolonged edema with longer repair delay
- **Late (>5 weeks)**
  - Presence of tendon edema and softening
  - Flexor tendon sheath becomes scarred, reducing likelihood of good tendon gliding within the tendon sheath.
  - Repair without advancement and extension deficit prohibited by significant muscular contraction
  - **Best treatments: Tendon graft or tendon transfer**

> **TIP:** The FDP tendon may be advanced up to, *but not more than,* 1 cm. Excessive advancement creates a *quadriga effect* in which a flexion deformity appears in the repaired digit, and the adjacent digits have limited active flexion.

## Tendon Grafting

**Segmental tendon loss or muscular contracture necessitates grafting for repair.**

- **Single-stage**
  - Requires adequate tendon sheath and pulleys, soft tissue coverage, and supple joints
  - **Common donors**
    - Palmaris longus (13 cm)
    - Plantaris (31 cm)
    - Extrinsic third or fourth toe extensor (30 cm)
- **Two-stage: Used when tendon sheath is scarred or unusable**
  - **First stage**
    - Native tendon is excised.
    - Pulleys are reconstructed as necessary.
    - A silicone rod **(Hunter rod)** is sutured to distal FDP tendon stump.
    - Rod induces formation of a **pseudosheath** with repetitive passive motion of the digit, within approximately 8 weeks.
  - **Second stage**
    - Tendon graft is sutured to the distal end of silicone rod and pulled through pseudosheath.
    - The **proximal** juncture to the native FDP (or FDS) tendon is made with a **Pulvertaft weave.**
    - The **distal** juncture is made with a **pull-out suture** or **suture anchor** to distal phalanx bone.
    - Tension is adjusted so that the cascade of fingers is slightly tighter in the grafted digit.
    - If the tendon graft is placed too loosely or if it is too long, it can result in a **lumbrical plus deformity.**

## Tendon Transfer

- Limited indications for flexor tendon repair
- Used when proximal muscle unusable because of denervation, direct injury, or contraction
- See Chapter 60 for more detailed information.

## Other Options

- For patients in whom normal active motion of DIP joint is not essential
  - DIP joint arthrodesis
  - Capsulodesis
  - Tenodesis

# OPERATIVE PRINCIPLES[15-19]

## General Technical Considerations

- Flexor tendon repair should be performed in the operating room with loupe magnification.
- Incisions should be designed to **maintain viability of skin flaps, permit wide exposure,** and **prohibit formation of scar contractures:** Midlateral, volar zigzag (Bruner), or combinations that incorporate traumatic laceration (Fig. 69-5).
- Minimal traumatic handling of the tendon surface limits subsequent adhesion formation.

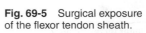

**Fig. 69-5** Surgical exposure of the flexor tendon sheath.

**TIP:** Recognize that the location of the skin laceration may be different than the location of the tendon laceration, based on the extension/flexion position of the digit at time of injury.

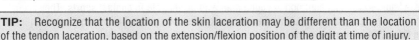

## Repair Strength and Technique

- **Initial strength of the repair is proportional to the size and number of suture strands crossing the repair site.**
- Multiple methods exist for placing core sutures.
  - The most popular methods are shown in Fig. 69-6.[15]
  - Locking sutures provide better repair strength than grasping sutures.[20]
  - A minimum of a **four-strand repair** is necessary for an early active motion rehabilitation protocol.
  - A running 6-0 epitendinous suture improves contour at the repair but also adds an average of **15%** strength to the core suture repair.
  - The recommended length of each core suture is 10 mm proximal and distal to the laceration site, if technically feasible.[21]
- **Pulvertaft weave**
  - Repair by weaving together the proximal and distal tendon ends.
  - As the strongest juncture, it is capable of immediate active motion.

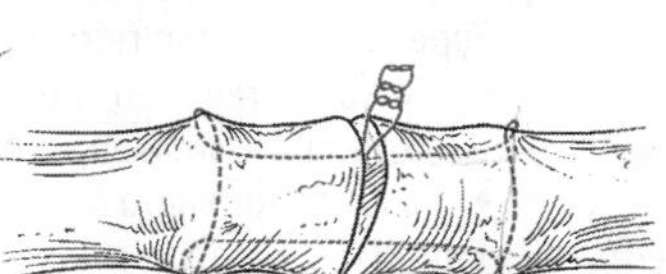

Modified Kessler technique

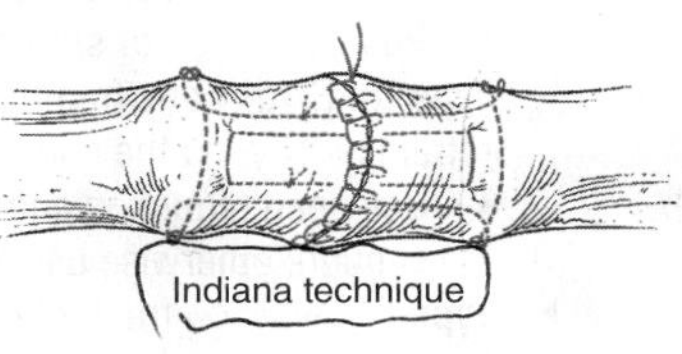

Indiana technique

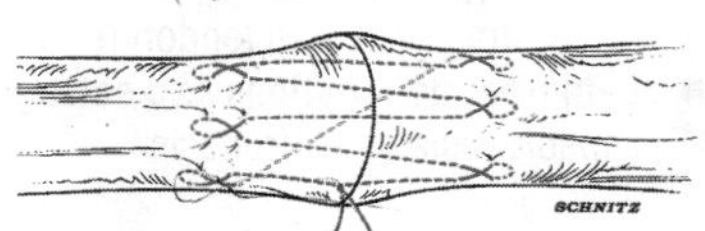


Six-strand technique

**Fig. 69-6** Popular core suture techniques for end-to-end tendon repair.

- Bulk prohibits use outside of zone III or zone V.
- Technique is suitable only for **tendon grafts** or **transfers** because of additional length requirement.

## Partial Tendon Lacerations

- Technique is controversial.
- Oblique or beveled lacerations can catch on a pulley and should be repaired with a few simple sutures.
- Most agree that tendon lacerations involving **more than 50% of tendon diameter** should be formally repaired with both core suture and epitendinous repair.
- Early mobilization is imperative.

## Zone I Injuries

- **Sharp injuries: Lacerations**
  - Vincula: Usually holds proximal tendon end within injured digit
  - DIP volar plate examined and repaired if necessary
  - Distal FDP tendon with 5 mm stump required to place adequate core sutures
  - If sufficient distal length not available, reinsert with a **pull-out suture** tied over a dorsal button, or use direct fixation to bone with **suture anchor(s)**

**TIP:** A monofilament pull-out suture is easier to remove and less susceptible to infection than braided suture material.

- **Avulsion injuries: "Rugger jersey finger"**

These injuries are most common in **young men who participate in contact sports.** They occur because of forced extension during maximal profundus contraction. This is most common in the **ring finger,** which is usually the longest digit when the PIP joints are fully flexed.

- **Types (Leddy classification)**
  - **Type I:** FDP tendon retracts into palm with rupture of both vincula.
    - Repair is required within 1 week, because the myotendinous unit will shorten and the tendon will weaken without the nutrition of either the vincula or synovial diffusion.
    - Treat as for sharp injuries.
  - **Type II:** FDP tendon avulses with small fragment of distal phalanx; the long vinculum remains intact, and the tendon retracts to the level of the PIP joint (A3 pulley).
    - Repair can be delayed up to 6 weeks.
    - Pull-out suture or suture anchor is used as for sharp injuries.
  - **Type III:** Large bony fragment is avulsed with the tendon and is prevented from retraction beyond the middle phalanx by the A4 pulley.
    - Use open reduction and K-wire fixation vs. screw fixation if the fragment is large enough; otherwise use a pull-out suture secured over dorsal button.
  - **Type IV:** Avulsion fracture of the distal phalanx combines with tendon avulsion from the fragment with tendon retraction.[22]
- **Late treatment options and salvage procedures:** Secondary tendon grafts, tenodesis, and DIP capsulodesis or arthrodesis

## Zone II Injuries

- **Historically associated with poor results,** acute repair used to be discouraged, given the name *no man's land.*
  - Acute repair now recommended because of improved techniques and results
- Repair of both FDP and FDS is advocated by most, except in cases of massive injury (e.g., replantation) when repair of only FDP is acceptable.
- Wide exposure is required.
- Neurovascular bundles are identified and protected.
- Transection of the A2 and A4 annular pulleys is avoided; instead windows can be made in tendon sheath by opening cruciate pulleys or the A1, A3, or A5 pulleys if necessary.
- **Tendon retrieval methods:**
  - Proximal to distal "milking" or use of reverse Esmarch's tourniquet
  - Skin hook, small-caliber clamp (Jake clamp), or tendon retriever passed retrograde into tendon sheath to grasp tendon end
  - Proximal (volar) incision made to expose proximal tendon end; small catheter used to pull tendon distally through pulley system to the repair site
- **Four-strand or six-strand core suture technique** of 3-0 or 4-0 braided or monofilament nonabsorbable suture is employed for repair.
- Strength and improved tendon gliding are added through use of **epitendinous suture** of running 5-0 or 6-0 monofilament polypropylene (increases repair strength by 15%-20%[23]).

## Zone III Injuries

- Repaired with same operative technique as for zone II
- **Prognosis better** than for zone II injuries
  - Repair bulk less important and postoperative adhesions less constricting (allows stronger six-strand repair routinely)
  - Functional results usually dictated by results of associated nerve repair

## Zone IV Injuries

- Exacting technique must be used, because tolerances within the carpal tunnel are similar to those for zone II.
- Operative technique is as for zone II.
- To prevent bowstringing, **transverse carpal ligament should be repaired** after tendon repair.

## Zone V Injuries

- Repair with core sutures as described previously, but epitendinous suture is *not* necessary.
- Outcomes are generally good, because stronger repairs in this area allow early active motion.
- Associated injuries in the median and ulnar nerves result in more disability than do tendon injuries themselves.

# POSTOPERATIVE CARE AND REHABILITATION[24-26]

## Extension Block-Splint

- Wrist at 30 degrees of flexion: Weakens the flexor tendons and minimizes risk of postoperative tendon rupture.
- MP joints at 45-70 degrees of flexion
- Should maintain IP joints in near-full extension or slight flexion (15 degrees)
- Sutures removed after 2 weeks

### Rehabilitation Protocols

- Early controlled mobilization protocols are now standard care, except with young children.
  - **Duran and Houser**[27]**:** Early controlled passive range of motion with goal of at least 2-4 mm of differential gliding between the FDS and FDP tendons.
  - **Kleinert et al**[28]**:** Elastic band traction for active extension, passive flexion
  - **Early active motion protocols**[29]**:** Requires a minimum of a four-strand repair, but results generally better.
  - Multiple variations and modifications of these protocols described

## COMPLICATIONS[27,30]

### Ruptures

- Occur in 5% of all repairs: Slightly more common for FPL than for other finger tendons
- **Immediate exploration and re-repair recommended**
- Recurrent rupture best treated with secondary tendon reconstruction, tendon transfer, or arthrodesis

### Adhesions

- Limited range of motion and function caused by postoperative and postinjury scars between tendon and surrounding structures
- **Increased likelihood of adhesions with prolonged immobilization and severe injury**
- **Consider tenolysis if:**
  - More than 3-6 months have elapsed since the tendon repair.
  - Tendon repair is intact, but there is a large discrepancy between total active range of motion (ROM) and total passive ROM.
  - Soft tissue is supple with normal or near-normal passive ROM.
  - There is no appreciable improvement in active ROM after 4-6 weeks of aggressive hand therapy.
- **Contractures**
  - Affect 17% of flexor tendon repairs[26]
  - Prevention and treatment primarily with splinting
  - Open or closed capsulotomy reserved for severe and recalcitrant cases

### Key Points

✓ The best results are associated with early repair.

✓ Flexor tendon repair should be performed in the operating room, with a tourniquet and loupe magnification.

✓ The FDP tendon should not be advanced more than 1 cm.

✓ Proper splint placement and postoperative rehabilitation are as important as operative technique.

## REFERENCES


1. Idler RS. Anatomy and biomechanics of the digital flexor tendons. Hand Clin 1:3-11, 1985.
2. Austin GJ, Leslie BM, Ruby LK, et al. Variations of the flexor digitorum superficialis of the small finger. J Hand Surg Am 14:262-267, 1989.
3. Doyle JR, Blythe WF. Macroscopic and functional anatomy of the flexor tendon sheath. J Bone Joint Surg Am 56:1094, 1974.
4. Doyle JR, Blythe WF. Anatomy of the flexor tendon sheath and pulleys of the thumb. J Hand Surg Am 2:149-151, 1977.
5. Doyle JR, Blythe WF. Anatomy of the flexor tendon sheath and pulley system: a current review. J Hand Surg Am 14:349-351, 1989.
6. Strickland JW. Development of flexor tendon surgery: twenty-five years of progress. J Hand Surg Am 25:214-235, 2000.
7. Townley WA, Swan MC, Dunn RL. Congenital absence of flexor digitorum superficialis: implications for assessment of little finger lacerations. J Hand Surg Eur Vol 35:417-418, 2010.
8. Kleinert HE, Lubahn JD. Current state of flexor tendon surgery. Ann Chir Main 3:7-17, 1984.
9. Strickland JW. Flexor tendon repair. Hand Clin 1:55-68, 1985.
10. Cohen MJ, Kaplan L. Histology and ultrastructure of the human flexor tendon sheath. J Hand Surg Am 12:25-29, 1987.
11. Strickland JW. Flexor tendon surgery. I. Primary flexor tendon repair. J Hand Surg Br 14:261-272, 1989.
12. Steinberg DR. Acute flexor tendon injuries. Orthop Clin North Am 23:125-140, 1992.
13. Strickland JW. Flexor tendon injuries. I. Foundations of treatment. J Am Acad Orthop Surg 3:44-54, 1995.
14. Schneider LH, Bush DC. Primary care of flexor tendon injuries. Hand Clin 5:383-394, 1989.
15. Seiler JG. Flexor tendon repair. J Am Soc Surg of the Hand 1:177-191, 2001.
16. Strickland JW. Acute flexor tendon injuries. In Green DP, Hotchkiss RN, Pederson WC, eds. Green's Operative Hand Surgery, 4th ed. Philadelphia: Churchill Livingstone, 1999.
17. Strickland JW. Flexor tendon injuries. II. Operative technique. J Am Acad Orthop Surg 3:55-62, 1995.
18. Strickland JW. Flexor tendon injuries. II. Flexor tendon repair. Orthop Rev 15:701-721, 1986.
19. Malerich M, Baird R, McMaster W, et al. Permissible limits of flexor digitorum profundus tendon advancement: an anatomic study. J Hand Surg Am 12:30-33, 1987.
20. Tanaka T, Amadio PC, Zhao C, et al. Gliding characteristics and gap formation for locking and grasping tendon repairs: a biomechanical study in a human cadaver model. J Hand Surg Am 29:6-14, 2004.
21. Tang JB, Zhang Y, Cao Y, et al. Core suture purchase affects strength of tendon repairs. J Hand Surg Am 30:1262-1266, 2005.
22. Henry SL, Katz MA, Green DP. Type IV FDP avulsion: lessons learned clinically and through review of the literature. Hand 4:357-361, 2009.
23. Papandrea R, Seitz WH Jr, Shapiro P, et al. Biomechanical and clinical evaluation of the epitenon-first technique of flexor tendon repair. J Hand Surg Am 20:261-266, 1995.
24. Wang AW, Gupta A. Early motion after flexor tendon surgery. Hand Clin 12:43-55, 1996.
25. Bainbridge LC, Robertson C, Gillies D, et al. A comparison of post-operative mobilization of flexor tendon repairs with "passive flexion–active extension" and "controlled active motion" techniques. J Hand Surg Br 4:517-521, 1994.
26. Chow JA, Thomes LJ, Dovelle S, et al. Controlled motion rehabilitation after flexor tendon repair and grafting. A multi-centre study. J Bone Joint Surg Br 70:591-595, 1988.

27. Duran RJ, Houser RG. Controlled passive motion following flexor tendon repair in zones two and three. In American Association of Orthopaedic Surgeons Symposium on Tendon Surgery in the Hand. St Louis: CV Mosby, 1975.
28. Kleinert HE, Kutz JE, Ashbell S. Primary repair of lacerated flexor tendons in "no man's land." J Bone Joint Surg Am 49:577, 1967.
29. Kitsis CK, Wade PJF, Krikler SJ, et al. Controlled active motion following primary flexor tendon repair: a prospective study over 9 years. J Hand Surg Br 23:344-349, 1998.
30. Taras JS, Gray RM, Culp RW. Complications of flexor tendon injuries. Hand Clin 10:93-109, 1994.

# 70. Extensor Tendon Injuries

**Bishr Hijazi, Michael S. Dolan, Blake A. Morrison**

## GENERAL CONSIDERATIONS[1]

- Concomitant neurovascular involvement is less common with extensor injuries.
  - Extensor tendons are relatively exposed, superficial structures.
  - The neurovascular bundles are guarded from dorsal injury by bone.
- Partial injuries are particularly common because of relatively flat extensor tendons in the digits.
- Penetrating injuries can easily involve underlying joints.
- Tendon repairs require proper splinting and postoperative therapy.

## ANATOMY[2,3]

### EXTRINSIC TENDONS

- Innervated by the **radial nerve**
- Cross the wrist under extensor retinaculum, which is divided into **six compartments** (Fig. 70-1)
  - **First compartment**
    - *Abductor pollicis longus* (APL)
      - Inserts into base of thumb metacarpal
      - Almost always multiple slips
    - *Extensor pollicis brevis* (EPB)
      - Inserts into base of thumb proximal phalanx
      - Rarely multiple slips
  - **Second compartment**
    - *Extensor carpi radialis longus* (ECRL)
      - Inserts into base of index finger metacarpal
    - *Extensor carpi radialis brevis* (ECRB)
      - Inserts into base of middle finger metacarpal
  - **Third compartment**
    - *Extensor pollicis longus* (EPL)
      - Inserts into base of thumb distal phalanx
      - Relative independence of action across all three joints because of multiple attachments to dorsal apparatus

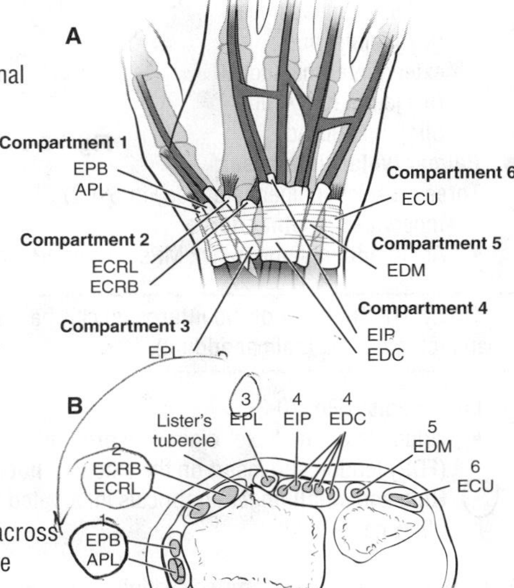


**Fig. 70-1** Extensor compartments. (*APL*, Abductor pollicis longus; *ECRB*, extensor carpi radialis brevis; *ECRL*, extensor carpi radialis longus; *EDC*, extensor digitorum communis; *ECU*, extensor carpi ulnaris; *EDM*, extensor digiti minimi; *EIP*, extensor indicis proprius; *EPB*, extensor pollicis brevis; *EPL*, extensor pollicis longus.)

- **Fourth compartment**
  - *Extensor digitorum communis* (EDC)
    - Often has two slips to ring finger
    - Slip to small finger absent in up to **56%** of population
  - *Extensor indicis proprius* (EIP)
    - Ulnar to EDC of index finger
    - **Most distal** myotendinous junction
- **Fifth compartment**
  - *Extensor digiti minimi* (EDM); also called *extensor digiti quinti* (EDQ)
    - Two slips in 80% of population
- **Sixth compartment**
  - *Extensor carpi ulnaris* (ECU)
    - **Only extensor tendon with a true sheath**
    - Tear of sheath: Leads to ulnar-sided wrist pain and popping sensation with subluxation of ECU

## INTRINSICS

- **Dorsal interossei:** Four muscles, bipennate (Fig. 70-2)
  - Innervated by **ulnar nerve**
  - Act to **abduct** fingers, flex metacarpophalangeal (MP) joints, and extend interphalangeal (IP) joints (only with MP joints flexed)

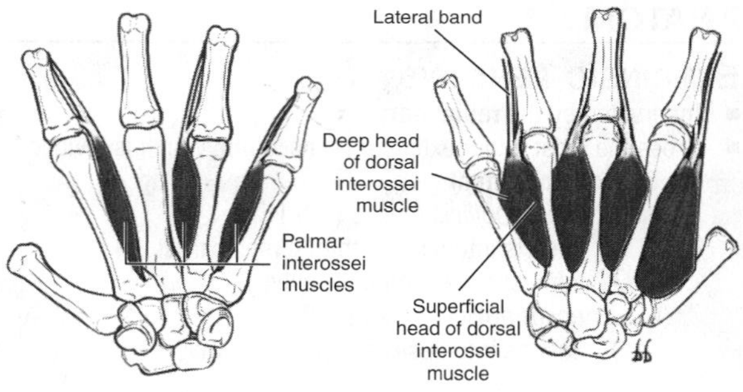


**Fig. 70-2** Anatomy of the interosseous muscles.

- **Palmar (volar) interossei:** Three muscles, unipennate (see Fig. 70-2)
  - Innervated by **ulnar nerve**
  - Act to **adduct** fingers, flex MPs, extend IPs (only with MP joints flexed)

> **TIP:** The function of the interossei can be remembered by the mnemonics DAB (dorsal abduct) and PAD (palmar adduct).

- **Lumbricals**[4] (Fig. 70-3)
  - Originate on the flexor digitorum profundus (FDP) tendon and insert on the extensor hood
  - **Ring** and **small** finger lumbricals innervated by **ulnar** nerve

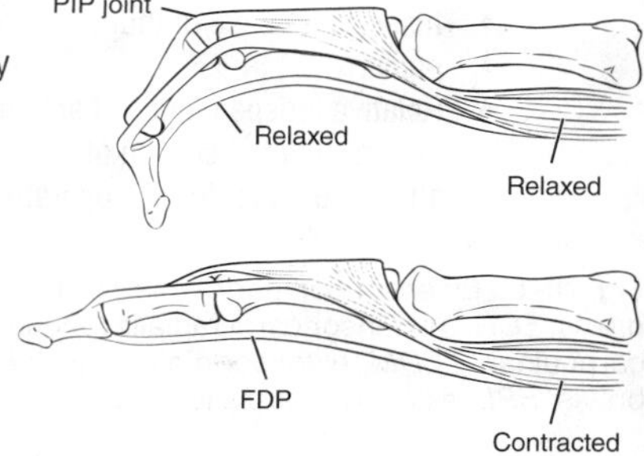


**Fig. 70-3** The lumbrical muscle originates from the FDP tendon. When the lumbrical muscle is relaxed and the flexor profundus muscle contracts, the IP joint flexes. When the lumbrical contracts, it extends the IP joint by relaxation of the profundus tendon distal to the lumbrical origin and by proximal pull on the lateral band and dorsal aponeurosis.

- **Index** and **middle** lumbricals innervated by **median** nerve
- Prime extensors of IP joints, weak flexors of MP joints

**NOTE: Lumbrical plus finger deformity occurs when the FDP shortens (classically from a finger amputation) and puts tension on the lumbrical. The result is paradoxical extension of the IP joint while attempting flexion.**

## Extensor Mechanism

- Complex structures balance synergistic and antagonistic actions of extrinsics and intrinsics.
- Extensor tendon trifurcates into central slip and two lateral slips.

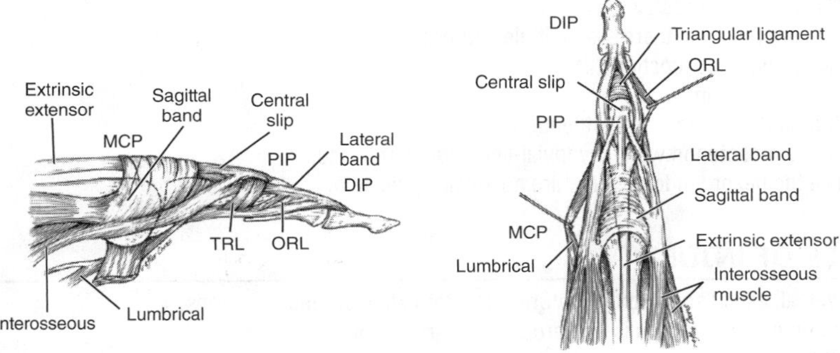


**Fig. 70-4** Dorsal view of the extensor mechanism of the finger. Extrinsic and intrinsic contributions of the dorsal aponeurosis.

- Central slip inserts into base of middle phalanx, with fibers from lumbricals and interossei.
- Lateral slips join with lateral bands of intrinsics to form conjoined lateral bands.
- Conjoined lateral bands reunite over distal portion of middle phalanx to form terminal extensor tendon, which inserts into base of distal phalanx[5] (Fig. 70-4).

## Juncturae Tendinum

- Interconnect EDC tendons
- **Most variable anatomy of extensor system**
  - Consistency varies: Fascial, ligamentous, or tendinous
- Can provide some cross-tendon motion in cases of lacerated EDC tendons proximal to the juncturae, leading to misdiagnosis

## Sagittal Bands

- Originate from intermetacarpal plate on either side of metacarpal head
- Form dorsal expansion, or hood
- Maintain central slip of extensors over MP joints, preventing lateral subluxation
- Prevent MP joint hyperextension

## Extensor Digitorum Brevis Manus (EDBM)

- **Anomalous muscle** located on dorsal wrist, with tendons inserting into extensors of hand
- Approximately **3%** incidence
- Occasionally can produce pain and a mass effect when wrist is flexed

- **Often misdiagnosed as ganglion or other tumor**
- Treatment of choice is excision

## PHYSIOLOGY OF TENDON HEALING

- See Chapter 69 for phases of tendon healing and tendon histology.

### Extensor Tendon Healing: Three Sources of Nutrition

- Endogenous circulation
- Synovial fluid diffusion (only under dorsal retinaculum)
- Exogenous circulation (from adhesions)

### Vascular Supply

- Like flexor tendons, there are multiple sources.
  - Myotendinous junction
  - Bony insertion
  - Paratenon along length of tendon
  - Long mesotenon within synovial-lined dorsal retinaculum
- Unlike the flexor tendons, there are **no vincular vessels.**

## ZONES OF INJURY[6]

- Universal, established nomenclature exists for extensor tendon injuries.
- Recommended techniques and prognoses vary by zone.
- **Nine zones:**
  - **Zone I:** Over distal IP joint
  - **Zone II:** Over middle phalanx
  - **Zone III:** Over proximal IP joint
  - **Zone IV:** Over proximal phalanx
  - **Zone V:** Over MP joint
  - **Zone VI:** Over metacarpals
  - **Zone VII:** Over carpus
  - **Zone VIII:** Distal forearm and retinaculum
  - **Zone IX:** Proximal forearm
- **Thumb zones** (Fig. 70-5)
  - **TI:** Over IP joint
  - **TII:** Over proximal phalanx
  - **TIII:** Over MP joint
  - **TIV:** Over metacarpal
  - **TV:** Over carpus

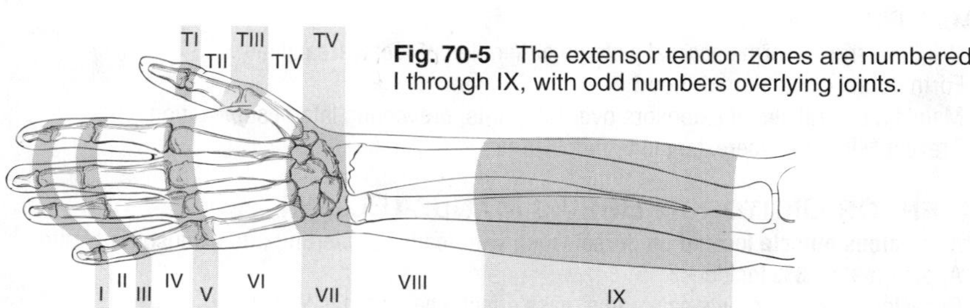


**Fig. 70-5** The extensor tendon zones are numbered I through IX, with odd numbers overlying joints.

**TIP:** Odd zones are over the joints; even zones are between joints.

## RECOMMENDED REPAIR TECHNIQUE BY ZONE[4]

### GENERAL CONSIDERATIONS

- Extensors are thin thus difficult to suture well.
- Kessler, Bunnell, and running horizontal mattress patterns are most popular for core sutures.
- Epitendinous sutures are usually 5-0 monofilament in a running cross-stitch, dorsal aspect only.
- Primary repair is preferred, except in cases of human bite or cellulitis.
- Injuries distal to the MP joints retract very little, because the adjacent juncturae limit proximal migration.

**TIP:** Avoid large knots of monofilament suture outside the tendon, because they may be palpable under the thin dorsal soft tissue coverage. Braided core sutures are less conspicuous.

### ZONE I (MALLET FINGER DEFORMITIES)

- Several **classification systems** have been proposed; the following was **described by Doyle.**[7]
  - **Type I:** Closed injury with loss of tendon continuity, with or without small avulsion fracture
  - **Type II:** Laceration at or proximal to distal interphalangeal (DIP) joint with loss of tendon continuity
  - **Type III:** Deep abrasion with loss of skin, subcutaneous cover, and tendon substance
  - **Type IV A:** Transepiphyseal plate fracture in children

**TIP:** Beware of Seymour fracture. This a serious open fracture with the nail bed trapped in the physis. It often presents with nail plate sitting on top of the nail fold and is often mistaken for a simple nail bed injury.

  - **Type IV B:** Fracture of 20%-50% of articular surface
  - **Type IV C:** Fracture of more than 50% of articular surface, and volar subluxation of distal phalanx
- **Treatment by type**
  - **Type I**
    - Nonsurgical
      - Immobilization of DIP joint only, in full extension
        - Dorsal- or volar-based aluminum foam splint, or plastic (Stack) splint
        - Requires at least 6 weeks of continuous extension followed by 2 weeks of splinting at night
        - Careful observation of skin to prevent necrosis or maceration

**TIP:** Inform patients that *even one episode of flexion* "starts the clock over."

    - Surgical
      - Percutaneous pinning across DIP joint in full extension
        - May be warranted in certain occupations (e.g., surgeons)
        - Option for patients **incapable of compliance** (e.g., children)

- **Type II**
  - Running monofilament suture, incorporating skin and tendon
  - Remove suture after 10-14 days
  - Splint as for type I
- **Type III**
  - Typically requires flap reconstruction of soft tissue
  - Terminal extensor reconstructed secondarily with tendon graft
- **Type IV**
  - Closed reduction and percutaneous K-wire fixation when possible
  - Open reduction with transarticular K-wire and pull-out suture or K-wire fracture fragment fixation
  - Fixation protected with splint for 6 weeks, then K-wires removed and progressive motion begun
- **Mallet thumb**
  - Closed injuries treated by splinting, as with fingers
  - Open injuries treated with direct repair
    - EPL is substantial and holds suture well.
    - Repair is protected with splinting for 6 weeks.

## ZONE II

- **Partial lacerations** *(less than 50% of surface)*
  - Repair is not required.
  - Debride frayed edges and provide closure or wound care.
  - Begin active motion after 7-10 days, or after wound is healed.
- **Lacerations greater than 50% of surface**
  - The tendon is often too thin for a core suture.
  - Repair with a running 4-0 suture, followed by 5-0 epitendinous cross-stitch.
  - Splint the DIP joint for 6 weeks, with DIP joint free.
- **Thumb**
  - The EPL can usually hold a core-type suture at this level.
  - Add an epitendinous suture.
  - Splint or pin the IP joint for 6 weeks, with the MP joint free.
  - Some advocate short, forearm-based thumb spica cast with thumb in full extension.

## ZONE III

- **Closed avulsion** *(boutonniere injury)*
  - Often misdiagnosed as a jammed or sprained finger
  - **Diagnosis**
    - Swelling and tenderness are observed at base of dorsal middle phalanx.
    - PIP joint extension exhibits weakness against resistance.
    - Extension function is preserved with only one lateral band intact.
    - MRI or ultrasound can confirm injury.
  - **Treatment**
    - Splint PIP in full extension for 6 weeks with MP and DIP joints free.
    - Follow with active PIP flexion and 2 weeks of splinting at night.
    - K-wire fixation of the PIP joint is an alternative.
    - Open reduction or reinsertion for avulsion fracture; fragment is viewed using radiographs.

- **Open injury**
  - Use Kessler pattern 4-0 core suture, followed by 5-0 epitendinous cross-stitch[4] (Fig. 70-6).
  - The PIP joint is violated easily; **irrigate thoroughly.**
  - Splint as for previously described closed injury.
  - Inadequate distal stump of tendon can be addressed by drilling a transverse hole through dorsal base of middle phalanx or by using a bone anchor.

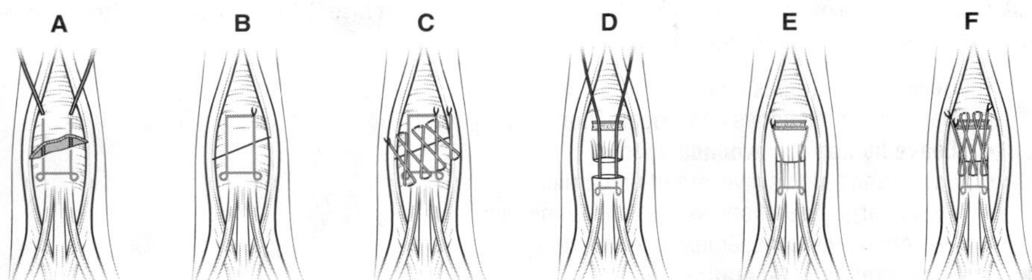


**Fig. 70-6** Techniques for repair of zone III lacerations. **A-C,** Central slip laceration with sufficient tendon to repair with core suture and oversew with Silfverskiöld epitendinous stitch. **D-F,** The core stitch can be passed through a trough in the base of the middle phalanx when the tendon laceration is distal, leaving a small stump of central slip.

- **Primary goal of treatment: Prevent development of boutonniere deformity** *(DIP hyperextension with flexion deformity of the PIP joint)* (Fig. 70-7)
  - Deformity can take weeks to develop, because **lateral bands slowly migrate volarly.**
  - Secondary reconstruction of chronic boutonniere is difficult.
  - Prevention is much easier than treatment.

- **Thumb**
  - Injury to one or both of the extensors (EPL or EPB) is possible.
  - Both tendons are large enough for core sutures.
  - Splint with wrist in 30 degrees of extension; thumb IP and MP joints are in extension for 3 weeks.
  - Establish progressive active motion over next 4 weeks.

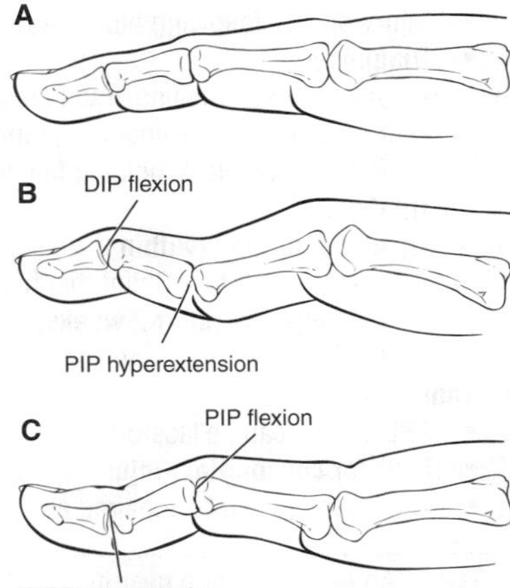


**Fig. 70-7** Characteristic swan neck and boutonniere deformities. **A,** Normal. **B,** Swan neck deformity. **C,** Boutonniere deformity.

## ZONE IV

- **Partial injuries** are common, because the tendon is broad at this level.
- Repair central tendon laceration with 4-0 core suture and 5-0 epitendinous cross-stitch.
- Maintain exact length relationships.
- Splint with wrist in 20- to 30-degree extension, MP joints in 70- to 90-degree flexion, and IP joints in full extension.

- Begin passive extension after 1 week and gentle active extension at 4 weeks.
- Isolated lateral band laceration can be repaired with a single 5-0 epitendinous cross-stitch.
- Thumb is treated as previously described for zone III injury.

## ZONE V

- **Open tendon lacerations**

**CAUTION: Beware of a wound from a closed-fist strike ("fight bite"). Victims of such altercations are notoriously evasive when interviewed.**

  - Review radiographs carefully.
  - Debride wound edges and irrigate thoroughly.
  - **Leave human bite wounds open.**
  - Lacerations at this level are often partial.
  - Repair large lacerations as for zone IV injuries.
  - Postoperative management is as for zone IV injuries.
- **Open sagittal band laceration**
  - This must be repaired to prevent subluxation of the tendon.
  - Use cross-stitch of 4-0 or 5-0 suture.
  - Splint with MP joints in full extension for 3-5 days, then follow with gentle flexion and extension exercises.
  - Prevent abduction or adduction by buddy-taping to the adjacent finger.
- **Closed sagittal band injury**
  - Injury occurs following blunt trauma, forceful extension, or flexion of digit.
  - **Diagnosis**
    - Tenderness, swelling, and inability to actively extend MP joint
    - Subluxation of extensor tendon (usually ulnar) with flexion
    - Patient capable of holding finger in extension once passively positioned
  - **Treatment**
    - **Acute injuries (within 2 weeks)**
      - Flexion block: Splint that holds MP joints in extension for 6 weeks
    - **Late injuries (after 2 weeks)**
      - Primary repair when possible, or one of many reconstructive procedures
- **Thumb**
  - APL or EPB can be lacerated.
  - **Look for concomitant injuries to the superficial radial nerve branches or the radial artery.**
  - Either tendon can be repaired as for zone III injury.

**TIP:** An APL laceration near its insertion can be treated with reinsertion into the metacarpal base.

## ZONE VI

- Tendons are substantial enough for core sutures.
- Prognosis tends to be very good in this zone, with adhesions uncommon.
- Use postoperative splint as for zone IV injury.

## ZONE VII

- Tendons are substantial enough for core sutures.
- Treatment of retinacular rent is controversial.
  - **Traditional approach**
    - Excise portion of the retinaculum adjacent to the repair.
    - Preserve a distal or proximal portion of retinaculum to prevent bowstringing.
  - **Alternative approach**
    - Repair the retinacular rent and use dynamic splint early (after 10 days).
    - Use postoperative splint as for zone IV injury.

## ZONE VIII

- **Associated neurovascular injuries are common;** document with a thorough examination.
- Lacerated tendons hold core sutures well.
- **Lacerations or avulsions at myotendinous juncture**
  - Approximate tendon to the fibrous septa of the muscle belly.
  - Splint statically with wrist in 40 degrees of extension, MP joints in 20 degrees of flexion, and fingers free for 5 weeks.
  - **These repairs are tenuous;** use tendon transfers as salvage procedures (see Chapter 71).

## ZONE IX

- Injuries are usually from penetrating trauma and require thorough exploration.
- **Nerve injuries are common** and should be repaired primarily.
- Repair muscle bellies with **multiple figure-of-eight absorbable sutures.**
- Immobilize with wrist in extension, MP joints in 20 degrees of flexion, and fingers free for 4 weeks.
- Follow with 2 weeks of night splinting.
- Immobilize elbow at 90 degrees if repaired muscles originate at or above the elbow.
- Use tendon transfers as salvage procedures.

# COMPLICATIONS

## RUPTURE

- As with flexor tendons, **explore immediately and repeat repair.**

## ADHESIONS

- Occurrence is less likely than with flexor repairs.
- Adhesions to the supple dorsal soft tissues can move and eventually break away with remodeling.
- When necessary, tenolysis can be performed with no need for pulley reconstruction.
- Preserve the sagittal bands.
- The dorsal retinaculum can be sacrificed when substantially involved.

## SEQUENCE OF EXTENSOR IMBALANCE

- Swan neck deformity
- Boutonniere deformity
- Extrinsic tightness
- Intrinsic tightness
- Extensor tendon subluxation with ulnar drift

## Key Points

- ✓ Partial injuries are common with extensor tendons. Involve a therapist early and remember that therapy protocols vary by patient.
- ✓ All extrinsic extensors are innervated by the radial nerve.
- ✓ The interossei are innervated by the ulnar nerve.
- ✓ The index finger and middle finger lumbricals are innervated by the median nerve, and the ring finger and small finger are innervated by the ulnar nerve.
- ✓ There are **six** dorsal wrist compartments.
- ✓ Extensor tendon lacerations may be camouflaged by the cross-tendon action of the juncturae tendinum.
- ✓ There are **nine zones** of the extensor tendon versus five of the flexor tendon. Odd zones are over joints, and even zones are over bones.
- ✓ A Bunnell suture technique frequently is the most useful because of the broad, flat nature of the extensor.
- ✓ Boutonniere and swan neck deformities can result from extensor tendon imbalance after subpunctural repair on neglected injuries.

## References

1. American Society for Surgery of the Hand. History and general examination. In American Society for Surgery of the Hand. The Hand: Examination and Diagnosis, 3rd ed. New York: Churchill Livingstone, 1990.
2. Agur AM, Dalley AF, eds. Grant's Atlas of Anatomy, 13th ed. Baltimore: Lippincott Williams & Wilkins, 2013.
3. el-Badawi MG, Butt MM, al-Zuhair AG, et al. Extensor tendons of the fingers: arrangement and variations—II. Clin Anat 8:391-398, 1995.
4. Wolfe SW, Hotchkiss RN, Pederson WC, et al, eds. Green's Operative Hand Surgery, 6th ed. Philadelphia: Churchill Livingstone, 2010.
5. Coon MS, Green SM. Boutonniere deformity. Hand Clinics 11:387-402, 1995.
6. Blair WF, Steyers CM. Extensor tendon injuries. Orthop Clin North Am 23:141-148, 1992.
7. Doyle JR. Extensor tendons—acute injuries. In Green DP, ed. Green's Operative Hand Surgery, 3rd ed. New York: Churchill Livingstone, 1993.

# 71. Tendon Transfers

**Purushottam A. Nagarkar, Bishr Hijazi,**
**Blake A. Morrison**

## GENERAL PRINCIPLES[1-3]

**Box 71-1** *Forearm and Hand Muscle Abbreviations*

**ADM:** Adductor digiti minimi
**APB:** Adductor pollicis brevis
**APL:** Adductor pollicis longus
**BR:** Brachioradialis
**ECRB:** Extensor carpi radialis brevis
**ECRL:** Extensor carpi radialis longus
**ECU:** Extensor carpi ulnaris
**EDC:** Extensor digiti communis
**EDM:** Extensor digiti minimi
**EDQ:** Extensor digiti quinti
**EIP:** Extensor indicis proprius
**EPB:** Extensor pollicis brevis
**EPL:** Extensor pollicis longus
**FCR:** Flexor carpi radialis
**FCU:** Flexor carpi ulnaris
**FDM:** Flexor digiti minimi
**FDP:** Flexor digitorum profundus
**FDS:** Flexor digitorum superficialis
**FPB:** Flexor pollicis brevis
**FPL:** Flexor pollicis longus
**ODM:** Opponens digiti minimi
**OP:** Opponens pollicis
**PL:** Palmaris longus
**PQ:** Pronator quadratus
**PT:** Pronator teres

### Basic Concept (Box 71-1)

- Partially or completely detach the insertion of a functioning muscle-tendon unit and reattach it to a nonfunctioning unit.
- Restore lost function and not just motion.
- **Supple joints**
  - Range of motion after transfer will not be greater than the passive range of motion before surgery.
  - Joints must be supple enough to provide adequate function at their passive range of motion.
- **Stable soft tissue**
  - Transferred tendon must be surrounded by healthy, noninflamed, stable soft tissue.
  - Prevents adhesions and poor results.
- **Appropriate donor tendon**
  - **Expendable**
    - Transferred tendon should have adequate backups so that no critical function is lost (e.g., use only one of the three wrist extensors or one of the two wrist flexors).
  - **One function**
    - Each transferred tendon should restore only one function.
    - Attempting to carry out multiple movements with a transferred tendon causes decreased strength and movement.

- **Adequate excursion**[4] (Table 71-1)
  - Transferred tendon should have excursion similar to the excursion being replaced.
  - More excursion is possible with dissection of fascia.
  - Wrist tenodesis increases excursion by 2.5 cm.

**Table 71-1** *Relative Excursion Potential of Muscle-Tendon Units*[4]

| Muscle-Tendon Units | Relative Excursion (cm) |
|---|---|
| PQ | 1.0 |
| PT | 1.6 |
| FPL, EPL, FCU | 1.9 |
| EDQ, EDC, PL, ECU, FCR, ECRB, EIP | 2.2 |
| FDP, FDS | 2.8 |
| ECRL | 3.3 |
| BR | 5.2 |

*BR,* Brachioradialis; *ECRB,* extensor carpi radialis brevis; *ECRL,* extensor carpi radialis longus; *ECU,* extensor carpi ulnaris; *EDC,* extensor digiti communis; *EDQ,* extensor digiti quinti; *EIP,* extensor indicis proprius; *EPL,* extensor pollicis longus; *FCR,* flexor carpi radialis; *FCU,* flexor carpi ulnaris; *FDP,* flexor digitorum profundus; *FDS,* flexor digitorum superficialis; *FPL,* flexor pollicis longus; *PL,* palmaris longus; *PQ,* pronator quadratus; *PT,* pronator teres.

**TIP:** Use the **3-5-7 rule** as a practical guide, based on the insertion of the various hand tendons.

- **Wrist level** (e.g., wrist extensors, flexors): **3.3 cm long**
- **Metacarpophalangeal (MP) joint level** (e.g., finger extensors): **5.0 cm long**
- **Fingertips** (e.g., FDP, FDS): **7.0 cm long**

- **Adequate power**[5] (Table 71-2)
  - Transferred muscle-tendon should have similar power to the unit being replaced.
- **Appropriate vector**
  - Transferred tendon vector of action should mimic vector of the original tendon.
- **Synergy**
  - Two tendon groups tend to act together.
    - Supination, wrist flexion, finger extension, and adduction
    - Pronation, wrist extension, finger flexion, and abduction
  - Ideally tendons within a synergistic group transferred to each other
  - Easier to retrain muscles within a group

**Table 71-2** *Relative Force Potential of Muscle-Tendon Units*[5]

| Muscle-Tendon Units | Relative Excursion (cm) |
|---|---|
| EDQ, EIP, PL | 1.0 |
| EDC, EPL | 1.5 |
| ECRL, BR | 2.2 |
| FDP, FPL, PQ, FCR | 3.1 |
| ECRB, ECU, FDS | 4.0 |
| FCU | 5.3 |
| PT | 6.4 |

*BR,* Brachioradialis; *ECRB,* extensor carpi radialis brevis; *ECRL,* extensor carpi radialis longus; *ECU,* extensor carpi ulnaris; *EDC,* extensor digiti communis; *EDQ,* extensor digiti quinti; *EIP,* extensor indicis proprius; *EPL,* extensor pollicis longus; *FCR,* flexor carpi radialis; *FCU,* flexor carpi ulnaris; *FDP,* flexor digitorum profundus; *FDS,* flexor digitorum superficialis; *FPL,* flexor pollicis longus; *PL,* palmaris longus; *PQ,* pronator quadratus; *PT,* pronator teres.

## ALTERNATIVES[5]

- **Correct the root cause**
  - Nerve injuries: Primary nerve repair, nerve graft, or nerve transfer
    - Theoretical advantages in rehabilitation
      - No adhesions to tendon junctions
      - Power, amplitude, and direction of pull all correct
    - Technically very demanding
  - Tendon injuries: Primary tendon repair, tendon graft
    - Primary repair is preferred when ends of injured tendon are suitable.
    - No task reeducation is required.
    - Muscles used are already correct in power, amplitude, and direction of pull.
  - Combined or muscle belly injuries: Free functional muscle transfer
- **External static or dynamic splinting**
  - Static: Fix the joint(s) involved in a static, but functional position.
  - Dynamic: Splint with devices (such as springs or rubber bands) that simulate function of the injured tendon and counteract opposing native forces dynamically.
- **Internal "splinting"**
  - Arthrodesis: Fuse the joint to provide functional joint position, similar to static splinting.
    - May provide adequate stability for desired function
    - Typically reduces number of muscle and tendon motors needed
  - Tenodesis: Fix the tendon origin to bone to provide functional joint position and tension, similar to dynamic splinting.
    - Consider this when prognosis for tendon transfer is poor.
    - Providing a fixed origin for a tendon may position a joint for acceptable movement.

## INDICATIONS

- **Nerve injury:** Most common indication
  - If repair or grafting is technically not possible (e.g., root avulsion) or if attempted repair or grafting has failed
  - If reinnervation will take so long that motor endplate fibrosis will occur
  - If presentation is delayed and motor endplate fibrosis has occurred
- **Tendon injury**
  - If tendon repair or grafting is not possible, or has failed
- **Combined tendon and nerve injury, or unrepairable muscle belly injury**
- **Spasticity**
  - If imbalance in forces across a joint (caused, for example, by cerebral palsy) causes a contracture, balance can be restored by tendon transfer.
  - Generally requires augmentation of wrist or digits extensors
    - FCU to ECRB
    - ECU to ECRB
    - FCU to EDC
    - BR to ECRB

**NOTE: Tendon transfers are less predictable for cerebral palsy patients.**

- **Medical disease**[2]
  - Tendon rupture associated with rheumatoid arthritis
    - Tendon rubbing over bone damaged by chronic synovitis attenuates and ruptures
  - Poliomyelitis
    - Muscles often regain function, particularly those affected early.
    - Delay tendon transfers until no recovery of weakness is documented for at least 6 months.
  - Leprosy (Hansen's disease)
    - Most common deficits requiring tendon transfer are clawing, loss of opposition, and key pinch.
    - Disease must be under control before surgery.

## CONTRAINDICATIONS

- Joint contractures or stiff joints
- Ongoing inflammation in the wound bed
- No appropriate donor tendon available
- Lack of specific functional deficit (i.e., lost motion does not result in a specific deficit, or patient does not have specific task difficulties)
- Lack of patient motivation or reliability (results are dependent on postoperative therapy and retraining)
- Ongoing systemic disease: Must first control root cause medically (e.g., rheumatoid arthritis in cases of tendon rupture)
- Athetoid movement
  - Involuntary movement that varies from spastic to flaccid
  - Tendon transfers typically too unpredictable to be useful
- Advanced age (relative contraindication) makes retraining more difficult

## PREOPERATIVE EVALUATION

- History
  - Timing of injury
  - Prior surgeries or therapies attempted
  - Specific functional deficit
  - Status of systemic disease
- Physical examination
  - Determine level and severity of nerve and tendon injuries with detailed neuromuscular examination
  - Assess range of motion of relevant joints
  - Assess scar maturity
  - Assess donor options (e.g., presence of palmaris longus)
- Psychosocial evaluation for patient motivation and reliability

## TREATMENT

### TIMING

- **Immediate**
  - Done when prognosis for nerve recovery poor
    - Destruction of large portion of muscle
    - Proximal destruction of nerve or large segmental loss
    - Advanced age
  - For temporary function while waiting for nerve repair
    - PT to ECRB transfer (e.g., after radial nerve palsy)
    - Serves as "internal splint"
      - Obviates need for external splint
      - Supplements extension once recovery begins
- **Delayed**
  - Perform after expected recovery period of injured nerve
    - Measure distance from point of injury to muscle in millimeters
    - *Distance in millimeters plus 30 provides the number of days in the expected recovery period.*
  - Perform only after the following requirements have been met:
    - Skeletal stability
    - Supple soft tissue coverage
    - Joint mobility
    - Adequate (i.e., at least protective) sensation
    - Correction of any contractures
- Options for specific functional deficits

### MEDIAN NERVE DISTRIBUTION[2,6,7]

- **Thumb opposition:** Combination of thumb abduction, flexion, pronation
  - Caused by median nerve injury at any level, or C8-T1 roots
  - Donor tendons
    - All options involve inserting donor tendon into the APB insertion (dorsoradial aspect of thumb metacarpal head).

- EIP
  - Tunnel subcutaneously around ulnar side of hand, across palm at level of pisiform.
  - Radial innervation, so generally available
- FDS ring finger
  - Loop around FCU as pulley
  - Unavailable in high median nerve injury
- Palmaris longus (Camitz)
  - PL + palmar fascia passed under APB origin as pulley
  - No loss of function, but weak motor action
- Abductor digiti minimi (Huber)
  - Insertion detached, turned over 180 degrees
  - Ulnar innervations, good power match, provides thenar bulk
  - Provides minimal abduction (mostly flexion and pronation)
- ECRL, ECU, EDQ
  - Routing similar to EIP, but may need tendon graft for length

- **Thumb flexion:** FPL
  - Caused by high median nerve injury, or C8-T1 roots
  - Also most common rupture in rheumatoid arthritis (attrition over the scaphoid)
  - Donors weaved to distal FPL tendon
  - Donor tendons
    - BR, ECRL, FDS to ring finger
      - Usually available: Radial and ulnar nerve innervations
      - Minimal donor site deficit
      - End-to-side transfer if native function expected to recover
      - FDS commonly used for ruptures associated with rheumatoid arthritis
- **DIP joint flexion:** Index FDP
  - Caused by high median nerve injury, or C8-T1 roots
  - Donors weaved to distal FPL tendon
  - Donor tendons
    - BR, ECRL, FDS to ring finger
      - Usually available: Radial and ulnar nerve innervations
      - Minimal donor site deficit
      - End-to-side transfer if native function expected to recover

## Ulnar Nerve Distribution[6-8]

- **Thumb adduction (key pinch):** Adductor pollicis and first dorsal interosseous
  - Caused by ulnar nerve injury at any level, or C8-T1 roots
  - Donors inserted into ulnar base of thumb proximal phalanx
  - Donor tendons
    - ECRB, BR
      - Passed between index finger/middle finger metacarpals into palm, around index finger metacarpal as pulley
      - Will need tendon graft to provide length
      - Good power match, minimal donor site deficit
    - FDS long/ring finger
      - Retrieved in the palm, passed deep to flexor tendons
      - FDS ring finger not available if high ulnar nerve injury (because FDP ring finger will be injured)
      - Weak power, and poor vector of pull

- **Ring, small finger DIP joint flexion:** Ring, small FDP
  - Caused by high ulnar nerve injury, or C8-T1 roots
  - Reconstruct by suturing these two tendons to the adjacent long finger FDP tendon
  - Reconstruction will make clawing worse
- **Clawing:** Ring, small MP joint flexors (lumbricals, interossei)
  - Caused by ulnar nerve injury at any level, or C8-T1 roots
  - Lack of MP joint flexors causes imbalance of forces with resultant MP joint hyperextension and PIP and DIP joint flexion
  - Reconstruction depends on whether PIP joint capsule and extensor mechanism are normal (i.e., Bouvier test positive) or abnormal
  - Donors passed along the path of the lumbrical, volar to the transverse metacarpal ligament, and then to a choice of insertion
    - Lateral band: Most anatomically accurate, ideal if Bouvier test is negative, but may add too much power to the extensor mechanism
    - Proximal phalanx: No power added to the extensor mechanism
    - Loop around A1 or A2 pulley and suture to itself
  - Donor tendons
    - Long finger FDS: Modified Stiles-Bunnell procedure
      - Divide tendon distally, split it into four slips to reconstruct each lumbrical.
      - Weakens grip, and can cause PIP joint hyperextension because PIP joint flexor has been removed
    - FCR, ECRL, ECRB, BR
      - Tendon graft weaved into donor, split into four slips to reconstruct each lumbrical
      - Improves grip strength, less chance of developing PIP joint hyperextension

## Radial Nerve Distribution[5]

- **Wrist extension:** ECRL, ECRB, ECU
  - ECRL lost with high radial nerve palsy, or C6-7 roots
  - ECRB, ECU lost with radial nerve palsy at any level, or C6-7 roots
  - ECRL, ECU generally not reconstructed
  - Donor tendons
    - Pronator teres to ECRB
      - Divide PT at insertion, route subcutaneously, superficial to the BR
      - End to side into ECRB if radial nerve recovery expected
      - End to end into divided ECRB if recovery not expected
- **Finger MP joint extension:** EDC
  - Caused by radial nerve palsy at any level, or C7 root
  - May also rupture in rheumatoid arthritis
    - Attrition over ulnar head
    - Often starts with small finger, followed by digits from ulnar to radial as intact tendons shift ulnarly
    - Perform dorsal tenosynovectomy, with or without distal ulnar excision.
    - Address MP joint with arthroplasty first if joints are diseased.
    - For one or two tendons, can suture to adjacent tendon
  - EDC tendons divided at myotendinous junction and woven into donor

- Donor tendons
  - FCU
    - Route around ulnar border of wrist subcutaneously
    - Disadvantage: Loss of ulnar deviation with flexion
  - FCR
    - Route around radial border of wrist subcutaneously
  - FDS of long finger
    - Used in cases of multiple tendon rupture in rheumatoid arthritis
    - Divide between A1 and A2 pulleys.
    - Route around the wrist, or through interosseous membrane
- **Thumb extension and abduction:** EPL, EPB, APL
  - Caused by radial nerve palsy at any level, or C7-8 roots
  - EPL rupture also common in rheumatoid arthritis
  - Donor tendons
    - Palmaris longus to EPL
      - Divide PL distally, EPL at myotendinous junction
      - Transpose EPL radial to Lister's tubercle and direct volarly
      - Used in conjunction with the FCU/FCR to EDC transfer
      - PL absent bilaterally in 9%, unilaterally in 16% of patients
    - FDS of ring finger to EPL
      - Divide between A1 and A2 pulleys.
      - Route around wrist or through interosseous membrane
      - Used in conjunction with the FDS to EDC transfer
    - FCR to EPB and APL
      - Provides independent radial abduction
      - Used in conjunction with the FDS to EDC, FDS to EPL transfers
    - EIP to EPL
      - Used in EPL rupture associated with rheumatoid arthritis
      - Also important to remove any bony spicules causing attrition

## POSTOPERATIVE CARE

- OR: Bulky splint to keep the transferred tendon at a no-tension length
- 1-2 weeks: Check incisions and change splint.
- 4 weeks: Start gentle active ROM of involved joints, place thermoplast splint.
- 6 weeks: Muscle retraining, activation of transferred muscle-tendon unit
- 8 weeks: Strengthening exercises, wean splint
- 12 weeks: Full activity

## COMPLICATIONS

- **Tendon adhesions**
  - Usually if tendon passes through inflamed tissue bed
  - Management with aggressive hand therapy
  - Tenolysis once inflammation resolved
- **Transfer rupture**
  - Excessive tension or inadequate immobilization
  - Immediate operative repair
- **Transfer weakness**
  - Poor power match/injured/atrophied donor muscle; inadequate tension; inadequate moment arm length
  - Operative repair: Reset tension or move insertion farther from joint axis of rotation to lengthen moment arm.

### KEY POINTS

✓ Tendon transfers are used when lost function cannot be restored by correcting the root cause (e.g., irreparable nerve palsies, or tendon injuries).

✓ The most common indication is nerve injury.

✓ Before tendon transfer, four requirements must be met: (1) supple joints, (2) stable soft tissue, (3) availability of appropriate donor tendon, and (4) control of any underlying medical disease.

✓ Donor tendon should match the power, excursion, and vector of the recipient, be expendable, and restore a single function.

✓ Multiple techniques and donor options are available for each functional goal. Appropriate donor choice and correct tension determine the functional result.

## REFERENCES


1. Beasley RW. Principles of tendon transfer. Orthop Clin North Am 1:433-438, 1970.
2. Phalen GS, Miller RC. The transfer of wrist extensor muscles to restore or reinforce flexion power of the fingers and opposition of the thumb. J Bone Joint Surg Am 29:993-997, 1947.
3. Richards RR. Tendon transfers for failed nerve reconstruction. Clin Plast Surg 30:223-245, 2003.
4. Lieber RL, Jacobson MD, Fazeli BM, et al. Architecture of selected muscles of the arm and forearm: anatomy and implications for tendon transfer. J Hand Surg Am 17:787-798, 1992.
5. Sammer DM, Chung KC. Tendon transfers. I. Principles of transfer and transfers for radial nerve palsy. Plast Reconstr Surg 123:169e-177e, 2009.
6. Brand PW. Tendon transfers for median and ulnar nerve paralysis. Orthop Clin North Am 1:447-454, 1970.
7. Sammer DM, Chung KC. Tendon transfers. II. Transfers for ulnar nerve palsy and median nerve palsy. Plast Reconstr Surg 124:212e-221e, 2009.
8. Mayer L. Operative reconstruction of the paralysed upper extremity. J Bone Joint Surg 21:377-383, 1939.

# 72. Hand and Finger Amputations

David S. Chang, Essie Kueberuwa, Prosper Benhaim

## GENERAL CONSIDERATIONS

- **Trauma** is the most common cause of emergency amputations.
- **Crush/avulsion** are the most common mechanisms of traumatic injury.
- Elective amputations can be performed for **malignancy, osteomyelitis, vasculitis, gangrene,** or **a painful, stiff, or nonfunctional digit of any cause.**
- Amputation can be performed for traumatic injuries when **no replant or salvage option exists.**
- In patients with severe vascular disease or other high-risk comorbidities, amputation is a quick, definitive treatment option.
- For patients whose primary goal is speedy recovery and expedited return to work, amputation may be the best option.

## INITIAL ASSESSMENT OF THE TRAUMATIC AMPUTATION PATIENT

- Level of amputation
- Complete vs. incomplete
- Mechanism of injury
- Structures involved in the injury and concomitant hand injuries
- Hand dominance of patient
- Occupation and hobbies of patient (assessment of level of function needed to perform activities of daily living)
- Preinjury functionality of the hand
- Patient's concerns, ideas, and expectations about amputation and rehabilitation
- Minimum three-view plain radiographs of the hand, with specific finger views if necessary.
- Wrist studies if indicated.

## GOALS OF AMPUTATION

- Preserve length (use reconstructive flaps if necessary to gain adequate soft tissue cover), especially in the thumb.
- Provide durable coverage
- Preserve sensation
- Prevent symptomatic neuromas
- Prevent adjacent joint contractures
- Minimize morbidity
- Early prosthetic fitting
- Early return to work and recreation

## INDICATIONS FOR AMPUTATIONS

- Nonsalvageable traumatic injury
- Poor replant candidate
- High likelihood of failed replant/salvage if performed (vascular disease, significant smoker)
- Multiple-level injury
- Medical comorbidities: High anesthetic risk
- Patient preference (manual laborers whose primary goal is expedited return to work)
- Tumor
- Infection (intractable osteomyelitis/severe necrotizing fasciitis)
- Severe burn contractures
- Vasculitis/ischemia/necrosis

## CONTRAINDICATIONS

- **There are no absolute contraindications to amputation.**
- Consider replantation if the patient is a good candidate and amputated part is in good condition (see Chapter 73).

## GENERAL SURGICAL PRINCIPLES FOR HAND AND FINGER AMPUTATIONS

### TECHNIQUE[1-2]

1. Administer adequate anesthesia.
2. Administer preoperative antibiotics and tetanus prophylaxis.
3. Remove gross wound contamination.
4. After field is prepared and draped, irrigate wound thoroughly with saline solution under tourniquet control.
5. Debride devitalized tissue.
6. Assess soft tissue coverage and shorten bone if necessary to allow primary closure.
7. Use volar skin for distal stump coverage if possible, or use a fishmouth incision (Fig. 72-1).
8. Cut back flexor and extensor tendons, depending on level of amputation. **Do not suture tendon ends to stump or extensor/flexor tendon stumps to each other (can cause a tethering quadriga effect).**
9. Identify digital nerves and transect proximal to amputation site to prevent symptomatic neuromas.
10. Close the stump with loosely approximated interrupted nonabsorbable sutures (e.g., 4-0 nylon). Avoid tight closure (can lead to amputation stump skin edge ischemia).
11. Ensure a rounded contour at amputation stump closure. Resect dog-ears at time of closure. These will generally not improve on their own postoperatively.
12. Place a splint and begin range of motion exercises 3-5 days postoperatively.

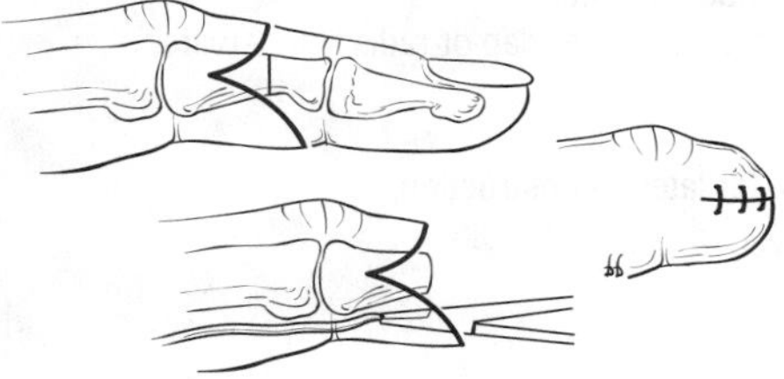

**Fig. 72-1** Use of volar and dorsal skin flaps for stump coverage. Volar flaps are preferable for greater sensibility.

**TIP:** Most traumatic finger amputations can be managed in the emergency department with a digital block and finger tourniquet.

- **Outcomes**
  - Primary digital amputation can result in better function and quicker return to work than complex reconstruction or replantation.[3]
  - Symptomatic neuromas can be prevented by transecting nerve proximal to the stump to allow retraction into uninjured tissue.
  - Early return to work can prevent symptomatic neuromas.[4]
  - Cold intolerance and dysesthesia are common complications that usually resolve, but may last up to 2 years.[5]

## Specific Amputations

- **Digital tip** (see Chapter 67)
- **Through distal interphalangeal (DIP) or proximal interphalangeal (PIP) joint**
  - Use skeletal shortening and primary closure.
  - Use rongeur to contour shape of stump, and **remove articular cartilage** to prevent pseudobursa formation.
  - Avoid lumbrical plus deformity.
    - Transection of flexor digitorum profundus (FDP) tendon and retraction proximally pulls on lumbrical. As finger is flexed, lumbrical puts tension on lateral bands of extensor mechanism, causing **paradoxical extension** of PIP joint.
    - Treat by sectioning lumbrical tendon (can be done later).
- **Through middle or proximal phalanx**
  - Use skeletal shortening and primary closure with dorsal and volar skin flaps (fishmouth incision).
- **Proximal to proximal phalanx:** Intrinsic muscles allow flexion up to 45 degrees unless amputation is at or near metacarpophalangeal (MP) joint, in which case preserving a very short proximal phalanx may impair function. *Consider ray amputation.*

CAUTION: ***Do not tether flexor tendons*** **to the bone distally or to the extensor tendons, because this can prevent excursion of flexors in the other remaining fingers (quadriga effect).**

**TIP:** If an injury to the middle phalanx is proximal to flexor digitorum superficialis (FDS) tendon, the need to preserve length is obviated because there will be no PIP joint motion without the FDS tendon.

- **Through thumb**
  - See Chapter 75 for algorithmic approach to thumb reconstruction.
  - Restoring sensibility is important for restoring function.
  - If no bone is exposed, allow to heal by secondary intention.
  - Coverage of exposed bone can be done with cross-finger flap or radially innervated sensory flap.
- **Multiple digits**
  - Preserve as much viable tissue as possible for later reconstruction.

## Hand

- **Ray amputation**
  - Amputation at or near MP joint is best treated with subtotal metacarpal resection.
  - Power grip, key pinch, and supination strength will be reduced, which must be weighed against disability associated with the gap created by the missing finger.
  - Small objects can fall through the gap created by the missing digit, especially with amputated long and ring fingers.

> **TIP:** Ray amputation can be performed electively and is rarely indicated at the time of initial trauma.

- **Technique**
  1. Make incision over dorsum of metacarpal.
  2. Divide extensor tendon.
  3. Dissect periosteum off metacarpal needing resection.
  4. Perform osteotomy at metacarpal base (metaphyseal flare).
  5. Third-ray amputations can be managed with index metacarpal transposition[6] or suture of deep intermetacarpal ligaments to close the space between the index and long fingers.[7]
  6. Fourth-ray amputations can be managed similar to third-ray amputations, with transposition of fifth metacarpal or suture of intermetacarpal ligaments.
  7. Fifth-ray amputations require preservation of metacarpal base because of insertions of flexor carpi ulnaris (FCU) and extensor carpi ulnaris (ECU) tendons. Second-ray amputations similarly should preserve the insertions of the extensor carpi radialis longus (ECRL) and flexor carpi radialis (FCR) tendons.
  8. Distract flexor tendons distally and transect proximally.
  9. Transect neurovascular bundles.
  10. Trim skin flaps and close wound primarily.
- **Outcomes**
  - Ray amputations result in **15%-20% loss of grip strength**[8-10] and narrowing of the palm.
  - **Index-ray amputations** also result in **50% loss of pronation strength.**[8]
  - Border-ray translocation to a central position can improve cosmetic results.

## Wrist

- **Through carpus**
  - Functional restoration results are worse than those for more distal amputations.
  - Initially preserve as much tissue as possible.
  - Preserve radiocarpal joint if possible; this may allow a functional prosthesis.
- **Wrist disarticulation**
  - This method is preferable to long, below-elbow amputations.
  - Preservation of distal radioulnar joint (DRU joint) and radial styloid allows full supination and pronation, as well as better-fitting prosthesis.
  - Ligate radial and ulnar arteries and transect nerves proximal to end of stump.
  - Pull flexor and extensor tendons distally and transect proximally; allow to retract proximally.
  - Use fishmouth incision with long volar flap and short dorsal flap.

## Forearm

- Transect the radius and ulna at the same level.
- Provide appropriate padding at the distal ends of the radius and ulna with muscle flap coverage.
- Minimum recommended length for useful forearm prosthesis use after surgery is 8-10 cm of residual radius and ulna length.
- If hand transplant is a significant consideration, minimize shortening of the tendons and neurovascular structures. Bury nerve ends deep in muscle to minimize neuroma formation.

**TIP:** Maintain as much length as possible.

## Key Points

- ✓ In traumatic amputations, address life-threatening injuries first (i.e., follow ABCs).
- ✓ Assess patient in emergency department for replantation.
- ✓ Prevent neuromas by cutting back ends of nerves and bury stump in soft tissue/muscle away from incision site.
- ✓ For digital amputations, do not suture flexor or extensor tendons to the stump or to each other.
- ✓ Preserve length.

## References

1. Adamson GJ, Palmer RE. Amputations. In Achauer BM, Erikson E, Guyuron B, et al, eds. Plastic Surgery: Indications, Operations, and Outcomes. St Louis: Mosby–Year Book, 2000.
2. Louis DS, Jebson PJ, Graham T. Amputations. In Green DP, Hotchkiss RN, Pederson WC, eds. Green's Operative Hand Surgery, 4th ed. Philadelphia: Churchill Livingstone, 1999.
3. Jones JM, Schenck RR, Chesney RB. Digital replantation and amputation: comparison of function. J Hand Surg Am 7:183-189, 1982.
4. Fisher GT, Boswick JA Jr. Neuroma formation following digital amputations. J Trauma 23:136-142, 1983.
5. Backman C, Nystrom A, Backman C. Cold-induced arterial spasm after digital amputation. J Hand Surg Br 16:378-381, 1981.
6. Carroll RE. Transposition of the index finger to replace the middle finger. Clin Orthop 15:27-34, 1959.
7. Steichen JB, Idler RS. Results of central ray resection without bony transposition. J Hand Surg Am 11:466-474, 1986.
8. Murray JF, Carman W, MacKenzie JK. Transmetacarpal amputation of the index finger: a clinical assessment of hand strength and complications. J Hand Surg Am 2:471-481, 1977.
9. Garcia-Moral CA, Putman-Mullins J, Taylor PA, et al. Ray resection of the index finger. Orthop Trans 15:71, 1991.
10. Melikyan EY, Beg MS, Woodbridge S, et al. The functional results of ray amputation. Hand Surg 8:47-51, 2003.

# 73. Replantation

Ashkan Ghavami, Kendall R. Roehl

## INDICATIONS AND CONTRAINDICATIONS[1-3]

### Indications

- Thumb
- Single digit distal to flexor digitorum superficialis (FDS) insertion (zone I)
- Multiple digits
- Hand amputation through palm
- Hand amputation (distal wrist)
- Any part in a child
- More proximal arm (sharp, clean injury pattern)

### Contraindications

- Single digits proximal to FDS insertion (zone II) (see next section)
- Severely crushed or mangled parts
- Multiple-level amputations
- Multiple traumas or severe medical problems (relative contraindication)

## SPECIFIC CASES

### Single-Digit Replantation

- **Distal to zone II** (distal to FDS tendon insertion)
  - Favorable outcomes
  - Fewer secondary operations
- **Within zone II**
  - Function after replantation, even after secondary operations (e.g., extensive tenolysis), is usually poor.
- **Exceptions**
  - Musician or other person requiring all 10 digits
  - Children
  - Thumb amputations (see later)
  - Cultural reasons (e.g., in Japan a missing digit has criminal connotations)

## Fingertip Amputations Distal to or at Distal Interphalangeal (DIP) Joint

- Expert technical skills and experience needed
- Main difficulties are venous paucity and venous repair
- **Tamai's fingertip classification**[4,5] (zones I and II not synonymous with tendon zones I and II) (Fig. 73-1)
  - **Zone I**
    - Distal to lunula
    - Volar venous plexus used for venous repair
    - Options when venous repair not possible: Arteriovenous (AV) shunting, nail bed bleed or heparin therapy, leech therapy
  - **Zone II**
    - DIP joint to lunula
    - Digital arteries and dorsal veins used

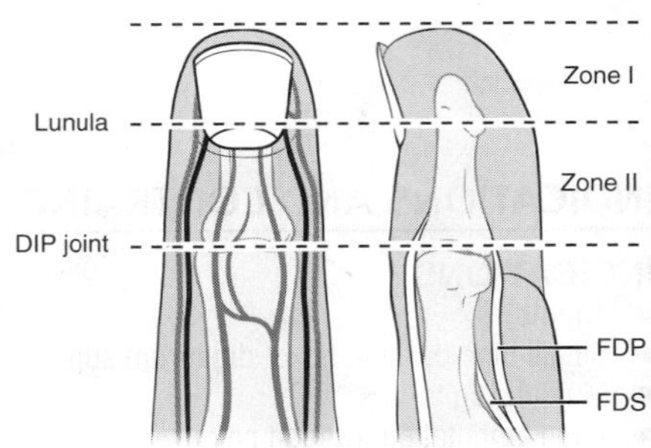


**Fig. 73-1** Tamai's classification of fingertip amputation. (*DIP joint,* Distal interphalangeal joint; *FDP,* flexor digitorum profundus; *FDS,* flexor digitorum superficialis.)

## Chung's Fingertip Classification[5] (Consistent With Tendon Zone I) (Fig. 73-2)

- **Zone IA**
  - Distal to lunula through sterile matrix
  - Artery: Very difficult
  - Vein: Impossible
  - Nerve: Impossible
- **Zone IB**
  - Between lunula and root of nail bed, through germinal matrix
  - Artery: Difficult
  - Vein: Very difficult
  - Nerve: Very difficult
- **Zone IC**
  - Between FDP insertion and neck of middle phalanx, periarticular
  - Artery: Easy
  - Vein: Difficult
  - Nerve: Easy
- **Zone ID**
  - Between neck of middle phalanx and FDS insertion
  - Artery: Easy
  - Vein: Easy
  - Nerve: Easy

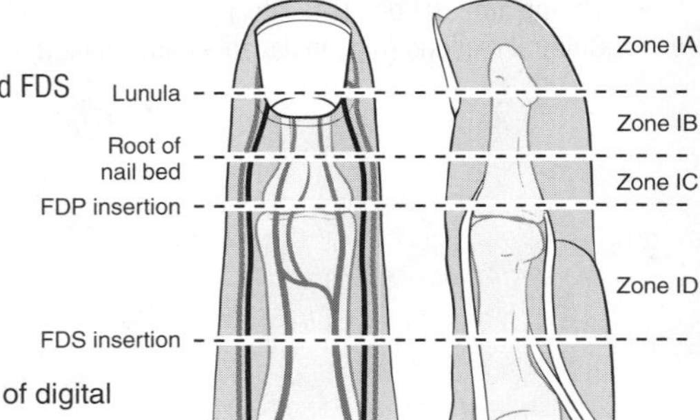


**Fig. 73-2** Chung's classification of digital amputations.

> **TIP:** Occupation should be considered in the decision-making process. Many laborers prefer revision amputations at this level to allow quick return to work with adequate functional results.

### Ring Avulsion Injuries

- **Ring finger classifications**[6]
  - **Type I:** Soft tissue injury *without* vascular compromise
    - *Treatment:* Standard neurovascular approach
  - **Type II:** Soft tissue damage *with* arterial and/or venous compromise
    - *Treatment:* May require coverage of vascular repairs using local flap or flow-through venous flap harvested as skin and soft tissue attached to underlying vein graft from forearm
  - **Type III:** *Complete degloving* of soft tissues; most controversial; function poor even with successful skin envelope revascularization
    - *Treatment:* Primary-ray amputation[6]
- **Thumb:** Similar to any other type of thumb injury or amputation, warrants every attempt at replantation

### Children

- **Every attempt should be made to replant no matter the type of amputation,** *except with severe crushes or multiple-level injuries.*
- **Distal amputations**
  - Such amputations may require only percutaneous needle for osteosynthesis.
  - Nerve repair is not always required.
  - Direct neurotization may allow normal two-point discrimination.[7]
  - Amputated part may survive as a "composite graft" without the need for microanastomosis *(only in children).* Neoepithelialization is often present under eschar.
- Better functional results are seen overall, likely because of greater neuronal regenerative capacity in children.
- Inform parents that a replanted finger can grow more slowly than other digits.[7]

> **TIP:** Avoid a running microvascular suture technique; this may increase the vessel stenosis rate as the child grows.[7]

## PREOPERATIVE WORKUP

### Before Transfer

- Stabilize patient.
- Wrap amputated part in moist gauze, place in ziplock bag or specimen container, and place on ice (4° C).
- Prevent warm ischemia.
  - Duration is preferably <6 hours.
  - >12-hour duration generally precludes digital replantation.
  - Sensitivity to warm ischemia increases in proportion to the amount of muscle mass in the amputated part (e.g., forearm amputation tolerates markedly less ischemia [maximum 4-6 hours] <volar amputation <digital level amputation—most tolerant because no muscle mass).

- Optimize cold ischemia.
  - Optimal cooling can allow up to 24 hours of cold ischemia.
  - Up to 30-40 hours of cold ischemia has been reported for digital replantation, with one report of 94 hours.[8]

**NOTE: These are rare cases and NOT recommended.**

  - More proximal injuries with more muscle mass tolerate 10-12 hours of cold ischemia.
- Alert other surgeons from replant team.
- OR is called to prepare staff, check microscope availability, create slush and warming fluid, obtain ICU bed, etc.

### On Arrival at ER

- Obtain thorough history.
  - Type of force, mechanism, machine, etc., resulting in amputation
  - Exact time of injury (to calculate accurate ischemia duration)
- Perform preliminary examination of stump and amputated parts.
  - **Avoid:**
    - Repeated manipulation of extremity (may increase vasospasm)
    - Digital blocks (decreases vascular flow)
- Assure hemodynamic stability.
- Obtain radiographs of stump and amputated parts (evaluation and planning for missing bone and parts).
- Start IV broad-spectrum antibiotics.
- Start tetanus prophylaxis.
- Points for consent:
  - Potential replant failure
  - Need for bone, nerve, and vein graft
  - Need for further surgery (e.g., secondary procedures such as tenolysis and capsulotomy)
  - Prolonged rehabilitation course
    - Realistic prognosis (e.g., sensation, mobility, and function)

> **TIP:** Always consider age, occupation, mental stability of patient, and presence of severe systemic injuries during the preoperative consultation and decision-making process.

## SURGICAL PRINCIPLES

### Anesthesia Adjuncts

- Brachial plexus blocks or axillary blocks may assist with vasodilation and postoperative patient comfort.

### General Preparation

- Well-padded operating table
- Foley catheter
- Tourniquets on upper extremity and leg for possible nerve, vein, or skin grafts

## Multiple-Digit Amputations

- Consider future function and replant position.
  - **Finger with highest chance of success is replanted first** (e.g., if index finger and middle finger are amputated and middle finger is not replantable, replant index finger in middle finger position to prevent a gap and help with grip).[9]

## Major Limb or Proximal Amputations

- **Reperfusion shunts** used for arterial inflow early in proximal level amputations
  - Fasciotomies
  - Nerve tunnel releases
  - Intrinsic compartment decompression
- High-volume blood transfusions
- Often several subsequent tissue (muscle) debridements required
- May require later free-functional muscle transfer for biceps function

## Hand Replantation

- Shunt for reperfusion to reduce ischemia duration
- Proximal and distal flexor and extensor tendons tagged before osteosynthesis
  - Flexor tendons need precise anatomic organization.
  - Repair as many tendons as possible.
- Wrist level approach
  - Bone shortening (proximal row carpectomy) may be required.

# Surgical Technique: Digital Replantation

## Operative Sequence

**TIP:** Optimize use of "spare parts" from nonsalvageable tissue. An example is harvesting a digital nerve from a nonreplantable digit to use for a nerve graft.

- **Two-team approach**
  - **First team**
    1. Brings amputated part(s) to OR as soon as possible (can precede patient's OR arrival)
    2. Examines part(s) thoroughly with loupes or under microscope; part(s) held on back table
    3. Obtains appropriate exposure (if possible, incorporating lacerations present)[10] (Fig. 73-3)
       - Bilateral longitudinal, midaxial incisions, or
       - Volar Bruner (zigzag) and dorsal longitudinal incisions

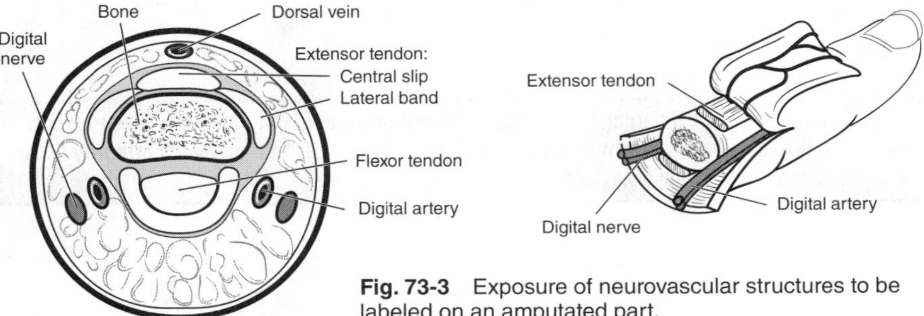


**Fig. 73-3** Exposure of neurovascular structures to be labeled on an amputated part.

4. Identifies and tags all neurovascular structures
   - Nerves: 6-0 black nylon
   - Arteries and veins: 6-0 Prolene
5. For bony preparation, places two K-wires in retrograde fashion

- **Second team**
  1. Works concurrently
  2. Begins with meticulous exploration, debridement, and irrigation of proximal part
  3. Identifies and tags all vital structures on proximal part
     - Nerves, arteries, and veins
     - Flexor and extensor tendons: May place core sutures before osteosynthesis to simplify later tendon coaptation
  4. Performs bony shortening as necessary (no more than 5-10 mm for digits)
     - Fractures through joints often require fusion.

**TIP:** Rigid fixation with low-profile plates, screws, or 90-90 intraosseous wiring allows earlier motion protocols and lower nonunion rates, which is especially important in more proximal amputations.

- **Vessel damage evaluation**
  - **Normal vessel:** Pearly gray with no petechiae ("paprika")
  - **Ribbon sign ("corkscrew"):** Tortuous-appearing vessel from avulsion or traction injury
  - **Red-line sign:** Red streak along neurovascular bundle implying distal vessel damage

**NOTE: Ribbon and red-line signs are poor prognostic indicators.**

- **Cobweb sign:** Intraluminal fibrin threads/webs[10] (Fig. 73-4)
- **Telescope sign:** Lumen telescopes away from outer vessel wall and past cut edge.
- **Terminal thrombus:** Indicates vessel wall disruption or damage
- **Measles sign:** Pinpoint (petechial) bruising along vessel wall
  - Result of high pressure from thrombus, usually after anastomosis complete
- **Sausage sign:** Ballooning of vessel from thrombus

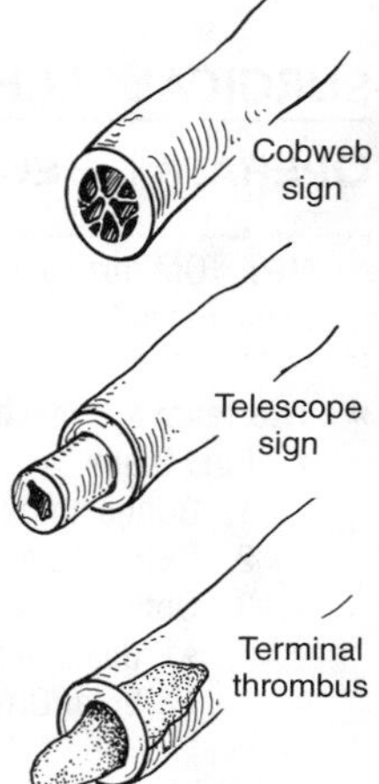


**Fig. 73-4** Signs of arterial damage should be appreciated, including the telescope, cobweb, and ribbon signs (terminal thrombosis), which require freshening of the vessel.

**TIP:** If signs of vessel damage are present, do not hesitate to cut back vessel as much as required. It is better to perform vein grafting than to be concerned for vessel integrity with replant failure postoperatively.

- **Perform the following after tourniquet deflation:**
  - **Spurt test:** Vessel must have strong pressure head.
    - Inadequate pressure necessitates more vessel resection.
  - **Patency test:** Milking of vessel to check back-bleeding and inflow patency

**TIP:** Performing all of the previous sequences during one tourniquet run (2 hours) expedites the operation. Blood pooling and clots can make later identification of vital structures, especially nerves, more challenging.

- **Vein graft harvest**
  - One surgeon (from either team, as soon as available) begins harvesting vein graft(s) from forearm or leg, if required.
  - Volar forearm veins and dorsal foot veins are good size-matches for digital vessels.
  - **Common vein graft indications:**
    - Thumb replants: Often require vein interposition graft from ulnar digital artery (larger caliber than radial side) to radial artery in anatomic snuffbox
    - Ring avulsions
    - Segmental tissue loss
- **Osteosynthesis completed**
- **Extensor and flexor tendon repair**
  - Use standard four-core suturing method of choice after edges are tidied up, e.g., modified Kessler-Tajima technique using 3-0 or 4-0 Ethibond.
  - Consider excision of FDS in zone II.
- **Primary digital nerve repair** (when possible)
  - Done under operative microscope
  - Epineurial suturing technique: 9-0 or 10-0 black nylon
  - Options if primary repair not feasible (see Chapter 68):
    - Autogenous nerve graft (preferred), polyglycolic acid conduit, vein graft (gap 2 cm)
    - Minimal joint repositioning to limit tension on repair once motion initiated
- **Microvascular artery repair**
  - A well-executed microsurgical technique is imperative.
  - Cut back artery to healthy intimal level.
  - One good artery is required.
  - Use 4% topical lidocaine (Xylocaine) and/or papaverine solution for vasospasm.

**TIP:** Allow at least 10 minutes for vasospasm to clear before manipulating anastomosis.

- **Microvascular venous anastomosis**
  - **Use at least two veins** to avoid venous congestion.
    - Dorsal veins are larger and do not interfere with repair of volar structures.
    - Procedure can be done before arterial repair.
  - **Without venous repair, approximately 80% of replants fail.**[4]
- **Closure**
  - Use skin closure, skin grafting, flow-through skin/vein flaps, or local flaps, if needed.
  - Prevent tension on the skin closure.
    - It is better to leave it loose and allow healing by granulation (or skin graft).

- **Dressing**
  - Antibiotic ointment
  - Nonadherent gauze **(avoid circumferential wrapping),** fluffy or bulky dressing
  - Accessibility to fingertips needed for postoperative monitoring
  - Protective splinting

> **TIP:** Perform Doppler assessment before leaving OR, and elevate extremity on foam pillow (e.g., Carter pillow).

- **Perioperative pharmacologic treatment**
  - 325 mg aspirin given per rectum before leaving OR
    - Aspirin inhibits platelet aggregation at the anastomosis at this dose level.
    - Heparin can be given during clamp removal of arterial anastomosis (1500-2500 units).

## POSTOPERATIVE MANAGEMENT

### ICU MONITORING

- 24-48 hours with frequent monitoring
- Clinical assessment
  - Capillary refill
  - Color
  - Turgor
  - Temperature
- Transcutaneous Doppler assessment every hour
- Laser-Doppler flowmetry
- Transcutaneous oxygen monitors
- Temperature probes
- Warm ambient temperature and warm extremity; use warming blankets (e.g., Bair Hugger [Arizant Healthcare, Eden Prairie, MN]) to keep digit warm
  - Aids in prevention of arterial spasm
  - Marked temperature decrease possibly a result of arterial inflow problem
- Adequate IV hydration

> **TIP:** The most practical and common monitoring tool is *temperature.* A well-perfused digit should be at or above 31° C.[3]

### PHARMACOLOGIC THERAPY

- **Antibiotics:** For skin flora coverage and as indicated by mechanism of injury
- **Aspirin:** 325 mg (or 81 mg) by mouth every day for approximately 3 weeks postoperatively
- **Chlorpromazine:** 25 mg by mouth three times per day
  - Antianxiety and vasodilation properties (for 3-5 days)
- **Indwelling axillary catheters:** Local anesthetics used for pain control and chemical sympathectomy
- **Other agents:** Calcium channel blockers and dipyridamole (Persantine)
  - For vasodilation or as antivasospastic agent

- **Systemic heparinization**
  - **Not** commonly required; some use low-dose continuous heparin and not full anticoagulation protocols
  - Used if anastomotic revision made or concern for thrombosis (severe crush injuries)
  - Used along with nail plate removal and heparin-soaked pledget if venous repair not done or tenuous
- **Leech therapy:** Valuable if signs of venous congestion not alleviated with other measures
  - *Hirudin,* an anticoagulant (thrombin inhibitor), is secreted by leeches during feeding; its use allows continued bleeding from site.
  - Leeches usually fall off patient 10-15 minutes after feeding.
  - **Prophylaxis against *Aeromonas hydrophila* infection is required.**
    - Third-generation cephalosporin, quinolones (avoid in children), or trimethoprim plus sulfamethoxazole (TMP/sulfa)
- **Smoking cessation:** At least 1 month after replantation

## REPLANT FAILURE AND SECONDARY PROCEDURES

Digits that undergo revision and "struggle to survive" show very poor function. They are often atrophic, have poor sensation, and move poorly, except for the thumb, which at minimum provides a usable post.[3]

> **TIP:** If there is a problem in the OR, do not leave until it is corrected. If a postoperative problem is not remedied by conservative measures, go back to the OR as soon as possible for reexploration. Use reasonable judgment in deciding for reexploration (limited benefit for severe avulsion/crush, more proximal amputations, and in patients with perioperative systemic complications).

### Arterial Insufficiency

- Accounts for up to **60%** of failures[11]
- **Signs**
  - Pale color
  - Poor turgor
  - Cool finger with slow capillary refill
  - Little to no bleeding from needle prick test
- **Treatment**
  1. **If doubts about patency, return to the OR immediately!**
  2. Warm finger.
  3. Loosen dressing.
  4. Use antispasmodic drugs.
  5. Improve pain control.
  6. Use bupivacaine (Marcaine) block (vasodilation).
  7. Use heparin.

### Venous Insufficiency

- Purple: Rapid capillary refill
- Congested, with dark bleeding from needle prick
- Increased tissue turgor

- **Treatment**
  1. Increase elevation of extremity.
  2. Loosen dressing and sutures.
  3. Use systemic heparin.
  4. Remove nail plate with heparin-soaked pledgets.
  5. Use leech therapy.
  6. **Return to OR for reexploration.**

## OUTCOMES

### Overall Success Rates

- Range from 54%-82%[12]
- Success rates for guillotine-type injuries: 77% versus 49% for crush amputations[11]
- Success is now measured based on function[3]
  - Often predicted by level of amputation
  - Single-finger distal replants (distal to FDS insertion) function well, even without DIP motion.
  - Hands proximal to the midpalm function well.
  - Replanted thumbs are almost always useful, even if just for opposition.
  - Proximal finger amputations and avulsion/crushed fingers have poorer function.

### Functional Outcomes

- Approximately 70% achieve two-point discrimination at <15 mm.[4]
  - **Factors affecting two-point discrimination**[12]
    - Patient age: **Best results with children**
    - Level and mechanism of injury (see previous sections)
      - Average thumb replant two-point discrimination is 11 mm. Average finger (sharply amputated) 2-point discrimination is 8 mm and 15 mm in crush-avulsion replants.[3]
    - Success of sensory reeducation
- **Total active motion**[13]
  - Approximately 50% total active motion (TAM) and 50% grip strength for average replant result.[14]
  - Injury distal to FDS tendon insertion gives better results.
  - TAM, when subtracting minor contribution of metacarpophalangeal (MP) joint, is 85.5 degrees at middle phalanx level and 80 degrees for proximal phalanx.
  - Therefore range of motion is improved significantly with joint preservation, especially with the proximal interphalangeal (PIP) and MP joints.
- **Largest major limb replant review**[15]
  - 11 of 24 had more than 50% TAM; 19 of 24 had protective sensation; and 22 of 24 were satisfied with function and appearance.
- **Largest review of distal digital amputation**[5]
  - Mean survival was 86%.
  - Outcomes were not different between Tamai zone I and zone II replantations.
  - Survival was significantly different between clean-cut and crush replants.
  - Repair of a vein improved survival in Tamai zone I and II replantations.
  - Mean two-point discrimination was 7 mm, and 98% returned to work.
  - Complications included pulp atrophy (14%) and nail deformity (23%).

## Complications and Secondary Procedures

- **Secondary surgery**[1]
  - Required in **60%** of cases
  - More common among replants proximal to FDS insertion
  - **Incidence of procedures**
    - Extensor and flexor tenolysis or release of joint contractures: 67%
    - Open reduction and internal fixation (ORIF) correction of nonunions: 22%
    - Digital replants proximal to FDS insertion: 93% with secondary surgery
    - Thumb amputations: 11%
- Flexor or extensor tenolysis
  - The average TAM improvement is **43%.**[14]
  - Thumb replants show less improvement.
- Neurolysis, with or without nerve grafting
- Nonunion, malunion
- Web space release, and soft tissue coverage
- Amputations (for poor function)

## Other Complications

- Cold intolerance: Often improves postoperatively over 2 years[9]
- Chronic pain (chronic regional pain syndrome)

### Key Points

✓ Every attempt must be made for replantation in children.
✓ Prompt arrival at the replantation center and a two-team approach are essential to decrease ischemia duration and improve success.
✓ Signs of vessel injury must be recognized, with resection of damaged vessel.
✓ All neurovascular structures and tendons must be delineated and tagged, preferably within one tourniquet run.
✓ When possible, rigid bony fixation should be performed to allow early motion-rehabilitation protocols.
✓ Close postoperative monitoring with multiple modalities and pharmacologic support (aspirin, vasodilation medications, analgesics, or anxiolytics) should be initiated.
✓ When conservative measures fail, return to the OR for reexploration as soon as possible.
✓ Often secondary procedures are required; these provide meaningful functional recovery when performed.
✓ Arm and hand replants often have good outcomes. Distal finger replants (beyond FDS insertion) often are more successful than proximal finger replants (tendon zone II) because of poor PIP function.

## References

1. Chao JJ, Castello JR, English JM, et al. Microsurgery: free-tissue transfer and replantation. Sel Read Plast Surg 9, 2000.
2. Goldner RD, Urbaniak JR. Replantation. In Green DP, Hotchkiss RN, Pederson WC, eds. Green's Operative Hand Surgery, vol 2, 4th ed. Philadelphia: Churchill Livingstone, 1999, pp 1139-1157.
3. Pederson WC. Replantation. Plast Reconstr Surg 107:823-841, 2001.
4. Tamai S. Twenty years' experience of limb replantation: review of 293 upper extremity replants. J Hand Surg 7:549-556, 1982.

5. Sebastin SJ, Chung KC. A systematic review of the outcomes of replantation of distal digital amputation. Plast Reconstr Surg 128:723-737, 2011.
6. Urbaniak JR, Evans JP, Bright DS. Microvascular management of ring avulsion injuries. J Hand Surg Am 6:25-30, 1981.
7. Merle M, Dautel G. Advances in digital replantation. Clin Plast Surg 24:87-105, 1997.
8. Wei FC, Chen HC, Chuang CC. Three successful digital replantations in a patient after 84, 86, and 94 hours cold ischemia time. Plast Reconstr Surg 82:346-350, 1988.
9. Buncke GM, Buncke HJ, Kind GM, et al. Replantation. In Russell RC, ed. Plastic Surgery: Indications, Operations, and Outcomes, vol 4. St Louis: Mosby–Year Book, 2000.
10. Callico CG. Replantation and revascularization of the upper extremity. In McCarthy JG, May JW Jr, Littler JW, eds. Plastic Surgery: The Hand and Upper Limb, vol 7. Philadelphia: WB Saunders, 1990.
11. O'Brien BM. Replantation surgery. Clin Plast Surg 1:405-426, 1974.
12. Wilhelmi BJ, Lee WP, Pagensteert GI, et al. Replantation in the mutilated hand. Hand Clin 19:89-120, 2003.
13. Chiu HY, Shieh SJ. Multivariate analysis of factors influencing the functional recovery after finger replantation or revascularization. Microsurgery 16:713-717, 1995.
14. Jupiter JB, Pess GM, Bour CJ, et al. Results of flexor tendon tenolysis after replantation of the hand. J Hand Surg Am 14:35-44, 1989.
15. Russell RC, O'Brien BM, Morrison WA, et al. The late functional results of upper limb revascularization and replantation. J Hand Surg Am 9:623-633, 1984.

# 74. Hand Transplantation

Tae Chong

## UNDERSTANDING THE PROBLEM

- **Disability:** Degree of disability affected by concomitant injury (blindness, lower extremity amputation), level of amputation, ability to use prosthetic, and amount of home/social support
- **Etiologic factors:** Some injuries are associated with poorer quality of the remaining soft tissue and functional structures
  - Ballistic
  - High-voltage burn
  - Avulsion injury
  - Sepsis
- **Level of amputation**
  - **Transmetacarpal:** Amputees are able to use their wrists to perform many activities of daily living.
    - Limited functional prosthetic options
  - **Radiocarpal:** Length preserved, but very little function without a prosthetic and difficult to fit a prosthetic at this level
  - **Midforearm:** Many options for prosthetic
  - **Proximal forearm:** Proximal to the myotendinous junction, which will affect transplantation
    - Limited prosthetic options
  - **Transhumeral:** Successful prosthetic use is dependent on mobile shoulder.[1]

## INDICATIONS

- **Functional loss** resulting from unreconstructable amputation of bilateral upper extremities or unilateral dominant upper extremity
- **Inclusion criteria**
  - Adults 18-69 years of age
  - Healthy with no coexisting medical or psychosocial problems
  - No history of malignancy within the past 10 years and no history of HIV
  - Amputation at least 9-12 months prior with an attempt at use of prosthetic[2]
- **Goal:** To restore independence in activities of daily living with psychological integration of the transplanted limb

## CONTRAINDICATIONS

- **Psychosocial contraindications**
  - Active psychiatric disorder
  - Substance abuse
  - Cognitive and perceptual inability to understand the problem and risks of the procedure
  - History of medical noncompliance
  - Inadequate support network

- **Medical conditions that would preclude safe transplantation**
  - Cancer: Active cancer diagnosis and high risk of recurrence
  - Active infectious disease: HIV, hepatitis
  - Hematologic and immunologic conditions: Hypercoagulable disorders, SLE, scleroderma
- **Pregnancy**
- **Congenital malformations**

## RISKS OF TRANSPLANTATION

### Immunosuppression

- Opportunistic infections: Bacterial, viral (cytomegalovirus [CMV]), fungal
- Malignancy: Skin cancers, virally associated (Epstein-Barr virus [EBV]), Kaposi's sarcoma
- Metabolic: Hypertension, diabetes, renal insufficiency/failure, and gastrointestinal intolerance
  - Most are transient and reversible with change in medications or decrease in dosage.[3]

### Loss of Hand Transplant

- Vascular compromise: Acute setting, low incidence overall
- Cessation of immunosuppression either because of complications from the medications or medical noncompliance
- Irreversible allograft rejection: Acute or chronic
  - One case in the Western literature in a medically compliant patient[4]
- Amputation of the transplanted hand would result in a more proximal stump and altered use of prosthetic.
  - This is particularly relevant in patients with a functional radiocarpal joint (metacarpal hand).

### Death

- Bilateral hand and face transplant recipient died from cerebral anoxia during reoperation.[5]
- Quadrimembral transplantation in Turkey

## BENEFITS OF TRANSPLANTATION

- Functional recovery
  - Return to independence with activities of daily living
  - Sensory return facilitating functional recovery and social interaction
- Restoration of sense of self and "wholeness"

## PREOPERATIVE EVALUATION

### Transplant Medical Clearance

- Physical health screening
- Infectious disease screening
  - CMV, EBV, herpes simplex virus (HSV), HIV, hepatitis virus (A, B, C), tuberculosis (Tb)
- Immunologic
  - ABO blood typing and HLA typing
  - Panel reactive antibodies
    - Reflect sensitization to potential donor antigens
    - Predict hyperacute rejection and may preclude transplant candidacy

### Psychiatric Clearance

- Rule out active psychiatric disorders.
- Assess medical compliance.
- Confirm that patient has cognitive understanding of transplant process and realistic expectations for outcome.
- Evaluate for postoperative regression and degree of coping skills.
- Assess and optimize the structure of home support.

### Occupational and Physical Therapy

- Evaluate candidacy based on level of engagement and ability to participate in postoperative hand therapy.
- Assess preoperatively needs for physical therapy after the surgery. This is especially relevant in quadrimembral amputees.

### Imaging of the Extremity

- Plain radiographs
- Vasculature: Angiography or CT angiography, venous ultrasound/mapping
- Soft tissue: MRI
  - To evaluate the degree of scarring and status of the myotendinous units and nerves

## TRANSPLANTATION

### Criteria for Match

- **Common criteria**
  - Immunologic
    - ABO blood type match
    - Negative crossmatch: Recipient's serum is tested against the donor's lymphocytes
      - A positive result indicates that the recipient has preformed antibodies against the donor and will likely have a hyperacute rejection after transplantation.
  - Infectious
    - Negative for mismatches against opportunistic viral infections: CMV and EBV
    - No active infections or history of malignancy
- **Specific criteria**
  - Matching of donor and recipient hand/forearm size, length, skin color, hair color
  - No evidence of arthritis, history of mixed connective tissue disease, paralysis, or any metabolic disorder that would preclude successful hand rehabilitation

### Anatomic and Technical Considerations

- In replantation, tissue availability is limited by the inciting trauma, and bone shortening may have to be performed.
  - However, tendon lengths are relatively intact, and de novo establishment of balanced tendon function is not necessary.
- In hand transplantation, the donor tissue is surgically procured so that abundant healthy donor tissue is available for reconstruction.
  - However, the surgeon must establish forearm lengths and the natural balance of flexor and extensor tendons.[6]

## Donor Operation

- Hand is procured after the solid organs have been isolated, but before cross clamping is performed.
- Begin procurement with a fishmouth incision at the humerus.
  - Cannulate the brachial artery for perfusion with University of Wisconsin solution or HTK solution (histidine-tryptophan-ketoglutarate).
  - Perform sharp amputation through the elbow.
  - Place hand in sterile transplantation bag on ice and transport to recipient team.
  - Place cosmetic prosthetic over the donor stumps.
- Prepare donor hand on the back table of the recipient OR.
  - Make volar and dorsal skin incisions, proceeding from proximal to distal.
  - Tag anatomic structures after identification[2] (Fig. 74-1).
    - *Flexor and extensor tendons:* Leave long for Pulvertaft weave
    - *Bone:* Coordinate with recipient team to plan the location of the osteotomy.
    - *Nerves:* Median, ulnar, and radial nerve
- In distal transplants, identify the volar cutaneous branch of the median nerve and the dorsal sensory branch of the ulnar nerve.
    - *Vasculature:* Remove indwelling access catheters, and perform on angiographic table if there is evidence of vessel injury.
      - Radial and ulnar arteries with venae comitantes
      - Dorsal superficial veins[7]

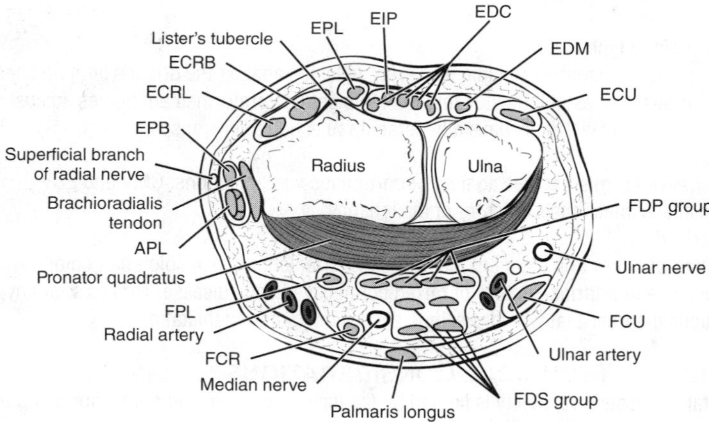


**Fig. 74-1** Cross-sectional anatomy at the level of radiocarpal amputation. Note the configuration of the flexor tendons (flexor digitorum superficialis *[FDS]* and flexor digitorum profundus *[FDP]* groups). *APL,* Abductor pollicis longus; *ECRB*, extensor carpi radialis brevis; *ECRL,* extensor carpi radialis longus; *ECU,* extensor carpi ulnaris; *EDC,* extensor digitorum communis; *EDM,* extensor digiti minimi; *EIP,* extensor indicis proprius; *EPB,* extensor pollicis brevis; *EPL,* extensor pollicis longus; *FCR,* flexor carpi radialis; *FCU,* flexor carpi ulnaris; *FPL,* flexor pollicis longus.

## Recipient Operation

- Recipient dissection is performed under tourniquet control.
  - Coordinated with donor dissection, same OR
  - Complicated by unpredictable anatomy and scarring, which can be worse in ballistic injuries, burns, and septic amputations
- Sequence of operation: Earlier revascularization is necessary in allografts with significant muscle to minimize ischemic fibrosis.
  - Proximal forearm (proximal two thirds)
    - Bony stabilization, revascularization, muscle and tendon repair, nerve, and then skin
  - Distal forearm (distal third)
    - Bony stabilization, extensor tendons, dorsal veins, nerve repair, revascularization, flexor tendons, and then skin
    - Takes advantage of the longer ischemia time to perform nerve repair (grouped fascicular) in a bloodless field without edema.
- **Specific details**
  - **Skin**[6] (Fig. 74-2)
    - Midlateral incisions are designed to create dorsal and ulnar skin flaps.
    - Final skin closure is a four-flap interposition with a zigzag scar pattern to prevent circumferential contracture.
  - **Bone:** Locking compression plates
  - **Tendon**
    - Pulvertaft weave to facilitate earlier, active motion
      - Disadvantage: Bulk of reconstruction
      - Tension is set for the extensors so that the fingers are extended when the wrist is flexed.
      - Flexor tendons are set thereafter to restore a natural cascade.
      - In proximal transplants, muscle belly repair or full functional myotendinous units may be transposed as a group.

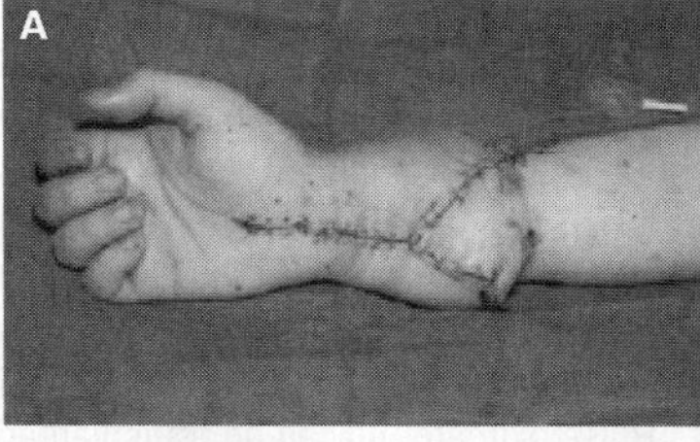

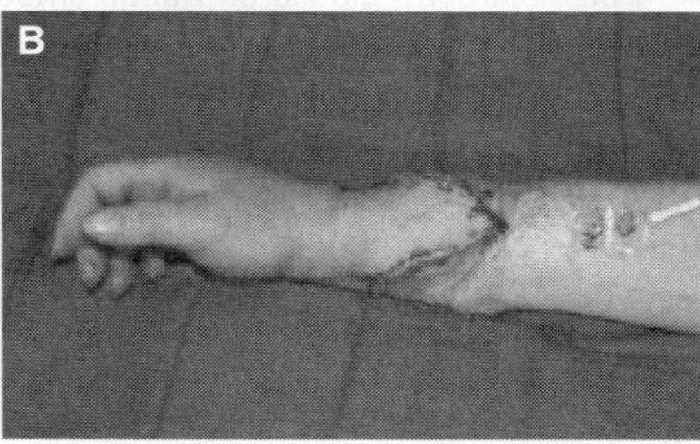

**Fig. 74-2 A and B,** Interdigitating skin flaps as final inset for hand transplant.

  - **Nerve:** Epineural in proximal-level transplants and group fascicular repair in distal level
    - Prophylactic carpal tunnel release
  - **Vasculature**
    - Radial and ulnar arteries along with the venae comitantes in end-to-end fashion
      - In proximal transplants, end-to-side to the recipient vessels to preserve native blood supply to forearm muscles
    - Superficial veins can be scarred and difficult to locate.
      - Consider preoperative venous mapping.[6]

## POSTOPERATIVE CARE

### IMMUNOSUPPRESSION

- **Induction:** Immunosuppression initiated before transplantation to prevent acute rejection of the transplant
  - Depleting agent: Decreases the lymphocyte count
    - Antithymocyte globulin or alemtuzumab (Anti-CD-52)
  - Calcineurin inhibitor: Prevents IL-2–dependent activation of lymphocytes
    - Tacrolimus or cyclosporine
  - Antiproliferative agent: Mycophenolate mofetil (MMF)
  - Steroid: General immunosuppressant with antiinflammatory properties[8-10]
- **Maintenance**
  - Most patients are on three-drug therapy with corticosteroids, tacrolimus, and MMF.
  - Many protocols today attempt to eliminate steroids and decrease the dose of tacrolimus or replace it with rapamycin.[11]
- **Prophylactic medications:** CMV, herpes virus, pneumocystis, and antifungal medications
- **Medications to treat metabolic complications**
  - Hypoglycemics, antihypertensives, and gastrointestinal prophylaxis
  - As the dosage of immunosuppressants is decreased or weaned, these medications can be discontinued.

### MONITORING

- Skin color, temperature, swelling, capillary refill
- Pulse oximeter placed on transplanted finger and nontransplanted finger (or toe in bilateral cases)
- External transcutaneous and implantable Doppler monitor

### REHABILITATION

- Daily hand therapy
- Focus on optimizing motor unit recovery, soft tissue pliability, and recovery with nerve regeneration.
- Early: Soft splint to minimize tissue trauma and allow close observation for vascular complications
  - Transition to intrinsic plus splint
  - Passive ROM and tenodesis
- First month: Place and hold and adaptive exercises
- Third month: Active ROM with wrists and digits
- Thereafter, strengthening, sensory reeducation, dynamic splints, and edema gloves as needed

## OUTCOMES

### MOTOR

Functional recovery depends on the level of transplantation.

- **Distal transplantation**
  - Improved functional recovery from reconstruction using Pulvertaft weave
  - Greater likelihood of intrinsic recovery because of shorter length for nerve regeneration
- **Proximal transplantation**
  - Reconstruction proximal to myotendinous junction requiring muscle repair or functional muscle unit transfer
  - Greater distance for nerve regeneration to the intrinsic muscles of the hand[12]

- **Data from International Registry on Hand and Composite Tissue Transplantation (IRHCTT)**[13]
  - 100% return of extrinsic hand function
  - Variable return of intrinsic hand function (<60%)
    - Delayed recovery possible, even several years after transplantation

## Sensory

- Protective, temperature, and pain: 100%
- Tactile sensation: 90%
- Discriminative sensation: 84%

## Scoring Systems

- Disability of Arm Shoulder and Hand (DASH): Patient-reported outcome measure that scores ability to perform ADLs and associated symptoms
  - Decrease of 15 points (scale of 100 points) suggests improvement.
  - Mean DASH score change of 27 points was reported in one series using the International Registry.
- Hand Transplantation Score System (HTSS): Only scoring system designed specifically for hand transplant[14]
  - **Six parameters:**
    1. Appearance
    2. Sensibility
    3. Movement
    4. Psychological and social acceptance
    5. Daily activities and work status
    6. Patient satisfaction

## Subjective Quality of Life Improvement

- >75%, despite rigorous medical regimen, side effects from medications, and intrusive therapy and monitoring schedule
- Most patients perform ADLs independently, and some have returned to full employment.

# COMPLICATIONS

- **Mortality**
  - Death of one patient after hand and face transplant
  - Death of a Turkish patient after quadruple limb transplant
- **Acute rejection:** Incidence 85% in the first year
  - All episodes treatable with topical immunosuppressants, adjustment of maintenance medications, steroid boluses, and depleting agents (severe and refractory cases only)
  - Banff classification for vascularized composite allograft (VCA) rejection: 4 mm punch with H&E and PAS staining[15]
    - **Grade 0:** No rejection
    - **Grade I:** Mild rejection—mild perivascular infiltrate (lymphocytic)
    - **Grade II:** Moderate rejection—moderate to dense perivascular inflammation, can include mild epidermal and adnexal involvement
    - **Grade III:** Severe rejection—dense inflammation with epidermal involvement, epithelial apoptosis/necrosis
    - **Grade IV:** Necrotizing rejection—necrosis of epidermis and/or other skin elements

- **Allograft loss**
  - Chinese series[16]
    - 7 of 15 transplanted hands were lost because of **medication noncompliance.**
  - Chronic rejection occurred in a medically compliant patient.
    - Recipient from Louisville who was on a steroid-sparing regimen developed chronic rejection 1 year after transplant.
  - Acute vascular compromise in a Polish patient[10]
- **Metabolic complications:** Incidence 69%
  - Hypertension, elevated creatinine, hyperglycemia, gastrointestinal intolerance[17]
- **Opportunistic infections:** Incidence 63%
  - Mostly CMV infections, herpes virus, and bacterial infections
- **Malignancy:** Rare case reports
  - Posttransplant lymphoproliferative disease: Managed with change in immunosuppression
  - Basal cell carcinoma: Treated with excisional biopsy

## KEY POINTS

- ✓ Hand transplantation is indicated in healthy adult patients with unreconstructable amputations of bilateral upper extremities or a unilateral dominant upper extremity who have functional disability from the amputation.
- ✓ Hand transplantation is contraindicated in patients who have medical contraindications to chronic immunosuppression, lack of psychosocial support, history of medical noncompliance, and patients with congenital malformations.
- ✓ Risks are related to the immunosuppression and include opportunistic infections, increased risk of malignancy, metabolic complications, and potential loss of the transplant, which may result in a more proximal amputation.
- ✓ Functional outcomes have been generally favorable compared with replants, and patients typically have return of extrinsic function, delayed and variable return of intrinsic hand function, and return of sensation.
- ✓ The anatomic level correlates with functional recovery. Distal transplants have improved outcomes because of the use of Pulvertaft weaves and nerve reconstruction closer to the target intrinsic musculature.
- ✓ Successful functional recovery is dependent on active participation in hand rehabilitation under the guidance of an occupational therapist, similar to replantation.
- ✓ Hand transplantation in combination with face or lower extremity transplantation should be approached cautiously because of an increased risk of complications and mortality.
- ✓ Uniform adoption and expansion of hand transplantation is dependent on the development of immunosuppression protocols that minimize or eliminate side effects.

## REFERENCES

1. Wright TW, Hagen AD, Wood MB. Prosthetic usage in major upper extremity amputations. J Hand Surg Am 20:619-622, 1995.
2. Gordon CR, Siemionow M. Requirements for the development of a hand transplantation program. Ann Plast Surg 63:262-273, 2009.
3. Schneeberger S, Gorantla VS, Brandacher G, et al. Upper-extremity transplantation using a cell-based protocol to minimize immunosuppression. Ann Surg 257:345-351, 2013.
4. Kaufman CL, Ouseph R, Blair B, et al. Graft vasculopathy in clinical hand transplantation. Am J Transplant 12:1004-1016, 2012.

5. Gordon CR, Zor F, Cetrulo C Jr, et al. Concomitant face and hand transplantation: perfect solution or perfect storm? Ann Plast Surg 67:309-314, 2011.
6. Azari KK, Imbriglia JE, Goitz RJ, et al. Technical aspects of the recipient operation in hand transplantation. J Reconstr Microsurg 28:27-34, 2012.
7. McDiarmid SV, Azari KK. Donor-related issues in hand transplantation. Hand Clin 27:545-552, 2011.
8. Cavadas PC, Landin L, Thione A, et al. The Spanish experience with hand, forearm, and arm transplantation. Hand Clin 27:443-453, 2011.
9. Kaufman CL, Breidenbach W. World experience after more than a decade of clinical hand transplantation: update from the Louisville hand transplant program. Hand Clin 27:417-421, 2011.
10. Jablecki J, Kaczmarzyk L, Domanasiewicz A, et al. First Polish forearm transplantation: final report (outcome after 4 years). Ann Transplant 15:61-67, 2010.
11. Brandacher G, Ninkovic M, Piza-Katzer H, et al. The Innsbruck hand transplant program: update at 8 years after the first transplant. Transplant Proc 41:491-494, 2009.
12. Ninkovic M, Weissenbacher A, Gabl M, et al. Functional outcome after hand and forearm transplantation: what can be achieved? Hand Clin 27:455-465, 2011.
13. Lanzetta M, Patruzzo P, Margreiter R, et al. The International Registry on Hand and Composite Tissue Transplantation. Transplantation 79:1210-1214, 2005.
14. Petruzzo P, Lanzetta M, Dubernard JM, et al. The international registry on hand and composite tissue transplantation. Transplantation 86:487-492, 2008.
15. Cendales LC, Kanitakis J, Schneeberger S, et al. The Banff 2007 working classification of skin-containing composite tissue allograft pathology. Am J Transplant 8:1396-1400, 2008.
16. Pei G, Xiang D, Gu L, et al. A report of 15 hand allotransplantations in 12 patients and their outcomes in China. Transplantation 94:1052-1059, 2012.
17. Breidenbach WC, Gonzales NR, Kaufman CL, et al. Outcomes of the first 2 American hand transplants at 8 and 6 years posttransplant. J Hand Surg Am 33:1039-1047, 2008.

# 75. Thumb Reconstruction

Wendy L. Parker, David W. Mathes

## GENERAL CONSIDERATIONS

- **Indication for thumb reconstruction:** Loss of functional tissue secondary to trauma, cancer resection, or congenital deformities
- In large, mutilation-type injuries, consider reconstruction as a delayed procedure.
  - Ensure that surrounding soft tissues have stabilized, bone healing is achieved, and neurovascular status is certain before reconstruction.

Reconstruction of the thumb can be assessed by dividing the first ray into proximal, middle, and distal thirds. The middle third can be further subdivided into proximal and distal halves[1-3] (Fig. 75-1).

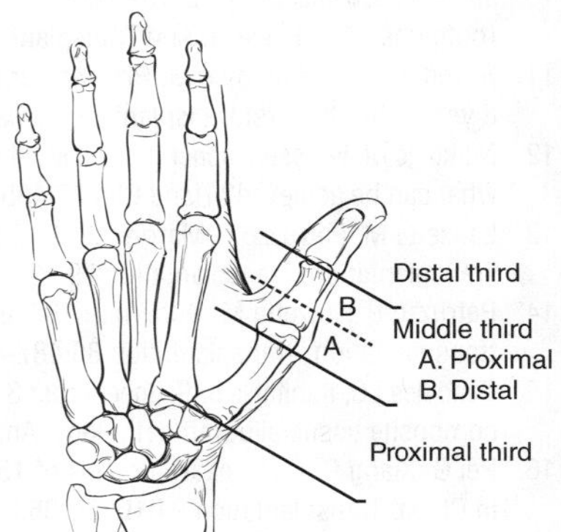


**Fig. 75-1** Areas of thumb loss: Distal third, middle third, and proximal third. The middle third is subdivided into proximal *(A)* and distal *(B)*.

## AMPUTATION THROUGH THE DISTAL THIRD

- This is a *compensated amputation.*
  - **Minimal functional impairment**
- **Efforts should be directed at:**
  - Restoring skeletal stability
  - Providing well-padded soft tissue coverage
  - Ensuring satisfactory sensory perception
- Choice of procedure depends on the **amount** and **depth** of tissue loss.
- An attempt should be made to salvage all viable tissue.
- Injuries to the volar pad surface can be reconstructed by the same coverage techniques used on the fingers, but the approach is modified to preserve length and provide sensibility.

> **TIP:** Completion amputation is the most common option for those seeking a rapid return to work. However, patients should be properly counseled, and revision amputation should not sacrifice significant function.

## Minimally Invasive Options

- **Secondary intention healing**
  - Useful for small soft tissue deficits <1 cm
  - Time to healing may be longer, but sensory result excellent with no donor deficit
- **Skin grafting**
  - Useful if underlying subcutaneous tissues are preserved (may be available from injured parts)
  - Full-thickness skin graft (FTSG) may be more durable but sensation return is not ideal.
  - Split-thickness skin graft (STSG) may be taken from hypothenar eminence under local anesthesia.[4]

## Volar Advancement Flap (Moberg Flap)[5] (Fig. 75-2)

- **Indications**
  - Use for avulsions of **less than 50%** of the volar surface
  - Can resurface as much as **1.5 cm$^2$**
  - Advantage of bringing **sensory-innervated skin** to resurface the pad of the thumb
  - Subcutaneous tissue and both neurovascular bundles included in volar flap
- **Technical tips**
  - Procedure is performed under tourniquet control.
  - Rongeur or file the distal phalanx to appropriate contour.
  - Midaxial incisions are made on the ulnar and radial side of the thumb and extended to the proximal thumb crease.
  - Do not disturb the underlying flexor tendon.
  - Flex the thumb at the metacarpophalangeal (MP) joint at 30 degrees and the interphalangeal (IP) joint at 45 degrees.
  - Distal edge of the flap is sutured to remaining nail, nail bed, or terminal skin remnant.
  - Proximal donor site management:
    - FTSG
    - Convert to V-Y[6]

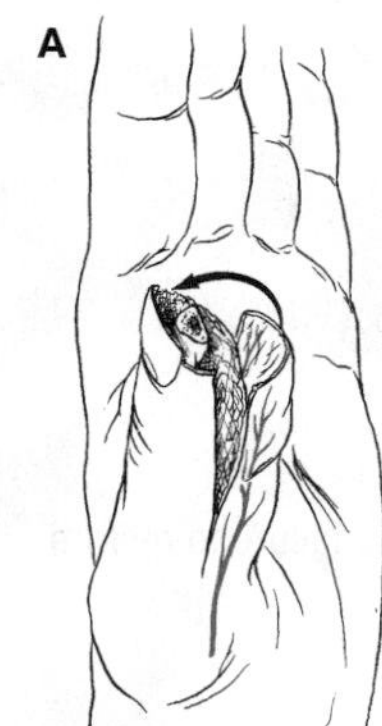


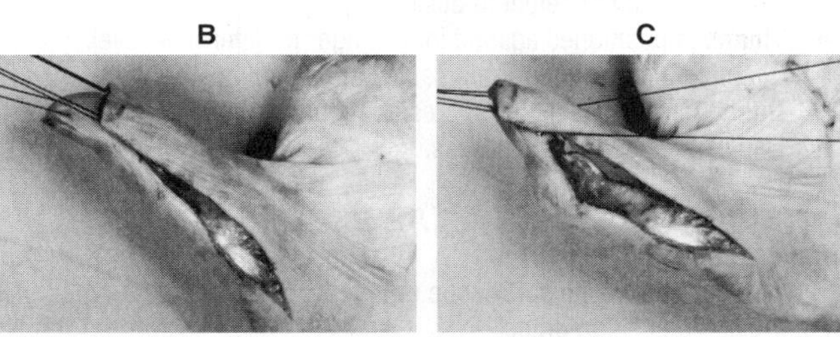


**Fig. 75-2** Volar advancement flap (Moberg flap). **A,** Arc to the distal phalanx of the thumb. **B,** Elevation of the flap. **C,** Coverage of the distal phalanx of the thumb.

## CROSS-FINGER FLAP (Fig. 75-3)

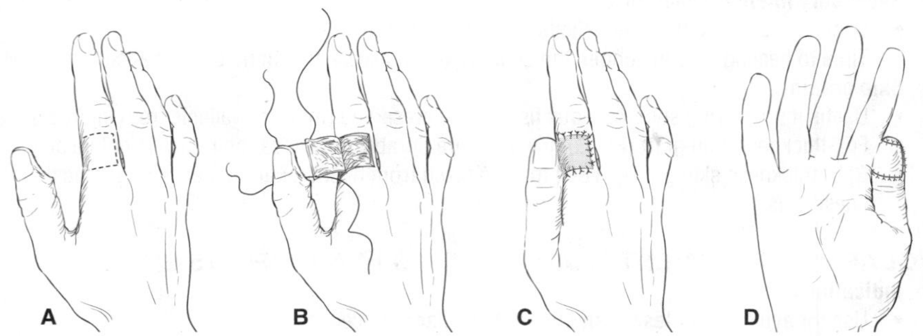


**Fig. 75-3** Cross-finger flap from the index finger to the thumb. **A,** Large defect involving most of the distal pulp of the thumb; outline the cross-finger flap on the proximal phalanx of the index finger. **B,** Placement of the flap on the thumb defect. **C** and **D,** Position of the thumb and cross-finger flap with a skin graft covering the donor defect.

- **Indications**
  - Use to resurface entire volar surface of the distal phalanx.
  - Use when skin grafting will not provide stable coverage.
  - Design cross-finger flap from proximal phalanx of the index finger.
  - Coverage and adequate sensory recovery are both provided.
- **Disadvantages**
  - Obvious dorsal donor site (requires skin graft)
  - Occasional problems with digital joint stiffness or thumb web contracture (avoid in elderly/arthritic)
- **Technical tips**
  - Perform under tourniquet control.
  - Use a template of defect to design flap.
  - Thumb is positioned against index finger to determine level.
  - Slightly oblique configuration aids in positioning.
  - During flap harvest, careful preservation of all small veins is essential.
  - Flap can be divided at 3 weeks.

## N/V ISLAND PEDICLED FLAPS[7]

- **Indications**
  - Ideal for composite **soft tissue and neurovascular bundle loss,** because failure to restore impairs pinch and grasp.
  - Amount of tissue harvested must match the defect.
- **Disadvantages**
  - Donor site morbidity
  - Technically demanding

- **Technical tips**
  - Perform under tourniquet control.
  - Donor tissue is designed from the ulnar pad of the middle finger.
    - Median nerve distribution makes cortical reintegration easier.
    - Pinch is not against ulnar side, so donor deficit is minimal.
  - If median nerve is lost, then donor is radial side of ring finger.

### Radial Sensory-Innervated Cross-Finger Flap (First Dorsal Metacarpal Artery Flap)[8]

This flap provides a large cross-finger pedicled flap that brings with it a sensory branch of the radial nerve.

- **Indications**
  - **For use when the defect requires:**
    - Substantial resurfacing (up to 4 cm)
    - Innervated skin (although sensory return is mostly protective and cortical reintegration more difficult)
- **Technical tips**
  - Defect of template is designed.
  - Suitable flap is designed over the dorsum of the proximal phalanx of the index finger with the base just volar to the midlateral line.
  - Flap design can be single, dual, or island flap.

## AMPUTATION THROUGH THE MIDDLE THIRD

- The **middle third** can be divided into **distal** and **proximal** components.
- **Functional deficits**
  - Loss of **fine pinch** and **strong grasp**
  - Acceptable carpometacarpal (CMC) joint rotation retained in most thumbs
  - Variable preservation of adequate thumb-index cleft
- **Functional requirements**
  - Length
  - Preservation of sensibility, mobility, and stability
  - Pain-free thumb
- **To achieve functional goals the procedures must:**
  - Create **relative ray lengthening** by deepening the first web space *(distal half of the middle third).*
  - **Add bone length** *(proximal half of the middle third).*
- **In mutilating injuries** preserve parts that may be useful for restoring soft tissue cover, adding bone length, or heterotopic replantation.[9,10]

> **TIP:** The best results for the proximal half are often obtained using free toe transfer techniques (great toe or second toe).

## Procedures That Deepen the First Web Space (Phalangization)

- **Web space Z-plasty (two or four flap)**[11] (Fig. 75-4)

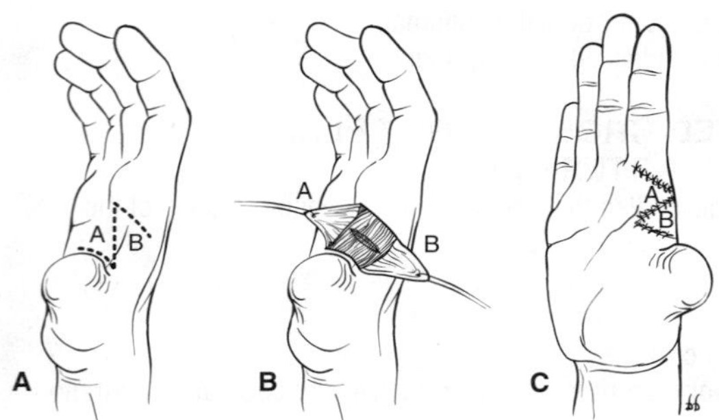


**Fig. 75-4** Simple Z-plasty of the thumb web. **A,** Design of the Z-plasty. Preferred angles are approximately 60 degrees. **B,** Flaps reflected with partial recession of the web space musculature. **C,** Appearance of the flap after reversal and suture. Corner sutures are preferred in the tips of the flaps.

- **Indications**
  - The skin must be pliable.
  - The first metacarpal must be mobile with no evidence of muscle contracture.
- **Advantage**
  - Simple procedure with little morbidity
- **Disadvantages**
  - Does not provide significant length; thus functional improvement is moderate.
  - Resulting cleft may look unnatural.
- **Technical tips**
  - The longitudinal axis of the Z-plasty should be on the **distal ridge of the first web space.**
  - Length gain is 1.5-2 cm.
  - Release of part of the first interosseous muscle and proximal transfer of the insertion of the adductor pollicis can be performed for additional length.

- **Dorsal rotation flap**[12,13] (Fig. 75-5)

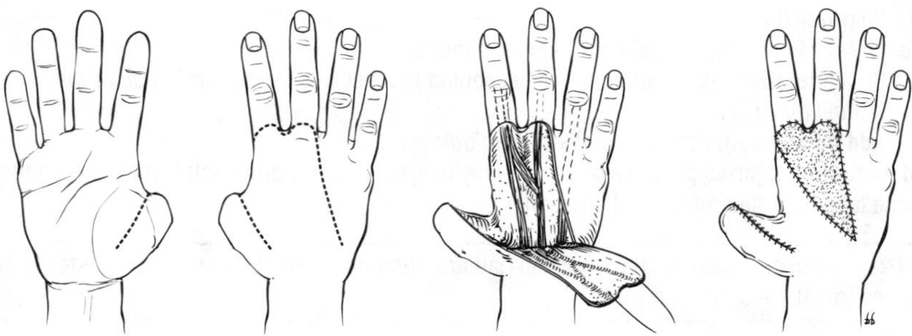

**Fig. 75-5** Dorsal rotation flap.

- **Indications**
  - Injury with thumb loss and adjacent tissue injury through the first web space **with contracture of the first metacarpal**
  - Need to restore the web space

- **Advantage**
  - Minimal morbidity
- **Disadvantages**
  - No direct improvement of thumb function
  - Need for skin graft to donor site
- **Technical tips**
  - Perform sequential division of all restraining skin, muscle, scar, and capsular adhesions.
  - Both the oblique and transverse heads of the adductor are divided.
  - Additional reconstructive procedures such as tendon transfer may be needed.

## PROCEDURES THAT ADD BONE LENGTH

These procedures are often used for reconstruction of the **proximal half** because of the need for length. **The addition of 2 cm of length can significantly improve the function of the thumb.**

- **Pollicization of an injured or normal digit (On-Top Plasty)**[14]
  - **Indications**
    - Can be performed acutely or in delayed fashion when the thumb is not replantable

**NOTE: Some make the argument to delay to allow patient to understand the functional deficit before reconstruction.**

  - **Advantages**
    - Minimal sacrifice of hand function
    - Excellent cosmetic and functional recovery
  - **Disadvantages**
    - Narrows the palm
    - May sacrifice a normal digit (if fails, then donor morbidity is high)
  - **Technical tips**
    - Use the nonfunctional injured finger (classically the index finger) for reconstruction, if applicable.
    - **Ring finger** is best **normal** digit to harvest and use for thumb reconstruction.
- **Metacarpal distraction osteogenesis**[15]

This simple and reliable technique increases length without sacrificing another digit or toe.

  - **Indications**
    - The patient must have:
      - Two thirds of the first metacarpal.
      - Adequate skin and subcutaneous coverage over the stump.
    - Procedure can increase the length up to 3-3.5 cm.
  - **Complications**
    - Infection, construct loosening, osteomyelitis
    - Nonunion
    - Tissue necrosis
    - Bone resorption
  - **Technical tips**
    - Distract the metacarpal gradually over several weeks (1 mm/day over a period of 25-40 days).
    - Bone grafting is needed in those older than 25 years and in cases of a gap larger than 3 cm.
    - Most need a subsequent web space deepening procedure.

- **Osteoplastic reconstruction**
  - **Indications**
    - Partial or distal subtotal amputations
    - Other fingers are either normal or too damaged to use.
    - Other lengthening procedures (such as toe transfer) are not an option.
  - **Advantage**
    - No digit is sacrificed.
  - **Disadvantages**
    - Multistage procedure
      - Option of composite iliac crest bone graft and tubed pedicled soft tissue flap[16,17]
    - Results may not be aesthetic.
    - Additional neurovascular flap is required for sensibility.
  - **Technical tips**
    - Iliac bone best source for bone graft
    - Soft tissue coverage of bone shaft
      - Tubed abdominal or groin flap
      - Reverse radial forearm flap
      - Anterolateral thigh flap

## AMPUTATION THROUGH THE PROXIMAL THIRD

- The entire thumb and at least the distal third of the first metacarpal are lost.
- Reconstruction must provide a **total thumb.**
- **Required length** will usually be >**5 cm.**

### Reconstruction Options

- **Pollicization of an injured index finger** (see previous discussion)
  - Best acute option at the time of injury
  - Can be performed as long as the neurovascular status of the index digit is adequate
    - **Be aware of structural changes** in converting index finger to thumb (Table 75-1).
- **Free toe transfer**

**Table 75-1** *Structural Changes During Pollicization*

| Initial Index Finger Structure | Reconstructed Thumb Structure |
|---|---|
| Metacarpal head | Trapezium |
| Proximal phalanx | Metacarpal |
| Middle phalanx | Proximal phalanx |
| Distal phalanx | Distal phalanx |
| Extensor digitorum communis | Abductor pollicis longus |
| Extensor indices proprius | Extensor pollicis |
| First dorsal interosseous | Abductor pollicis brevis |
| First palmar interosseous | Adductor pollicis |

## TOE-TO-THUMB TRANSFER[18,19]

- Complete or partial toe transfer is an effective way to reconstruct an absent or deficient thumb.

### WHY A TOE TRANSFER?

- Can restore certain attributes of a functional thumb in a single operation (Fig. 75-6)
  - Excellent cosmetic appearance (glabrous skin and nail support)
  - Strength
  - Stability
  - Movement (restores pinch and grasp)
  - Sensation
  - Growth (critical importance for children)

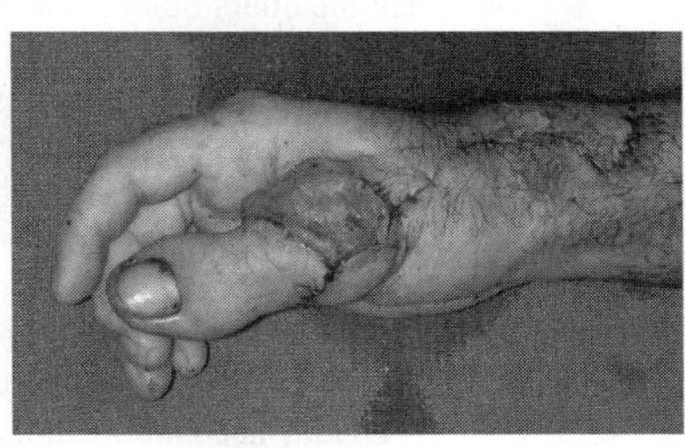

**Fig. 75-6** Immediate postoperative result of a great-toe transfer.

- **Disadvantages**
  - Donor site morbidity: Decreased balance and push-off
  - Lengthy operation: Requires microvascular expertise
    - Consider preoperative donor and recipient angiograms.
- **Foot donor site anatomy**
  - First dorsal metatarsal artery supplies the great and second toes and usually arises from the dorsalis pedis artery.
  - Venous drainage is by the superficial dorsal veins to the greater saphenous vein.
  - Volar digital nerves arise from the medial plantar nerve.
- **There are three central questions to be addressed before performing a toe-to-thumb transfer.**
  1. **Is toe transfer the best surgical option?**
     - Patient considerations
       - Age
       - Motivation
       - Handedness
       - Functional requirements at work
       - Bilateral
     - Better discriminative sensation and fine motor control with pollicization
     - Better strength with toe transfer
     - Possibility of local reconstructive options
     - Contraindications
       - Vascular abnormalities/smoker
       - Significant comorbidity precluding extended anesthesia time
       - Cultural footwear preferences
  2. **What is the ideal timing of transfer?**
     - **Urgent** toe-to-thumb transfer
       - Thumb salvage after soft tissue avulsion can be treated with an urgent wraparound flap.
     - **Delayed** toe-to-thumb transfer
       - Functional capability of a hand with a shortened or absent thumb is not immediately apparent.
       - Patient may find new length more or less functional.
       - Patient needs to understand donor site morbidity in foot.

**3. Which toe transplant procedure is indicated?**

- **Whole great-toe transfer** (Fig. 75-7).
  - Great toe offers optimal mobility and excellent strength.
  - Use the **ipsilateral** great toe, because it orients the vascular pedicle to the radial artery at the dorsal first web space.
  - Appearance is somewhat compromised.
    - Great toe is **20% larger** than the thumb.
    - Great toenail is broader and shorter.
    - Donor site is not aesthetic and often requires skin graft for closure.
  - Neurovascular bundles of the toe are plantar to midaxial line.
    - Lateral bundle is larger than the medial bundle.
      - May need intraneural dissection into common digital nerve for length
    - Arterial system may be variable, with first MT artery not arising directly off dorsalis pedis.
    - Two levels of veins are available.
    - An **oblique osteotomy** of the MT to bring the joint into hyperextension for improved arc of motion

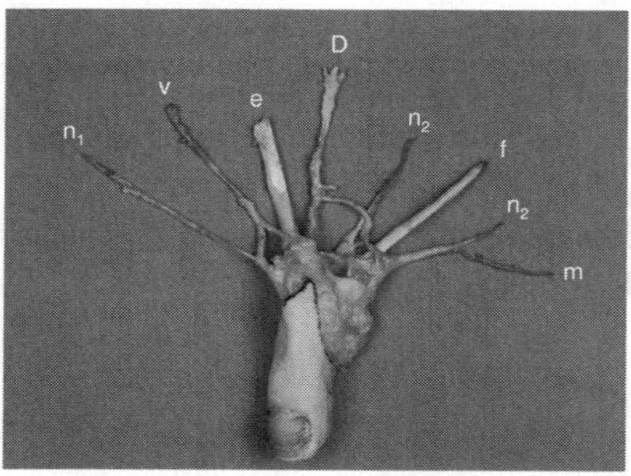


Dorsal surface of flap

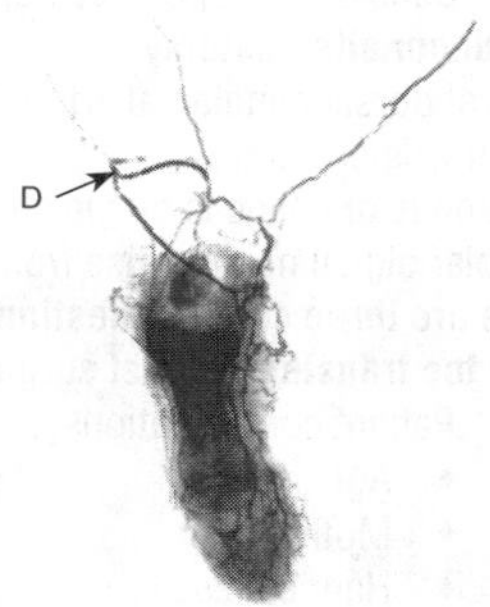


Radiographic view

**Fig. 75-7** Surgical anatomy of the great toe. *D,* First dorsal metatarsal artery (dominant pedicle); *e,* extensor pollicis longus; *f,* flexor pollicis longus; *m,* first metatarsal artery (minor pedicle); $n_1$, dorsal digital nerve; $n_2$, plantar digitial nerve; *v,* superficial vein.

- **Second-toe transfer**
  - Second toe is thinner, nail is shorter
  - **Advantages**
    - Second metatarsal and MP joints can be harvested
    - Offers a good donor site and good sensation after transfer
    - Favored in children
    - Can usually close donor primarily with MT resection
  - **Disadvantages**
    - Reconstructed thumb can be narrower than native thumb
    - Not as strong as great toe
    - Skin problems and need for skin grafts
- **Wraparound procedure**
  - Soft tissue flap and nail from great toe transferred

- Osseous support provided by iliac bone graft
- **Advantages**
  - Good sensation
  - Adequate strength
  - Excellent aesthetic replacement for missing thumb
- **Disadvantages**
  - No motion at IP joint
  - Technically demanding
  - Bone resorption

**TIP:** The wraparound procedure should not be used for children (because of growth restriction).

- **Trimmed toe technique**
  - Smaller structure that is capable of movement
  - Great toe trimmed to size of thumb
  - **Advantages**
    - Good sensation, strength, and appearance
    - Excellent mobility
  - **Disadvantages**
    - Complicated procedure
    - Cannot be used in children
- **Partial toe transfer (pulp, nail, or joint used)**
  - Second MP joint
  - Skin of first web site
  - Pulp skin
  - Nail and dorsal skin

## Site-Specific Selection of Toe Transfer

- **At or distal to interphalangeal joint**
  - No need for toe transplant
- **Through proximal phalanx with intact MP joint**
  - Wraparound transfer (better appearance than great toe)
  - Trimmed toe is better with mobility intact.
  - Great toe provides best strength.
- **Distal half of metacarpal**
  - Great toe is the best option.
  - Harvested at MP joint.
  - Thenar muscle should be reconstructed, or opposition transfer should be done.
  - If the great toe is too short, then the second toe can be harvested.
- **Proximal half of metacarpal to MP joint**
  - Second toe is best option.
  - Second toe is skin deficient, and muscle must be covered by skin grafts.
  - An opposition transfer should be done.
- **Proximal to the metacarpal**
  - Reconstruction is difficult because of lack of metacarpal bone.
  - Pollicization of the index finger is often the best option.
    - Standard of care for Blauth IV and V congenital thumb absence
  - If other fingers are injured, then toe transfer is indicated.

## Key Points

- ✓ A useful algorithm for evaluating thumb defects is to divide the thumb into thirds.
- ✓ The choice of the correct procedure depends on the *defect, location, size, and requirements for sensibility and durability.*
- ✓ The goals of reconstruction are *primary stable wound healing and early active use with preservation of functional length.*
- ✓ Toe transfers provide strong functional results in patients willing to undergo the procedure and accept the donor deficit.

## References


1. Azari KK, Lee WPA. Thumb reconstruction. In Wolfe SW, Hotchkiss RN, Pederson WC, eds. Green's Operative Hand Surgery, vol 2, 6th ed. Philadelphia: Churchill Livingstone, 2011.
2. Eaton CJ. Thumb reconstruction. In Aston SJ, Beasley RW, Thorne CH, eds. Grabb and Smith's Plastic Surgery, 5th ed. Philadelphia: Lippincott-Raven, 1991.
3. Lister G. The choice of procedure following thumb amputation. Clin Orthop Relat Res 195:45-51, 1985.
4. Grossman JA, Robotti EB. The use of split-thickness hypothenar grafts for coverage of fingertips and other defects of the hand. Ann Chir Main Memb Super 14:239-243, 1995.
5. Keim HA, Grantham SA. Volar-flap advancement for thumb and finger-tip injuries. Clin Orthop Relat Res 66:109-112, 1969.
6. Elliot D, Wilson Y. V-Y advancement of the entire volar soft tissue of the thumb in distal reconstruction. J Hand Surg Br 18:399-402, 1993.
7. Foucher G, Khouri RK. Digital reconstruction with island flaps [review]. Clin Plast Surg 24:1-32, 1997.
8. El-Khatib HA. Clinical experiences with the extended first dorsal metacarpal artery island flap for thumb reconstruction. J Hand Surg Am 23:647-652, 1998.
9. Haddock NT, Ehrlich DA, Levine JP, et al. The crossover composite filet of hand flap and heterotopic thumb replantation: a unique indication. Plast Reconstr Surg 130:634e-636e, 2012.
10. Weinzweig N, Chen L, Chen ZW. Pollicization of the mutilated hand by transposition of middle and ring finger remnants. Ann Plast Surg 34:523-529, 1995.
11. Eaton CJ, Lister GD. Treatment of skin and soft-tissue loss of the thumb. Hand Clin 8:71-97, 1992.
12. Canale ST. Campbell's Operative Orthopedics, vol 4, 10th ed. St Louis: Elsevier, 2003.
13. Emerson ET, Krizek TJ, Greenwald DP. Anatomy, physiology, and functional restoration of the thumb [review]. Ann Plast Surg 36:180-191, 1996.
14. Foucher G, Rostane S, Chammas M, et al. Transfer of a severely damaged digit to reconstruct an amputated thumb. J Bone Joint Surg Am 78:1889-1896, 1996.
15. Moy OJ, Clayton PA, Sherwin DS. Reconstruction of traumatic or congenital amputation of the thumb by distraction-lengthening [review]. Hand Clin 81:57-62, 1992.
16. Parmaksizoglu F, Beyzadeoglu T. Composite osteocutaneous groin flap combined with neurovascular island flap for thumb reconstruction. J Hand Surg Br 28:399-404, 2003.
17. Reinisch JF, Winters R, Puckett CL. The use of the osteocutaneous groin flap in gunshot wounds of the hand. J Hand Surg Am 9:12-17, 1984.
18. Morrison WA. Thumb reconstruction: a review and philosophy of management. J Hand Surg Br 17:383-390, 1992.
19. Lister GD, Kalisman M, Tsai TM. Reconstruction of the hand with free microneurovascular toe-to-hand transfer: experience with 54 toe transfers. Plast Reconstr Surg 71:372-386, 1983.

# 76. Soft Tissue Coverage of the Hand and Upper Extremity

**Sam Fuller, Grant M. Kleiber**

## GENERAL CONCEPTS

### Secondary Healing

- **Indications**
  - Small fingertip wounds
    - Excellent cosmetic and functional result
- **Contraindications**
  - Exposed bone in wound
  - Wounds greater than 1 $cm^2$
  - More proximal wounds (may result in hook-nail deformity)

### Skin Grafts

- **Indications**
  - Defects with a well-vascularized wound bed
    - Volar or dorsal aspect
  - Surgically created defects (usually donor site from a local flap)
- **Contraindications**
  - Exposed bone or tendon without periosteum or paratenon
  - Wounds crossing flexion creases (may lead to flexion contracture)
- **Types of grafts**
  - Split-thickness: Epidermis and partial-thickness dermis
    - May be harvested from anywhere, typically taken from areas of thick dermis and low sensitivity
    - Higher rate of secondary contraction
  - Full-thickness
    - Harvested from area of redundant skin: Groin, supraclavicular area, upper arm
    - More primary contraction (graft shrinking after harvest) but less secondary contraction
  - Glabrous: For palmar defects
    - Harvested from hypothenar skin or sole of foot

**TIP:** Split-thickness skin grafts, if necessary, should be placed as sheet grafts rather than as meshed grafts to achieve better cosmesis and less secondary contraction.

- Glabrous grafts will slough their thick stratum corneum after 1-2 weeks. This will regrow.

## LOCAL COVERAGE OF THE FINGERS AND HAND[1]

### LOCAL FLAPS FOR FINGER RECONSTRUCTION

- **Covered in depth in Chapter 67**
- **Revision amputation**
  - Indications: Acute fingertip amputation, failed replantation
  - Exposed bone shortened; rough portions removed with rongeur
  - Soft tissue closed over bone
  - Advantages
    - Easy to perform in emergency department in acute setting
    - Usually good functional and cosmetic result
  - Disadvantages
    - Flexor digitorum profundus (FDP) tendon adhesions may lead to *quadriga effect.*
    - Many patients experience hypersensitivity in fingertip.
- **Atasoy-Kleinert flap**
  - Volar V-Y flap
  - Sensation and soft tissue pulp preserved
  - Best for dorsal-oblique fingertip amputations

**TIP:** The tissue plane is just above the periosteum.

**TIP:** If in OR, use glove with hole cut out of finger as digit tourniquet.

- **Kutler flaps**
  - Bilateral lateral-based V-Y flaps
  - Neurovascular bundles preserved to flaps
  - Flaps mobilized and brought together in midline of defect

**TIP:** These are good for defects 1-1.5 cm in size.

- **Homodigital island flap**
  - Indications: Fingertip wound requiring flap coverage, no gross contamination
  - Contraindications: Injury to either digital artery of affected digit
    - Requires two patent digital vessels to digit, because one will be sacrificed to supply the flap
    - Allows advancement of flap
  - Flap designed proximal to defect (either V-Y design or step-cut design)
    - Based on single digital vessel
    - Sensation to flap preserved
  - Neurovascular bundle dissected proximally into palm to bifurcation of common digital vessels
  - Flap advanced into defect; may require finger flexion
    - May be advanced up to 2 cm with finger flexion
- **Thenar/hypothenar flap**
  - Indications: Fingertip wounds with exposed bone or tendon, requiring flap closure
  - Contraindications: Elderly patients, arthritic patients, noncompliant patients
  - Two-stage flap raised from either thenar or hypothenar eminence
    - Flap divided at 10-14 days
    - Donor site closed primarily or with local tissue rearrangement
  - May result in finger stiffness because it requires 2 weeks of immobilization

- **Cross-finger flap**
  - Indications: Defects of fingertip or volar surface of finger, defects of thumb tip
    - Defect usually has exposed bone or tendon and would not support a skin graft
  - Contraindications: Elderly patients, arthritic patients, noncompliant patients
  - Flap designed on dorsum of middle phalanx on adjacent digit
  - Flap is based on its closest border to the defect and left attached as pedicle
  - Elevated as full-thickness skin with paratenon left intact on flap donor site
  - Flap turned over and sutured to volar defect
  - Donor site closed with skin graft
  - Flap divided at 8-14 days
  - Disadvantages: Insensate, cold intolerance, stiffness may result (especially in elderly)
- **Reverse cross-finger flap**
  - Indications: Defects of dorsal finger that would not support a skin graft
  - Contraindications: Same as cross-finger flap
  - Flap designed on dorsum of middle phalanx on adjacent digit, similar to cross-finger flap
  - Flap raised with dermis and fat only (epidermis is deepithelialized)
    - Paratenon left on donor site so it may be covered with skin graft
  - Flap flipped onto donor site, deepithelialized dermal side facing down
  - Flap and donor site skin grafted
  - Flap divided at 8-14 days

## Local Flaps for Thumb Reconstruction

- **Moberg volar advancement flap**
  - Indications: Defects of volar distal thumb (generally up to 1.5 cm in size)
  - Contraindications: Injury to princeps pollicis artery (dorsal blood supply to thumb)
  - Flap raised, including both neurovascular bundles just over flexor sheath
  - Flap advanced as thumb interphalangeal (IP) joint flexed, sutured into place
    - Additional advancement possible by dividing skin of thumb at metacarpophalangeal (MP) crease
    - Neurovascular bundles preserved, defect grafted
  - Moberg flap only possible in **thumb,** because it is the only digit with an additional dorsal blood supply
  - Thumb typically has flexion contracture at IP joint, which resolves with time and therapy.

**TIP:** Extension into the thenar eminence adds length to the flap.

- **First dorsal metacarpal artery flap**
  - Indications: Defects of thumb tip, thumb dorsum, volar thumb, degloving injuries, first web space defects
  - First dorsal metacarpal artery is reliably present with adequate venae comitantes and cutaneous nerves.
    - Direct branch of radial artery
  - Most commonly based proximally but may also be distally based
  - Proximally based flap usually designed on dorsum of proximal phalanx of index finger
    - Incision extended proximally to facilitate pedicle dissection
    - Dorsal metacarpal artery dissected proximal to bifurcation
  - Sensory branches of radial nerve may be dissected along with pedicle for innervated flap.
  - Donor site skin grafted

- **Neurovascular island flap (Littler flap)**
  - Indications: Defects of thumb tip requiring innervated coverage
    - Innervation of thumb tip vital for normal tactile pinch
  - Contraindications: Injury to EITHER digital artery to the long finger or ulnar digital artery to ring finger
    - Radial digital artery to ring finger ligated to allow adequate pedicle mobilization
  - Flap harvested from ulnar side of long finger
    - Neurovascular bundle harvested with flap, dissected proximal to bifurcation into palm
  - Flap tunneled into defect
  - Donor site skin grafted
  - Advantages
    - Provides innervated tissue on tip of thumb for tactile feedback
    - Ulnar long finger donor site less vital for tactile feedback during grip and pinch than on radial side

### LOCAL FLAPS FOR HAND RECONSTRUCTION

- **Distally based dorsal hand flap (Quaba flap)**[2]
  - Indications: Smaller dorsal hand defects <2 cm diameter, web space defects, dorsal proximal phalanx defects
  - Flap based on recurrent cutaneous branch of dorsal metacarpal artery
    - Perforators located between metacarpals 5-10 mm proximal to MP joints
    - Vessels diminish in caliber moving radial to ulnar
  - Flap rotated into defect in propeller transposition fashion
    - Donor site can be closed primarily up to 2.5 cm
    - Larger flaps require skin graft to donor site
- **Kite flap**
  - Indications: Distal dorsal hand defects, first web space
  - Variant of the first dorsal metacarpal artery flap, includes rhomboid flap to close donor defect
  - Flap designed as proximally based transposition flap on first dorsal metacarpal artery
    - Donor site closed with modified rhomboid flap
  - Ideal for first web space deepening or coverage of base of thumb

## LOCAL HAND, WRIST, AND FOREARM COVERAGE

### RADIAL FOREARM FLAP

- **Indications**
  - Small and large defects almost anywhere on the hand
    - Volar or dorsal aspect
- **Contraindications**
  - Abnormal Allen's test
  - Injury to radial artery
    - Up to **15%** of patients do not have a complete palmar arch
  - Cosmetically unacceptable donor site scar
- **Flap variations**
  - Can be free or pedicled
  - Can include skin and/or fascia
  - Can include sensory nerves to preserve innervation

- Can include distal radius bone
- Can include palmaris longus and/or flexor carpi radialis (FCR) tendon for reconstruction

■ **Anatomy**
- Radial artery and venae comitantes lie in intermuscular septum between FCR and brachioradialis.
- Preserve nerve fibers from radial nerve and median nerve.
- May approach ulnarly or radially, making sure to preserve pedicle within septum.
- Venous drainage of flap
  - ▸ Venae comitantes (often small)
  - ▸ Can incorporate cephalic vein and/or basilic vein for larger free flap to ensure sufficient venous drainage

**TIP:** Perform an Allen's test preoperatively to confirm satisfactory ulnar artery perfusion of the entire hand.

- Place a pulse oximeter on the thumb and visualize return of the pulse while the radial artery is compressed and the ulnar artery is released.
- Map the course of cephalic vein and radial artery before making the incision to incorporate these into the flap design.
- A tourniquet may facilitate dissection.
- Leave the skin graft unmeshed to improve the donor site appearance.
- Splint the wrist postoperatively to aid with skin graft adherence and healing.
- The radial artery can be reconstructed (ideally with a nearby cephalic vein graft) if hand perfusion becomes a concern.
- After the radial artery is palpated distally, a line can be drawn to the middle of the antecubital fossa to mark the approximate path of the radial artery.

## Reverse Radial Artery Forearm Flap

■ **Based on retrograde flow of radial artery**
- Large skin paddle can be used (nearly entire volar forearm skin).
  - ▸ Use template to ensure that the flap is able to rotate into defect.
  - ▸ Use pencil Doppler device to locate and include perforators from radial artery in flap design.
- Design flap using template based on a pivot point approximately at the radial styloid.

**TIP:** Most perforators are located in the distal or proximal forearm. The central portion of the forearm has a paucity of perforators.

- For subfascial elevation, incise and elevate antebrachial fascia with skin paddle.
- For suprafascial elevation, raise flap above antebrachial fascia medially and laterally, then incise fascia at brachioradialis and FCR tendons to protect pedicle.
- Attempt to preserve neurosensory fibers when possible.
- Close donor defect partially and use skin to graft remaining portion.
  - ▸ Full-thickness skin graft (FTSG) may have better cosmesis.
  - ▸ Defects smaller than 5-6 cm in width may be closed primarily.

## POSTERIOR INTEROSSEOUS FLAP[3,4] (Fig. 76-1)

- Based on posterior interosseous artery (PIA), a branch of ulnar artery
- **Indications**
  - Now generally used for proximal dorsal hand defects: (i.e., first web space injuries, metacarpophalangeal [MP] joints)
  - Other flaps contraindicated
- **Advantage**
  - No major arteries sacrificed
- **Contraindications**
  - Risk of PIA thrombosis if significant wrist or forearm injury (avoid if near zone of injury)
  - Questionable viability
  - Risk of injury to posterior interosseous nerve
- **Technical tips**
  - A line is marked from distal radioulnar joint (DRU joint) to lateral epicondyle with elbow completely flexed.
    - ▸ Skin paddle may be up to 6-7 cm wide.
  - PIA courses between extensor carpi ulnaris (ECU) and extensor digiti minimi (EDM) tendons, giving off perforators.
  - PIA arises dorsally deep to anconeus from the interosseous membrane, approximately 5-6 cm distal to lateral epicondyle, just below supinator.
  - Pivot point for flap is 2 cm proximal to ulnar styloid.
  - Raise radial margin of flap, and extend it to distal DRU joint.
  - Incise fascia over extensor digiti minimi 5 mm radial to thick fascial septum.
  - Divide muscular branches.

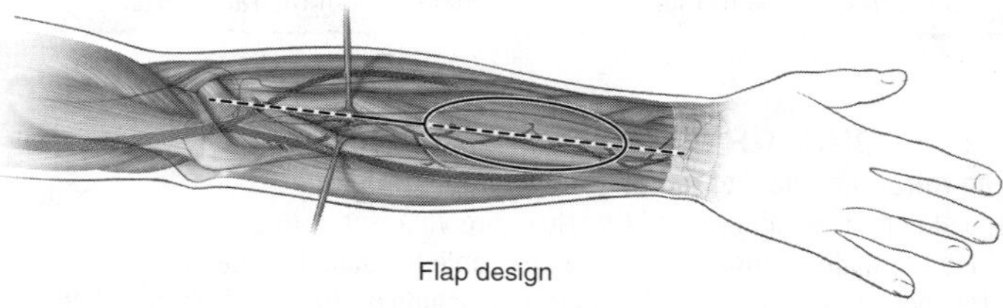

Flap design

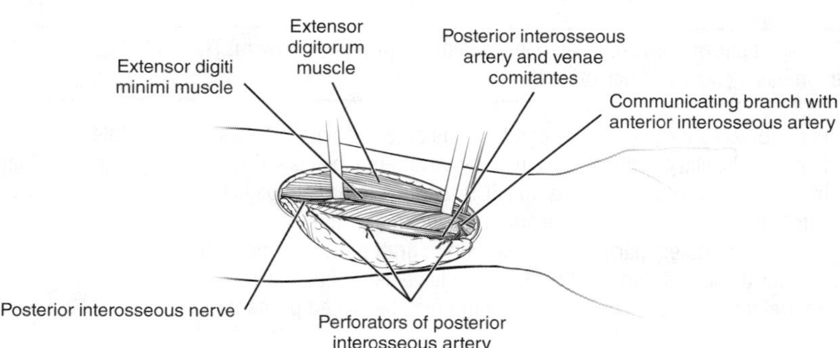


Approach to PIA

**Fig. 76-1** Bony landmarks and locations of skin paddle for the posterior interosseous artery flap.

**TIP:** There is a risk of partial flap loss if it is used to cover more distal flaps (proximal interphalangeal [PIP] joint).

### Reverse Ulnar Artery Forearm Flap

- **Indication**
  - Elbow defects
- **Disadvantages**
  - Dominant blood supply to the hand commonly from ulnar artery
  - Risk of ulnar nerve injury
- **Technical tips**
  - Ulnar nerve is deep to artery.
  - Vessels can be found between flexor carpi ulnaris (FCU) and flexor digitorum superficialis (FDS).

## LOCAL ELBOW COVERAGE

- Evaluate defect and what is needed for reconstruction.
  - **Consider what is exposed (i.e., joint, nerve, bone).**

## SMALL ELBOW DEFECTS

### Flexor Carpi Ulnaris Flap

- **Indication**
  - Small anterior elbow defects (muscle belly on average is 5 cm wide and 20 cm long)
- **Advantages**
  - Can be myocutaneous or muscle only
  - Better overall cosmesis than radial forearm flap
  - Excellent for elderly patients with thin skin and large dorsal defects (skin cancer or chemotherapy/chemical burns)
- **Disadvantages**
  - Major wrist flexor and ulnar deviator
  - Difficult to rotate and cover posterior defects
  - Adjacent ulnar nerve is at risk for injury.
- **Technical tips**
  - Blood supply based on posterior ulnar recurrent artery
  - Vascular branch can be found near bicipital tuberosity of the radius. It enters FCU roughly 6 cm distal to medial epicondyle.
  - Skin paddle up to 6 by 10 cm can be included.

**TIP:** Skin grafting over a rotated FCU may improve elbow contour, compared with a skin paddle.

## Brachioradialis Flap

- **Indication**
  - Small anterolateral or posterolateral elbow defects
- **Advantages**
  - Minimal donor site morbidity or functional loss
  - Muscular or myocutaneous flap
- **Disadvantages**
  - Should be preserved in absence of other elbow flexors
  - Donor site of skin paddle is disfiguring.
- **Technical tips**
  - Blood supply based on branch of radial recurrent artery (average pedicle length 3 cm, 1 mm diameter)
  - Branch to brachioradialis is near origin of radial recurrent artery.
  - Skin paddle of up to 6 by 10 cm can be included.

**TIP:** Locate and preserve sensory nerves during the flap harvest.

**TIP:** Though the tendon does not contour to fill defects, include it in flap transfers to aid in flap insetting and suturing to surrounding tissue. (Tendon holds suture better than muscle fibers.)

## Reverse Lateral Arm Flap (Fig. 76-2)

- **Indication**
  - Posterior elbow defects
- **Contraindications**
  - Overweight patients: Flap can be excessively bulky
  - Epicondylitis or other inflammatory elbow disease
- **Advantage**
  - Donor site in same operative field as defect
- **Disadvantage**
  - Arc of rotation may not allow complete coverage of defect.
- **Technical tips**
  - Blood supply: Radial recurrent artery when based distally
  - Include skin over lateral epicondyle to better preserve vascular network to distally based flap.
  - Often requires skin graft for closure of donor site.

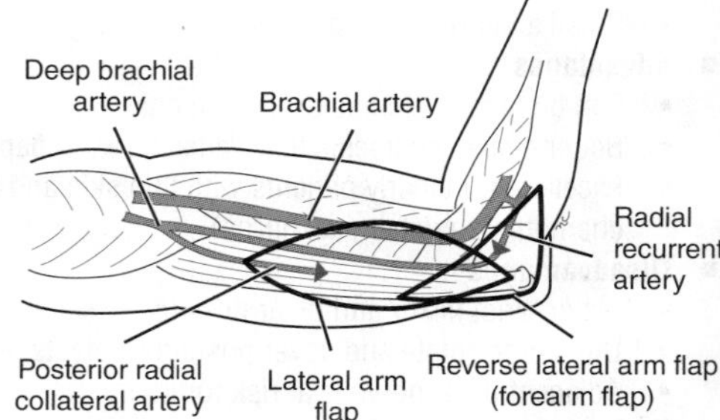


**Fig. 76-2** Reverse lateral arm flap (forearm flap) and lateral arm flap.

**TIP:** Use template to ensure that rotation will allow inset over the defect.

## DISTANT FLAPS: PEDICLED

**TIP:** Except for the epigastric and abdominal flaps (true random flaps), all can be used as free tissue transfers.

### Groin Flap

- Flap is less commonly used today
- **Indication**
  - Large amount of soft tissue coverage needed without better donor site options
- **Advantage**
  - Cosmetically appealing donor scar
- **Disadvantage**
  - Requires joint positioning and prolonged immobilization
- **Anatomy**
  - Blood supply based on superficial circumflex iliac artery
  - Run approximately 1-2 cm inferior to inguinal ligament
  - Can design flap based on coverage needed

## DISTANT FLAPS: FREE TISSUE TRANSFER[5,6]

### Lateral Arm Flap (see Fig. 76-2)

- **Indication**
  - Volar or dorsal hand defects
- **Contraindication**
  - Previous elbow trauma or surgical procedures
- **Advantages**
  - Bone can be taken with flap
  - Can be as large as 8 by 15 cm
  - Out of zone of injury, but may keep surgical sites on same field/extremity
- **Disadvantage**
  - Hypersensitivity of donor site, prolonged elbow pain, numbness in the forearm, and excessive flap bulk
- **Technical tips**
  - Blood supply based on posterior radial collateral artery (PRCA) when based proximally
  - Center flap over lateral intermuscular septum.

**TIP:** The midpoint of the flap (intermuscular septum) is created by drawing a line from the lateral epicondyle to the insertion point of the deltoid.

**TIP:** Doppler ultrasonography helps to confirm vessel location. Preserve the paratenon on the base of the wound to ensure skin graft take at the donor site.

## OTHER FREE TISSUE TRANSFER OPTIONS

### Anterolateral Thigh Flap

- Offers abundant and pliable tissue for small and large surface areas
- Acceptable donor site morbidity
- Based on lateral femoral circumflex vessels

### Omental Flap

- Based on gastroduodenal vessels
- Offers abundant and pliable tissue for larger surface area coverage
- Skin graft over omentum
- Useful in severe vascular compromise (increases vascularity to hand)
- Disadvantage: Intraabdominal dissection

### Gracilis Muscle Flap

- Based on medial femoral circumflex system
- Minimal donor site morbidity but short pedicle length (usually 6 cm)
- Good for very lengthy arm defects and for limb salvage
- Can be used for free functional tissue transfer (obturator nerve)

### Temporoparietal Fascia Flap

- Well-vascularized, blood supply based on superficial temporal artery and vein
- Thin, may close donor site primarily

### Dorsalis Pedis Flap

- Based on dorsalis pedis artery (underlying extensor tendon can be included with flap harvest)
- Problems with healing of donor site

### Serratus Anterior Flap

- Blood supply based on thoracodorsal artery and lateral thoracic artery
- Able to fit muscle fibers over different defects on digits

### Latissimus Dorsi Flap

- Based on thoracodorsal artery
- Used to cover large defects
- Skin graft rather than skin paddle will make flap less bulky.

### Scapular/Parascapular Flaps

- Can be based on angular branch of thoracodorsal artery or circumflex scapular arterial systems
- Lateral border of scapula may be harvested if bone needed
- Donor site usually closed primarily
- Often very bulky

## Key Points

- ✓ Adequate debridement, fracture stabilization, and revascularization should be achieved before soft tissue coverage is performed.
- ✓ Each patient's preoperative function, job status, and psychological assessment are critical in managing expectations, establishing rehabilitation goals, and assuring adherence to postoperative care.

## References


1. Lemmon JA, Janis JE, Rohrich RJ. Soft-tissue injuries of the fingertip: methods of evaluation and treatment. An algorithmic approach. Plast Reconstr Surg 122:105e-117e, 2008.
2. Quaba AA, Davison PM. The distally based dorsal hand flap. Br J Plast Surg 43:28-39, 1990.
3. Rayan GM. First dorsal metacarpal artery flap. In Rayan GM, Chung KC, eds. Flap Reconstruction of the Upper Extremity. Chicago, IL: American Society for Surgery of the Hand, 2011.
4. Gilbert A, ed. Pedicle Flaps of the Upper Limb: Vascular Anatomy, Surgical Technique, and Current Indications. Philadelphia: Lippincott Williams & Wilkins, 1992.
5. Netscher DT, Schneider A. Homodigital and heterodigital island pedicle flaps. In Rayan GM, Chung KC, eds. Flap Reconstruction of the Upper Extremity. Chicago, IL: American Society for Surgery of the Hand, 2011.
6. Buntic RF. Microsurgery Atlas, Techniques and Principles. Available at: *http://www.microsurgeon.org.*

# 77. Compartment Syndrome

Alison M. Shore, Benjamin T. Lemelman

## DEFINITION

- **Acute Compartment Syndrome (ACS)** is a limb-threatening condition in which increased pressure within a closed space (compartment) compromises nutrient blood flow to muscles and nerves.[1]
  - Occurs when **tissue pressure exceeds perfusion pressure**
  - Results in tissue ischemia
- Untreated compartment syndrome leads to tissue necrosis, permanent functional impairment, and if severe, renal failure and death.

## DEMOGRAPHICS

- ACS can occur in any anatomic compartment: hand, forearm, upper arm, buttock, abdomen, and entire lower extremity (thigh, leg, foot).

### INCIDENCE[2-6]

- Anterior lower extremity (secondary to frequency of injury) is most common.
- Ranges of 2%-12% have been published.
- 30% of limbs develop compartment syndrome after vascular injury; however, this is not well documented.
- McQueen et al[3] retrospectively studied 164 patients diagnosed with compartment syndrome: 69% were associated with a fracture, half of which were the tibia.
- The most commonly affected leg compartments are the **anterior compartment,** followed by the **deep posterior compartment** (Masquelet).[6]
- In the forearm, ACS most commonly affects the **deepest compartment muscles** (flexor pollicis longus and flexor digitorum profundus) because of their proximity to bone.

### SEX

- Affects **males** more than females, which likely represents selection bias, because men are more often patients with traumatic injuries.

## CAUSES

- ACS results from either an increase in volume of compartment contents or a reduction in the volume or expansion capacity of a compartment.
- Specific causes are listed in Box 77-1.[7,8]

**Box 77-1** *CAUSES OF COMPARTMENT SYNDROME*

| Increased Compartment Volume | Reduced Compartment Volume |
|---|---|
| Fractures/dislocations* | Burns (e.g., circumferential) causing constriction |
| Ischemia-reperfusion injury (e.g., vascular injury) | Tight dressings/casts |
| Soft tissue (e.g., crush) injury | Prolonged limb positioning (e.g., in paralytics, during surgery)[7,8] |
| Hemorrhage | |
| Strenuous muscle use (e.g., exercise, seizures, tetany) | |
| Envenomation | |
| Burns (e.g., electrical) causing edema | |
| Postviral rhabdomyolysis | |

*Most common cause.

## PATHOPHYSIOLOGY[2,3,9-11]

- ACS follows the path of ischemic injury.
  - "Container" pressure rises as more fluid is introduced into a fixed volume, and various fascial compartments have relatively fixed volumes.
  - Excess fluid or extraneous constriction increases pressure and decreases tissue perfusion until no oxygen is available for cellular metabolism.
  - Elevated perfusion pressure is the physiologic response to rising intracompartmental pressure (ICP).
  - As ICP rises, compensatory mechanisms are overwhelmed, and a cascade of injury occurs.
- **Tissue perfusion** is determined by measuring **capillary perfusion pressure (CPP) minus the interstitial fluid pressure.**
- Normal cellular metabolism requires oxygen tension of **5-7 mm Hg.**
  - This tension is easily maintained when the CPP averages 25 mm Hg and the interstitial pressure averages 4-6 mm Hg.
  - In ACS, rising interstitial pressure overwhelms perfusion pressure.
- As ICP rises, venous pressure rises, and when venous pressure is higher than CPP, capillaries collapse.
  - The pressure at which collapse occurs is debated; however, **ICP >30 mm Hg requires intervention.** At this pressure, blood flow through the capillaries stops.
- Hypoxia causes tissues to undergo anaerobic metabolism.
  - Lactic acid accumulates, and with continued hypoxia, energy requirements are not met.
  - The ATP-dependent $Na^+/K^+$ pump fails, and the cellular membrane is unable to maintain the osmolar gradient.
  - The resulting edema causes more ischemia as pressure rises, and a self-perpetuating cycle leads to compartment syndrome.

- Continued compression of nutrient capillaries exacerbates anoxia, which induces lipid peroxidation of the cell membrane, stimulates the inflammatory cascade, activates neutrophils, and generates hypoxanthine (a product of ATP breakdown that forms the oxygen free radical superoxide).
- The process eventually results in permanent damage, and the "no-reflow" phenomenon occurs. (Reversal and correction of existing metabolic and structural deficits are not possible even if flow is reestablished.)

■ Reperfusion of an ischemic compartment brings an abundant supply of oxygen that reacts with hypoxanthine to produce superoxide.
  - Iron from red blood cells reacts with hydrogen peroxide to form the highly toxic hydroxyl radical and other free radicals that potentiate the insult to the already damaged cell membranes.
  - These radicals also promote platelet aggregation and microvascular clotting, resulting in renewed ischemia.

## INDICATIONS/PATIENT SELECTION

Diagnosis is usually made by history and physical examination and confirmed with measurement of ICP.

### History

- **Suspect ACS whenever there is disproportionate or significant pain in an extremity after injury, either at rest or with passive stretch.**
- Ask about mechanism of injury (high- vs. low-energy).
- Identify medical comborbidities (i.e., anticoagulation).
- **Classic features: The six Ps:**
  - **P**ain
  - **P**allor
  - **P**oikilothermia (coldness)
  - **P**ressure
  - **P**aralysis/paresthesias (sensory nerves affected first, followed by motor nerves)
  - **P**ulselessness
- **Each symptom on its own is a poor indicator of ACS.** However, the likelihood of ACS increases when more than one feature is present (two: 68%; three: 93%; four: 98%).[12]

### Maintain Suspicion

- High-velocity injuries
- Long-bone fractures
- High-energy trauma
- Penetrating injuries (e.g., gunshot wounds, stabbings) may cause arterial injury that can quickly lead to ACS.
- Venous injuries may cause compartment syndrome, but do not be misled by palpable pulses.
- Crush injuries
- Anticoagulation therapy: Compartment syndrome requiring fasciotomy has occurred after simple venipuncture in patients undergoing anticoagulation therapy.
- Intense physical activity (e.g., in soldiers and athletes without trauma)
- Children: Delay in diagnosis because of communication difficulties[13]

## Physical Examination

- Perform serial examinations to detect progression to a more severe clinical state and initiate timely intervention.

**TIP:** Always compare the affected limb with the unaffected limb.

- **Pain with passive stretch is one of the earliest and most sensitive indicators of ACS.**
- Paresthesia indicates early nerve ischemia.
- Paralysis is a late finding that indicates both nerve and muscular dysfunction.

**CAUTION: Pulselessness is a late sign. (Too late!)**

# PREOPERATIVE WORKUP

## Laboratory Studies

- Less helpful in the **diagnosis** of ACS
- Chemistries: Elevated potassium and creatinine levels
- Complete blood count (can see decreased m/m from hemorrhage)
- Elevated creatine phosphokinase (CPK) and urine myoglobin: Indicate rhabdomylosis
- Elevated serum myoglobin
- Positive result to urine toxicology screen
- Urinalysis: Positive for blood but negative for RBCs (indicates myoglobinuria)
- Prothrombin time (PT) and activated partial thromboplastin time (aPTT)

## Imaging Studies

- **Plain radiographs** of affected extremity (look for fracture)
- **Ultrasonography** to evaluate arterial flow and presence of deep venous thrombosis (DVT)

**NOTE: Ultrasound is not helpful for the diagnosis of compartment syndrome; however, it aids in the elimination of differential diagnosis.**

## Compartment Pressure Measurement

- Normal ICP is <10 mm Hg.
- **In general, decompression is recommended for ICP >30 mm Hg.**

**TIP:** Some argue than the differential between ICP and diastolic blood pressure (Δp 30-45 mm Hg) is more accurate.[14]

- Various products are commercially available for direct pressure measurements through ACE Medical Equipment, Inc. (Clearwater, FL) and Stryker (Kalamazoo, MI).
- Other noninvasive imaging techniques to determine ICP include near-infrared spectroscopy (NIRS) and laser Doppler flowmetry. However, their benefit is unclear.[15]
- McQueen et al[3] recommend ICP measurements for:
  - Tibial diaphysis fracture.
  - High-energy injuries to forearm diaphysis or distal radius.
  - High-energy fractures of the tibial metaphysis.
  - Young men with injury to the soft tissues or those with bleeding diathesis.

**NOTE: Try to get ICP measurement within 5 cm of fracture site for most accurate pressure diagnosis.**

## …EATMENT

Many cases of compartment syndrome result from trauma. Follow advanced trauma life support (ATLS) guidelines to stabilize patient before attempting to treat compartment syndrome.

### PRINCIPLES

- **Early intervention is critical.**
  - The most important determinant of a poor outcome from ACS is *delay in diagnosis* (McQueen et al).[3]
  - Irreversible tissue injury and muscle necrosis *may start as early as 3 hours after the onset of compartment syndrome.*[1] **Six hours is the upper limit of muscle viability.**[9]
- **Surgical decompression (fasciotomy)** remains the definitive therapy for compartment syndrome.
  - **Goals**
    - To achieve expedient, complete opening of all tight fascial envelopes
    - In the case of fracture, perform decompression without or with limited fracture fragment exposure.
  - Consider **prophylactic fasciotomies** in high-risk patients (e.g., those undergoing limb reperfusion following prolonged ischemia times).
- **Envenomation**
  - Myonecrosis likely results primarily from direct venom toxicity rather than from compartment syndrome.
    - Fasciotomies may **not** help prevent myonecrosis; however, they should still be performed if compartment pressure is elevated (Fig. 77-1 through Fig. 77-8).[16,17]
  - Should treat with antivenin and IV antibiotics.

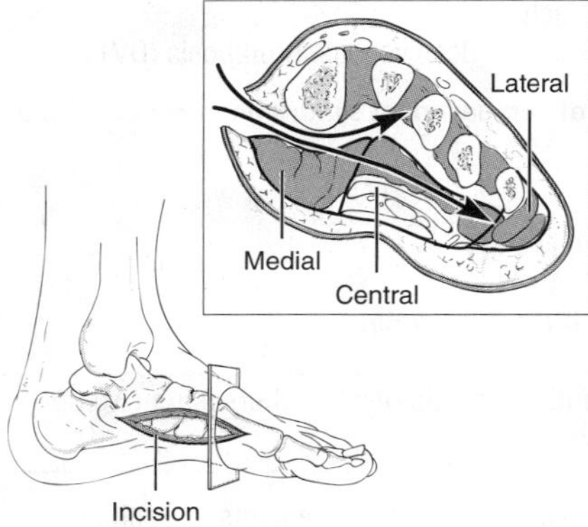


**Fig. 77-1** Foot fasciotomy by medial incision. To decompress the four compartments of the foot using a medial approach, an incision is made along the plantar border of the first metatarsal, allowing access to all four compartments. The incision can be extended proximally if the posterior tibial neurovascular bundle requires decompression as well.

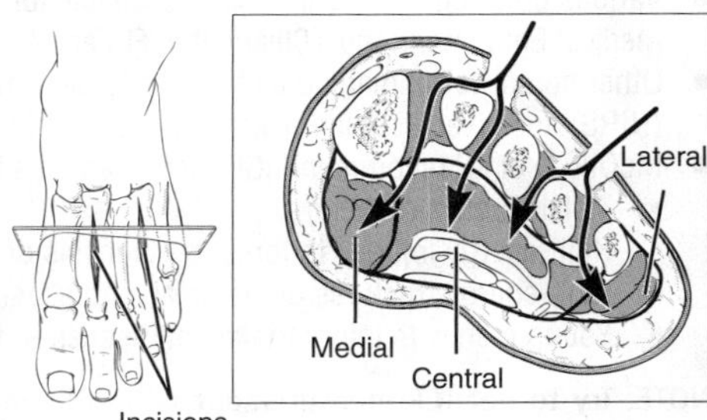


**Fig. 77-2** Foot fasciotomy by dorsal incision. The dorsal approach to compartment decompression is performed along the second and fourth interspaces.

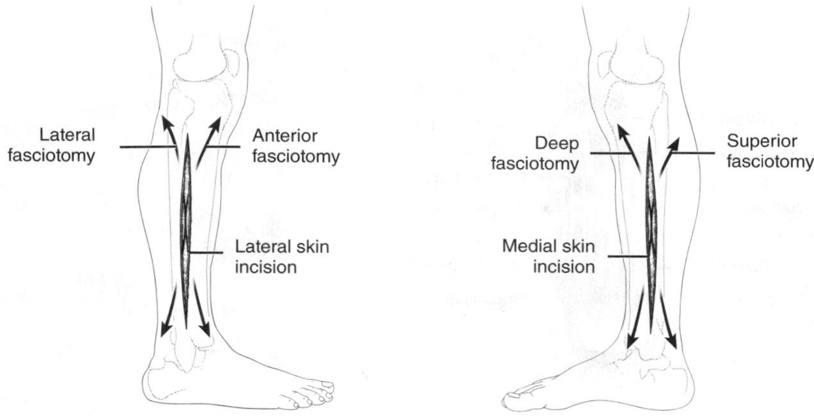


**Fig. 77-3** Leg fasciotomy. Lateral and medial leg incisions for a four-compartment fasciotomy. The lateral and anterior compartments are decompressed through a lateral incision and the superficial and deep posterior compartments through a medial incision.

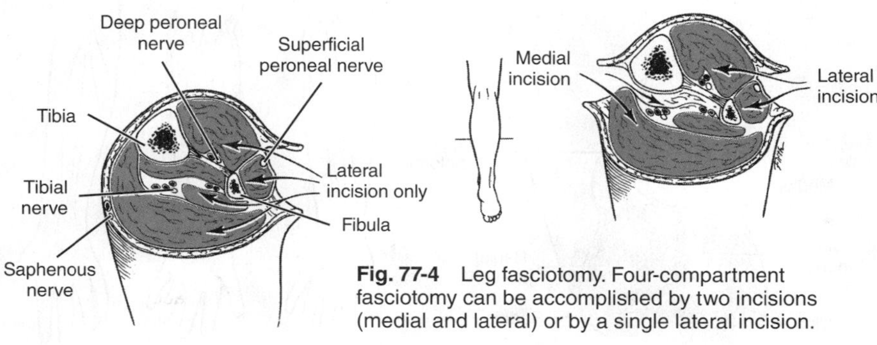


**Fig. 77-4** Leg fasciotomy. Four-compartment fasciotomy can be accomplished by two incisions (medial and lateral) or by a single lateral incision.

**Fig. 77-5** Thigh fasciotomies. The anterior and posterior compartments can be decompressed using a lateral incision, and the medial compartment is decompressed through a medial incision.

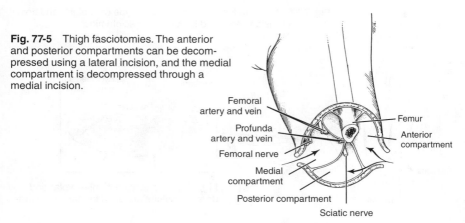

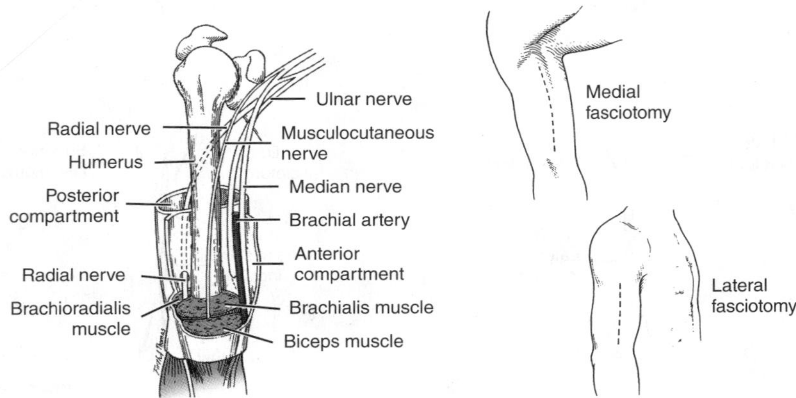


**Fig. 77-6** Arm fasciotomies. The anterior compartment is decompressed using a medial incision, and the posterior compartment is decompressed through a lateral incision. The ulnar and radial nerves travel in both compartments; therefore increased pressure in either produces symptoms along the distribution of both nerves.

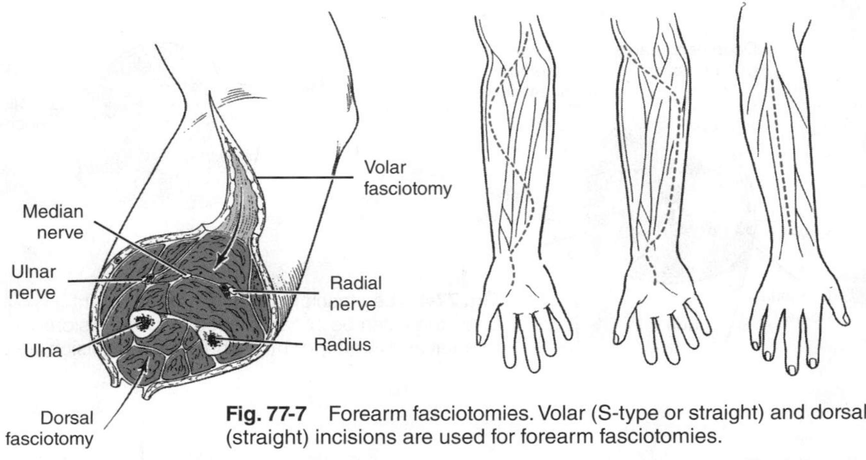


**Fig. 77-7** Forearm fasciotomies. Volar (S-type or straight) and dorsal (straight) incisions are used for forearm fasciotomies.

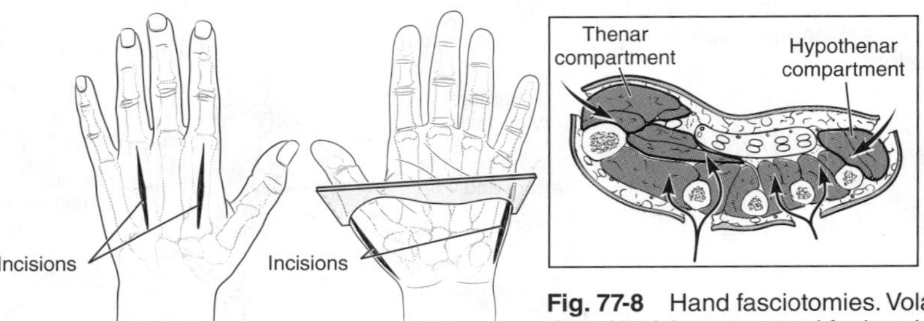


**Fig. 77-8** Hand fasciotomies. Volar and dorsal incisions are used for hand compartment releases.

## POSTOPERATIVE CARE

- **Supportive care**
  - Pain control
  - Wet-to-dry dressings
- **Wound closure (Ojike)**[18]
  - Rarely done primarily
  - Most have delayed primary closure (59%), followed by skin grafts (26%).[18]
  - Adjuncts to expedite wound edge approximation include vacuum-assisted closure devices and shoelace suturing techniques.[15]
- **Treatment of rhabdomyolysis**
  - A urine output goal should be **1-2 ml/kg/hr** to prevent accumulation of myoglobin and subsequent renal dysfunction.[15]
  - Mannitol has been shown to help treat rhabdomyolysis, and may also directly treat ACS. Further investigation is warranted.[19]

## COMPLICATIONS

Most are improved or prevented with expedient diagnosis and treatment; however, if the diagnosis is missed and fasciotomy is delayed or not performed, the following may result:

- **Volkmann's contracture:** Myonecrosis and secondary contracture after prolonged muscle ischemia[20]
  - Late contracture in upper extremity injuries often results in fibrosis of flexor muscles.
  - First step in management of known contracture is **occupational therapy.**
- Limb loss
- Permanent nerve damage
- Renal failure
- Death
- Scarring, cosmetic deformity from fasciotomies

## OUTCOMES

- Outcome depends on both the diagnosis and the time from injury to intervention.
  - Rorabeck and Macnab[10] reported almost complete recovery of limb function if fasciotomy was performed **within 6 hours.**
  - Matsen et al[9] found necrosis **after 6 hours** of ischemia, which currently is the accepted upper limit of viability.
- The prognosis is excellent to poor, depending **on how quickly compartment syndrome is treated** and whether complications develop.
- Fitzgerald et al[21] reported the results of a retrospective study over an 8-year period of patients requiring fasciotomies of either upper or lower limbs. Results for long-term morbidity are as follows:
  - Pain (10%)
  - Altered sensation within margins of wound (77%)
  - Dry, scaly skin (40%)
  - Pruritis (33%)
  - Discolored wounds (30%)

- Swollen limbs (25%)
- Tethered scars (26%)
- Recurrent ulceration (13%)
- Muscle herniation (13%)
- Tethered tendon (7%)

## Key Points

- ✓ ACS results from either a decrease in volume capacity of a myofascial compartment or an increase in the volume of its contents.
- ✓ Pain that is disproportionate to injury and pain with passive stretch are the earliest and most sensitive indicators of ACS. (Pulselessness is a late finding—too late!)
- ✓ In general, decompression is recommended for ICP >30 mm Hg.
- ✓ Early intervention is critical. The prognosis for limb function is best if fasciotomy is performed within 6 hours of injury.
- ✓ Maintain a high level of suspicion for rhabdomyolysis and treat accordingly.
- ✓ "Missed" compartment syndrome leads to Volkmann's contracture.

## References


1. Vaillancourt C, Shrier I, Vandal A, et al. Acute compartment syndrome: how long before muscle necrosis occurs? CJEM 6:147-154, 2004.
2. Velmahos GC, Toutouzas KG. Vascular trauma and compartment syndrome. Surg Clin North Am 82:125-141, 2002.
3. McQueen MM, Gaston P, Court-Brown CM. Acute compartment syndrome. Who is at risk? J Bone Joint Surg Br 82:200-203, 2000.
4. McQueen MM, Court-Brown CM. Compartment monitoring in tibial fractures. The pressure threshold for decompression. J Bone Joint Surg Br 78:99-104, 1996.
5. Styf J, Wiger P. Abnormally increased intramuscular pressure in human legs: comparison of two experimental models. J Trauma 45:133-139, 1998.
6. Masquelet AC. Acute compartment syndrome of the leg: pressure measurement and fasciotomy. Orthop Traumatol Surg Res 96:913-917, 2010.
7. Kavouni A, Ion L. Bilateral well-leg compartment syndrome after supine position surgery. Ann Plast Surg 44:462-463, 2000.
8. Pollard RL, O'Broin E. Compartment syndrome following prolonged surgery for breast reconstruction with epidural analgesia. J Plast Reconstr Aesthet Surg 62:648-649, 2009.
9. Matsen FA III, Winquist RA, Krugmire RB Jr. Diagnosis and management of compartmental syndromes. J Bone Joint Surg Am 62:286-291, 1980.
10. Rorabeck CH, Macnab I. The pathophysiology of the anterior tibial compartmental syndrome. Clin Orthop Relat Res 113:52-57, 1975.
11. Seiler JG III, Casey PJ, Binford SH. Compartment syndromes of the upper extremity. J South Orthop Assoc 9:233-247, 2000.
12. Ulmer T. The clinical diagnosis of compartment syndrome of the lower leg: are clinical findings predictive of the disorder? J Orthop Trauma 16:572-577, 2002.
13. Erdös J, Dlaska C, Szatmary P, et al. Acute compartment syndrome in children: a case series in 24 patients and review of the literature. Int Orthop 35:569-575, 2011.

14. Whitesides TE, Haney TC, Morimoto K, et al. Tissue pressure measurements as a determinant for the need of fasciotomy. Clin Orthop Relat Res 113:43-51, 1975.
15. Mabvuure NT, Malahias M, Hindocha S, et al. Acute compartment syndrome of the limbs: current concepts and management. Open Orthop J 6:535-543, 2012.
16. Aston SJ, Beasley RW, Thorne CH, eds. Grabb and Smith's Plastic Surgery, 6th ed. Philadelphia: Lippincott Williams & Wilkins, 2006.
17. Velmahos GC, Toutouzas KG. Vascular trauma and compartment syndromes. Surg Clin North Am 82:125-141, 2002.
18. Ojike NI, Roberts CS, Giannoudis PV. Compartment syndrome of the thigh: a systematic review. Injury 41:133-136, 2010.
19. Better OS, Zinman C, Reis DN, et al. Hypertonic mannitol ameliorates intracompartmental tamponade in model compartment syndrome in the dog. Nephron 58:344-346, 1991.
20. Volkmann R. Die ischäemischen Muskellähmungen und Kontrakturen. Zentralbl Chir 8:801-803, 1881.
21. Fitzgerald AM, Gastron P, Wilson Y, et al. Long-term sequelae of fasciotomy wounds. Br J Plast Surg 53:690-693, 2000.

# 78. Upper Extremity Compression Syndromes

Prosper Benhaim, Edward M. Reece, Joshua A. Lemmon

## ANATOMY[1-6] (Table 78-1)

**Table 78-1** *Physiologic Anatomy of the Upper Extremity*

| Nerves | Motor | Sensory |
|---|---|---|
| Median nerve | Pronator teres<br>Pronator quadratus<br>Palmaris longus<br>Flexor carpi radialis<br>Flexor digitorum superficialis (×4)<br>Flexor digitorum profundus (×2) (index, middle)<br>Flexor pollicis longus<br>Index and middle finger lumbrical muscles<br>*Thenar muscles:*<br>Abductor pollicis brevis<br>Opponens pollicis<br>Superficial belly of flexor pollicis brevis | Volar part of the wrist, thumb, index, middle and radial side of ring finger extending to the dorsal DIP joint on all of them |
| Ulnar nerve | Flexor carpi ulnaris<br>Flexor digitorum profundus (×2) (ring, small)<br>Palmaris brevis<br>Dorsal interosseous muscles<br>Palmar interosseous muscles<br>Ring and small finger lumbrical muscles<br>Adductor pollicis<br>Deep belly of flexor pollicis brevis<br>*Hypothenar muscles:*<br>Abductor digiti minimi<br>Flexor digiti minimi brevis<br>Opponens digiti minimi | Dorsal and volar aspect of small finger, ulnar side of ring finger<br>Ulnar dorsal half of the hand |
| Radial nerve | Triceps<br>Anconeus<br>Brachioradialis<br>Supinator<br>Extensor carpi radialis brevis<br>Extensor carpi radialis longus<br>Extensor carpi ulnaris<br>Extensor digitorum communis<br>Extensor indicis proprius<br>Extensor digitorum minimi<br>Abductor pollicis longus<br>Extensor pollicis longus<br>Extensor pollicis brevis | Dorsal thumb, index, middle, and radial side of ring fingers up to PIP joints<br>Dorsal radial half of the hand<br>Dorsal wrist capsule (posterior interosseous branch) |

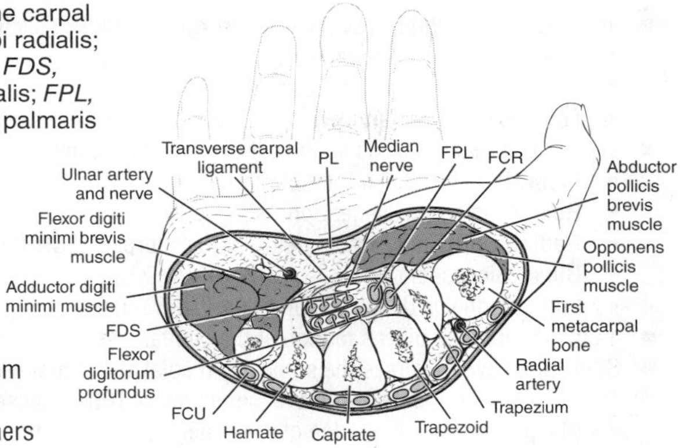

**Fig. 78-1** Anatomy of the carpal tunnel. (*FCR*, Flexor carpi radialis; *FCU*, flexor carpi ulnaris; *FDS*, flexor digitorum superficialis; *FPL*, flexor pollicis longus; *PL*, palmaris longus.)

## Median Nerve (C5-C7)

- Formed from **medial** and **lateral cords** of brachial plexus
- Courses between the brachialis muscle and intermuscular septum
  - Medial to the brachial artery
- Passes under ligament of Struthers at the supracondylar rim
  - Ligament associated with humeral head of the pronator teres muscle
- Crosses the antecubital fossa under the bicipital aponeurosis (lacertus fibrosis)
- Separates from artery to pass between heads of the pronator teres muscle
  - Anterior interosseous nerve descends on the volar surface of the interosseous membrane
- Continues between the flexor digitorum profundus (FDP) and the flexor pollicis longus (FPL) muscle and behind pronator quadratus
- Distally in the forearm, it is found between the flexor digitorum profundus (FDP) and flexor digitorum superficialis (FDS)
- Median trunk continues deep to tendinous FDS arch
- Travels distally under the palmaris longus (PL) tendon to enter the carpal tunnel
- Palmar cutaneous branch of the median nerve branches off the main nerve approximately **5 cm** proximal to the carpal tunnel
  - Provides sensory innervation to the thenar eminence
- **Carpal tunnel**[5]
  - **Floor:** Carpal bones
  - **Ulnar:** Hamate hook, triquetrum, pisiform
  - **Radial:** Scaphoid, trapezium, fascial septum
  - **Roof:** Transverse carpal ligament from scaphoid tuberosity/trapezium to pisiform and hamate hook
  - Nine tendons (FPL, 4 FDS, 4 EDP) and the median nerve
  - **Variant branches of the median recurrent motor nerve:** Beyond the transverse carpal ligament, below the ligament, or through the ligament6 (Fig. 78-1)
  - **Anterior interosseous nerve:** Reliably innervates radial side of FDP (index and middle finger FDP), FPL, pronator quadratus muscle, and radiocarpal, radioulnar, and carpometacarpal (CMC) joints
  - **Median nerve:** Reliably innervates thenar hand musculature (abductor pollicis brevis, opponens pollicis, superficial belly of flexor pollicis brevis). Also innervates the index and middle finger lumbrical muscles.

## Radial Nerve (C5-C7)

- Terminal branch **posterior cord**
- Bifurcates from axillary nerve running posterior to axillary/brachial artery
- Travels posterior to brachial artery, anterior to triceps/subscapularis muscle
- Proceeds posterior to profunda brachii artery between lateral/medial heads of triceps

- Transects lateral intermuscular septum with the radial collateral artery
  - 10 cm proximal to distal humerus
  - Between brachialis and brachioradialis muscle
  - Further distally, enters between the brachialis and extensor carpi radialis longus (ECRL) muscle
- Traverses radial tunnel as soon as it overlies the tunnel floor
  - **Floor:** Radiocapitellar joint bursa
  - **Roof:** Brachioradialis tendon
  - **Radial:** ECRL and extensor carpi radialis brevis (ECRB) tendons
  - **Ulnar:** Biceps tendon
  - End of tunnel is distal border of supinator muscle
- 1 cm lateral to the biceps tendon at the cubital fossa
- Splits at elbow, traverses the supinator medial and lateral heads
  - Deep branch **(posterior interosseous nerve [PIN])** passes under the arcade of Frohse (the proximal leading edge of the superficial layer of the supinator muscle) and is distally adjacent to the extensor digitorum communis tendon.
  - Superficial radial nerve branch is a sensory branch to the dorsal radial aspect of the hand.
  - PIN branch enters the fourth compartment of the dorsal forearm
  - **Four areas of radial nerve compression** cross the elbow[3] (Fig. 78-2)
    1. Proximal to the radial tunnel (fibrous bands anterior to the radiocapitellar joint)
    2. Vascular leash of Henry (radial recurrent artery)
    3. Proximal tendinous margin of extensor carpi radialis brevis
    4. Arcade of Frohse (proximal edge of the superficial supinator muscle): *Most common site of compression*
  - **PIN reliably supplies** extensor indicis proprius muscle and extensor pollicis longus muscle; supplies sensation to the dorsal wrist capsule (no skin representation)

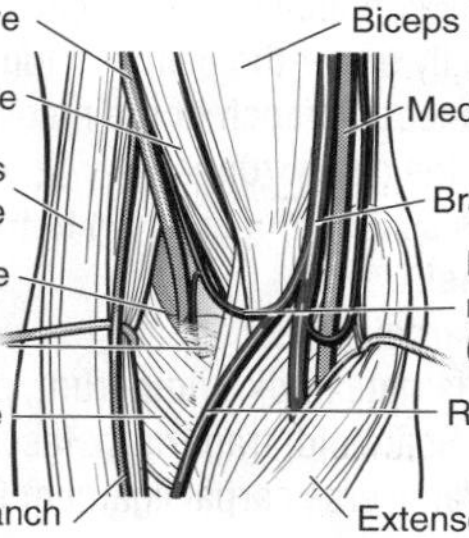

**Fig. 78-2** Sites of compressions of the radial nerve at the radial tunnel.

## Ulnar Nerve (C8-T1)

- **Medial cord** terminal branch, medial and posterior to brachial artery
- Transects medial intermuscular septum in middle arm 10 cm proximal to medial epicondyle to enter posterior arm
- Covered by arcade of Struthers **8 cm** proximal to medial epicondyle
- Passes medial to medial head of triceps and posterior to medial epicondyle
- **Cubital tunnel**
  - Nerve is covered by the flexor carpi ulnaris (FCU) tendon/arcuate ligament of Osborne.
  - Tunnel floor is composed of the capsule/medial collateral ligament.
  - Joint capsule/bursa of elbow is innervated by ulnar nerve.
- Innervates the FCU heads, passing between them
- Distally lies between the FDP/FDS muscle bellies
- Nerve tracks radial to FCU tendon and ulnar to hook of hamate to enter **Guyon's canal** (Fig. 78-3)

- Canal begins at proximal volar carpal ligament, ending with fibrous hypothenar origin radial to pisiform bone.
- **Roof:** Volar carpal ligament.
- **Ulnar border:** Pisiform/FCU, pisohamate ligament, abductor digiti muscle.
- **Radial border:** Hook of hamate.
- **Floor: Transverse carpal ligament and hypothenar muscles.**
- Neurovascular bundle and fatty tissue run below abductor and flexor digiti minimi within the canal, separated by the transverse carpal ligament.
- Neurovascular motor bundle runs midvolarly after leaving canal (61%). The motor branch travels beneath the pisohamate ligament (arcuate ligament).
- Canal exit is bound by fascial arcade.

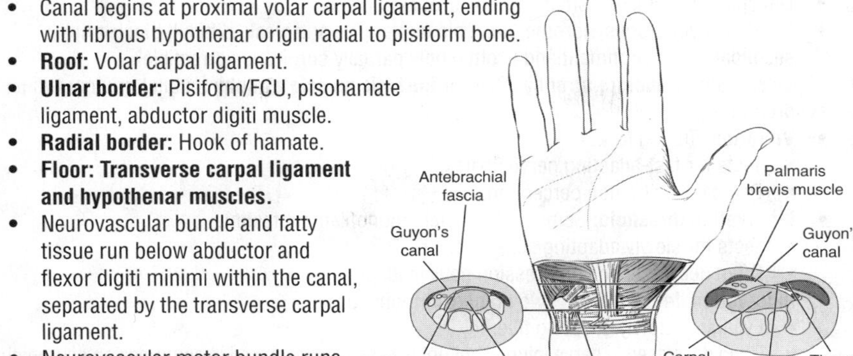


**Fig. 78-3** Relationships of the ulnar nerve at the wrist.

- **Reliably innervates** the palmaris brevis, dorsal interossei, palmar interossei, the ring/small finger lumbricals, adductor pollicis, deep belly of flexor pollicis brevis, and the hypothenar muscles (abductor digiti minimi, flexor digiti minimi brevis, and opponens digiti minimi).
  - **Ulnar nerve palsy** is demonstrated by inability to deviate the extended middle finger ulnarly or radially while the hand is on a flat surface, or inability to cross the index/middle fingers over each other.

## NERVE COMPRESSION PHYSIOLOGY[4]

### BACKGROUND

- Compression may be acute or chronic.
- Compression of **20 mm Hg or more** interferes with nerve vasculature and has adverse effects on protein synthesis, axonal transport, saltatory conduction, and myelin sheath integrity.
- **Exacerbating factors** are vibration, prolonged stress loading, and prolonged non-neutral tendon excursion. Extraneural pressure can accelerate nerve damage additively.
- Motor system manifestations occur first as weakness, followed by numbness and tingling, and finally as muscle atrophy.[5]
- Chronic nerve compression does not typically result in axonal damage in the early stages.[7]
- **Associated comorbidities** are thyroid disorders, collagen vascular disease, obesity, pregnancy, amyloidosis, and diabetes.

### DIAGNOSIS[6]

- **History**
  - Determine patterns of paresthesias, pain, and weakness; location and direction of radiation of pain and paresthesias
  - Determine duration and rate of symptom progression
  - Identify relationship of symptoms to activities or extremity position
  - Nocturnal disturbance
  - Presence or absence of neck pain
  - Work environment

- Difficulty manipulating small objects, dropping items
- Hand-arm vibratory syndrome (i.e., cold intolerance and weak, difficult pinch-grip) is secondary to environment and is often only partially surgically correctible[8]

■ Physical exam for **themor atrophy** (CTS) or **intrinsic muscle atrophy** (cubital or ulnar tunnel syndrome)
- **Vibration:** Tuning fork
  - Tests for fast-adapting nerve fibers
  - Decreased vibration perception
- **Innervation threshold:** Semmes-Weinstein monofilament testing
  - Tests for slowly adapting sensory fibers
  - Often decreased in compression neuropathies
- **Innervation density:** Static two point discrimination
  - Evaluates slowly adapting fibers
  - Often decreased in nerve injuries but not necessarily decreased in compression neuropathies
- **Provocative examination:** Phalen's sign, Tinel's sign, Durkan's compression test

■ Imaging
- Plain radiographs
- Ultrasound: Carpal tunnel syndrome creates an increased cross-sectional area of the median nerve[9]
- Magnetic resonance imaging
  - Indicated for soft tissue etiologic factors of neuropathy, mass, or suspected bone fracture

■ Testing
- Electrodiagnostic testing
  - Examines lower motor neurons; two components:
    1. Nerve conduction study (NCS)
    2. Needle electrode examination (NEE) or electromyogram (EMG)
- Nerve conduction velocities (NCV)
  - Latencies provide objective measurement of neuropathy; sensory changes occur before motor changes
    - Sensory NCS: Stimulation and recording over sensory nerve generates a sensory nerve action potential (SNAP)
    - Motor NCS: Stimulation over nerve, recording over muscle; generates a compound muscle action potential (CMAP)

## MEDIAN NERVE COMPRESSION

### Carpal Tunnel Syndrome (CTS)[8,10-13]

■ **Most common upper extremity compression neuropathy.**

■ Prevalence of CTS is estimated to be as high as 3.72%.[14]

■ Pain (worse at night) and numbness over the volar hand with dose-dependent aggravation from repetitive movements; thenar eminence is often spared of tingling (palmar cutaneous branch)

■ **Diagnosis**
- NCV shows **motor latencies are usually greater than 4.5 msec** and **sensory latency is greater than 3.5 msec.**
- **Pediatric CTS** commonly presents with **thenar atrophy** and is **often bilateral**—it is treated with the same algorithm as adult CTS.
- Lumbrical musculature can occasionally violate the carpal tunnel, increasing the resting pressure.
- Decreased light touch sensation in median nerve distribution (thumb, index, middle, and radial half of ring finger).

- Weakness of thumb opposition; thenar eminence atrophy is a late sign.
- Normal thumb interphalangeal (IP) joint flexion strength (FPL).

■ **Treatment**

- **Nonsurgical**
  - Wrist cock-up splint
  - Activity modification, ergonomic workstation
  - Nonsteroidal anti-inflammatory medications
  - Steroid injection into carpal tunnel
  - Approximately 20% of patients are symptom free 1 year after steroid injection, particularly if NCV is normal/mild and symptoms have been present less than 1 year.
  - Patients with mild symptoms respond more reliably.
- **Surgical**
  - Surgical release of the transverse carpal ligament (roof of the carpal tunnel)
  - Neurolysis/epineurotomy/flexor tenosynovectomy *not* indicated in open release
  - Symptomatic improvement of sensation within 2 weeks
  - Nerve conduction improvement by 3 months
  - Strength improvement by 6 months, but thenar atrophy may persist for 2 years or longer
  - Reexploration indicated if postoperative symptoms persist
  - **Sensitive palmar scar** most common complication (62%)
  - **Open carpal tunnel release**
    - **Advantages**
      - Critical structures/anatomic variance made directly visible
      - Complete transverse carpal ligament release
      - Concomitant Guyon's canal decompression

**TIP:** 93% of patients improve after nerve dissection and decompression.

    - **Disadvantages**
      - Bowstringing of flexor tendons
      - Longer and more tender scar
      - Traction neuritis
  - **Endoscopic carpal tunnel release**
    - **Advantages**
      - Smaller and less tender scar
      - Faster return to work
    - **Disadvantages**
      - Higher rates of neurapraxia
      - Higher incidence of recurrent CTS, most often caused by incomplete transverse carpal ligament release; also adhesions and flexor tendon synovitis
      - Inability to view anatomic variants
        - ❖ Median recurrent motor nerve branches 50%-90% of the time beyond the transverse carpal ligament, 30% below the ligament, and approximately 23% through the ligament[2] (Fig. 78-4)

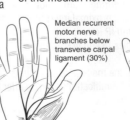

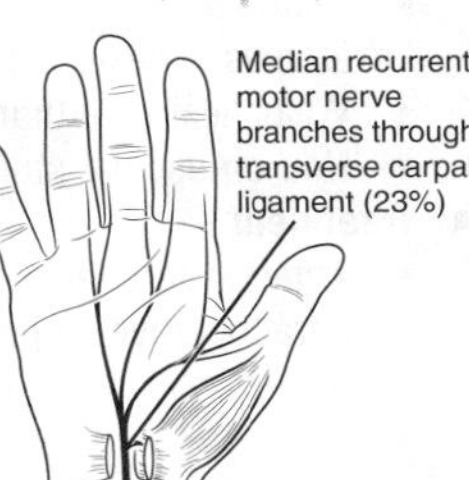


**Fig. 78-4** Normal variation of the recurrent motor branch of the median nerve.

## Pronator Syndrome[15]

Proximal forearm pain, paresthesia, and hypoesthesia occur over pronator teres, extending distally onto the thenar eminence and into thumb, index, middle, and ring fingers. There is often no median nerve distribution weakness.

- **Causes**
  - Median nerve adherence/compression at:
    - Lacertus fibrosus
    - Pronator teres
    - Arch of the flexor digitorum superficialis
  - Anomalies or vascular branches in the distal forearm
  - Entrapment beneath the ligament of Struthers between the supracondylar process of the distal humerus and fascia of the pronator teres
- **Diagnosis**
  - Tingling
    - Tapping over the pronator teres
    - Elbow flexion
    - Forearm pronation
    - Active resistance to finger flexion
    - Symptoms of tingling over the thenar eminence (palmar cutaneous branch) and within median nerve distribution in the fingers
    - Weakness of thumb IP joint flexion (FPL) and index finger distal interphalangeal (DIP) joint flexion (index FDP)
  - Neuromuscular studies of limited benefit for diagnosis
- **Treatment**
  - Surgical release indicated, with excellent results
  - Release ligament of Struthers, bicipital aponeurosis, and tendinous arch of the flexor digitorum superficialis

## Anterior Interosseous Nerve Syndrome[1,3,16]

Loss of function of the flexor pollicis longus, index/middle flexor digitorum profundus, and pronator quadratus.

- **Sensation unaffected**
- **Causes**
  - Entrapment of median nerve by the tendinous edge of deep head of the pronator teres muscle or tendinous origin of FDS
- **Diagnosis**
  - Characteristic finding during examination is index finger extension at DIP joint and increased flexion at the proximal interphalangeal (PIP) joint, generating a **pinch deformity**
  - Weak flexion of thumb IP joint (FPL)
  - Neuromuscular studies useful in diagnosis
- **Treatment**
  - Anterior approach to the median nerve at the antecubital fossa with neurolysis using intraoperative loupe magnification is highly effective in treatment

## RADIAL NERVE COMPRESSION

### RADIAL TUNNEL SYNDROME (POSTERIOR INTEROSSEOUS NERVE)

Pain during movement at the elbow (tennis elbow) radiating distally to the dorsal hand, accompanied by tingling of the hand and weakness of grip.[3,8]

- **Causes**
  - Repetitive elbow extension/rotation (weakness is a result of pain)
- **Diagnosis**
  - Radial nerve block is diagnostic and prognostic for surgical repair
  - **Middle finger test:** Pain over ECRB during forceful extension of the middle finger, with the elbow held at full extension
  - Electrodiagnostic studies not typically helpful
  - Lidocaine injection into the compartment temporarily alleviates symptoms; proper placement confirmed by temporary radial nerve palsy
- **Treatment**
  - Radial nerve release using the anterolateral approach (between brachioradialis and brachialis muscles)
  - Results only marginally beneficial and up to 50% of cases recalcitrant to surgery

> **TIP:** Nonoperative management of radial tunnel syndrome always should be pursued initially with NSAIDs, resting splints, and avoidance of inciting activity.

### POSTERIOR INTEROSSEOUS NERVE SYNDROME

Weakness and pain during finger/wrist extension without sensory involvement.

- **Causes**
  - Trauma
  - Acute bleeding from arteriovenous malformation
  - Rheumatoid arthritis inflammation at the elbow or radial head involvement
  - Soft tissue growing mass (e.g., lipoma)
  - Traction neurapraxia
- **Diagnosis**
  - Plain films of elbow to assure no radial head displacement
  - Electrodiagnostic testing
  - Ultrasound evaluation of soft tissue masses
  - MRI: Operative planning if PIN etiologic factors involve soft tissue masses
  - May see index finger extension failure with paresthesia
    - Tendinous compression of the nerve at the arcade of Frohse can result in hand paresthesia at the wrist and loss of distal hand extension
- **Treatment**
  - **Nonoperative treatment**
    - Considered with new, sudden onset of symptoms
    - Up to 3-month trial resting splint
    - Steroid injections for patients with rheumatoid arthritis (RA), but with risk of injuring the posterior interosseous nerve
  - **Operative treatment**
    - **Anatomic sites**
      - Radiocapitellar joint fascia
      - Leash of Henry (radial recurrent vessel bundle)

- ECRB lateral edge
- Arcade of Frohse (proximal leading edge of superficial layer of supinator muscle)
- Anterolateral approach to expose radial tunnel inlet (between brachioradialis and brachialis muscles)
- Posterior approach to the arcade of Frohse (incision between the EDC and ECRB muscles)

### Wartenberg's Syndrome

Compression of the superficial radial nerve at point of exit from beneath brachioradialis muscle.

- **Clinical findings**
  - Pain and possible numbness at dorsal radial aspect of distal forearm and hand
  - Positive Tinel's sign over superficial radial nerve proximal to radial styloid process
  - Differential diagnosis: deQuervain's tenosynovitis, intersection syndrome, lateral antecubital cutaneous nerve compression
- **Treatment**
  - Nonoperative: Splinting, activity modification, NSAID, steroid injection
  - Surgical: Release of superficial radial nerve as it passes beneath the brachioradialis muscle

## ULNAR NERVE COMPRESSION

### Cubital Tunnel Syndrome[3]

Ulnar-sided forearm tingling and pain extending to the ulnar half of the ring finger, the entire small finger, and ulnar dorsal half of the hand that may involve weakness and atrophy.

- **Causes**
  - Aponeurotic compression
  - Tumor
  - Trauma
  - Ulnar nerve subluxation at the medial epicondyle level
  - Anatomic variation
- **Diagnosis**
  - Provocative testing: Percussion and compression testing over the cubital tunnel
  - Increased paresthesias with elbow flexed and forearm supinated (elbow flexion test)
  - Late motor signs: Froment's sign, Wartenberg's sign, ring/small finger clawing
  - Neuromuscular conductivity testing of limited use for diagnosis (up to 30% false-negative rate)
  - Decreased sensation in the ulnar half of ring finger, entire small finger, and ulnar dorsal half of hand
  - Decreased small finger DIP flexion strength (small finger FDP weakness)
  - Intrinsic muscle weakness with or without interosseous atrophy
- **Treatment**
  - Nonsurgical: Anterior elbow splint with elbow at 30 degrees of flexion
  - Medial approach: Decompression of the cubital tunnel, avoiding damage to the medial antebrachial cutaneous nerves of the arm
  - Posterior/medial approach: Decompression of the cubital tunnel, avoiding damage to the medial antebrachial cutaneous nerves of the arm
  - **Five sites of surgical decompression:** Arcade of Struthers, ligament of Osborne, medial intermuscular septum, proximal fascia between the two heads of the FCU, and fascial bands within the FCU tunnel

- Five surgical treatment options:
  - In situ decompression (open or endoscopic)
  - Medial epicondylectomy and in situ decompression
  - Anterior subcutaneous transposition
  - Anterior intramuscular transposition
  - Anterior submuscular transposition
- Results somewhat unpredictable; ulnar neuropathy may only partially improve after decompression
- Submuscular ulnar nerve transposition indicated for recurrent cases[17,18]

## Ulnar Tunnel Syndrome (Guyon's Canal)[1,3]

Wrist pain with numbness, tingling, and burning in the small finger and ulnar half of the ring finger.

- **Three zones** (Fig. 78-5)
  - **Zone I** is proximal to the ulnar nerve bifurcation.
  - **Zone II** surrounds the ulnar nerve deep motor branch as it passes the hamate hook.
  - **Zone III** surrounds the superficial sensory ulnar nerve sensory branch.

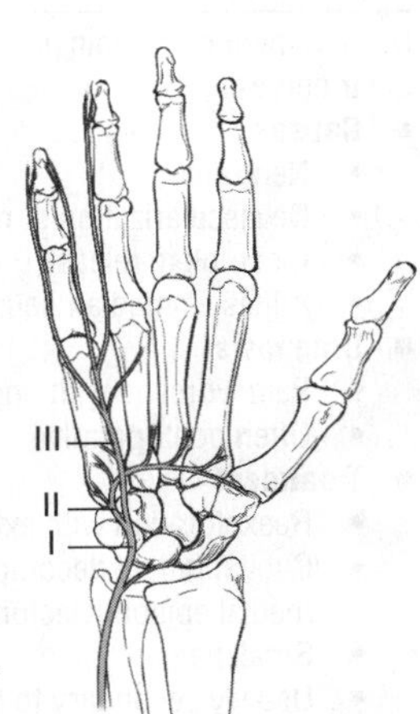

**Fig. 78-5** Zones of ulnar nerve compression within Guyon's canal.

- **Causes**
  - Carpal ganglion cyst arising from the triquetrohamate joint
  - Occupational trauma (e.g., hypothenar hammer syndrome)
  - Vascular thrombosis/ulnar artery aneurysm
  - Synovial inflammation
  - Anomalous muscles
- **Diagnosis**
  - Symptoms correlate with location of compression
    - Proximally, motor and sensory deficits occur (zone I).
    - Distal to the canal, motor deficits frequently occur (zone II).
    - Rarely isolated sensory deficits occur, which are distal (zone III).
    - Sensation is classically intact on the dorsal/ulnar hand because dorsal cutaneous branch originates proximal to Guyon's canal.

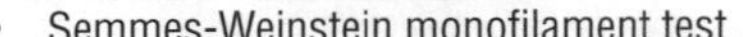

  - Semmes-Weinstein monofilament test
  - Two-point discrimination
  - Bedside intrinsic muscle motor testing
  - Normal small finger DIP flexion strength (no weakness of the small finger FDP muscle)
  - Clawing of the fingers is typically absent
  - Normal elbow flexion test
  - Plain films of the wrist and hand
  - CT scan of the wrist and hand if fracture suspected (e.g., hook of hamate fracture)
  - Electrodiagnostic examination to help determine zone of injury
- **Treatment**
  - **Nonoperative**
    - NSAID medical therapy
    - Resting splint immobilization
    - Reduction of repetitive hand motion

- **Operative**
  - Indicated with identifiable lesions
  - Release of the nerve requires both release of Guyon's canal and release of the motor branch running beneath the fascial arcade at the deep distal hiatus (also called the pisohamate ligament or arcuate ligament).[19]
  - Complete release of the nerve from Guyon's canal

**TIP:** Pursue immediate ulnar nerve decompression after any wrist fracture with ulnar neuropathy or after ulnar neuropathy that persists longer than 24 hours.

## TRACTION NEURITIS

Development of chronic pain following open carpal ligament release or transposition of the ulnar nerve.

- **Causes**
  - Neuroma
  - Devascularization of nerve
  - Incomplete release during decompression or transposition
  - Adhesive median neuritis
- **Diagnosis**
  - Pain worsens with finger motion or during increased pressure over the site[20]
  - Often postoperative
- **Treatment**
  - Reexploration with external and internal neurolysis
  - Cubital tunnel decompression, treating persistent pain with submuscular transposition or medial epicondylectomy
  - Small percentage of patients do not improve after reexploration
  - Usually secondary to scar formation; may progressively worsen
  - End-stage traction neuritis
    - External and internal neurolysis, epineurectomy, wrapped with free or local flap coverage (e.g., ulnar tunnel fat pad)

### KEY POINTS

✓ History of the work environment is critical to compression neuropathy treatment.
✓ Operative intervention for carpal tunnel syndrome is indicated with **median nerve sensory latencies greater than 3.5 msec** and/or **median nerve motor latencies greater than 4.5 msec.**
✓ Nonoperative treatment of carpal tunnel syndrome has an **80%** rate of recurrent symptoms.
✓ Carpal tunnel syndrome release procedures must avoid injury to the median recurrent nerve.
✓ Testing the sensory distribution of the thenar eminence determines median nerve compression proximal or distal to the carpal tunnel.
✓ Inability to extend index finger with paresthesia is indicative of PIN syndrome.
✓ Ulnar nerve transposition is required if symptoms persist after cubital tunnel release.
✓ Traction neuritis mandates operative reexploration.

## REFERENCES


1. Eversmann WW Jr. Entrapment and compression neuropathies. In Green DP, Hotchkiss RN, Pederson WC, eds. Green's Operative Hand Surgery, 4th ed. Philadelphia: Churchill Livingstone, 1998.
2. Lanz U. Anatomical variations of the median nerve in the carpal tunnel. J Hand Surg 2:44, 1977.
3. Eversmann WW Jr. Compression and entrapment neuropathies of the upper extremity. J Hand Surg 8:759, 1983.
4. Rempel D, Dahlin L, Lundborg G. Pathophysiology of nerve compression syndromes: response of peripheral nerves to loading. J Bone Joint Surg Am 81:1600, 1999.
5. Spinner M, Spencer PS. Nerve compression lesions of the upper extremity: a clinical and experimental review. Clin Orthop 104:46, 1974.
6. Dellon AL. Patient evaluation and management considerations in nerve compression. Hand Clin 8:229, 1992.
7. Pham K, Gupta R. Understanding the mechanisms of entrapment neuropathies. Neurosurg Focus 26:E7, 2009.
8. Stromberg T, Dahlin LB, Lundborg G. Vibrotactile sense in the hand-arm vibration syndrome. Scand J Work Environ Health 24:495, 1998.
9. Karadağ YS, Karadağ O, Çiçekli E, et al. Severity of carpal tunnel syndrome assessed with high frequency ultrasonography. Rheumatol Int 30:761, 2010.
10. Mackinnon SE, McCabe S, Murray JF, et al. Internal neurolysis fails to improve the results of primary carpal tunnel decompression. J Hand Surg Am 16:211, 1991.
11. Singh I, Khoo KMA, Krishnamoorthy S. The carpal tunnel syndrome: clinical evaluation and results of surgical decompression. Ann Acad Med Singapore 23:94, 1994.
12. Shurr DG, Blair WF, Bassett G. Electromyographic changes after carpal tunnel release. J Hand Surg Am 11:876, 1986.
13. Botte MJ, von Schroeder HP, Abrams RA, et al. Recurrent carpal tunnel syndrome. Hand Clin 12:731, 1996.
14. Papanicolaou GD, McCabe SJ, Firrell J. The prevalence and characteristics of nerve compression symptoms in the general population. J Hand Surg Am 26:460, 2001.
15. Olehnik WK, Manske PR, Szerzinski J. Median nerve compression in the proximal forearm. J Hand Surg Am 19:121, 1994.
16. Hill NA, Howard FM, Huffer B. The incomplete anterior interosseous nerve syndrome. J Hand Surg Am 10:4, 1985.
17. Learmonth JR. A technique for transplanting the ulnar nerve. Surg Gynecol Obstet 75:792, 1942.
18. Amadio PC, Beckenbaugh RD. Entrapment of the ulnar nerve by the deep flexor-pronator aponeurosis. J Hand Surg Am 11:83, 1986.
19. Konig PS, Hage JJ, Bloem JJ, et al. Variations of the ulnar nerve and ulnar artery in Guyon's canal: a cadaveric study. J Hand Surg Am 19:617, 1994.
20. Jones NF, Shaw WW, Katz RG. Circumferential wrapping of a flap around a scarred peripheral nerve for salvage of end-stage traction neuritis. J Hand Surg Am 22:527, 1997.

# 79. Brachial Plexus

Rey N. Ramirez, Ashkan Ghavami

## ANATOMY[1] (Fig. 79-1)

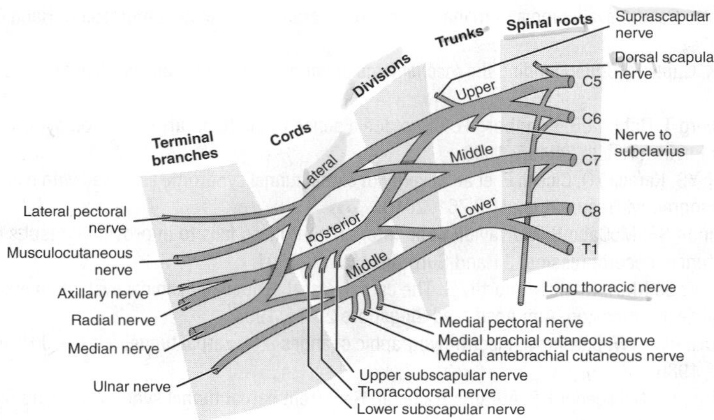


**Fig. 79-1** Brachial plexus.

- **Spinal roots:** Generally C5, C6, C7, C8, and T1
  - Between anterior and middle scalene muscles
  - *Prefixed plexus:* C4 significant contributor
  - *Postfixed plexus:* Contains T2 contribution
  - Long thoracic nerve and dorsal scapular nerve arise at this level.
- **Trunks:** Upper, middle, and lower
  - In posterior cervical triangle
  - Suprascapular nerve and nerve to subclavius arise at this level.
- **Divisions:** Each trunk gives off an **anterior** and **posterior** division.
  - Under clavicle and pectoralis minor
  - **No** peripheral nerves arise at this level.
- **Cords:** Lateral, posterior, and medial (named for position **relative to axillary artery**)
  - **Lateral** cord consists of anterior divisions of upper and middle trunks. **Lateral pectoral nerve** arises here.
  - **Posterior** cord consists of posterior divisions of all three trunks. It gives off (proximal to distal) **upper subscapular nerve, thoracodorsal nerve, lower subscapular nerve.**
  - **Medial** cord consists of anterior division of lower trunk. It gives off (proximal to distal) **medial pectoral nerve, medial antebrachial cutaneous nerve, medial brachial cutaneous nerve.**

- **Terminal branches:** Cords divide into major peripheral nerves of the upper extremity: **myocutaneous nerve, axillary nerve, radial nerve, ulnar nerve, median nerve.**
- Injuries may be classified into **supraclavicular** or **infraclavicular** to assist in planning approach.
  - **Supraclavicular** (75% of patients)[2]
    - Involves cervical roots or trunks
    - **Erb's point:** Convergence of C5 and C6 roots as they form upper trunk
      - Injury here (or proximally, to the C5 and C6 roots) forms the classic *Erb's palsy* or *waiter's tip:* lack of deltoid (axillary nerve), supraspinatus (suprascapular nerve), biceps (myocutaneous nerve), causing the arm to hang straight down at the side, with the forearm pronated.
  - **Infraclavicular**
    - Shoulder dislocations
    - Fractures often present
    - Cords or branches affected

## INJURIES MAY BE PREGANGLIONIC OR POSTGANGLIONIC (Fig. 79-2)

- **Root avulsions** (preganglionic or supraganglionic)
  - Occur **proximal** to intraforaminal dorsal root ganglion (DRG)
  - **No Wallerian degeneration** of sensory nerves, because cell bodies still in continuity with axons; thus:
  - Sensory Nerve Action Potentials (SNAPs) are present (pathognomonic).
  - **It cannot be repaired with primary repair or nerve grafting** (often requires *neurotization* [nerve transfer]).
    - Largely for technical reasons (It is not possible to suture nerves back to the spinal cord itself.)
  - Physical examination findings
    - Denervation of paracervical muscles
    - Severe pain (deafferentation) in nerve distribution
    - **Horner's syndrome:** Evidence of C8 or T1 level injury that is also highly associated with preganglionic injury
      - Ptosis (drooping of upper eyelid)
      - Miosis (pupillary constriction)
      - Enophthalmos (posterior recession of the eye)
      - Anhidrosis (lack of sweat)

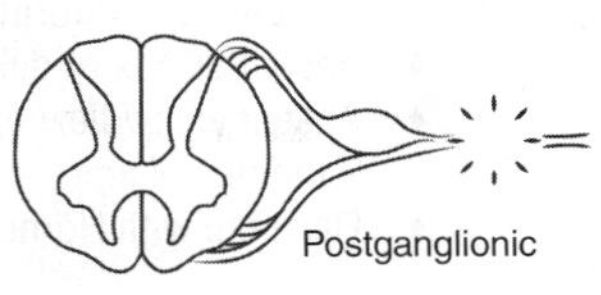


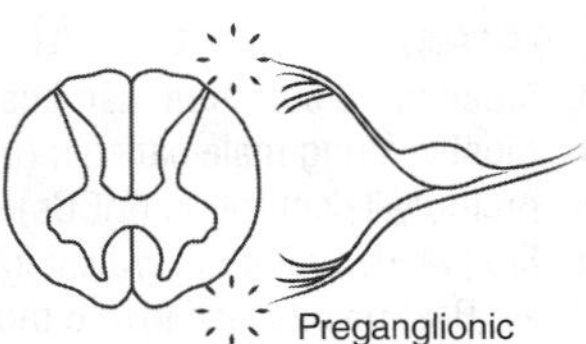


**Fig. 79-2** Preganglionic versus postganglionic injury. The lower image demonstrates root avulsion.

- **Postganglionic or infraganglionic**
  - Injury **distal** to DRG
  - Paracervical muscles intact
  - Rami communicans to sympathetic ganglion intact (no Horner's syndrome)
  - **Wallerian degeneration** in peripheral nerve fibers (absence of SNAPs)
  - No action potentials recordable
  - **Surgical repair with nerve grafts or primary repair possible** because a proximal portion is intact and present

## EPIDEMIOLOGY

### Brachial Plexus Birth Palsy (BPBP)[3,4]

- **Incidence:** 1.5 per 1000 full-term births
- **Risk factors**
  - Shoulder dystocia

> **TIP:** Clavicle fracture during delivery should raise concern for brachial plexus injury.

  - Gestational diabetes
  - Forceps delivery
  - Vacuum extraction
  - Breech delivery
  - Macrosomia
  - Multiparity
- **Clinical presentation**[3]
  - Most patients (73%) present with upper root cervical injury **(Erb-Duchenne palsy)**
    - 4%-5% are bilateral
  - Indications for surgical exploration are controversial. Up to 90% of patients will have spontaneous recovery within first 2 months.[5]
    - **Indications for exploration**[4]**:**
      - Absent biceps or deltoid function by 3-6 months
      - Absent elbow flexion and extension, wrist extension, or thumb/finger extension at 9 months of age
      - Flail limb with Horner's syndrome is a relative indication for early exploration.

### Traumatic Brachial Plexus Injury[1]

- **Much more common** than obstetrical injuries
- Mostly young male patients (up to 90% of cases), often from motor vehicle collision (MVCs) or motorcycle collisions (MCCs)
- Frequently requires surgical intervention
  - Best results less than 6 months after insult, after 1-2 years results are poorer

**NOTE: Many surgeons do not attempt nerve reconstruction more than 1 year after injury because of irreversible muscle changes and neuronal cell body changes. Patients may still benefit from distal nerve transfers or other reconstructive options, including free muscle transfer and tendon transfer.**

## MECHANISM OF INJURY

### Traction

- Most common
- Downward direction (e.g., MCCs, skiing) from **forceful neck flexion** to contralateral side causing upper root or trunk injury
- Forceful shoulder abduction >90 degrees causing damage in lower plexus
- Iatrogenic from surgical retraction or positioning causing extreme shoulder abduction
- Young male patients (approximately 90%-95% of cases)
- **High-velocity causes**
  - MVCs, MCCs more than 80% of cases, with greater traction forces
  - Root avulsions more common

- Reevaluate with examination and electrodiagnostics after 3 months of observation
- If evidence of recovery, then periodic reevaluation every 6-12 weeks

- **Low-velocity causes**
  - Sports injuries, bicycling, skiing, or falling from a height
  - Require same reevaluation and electrodiagnostic protocol as high-velocity injuries if no evidence of recovery
  - Explore if inadequate reinnervation at 3-6 months

### CRUSH/COMPRESSION

- In costoclavicular region, between first rib and clavicle
- Often from direct trauma (MVCs), occupational injury (heavy object falling on shoulder), or football injury
- Adjacent tissues (bony fragments)
- Hematoma or pseudoaneurysm
- Cervical rib(s)
- Fibrous bands
- Prominent transverse process(es)
- Iatrogenic from positioning

### OPEN INJURY

- Most amenable to immediate exploration and repair
- Less common than closed traction-type injury patterns
- Concomitant vascular injury can increase injury severity.
- Gunshot wounds (GSWs)
- Rule out vascular injury.
- Often **mixed injury pattern** with neurapraxic component (Mackinnon sixth-degree stage)
- Most gunshots are low velocity and will be largely neurapraxic. Observe these and expect recovery.
- High-velocity gunshots have higher potential for neurotmesis and should be explored earlier.
- **Sharp injuries (e.g., knife wounds)** *are more amenable to immediate repair.*
  - **Primary repair:** Along with repair of vascular or limb-threatening injury
    - Only if area of nerve injury can be clearly delineated (minimal crush component)
  - **Delayed repair:** When zone of injury may be unclear
    - Explore and tag nerves out to length and reexplore in approximately 3-4 weeks with better wound conditions and when patient is stable.

> **TIP:** In blast, crush, or stretch injuries, allow the injury to mature for several weeks. This may help to identify the true zone of injury.

## PATIENT EVALUATION[1,4,6-8]

### PRINCIPLES

- The injury will generally involve multiple nerves, with different degrees of injury to each. Detailed examination of the entire affected extremity is crucial to identify injury and determine candidate nerves available for transfer.
- **Time interval from injury is most important determinant of outcome.**
  - Exact time threshold for evaluation and treatment is debatable, but less than 6 months is optimal, and no later than 12-18 months.
  - Chance of end-organ denervation, muscle atrophy, and cell loss is decreased if treatment starts less than 6 months from initial injury.

- **Age vital to functional outcome**
  - **20 years old or younger:** Significantly better outcomes than older patients
  - Older than 40 years: Prognosis worsens
- **Details of initial injury:** Help direct examination and diagnosis of injury pattern
  - **MVC:** Speed, seat belt, helmet, airbag, distance thrown
  - **Occupational:** Type of machine, force and direction of pull, weight and location of impact, head and neck, height of fall
  - **GSW:** High versus low velocity, associated vascular injury

## PHYSICAL EXAMINATION

- Note: Brachial plexus birth palsy (BPBP) is generally evaluated by different criteria than traumatic. For these patients assess the Mallet score[4] (Table 79-1) or the Active Movement Scale.

**Table 79-1** *Mallet Score*

| | 1 | 2 | 3 | 4 | 5 |
|---|---|---|---|---|---|
| Global abduction at shoulder | No function | <30 degrees | 30-90 degrees | >90 degrees | Normal |
| Global external rotation of arm | No function | <0 degrees | 0-20 degrees | >20 degrees | Normal |
| Hand to neck | No function | Not possible | Difficult | Easy | Normal |
| Hand to spine | No function | Not possible | Hand reaches S1 | Hand reaches T12 | Normal |
| Hand to mouth | No function | With marked shoulder abduction | With shoulder abduction 45 degrees | With <40 degrees of shoulder abduction | Normal |
| Supination | No function | Not possible | <90 degrees | >90 degrees | Normal |

  - **Active Movement Scale[4]:**
    - Test: Shoulder abduction, shoulder adduction, shoulder flexion, shoulder internal/external rotation, elbow flexion/extension, forearm pronation/supination, wrist flexion/extension, finger extension, thumb flexion/extension
    - Score each muscle group by the following criteria:
      - Gravity eliminated:
        - 0: No contraction
        - 1: Twitch without motion
        - 2: <50% motion
        - 3: >50% motion
        - 4: Full motion
      - Against gravity
        - 5: <50% motion
        - 6: >50% motion

**TIP:** Examine **all** muscle groups in upper extremity and shoulder. Injuries may spare portions of a nerve.

- **Document**
  - Muscle grades
  - Atrophy
  - Joint mobility
  - Passive or active function

**TIP:** Compare results with those on the contralateral side.

- **Muscle/innervations**[1,9] (Table 79-2)

**Table 79-2** *Root Innervations of Key Muscles*

<table>
<tr><th colspan="2">C6</th><th colspan="2">C8</th></tr>
<tr><th>C5</th><th colspan="2">C7</th><th>T1</th></tr>
<tr><td colspan="2">Serratus anterior</td><td colspan="2">Flexor digitorum superficialis</td></tr>
<tr><td>Deltoid</td><td rowspan="2">Pronator</td><td rowspan="2">Palmaris longus</td><td rowspan="2">Flexor digitorum profundus</td></tr>
<tr><td>Supraspinatus</td></tr>
<tr><td>Infraspinatus</td><td>Flexor carpi radialis</td><td>Extensor pollicis brevis</td><td>Abductor pollicis brevis</td></tr>
<tr><td>Biceps</td><td colspan="2">Latissimus dorsi</td><td>Opponens</td></tr>
<tr><td>Brachialis</td><td colspan="2">Triceps</td><td>Flexor pollicis longus</td></tr>
<tr><td>Brachioradialis</td><td>Extensor carpi radialis</td><td>Abductor pollicis longus</td><td>Adductor pollicis</td></tr>
<tr><td>Supinator</td><td rowspan="2">Extensor digitorum communis</td><td>Extensor pollicis longus</td><td>Palmar interossei</td></tr>
<tr><td>Teres major</td><td>Flexor carpi ulnaris</td><td>Dorsal interossei</td></tr>
<tr><td colspan="4">Pectoralis major</td></tr>
</table>

  - Graded by British Medical Research Council Grading System[10] (Table 79-3)

**Table 79-3** *British Medical Research Council Grading System*

| Grade | Degree of Strength |
|---|---|
| 1 | Muscle contracts, but part does not move |
| 2 | Movement with gravity eliminated |
| 3 | Movement through full range of motion against gravity |
| 4 | Movement through full range of motion against resistance |
| 5 | Normal strength |

  - A few key muscles:
    - Trapezius to confirm spinal accessory nerve function for transfer
    - Serratus muscle/long thoracic nerve (C5-C7), very proximal, injury may suggest preganglionic lesion
    - Supraspinatus and infraspinatus muscles/suprascapular nerve (C5-C6)
    - Biceps/myocutaneous nerve (C5-C6)
    - Pectoralis major muscle/lateral and medial pectoral nerves (medial and lateral cords)
    - Latissimus/thoracodorsal nerve (posterior cord)
    - Triceps/radial nerve (C7)
    - Interossei/ulnar nerve (C8/T1)
- **Vascular**
  - Peripheral pulses, including Allen's test and Doppler testing
  - Consider angiography (e.g., magnetic resonance angiography)

**TIP:** Vascular injury can suggest severe nerve injury.

- **Sensory**
  - Touch, pain, two-point discrimination, and vibratory tests
  - **Tinel's sign:** Positive if paresthesias produced from percussion over most distal point of viable nerve fibers
    - It suggests most distal point of nerve regeneration.
    - *It does **not** provide status of motor component.*
    - Absence in supraclavicular region suggests total plexus avulsion with grave prognosis.[11]

**TIP:** Estimate the specific area of injury by conducting a detailed motor examination and by charting motor and sensory deficit patterns.

## Electrodiagnostic Tests

- **Electromyography (EMG)**
  - Delay 3-6 weeks to allow changes to develop.
  - Denervated muscles show **fibrillation** and **decreased motor unit potentials** with voluntary effort.
  - **Serial EMGs** for presence of reinnervation
    - Decreased fibrillations
    - Increased voluntary motor unit potentials (MUPs)
    - Positive polyphasic low-amplitude potentials
- **Nerve conduction study (NCS)** to demonstrate continuity or sensory nerve action potentials (SNAPs)
  - Combined presence of SNAP, normal sensory conduction velocity in peripheral nerve, and paralyzed muscle (absent motor nerve)
    - Indicates **root avulsion** (preganglionic injury) with preservation of DRG
    - Absence of SNAP does not imply lack of preganglionic injury, because nerve can have double lesion (nerve rupture and root avulsion).[11,12]

## Imaging

- **Plain radiographs:** Indicated in acute setting
  - Cervical spine
  - Shoulder
  - Clavicle
  - Chest
  - Possible correlations
    - **Transverse process of cervical spine fracture:** *Root lesion*
    - **Hemidiaphragm elevation:** *Preganglionic injury*, *phrenic nerve* involved (phrenic and ipsilateral intercostal nerves as donor nerves risky)
    - **Rib fractures:** *Intercostal nerves may not be usable as donors*
    - **Scapula and clavicle fractures:** *Compression, high-energy injury,* and *supraclavicular injury*

- **CT cervical myelogram**[11]
  - Helps diagnose **pseudomeningoceles** and **root deviations,** which suggest presence of root avulsions
  - *Key point: Perform at least 1 month after injury to allow pseudomeningocele formation*
  - Excellent sensitivity (95%) and specificity (98%)[6]
- **MRI**
  - Noninvasive
  - No need to wait 4 weeks
  - Can suggest areas of plexal injury
  - Equivalent to CT/myelogram for root avulsions; less effective for lower root injury
- **Angiography**
  - Indicated in acute setting if vascular injury suspected
  - Can acutely explore open injuries without angiogram

**TIP:** Standard evaluation of all brachial plexus patients should include physical examination, electrodiagnostic tests, cervical spine/chest/shoulder radiographs, MRI, and possible CT myelogram or MR angiogram.

## PREOPERATIVE MANAGEMENT[1,4,5,7,12-14]

### Physical Therapy

- This is crucial for management in all phases of care.
- Maintain passive joint motion and appropriate splinting both preoperatively and postoperatively.
- This is especially crucial in BPBP, because preservation of range of motion is paramount.
- Motor reeducation and strengthening exercises are important if nerve transfers are undertaken.
- Electrical stimulation of nonfunctioning muscles to maintain the motor endplates is controversial.

### Pain Management

- Severe with total plexus avulsion
- Trial of gabapentin (Neurontin) and referral to pain specialist for multipharmaceutical therapy
- Neurosurgical referral last resort for *intraspinal dorsal root coagulation*

## TREATMENT PRINCIPLES: TRAUMATIC BRACHIAL PLEXUS INJURIES*

### General Principles

*"To someone who has nothing, a little is a lot"* – Sterling Bunnell, MD

- Patients will require long-term longitudinal, comprehensive care from a team.
- Initial management is conservative unless exact injury level is known.
- Lower trunk (C8 and T1) is not reconstructed, because distance to target muscles is so long that muscle atrophy before nerve regeneration is expected.
- Evaluate whether nerve is in continuity (indication for neurolysis) or nonviable/discontinuous (excision and nerve grafting).

*References 1, 2, 5, 8, 9, 11, 14, 15.

**TIP:** Treatment decisions for brachial plexus injuries are extremely complex. In general, consider what is missing, prioritize the arm functions to restore, and inventory available axons to power muscles to restore those functions.

### Goals of Reconstruction

- **Reconstitute elbow flexion:** First priority is to allow hand-to-mouth function.
- **Stabilize shoulder** to prevent subluxation and to support power across elbow.
- Allow shoulder **external rotation.**
- **Perform later reconstruction of wrist extension and finger flexion** through muscle/tendon unit transfers.
- **Reestablish sensation** through neurotization of median and ulnar nerves.
- Often a **combination** of nerve grafts and nerve transfers will ultimately be used.
- Though controversial, shoulder arthrodesis can simplify the upper extremity and allow donors to be used for distal targets.

### Acute Brachial Plexus Reconstruction or Repair During Exploration[5,13,14]

- Primary nerve repair or use of shorter grafts is allowed, because there is less nerve retraction.
  - More scarring is present during secondary operations.
- If arm ischemia or vascular compromise with open injury:
  - Explore plexus at time of repair.
  - Define injury level.
  - Decompress lesions (e.g., evacuation of hematoma and bony reduction).
- Perform primary repair or if concern for crush, tag nerves and repair after zone of injury declares.
- Intraoperative nerve conduction testing is used to confirm nerve function.
  - If nerve is in continuity but does not conduct, there is a neuroma that must be resected and grafted.

### Delayed Repair

- 4-6 weeks
- Lesion more accurately identified because of Wallerian degeneration and neuroma formation
- Noncontaminated wound
- Allows time for skeletal stability

## NERVE GRAFTS AND TRANSFERS[1,5,10-12,14,15]

### Nerve Grafts[5,14]

- In this type of treatment, brachial plexus nerves are used as sources of axons.
- Resect all injured nerve to healthy fascicles.
- Reconstruct with nerve graft.
- Donor nerves are commonly used as source of graft.
  - Sural nerve (most common)
  - Medial antebrachial cutaneous (MABC)
- Consider grafting either to cords or directly to terminal nerve branches.

**NOTE: Intraoperative visualization or palpation is not a reliable means of predicting preganglionic versus postganglionic injury or of detecting neuromas-in-continuity.**

- Nerve function is confirmed by a variety of methods:
  - **Somatosensory evoked potentials** (SSEPs) and **motor evoked potentials** (MEPs)[1]
    - These function by the principle that low-amplitude potentials can be detected through the scalp with contralateral nerve stimulation.
    - SSEPs do not confirm motor axon function, and MEPs do not confirm sensory axon function.
    - Presence of SSEPs and MEPs confirms lack of preganglionic injury.
  - Histopathologic examination for **choline acetyltransferase** activity can confirm nerve function.
    - Its presence confirms motor axon availability of sufficient function for use.
  - **Nerve action potentials**
    - Areas of suggested injury are tested directly for electrical conduction.
    - Nerves that conduct may be functioning but may not have regenerated all the way to the muscle.
      - These nerves should undergo neurolysis.
    - Nerves that do not conduct need resection of the neuroma and grafting.

**TIP:** Perform *intraoperative nerve testing.* The exact operative plan is determined *intraoperatively.*

## Nerve Transfers[5,10,12,15]

- An important part of reconstruction of brachial plexus injuries
- May allow neurotization closer to the target muscle than would be obtained by intraplexal repair or grafting
  - Important because motor endplates begin to **permanently degenerate** after 1 year
- Allow donation of motor axons only
- **Indications**
  - Adjunct to brachial plexus grafting or repair
  - Nonreconstructible injury (e.g., preganglionic root avulsions)
  - Very proximal postganglionic injury
- **Motor nerve transfers**
  - Inventory available nerves.
    - Synergistic (moving in concert, as in flexors with flexors) donor or recipient muscles are preferable.
    - Nonsynergistic transfers will be futile (e.g., radial nerve powering both triceps and biceps).
    - Muscles that can be sacrificed without causing disability are preferred.
    - Donor muscle should be grade 4 strength or better.
  - Use intraoperative nerve stimulation to confirm lack of recipient function and to selectively select fascicles for donation.
- **Sensory nerve transfers**
  - Hand sensation in critical areas (e.g., thumb and index fingers) is important.
  - Timing is not as important as for motor end targets.
    - Because of this, protective sensation may be regained with repair of median or ulnar nerve despite lack of motor recovery.

- Donors can be classified as **intraplexal, extraplexal,** or **distal.**
  - **Intraplexal donors:** Ulnar nerve fascicle, median nerve fascicle, thoracodorsal nerve, medial pectoral nerve, radial nerve branch to triceps, myocutaneous nerve branch to brachialis, pectoral branch of C7
  - **Extraplexal donors:** Spinal accessory nerve, intercostal nerve (up to seven may be taken), phrenic nerve, contralateral C7 nerve root (all or partial)
  - **Distal donors:** Distal anterior interosseous nerve, radial nerve branch to extensor carpi radialis brevis (ECRB), posterior interosseous nerve branches to supinator, radial nerve branch to brachioradialis
- **Contralateral C7**
  - Commonly used as donor to median or myocutaneous nerve.
  - Generally considered if other donors are lacking (e.g., complete C5-T1 root avulsions).
  - Inconsistent results reported, **some authors recommend against use.**[5]
- Donor nerves should be selected by determining what function to restore and choosing a donor that will allow nerve coaptation **close to the target** and **without use of interpositional graft.** A large variety of transfers are possible; the following are the most common.

## SPECIFIC PROCEDURES[15] (Tables 79-4 through 79-6)

**Table 79-4** *Common Intraplexal Motor Transfers*

| Motor Deficit | Recipient Nerve or Nerves | Donor Nerve or Nerves | Comment |
|---|---|---|---|
| Elbow flexion | Myocutaneous nerve: biceps and brachialis branches dual transfer | Ulnar nerve fascicle and median nerve fascicle | Primary choice, if possible, in upper nerve root brachial plexus injury (C5-C6, C5-C7) |
| | Myocutaneous nerve | Medial pectoral nerve | Secondary choice |
| | Myocutaneous nerve | Thoracodorsal nerve | Secondary choice |
| Shoulder stabilization/abduction/external rotation | Suprascapular nerve and axillary nerve dual transfer | Spinal accessory nerve and triceps branches | Primary choice, if possible, combination intraplexal and extraplexal |
| Shoulder stabilization/abduction | Axillary nerve | Medial pectoral nerve | Secondary choice |
| | Axillary nerve | Thoracodorsal nerve | Secondary choice |
| Scapular stabilization/antiwinging | Long thoracic nerve | Thoracodorsal nerve | Primary choice if possible |
| | Long thoracic nerve | Pectoral fascicle from middle trunk from C7 | Secondary choice |
| Thumb and index finger flexion | Posterior fascicle of median nerve in arm, which corresponds to anterior interosseous nerve | Brachialis branch of myocutaneous nerve or extensor carpi radialis brevis supinator branches of radial nerve | For lower trunk plexus injury or high median nerve injury<br>Coupled with tenodesis of four flexor digitorum profundus tendons in forearm |
| Elbow extension | Triceps branch of radial nerve | Ulnar nerve fascicle to flexor carpi ulnaris or median nerve fascicle to flexor digitorum superficialis | — |

**Table 79-5** *Common Extraplexal Motor Transfers*

| Motor Deficit | Recipient Nerve or Nerves | Donor Nerve or Nerves | Comment |
|---|---|---|---|
| Elbow flexion | Myocutaneous nerve | Intercostal nerves | Primary choice if intraplexal nerve transfers not possible |
| | Myocutaneous nerve | Spinal accessory nerve | Secondary choice |
| | Myocutaneous nerve | Phrenic nerve | Infrequently performed given decreased exercise tolerance |
| Shoulder stabilization/ abduction/external rotation | Suprascapular nerve | Spinal accessory nerve | Primary choice as part of dual nerve transfer with triceps branches to axillary nerve |
| | Suprascapular nerve | Intercostal nerves | Secondary choice |
| Shoulder stabilization/ abduction | Axillary nerve | Intercostal nerves | Secondary choice if triceps branch is not available |
| Scapular stabilization/ antiwinging | Long thoracic nerve | Intercostal nerves | Secondary choice if thoracodorsal nerve is not available |
| Elbow extension | Triceps branch of radial nerve | Intercostal nerves | — |
| Elbow flexion, hand function | Myocutaneous nerve<br>Median nerve | Contralateral C7 | For five-root avulsion in a young patient, less commonly performed |

**Table 79-6** *Common Distal Motor Transfers*

| Motor Deficit | Recipient Nerve or Nerves | Donor Nerve or Nerves | Comments |
|---|---|---|---|
| Intrinsic hand | Ulnar nerve motor branch | Distal anterior interosseous nerve | For high ulnar nerve lesions |
| Thumb, finger extension | Posterior interosseous nerve branches of radial nerve | Nerve to supinator | For C7-T1 plexus injuries |
| Wrist, finger extension | Radial nerve branch to extensor carpi radialis brevis and posterior interosseous nerve | Median nerve fascicles to flexor digitorum superficialis and median nerve fascicles to flexor carpi radialis | Dual transfer |
| Thumb, finger flexion | Anterior interosseous nerve | Radial nerve branch to brachioradialis | Indicated for lower trunk plexus injury or high median nerve injury<br>Coupled with tenodesis of four flexor digitorum profundus tendons in forearm |

**TIP:** When injury is severe and donor availability is scarce, consider shoulder fusion.

### Hand Sensation[1,7]

- May be restored by neurotization of median or ulnar nerves
- Donor nerves for transfer
  - Intercostobrachial nerve
  - Intercostal sensory nerve
  - Supraclavicular nerve branches
  - Superficial radial nerve
- Recipient nerves
  - Ulnar nerve in upper arm
  - Lateral cord contribution to median nerve for thumb and radial digits
  - Transfer of fourth web space sensory nerve to first web space[10]

## PALLIATIVE PROCEDURES/ADJUNCTIVE PROCEDURES[5]

> **TIP:** Consider palliative and adjunctive procedures if injury is older than 6-12 months and no recovery is seen.

### Tendon Transfer

- Commonly indicated for **older patients** (>40 years)
- **Restoration of elbow flexion most common indication**
- Restoration of hand intrinsic function and thumb opposition regardless of time from injury
- **Operations**
  - Upper trapezius transfer to the humerus to stabilize shoulder
  - Steindler flexorplasty using flexor pronator muscle to restore elbow flexion
  - Pectoralis major for shoulder abduction
  - Latissimus dorsi/teres major rerouting to restore shoulder abduction and external rotation

### Functional Free-Muscle Transfer

- Usually indicated for elbow flexion, wrist flexion/extension, and digital flexion/extension
- Tendon transfers often preferred unless total plexus avulsion is present, requiring extraplexal neurotization (nerve transfers)[5,9]
- **Donor muscles:** Gracilis, rectus, or contralateral latissimus dorsi
- Double gracilis transfer (Doi procedure) provides shoulder stability and function, as well as elbow flexion and extension, hand sensation, and grasp.

### Arthrodesis

- Shoulder fusion
- Small-joint arthrodesis and tendon transfers to improve hand prehensile function, wrist fusion, and thumb fusion

## POSTOPERATIVE CARE[1]

- Immobilization is limited to minimize joint stiffness and scars or adhesions.
- Prefabricated splint is used for immobilization based on specific surgery.
  - Timing varies from 10-14 days (take tension off of nerve grafts).
  - It is worn for 14-21 days with direct nerve repair.
  - Protective splint is used for 6-8 weeks, then a sling for 1 more month.

- Initiate progressive therapy program based on surgery to increase passive range of motion (PROM) followed by increasing active range of motion (AROM) protocols.
- Tendon transfers require longer immobilization to allow healing of the tendon repair.

## TREATMENT OF BRACHIAL PLEXUS BIRTH PALSY[4,13,16,17]

### INITIAL

- Assess passive and active range of motion.
- Imaging is generally **not needed.**
- Assess shoulder stability: Patients may develop posterior humeral subluxation.
- Primitive reflexes (Moro, asymmetrical tonic neck, symmetrical tonic neck) may be used to assess motor function.
  - Moro reflex: Lifting then rapidly lowering baby on back will cause spreading of the arms following by unspreading.
  - Symmetrical/asymmetrical tonic neck: Turning the head to the side will cause the arm/leg on that side to straighten and the arm/leg on the opposite side to flex (also known as the *fencing reflex*).
- Focus on physical therapy to preserve range of motion and prevent contracture.
  - Scapular stabilization
  - Passive glenohumeral mobilization
  - Requires supervised home program with professional monitoring

### INDICATIONS FOR SURGERY

- For global lesions and infants with Horner's syndrome, perform surgery by 3 months of age.
- With absence of antigravity biceps function, perform surgery by 3-6 months (exact age is controversial).
- With partial recovery, decision to perform nerve grafting versus tendon transfers is controversial.
- Patients need to be followed longitudinally, because they may require tendon transfer or shoulder treatment at later ages.

### SURGICAL PROCEDURES

- Exploration with neurolysis, resection of neuroma, and nerve grafting (using sural nerve) is the standard treatment.
- Direct repair is generally not possible.
- Depending on surgeon preference, nerve transfers may be used.
  - Provides advantage of being closer to target muscle, allowing earlier innervations
  - Requires only a single microsurgical interface
- Priorities include shoulder stabilization and elbow function. There are a variety of options.
  - Spinal accessory nerve to suprascapular nerve
  - Long head of triceps motor branch to axillary nerve
  - Flexor carpi ulnaris branch of ulnar nerve to biceps motor (Oberlin transfer)
  - Intercostal nerve transfer
  - Medial pectoral nerve to myocutaneous nerve
  - C7 nerve transfer from same or opposite side
  - Unlike in adults, repairs to the lower trunk have a much higher chance of success. Some advocate repair of the median nerve to restore hand function.

## Shoulder Problems in BPBP[17]

- Up to 35% of infants with BPBP will develop shoulder weakness, contracture, or joint deformity.
- Internal rotation contractures are common and caused by **weakness in infraspinatus and teres minor.**
- Internal rotators receive dual innervation and are less affected.
- Glenohumeral joint dysplasia and joint instability may develop.
  - Glenoid retroversion
  - Humeral head flattening and posterior subluxation
    - **Waters classification**[4]
      - **Grade 1:** Normal
      - **Grade 2:** Posterior glenoid deformity
      - **Grade 3:** Humeral head subluxation
      - **Grade 4:** Formation of a posterior false glenoid
      - **Grade 5:** Flattening of both glenoid and humeral head
  - Imaging may be used when joint dysplasia suspected.
    - MRI is most commonly used.
    - CT has drawback of radiation exposure.
    - Ultrasound is fast, cheap, and can assess dynamic stability, but requires skilled operator.
    - Radiographs are generally less useful because of the cartilaginous nature of the pediatric humeral head.
- **Surgical management**
  - **Indications**
    - Dislocation
    - Persistent internal rotation contracture
    - Limitation of abduction or external rotation
    - Glenohumeral deformity
  - **Principles**
    - Release contracture
    - Rebalance muscles
    - Joint reduction
  - **Treatment options**
    - Botulinum toxin A
      - Used after tendon lengthening or alone with serial casting
    - Myotendinous lengthening or capsular release
      - Indication: Contracture
      - May be performed open or arthroscopically
    - Transfer of the teres major and latissimus dorsi to rotator cuff **(Hoffer/Sever-L'Espiscopo transfer)**
      - Will improve both external rotation and shoulder abduction
    - Derotational humeral osteotomy
      - Indicated for older patients with advanced shoulder deformity

**TIP:** Intraarticular release, combined with tendon transfers, may allow glenohumeral joint remodeling.

## OUTCOMES

### ADULT TRAUMATIC BRACHIAL PLEXUS*

- With traumatic brachial plexus injury, some degree of arm impairment is expected even in the best cases.
- Better results are seen with more distal lesions (closer to target muscle).
- Motor nerve transfers are commonly superior to nerve grafts, especially proximal lesions, with muscle grades ranging from 4 to 5 on the British Medical Research Council (MRC) scale for biceps flexion.[18]
- Outcomes are better for postganglionic lesions over avulsion injuries (outcomes for injuries involving upper roots even better).
- Postoperative muscle strength is higher in younger patients (≤20 years).
- 78% of patients (compared with 90% of general population) are content with quality of life after reconstruction, although some reported a negative impact in the workplace.[7]
- Job satisfaction was rated as moderate to high in 75% of this group.

### INFANTS WITH BPBP[4,13,16]

- Infants with BPBP who recover antigravity strength in first 2 months of life should have full neurologic recovery by 2 years of age.
- Infants with BPBP who recover biceps function by 6 months with later tendon transfers should be expected to reach grade 4 for all Mallet classes.

**TIP:** Good functional recovery requires a motivated patient; an expert surgical team that performs properly indicated, timely, and well-executed procedures; and appropriate postoperative rehabilitation.

## KEY POINTS

- ✓ Treatment of brachial plexus injuries requires a team-based approach by experienced practitioners. Early referral is essential, especially given the time-sensitive nature of many of the reconstructive options.
- ✓ Most causes of brachial plexus problems are nonobstetric, closed injuries from MVCs or MCCs in young adult men.
- ✓ An initial observation period of 3 months for closed injuries is acceptable. If positive recovery is observed, then continue periodic reevaluation with physical examination and electrodiagnostic testing.
- ✓ Patients must be carefully selected (i.e., highly motivated, compliant, and cognitively aware of lengthy rehabilitation protocol and limitations of functional outcomes).
- ✓ The primary functional goal should be elbow flexion, followed by shoulder abduction.
- ✓ Tendon transfers, functional free-tissue transfers, and small- and large-joint arthrodesis (shoulder and wrist) play significant roles in treatment when functional recovery is poor.

*References 1, 5, 8, 14, 15, 18.

## REFERENCES


1. Spinner R, Shin AY, Hebert-Blouin M, et al. Traumatic brachial plexus injury. In Wolfe SW, Hotchkiss RN, Pederson WC, et al, eds. Green's Operative Hand Surgery, 6th ed. Philadelphia: Elsevier, 2010.
2. Alnot JY. Traumatic brachial plexus lesions in the adult. Indications and results. Hand Clin 11:623-631, 1995.
3. Brunelli GA, Brunelli GR. Preoperative assessment of the adult plexus patient. Microsurgery 16:17-21,1995.
4. Waters PM. Pediatric brachial plexus palsy. In Wolfe SW, Hotchkiss RN, Pederson WC, et al, eds. Green's Operative Hand Surgery, 6th ed. Philadelphia: Elsevier, 2010.
5. Giuffre JL, Kakar S, Bishop AT, et al. Current concepts of the treatment of adult brachial plexus injuries. J Hand Surg 35:678-688, 2010.
6. Roger B, Travers V, Laval-Jeantet M. Imaging of posttraumatic brachial plexus injury. Clin Orthop Relat Res 237:57-61, 1988.
7. Terzis J, Vekris MD, Soucacos PN. Brachial plexus. In Achauer BH, Eriksson E, Guyuron B, et al. Plastic Surgery: Indications, Operations, and Outcomes, vol 4. St Louis: Mosby–Year Book, 2000.
8. Tung TH, Mackinnon SE. Brachial plexus injuries. Clin Plast Surg 30:269-287, 2003.
9. Terzis JK, Papakonstantinou KC. The surgical treatment of brachial plexus injuries in adults. Plast Reconstr Surg 106:1097-1122, 2000.
10. Mackinnon SE, Dellon AL. Surgery of the Peripheral Nerve. New York: Thieme, 1988.
11. Chuang DC. Neurotization procedures for brachial plexus injuries. Hand Clin 11:633-645, 1995.
12. Merrell GA, Barrie KA, Katz DL, et al. Results of nerve transfer techniques for restoration of shoulder and elbow function in the context of a meta-analysis of the English literature. J Hand Surg 26:303-314, 2001.
13. Shenaq SM, Kim JY, Armenta AH, et al. The surgical treatment of obstetric brachial plexus palsy. Plast Reconstr Surg 113:54E-67E, 2004.
14. Shin AY, Spinner RJ, Steinmann SP, et al. Adult traumatic brachial plexus injuries. J Am Acad Orthop Surg 13:382-396, 2005.
15. Lee SK, Wolfe SW. Nerve transfers for the upper extremity: new horizons in nerve reconstruction. J Am Acad Orthop Surg 20:506-517, 2012.
16. Hale HB, Bae DS, Waters PM. Current concepts in the management of brachial plexus birth palsy. J Hand Surg 35:322-331, 2010.
17. Pearl ML. Shoulder problems in children with brachial plexus birth palsy: evaluation and management. J Am Acad Orthop Surg 17:242-254, 2009.
18. Tomaino MM. Nonobstetric brachial plexus injuries. J Am Soc Surg Hand 1:135-153, 2001.

# 80. Nerve Injuries

Ashkan Ghavami, Prosper Benhaim, Charles F. Kallina IV

## ANATOMY AND PHYSIOLOGY[1] (Fig. 80-1)

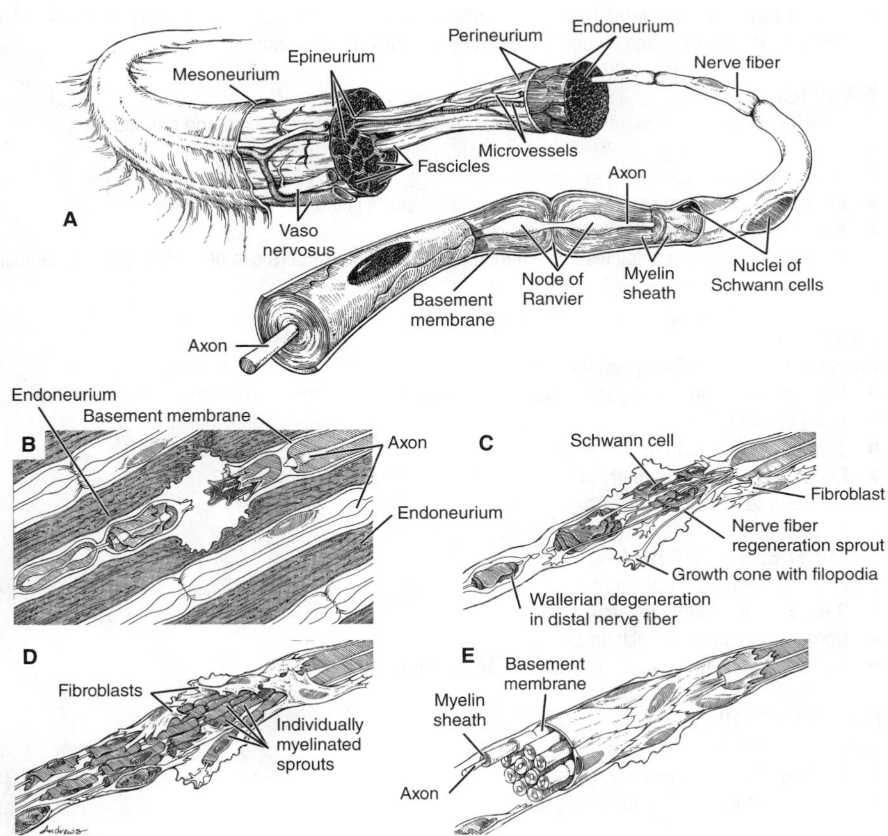


**Fig. 80-1** Nerve anatomy and regeneration. **A,** The normal nerve consists of myelinated and unmyelinated axons. **B,** When a myelinated axon is injured, degeneration occurs distally and for a variable distance proximally. **C,** Multiple regenerating fibers sprout from the proximal axon, forming a regenerating unit. A growth cone at the tip of each regenerating fiber samples the environment and advances the growth process distally. **D,** Schwann cells eventually myelinate the regenerating fibers. **E,** Because it is from a single nerve fiber, a regenerating unit that contains several fibers is formed, and each fiber is capable of functional connections.

## Axons

- Peripheral nerve axons are surrounded by **endoneurium;** loose gelatinous collagen matrix, minimal tensile strength

## Schwann Cell

- Surrounds individual **myelinated** axons (produces myelin), or surrounds several unmyelinated axons

## Node of Ranvier

*Gap at junction between Schwann cells*

- Allows **rapid nerve conduction:** Action potential depolarization jumps from one node of Ranvier to the next (3-150 m/sec versus 2-2.5 m/sec for unmyelinated axons)

## Fascicles

*Grouped arrangement of axons with endoneurium surrounding each axon and perineurium surrounding each fascicle*

- Invested by internal (inner) epineurium
- Logistically the smallest unit that can be treated surgically
- Interconnect and branch proximally[2]
  - Makes matching fascicles more difficult proximally, but fibers can be adjacent in a fascicular group

## Perineurium

*Connective tissue encircling each fascicle*

- Selective permeability (tight junctions that create a blood-nerve barrier, similar to the blood-brain barrier)
- Thin but dense; high tensile strength
- Encircled by internal (inner) epineurium
  - Sutured in *fascicular repair*

## Outer Epineurium

*Outer sheath of peripheral nerve*

- Sutured in *epineurial repair*
- Contains collagen and elastin fibers
- Surrounded by loose areolar tissue (mesoneurium)

## Mesoneurium

*Outer adventitial layer of nerve*

- Incorporated in epineurial repair
- Critical for nerve excursion and gliding

## Blood Supply

- **Arteriae nervosum (vaso nervosus)**
  - Enter nerve segmentally
  - Divide into longitudinal superficial branches in epineurium
  - Help guide proper orientation of nerve ends during repair
- **Extrinsic vessels** supply intrinsic longitudinal vessels in epineurium, which communicate with capillary plexus in perineurium

- **Capillary plexus**
  - Enters the endoneurium obliquely
  - Becomes occluded if endoneurial pressure rises because of injury (crush, edema)

### MARTIN-GRUBER ANASTOMOSIS

- **Motor connections between median and ulnar nerves in forearm,** or distally between anterior interosseous nerve and ulnar branches
- Present in up to **17%** of the population
- **May mask the actual site of nerve injury** (e.g., a median nerve injury at elbow level with loss of all intrinsic muscle function, even though the ulnar nerve is intact)

### RICHE-CANNIEU ANASTOMOSIS

- **Motor connections between median and ulnar nerves in *palm***
- Present in up to **70%** of the population[3]
- **Can mask injury pattern**

### FROMENT-RAUBER ANASTOMOSIS

- **From radial nerve (either posterior interosseous nerve or superficial radial nerve) to ulnar motor branches innervating the first, second, or third dorsal interosseous muscles**
- Rare
- Can mask injury pattern

### BERRETTINI CONNECTION

- **Sensory connections between the ulnar and median nerves in the palm**
- Usually travels deep to the superficial volar arch or immediately distal to the carpal tunnel
- Present in approximately **80%** of all cadaver specimens
- Can produce confusing findings in physical examination for nerve injury

## PATHOPHYSIOLOGY[4]

### WALLERIAN DEGENERATION

- Nerve stump undergoes degeneration **distal** to axonotomy.
- Cytoplasmic calcium increases.
- Macrophages proliferate; myelin phagocytosis.
- Schwann cells proliferate and myelin breaks down.
- Schwann cells and macrophages replace neural tube and organize into ***bands of Bunger,*** providing a scaffold for regenerating axons.

### CHROMATOLYSIS

- Mechanism of **proximal** neuronal cell body damage
- Axonal degeneration of axons in proximal stump
- **Growth cone** formed by individual axons creating numerous axonal sprouts (5-24 hours after injury)

## Growth Cone

- Filopodia in cone explore neural tube and find correct distal stump by contact guidance and neurotropic factors.
- If incorrect distal stump and target organ are reached, sprouts are denied factors necessary for maturation.
- Approximately **50%** of axonal sprouts make incorrect connections.

## Neurotropism

- Chemotactic gradient toward proper distal stump that attracts regenerating axon toward correct end target.
- Neurotropic factors are released from distal target.

## Neurotrophism

- Trophic (nutritional) support provided to axons connecting with correct distal stump: Nerve growth factor (NGF), epidermal growth factor (EGF), insulin-like growth factor (IGF) I and II, etc.

## Double Crush Syndrome

- Nerve entrapment at one location can predispose to clinical nerve compression more distally.
- Endoneurial edema at a proximal level can affect axonal transport and blood supply to nerve distally.

## Etiologic Factors in Nerve Injuries

- Compression
- Tension, stretch
- Laceration

## Muscle Denervation

- Results in atrophy and interstitial fibrosis that is complete by 2-3 years after injury
- **Best reinnervation within 3 months of injury**
- Denervated muscles lose **1% of motor endplates per week.** A minimum of **25%** of motor endplates are required for functional muscle contraction.
  - A repaired nerve will regenerate at **1 mm/day** or roughly **1 inch/month.**
- Time for regenerating nerve to reach target muscle must be calculated in context of motor endplate degeneration.
- Functional reinnervation possible up to **1 year after injury**
- **No reinnervation possible 2-3 years after injury**
- Outcome worse with **advanced age** (>40 years old) and **disuse**

## Sensory End Organs

- Best results seen in patients **less than 20 years old,** as with all nerve injuries
- **Mechanism**
  - Native nerve regeneration not required
  - Axonal collateral sprouting from adjacent axons present, allowing increased chance of successful reinnervation

- Delayed repairs (after more than 1 year): Only protective sensation achieved
- **Sunderland and Seddon classifications**[5] (Table 80-1)

**Table 80-1** *Two Classification Systems of Nerve Injuries*

| Seddon | Sunderland | Disrupted Structure | Prognosis |
|---|---|---|---|
| Neurapraxia | 1st degree | Axon (minimal) | Complete return in days or months |
| Axonotmesis | 2nd degree | Axon (total, Wallerian degeneration) | Complete return in months |
| Neurotmesis | 3rd degree | Axon, endoneurium | Mild/moderate reduction in function |
| Neurotmesis | 4th degree | Axon, endoneurium, perineurium | Moderate reduction in function |
| Neurotmesis | 5th degree | All structures | Marked reduction in functional return |

## DIAGNOSIS

Diagnosing nerve injuries requires taking a complete history of the injury, performing accurate testing, and recording sensory and motor deficits.

### Tinel's Sign

- Tapping over distal area of injury produces paresthesia.
- Axonal regeneration is suggested.

### Two-Point Discrimination (2PD)

- **Test of innervation density; most applicable for nerve injuries, less reliable in compression neuropathies**
- **Static 2PD:** Up to 6 mm is normal for volar fingertip.
- **Moving 2PD:** 2-3 mm is normal when testing perpendicular to digit, moving longitudinally (proximal to distal).
- Must stay on ulnar and radial sides *without crossing over,* otherwise false results may occur from contralateral side of digit.

### Vibration Thresholds

- Very sensitive test

### Semmes-Weinstein Monofilament

- Measures pressure thresholds; most applicable for compression neuropathies, but also abnormal in complete nerve injuries
- Expensive and time-consuming, but very sensitive
- Can be performed early

### Pick-Up Test

- Performed during sensation reeducation

### Daily-Living Task Performance

- Used in rehabilitation protocols

### Electrodiagnostic Studies

- Electromyogram (EMG) and/or nerve conduction velocity (NCV)
  - When unable to arrive at accurate diagnosis
  - NCV testing early after a nerve injury cannot distinguish neurapraxia from complete nerve injury; recommendation is to wait at least 2-6 weeks before obtaining NCV[6]

## SURGICAL PRINCIPLES[7]

### Open Injury Repair

- **Primary**
  - Within first 24 hours
  - Best for sharp lacerations, clean wounds, minimal to no crush component, no significant soft tissue damage
- **Delayed primary**
  - Within 1 week
  - Initial exploration to reveal previously listed contraindications for primary repair
  - Zone of injury allowed sufficient time to declare itself
- **Secondary**
  - Delay of more than 1 week
  - Unstable skeletal extremity
  - Significant vascular compromise
  - Associated life-threatening injuries
  - Delayed repair may eliminate possibility for direct nerve repair (nerve fibrosis, retraction, loss of compliance); may require nerve grafting

### Closed or Blunt Injury

- **Unexplored, closed injuries**
  - Waiting period of more than 6 weeks before electrodiagnostics employed
  - Reevaluation at 12 weeks with repeat of tests; expectation of regeneration at approximately 1 mm/day; if recovery still incomplete, tests repeated
- **Operative exploration**
  - Indicated at 3 months when no clinical or electrical signs of reinnervation present (e.g., motor unit potentials)

## NERVE REPAIR: TECHNICAL CONSIDERATIONS

### Principles of Nerve Repair[8]

- Quantitative preoperative and postoperative assessment of sensory and motor function
- Microsurgical technique
- Primary repair when possible
- Tension-free repair
- Interpositional nerve grafts, nerve allografts, vein conduits, or synthetic nerve conduits (when necessary)
- Avoidance of excessive postural movement
- Secondary repair if zone of injury indeterminate
- Sensory and motor reeducation

## Microsurgical Principles

- Adequate magnification is required.
  - An operative microscope is preferred over surgical loupes (microscope up to 25×, loupes up to 2.5-6× magnification).
  - Use 8-0, 9-0, or 10-0 interrupted monofilament nylon sutures.
- Cut back nerve ends to healthy tissue with a No. 15 or No. 11 blade against a rigid background (sterile tongue-blade works well).
- For soft end-to-end fascicle contact, trim fascicles that protrude outward.
- When motor-sensory topography is unclear:
  - Can use electrical stimulation tests of distal nerve stump (motor) or proximal nerve stump (sensory) intraoperatively if injury is acute
  - Immunohistochemical staining: Rarely clinically feasible—time-consuming and expensive
- Proximal and distal nerve can be safely mobilized for 1-2 cm (4%-25% of nerve length) to allow increased length and decreased tension on repair.[2,4]
  - Less mobilization is feasible in digits.
- Avoid excessive postural maneuvering to release tension.
  - Do not hesitate to use other options (e.g., nerve autograft, nerve allograft, vein graft, conduit) as indicated.

# NERVE REPAIR OPTIONS[9] (Fig. 80-2)

## Perineurial (Fascicular) Repair

**NOTE: The superiority of perineurial repair over epineurial repair is not established.[1,5] However, it is more appropriate for nerves with fewer than five fascicles and for nerve grafting.**

- **Advantages**
  - More nerve stump myelination potential
  - Better perineurial tube alignment, more regenerating axons enter distal nerve, greater sensory and motor end-organ recovery[2]

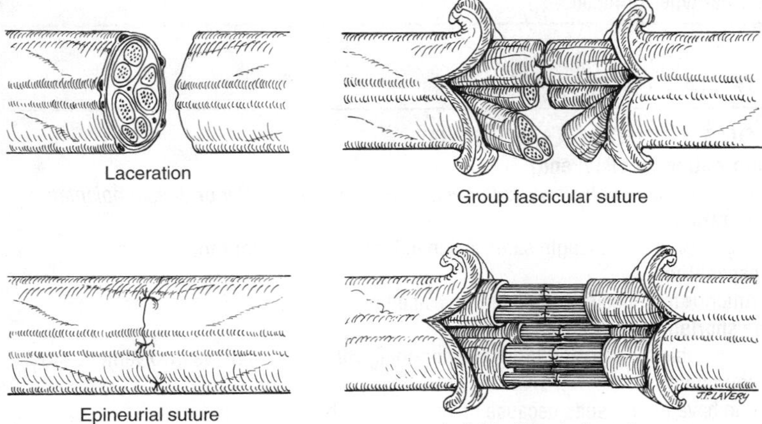


**Fig. 80-2** Nerve suturing techniques.

- **Disadvantages**
  - Longer operative times
  - Increased fibrosis at repair
  - Potential vascular compromise
  - Suture crowding
  - Potential for fascicular mismatch

### Group Fascicular Repair

- **Indicated when nerve transection is at level where well-formed sensory and motor branches are easily identified**
- **Examples**[2]:
  - **Median nerve:** 5 cm above wrist crease to end point in palm and several centimeters below elbow
  - **Ulnar nerve:** 7-8 cm proximal to wrist crease

### Epineurial Repair

- **Best for digital nerves**
- Outcomes similar to other types of nerve repair[10]
- **Advantages**
  - Short operative time
  - Technically simple
  - Less magnification requirement
  - Intraneural tissue not violated; less scarring
  - Good for primary and secondary repairs
- **Disadvantages**
  - May compromise specific fascicular alignment
  - Tension from retraction of cut nerve ends
  - Multiple sutures may be needed

> **TIP:** In general, no differences in outcomes have been seen when comparing epineurial repair with other types of repair.

## NERVE GAP OPTIONS[11]

### Options Without Grafting[5]

- **Neurotization (of distal end)**
  - *Direct implantation closer to target muscle by nerve transfer or direct implantation*
- **Mobilization**
  - 4%-25% of nerve length safe[5,12]; general rule of 1-2 cm for most nerves
- **Transposition**
  - Anterior transposition of ulnar nerve at elbow
- **Bone shortening**
  - Acceptable for digit and humeral shortening with multiple nerve involvement and comminution
  - Can have poor results because of alterations in biomechanics

## Nerve Grafting

- **Autografts**
  - *Gold standard*
  - **Indication**
    - When end-to-end coaptation is under tension
  - **Ideal donor nerve**
    - Produces noncritical sensory deficit
    - Contains long, unbranched segments
    - Easily accessible
    - Overall, small diameter with large fascicles and few interfascicular connections
  - **Common donor nerves**
    - **Sural nerve** (30-40 cm)
      - **Most commonly used purely sensory nerve**
    - **Lateral antebrachial cutaneous nerve** (5-8 cm)
      - Preferred over medial antebrachial branch
    - Anterior branch of **medial antebrachial cutaneous nerve** (10-20 cm)
      - Good for digital nerve gaps longer than 1 cm
      - Can have hypersensitivity, dysesthesia of donor site
    - **Posterior interosseous nerve** (distal segment, terminal filament purely sensory)
      - Easily accessible on same extremity

## Vascularized Nerve Grafts[13]

- Best for **extensive recipient bed scarring** and devascularity (e.g., radiation injury)
- Very large donor nerve needed
  - Examples: Nonfunctional ulnar nerve sensory branch in proximal forearm or deep peroneal nerve

## Autogenous Interpositional Vein Graft

- Less 2PD than with direct repair or nerve autograft
- **Common indication:** Small gaps of **less than 3 cm** in nonessential peripheral sensory nerves
  - Good for zone II injuries
- Can collapse in center, leading to mechanical obstruction of regenerating nerve fibers

## Muscle Graft

- Muscle fascicles used directly as interposition graft
- Not commonly used
- Good results for sensory nerves in acute settings[5]

## Allografts

- Require appropriate pretreatment, preservation, and host immunosuppression
- When neural regeneration complete, elements within allograft are entirely of host origin, therefore immunosuppression needed only temporarily

## Processed Nerve Allografts[14]

- Decellularized and predegenerated human nerve tissue, so immune response is absent
- Maintenance of microarchitecture of nerve tissue and is rapidly revascularized
- Outcomes superior to conduit use
- Good to excellent results in 75% of cases, particularly for sensory deficits, with gaps between 5 and 50 mm

### Synthetic Nerve Conduits

- **Short distances (<3 cm)**
- Noncritical sensory areas
- Patients who decline autogenous harvest[12]
- Preliminary results good

### Nerve Transfers

- Noncritical motor or sensory unit used to reconstruct important missing function
- **Indications**[12,15,16]
  - Brachial plexus injuries with no proximal nerve for grafting
  - Proximal nerve injuries requiring long distance for regeneration
  - Scarred bed in area with critical neurovascular structures
  - Major limb trauma with loss of nerve segment
  - Older injury and/or older patient
- Common nerve transfers: See Chapter 79

### End-to-Side Repair

- For sensory nerve injury having distal end without proximal neuronal source
- Worse outcomes than for primary repair and autograft
- Not indicated for motor nerves

## POSTOPERATIVE CARE

- To protect the repair, the splint is placed in the OR without excessive postural positioning.
- Wounds should be examined within 1 week.
- Immobilization is continued for 2-4 weeks; then the splint is readjusted for protection, with joint position as close to optimal as possible.

### Rehabilitation

- **Early (2-4 weeks)**
  - Mobilization proceeds with active, active-assisted, then passive range-of-motion exercises to avoid joint stiffness.
- **Late**
  - Seek sensory and motor reeducation.
  - Begin as soon as patient is able to perceive any type of sensory stimulus.
- **Sensory reeducation stages**
  1. Desensitization
  2. Early phase discrimination and localization
  3. Late phase discrimination and tactic gnosis

## SECONDARY PROCEDURES[15]

- Internal neurolysis
- Recoaptation of the nerve
- Bypass nerve grafting
- Neuroma excision[13,15]
  - Usually at 3-4 months
  - Electrodiagnostic studies and clinical examination: Can include **nonprogressing Tinel's sign,** lack of functional recovery

- Exploration indicated with or without intraoperative stimulation testing
- Painful neuromas: If critical sensory region and distal nerve available, consider nerve autograft rather than excision with intramuscular or intraosseous transposition
  - Transposition (into bone, muscle) away from contact surface preferred with complete transections
- Neuroma-in-continuity[5,17]
  - Lateral neuromas: Consider partial resection and perineurial repair of involved fascicles
  - Spindle-shaped neuromas: If fascicles in continuity, internal neurolysis required; if complete transection, resection and coaptation warranted

# OUTCOMES

## EVALUATION OF MOTOR AND SENSORY FUNCTION

- British Medical Research Council (MRC) grading system very useful

**Box 80-1** *HIGHET'S METHOD OF END-RESULT EVALUATION AS MODIFIED BY DELLON ET AL*

| | |
|---|---|
| **Motor Recovery** | |
| M0 | No contraction |
| M1 | Return of perceptible contraction on both proximal muscles |
| M2 | Return of perceptible contraction in both proximal and distal muscles |
| M3 | Return of function in both proximal and distal muscles to degree that all important muscles are sufficiently powerful to act against gravity |
| M4 | Return of function as with stage M3; in addition, all synergistic and independent movements possible |
| M5 | Complete recovery |
| **Sensory Recovery** | |
| S0 | Absence of sensory recovery |
| S1 | Recovery of deep cutaneous pain sensibility within autonomous area of nerve |
| S2 | Return of some degree of superficial cutaneous pain and tactile sensibility with autonomous area of nerve |
| S3 | Return of superficial cutaneous pain and tactile sensibility throughout autonomous area, with disappearance of any previous overresponse |
| S3+ | Return of sensibility as with stage S3; in addition, discrimination within autonomous area (7-15 mm) |
| S4 | Complete recovery (2-point discrimination, 2-6 mm) |

In the hand, proximal muscles are defined as extrinsic and distal muscles are intrinsic.

## SPECIFIC NERVES

- **Median:** Good to excellent results of motor component and sensation at wrist level; good to excellent results seen in more than one third of forearm-level repairs
  - Grafting: Fair to good results

- **Ulnar:** Less favorable, especially the motor component because need accurate reinnervation of distal intrinsics
  - Sensory recovery better than motor function recovery
- **Radial:** Poor results, with motor function poorer than sensation
  - M4 recovery in 20%-40% of patients[15]
- **Digital:** 2PD variable
  - Up to 95% of patients are S3 or better with autogenous nerve grafting[15]

## Key Points

- ✓ Presence of Martin-Gruber and/or Riche-Cannieu connections can mask injury and confuse diagnosis. Explore laceration or wound when in doubt.
- ✓ Epineurial repair provides equivalent results in most situations, compared with other types of repair.
- ✓ Avoid tension on repair and be prepared to perform nerve autograft (or conduit/processed allograft, if appropriate) when gap exceeds 1-3 cm.
- ✓ Criteria for optimal results:
  - Age, less than 20 years old
  - Early repair—less than 3 months best
  - Distal injury
- ✓ Immobilization for 2-3 weeks, followed by a consistent rehabilitation program is key for successful treatment.
- ✓ Sensory recovery is often better than motor recovery.
- ✓ Follow results with clinical and electrophysiologic testing.
- ✓ If motor recovery is poor by 6 months to 1 year, consider appropriate tendon transfer(s).

## References


1. Brandt KE, Mackinnon SE. Microsurgical repair of peripheral nerves and nerve grafts. In Aston JS, Beasley RW, Thorne CM, eds. Grabb and Smith's Plastic Surgery, 5th ed. New York: Lippincott-Raven, 1997.
2. Jabaley ME. Current concepts of nerve repair. Clin Plast Surg 8:33-44, 1981.
3. Harness D, Sekeles E. The double anastomotic innervation of thenar muscles. J Anat 109:461-466, 1971.
4. Maggi SP, Lowe JB III, Mackinnon SE. Pathophysiology of nerve injury. Clin Plast Surg 30:109-126, 2003.
5. Gutowski KA. Hand II: peripheral nerve and tendon transfers. Sel Read Plast Surg 9:1-19, 2003.
6. Parry GJ. Electrodiagnostic studies in the evaluation of peripheral nerve and brachial plexus injuries. Neurol Clin 10:921, 1992.
7. Novak CB. Evaluation of the nerve-injured patient. Clin Plast Surg 30:127-138, 2003.
8. Watchmaker GP, Mackinnon SE. Advances in peripheral nerve repair. Clin Plast Surg 24:63-73, 1997.
9. Brushart T. Nerve repair and grafting. In Green DP, Hotchkiss RN, Pederson WC, eds. Green's Operative Hand Surgery, vol 2, 4th ed. Philadelphia: Churchill Livingstone, 1998.
10. Young L, Wray RC, Weeks PM. A randomized prospective comparison of fascicular and epineural digital nerve repairs. Plast Reconstr Surg 68:89-93, 1981.

11. Millesi H. The nerve gap: theory and clinical practice. Hand Clin 2:651-663, 1986.
12. Dvali L, Mackinnon SE. Nerve repair, grafting, and nerve transfers. Clin Plast Surg 30:203-221, 2003.
13. Taylor GI, Ham FJ. The free vascularized nerve graft. A further experimental and clinical application of microvascular techniques. Plast Reconstr Surg 57:413-426, 1976.
14. Cho MS, Rinker BD, Weber RV, et al. Functional outcome following nerve repair in the upper extremity using processed nerve allograft. J Hand Surg Am 37:2340-2349, 2012.
15. Mackinnon SE, Dellon AL. Surgery of the Peripheral Nerve. New York: Thieme, 1988.
16. Maser BM, Vedder N. Nerve repair and nerve grafting. In Achauer BM, Eriksson E, Guyuron B, et al, eds. Plastic Surgery: Indications, Operations, and Outcomes, vol 4. St Louis: Mosby, 2000.
17. Vernadakis AJ, Koch H, Mackinnon SE. Management of neuromas. Clin Plast Surg 30:247-268, 2003.

# 81. Hand Infections

**Tarik M. Husain, Bishr Hijazi, Blake A. Morrison**

## MICROBIOLOGY

- *Staphylococcus aureus* is the most common pathogen.
- *Streptococcus* spp are the next most common pathogens.
- **Immunocompromised hosts** are more likely to have gram-negative anaerobes or unusual organisms cultured.

> **TIP:** Before initiating antibiotic treatment, **obtain cultures** using careful antiseptic techniques. Include aerobic, anaerobic, mycobacterial, and fungal cultures.

- Mycobacterial and fungal infections are relatively common in chronic infections.

> **TIP:** If possible, avoid aspirating through an area of erythema to minimize risk of seeding a potentially sterile environment.

- **Methicillin-resistant *S. aureus* (MRSA)** is the most common community-acquired organism in *S. aureus* infections (60%).[1] If resistance is common in your area, **treat for MRSA until cultures are identified.**

> **TIP:** Many strains of MRSA are susceptible to trimethoprim/sulfamethoxazole, clindamycin, doxycycline, rifampin, tetracycline, and erythromycin, among others.

## MEDICAL CONDITIONS WITH INCREASED RISK

- **Diabetes mellitus**
  - 7% of adults in United States have diabetes.[2]
  - 17% incidence of undiagnosed diabetes in patients treated for infections of the extremities[3]
  - Higher rates of deep space infections, amputations, and necrotizing fasciitis
  - Hyperglycemia impairs polymorphonuclear (PMN) cell function and favors bacterial proliferation.
  - Peripheral neuropathy may delay presentation.
  - Mechanism for increased susceptibility
    - Lymphocyte dysfunction: Less capable of fighting infection
    - Decreased chemotaxis
    - Decreased phagocytosis
    - Decreased intracellular bactericidal activity

**NOTE: Diabetes with renal failure is especially morbid, with up to 100% amputation rates reported for extremity infection.[4]**

- **Immunosuppressive conditions**
  - AIDS
  - Major debilitating medical conditions (e.g., liver disease, hematologic disease, or neoplasms)
  - Transplant patients
  - Patients with autoimmune disorders
- **Alcohol and drug abuse**
- **Malnutrition**
- **Renal failure**
- **Occupational or other behavioral factors that increase risk**
  - Dentists, dental hygienists, or others exposed to oral secretions: **Herpetic whitlow**
  - Dishwashers: **Chronic paronychia**
  - Nail biting: **Paronychia**

## EVOLUTION AND BASICS OF TREATMENT

### HISTORY

- There is almost always a history of minor trauma, such as a splinter, penetrating injury, or a bite.
- Look for a history of systemic disease such as diabetes.
- Determine tetanus status.

### PHYSICAL EXAMINATION

- Expose and examine the entire upper extremity.
  - Notice discoloration, edema, discharge, or lymphatic streaking; palpate for swelling, lymph node enlargement, or temperature change.
  - Compare results with opposite extremity, using it as a control.

### RADIOLOGY

- At minimum, obtain radiographs.
- Ultrasound, CT scan, and/or bone scan may be considered in specific situations.
- MRI (with contrast) is most useful to evaluate for fluid collection.
- Review for possible foreign bodies.
- Review for signs of osteomyelitis (periosteal reaction).
- Review for gas in the soft tissues (gas gangrene or necrotizing fasciitis).

### SURGICAL PRINCIPLES

- Tourniquet should be used but **only with gravity exsanguinations,** because Esmarch wrapping may predispose to bacteremia.
- Surgical drainage is performed through large incision(s) that may be extended in almost any direction.
- Avoid longitudinal incisions across a flexion crease.
- Minimize exposure of blood vessels, nerves, and tendons if possible.
- Excise all necrotic tissue.
- Intraoperative cultures (Gram stain, aerobic/anaerobic/acid-fast bacilli [AFB]/fungal cultures)
- Copious irrigation: Best done with large saline bag via gravity and cystoscopy tubing
- Most wounds left open with moist gauze and/or wick
- Loose dressings and splint
- Early mobilization

## SPECIFIC INFECTIONS[5-7]

### CELLULITIS

Acute inflammation of the skin and subcutaneous tissues

- **Etiologic factors**
  - Usually caused by minor trauma such as a scratch or splinter
  - Usually by *S. aureus* or group A streptococcus
- **Diagnosis:** Pain, swelling, and erythema, without abscess formation
- **Treatment**
  - IV vancomycin as first-line antibiotic, given prevalence of MRSA[8,9]
  - Consider inpatient admission. Study investigating rate of admission for cellulitis after 24-hour observation period in emergency department has demonstrated a hand infection to be a significant risk factor (odds ratio 2.9).[10]
  - Consider IV antibiotics for diabetics or when complicated by lymphangitis.

> **TIP:** Monitor antibiotic treatment by encircling the visible cellulitic area using an indelible marker; erythema should retreat from the line centrally. Record date and time of marking.

    - Consider changing antibiotic therapy to a more aggressive second line if no response.
    - Obtain cultures in an area of fluctuance by aspiration.
    - Consider the possibility of deep abscess and the need for surgical drainage if antibiotic therapy is unsuccessful.
  - Warm soaks, splinting, and elevation are important adjuncts.

### PARONYCHIA[11,12]

An infection, including abscess, of the soft tissues surrounding the nail; occurs in acute and chronic forms

- **Acute infection**
  - **Etiologic factors**
    - **Most common infection type of the hand**
    - Associated with nail biting, poor manicure technique, or minor trauma
    - Usually *S. aureus,* occasionally anaerobes
  - **Diagnosis**
    - Patients present with pain, redness, and swelling around the nail.
    - Patients occasionally report drainage of pus.
  - **Treatment**
    - Early treatment: Warm soaks, oral antibiotics, rest.
    - Later treatment: Drainage of abscess.
    - Incise perionychial fold with blade directed away from nail bed and matrix.
    - Culture and place a small wick of gauze under the nail fold.
    - Prescribe oral antibiotics for 5-7 days (Bactrim, clindamycin, or doxycycline).
    - If unresponsive to oral antibiotics, consider IV antibiotics (vancomycin or clindamycin).
    - Start hydrotherapy in 24 hours at least twice a day.
    - If purulence is below nail plate, partial or complete nail plate removal may be required.
    - Pack to prevent premature closure.

- **Chronic infections**
  - **Etiologic factors**
    - **Usually fungal** *(Candida albicans),* occasionally *Pseudomonas* spp, or atypical mycobacteria
    - Associated with diabetes and chronic exposure to moisture (dishwashers, cafeteria workers)
  - **Diagnosis**
    - Indurated, erythematous eponychium
    - May have intermittent drainage, often a cheesy consistency
  - **Medical treatment**
    - Topical antifungals tried first
    - Eponychial marsupialization when conservative treatment fails
  - **Surgical treatment**[13] (Fig. 81-1)
    - A crescent-shaped portion of skin, proximal to eponychial fold, is excised.
    - Granulated tissue is removed.
    - Wound is allowed to close by secondary intention.

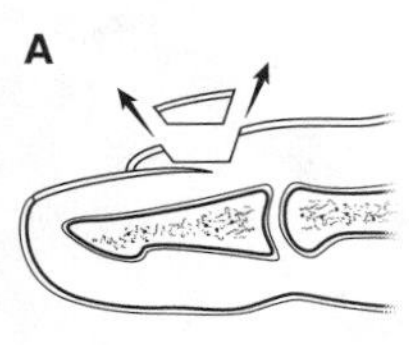


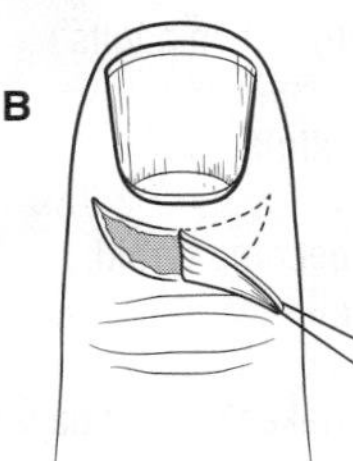


**Fig. 81-1** Eponychial marsupialization for chronic paronychia. **A,** Lateral view showing the area of wedge-shaped excision. Undisturbed matrix is stippled. **B,** Dorsal view of the crescent-shaped area of excision extending to the margins of the nail folds on each side.

## FELON[11,12]

An abscess of the pulp of the thumb or fingertip

- **Etiologic factors**
  - Typically, a felon occurs after a puncture wound.
  - *S. aureus* is the most common pathogen.
  - Gram-negative microbes are possible, particularly in immunocompromised patients.
- **Diagnosis**
  - Patients have a **red, swollen, fluctuant fingertip** that is exquisitely tender.
  - Patients often have throbbing pain that keeps them up at night.
- **Surgical treatment**
  - For an obvious pointing abscess, **open longitudinally over the point of maximum fluctuance.**
  - Otherwise use a **lateral incision over the midaxial line:** Ulnar for the index, middle, and ring fingers, but radial for the small finger and thumb.

**TIP: Avoid a fishmouth incision, because this may cause vascular compromise.**

- Pack loosely with gauze.
- Start sink hydrotherapy and daily dressing changes after 24-48 hours.
- Adjust antibiotics to culture results, when obtained.

**TIP:** Divide enough septa for thorough drainage, and stay dorsal to the neurovascular bundles.

## HERPETIC WHITLOW[14]

A **herpes simplex** infection of the hand

- Usually self-limited, 2- to 3-week course
- Anti-HSV antibodies present
- Unroofing vesicles may improve patient comfort
- **Etiologic factors**
  - Herpes simplex virus types 1 and 2
    - **HSV type** 1 more commonly affects young children and the medical and dental professionals in contact with saliva.
    - **HSV type 2** infections have been more common in adults.
- **Diagnosis**
  - Patients present with a **red, swollen, painful digit.**
  - The pulp is not as tense as with a felon.
  - **Clear vesicles** form, which may coalesce or become turbid.
  - Early diagnosis depends on clinical suspicion.
  - Perform Tzanck smear on fresh vesicles.
  - Viral cultures definitively establish diagnosis (takes several days).

**NOTE: A whitlow tends to mimic a felon.**

**TIP:** Whitlows and felons can usually be differentiated based on history. Whitlows have a prodromal phase of 24-72 hours of burning pain before skin changes develop.

**CAUTION: DO NOT incise these lesions (unless secondary bacterial infection is strongly suspected); there is risk of viral encephalitis or death.**

- **Treatment**
  - Unroofing a vesicle is acceptable to obtain viral cultures or a Tzanck smear, if the diagnosis is in doubt.
  - Treatment is nonsurgical. Keep digit covered with a dry dressing and avoid contact.
  - IV, oral, or topical antivirals may shorten course.
  - **Acyclovir** is used in severe cases, or for immunocompromised patients at risk for a life-threatening viremia.
  - **Advise patients that about 20% recur,** but these are typically less severe than the primary attack.
  - Misdiagnosis may lead to surgical intervention, which can result in viral encephalitis and/or death.
  - HIV-associated viral infections typically do not self-resolve.

## VOLAR/DEEP SPACE ABSCESSES

Abscess formation within one of the potential deep spaces of the hand. *Knowledge of anatomy is essential to treatment.*

- **Anatomy**
  - **Thenar**[15] (Figs. 81-2 and 81-3)
    - Floor (dorsal boundary): Adductor pollicis fascia
    - Superficial (volar boundary): Tendon sheath of index finger (IF) and volar fascia
    - Radial border: Adductor insertion on thumb P1
    - Ulnar border: Vertical midvolar septum

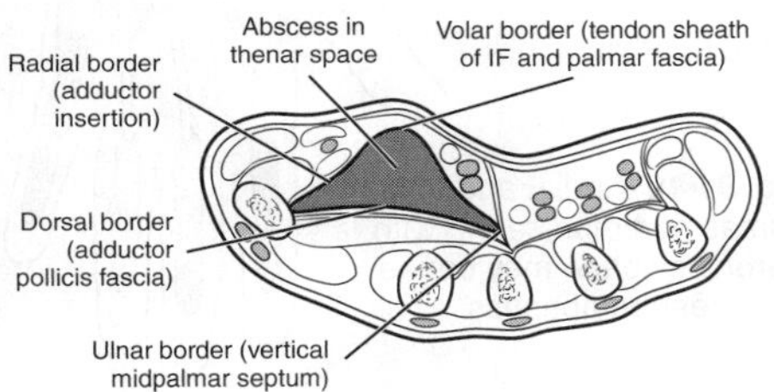


**Fig. 81-2** Thenar deep space abscess (deep to volar fascia).

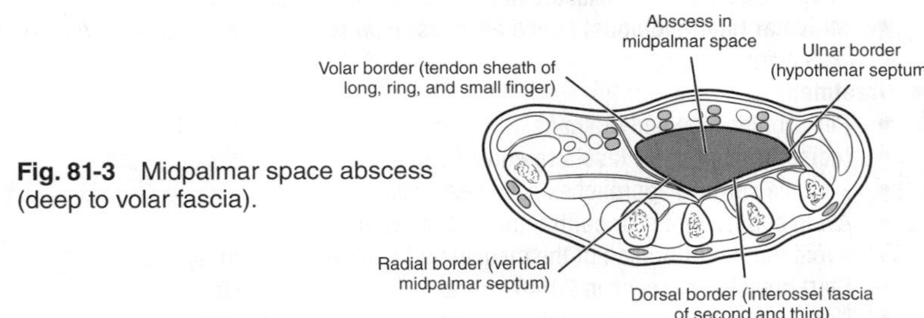


**Fig. 81-3** Midpalmar space abscess (deep to volar fascia).

  - **Midvolar**
    - Characterized by loss of volar concavity in area of midpalm between the thenar and hypothenar eminence
    - Floor (dorsal boundary): Interossei fascia of second and third
    - Superficial (volar boundary): Tendon sheath of long finger, ring finger, small finger
    - Radial border: Vertical midvolar septum
    - Ulnar border: Hypothenar septum
  - **Hypothenar** (least frequently seen)
    - Area between hypothenar septum and hypothenar muscles
    - Floor (dorsal boundary): Periosteum of fifth metacarpal and fascia of deep hypothenar muscles
    - Superficial (volar boundary): Volar fascia of superficial hypothenar muscles
    - Radial border: Hypothenar septum
    - Ulnar border: Hypothenar muscle/fascia
  - **Parona's space**
    - Located in distal forearm between the pronator quadratus and FDP tendon sheaths.

    - Infection of the thumb flexor tendon sheath may propagate proximally to the radial bursa, and infection of the small finger flexor tendon sheath may propagate proximally to the ulnar bursa.
    - Communication between radial bursa and ulnar bursa via Parona's space is known as a *horseshoe abscess*[16] (Fig. 81-4).

- **Collar button abscess**
  - Occurs in interdigital web space
  - Use dorsal and volar incisions
  - Preferred not to cross web space to prevent contracture
- **Etiologic factors**
  - These typically occur after a puncture wound or other penetrating injury.
  - *S. aureus* is the most common pathogen.
- **Diagnosis**
  - Presentation with pain, redness, and swelling over affected area
  - **Interdigital web space abscess:** *Abducted posture of adjacent fingers*
  - **Thenar abscess:** *Pain exacerbated by flexion or opposition of the thumb*
  - **Midvolar (subtendinous) space abscess:** *Pain on flexion of ulnar three fingers, loss of volar concavity*
- **Treatment**
  - Perform incision and drainage in the operating room with tourniquet control.
  - **Incise through volar fascia to enter deep space.**
  - Multiple surgical approaches have been described.
  - Avoid subsequent scar contractures in the web spaces.
  - Avoid the motor branch of the median nerve to the thenar muscles.
  - Start dressing changes in 24-48 hours.
  - Use elevation, splinting, and IV antibiotics.
  - **Antibiotic choice: IV vancomycin or clindamycin. Consider Piperacillin/Tazobactam for broad-spectrum coverage if gram-negative organisms are suspected.**[15]

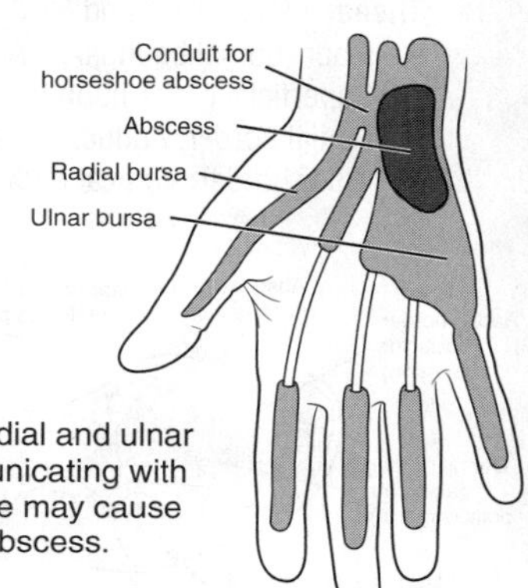


**Fig. 81-4** Radial and ulnar bursas communicating with Parona's space may cause a horseshoe abscess.

## Flexor Tenosynovitis[17]

An abscess within the flexor tendon sheath

- **Etiologic factors**
  - *S. aureus* is the most common pathogen.
  - Usually a history of penetrating trauma; may occur as extension of a felon
  - Rarely caused by hematogenous spread (suspect gonococci)
- **Diagnosis: Kanavel's four cardinal signs**
  1. Pain on passive extension of the finger (earliest and most reliable sign of the four)
  2. Fusiform swelling of digit
  3. Tenderness over flexor tendon sheath
  4. Partially flexed posture of digit (added later to original description)
- **Treatment**
  - Very early cases *(symptoms <48 hours)*
    - Splinting
    - Elevation

- IV antibiotics (Ampicillin/Sulbactam and consider adding cefoxitin, a second-generation cephalosporin)
- May discharge home on oral antibiotics, consider Amoxicillin/clavularic acid; if penicillin (PCN)-allergic, then use a fluoroquinolone and clindamycin

**CAUTION: Patients must be reassessed after 24 hours and operated on emergently if they fail to improve. Keep patients NPO after midnight when admitting so that they may be operated on the next day.**

- **Emergency incision and drainage** in the operating room required for most cases
  - **Surgical principles**
    - Perform with tourniquet control. If pus in the sheath is thin enough to be flushable, make limited incisions at the proximal and distal ends of the sheath, irrigate copiously with saline, and leave a catheter in place for 24-48 hours of irrigation postoperatively[13] (Fig. 81-5).
    - **If the pus is thick,** open widely with a midlateral or Bruner incision, debride while preserving the pulleys, and pack wound with gauze. Close wound loosely once infection subsides, usually after 5-7 days of dressing changes.

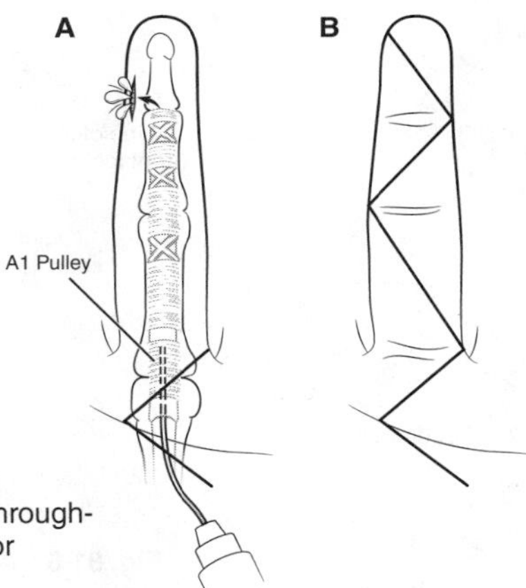


**Fig. 81-5** Drainage of tendon sheath infections. **A,** Incision for intermittent through-and-through irrigation. **B,** Technique for closed tendon sheath irrigation.

- **Treatment for all cases**
  - Rest in a splint
  - Heat and pain control
  - IV antibiotics
  - **Aggressive hand therapy as soon as feasible**
- **Outcomes**
  - Pang et al[18] published level II evidence identifying risk factors with poor outcomes with regards to amputation rates and total active motion. Those at higher risk were identified as:
    1. Age >43 years
    2. Presence of diabetes, peripheral vascular disease, or renal disease
    3. Presence of subcutaneous purulence
    4. Presence of digital ischemia
    5. Polymicrobial infection
  - Fusiform swelling was present in 97% of patients, pain on passive extension in 72%, semiflexed posture in 69%, subcutaneous purulence in 68%, tenderness along the flexor sheath in 64%, and fever in only 17%.

## BITES

Classified according to source: Human or animal

- **Human**
  - Etiologic factors
    - Bites are most common over the ring and small-finger metacarpal head *(fight bite)*[15] (Fig. 81-6).
    - Organisms include the relatively virulent flora of the human mouth.
      - *Streptococcus viridans*
      - *S. aureus, Bacteroides* spp
      - *Eikenella corrodens*
  - **Diagnosis**
    - Maintain a high index of suspicion for what may be a very unimpressive external wound.

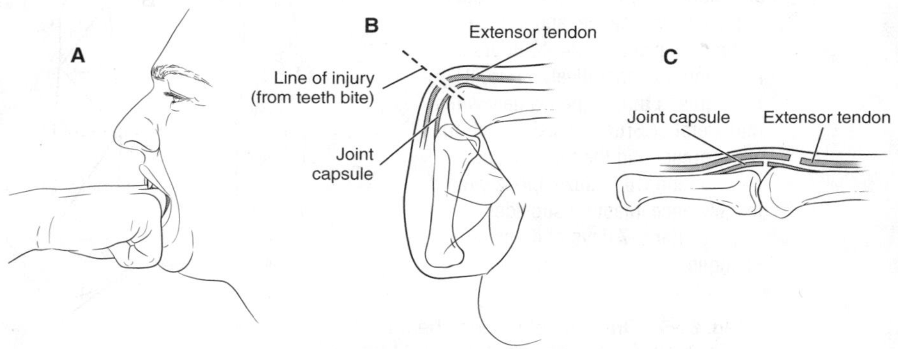


**Fig. 81-6 A-C,** Fight bite mechanism.

**TIP:** Patients involved in fights are notoriously evasive during initial questioning.

- **The hand must be examined with the fingers fully flexed** to reproduce the orientation of skin, tendons, and joints at the time of impact.
- **Radiographs are essential.** Look for a tooth fragment, metacarpal head fracture, or air in the joint.

- **Treatment**
  1. Explore wound in the operating room.
     - Patzakis et al[19] described surgical findings in 191 patients with clenched fist injuries.
       - 75% had injury to deep tissue layers, including tendon, capsule, and bone.
       - 22% had cartilage and bone involvement.
       - Findings stress importance of surgical exploration and debridement.
  2. Irrigate the joint and debride wound edges.
  3. Allow to close by secondary intention or after 7 days of dressing changes.
  4. IV antibiotics (Unasyn or if PCN-allergic clindamycin plus Cipro), splinting, and elevation[15]
  5. Start hand therapy after 48-72 hours.
  6. Send patient home on PO antibiotics (Augmentin).[15]

- **Animal** (dog and cat bites)
  - 1 million dog bites are reported annually (90% of all animal bites).
  - In >70% of cases the dog is known by the victim.
  - 50% of all dog bites occur in children <5 years old.
  - Cat bites represent 5% of all animal bites.
  - Cat bites represent 76% of infected bites.
  - Ascertain rabies immunization status of animal.
  - Vaccinate patient if necessary to prevent fatal viral encephalitis.
  - **Etiologic factors**
    - **Dog bites are the most common.**
    - **Cat bites are more likely to cause an abscess,** because their long, thin teeth are more likely to cause puncture wounds.
    - Both bite types require coverage for *Pasteurella multocida,* as well as *Staphylococcus* spp, *Streptococcus* spp, and anaerobes.
  - **Diagnosis**
    - Determine tetanus status and investigate the possibility of rabies.
    - Cat bites may cause **cat-scratch fever.**
      - Patient presents with a small pustule at wound site and painful lymphadenopathy proximally.
      - The process is self-limiting. Treat with nonsteroidal antiinflammatory drugs (NSAIDs).
  - **Treatment**
    - Irrigate all wounds thoroughly.
    - Explore joints, when indicated, as for human bites.
    - For dog bites, loosely approximate and sharply debride skin edges.
    - Substantial bite injuries may benefit from splinting and hand therapy.
    - Cat bites rarely require closure.
    - Antibiotics: IV Unasyn or if PCN-allergic clindamycin plus Cipro.
    - May send home with PO antibiotics (Augmentin).

## Septic Arthritis

Infection of the joint space

- May degrade articular surface, leading quickly to irreversible arthritic changes
- Can progress to osteomyelitis
- May aspirate joint to confirm diagnosis, but somewhat difficult in smaller joints
  - Concern of inoculating joint fluid: Do not aspirate through area of erythema.
- Synovial fluid analysis: *WBC >50,000/mm$^3$ strongly suggests joint sepsis.*
- **In general send all fluid for following: Gram stain, aerobic, anaerobic, AFB, fungal cultures; crystals; cell count**
- **Etiologic factors**
  - Typically secondary to a penetrating trauma; *S. aureus* is the most common pathogen.
  - The infection may occur from hematogenous seeding.
    - In **children,** search for an infectious source elsewhere in the body. *Streptococcus* spp, *Staphylococcus* spp, and *Haemophilus influenzae* are the most common pathogens.
    - In **adults,** particularly a single-joint arthritis in an otherwise healthy individual, suspect gonococci.

- **Diagnosis**
  - A septic joint appears hot, swollen, erythematous, and tender, with marked pain during passive movement.
    - **Hallmark examination finding: Painful and limited range of motion in affected joint**

> **TIP: Crystalline arthropathies can mimic septic arthritis or occur simultaneously. Always send aspirate of joint for crystal analysis.**

  - In the absence of a clear history of traumatic penetration, aspirate to confirm diagnosis. Send the aspirate for a Gram stain, culture, antibiotic sensitivity, and analysis for crystals.
- **Treatment**
  - All septic joints must be explored in the operating room via an arthroscopic or open procedure.
  - The joint space is irrigated copiously and gently debrided.
  - Status of cartilage surfaces is documented after inspection.
  - The wound is packed open, with daily dressing changes until it closes by secondary intention.
  - Alternatively, the joint is closed over an irrigation catheter and drain and irrigated for 48-72 hours.
  - IV antibiotics (vancomycin, add ceftriaxone if gonococcal infection is suspected), splinting, and elevation.
  - Hand therapy is started as soon as it is tolerated (after the drain is removed, if used).

## NECROTIZING FASCIITIS[20]

**Life- and limb-threatening,** rapidly progressive infection of the subcutaneous tissue and fascia

- Mortality rates range from 9%-75%.
- Early deaths within 10 days after initial debridement are usually from sepsis.
- Late death is attributable to multiple organ system failure.
- **Etiologic factors**
  - Commonly follows major or minor trauma
  - **Patients most at risk**
    - Diabetics
    - Elderly
    - Immunocompromised
  - Classically attributed to group A *Streptococcus* spp, but polymicrobial infections of aerobes and anaerobes in most cases
  - Closely related to gas gangrene caused by *Clostridium* spp
    - Demonstrates **crepitus** during physical examination and air in fascial planes on radiographs
- **Diagnosis**
  - Initial presentation is a low-grade cellulitis; rapidly followed by cyanosis or bullae in the skin.
  - Patients typically appear diaphoretic, obtunded, and pale, with tachycardia (i.e., toxic/septic shock).
  - An area of cutaneous anesthesia often follows the spread of the underlying infection.
  - **Foul-smelling, "dishwater" pus is evident.**
- **Treatment**
  - **Perform emergency, aggressive debridement of all nonviable tissue.**
  - Leave wounds open.

> **TIP:** Silver sulfadiazine (Silvadene) cream is an excellent local antibiotic and helps prevent tendons and other critical structures from desiccating.

- **Monitor in the ICU.** Sepsis associated with necrotizing fasciitis can cause significant hemodynamic instability.
- **Repeat debridement** every 24 hours until the infection is under control. Some patients may require life-saving amputations.
- Give **high-dose, broad-spectrum IV antibiotics** (IV vancomycin and Zosyn, may add PCNG or clindamycin for synergistic effect), but surgical debridement is the cornerstone of treatment.
- **Infectious disease consult**
- Consider hyperbaric treatment, particularly for clostridial infections. Once infection is controlled, skin graft wounds or perform other form of secondary reconstruction as indicated.
- Prolonged OT is required for functional recovery.

## Gas Gangrene

Uncommon infection of the upper extremity

- May be rapidly fatal.
- Death can occur within 12 hours after onset of infection.
- **Mortality rate is 25%.**
- **Etiologic factors**
  - >60 types of *Clostridium,* but six types cause gas gangrene
  - ***C. perfringens* most common**
  - **Alpha toxin** causes myonecrosis, hemolysis, and myocardial depression by inhibition of the calcium pump.
  - **Theta toxin** is a hemolysin and is cardiotoxic.
  - **Kappa toxin** destroys blood vessels through collagenase activity.
  - Devitalized tissue provides excellent environment for clostridial growth.
  - Toxins quickly produce muscle, subcutaneous, and fat necrosis.
  - Hydrogen sulfide and carbon dioxide gas are produced.
  - Severe hemolysis, hemoglobinuria, and ultimately renal failure occur.
- **Diagnosis**
  - Differential diagnosis includes necrotizing fasciitis, but gas gangrene proceeds more rapidly.
  - *C. perfringens* is difficult to culture and must be grown in an anaerobic environment in a medium with a reducing agent such as sodium thioglycolate.
- **Treatment**
  - **Requires rapid recognition and emergent surgical debridement**
  - Imperative to leave wounds open
  - Frequent dressing changes shortly after surgery
  - IV antibiotics: Vancomycin, Zosyn, including high-dose penicillin and clindamycin[15]

## Osteomyelitis[21]

A destructive infection of bones

- **Etiologic factors**
  - Usually develops as a local extension of an adjacent felon, septic arthritis, flexor tenosynovitis, or after an open fracture.
  - Occasionally caused by hematogenous spread.
  - *Staphylococcus* spp and *Streptococcus* spp most common pathogens.
    - Gram-negative, anaerobic, and polymicrobial infections are possible, particularly in immunocompromised patients.

- Cierney et al[22] (1985) developed classification for osteomyelitis (12 clinical types of osteomyelitis).
  - **Physiologic class (host characteristics)**
    - **A host:** Normal host with good immune system
    - **B host:** Local or systemic compromise
    - **C host:** Markedly compromised host. Treatment of disease is worse than disease itself.
  - **Anatomic location**
    - **Type I:** Medullary osteomyelitis—limited to endosteum, most common is hematogenous cause or intramedullary fixation
    - **Type II:** Superficial osteomyelitis—involves surface of bone
    - **Type III:** Localized infection—both medullary and superficial; full-thickness sequestrum
    - **Type IV:** Diffuse; bony instability

- **Diagnosis**
  - Patients have pain, swelling, and erythema over the affected bone, and may have a **chronically draining sinus.**
  - It may be difficult, in early radiographs, to distinguish demineralization from periosteal reaction of overlying wound infection without bone involvement.
  - A **bone scan or MRI** supports the diagnosis, when in doubt. MRI with contrast is most sensitive.
- **Treatment**
  - Prescribe **antibiotics for a minimum of 4-6 weeks,** continuing as long as symptoms persist.
  - **Antibiotic choice must be based on a bone biopsy and microbial culture.**
  - Nonviable bone must be curetted back to bleeding, viable bone stock.
  - Bone loss may require bone grafting and/or fracture fixation.
  - Amputation rates as high as **39%** have been reported.

## FUNGAL INFECTIONS

Common fungal infections of the upper extremity include **onychomycosis** (fungal infection of the nail) and **sporotrichosis** (granulomatous fungal infection of the subcutaneous tissue).

- **Onychomycosis *(tinea unguium)***
  - **Etiologic factors**
    - *Trichophyton rubrum* is the most common cause in the United States.
    - *C. albicans* is common in diabetics.
  - **Diagnosis**
    - Thickened, discolored nail
    - Occasionally, flaky nail plates may separate from nail bed.
    - Fungal cultures are obtained before initiating therapy, because different antifungal agents are used for each organism.
  - **Treatment**
    - *T. rubrum:* Oral terbinafine
    - *C. albicans*
      - **Topical:** Nystatin, miconazole, or econazole
      - **Oral:** Ketoconazole, itraconazole, or griseofulvin
    - **Removal of a thickened nail plate** can reduce the duration of oral therapy by 50%.

- **Sporotrichosis**
  - **Etiologic factors**
    - *Sporothrix schenckii* is the most common fungus on rose thorns, moss, and other plants.
    - Typically, this infection develops after a puncture wound occurs while handling plants or soil.
  - **Diagnosis**
    - Patients present with a nodule at a puncture site, which later ulcerates.
    - This is followed by **nodule formation** along lymphatic channels, which also ulcerate.
    - Definitive diagnosis is made by **fungal culture** of a nodule aspirate.
  - **Treatment**
    - Classic treatment is the use of a **saturated solution of potassium iodide.**
    - **Currently, potassium iodide is supplanted by itraconazole or fluconazole.**
    - All oral antifungal regimens require **long-term treatment** for 3-6 months (at least 4 weeks after resolution of symptoms).

## Atypical Mycobacterial Infections

Relatively rare infections caused by nontubercular *Mycobacterium* spp

- **Etiologic factors**
  - Most cases in the hand are caused by *Mycobacterium marinum, M. kansasii,* and *M. terrae.*
  - *M. marinum* is indigenous to fresh and salt water.
  - Patients with any break in the skin can become infected after contact with fish, contaminated water, or other sources of the organism.
- **Diagnosis**
  - Suspect mycobacteria when a chronic skin lesion, draining sinus tract, or other infection fails to heal as expected.
  - A biopsy will show granulomas with negative fungal staining.
  - Culture in **Lowenstein-Jensen medium** at 31° C for up to 8 weeks.
- **Treatment**
  - Surgical debridement of lesions
  - Long-term antibiotics (2-6 months) specific for the organism

## Prosthetic/Implant Infections

- Infections after prosthetic implants in hand range from 0.5%-3%.
- **Treatment**
  - Removal of implant
  - Irrigation and debridement
  - Cultures
  - Antibiotics
  - Resection arthroplasty
  - Joint fusion
  - Antibiotic spacer
  - Before reimplantation, patient should have normal WBC, erythrocyte sedimentation rate (ESR), and C-reactive protein (CRP).
  - At time of surgery obtain Gram stain and frozen section with $<5$ PMNs/high-power field before proceeding to reimplantation.

## Bacterial Biofilms[23,24] (Fig. 81-7)

- Recognized in 1970s.
- Bacterial colonies adhere to inert surfaces such as plastic, metal, or nonviable bone.
- **Exopolysaccharide matrix** is secreted, isolating the bacterial colonies from surrounding tissues and protecting them from host defense mechanisms.
- The biofilm may release bacteria, resulting in a "planktonic state."
- Antibiotic concentrations 1000 times higher than normal may be required to penetrate biofilm. (Antibiotic cement often is used, because it allows 1000 times higher local concentration compared with systemic antibiotics.)
- Aseptic loosening may be a misnomer.[23]

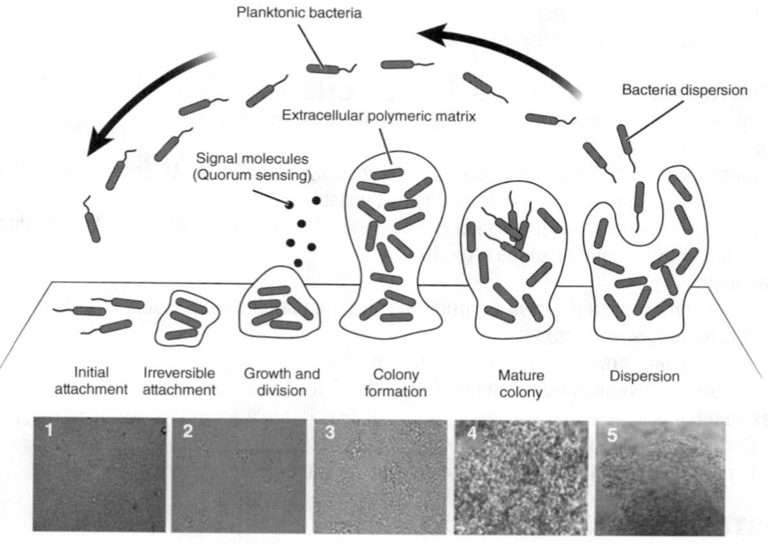


**Fig. 81-7** Biofilm.

## Shooter's Abscess

IV drug abuse abscesses of the forearm and hand

- Incidence of Hep B is 29%.
- Hep C incidence may be higher.
- HIV incidence range is 9%-50%.
- It usually is more associated with subcutaneous or intramuscular injection than with intravenous injection.
- MRSA accounts for 82%.
- Gram-negative isolates are more common in patients older than 40 years.
- Prolonged hospitalizations: Social concerns, noncompliance.
- Patients cannot be discharged from hospital with indwelling IV catheter (PICC line).
- Cardiac issues include murmur and endocarditis.

## High-Pressure Injections

- Soft tissue damage is extensive despite benign appearance of entry wound.
- Material is injected through the skin at pressures of up to 7000 psi.
- **Nondominant index finger is most common site.**
- **Oil-based solvents** cause more damage than water-based.
- Amputation rates of up to **50%** are reported with oil-based paints.
- **Emergent surgical decompression and debridement are required.**
- Removal of all foreign material is sometimes impossible.

## Mimickers of Infection: Do Not Be Fooled

- Gout
- Pseudogout
- Acute calcific tendinitis
- Pyogenic granuloma
- Pyoderma gangrenosum
- Retained foreign body: Inflammatory response
- Metastatic or primary tumors

## Key Points

- ✓ Comorbidities can predispose to hand or finger infections.
- ✓ *Staphylococcus* spp and *Streptococcus* spp are usually the most common pathogens.
- ✓ MRSA is the most prevalent community-acquired pathogen.
- ✓ Paronychia (acute) is the most common hand infection.
- ✓ Chronic paronychia is a common fungal infection.
- ✓ Plan your incisions carefully, in general, to prevent exposure of underlying vital structures while allowing adequate drainage.
- ✓ When obtaining cultures, obtain a Gram stain, aerobic, anaerobic, AFB, and fungal cultures.
- ✓ When submitting synovial fluid for analysis, request cell count and analysis for crystals, in addition to a Gram stain and cultures. A WBC count of >50,000 is likely to be septic arthritis.
- ✓ Whitlows resemble felons, although they can be differentiated by the patient's history and the presence of clear vesicles. Do not incise whitlows, because this can lead to dissemination of the virus.
- ✓ Watch for Kanavel's four signs to diagnose flexor tenosynovitis.
- ✓ Include antibiotic coverage for *Eikenella* infections that originate from human bites.
- ✓ Include antibiotic coverage for *Pasteurella* infections that originate from cat and dog bites.
- ✓ Suspect necrotizing fasciitis if "dishwater" drainage and rapidly progressing cellulitis are present.

## References

1. Crum N, Lee R, Thornton S, et al. Fifteen year study of the changing epidemiology of methicillin resistant *Staphylococcus aureus.* Am J Med 119: 943-951, 2006.
2. Calvet H, Yoshikow T. Infections in diabetes. Infect Dis Clin North Am 15:407-421, 2001.
3. Cohen M, Schnall S, Holtom P. New onset diabetes mellitus in patients presenting with extremity infections. Clin Orthop Relat Res 403:45-48, 2002.

4. Francel T, Marshall K, Savage R. Hand infections in the diabetic renal transplant patient. Ann Plast Surg 24:304-309, 1990.
5. Leddy J. Infections of the upper extremity. J Hand Surg Am 11:294-297, 1986.
6. Mann R, Peacock J. Hand infections in patients with diabetes mellitus. J Trauma 17:376-380, 1977.
7. Milford LW, ed. The Hand, 2nd ed. St Louis: CV Mosby, 1982.
8. LeBlanc DM, Reece EM, Horton BJ, Janis JE. Increasing incidence of MRSA in hand infections: a three year county hospital experience. Plast Reconstr Surg 119:935-940, 2007.
9. Janis JE, Reece EM, Hatef DA, Wang C. Does empiric antibiotic therapy change hand infection outcomes: a randomized prospective trial in a county hospital. (Accepted by Plast Reconstr Surg 2013.)
10. Volz KA, Canham L, Kaplan E, et al. Identifying patients with cellulitis who are likely to require inpatient admission after a stay in an ED observation unit. Emerg J Am Med 31:360-364, 2013.
11. Canales F, Newmeyer W, Kilgore EJ. The treatment of felons and paronychias. Hand Clin 5:515-523, 1989.
12. Jebson P. Infections of the fingertip: paronychias and felons. Hand Clin 5:547-555, 1998.
13. Wolfe SW, Hotchkiss RN, Pederson WC, et al, eds. Green's Operative Hand Surgery, 13th ed. Philadelphia: Churchill Livingstone, 2005.
14. Carter SJ. Herpetic whitlow: herpetic infections of the digits. J Hand Surg Am 4:93-94, 1979.
15. Stevanovic MV, Sharpe F, Wolfe SW. Acute infections. In Wolfe SW, Hotchkiss RN, Pederson WC, et al, eds. Green's Operative Hand Surgery, 6th ed. St Louis: Elsevier, 2011.
16. Netter FH. Atlas of Human Anatomy. Rye, NY: Novartis, 1997.
17. Neviaser RJ, Gunther SF. Tenosynovial infections in the hand: diagnosis and management. I. Acute pyogenic tenosynovitis of the hand. In AAOS Instructional Course Lectures. St Louis: CV Mosby, 1980.
18. Pang HN, Teoh L, Yam A, et al. Factors affecting the prognosis of pyogenic flexor tenosynovitis. J Bone Joint Surg Am 89:1742-1748, 2007.
19. Patzakis M, Wilkins J, Bassett R. Surgical findings in clenched fist injuries. Clin Orthop Relat Res 220:237-240, 1987.
20. Giuliano A, Lewis F Jr, Hadley K, et al. Bacteriology of necrotizing fasciitis. Am J Surg 134:52-57, 1977.
21. Reilly KE, Linz JC, Stern PJ, et al. Osteomyelitis of the tubular bones of the hand. J Hand Surg Am 22:644-649, 1997.
22. Cierney G III, Mader J, Penninck J. A clinical staging system for adult osteomyelitis. Contemp Orthop 10:17-37, 1985.
23. Costerton J. Biofilm theory can guide treatment for device-related orthopaedic infections. Clin Orthop Relat Res 437:7-11, 2005.
24. Davies DG. Microbiology, bacterial physiology, biofilm research. Available at: *http://www2.binghamton.edu/biology/faculty/davies/research.htm.*

# 82. Benign and Malignant Masses of the Hand

**Russell A. Ward, Melissa A. Crosby**

## BENIGN SOFT TISSUE TUMORS[1-5]

### Ganglion Cysts

- **Demographics**
  - **Most frequent benign mass in the hand** (33%-69% of all hand masses)
  - Two to three times more common in women, second to fourth decades
- **Pathologic conditions and etiologic factors**
  - Mucoid degeneration of fibrous connective tissue occurs in joint capsules or tendon sheaths.
  - 10% of cases present after a specific, traumatic, antecedent event.
  - Repeated minor trauma may be an etiologic factor in development.
- **Diagnosis**
  - May present with or without pain, or waxing and waning size
  - Mobile, **transilluminate,** may move with tendon
  - Radiographs **not** helpful to diagnose a ganglion cyst but needed to rule out underlying articular pathology or soft tissue calcification
  - Histology
    - Compressed collagen
    - No synovial or epithelial cells
  - Cysts contain glucosamine, albumin, globulin, and hyaluronic acid
- **Types**
  - **Dorsal carpal ganglion**
    - Overlies scapholunate ligament
    - **70%** of all ganglia
    - Often occurs between third and fourth extensor compartments
  - **Volar carpal ganglion**
    - **Most frequent site in children** <10 years old and in 15%-20% of adult cases
    - Originates from flexor carpi radialis (FCR) tendon sheath, radiocarpal, or scaphotrapezial joints
    - **Adjacent to radial artery**
  - **Flexor tendon sheath ganglion (volar retinacular)**
    - Often at **A1 pulley** (or between A1 and A2 pulleys), base of digit
    - 3-8 mm diameter
    - Attached to tendon sheath and **does not move with tendon**
    - Result of direct damage to fibrous sheath
    - Possibly delay or obviate need for surgery by using needle aspiration, steroid injection, and massage until rupture

- **Mucous cysts**
  - **Dorsal aspect of P3** (digital phalanx) is associated with extensor tendon, joint, or joint capsule.
  - Longitudinal grooving of the nail is possible.
  - Cysts are found mostly in older women, associated with degenerative changes in the distal interphalangeal (DIP) joint.
  - Radiographs show narrow space and osteophytes.
  - Skin is thin and may rupture.
  - **Always remove osteophytes at the time of excision, and look for occult cysts on the contralateral side.**
- **Carpal bosses**
  - Painful masses on dorsal IF or MF metacarpal bases
  - Associated with arthritis
  - More common in the right hands of women in the third or fourth decades
  - Ganglia present 30% of the time

- **Medical management**
  - **Children:** Rosson and Walker,[6] 22 of 29 cases resolved spontaneously
  - **Adult regression:** Approximately 38%-58% incidence
  - **Treatment**
    - Aspiration
    - Injection of enzymes, sclerosing agents, or cortisone
- **Surgical management**
  - Indicated for pain, deformity, or limitation of function
  - Resection must include entire cyst wall, stalk, and joint surface
  - Do **not** need to close joint capsule
  - No splint postoperatively, if uncomplicated
  - Most return to work in a few days
- **Recurrence:** Treatment associated with 1%-50% recurrence **(mean 24%)**

## Giant Cell Tumor of Tendon Sheath[7-9]

- **Demographics**
  - **Second most common hand tumor**
  - Generally in fourth to sixth decades
  - Also called *pigmented villonodular synovitis* (PVNS)
  - Occurs most commonly in radial three digits
- **Pathologic conditions and etiologic factors**
  - May be reaction to injury
  - Growth interferes with functioning of hand
  - Often confused with ganglion, but giant cell tumors fixed to deeper tissues and may erode bone
- **Diagnosis**
  - Yellow-brown subcutaneous mass usually evident
  - Fine-needle aspiration (FNA) may help in difficult cases
  - Histology: Cells of fibrous xanthoma, spindle cells, foam cells
  - **May erode into bone,** infiltrate dermis
- **Treatment:** Marginal excision

- **Recurrence**
  - Common (5%-50%) because of incomplete excision or satellite lesions
  - Reexcise; may need arthrodesis; amputation rare
  - Postoperative radiotherapy: Possible role after excision of recurrent lesions or lesions not able to be completely excised[10]

## Epidermal Inclusion Cyst

- **Demographics**
  - **Third most common tumor in the hand**
  - Most on palm and fingertips of people with occupations that predispose them to penetrating injuries
  - Evolution may take months to years
- **Pathologic conditions and etiologic factors**
  - Penetrating injury causes implantation of epidermal cells in the dermis.
- **Diagnosis**
  - Firm, spherical, nontender mass
  - Cyst material: Protein, cholesterol, and fat
  - May cause bone erosion
- **Treatment:** Must excise completely to avoid recurrence
- **Recurrence:** Low recurrence rate if excised completely

## Glomus Tumor

- **Demographics**
  - 1%-2% of all hand tumors
  - Malignant glomus tumor is a rare variant (<1%)
- **Pathologic conditions and etiologic factors**
  - Benign hamartoma of glomus apparatus (arteriovenous anastomosis involved in regulation of cutaneous circulation)
- **Diagnosis**
  - **Triad of symptoms**
    1. **Pain**
    2. **Pinpoint tenderness**
    3. **Cold sensitivity**
  - **Subungual** most common site
  - Multiple tumors in up to 10% of cases
  - **Nail-ridging** and red to bluish discoloration
  - Tumor less than 1 cm in diameter
  - Ultrasound with high-frequency transducer detects lesion
  - MRI: High-signal intensity on T2-weighted and STIR images
- **Treatment:** Local complete excision through sterile matrix
- **Recurrence:** Low incidence of recurrence if completely excised

## Ulnar Artery Aneurysm

- **Demographics**
  - Commonly seen in **carpenters** using hammers or in other laborers
  - Mostly in **men**
- **Pathologic conditions and etiologic factors**
  - Posttraumatic repetitive motion **(hypothenar hammer syndrome)** near ulnar artery
- **Diagnosis**
  - Pulsatile mass
  - Digital ischemic changes
  - Emboli
  - *Tinel's sign* of ulnar nerve often present
    - Allen's test to determine patency
  - Arteriogram results
- **Treatment**
  - Resection and ligation
  - Interposition, if collateral circulation inadequate
  - Consider lysis for emboli
- **Recurrence:** Rare

## Peripheral Nerve Tumors

- **Demographics**
  - 1%-5% of all hand tumors
- **Pathologic conditions and etiologic factors**
  - Originate from Schwann cells
- **Diagnosis:** Evaluation with CT scan and MRI
- **Five types of peripheral nerve tumors**
  1. **Neurilemmoma (also called *schwannoma*)**
     - *Most common nerve tumor*
     - Prevalent in middle age
     - Asymptomatic nodular swellings extrinsic to nerve
     - Treatment: Enucleate
     - Recurrence: Rare
  2. **Neurofibroma**
     - Can proliferate within fiber
     - Functional abnormality possible, including paresthesias
     - Lesions seen before age 10 years
     - Can cause gigantism in affected part
     - Histology demonstrates mast cells
     - Treatment: Consider resection if primary repair possible
  3. **Neurofibromatosis (von Recklinghausen's disease)**
     - Autosomal dominant
     - Acoustic neuromas
     - Optic gliomas
     - Meningiomas
     - Gigantism of limb
     - >6 café-au-lait spots
     - Plexiform pattern
     - Sarcomatous degeneration in 10%-15% of cases

4. **Malignant peripheral nerve sheath tumor**
   - 2%-3% of malignant hand tumors
   - Associated with von Recklinghausen's disease
   - Local extension or metastasis common
   - 90% mortality
   - Treatment: Wide excision if possible; if not, amputation recommended
5. **Intraneural nonneural tumors:** Lipoma, hemangioma, lipomatosis of nerve
   - May see macrodactyly
- **Recurrence:** Rare with complete excision

## MALIGNANT SOFT TISSUE TUMORS[2-4,11]

### Basal Cell Cancer

- **Demographics**
  - **Second most common cutaneous malignancy of hand**
  - 2%-3% of all basal cell cancers
  - Occur in middle-aged and elderly light-skinned individuals
- **Pathologic conditions and etiologic factors**
  - Does not arise from malignant changes in preexisting structures
  - Occur most often at sites with greatest concentration of pilosebaceous follicles
  - Up to 26 histologic variants described
  - Volar variants associated with *Gorlin's syndrome,* also subungual
- **Diagnosis**
  - Diagnosis assisted by biopsy
  - Slow-growing tumors with skin atrophy, pink to red discoloration, telangiectasias, and ulceration in pearly lesions
  - Metastases uncommon, but may be locally aggressive
- **Treatment**
  - Primary excision or Mohs' excision best treatment
  - Electrodesiccation and curettage, cryosurgery, and laser phototherapy for superficial lesions or high surgical risk patients
  - Medical treatment may include:
    - Intralesional interferon injection
    - Chemotherapy
    - Radiotherapy
- **Recurrence**
  - Increases with larger lesions
  - Increased rate with infiltrative nodular variants that have poorly defined borders, sclerosing, and morpheaform variants

### Squamous Cell Cancer

- **Demographics**
  - **Most common malignant cutaneous tumor of hand**
  - **Most common malignancy of nail bed**
  - 11% of all squamous cell tumors
  - **Dorsum of hand** most common location
  - Elderly patients
  - Mostly in men

- **Pathologic conditions and etiologic factors**
  - Originate from spindle cell layer of epithelium
  - Originate in areas of premalignant conditions
    - Sun damage (solar radiation) main factor
    - Actinic keratosis
    - Leukoplakia
    - Radiation keratosis
    - Scars
    - Chronic ulcers or draining sinuses (Marjolin's ulcer)
- **Diagnosis**
  - Diagnosis assisted by biopsy
  - Appearance
    - Smooth
    - Verrucous
    - Papillomatous
    - Ulcerative
  - Aggressive metastatic rate more common in hand than any other part of body, especially if digital web space involved
- **Treatment**
  - Wide local surgical excision or Mohs' excision is mainstay of treatment.
  - Consider sentinel lymph node biopsy for high-grade lesions.
  - Destruction by electrodesiccation and curettage; cryosurgery limited to very superficial lesions
  - Medical interventions
    - Radiotherapy
    - Topical 5-fluorouracil for premalignant lesions
    - Systemic chemotherapy
- **Recurrence**
  - Depends on degree of cellular differentiation, depth of tumor invasion, and perineural invasion
  - 7% for well-differentiated tumors versus 28% for poorly differentiated tumors

## MELANOMA

- **Demographics**
  - 10%-20% of all melanomas found in the hand
  - Volar or subungual locations common
- **Pathologic conditions and etiologic factors**
  - Sun exposure important etiologic factor
  - Consider dysplastic nevus syndrome
  - **Types**
    - Superficial spreading
    - Nodular
    - Acral-lentiginous
    - Lentigo maligna
- **Diagnosis**
  - Biopsy important to diagnosis: **Complete excisional biopsy preferred**
  - **Tumor thickness** only prognostic indicator

- **Treatment:** Wide local excision (WLE) or amputation; level not definitively determined, but **most agree with joint proximal to lesion**
  - Regional lymphadenectomy and sentinel lymph node biopsy controversial; most often for intermediate-depth tumor
- Recurrence more common with increased tumor thickness

## SOFT TISSUE SARCOMA

- **Demographics**
  - Uncommon in hand
  - ~50 distinct histiotypes arising from virtually all mesencymal tissues
  - 15% in upper extremity
  - Young patients
- **Pathologic conditions and etiologic factors**
  - Share common mesodermal origin
  - Increased risk with previous exposure to radiation and herbicides
  - Increased risk in patients with neurofibromatosis and Li-Fraumeni syndrome
- **Diagnosis**
  - Painless mass with recent growth
  - Innocuous at presentation (may mimic ganglion cyst)
  - Plain radiographs may demonstrate:
    - Soft tissue calcification
    - Fat density
    - Bony involvement
  - MRI helpful for defining pathologic anatomy and local extent of disease, and for preoperative planning
  - **Biopsy important**
    - Plan in line with limb salvage or amputation procedure, because the biopsy tract must be excised *en bloc.*
  - Prone to local recurrence
  - High incidence of metastasis, lungs > bone > regional lymph nodes
- **Seven types of sarcoma**
  1. **Epithelioid sarcoma**
     - **Most common subtype in the hand**
     - Possibly posttraumatic
     - Insidious
     - Originates on palm or volar surface of digits
     - Local recurrence common
     - Distant metastases common with increased incidence of nodal metastasis
  2. **Undifferentiated pleomorphic sarcoma**
     - Variable lesions
       - Superficial
       - Deep
       - Single
       - Multinodular
     - Extend along tissue planes
     - Metastasis through hematogenous spread

3. **Alveolar rhabdomyosarcoma**
   - Thenar or hypothenar musculature
   - Highly malignant and devastating tumor
   - Rapidly growing deep mass when in palm of children
   - Prognosis poor even with multimodal treatment
4. **Synovial sarcoma**
   - Originates in juxtaarticular soft tissues (tendon, tendon sheath, bursa)
     - Commonly show soft tissue calcification on plain radiographs
   - Poor prognosis
   - High incidence of metastases with increased risk of nodal metastasis
   - **Treatment multimodal**
     - Wide resection
     - Radiotherapy
     - Chemotherapy
5. **Fibrosarcoma**
   - **Origin**
     - Deep subcutaneous space
     - Facial septa
     - Muscle
   - Insidious
   - Hematogenous spread
6. **Clear cell sarcoma**
   - Uncommon
   - Slow-growing
   - Deep mass attached to tendons and aponeuroses or fascia
   - Poor prognosis
   - Local recurrence high
   - **Treatment**
     - Surgery with node dissection
     - Radiotherapy
     - Chemotherapy
7. **Kaposi's sarcoma**
   - Prevalent in fourth or fifth decade
   - Male/female ratio 10:1
   - Associated with **AIDS**
   - Dark-blue to violaceous macules replaced by infiltrative plaques
   - Diameter of 0.5-3 cm
   - Treatment includes: Radiotherapy and chemotherapy
   - Fulminating lesions, 6-12 month life expectancy
   - If slower growing, up to 20-year life expectancy

- **Treatment principles for sarcoma**
  - Surgical excision is wide and includes 2-3 cm of normal tissue, with or without adjunctive radiotherapy and/or chemotherapy.
  - Biopsy tract must be excised *en bloc*, therefore biopsy of suspicious lesions should be performed by definitively treating surgeon.
  - For all histiotypes combined, overall 5-year survival is 65%-70% with multimodal treatment.
- **Local recurrence:** Rare if excised completely with adequate margins

## BENIGN BONE TUMORS[12,13]

### ENCHONDROMA

- **Demographics**
  - *Most common benign bone tumor of the hand*
- **Pathologic conditions and etiologic factors**
  - Most result from aberrant focus of cartilage
- **Diagnosis**
  - Plain radiography often helpful
  - CT scan and MRI useful
  - May be asymptomatic or present with pain from pathologic fracture or remodeling
    - Favor the **tubular bones** of the hand
    - Well-demarcated, round, expansile lesions with flocculent matrix calcification on radiographs
    - **Pathologic fracture may occur**
- **Treatment:**
  - Observation if asymptomatic
    - Curettage with or without cancellous bone grafting
    - If fracture present, allow to heal before curettage
  - Multiple enchondromas
    - Rare
    - May be unilateral or mosaic
    - Known as *Ollier's disease*
    - *Maffucci's syndrome* is associated with soft tissue vascular malformations.
    - 20% degenerate into chondrosarcoma in *Ollier's disease.*
    - **Treatment for secondary chondrosarcoma:** Wide excision or amputation

### OSTEOCHONDROMA

- **Demographics**
  - **Most common cartilaginous neoplasm overall**
  - Present in young patients
- **Pathologic conditions and etiologic factors**
  - Originate from the physis and maintain a cartilaginous cap
  - May be seen in the setting of *hereditary multiple exostosis,* 15% of cases, AD inheritance
- **Diagnosis**
  - Bony protuberances extending beyond metaphyseal cortex on stalk seen on diagnostic radiographs
  - May be sessile (broad-based) or pedunculated (with narrow stalk)
  - May be subungual (also called *subungual exostosis*)
  - Medullary contents shared with the host bone
  - <1% risk of malignant transformation
- **Treatment**
  - Excision flush with cortex of host bone for symptomatic lesions
- **Recurrence:** Rare with complete excision

## Periosteal Chondroma

- **Demographics**
  - Only 2% of chondromas
  - Seen in adults and children with equal sex distribution
- **Pathologic conditions and etiologic factors**
  - Surface lesion arising from the periosteum of the tubular bones
  - Benign hyaline cartilage neoplasm
- **Diagnosis**
  - Palpable, slow-growing, often painful mass
  - Saucerization of underlying cortex on radiographs with adjacent buttress of cortical bone
  - CT or MRI may be useful in surgical planning
- **Treatment:** Complete excision with margin expansion using a high-speed burr
- **Recurrence:** Rare with complete excision

## Aneurysmal Bone Cyst

- **Demographics**
  - 5% of all benign bone tumors
  - Equal sex distribution
  - Most common in second decade of life before closure of epiphyseal plate
- **Pathologic conditions and etiologic factors:** Unknown
- **Diagnosis**
  - Eccentric in metaphysis or diaphysis
  - Expansile
  - Multiloculated lucent lesion on radiographs
- **Treatment**
  - Curettage with adjuvants and bone grafting
  - Radical excision for highly aggressive lesions
- **Recurrence:** Up to 60% after curettage and bone grafting

## Osteoid Osteoma

- **Demographics**
  - Uncommon osteoblastic tumor in hand: 10% of all benign bone tumors
  - Two to three times more prevalent in males than females
  - Most prevalent in first and third decades
- **Pathologic conditions and etiologic factors:** Nidus of abnormal bone $<$1.5 cm in diameter
- **Diagnosis**
  - Distal phalanx most commonly affected
  - Painful, localized area over tubular bone
  - **Pain worse at night**
  - Relief of pain with nonsteroidal antiinflammatory drugs (NSAIDs)
  - Central area of lucency surrounded by zone of sclerotic bone on radiographs
  - Bone scintigraphy and CT scan useful
- **Treatment**
  - Radiofrequency ablation
  - Curettage with cancellous bone grafting
- **Recurrence:** Rare after complete excision of the nidus

## Osteoblastoma

- **Demographics**
  - Rare in hand
  - Second to third decade
  - No sex predilection
- **Pathologic conditions and etiologic factors**
  - Poorly mineralized immature bars of neoplastic osteoid
- **Diagnosis**
  - Localized to carpus, especially scaphoid and tubular bones such as metacarpal
  - Larger than 1.5-2 cm
  - Localized swelling and pain
- **Treatment:** Curettage with adjuvants and bone grafting
- **Recurrence:** Recurrence rare with complete excision

## Bizarre Parosteal Osteochondromatous Proliferation (Nora Lesion)[14,15]

- **Demographics**
  - Rare lesion usually affecting tubular bones of the hand
  - Peak incidence in third and fourth decade with no sex predilection
- **Pathologic conditions and etiologic factors**
  - Thought to be a reactive lesion
  - Surface lesion composed of bone, cartilage, and fibrous tissue
- **Diagnosis**
  - Painful growing (sometimes rapidly) mass
  - May cause mechanical symptoms by location
  - Heavily calcified juxtacortical mass on plain radiographs
  - Medullary contents not shared with the host bone
- **Treatment:** Complete excision with saucerization of underlying cortex by high-speed burr
- **Recurrence:** Recurrence rates vary from 25%-65%; reexcision not always required

## Giant Cell Tumor of Bone[9]

- **Demographics**
  - 2%-5% occur in hand
  - Prevalent in third to fifth decades
  - Incidence greater in females than in males
- **Pathologic conditions and etiologic factors**
  - Benign lesions based on histology, but behave in locally aggressive fashion; can metastasize to the lungs in up to 5% of cases
- **Diagnosis**
  - Solitary lesion
  - Dull, constant pain, osseous expansion
  - Metaphyseal lesion with extension into the epiphysis
  - Radiolucent with thin cortex on radiographs
- **Treatment**
  - Curettage with adjuvants and cementation
  - Wide resection in very aggressive lesions

- **Recurrence**
  - Variable depending on treatment
  - May be reduced to below 20% by meticulous curettage with or without adjuvants
  - Decreased risk with wide resection

## MALIGNANT BONE TUMORS

### Ewing's Sarcoma

- **Demographics**
  - Rare in hand, 10% of all primary malignant bone tumors
  - Metacarpal most common site of involvement
  - Male/female incidence 2:1
  - Young patients (second and third decade)
- **Pathologic conditions and etiologic factors**
  - Neuroectodermal origin
- **Diagnosis**
  - Focal, permeating bone lesion with periosteal elevation and soft tissue extension on radiographs
  - Workup includes MRI, CT chest, total body bone scan, and bone marrow biopsy
- **Treatment**
  - Chemotherapy and wide excision
  - Radiotherapy effectively augments local control when needed.
- **Recurrence:** Uncommon with complete excision and multimodal therapy

### Chondrosarcoma

- **Demographics**
  - **Most common primary malignant bone tumor that occurs in the hand**
  - Most prevalent in sixth to eighth decades
- **Pathologic conditions and etiologic factors**
  - Occasionally associated with osteochondromas and multiple enchondromatosis
- **Diagnosis**
  - Epiphyseal area of proximal phalanx or metacarpal
  - Clinical course slow
  - May have late metastasis
  - Painful large mass near metacarpophalangeal joint
  - Destructive bone lesion with coarse calcifications on radiographs
  - Work-up includes MRI, CT chest, and total body bone scan
- **Treatment**
  - Wide resection or amputation
  - Radiotherapy and chemotherapy are ineffective.
- **Recurrence:** Rare after complete excision; may recur locally or present with metastases several years later

## Osteosarcoma

- **Demographics**
  - Rare tumor of hand: 0.18% incidence
  - Peak incidence in fourth to seventh decades, when hand involved
  - Male/female incidence 2:1
- **Pathologic conditions and etiologic factors**
  - Mesenchymal origin: Immature, neoplastic osteoid directly produced by proliferating cellular stroma
  - More frequent in irradiated bone, or in Paget's disease
- **Diagnosis**
  - Persistent, increasing pain from rapidly growing mass
  - Sunburst pattern seen in plain radiographs
  - Workup includes MRI, CT chest, and total body bone scan
  - Histology: Malignant spindle cells producing immature osteoid
- **Treatment**
  - Chemotherapy and wide excision
  - Five-year survival rate 70% if no metastasis, 10%-20% with metastasis
- **Recurrence:** Uncommon with complete excision and no metastasis

### Key Points

✓ The most common hand mass is a ganglion cyst.

✓ The most common bone tumor of the hand is an enchondroma (benign).

✓ The difference between Ollier's disease and Maffucci's syndrome is that Maffucci's syndrome is associated with soft tissue hemangiomas and lymphangiomas; both involve multiple enchondromas.

✓ Osteoid osteoma (benign) symptoms are relieved by NSAIDs.

✓ Pathologic fractures often are seen with enchondromas. These fractures should be allowed to heal before curettage and bone grafting.

✓ The glomus tumor triad of symptoms includes pain, pinpoint tenderness, and cold sensitivity in the subungual location.

## References

1. Athanasian EA. Bone and soft tissue tumors. In Green DP, Hotchkiss RN, Pederson WC, eds. Green's Operative Hand Surgery, 4th ed. Philadelphia: Churchill Livingstone, 1998.
2. Fleegler EJ. Skin tumors. In Green DP, Hotchkiss RN, Pederson WC, eds. Green's Operative Hand Surgery, 4th ed. Philadelphia: Churchill Livingstone, 1998.
3. Mankin HJ. Principles of diagnosis and management of tumors of the hand. Hand Clin 3:185-195, 1987.
4. Masson JA. Hand I: fingernails, infections, tumors and soft-tissue reconstruction. Sel Read Plast Surg 8, 1999.
5. Nahra ME, Bucchieri JS. Ganglion cysts and other tumor related conditions of the hand and wrist. Hand Clin 20:249-260, 2004.
6. Rosson JW, Walker G. The natural history of ganglia in children. J Bone Joint Surg Br 71:707-708, 1989.

7. Adams EL, Yoder EM, Kasdan ML. Giant cell tumor of the tendon sheath: experience with 65 cases. Eplasty 12:e50, 2012.
8. Garg B, Kotwal PP. Giant cell tumor of the tendon sheath of the hand. J Orthop Surg (Hong Kong) 19:218-220, 2011.
9. Errani C, Ruggieri P, Asenzio MA, et al. Giant cell tumor of the extremity: a review of 349 cases from a single institution. Cancer Treat Rev 36:1-7, 2010.
10. Coroneos CJ, O'Sullivan B, Ferguson PC, et al. Radiation therapy for infiltrative giant cell tumor of the tendon sheath. J Hand Surg Am 37:775-782, 2012.
11. TerKonda SP, Perdikis G. Non-melanotic skin tumors of the upper extremity. Hand Clin 20:293-301, 2004.
12. Feldman F. Primary bone tumors of the hand and carpus. Hand Clin 3:269-289, 1987.
13. Young L, Bartell T, Logan SE. Ganglions of the hand and wrist. South Med J 81:751-760, 1988.
14. Gruber G, Giessauf C, Leithner A, et al. Bizarre parosteal osteochondromatous proliferation (Nora lesion): a report of 3 cases and a review of the literature. Can J Surg 51:486-489, 2008.
15. Flint JH, McKay PL. Bizarre parosteal osteochondromatous proliferation and periosteal chondroma: a comparative report and review of the literature. J Hand Surg Am 32:893-898, 2007.

# 83. Dupuytren's Disease

Douglas M. Sammer

## DEFINITION

**Dupuytren's disease (DD)** is a benign fibroproliferative disorder that occurs in the fascia of the palm and digits, resulting in nodules, cords, and contractures of the fingers. Guillaume Dupuytren, a French surgeon, clarified the nature of this disease in 1831.

## DEMOGRAPHICS

- DD can affect individuals of any ethnic background.
- The highest incidence is in **white males of northern European ancestry.**
- It is rare in blacks.
- It is common in Japan, but not in the rest of Asia.
- There is a greater prevalence in men until age 70-80.
- Incidence increases with age.
- Proposed mode of inheritance is **autosomal dominant with variable penetrance and variable expression.**
- Bilateral involvement is common.
- The **ulnar rays** of the hand are most commonly affected.
    - Ring finger, followed by small and long fingers. Thumb and index involvement less common.
- **Dupuytren's diathesis** is an aggressive presentation of the disease with earlier and more rapid progression, and increased likelihood of recurrence after treatment. Risk factors for Dupuytren's diathesis include:
    - Male sex
    - Early onset of disease
    - Bilateral involvement
    - Family history
    - Ectopic disease (e.g., dorsal knuckle pads **[Garrod's pads]**)
- Other diseases in the Dupuytren's family are:
    - Penile fibromatosis **(Peyronie's disease)**
    - Plantar fibromatosis **(Ledderhose disease)**
    - Frozen shoulder

## ETIOLOGIC FACTORS AND PATHOPHYSIOLOGY

No single causative factor has been described. Many associated conditions have been implicated, but the ***data for these associations are still conflicting.***

- **Alcohol**
  - **DD occurs more often in alcoholics,** with a possible liver-related mechanism, although this connection is controversial.
- **Manual labor**
  - **No clear correlation;** possible microtrauma mechanism leading to myofibroblast contracture
- **Smoking**
  - Smoking may have a **role in causation and progression of DD.**
  - Association with drinking may explain high prevalence in alcoholics.
- **Diabetes**
  - **More common in diabetics,** an association not found in all epidemiologic studies
- **Epilepsy**
  - No clear mechanism; possible relation to anticonvulsants

## ANATOMY/HISTOLOGY/PATHOLOGY[1,2]

- Dupuytren's fascia has a higher percentage of **type III collagen** than normal fascia (40% compared with 5%).
- **Three stages of disease**
  1. Nodule formation (type III collagen, disorganized, high cellular density, myofibroblasts)
  2. Cord formation without contracture (decreasing cellularity, more organization to collagen)
  3. Mature cords with finger contractures (organized collagen, hypocellularity)
- **Bands are normal** fascial structures, **cords are pathologic.**
- Fascial structures that can become affected:
  - Spiral bands
  - Lateral digital sheets
  - Natatory ligaments
  - Pretendinous bands
  - Grayson's ligaments
- **Cleland's ligaments** (dorsal to the neurovascular bundle) do **not** become involved.
- For every band that becomes diseased, there is a corresponding cord of diseased tissue.
- Specific cords result in specific joint contractures.
  - **Metacarpophalangeal (MP) joint:** *Pretendinous cord, or pretendinous portion of spiral cord*
  - **Proximal interphalangeal (PIP) joint:** *Central, spiral, and lateral cords*
    - **Spiral cord:** Made up of pretendinous band, spiral band, lateral sheet, and Grayson's ligament; displaces the neurovascular bundle centrally and superficially in the finger
    - **Central cord:** Continuation of the pretendinous fibers in the palm to the digit
    - **Lateral cord:** Runs from natatory ligament to the lateral digital sheet
  - **Web space contracture:** *Natatory cord*
  - **Distal interphalangeal (DIP) joint:** *Retrovascular cord*

## INDICATIONS FOR SURGERY AND PATIENT SELECTION

- **Surgery will not cure the disease.** Patients with unrealistic expectations should be treated with caution. **Recurrence is common.**
- In general, surgery is indicated for contractures that lead to loss of function or difficulty with hygiene.
- MP joint flexion contractures can be treated much more successfully than PIP joint contractures. Therefore significant contractures are an indication for surgery.
  - **MP joint contracture >30 degrees** is often cited as the threshold for surgery, but patients must be evaluated individually.
- **PIP joints** are more difficult to fully correct, so earlier intervention is advisable. *Any degree of PIP contracture is considered an indication for surgery.*
- **Rapidly progressive** cases warrant **earlier operative treatment** than slowly progressive forms.

> **TIP: Hueston's tabletop test** can indicate need for surgical intervention. Result is positive if the patient is unable to place all fingers in a flat position on a flat tabletop simultaneously.

## CONTRAINDICATIONS TO SURGERY

- Mild MP joint contracture without functional consequence (usually <30 degrees)
- Nodules or cords without contracture
- Unrealistic patient expectations

## PREOPERATIVE WORKUP

**Dupuytren's disease is a clinical diagnosis.** No confirmatory lab work or studies are indicated.

### HISTORY

- Progression of the disease
- Specific tasks that are compromised by contractures
- Family history of DD
- General medical history (including associations listed above)

### PHYSICAL EXAMINATION

- Visually inspect and palpate for:
  - **Cords:** Type and location
  - **Nodules**
  - **Tethered skin**
- **Boutonniere's deformity** (PIP flexion and DIP extension) indicates an attenuated central slip, and poor outcome after contracture release.
- Attempt to determine how much of PIP contracture is joint capsular/ligamentous contracture, and how much is from DD cord.
  - Passively flex the MP joint fully to take tension off the cord, then passively extend the PIP joint.
  - If the PIP joint still will not extend with tension taken off the cord, **capsular/ligamentous contracture** of the joint is possible.
- Presence and severity of joint contractures: Measure degrees
- Ectopic disease (Garrod's pads)

## TREATMENT

### NONOPERATIVE

- Many modalities have been tried without consistent success (radiation, ultrasound, colchicine, interferon).
- **Steroid injections** may help to reduce pain in **isolated, painful volar nodules,** but will not change the natural history of the disease.
- **Collagenase injections**[3-5]
  - **Collagenase–*Clostridium histolyticum:*** Mixture of two enzymes that target different sites of collagen molecule
  - Injected into cord on treatment day 1
  - 24 hours later, the finger is **manually extended,** breaking the cord and straightening the finger.
  - Splint is worn nocturnally for 3 months (no formal therapy needed).
  - Only **one cord can be treated at a time.**
    - May inject an individual cord up to three times if necessary to achieve maximum straightening
    - Must wait 30 days between treatments
  - **Complications**
    - Injection site tenderness: Common
    - Injection site swelling and ecchymosis: Common
    - Skin tear: Common, but heals quickly with dressing changes
    - Tendon rupture: Very uncommon, but severe complication
  - **Results**
    - **45%-65%** achieve **near-full extension**; more achieve incomplete improvement.[3,4]
    - Results at **MP joint are much better** than those at PIP joint (true for any treatment, surgical or nonsurgical).
  - **Recurrence**
    - **35%** of those who achieve full extension at initial treatment have some degree of recurrence 3 years later.[5]
    - Recurrence is **more common at the PIP joint** than at the MP joint.

> **TIP:** Collagenase injection is only indicated for **adults** with **Dupuytren's contractures** with a **palpable cord.** It should not be used in children (or nursing mothers), or if there is disease without a contracture, and if the cord is not palpable.

- **Needle fasciotomy (percutaneous aponeurotomy)**
  - A needle is inserted through the skin at multiple locations along the cord, and used to cut the cord.
  - The finger is extended, and straightened as the cord is cut at multiple locations.
  - Nocturnal splinting is needed for 3 months, but no formal therapy.
  - Results not as well studied as those of collagenase treatment.
  - Multiple cords can be treated at one time.

- **Complications**
  - **Skin tear:** Not uncommon, heals quickly with dressing changes
  - **Digital nerve injury:** Uncommon, must be careful, particularly when treating a spiral cord
  - **Tendon injury:** Uncommon
- **Results**
  - Near-full extension is often achieved at MP joint.
  - Results at PIP joint are not as good.
- **Recurrence**
  - At 5 years, recurrence rate substantially higher (85%) than after limited fasciectomy (21%).[6]

- **Fat grafting**[7,8]
  - Recent increased interest in fat grafting after percutaneous needle fasciotomy
  - May reduce recurrence (unproven, and mechanism of action unclear)
  - May soften scar and overlying skin (unproven, and mechanism of action unclear)
  - Potential benefits possibly related to physical barrier to recurrent cord formation, presence of adipose-derived stem cells in fat graft material, or another mechanism[8]

> **TIP:** Nonsurgical options such as injectable collagenase and percutaneous fasciotomy are becoming more popular because of convenience, ease, and patient tolerance of these clinic procedures. For many patients, these factors outweigh the *likely* higher recurrence rate associated with nonsurgical options, compared with limited fasciectomy.

## SURGICAL

- **Open fasciotomy**
  - Skin incisions are made, usually more than one, and usually small (1-1.5 cm), and the *cord is divided but not removed.*
  - **Recurrence rate is likely higher than with fasciectomy** (removal of fascia), but this has not been definitively demonstrated.
- **Limited fasciectomy**
  - **Grossly diseased fascia is removed** from involved areas of palm and fingers, leaving **normal fascia intact.**
  - **It is the most commonly used technique.**
  - **McCash technique** is a variant of limited fasciectomy that involves transverse incisions in distal palm, base of finger, and PIP flexion crease.
    - Limited fasciectomy then performed
    - Incisions left open, and skin allowed to heal secondarily over 2-3 weeks
    - Prevents hematoma
- **Radical fasciectomy**
  - Extensive resection of volar and digital fascia, including diseased and **normal fascia**
  - **Does not decrease recurrence rate, higher complications than limited fasciectomy**
- **Dermatofasciectomy**
  - Removal of the fascia **and overlying skin**
  - Used most often for extensive skin involvement or recurrent cases
  - Skin left open to heal secondarily or closed with a skin graft

## Incisions for Limited Fasciectomy (Fig. 83-1)

- **Longitudinal incisions** over the cords, closed with multiple Z-plasties
  - Allows skin lengthening. This is important, because the volar skin contracts and skin domain is lost over time with DD.
- **Transverse incisions**
  - Commonly used in the palm
  - May leave portions open to close by secondary intention, reducing the risk of hematoma or skin flap ischemia
  - **Limited exposure** when multiple transverse incisions are used in the digits
- **Bruner incisions**
  - Can allow skin lengthening by closing with V-Y flaps in each limb
  - May be more ischemic than longitudinal incisions, particularly at the flap tips

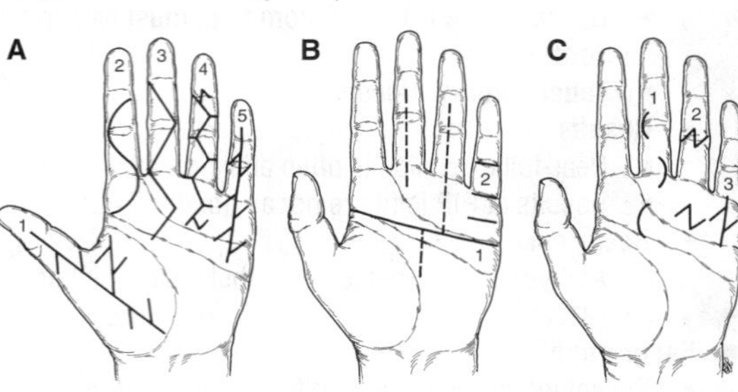


**Fig. 83-1 A,** Longitudinal incisions. (*1,* T-shaped; *2,* lazy S [NOT recommended]; *3,* Bruner incisions; *4,* multiple V-Y with Z-plasties on either end; *5,* midline longitudinal incision.) **B,** Transverse incisions. (*1,* Most commonly used; *2,* multiple short transverse incisions.) **C,** minimal exposure. *1,* Moerman's short, curved incisions; *2,* fasciotomy incisions; *3,* limited fasciotomy incisions.)

## PIP Joint Capsular/Ligamentous Contracture

- Stiffness at the PIP joint may limit straightening even after all abnormal Dupuytren's tissue has been removed.
- This is addressed with the following sequential steps. If the joint extends after any step, the subsequent step(s) are not completed.
  1. Check rein ligament release
  2. Volar capsulotomy
  3. Collateral ligament release
- There is evidence that a capsuloligamentous release in addition to fasciectomy does **not** provide advantage and may lead to increased complications.[9]

## Failure to Correct the Contracture

- Inadequate resection of the involved fascia
- Failure to address contracture of the joint itself (PIP joint most problematic)
- Failure to recognize attenuation of central slip of the extensor tendon
- Poor compliance with hand therapy
- Contracture of the digital vessels over time can limit the amount of extension that can be achieved intraoperatively.

# ROUTINE POSTOPERATIVE CARE

## Dressing

- Postoperative dressings or splint should be changed at 2-4 days to check wounds.
- Sutures are removed at 2-3 weeks.
- Daily dressing changes are initiated for wounds left open.

### Splinting

- Plaster splint placed in OR is changed to thermoplastic splint at first postoperative visit.
- Involved fingers should be splinted in full extension.
- **Splinting at night** may continue for up to **3 months** depending on the severity of the contracture.
- **Serial splinting** may be required if vascular compromise does not allow full intraoperative extension.
- **Dynamic extension splinting** postoperatively can improve and maintain postoperative results.[10]

### Mobilization

- **Begin mobilization at the first postoperative visit** with therapist.

## COMPLICATIONS

### Hematoma

- Risk is reduced when incision is left open (McCash technique).
- Remove the tourniquet before closing, and establish hemostasis.

### Digital Nerve or Artery Injuries

- The neurovascular bundle typically will be displaced superficially and toward the midline if spiral cords are present.

> **TIP:** Dissection should start in the palm and proceed distally. A tight piece of the diseased fascia can look like a nerve and vice versa; proceed with caution.

### Flap Necrosis

- Reduce risk with careful choice of incisions.
- If there is any excessive tension on skin closure, have a low threshold for leaving portions of incision open.

### Dupuytren's Flare Response

- There is an inordinate amount of swelling, redness, and stiffness after Dupuytren's surgery.
- Contractures may worsen.
- This may be a form of **complex regional pain syndrome** (CRPS).
- Institute early, aggressive hand therapy.
- Consider methylprednisolone (Medrol) dose pack, or other pharmacologic treatment.
- Sympathetic blockade is advocated by some.

## OUTCOMES

- Restoration of motion after extended follow-up is good.
- Durability of PIP joint capsular/ligamentous contracture correction is marginal.
- **Recurrence is common.**
  - Recurrence rate after surgery is extremely variable in the literature, ranging from about 20%-100%.

## Key Points

- ✓ DD most commonly affects older males of northern European descent.
- ✓ The ring and small rays are most commonly affected.
- ✓ DD is associated with alcoholism, smoking, diabetes, epilepsy, and other comorbidities. However, the associations are controversial and poorly supported in the literature. It is inherited in an autosomal dominant fashion with variable penetrance and expression.
- ✓ Dupuytren's diathesis is an aggressive form of the disease characterized by male gender, bilateral involvement, young age, ectopic involvement, and family history.
- ✓ Cleland's ligament is **not** affected by DD.
- ✓ Watch out for the neurovascular bundle when a spiral cord is present, because it is displaced volarly, proximally, and toward midline.
- ✓ Indications for surgery include >30 degrees of MP joint contracture, any PIP joint contracture, or if the disease is causing functional or hygiene problems.
- ✓ Injectable collagenase is indicated for adult Dupuytren's patients with a finger contracture and a palpable cord.

## References

1. McFarlane RM. Patterns of the diseased fascia in the fingers in Dupuytren's contracture. Plast Reconstr Surg 54:31-44, 1974.
2. McFarlane RM. On the origin and spread of Dupuytren's disease [review]. J Hand Surg Am 27:385-390, 2002.
3. Hurst LC, Badalamente MA, Hentz VR, et al. Injectable collagenase clostridium histolyticum for Dupuytren's contracture. N Engl J Med 361:968-979, 2009.
4. Gilpin D, Coleman S, Hall S, et al. Injectable collagenase clostridium histolyticum: a new nonsurgical treatment for Dupuytren's disease. J Hand Surg Am 35:2027-2038, 2010.
5. Peimer CA, Blazar P, Coleman S, et al. Dupuytren contracture recurrence following treatment with collagenase clostridium histolyticum (CORDLESS study): 3-year data. J Hand Surg Am 38:12-22, 2013.
6. van Rijssen AL, ter Lindan H, Werker PM. Five-year results of a randomized clinical trial on treatment in Dupuytren's disease: percutaneous needle fasciotomy versus limited fasciectomy. Plast Reconstr Surg 129:469-477, 2012.
7. Hovius SER, Smit X, Khouri RK. Fat grafting of Dupuytren's contracture after complete percutaneous release. In Coleman SR, Mazzola RF, eds. Fat Injection: From Filling to Rejuvenation. St Louis: Quality Medical Publishing, 2009.
8. Hovius SE, Kan HJ, Smit X, et al. Extensive percutaneous aponeurotomy and lipografting: a new treatment for Dupuytren's disease. Plast Reconstr Surg 128:221-229, 2011.
9. Weinzweig N, Culver JE, Fleegler EJ. Severe contractures of the proximal interphalangeal joint in Dupuytren's disease: combined fasciectomy with capsuloligamentous release versus fasciectomy alone. Plast Reconstr Surg 97:560-566, 1996.
10. Rives K, Gelberman R, Smith B, et al. Severe contractures of the proximal interphalangeal joint in Dupuytren's disease: results of a prospective trial of operative correction and dynamic extension splinting. J Hand Surg Am 17:1153-1159, 1992.

# 84. Rheumatoid Arthritis

Douglas M. Sammer

Rheumatoid arthritis (RA) is a chronically progressive, systemic, autoimmune inflammatory disease.
The primary target of the disease is **synovium.**

## INCIDENCE AND DEMOGRAPHICS

- 1% of population affected, but varies in subpopulations
- 6% of Pima Indians affected
- More common in women than men at 2:1 to 3:1 ratio
- Onset in third to sixth decade

## ETIOLOGIC FACTORS

- RA is **idiopathic.**
- Twin studies show 20% concordance in identical twins, 5% concordance in fraternal twins.
  - There is a genetic component to RA, but there is also an unknown environmental trigger.
  - The environmental trigger may be a bacterium or virus.
- Gene called *HLA* (human leukocyte antigen) *DR4* is strongly associated with development and increased severity of RA.
- Smoking and caffeine are epidemiologically associated with RA.

## PATHOPHYSIOLOGY[1,2]

- An antigen triggers an inflammatory response within the synovium.
- A complex interaction between T cells, B cells, and macrophages occurs within the synovium.
  - A systemic inflammatory response occurs, with upregulation of TNF-alpha, IL-1.
- The synovium produces matrix metalloproteinases, collagenases, and cathepsins that destroy cartilage and bone.
- Local cytokines upregulate osteoclasts in adjacent bone.
- The end result is a thickened, inflamed synovium called ***pannus*** that erodes cartilage, bone, and soft tissue.

## DIAGNOSIS

### Diagnostic Criteria

- **Four of the following seven criteria** must be present for diagnosis.
- Criteria 1 through 4 must be present for at least 6 weeks.
  1. **Morning stiffness** in joints
  2. **Soft tissue swelling** at three or more joints
  3. **Symmetrical involvement** of joints

4. Involvement of **metacarpophalangeal (MP), proximal interphalangeal (PIP), or wrist** joints
5. **Rheumatoid nodules**
6. Seropositive for **rheumatoid factor** (RF)
7. Typical **radiographic findings** (see below)

## Laboratory Tests

- **Rheumatoid factor** (RF)
  - RF seropositivity is present in **70%-80%** of RA patients.
  - Some patients become seropositive before development of symptoms.
  - Some patients convert to seropositivity late in disease process.
  - Some patients with RA always remain seronegative.
- **Anticitrullinated peptide antibody has** high specificity for RA (88%-96%)

## Imaging

- **Radiographs**
  - Periarticular osteoporosis and soft tissue swelling
  - Joint space narrowing
  - **Marginal erosions**
  - Symmetrical bilateral involvement
  - Carpal ankylosis
  - Characteristic deformities (e.g., ulnar translocation of carpus, ulnar deviation at MP joints) (Fig. 84-1)

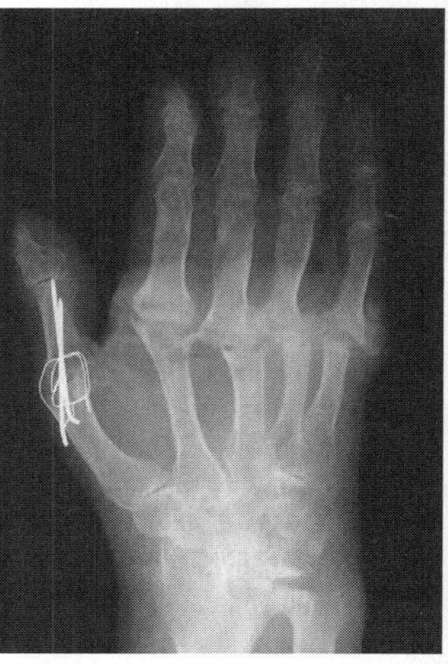

**Fig. 84-1** Characteristic ulnar deviation of metacarpophalangeal joints. Joint destruction is severe, particularly at the MP joints. This patient has had previous thumb MP joint arthrodesis with the tension band technique.

> **TIP:** Bony erosions occur first at unprotected sites such as at the margins of the joint, where there is no cartilage, or at sites of nutrient vessels. These unprotected areas are more susceptible to ingrowth of the erosive inflammatory pannus.

## JOINT AND TENOSYNOVIAL INVOLVEMENT

- **Wrist joint and distal radioulnar joint (DRU joint)**
  - **Early sites of involvement**
    - Scaphoid waist, scapholunate ligament, ulnar styloid, DRU joint
  - **Late findings**
    - Radiocarpal and midcarpal involvement: Radiocarpal joint tends to be more severely involved.
    - Erosion of volar rim of radius, with volar subluxation of the carpus
    - Ulnar translocation and radial deviation of carpus
    - Dorsal subluxation of ulna, and carpal supination **(caput ulnae)**

- **MP joints**
  - Volar subluxation
  - Ulnar deviation is from multiple factors.
    - Radial deviation of carpus results in ulnar approach of extensor tendons to MP joints.
    - Pinch forces between thumb and fingers push fingers in an ulnar direction.
    - Pannus stretches and erodes dorsoradial joint capsule, radial sagittal band, and collateral ligament early.
    - Extensor tendons subluxate ulnarly into valley between MP joints, acting as ulnar deviators.
- **Interphalangeal (IP) joints**
  - PIP joints more severely affected than distal interphalangeal (DIP) joints
  - Can take on flexion or extension deformity
- **Finger and thumb deformities**
  - **Boutonniere deformity:** *PIP flexion, DIP hyperextension* (Fig. 84-2)[3]
    - Pathology originates at the PIP joint in all cases.
    - Pannus erodes dorsally, rupturing central slip insertion, and PIP cannot extend.
    - Lateral bands subluxate volarly and act as PIP flexors and DIP extensors.
  - **Swan neck deformity:** *PIP hyperextension, DIP flexion* (see Fig. 84-2)
    - *Unlike boutonniere deformity,* can result from pathology at MP, PIP, or DIP joint
    - DIP joint: Pannus erodes terminal tendon, and mallet finger develops. PIP hyperextension is secondary.
    - PIP joint: Pannus erodes volarly, stretching volar plate. Flexor digitorum superficialis (FDS) insertion can rupture, resulting in PIP hyperextension.
    - MP joint: Volar subluxation results in intrinsic muscle/tendon tightening over time, and secondary PIP hyperextension.

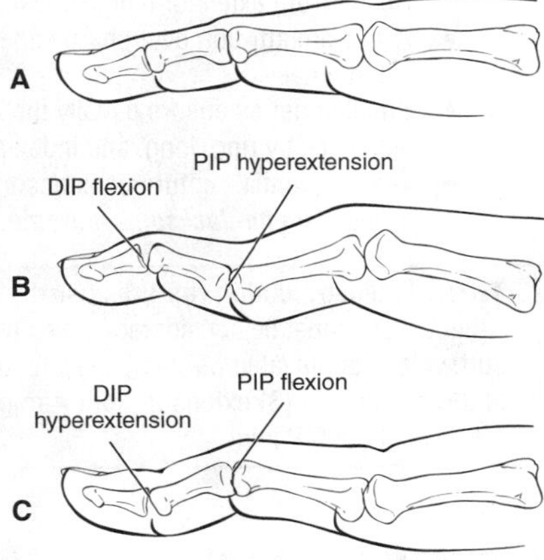


**Fig. 84-2** Characteristic swan neck and boutonniere deformities. **A,** Normal. **B,** Swan neck. **C,** Boutonniere deformity.

> **TIP:** When stiff or fixed, swan neck deformities are much more debilitating than boutonniere deformities. With boutonniere, patients can grip and pinch. With a swan neck, these motions are difficult or impossible.

  - **Thumb deformity**
    - **Five types:** The most common two are described below.
      - **Type I is most common: Boutonniere deformity**
        - MP flexion, IP hyperextension, radial abduction of metacarpal
        - Pannus at MP erodes dorsally and ruptures extensor pollicis brevis (EPB) insertion, and extensor pollicis longus (EPL) subluxates volarly.

- ♦ **Type III is second most common: Swan neck deformity**
  - – MP hyperextension, IP flexion, adduction contracture of metacarpal
  - – Carpometacarpal (CMC) joint subluxates radially and proximally, and metacarpal adducts.
  - – Pannus erodes volarly through capsule and volar plate at MP joint, causing hyperextension.

- **Tendon problems and pathology resulting from tenosynovitis**
  - **Carpal tunnel syndrome**
    - Results from mass effect of thick tenosynovitis/pannus within the carpal tunnel
  - **Trigger finger**
    - Results from focal tenosynovitis or rheumatoid nodule within sheath or tendon
    - Pathology not necessarily located at A1 pulley; can have offending nodule or focal tenosynovitis anywhere within flexor sheath
  - **Flexor pollicis longus (FPL) rupture**
    - Attrition rupture that occurs over sharp bony edge at scaphoid
    - Most common flexor tendon rupture, called the ***Mannerfelt lesion***
  - **Extensor tendon ruptures**
    - Result from extensor tenosynovitis within extensor retinaculum
    - Also from attrition over sharp edges caused by DRU joint and radiocarpal arthritis, and caput ulnae
    - Small finger extensors usually the first to rupture, and are often followed shortly in sequence by ring, long, and index extensors
    - This sequential rupture of extensor tendons, in ulnar to radial direction over time, is called ***Vaughn-Jackson syndrome.***

**TIP:** Extensor tendon ruptures usually present with sudden-onset loss of MP extension. Other causes must be considered in the differential diagnosis in RA patients. These include (1) stiff, volarly subluxated MP joints, (2) posterior interosseous nerve (PIN) palsy from synovitis at the elbow, and (3) extensor digitorum communis (EDC) tendon ulnar/volar subluxation at the level of the MP joint.

## SYSTEMIC DISEASE

- Although RA primarily affects synovium and joints, it is a **systemic disease.**
  - **Respiratory**
    - Rheumatoid nodules
    - Pleuritis
    - Effusions
  - **Cardiac**
    - Rheumatoid nodules
    - Pericarditis
    - Myocarditis
  - **Hematologic**
    - *Felty's syndrome:* Splenomegaly and leukopenia
  - **Ocular**
    - Uveitis
    - Iritis
    - Keratoconjunctivitis

- **Neurologic**
  - Polyneuropathy
- **Vascular**
  - Vasculitis
- **Cutaneous**
  - Rheumatoid nodules

## MEDICAL MANAGEMENT

### PHARMACOTHERAPY

*Medical management of RA has advanced dramatically over the last two decades, resulting in much better control of the disease. Therefore fewer patients with RA are requiring surgery.*

- **Three main categories** of medications are used to treat RA: **NSAIDs, corticosteroids,** and **disease-modifying antirheumatic drugs** (DMARDs)
  1. **NSAIDs:** e.g., aspirin, naproxen, indomethacin
     - Do not modify or alter the course of the disease; provide symptomatic relief only, but are very helpful
  2. **Corticosteroids**
     - Helpful as local injection to reduce joint inflammation and pain
     - With systemic administration (typically oral prednisone), a minimal effective dose used to prevent side effects
     - Often only used during flare-ups
  3. **DMARDs**
     - Actually modify the course of the disease; slow or halt progression in some cases
     - **Two types:** Conventional and biologic
       - **Conventional**
         - Examples: Methotrexate, azathioprine, Plaquenil, sulfasalazine, and gold
         - **Methotrexate often the first-line** agent for RA, and often used in combination with one or more other medications
       - **Biologic**
         - Specifically **target TNF-alpha, IL-1, or specific immune cells** such as B cells or T cells
         - Examples: Etanercept, infliximab, anakinra, and others

**TIP:** *Always discuss perioperative management of rheumatoid medications with the rheumatologist.* Some medications can impair healing and increase infection rate. However, stopping medications perioperatively can result in a severe rheumatoid flare that limits the patient's ability to participate in postoperative rehabilitation. In general, corticosteroids and methotrexate can be continued perioperatively. Biologic DMARDs should be withheld 2-4 weeks before and after surgery.

### INTRAARTICULAR STEROID INJECTIONS

- Indicated for severe joint pain
- Provide transient benefit
- Limited by multiple joint involvement

### Joint Protection and Splinting

- Decreases excess wear of joints and tendons; counteracts deforming forces
- Decreases deformity severity and can simplify surgical plan
- Does not prevent disease progression
- Must include non-weight-bearing exercise program

## PREOPERATIVE WORKUP

- Must consult anesthesiologist preoperatively
  - **Temporomandibular joint (TMJ)** can be stiff or ankylosed, causing difficult airway.
  - **Cricoarytenoid inflammation** can cause difficult intubation or loss of airway.
  - **Atlantoaxial instability** can inhibit neck extension during intubation.
  - Electrolyte, hematologic, hepatic, pulmonary, or cardiac problems (e.g., neutropenia, pericarditis, interstitial disease) are possible.
- Electrolytes, liver enzymes, CBC, EKG, chest radiographs, C-spine series

## SURGICAL PRINCIPLES[3]

### General Principles

- **6-12 months of medical management before surgery**
  - Exceptions include urgent operations (e.g., tendon ruptures).
- **Indications for surgery**
  - Progressive deformities that are **functionally limiting** or **painful** and have become **unresponsive to conservative therapy**

> **TIP:** *Deformity alone is not an indication for surgery.* Many patients have severe deformity, but they are functional and have little pain. These patients should not have surgery.

- **Surgical goals** (in order of decreasing importance)
  - Treat painful joints.
  - Restore function, and provide stability and mobility.
  - Prevent further progression (debatable whether this is possible).
  - Aesthetic improvement is important to patients, but should never be the reason for operating.

## SURGERY FOR TENDON PROBLEMS OR PATHOLOGY CAUSED BY TENOSYNOVITIS

### Extensor Tendon Rupture (Vaughn-Jackson Syndrome)[4,5]

- **Caused by extensor tenosynovitis and attrition over sharp bony edges at DRU joint and radiocarpal joint**
  - Must rule out other causes of loss of MP extension:
    - Tendon ulnar subluxation at MP joints
    - MP joint dislocation
    - Extensor paralysis (PIN palsy)
- **Treatment and surgical principles**
  - Full exposure of the extensor compartments at the wrist
  - Full extensor **tenosynovectomy**
  - Debride sharp osteophytes or bony edges; perform **Darrach** procedure for prominent ulna.
    - Use strip of extensor retinaculum to pad the debrided area.

- Perform appropriate **tendon transfer.** *Repair* of ruptured tendons is not possible, so tendon transfer is required.
  - **Tendon transfers**
    - **Small finger extensor rupture:** Transfer EDC/extensor digiti quinti (EDQ) of small finger end-to-side into adjacent ring EDC.
    - **Small and ring finger extensor ruptures:** Extensor indicis proprius (EIP) transfer to ring and small extensors
    - **Small, ring, long extensor ruptures:** EIP transfer to ring and small extensors, and end-to-side transfer of long EDC into index
    - **Extensor ruptures of all four fingers:** Ring FDS transfer to ring/small extensors, and long FDS transfer to index/long extensors
    - **Isolated EPL rupture:** EIP to EPL transfer

**TIP:** The underlying cause of the tendon rupture must be treated at the time of tendon reconstruction. It is futile to perform tendon transfers without treating the sharp bony edges and tenosynovitis that caused the rupture.

## Flexor Tendon Rupture

- **FPL rupture** *(Mannerfelt lesion)*
  - Remove bony osteophyte at level of scaphoid.
  - Pad with flap of volar wrist capsule.
  - Perform flexor tenosynovectomy.
  - Treat tendon rupture with one of the following options:
    - Index FDS tendon transfer into FPL
    - Tendon graft of FPL
    - Arthrodesis of thumb IP joint
- **Flexor digitorum profundus (FDP) and FDS ruptures**
  - **Isolated FDS rupture**
    - Tenosynovectomy
    - If rupture occurred in palm, suture FDS stump to adjacent finger FDS.
    - If rupture occurred in flexor tendon sheath, excise remaining FDS and leave finger with FDP only.
  - **Isolated FDP rupture**
    - Tenosynovectomy
    - If rupture occurred in palm, suture FDP stump to adjacent finger FDP.
    - If rupture occurred in flexor tendon sheath, excise remaining FDP and leave finger with FDS only.
  - **Rupture of both FDS and FDP is difficult problem with poor outcomes.**
    - Tenosynovectomy
    - If rupture occurred in palm, suture FDS and FDP stumps to adjacent finger FDS and FDP.
    - If rupture occurred in flexor tendon sheath, staged flexor tendon reconstruction with Hunter rod (poor outcomes in RA).
    - Alternatively, DIP and PIP can be fused in functional position, with preserved flexion at MP joint through the intrinsic muscles.

### Trigger Finger

- **Do not perform A1 pulley release.**
- Extensile flexor tendon sheath exposure
  - **Remove all tenosynovitis and nodules** that may cause triggering.
  - Pathology can occur at **any level** within sheath, not only at A1 pulley.

### Carpal Tunnel Syndrome

- **Do not perform standard limited-incision carpal tunnel release.**
  - Extensile exposure from distal forearm into midpalm
  - Perform extensive **flexor tenosynovectomy** to decompress carpal tunnel.

## SURGERY FOR FINGER AND THUMB DEFORMITIES (JOINT SURFACES PRESERVED)

### Swan Neck Deformities (Joint Surfaces Preserved)

- **Surgery indicated if splinting has failed**
  - **Early stages (supple PIP joint)**
    - Intrinsic release allows MP joint to extend and takes extension force off PIP joint.
    - Block PIP hyperextension (sublimis sling). A slip of FDS is used to create a static block to PIP hyperextension.
  - **Late stage (stiff PIP joint)**
    - Step 1: Increase PIP joint suppleness with serial splinting or casting, or surgical release if required.
    - Step 2: Once PIP joint is supple, treat deformity like an early-stage swan neck.

### Boutonniere Deformities (Joint Surfaces Preserved)

- **Surgery indicated if splinting has failed**
  - **Early stages (supple joints, mild PIP extension lag)**
    - Extensor tenotomy
    - Divide entire extensor mechanism at level of middle of middle phalanx.
    - This decreases pull at DIP joint, and increases pull at PIP joint.
  - **Late stages (significant extensor lag at PIP joint, PIP joint stiffness)**
    - Step 1: If stiff, increase PIP joint suppleness with serial splinting or casting, or surgical release.
    - Step 2: Perform surgery to shorten central slip (increases extension at PIP joint) and dorsalize the volarly subluxated lateral bands.

### Thumb Deformities (Joint Surfaces Preserved)

- **Type I: Boutonniere deformity**
  - **Early, mild deformity:** EPL is rerouted and EPB reinserted.
  - **Late, moderate deformity:** EPL is divided distal to MP joint. EPL and EPB are inserted at base of proximal phalanx to release extension force at IP joint and increase extension force at MP joint.
  - **Late, severe deformity:** MP arthrodesis with or without EPL release

- **Type III: Swan neck deformity**
  - Treatment in some ways similar to that for thumb CMC osteoarthritis
  - Ligament reconstruction tendon interposition **(LRTI)** to treat CMC joint
  - If MP hyperextension is severe, **MP arthrodesis**
  - If adduction contracture is severe, **adductor pollicis release**

### Metacarpophalangeal Joint Subluxation and Ulnar Deviation (Joint Surfaces Preserved)

- Soft tissue reconstruction is performed, which will likely wear out over time, with recurrence of deformity.
  - Intrinsic release: Allows MP extension
  - Cross-intrinsic transfer: The tight intrinsic tendon on ulnar side is sutured to the radial side of the adjacent digit to correct ulnar deviation.
  - Ulnar-sided sagittal band (which is tight) is released: Helps centralize subluxated extensor tendon
  - Radial-sided sagittal band (with is attenuated) is tightened: Helps centralize subluxated extensor tendon
  - Radial collateral ligament is tightened or reconstructed: Helps correct ulnar deviation

> **TIP:** The soft tissue reconstruction described for MP joints can be performed in isolation when the articular cartilage is preserved, with the goal of improving joint alignment and motion. It can also be performed along with an MP arthroplasty when the joint cartilage is not salvageable, and will prolong results of arthroplasty.

## SURGERY FOR METACARPOPHALANGEAL AND PROXIMAL INTERPHALANGEAL JOINTS (ARTHRITIC JOINTS, NOT SALVAGEABLE)

### Proximal Interphalangeal Joint Arthritis (Joint Surface Not Salvageable)

- **Index PIP joint**
  - **Arthrodesis:** Because of pinch forces, *arthroplasty is not an option;* it would be unstable.
- **Long, ring, or small PIP joint**
  - **Arthrodesis versus arthroplasty**
    - Both arthrodesis and arthroplasty treat pain effectively (primary goal of operation).
    - **Arthrodesis** is more predictable with **fewer complications**, but **sacrifices motion.**
      - All cartilage and subchondral bone removed from joint, exposing cancellous bone
      - Multiple fixation options: K-wires, tension band most common
    - **Arthroplasty** is less predictable with **higher complication rates**, but **preserves motion.**
      - Cartilage and bone removed from joint surfaces
      - Medullary canals broached to accept implant stems
      - Silicone prosthesis placed in joint
      - Pyrolytic carbon or surface replacement arthroplasties not a good option in RA because of poor soft tissue support

### Metacarpophalangeal Joint Arthritis (Joint Surface Not Salvageable)

- **Arthrodesis versus arthroplasty**
  - As above, both arthrodesis and arthroplasty treat pain effectively.
  - Arthrodesis has fewer complications, but motion is sacrificed.
  - Arthroplasty has higher complication rate, but preserves motion.
  - *However, compared with PIP arthroplasty, MP arthroplasty is very reliable.*
    - **Arthroplasty** usually **performed with soft tissue stabilization** described above
      - Joint surfaces prepared, cartilage and some bone removed
      - Medullary canals broached to accept implant stems
      - Implant placed
      - Soft tissue stabilization performed
    - Silicone prosthesis preferred in RA

## SURGERY FOR WRIST AND DISTAL RADIOULNAR JOINT (ARTHRITIC JOINTS, NOT SALVAGEABLE)

**TIP:** Wrist surgery, if needed, should be performed before finger surgery. If the "platform" of the wrist is not corrected before surgery is performed on the fingers, finger deformity is likely to recur.

### Wrist Arthritis

- **Wrist arthrodesis**
  - **Radioscapholunate arthrodesis**
    - The midcarpal joint is often relatively preserved in RA, compared to the radiocarpal.
    - The radius is fused to the lunate and scaphoid.
    - Some wrist motion (often $<50\%$) is preserved at the midcarpal joint.
    - The articular surface of the distal radius and the proximal articular surfaces of the lunate and scaphoid are prepared.
    - The distal pole of the scaphoid is removed to "unlink" the distal and proximal rows and allow better midcarpal motion.
    - Bone graft is packed into fusion site, and fixation is performed with K-wires, compression screws, or plate.
  - **Complete wrist fusion**
    - Performed when both radiocarpal and midcarpal joints are arthritic
    - Radiocarpal (radiolunate at minimum), midcarpal (capitolunate at minimum), and long finger CMC joints fused
    - Often performed with Steinmann pins in RA patients, but plate can be used if bone stock is adequate
- **Wrist arthroplasty**
  - *High complication and revision rate must be accepted, with the goal of treating pain and preserving motion.*
  - Many implants have been developed and discarded, beginning in the 1970s with a silicone total wrist implant.
    - Modern wrist implants are made of cobalt-chromium-molybdenum and ultrahigh-molecular-weight polyethylene (UHMWPE).
    - Proximal carpal row and part of the distal carpal row are removed, and the radius is broached.

  - The proximal (radius) component is placed into the radius, and the distal (carpal) component is secured distally.
  - The proximal component stem is covered with a plasma spray of titanium to help osseointegration.
  - Its articular surface is highly polished cobalt-chrome.
  - The distal component has pegs or screws that provide fixation in the distal carpal row and metacarpals.
  - The articular surface of the distal component is made of UHMWPE.
- Indicated for patients who have pain and must preserve some motion (e.g., contralateral wrist arthrodesis)

## Distal Radioulnar Joint Arthritis/Caput Ulnae

- **Darrach** procedure (Fig. 84-3)
  - Ulnar head is resected.
  - Transverse osteotomy is made in ulnar neck, just proximal to level of sigmoid notch of radius.
  - Dorsal edge is rasped smooth to prevent tendon irritation or rupture.
  - Complications such as forearm instability, or radioulnar convergence leading to impingement can occur.
    - The stump of the ulna converges on and impinges on the radius during grip, causing pain.
  - Multiple methods for stabilizing the ulnar stump have been described, with the goal of preventing these complications.
- **Sauve-Kapandji** procedure[6] (Fig. 84-4)
  - Two transverse osteotomies are made in the distal shaft/neck of the ulna, and a disc of ulna removed.
  - The ulnar head is fused to the sigmoid notch of the radius.
  - The segmental defect in the ulnar neck made by the removal of a disc of bone results in a pseudarthrosis and allows forearm rotation.

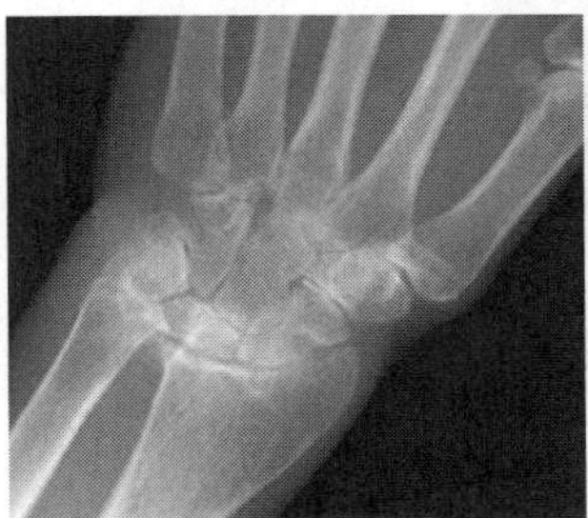
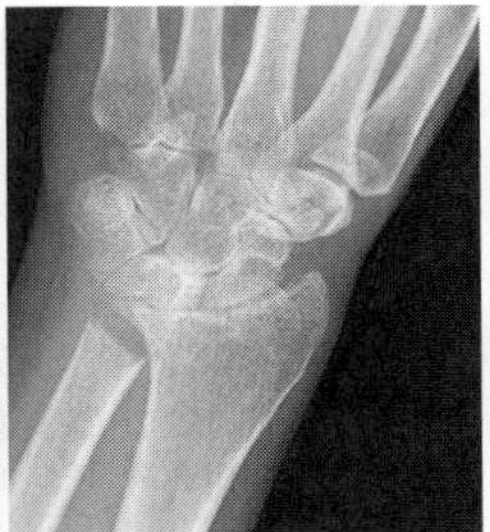

**Fig. 84-3** Preoperative *(left)* and postoperative *(right)* PA wrist radiographs demonstrate resection of the ulnar head (Darrach procedure) in a patient with caput ulnae.

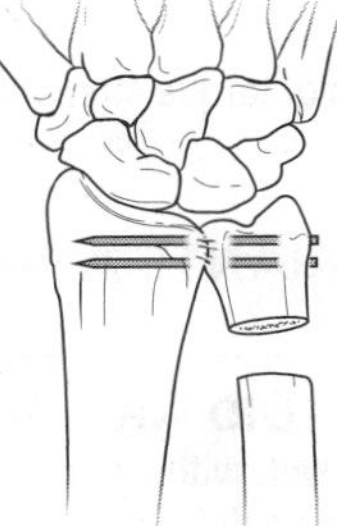
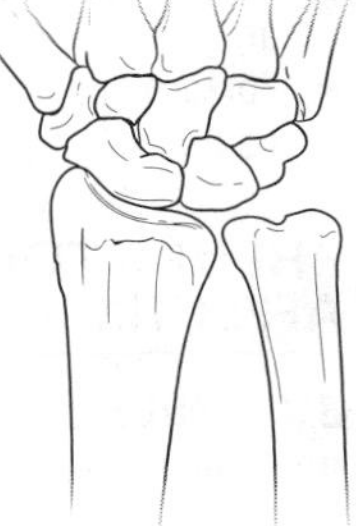

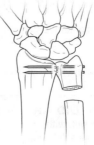

**Fig. 84-4** Sauve-Kapandji procedure *(left)* and Darrach procedure *(right)*. Both procedures can be used to treat DRUJ arthritis or caput ulnae. However, with the Darrach procedure, support for the ulnar side of the carpus is lost and may accelerate ulnar translocation that occurs in RA patients.

- The fusion of the ulnar head to the sigmoid notch treats the arthritis pain.
  - Sauve-Kapandji may be a better option than the Darrach procedure in RA patients with carpal translocation, because the preserved ulnar head provides support to the ulnar side of the carpus, and theoretically resists carpal translocation.
  - As with the Darrach procedure, forearm instability and radioulnar impingement are possible complications.

## OUTCOMES

### Tenosynovectomy

- Does **not** alter course of joint disease progression
- May prevent tendon ruptures
- Improves pain, but likely temporary

### Tendon Transfers

- Variable reports
- Difficult to study because of different rupture combinations with varied stages of joint disease
- Less favorable outcomes when multiple ruptures

### Metacarpophalangeal Arthroplasty

- Short term: Strength improved
- Long term: Strength not maintained, but pain generally does not recur
- Correction of ulnar drift improves the gripping and pinching mechanism
- Total ROM not as improved as arc of motion
- Short-term daily hand function improvements good (few long-term studies)
- Late fractures often seen on radiographs, but not significant

### Wrist Arthroplasty

- Effective for treating pain
- High complication and revision rate
- Preserve wrist motion, but do not reliably improve motion
- If problems occur, usually related to the distal carpal component—subsidence, loosening, perforation

### Wrist Arthrodesis

- Very reliable for treating pain
- Lower complication and revision rate compared with arthroplasty

### Distal Radioulnar Joint

- Darrach and Sauve-Kapandji procedures are effective at treating pain related to DRU joint arthritis.
- Forearm instability, loss of torque strength, and radioulnar impingement are potential complications.

## RHEUMATOID VARIANTS AND AUTOIMMUNE DISEASES AFFECTING HANDS[7,8]

### Juvenile Rheumatoid Arthritis

- **Z deformities are reversed,** with ulnar deviation of metacarpals and radial deviation of digits.
- Swan neck and boutonniere deformities, tendon ruptures, and nerve compression are rare.

## Psoriatic Arthritis

- Seronegative spondyloarthropathy
- **DIP** joints involved more than other joints (unlike RA)
- Nail changes (pitting, other findings)
- Pencil-in-cup radiographic changes
- Can have arthritis mutilans

## Systemic Lupus Erythematosus

- **Multisystem disease** in young women
    - Renal
    - Cardiac (pericarditis)
    - Respiratory, integument "butterfly" (malar) rash
- Commonly involves multiple joints, including hands
- **Hand findings**
    - Joints involved, but **no cartilage destruction** with **normal joint spaces**
    - **Hallmark:** Ligamentous and volar plate laxity; tendon subluxation
    - Deformity similar to RA, but with preservation of articular surfaces
    - **Mainstay treatment**
        - Pharmacologic
        - Splinting
        - Exercise

## Scleroderma

- Can involve multiple organ systems
- Two main forms: Systemic and CREST (**c**alcinosis, **r**aynaud's phenomenon, **e**sophageal dysfunction, **s**clerodactyly, and **t**elangiectasias)
- Small vessel vasculitis can result in **fingertip ulceration, chronic wounds, amputations.**
- Contractures usually result from skin and soft tissue changes.
    - **MP hyperextension, PIP flexion contractures common**
- **Arthritic changes are secondary.**

## Key Points

- ✓ In RA patients, the primary indication for surgery is pain, followed by loss of function.
- ✓ Patients who have severe deformity with no pain and good function should not have surgery.
- ✓ Unless surgery is urgent (e.g., pending tendon rupture), patients should have 6-12 months of medical management before considering surgical intervention.
- ✓ Always discuss perioperative management of medications with the rheumatologist. In general, steroids and methotrexate can be continued perioperatively. Biologic DMARDs should usually be withheld 2-4 weeks before and after surgery.
- ✓ RA is very common! Plastic surgeons and hand surgeons may be the first to diagnose patients with RA. This is important to remember for patients who have carpal tunnel syndrome, trigger fingers, joint pain, or swelling.

## REFERENCES


1. Brown FE, Collins ED, Harmatz AS. Rheumatoid arthritis of the hand and wrist. In Achauer BM, Elof E, Guyuron B, et al, eds. Plastic Surgery: Indications, Operations, and Outcomes, vol 4. St Louis: Mosby–Year Book, 2000.
2. Feldon P, Terrono AL, Nalebuff EA. Rheumatoid arthritis in the hand and wrist. In Green DP, Hotchkiss RN, Pederson WC, eds. Operative Hand Surgery, vol 2, 6th ed. Philadelphia: Churchill Livingstone, 2011.
3. Lister G. Rheumatoid arthritis, its variants, and osteoarthritis. In Smith P, ed. Lister's the Hand: Diagnosis and Indications, 4th ed. London: Churchill Livingstone, 2002.
4. Masson JA. Hand IV: Extensor tendons, Dupuytren's disease, and rheumatoid arthritis. Sel Read Plast Surg 35:23-34, 2003.
5. Richards RA, Wilson RL. Management of extensor tendons and the distal radioulnar joint in rheumatoid arthritis. J Am Soc Surg Hand 3:132-144, 2003.
6. Flatt AE, ed. The Care of the Arthritic Hand, 5th ed. St Louis: Quality Medical Publishing, 1995.
7. O'Brien ET. Surgical principles and planning for the rheumatoid hand and wrist. Clin Plast Surg 23:407-419, 1996.
8. Sammer DM, Chung KC. Rheumatologic conditions of the hand and wrist. In Neligan PC, ed. Plastic Surgery, vol 6, 3rd ed. London: Elsevier, 2013.

# 85. Osteoarthritis

Wendy L. Parker, Ashkan Ghavami

## INCIDENCE AND ETIOLOGIC FACTORS[1,2]

- Population affected by osteoarthritis (OA)
  - Younger than 45 years: 2%; 45-64 years: 30%; older than 65 years: >60%
- The incidence is much greater for **women.** This is thought to be related to hormonal influence on ligamentous support of joints, leading to laxity.
- OA can be **primary** or **secondary.**
  - **Primary** (idiopathic): Genetic factors combined with aging of cartilage from mechanical forces
  - **Secondary** (causative factor): Trauma (major or repetitive minor) leads to joint instability and wear or direct cartilaginous injury.

## DIAGNOSIS

### CLINICAL HISTORY

- **Joints involved**
  - Hand
    - Distal interphalangeal (DIP) joints
    - Proximal interphalangeal (PIP) joints
    - Metacarpophalangeal (MP) joints
  - Wrist
    - First carpometacarpal (CMC) joint
    - Intercarpal joints
    - Radiocarpal (RC) and ulnocarpal (UC) joints
    - Distal radioulnar joint (DRU joint)
- **Pain typically occurs with joint loading, use, and repetitive motion.**
  - In contrast to those with rheumatoid arthritis (RA), OA patients have **less pain in the morning** and **more pain during the day or with use.**
  - OA often interferes with sleep.
  - Pain can be dull, aching, and constant to sharp, intermittent, and radiating.
- **Subjective weakness is common.**
  - Pain and loss of motion lead to weakness.
- **Determine aggravating and alleviating factors and associated symptoms.**
- **Rule out underlying pathology and treat accordingly.**
  - Seropositive arthritis: RA, scleroderma, lupus, Sjögren's syndrome
  - Seronegative arthritis: Psoriatic, inflammatory bowel disease, infectious, gout/pseudogout

## Physical Examination

- Comprehensive motor and sensory examination
- Identify other factors suggestive of non-OA disease process (triggering, synovitis, skin changes)
- Joint examination
  - Appearance, swelling, angulation deformity
  - Motion: Active and passive
  - Pain: Loading and distraction
  - Associated findings
    - Ligament laxity and instability
    - Nodules: **Heberden** (DIP) and **Bouchard** (PIP)
    - Ganglia and mucous cysts

> **TIP:** Carpal tunnel syndrome is diagnosed in up to 45% of patients with first CMC OA.

## Imaging

- **Radiographic findings (standard views: AP/lateral/oblique)**
  - Bone changes and ligament laxity
  - Early: Joint space widening secondary to inflammation
  - Late: Joint space narrowing, subchondral sclerosis/eburnation, bone spurs
  - Special views
    - **Robert's view:** AP in hyperpronation allows ideal visualization of all four trapezial articulations
    - **Eaton stress:** A CMC stress PA view in which the patient presses thumbs together; may indicate increased joint laxity
    - **Bett's/Gedda's view:** PA in pronation and flexion
- **Bone scan (third phase, delayed/metabolic phase):** Very sensitive, a negative result excludes erosive arthritis
- **CT:** Useful to determine site of cortical disruption related to cysts
- **MRI:** Sensitive for cartilage erosion if diagnosis is unclear

> **TIP:** Patients' symptoms do not necessarily correlate with radiographic findings.

## CONSERVATIVE/NONOPERATIVE TREATMENT

Aimed at all OA-involved joints

Always the first line of treatment

- **Rest**
- **Heat**
  - 10 minutes twice daily in water/wax
- **Pain relief medications**
  - Acetaminophen
  - Antiinflammatories: Ibuprofen, COX inhibitors (meloxicam)
- **Splinting and therapy**
  - Night/resting splints in safe position to offload involved joints
  - ROM activities to maintain joint movement, plus activity modification

- **Injections**
  - Corticosteroids
    - With a treatment of one injection for thumb CMC arthritis, 80% of patients with stage I disease had pain relief beyond 18 months.[3]
    - A prospective rheumatology series showed significant improvement in the visual analog pain scale at 1 month, and 5 patients were pain free at 1 year.[4]
  - Other
    - Hylan G-F 20 (Synvisc): 32 patients treated in a small, open-label study were reviewed at 26 weeks and seemed to have less pain and improved function.[5]

## WRIST

- **Joints**
  - Intercarpal: Proximal and distal rows
  - RC/UC
  - DRU joint
- OA more commonly secondary (posttraumatic)
  - Distal radius fracture ± ulnar styloid fracture, triangular fibrocartilage complex (TFCC) injury, intercarpal ligament injury (scapholunate, lunotriquetral)
  - Leads to joint misalignment and ensuing wear
- **Clinical history**
  - Pain
  - Swelling
  - Crepitus
  - Ganglia
- **Physical examination**
  - Localize points of maximal tenderness through loading, often diffuse
  - Instability
    - Intercarpal: Watson's scaphoid shift
    - DRU joint: AP translation and pain with compression
- **Radiology**
  - Obtain dedicated wrist views (PA, lateral, oblique ± clenched fist).
  - Look for classic patterns.
    - **s**capholunate **a**dvanced **c**ollapse (SLAC) and **s**caphoid **n**onunion **a**dvanced **c**ollapse (SNAC) wrist deformity
    - DRU joint misalignment and spurs
    - RC/UC collapse and articulation steps

### SURGICAL OPTIONS

Manage each involved joint.

Patient considerations: Age, hand dominance, occupation, functional demands, and involvement of contralateral wrist

- **Isolated pisotriquetral joint**
  - Responds well to pisiform excision (if conservative management was unsuccessful)
- **Isolated RC joint**
  - Radioscapholunate (RSL) fusion (partial arthrodesis)
- **Isolated midcarpal joint**
  - Midcarpal fusion (partial arthrodesis)

- **Isolated DRU joint**
  - Ulnar head arthroplasty (hemiarthroplasty or constrained): Preserves forearm rotation
- **Total wrist involvement**
  - Total wrist arthrodesis/fusion (TWF) in 20 degrees of extension (prebent dorsal plates)
  - Total wrist arthroplasty
  - Both options can be combined with Darrach resection (distal ulna) or ulnar head arthroplasty.

**TIP:** TWF is a reliable option in all patients to achieve pain-free strength and stability.

# HAND

## First CMC Joint/Thumb Basilar Joint

- Biconcave saddle joint that allows flexion, extension, and opposition
- **Second most commonly involved joint in OA**
- 16 ligaments support the first CMC joint.[6]
  - Primary stabilizers are the dorsoradial and deep anterior oblique ligaments.
  - **Primary OA:** Ligament laxity and attenuation with advancing age or hormonal influence
  - **Secondary OA:** Posttraumatic ligament injury or direct cartilage injury
  - Both lead to misalignment of the joint and wear
- **Clinical history**
  - Pain ± swelling
  - Weak lateral pinch (pulling pants up or holding large objects/book)
  - Weak grip (opening jars/door knobs)
- **Physical examination**
  - Pain with distraction and torque, often early finding
  - Pain with joint loading ± crepitus
  - Visible dorsal CMC joint subluxation ± ganglion
  - MP joint compensatory hyperextension
  - Thumb adduction into palm
  - Pain with palpation of STT joint critical in determining responsiveness to surgical approaches
- **Eaton's radiographic stages of CMC joint degeneration**[7,8] (Table 85-1 and Fig. 85-1)

**Table 85-1** *Radiographic Staging*

| Stage | Radiographic Findings |
|---|---|
| I | Normal articulations with widening of joint space suggestive of an effusion, less than a third CMC joint subluxation |
| II | Slight narrowing of the thumb CMC joint, minimal subchondral sclerosis, debris/osteophytes <2 mm diameter, more than a third CMC joint subluxation |
| III | As per stage II, increased sclerosis, subchondral cysts, debris/osteophytes >2 mm diameter |
| IV | As per stage III, with narrowed ST joint demonstrating sclerosis and cysts |
| V | Pantrapezial arthritis |

*CMC,* Carpometacarpal; *ST,* scaphotrapezial.

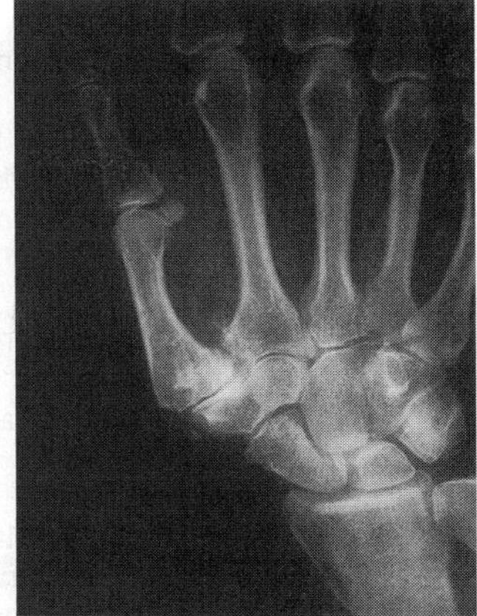

**Fig. 85-1** Eaton stage III CMC osteoarthritis shows significant joint narrowing, subchondral sclerosis, large osteophytes, and bony cysts.

## THUMB CMC JOINT[8-11]

- **Indications for surgery**
  - Pain, deformity, and dysfunction that do not respond to conservative measures
- **Goals of surgical treatment**
  - Excision/replacement of involved arthritic surfaces
  - Creation of a stable joint
- **Options** (Box 85-1)

**CAUTION: Surgeons should beware of failure if arthritic surfaces are not treated.**

**Box 85-1** *SURGICAL OPTIONS FOR THUMB CARPOMETACARPAL OSTEOARTHRITIS*

- Isolated trapezial resection (with or without K-wire fixation)
- Isolated volar ligament reconstruction
- Closing wedge/metacarpal extension osteotomy
- Soft tissue interposition
  - Without trapezial resection
  - Autogenous cartilage or other material
  - Open or arthroscopic
- Soft tissue interposition
  - With trapezial resection
  - With or without ligament reconstruction or metacarpal suspension
- Carpometacarpal fusion
- Hemiarthroplasty, total arthroplasty

- **Trapezial resection**
  - Alone leads to proximal migration of the MC, resulting in weakness, instability, and potential scaphometacarpal OA
  - Combined with K-wire fixation shows similar outcomes to ligament reconstruction and tendon interposition (LRTI) at 1 year[12]
- **Volar beak ligament reconstruction**
  - For hypermobile CMC joints and beak ligament laxity in Eaton stage I and II disease, use distally based half of flexor carpi radialis (FCR) strip or FRC.
- **Extension osteotomy**
  - MC extension osteotomy of 30 degrees is dependent on minimal OA changes at the joint and the concept of load transfer.
  - Long-term follow-up at 6-13 years demonstrated excellent functional outcomes.[13]

- **Soft tissue interposition**[7]
  - LRTI[9,12] long-term outcomes (6 years) showed pain relief and improved grip strength for 95% of patients.[14]
  - Weilby or modifications (Fig. 85-2) involve weaving a third to half of the FCR tendon around the abductor pollicis longus (APL) and suturing the APL over the imbrications.
    - Overall, results are similar to other series, but time for completed recovery is up to 6 months.[15,16]
- **Fusion**
  - Nonunion has been reported in up to 13% of patients,[10,17,18] pain from hardware, and a higher rate of complications.
- **Arthroplasty**
  - Pyrocarbon hemiarthroplasty showed 80% implant survival.[19]
  - A recent series of cemented total joint arthroplasty for stage III and early stage IV disease reported favorable results.[20]

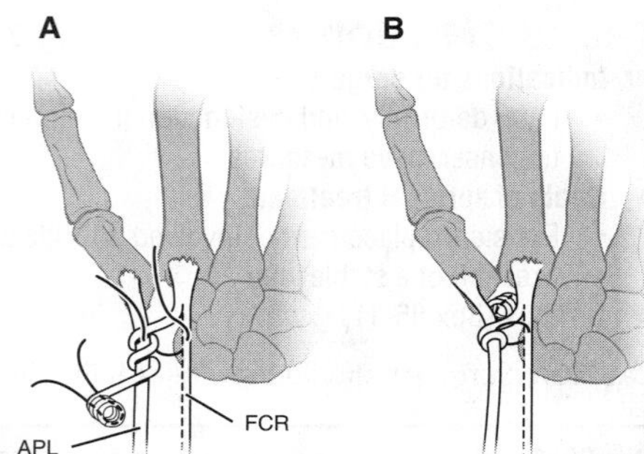


**Fig. 85-2** The author's preferred modified Weilby suspension arthroplasty. **A,** The FCR tendon is split longitudinally, freeing up the radial side. This is woven around the APL tendon and secured with 2-0 Fiberwire. The free end is rolled and similarly secured. **B,** A Fiberwire suture is then passed through the FCR tendon (running across the floor of the trapezial void) and secured to the FCR-APL construct, drawing it into the defect to correct the MC base dorsal subluxation. Finally, the rolled end is positioned in the void as a cushion.

**TIP:**
1. Choose a technique with which you are comfortable and have had predictable results.
2. Arthrodesis does not necessarily provide an advantage over other techniques.
3. Beware of subluxation/dislocation with arthroplasty techniques.

## MP Joints

- OA is **uncommon** except after trauma.
- **Surgical option is arthroplasty.**
  - Pyrocarbon: Excellent outcomes with good motion
  - Silastic: Better if poor soft tissue stability
- Fusion is a last resort. Patients likely will fair better with ray amputation.

## Thumb MP Joint

- **Most common digit to require surgical intervention for OA**
- **Mechanism**
  - MC base subluxation caused by MP joint degeneration
  - First web space narrowed by MC adduction deformity
  - Hyperextension deformity or instability

- **Treatment goals**
  - Provide good pinch grip, resistance, and stability
- **Surgical option is arthrodesis.**
  - Neutral to 15 degrees of flexion with 10 degrees of pronation
  - K-wires ± tension-band wires, cannulated screw

## PIP Joints

- **Mechanism**
  - Often posttraumatic
    - Dislocations, isolated central slip injuries (chronic boutonniere), untreated mallet finger resulting in swan neck deformity
- Debilitating: Loss of motion and pain
- **Surgical options**
  - **Arthrodesis**
    - Reliable
    - 20 degrees of flexion at index to 40 degrees at small
    - K-wires ± tension-band wires, cannulated screw
  - **Arthroplasty**
    - Requires adequate bone stock and intact, balanced flexion and extension mechanism
    - Expected motion 40-75 degrees of total flexion
    - Metallic/polyethylene combinations, pyrocarbon, silastic prebent to 30 degrees
    - Higher revision rates with nonconstrained implants because of lateral instability
    - Risk of failure from fracture with constrained implants

**TIP:**
1. Avoid arthroplasty on border digits, because instability from lateral forces can result in implant failure.
2. Fusions are very reliable, regardless of fixation method, if joint surfaces are properly debrided of cartilage and sclerotic margins and are adequately immobilized.

## DIP Joints

- **Most commonly affected joint in OA**
- Can develop severe deformity without symptoms
- Significant heredity
- Frequently accompanied by **mucous cyst** (secondary to osteophyte irritation of joint capsule)
  - Avoid manipulation, because infection can lead to joint sepsis.
  - May compress germinal matrix (nail grooving or deformity)
  - **Treatment**
    - **Excision:** For pain or impending rupture or cosmetic deformity (nail deformity often permanent)
      - Preserve at least half of the terminal tendon.
      - Excise osteophytes and debride capsule to promote scarring (decreases recurrence).
      - Skin healing is very reliable **without** the use of local flaps or skin grafts.

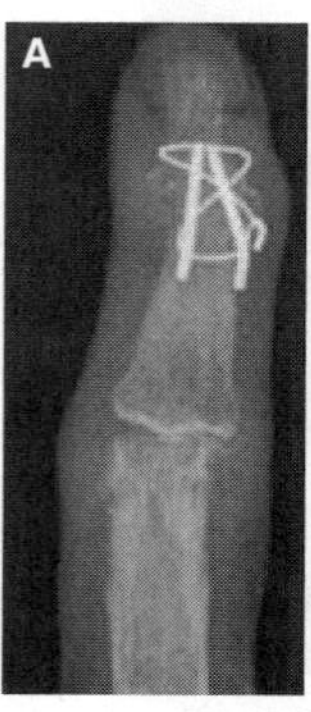

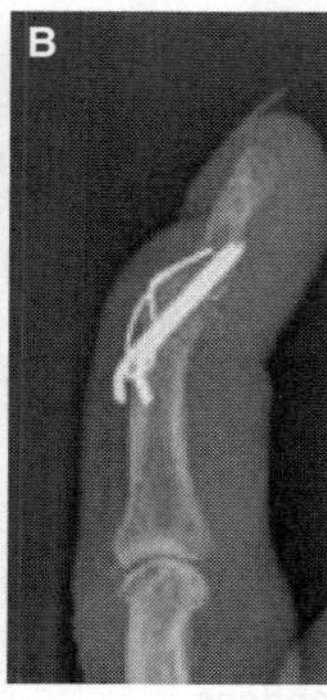

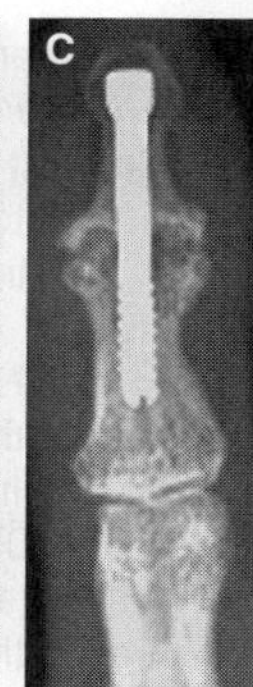


**Fig. 85-3** Index finger DIP fusion. **A** and **B,** Using K-wires and tension-band wiring. **C,** Using cannulated screw fixation.

- **Surgical option is arthrodesis.**
  - Reliable and definitive treatment of cysts and Heberden's nodes
  - Neutral to 10 degrees of flexion
  - K-wires ± tension-band wires, cannulated screw (Fig. 85-3)

**TIP:** Do not cross K-wires at the fusion site. Use an H-shaped or a Y-shaped incision or small rotation flap for better skin healing, and leave the germinal matrix intact to prevent nail growth problems.

## Key Points

- ✓ Rule out underlying conditions or trauma.
- ✓ Always consider conservative nonsurgical care as the first line of treatment.
- ✓ For the treatment of large joints with OA, consider the patient's goals and needs in determining arthroplasty versus arthrodesis.
- ✓ Successful treatment of OA in the first CMC requires removal of involved surfaces and stabilization of joints. Currently LRTI and suspension techniques are the best options.
- ✓ For small joints, fusions are reliable, despite loss of motion, and provide patient satisfaction and excellent outcomes.

## References


1. Armstrong AL, Hunter JB, Davis TR. The prevalence of degenerative arthritis of the base of the thumb in post-menopausal women. J Hand Surg Br 19:340-341, 1994.
2. Bednar MS, Light TR. Degenerative arthritis. In Achauer BM, Eriksson E, Guyuron B, et al, eds. Plastic Surgery: Indications, Operations, and Outcomes, vol 4. St Louis: Mosby–Year Book, 2000.
3. Day CS, Gelberman R, Patel AA, et al. Basal joint osteoarthritis of the thumb: a prospective trial of steroid injection and splinting. J Hand Surg Am 29:247-251, 2004.
4. Joshi R. Intraarticular corticosteroid injection for first carpometacarpal osteoarthritis. J Rheumatol 32:1305-1306, 2005.
5. Mandl LA, Hotchkiss RN, Adler RS, et al. Injectable hyaluronan for the treatment of carpometacarpal osteoarthritis: open label pilot trial. Curr Med Res Opin 25:2103-2108, 2009.
6. Bettinger PC, Linscheid RL, Berger RA, et al. An anatomic study of the stabilizing ligaments of the trapezium and trapeziometacarpal joint. J Hand Surg Am 24:476-482, 1999.
7. Eaton RG, Glickel SZ. Trapeziometacarpal osteoarthritis: staging as a rationale for treatment. Hand Clin 3:455-471, 1987.
8. Lister G. Rheumatoid arthritis, its variants, and osteoarthritis. In Smith P, ed. Lister's the Hand: Diagnosis and Indications, 4th ed. London: Churchill Livingstone, 2002.

9. Burton RI, Pellegrini VD Jr. Surgical management of basal joint arthritis of the thumb. Part II. Ligament reconstruction with interposition arthroplasty. J Hand Surg Am 11:324-332, 1986.
10. Tomaino MM. Ligament reconstruction tendon interposition arthroplasty for basal joint arthritis: rationale, current technique, and clinical outcome. Hand Clin 17:207-221, 2001.
11. Tomaino MM, Pellegrini VD, Burton RI. Arthroplasty of the basal joint of the thumb: long-term follow-up after ligament reconstruction with tendon interposition. J Bone Joint Surg Am 77:346-355, 1995.
12. Davis TR, Brady O, Dias JJ. Excision of the trapezium for osteoarthritis of the trapeziometacarpal joint: a study of the benefit of ligament reconstruction or tendon interposition. J Hand Surg Am 29:1069-1077, 2004.
13. Parker WL, Linscheid RL, Amadio PC. Long-term outcomes of first metacarpal extension osteotomy in the treatment of carpal-metacarpal osteoarthritis. J Hand Surg Am 33:1737-1743, 2008.
14. Young SD, Mikola EA. Thumb carpometacarpal arthrosis. J Am Soc Surg Hand 4:73-93, 2004.
15. Vadstrup LS, Schou L, Boeckstyns ME. Basal joint osteoarthritis of the thumb treated with Weilby arthroplasty: a prospective study on the early postoperative course of 106 consecutive cases. J Hand Surg Eur Vol 34:503-505, 2009.
16. Vermeulen GM, Brink SM, Sluiter J, et al. Ligament reconstruction arthroplasty for primary thumb carpometacarpal osteoarthritis (Weilby technique): prospective cohort study. J Hand Surg Am 34:1393-1401, 2009.
17. Bamberger HB, Stern PJ, Kiefhaber TR, et al. Trapeziometacarpal joint arthrodesis: a functional evaluation. J Hand Surg Am 17:605-611, 1992.
18. Goldfarb CA, Stern PJ. Indications and techniques for thumb carpometacarpal arthrodesis. Tech Hand Upper Extrem Surg 6:178-184, 2002.
19. Martinez de Aragon JS, Moran SL, Rizzo M, et al. Early outcomes of pyrolytic carbon hemiarthroplasty for the treatment of trapezial-metacarpal arthritis. J Hand Surg Am 34:205-212, 2009.
20. Badia A, Sambandam SN. Total joint arthroplasty in the treatment of advanced stages of thumb carpometacarpal joint osteoarthritis. J Hand Surg Am 31:1605-1614, 2006.

# 86. Vascular Disorders of the Hand and Wrist

**Kevin Shultz, Robert A. Weber**

## DIAGNOSIS

- Patients with vascular disorders of the hand typically present in one of three general categories:
  1. **Trauma**
     - Acute, such as an arterial laceration
     - Delayed, such as a posttraumatic aneurysm
  2. **Ischemia**
     - Acute, such as arterial embolism
     - Chronic, such as Raynaud's phenomenon, inflammatory arteritis, atherosclerosis, or thoracic outlet syndrome
  3. **Tumors**
     - Congenital, such as an arteriovenous malformation
     - Acquired, such as a glomus tumor or malignancy
- **History**
  - Episodes of cold intolerance
  - Whole hand and/or fingertip numbness
  - Hand cramping with fine motor activities
  - Color changes in the hand
  - Previous fingertip wounds
  - Use of tobacco or other nicotine sources should be noted.

**TIP:** Patients may be referred for an "infection" of a fingertip or nail.

- **Physical examination**
  - Vascularity
    - Assess: Skin color, temperature, turgor, capillary refill, peripheral pulses by palpation or Doppler evaluation
    - Palpate for masses, bruits, thrills.
    - Allen's test[1]
  - ROM
  - Musculature
- **Noninvasive studies:** Doppler imaging
- **Invasive imaging studies**[2] (Table 86-1)
  - CT angiography (CTA)
  - MR angiography (MRA)
    - Not as effective as CTA at allowing appreciation of spatial relationships between anatomic structures.

---

The opinions or assertions contained herein are the private views of the authors and are not to be construed as official or as reflecting the views of the Department of the Army or the Department of Defense.

**Table 86-1** *Imaging Studies*

| Test Name | Purpose | Comment |
|---|---|---|
| Magnetic resonance imaging (MRI) | Leading imaging modality in the diagnosis and follow-up of patients with vascular malformations. MRI should include T1- and T2-weighted spin-echo imaging in multiple planes, fat-saturated T1-weighted imaging with the intravenous administration of a gadolinium-based contrast agent, and gradient-recalled echo (GRE) imaging. First evaluate fat-suppressed T2-weighted images to determine the extent of the anomaly, and then to evaluate the GRE images to decide whether the anomaly is a high-flow lesion. | Commonly performed without a gradient-echo sequence or without the intravenous administration of contrast material. T2-weighted images are mainly used to evaluate the extent of the abnormality; GRE images are used to identify high- versus low-flow lesion. Contrast-enhanced images are used to determine the extent of the malformation and to distinguish slow-flow vascular anomalies (VM versus LM). |
| Magnetic resonance angiography (MRA) | Contrast-enhanced MRA has been gaining widespread clinical use. Allows the production of multiangular reprojections; it uses no ionizing radiation, and its contrast materials are less toxic than those of other modalities. | The technique is not yet standardized, and imaging characteristics are not well documented. |
| Magnetic resonance venography (MRV) | MRV is commonly used for patients with low-flow vascular anomalies to identify those involving the venous system. Can be performed with either flow-dependent angiographic techniques or contrast-enhanced angiographic techniques. | Commonly used to demonstrate the patency of the deep veins in the extremities before surgical debulking procedures. |
| Magnetic resonance lymphangiography (MRL) | MRL is used to demonstrate malignant lymph nodes by using special contrast agents or to evaluate the lymphatic system by using presaturated, heavily T2-weighted sequences without the administration of contrast material. | Promising as an adjunct to the conventional MRI protocol for vascular anomalies and edematous extremities; however, the technique has not been fully integrated into mainstream practice. |
| Ultrasound (US) | Portability and availability are the main advantages of US. Duplex US, continuous-wave Doppler US, color Doppler US, and Doppler spectral analyses all are useful in the evaluation of vascular malformations. | Doppler spectral analysis can be used to differentiate arterial from venous flow. An experienced sonographer or radiologist is necessary for appropriate sonographic evaluation. |
| Computed tomography (CT) | Particularly useful for detecting phleboliths in VMs and evaluating bone overgrowth or lysis that may accompany vascular anomalies. | Can also be used for patients who cannot be sedated for MRI or for patients in whom MRI is contraindicated (e.g., presence of a pacemaker or aneurysm clip). |

*AVF,* Arteriovenous fistula; *AVM,* arteriovenous malformation; *LM,* lymphatic malformation; *VM,* venous malformation.

*Continued*

**Table 86-1** *Imaging Studies—cont'd*

| Test Name | Purpose | Comment |
|---|---|---|
| Angiography | Includes arteriography, venography, and direct intralesional contrast agent injection. Arteriography is the standard for evaluation of high-flow vascular anomalies, particularly for AVMs and AVFs. | Arteriography has no diagnostic value for assessing low-flow anomalies. However, venography and direct intralesional contrast material injections usually are performed during interventional procedures for low-flow vascular anomalies (particularly VMs) to confirm the diagnosis and to tailor the procedure (sclerotherapy). Occlusive venography can be helpful for assessing the extent of low-flow vascular anomalies. |
| Radiography | Plain radiographs have limited value in the diagnostic workup for vascular anomalies. | Plain radiographs can demonstrate phleboliths (characteristic of VMs), and they are helpful for evaluating leg-length discrepancies and/or osseous involvement. |

*AVF,* Arteriovenous fistula; *AVM,* arteriovenous malformation; *LM,* lymphatic malformation; *VM,* venous malformation.

# TRAUMA

## TRAUMATIC ARTERIAL INJURIES[3,4]

- **Seven physical findings** indicate possible arterial injury:
  1. Decreased or absent pulse
  2. History of persistent arterial bleeding
  3. Large or expanding hematoma
  4. Major hemorrhage with hypotension
  5. Bruit at or distal to the artery
  6. Injury to an anatomically related nerve
  7. Anatomic proximity of a wound to a named artery
- If physical findings are equivocal for an arterial injury, but the wound is near a named artery, angiography is indicated. Direct exploration may be feasible if injury is distal to midforearm.
- If audible Doppler signal is different between two paired extremities, angiography is also indicated.
- The **radial artery** is the most commonly used arterial cannulation site.
- In a review of the literature published from 1978 to 2001,[5] a total of 19,617 patients had radial artery cannulation, and the incidences of permanent ischemic damage and pseudoaneurysm were each **0.09%.**
  - It is difficult to estimate the exact percentage, because many likely go unreported.
  - The most common complications of radial artery cannulation are temporary thromboembolism (23%) and hematoma (14.4%).[6]

- **Treatment**
  - Table 86-2 summarizes different injury scenarios and recommended treatment strategies.[7,8]

**TIP:** One can never go wrong in safely repairing normal anatomy.

**Table 86-2** *Treatment Strategies for Arterial Injuries*

| Injury | Treatment | Comment |
|---|---|---|
| Forearm vessel: Single with no nerve injury | Ligation | Gelberman et al[4] found that single, unrepaired arterial injuries caused modest consistent changes in hand vascularity but few clinical signs of ischemia or cold intolerance. |
| Forearm vessel: Single with nerve injury | Repair | Gelberman et al[4] found that an arterial injury combined with a nerve injury (especially the median nerve) resulted in decreased vascularity of the hands (which could be disabling). Repair of the artery had no effect on nerve recovery.<br>Leclercq et al[8] had a different result. In a study of ulnar nerve and artery injuries, nerve recovery (both motor and sensory) was superior when the artery was repaired, compared with a ligated or thrombosed artery. |
| Radial and ulnar artery | Repair | At a minimum, attempt to repair at least one artery, preferably the ulnar, and suture ligate the other ends of the other vessel. |
| Superficial volar arch | Ligation | If there is brisk flow from both cut ends |
| Superficial volar arch | Repair | If there is sluggish or no flow from one end or the other |

## Upper Extremity Aneurysms[3,9]

- Most caused by **trauma**
- **Mycotic aneurysms** generally caused by injection of drugs into hand with dirty needle, but also can be caused by septic emboli
- Atherosclerotic aneurysms very rare
- More common in the wrist and digital arteries
- **True versus false (pseudo) aneurysms**
  - **True aneurysms**
    - **All three layers** of arterial wall are involved.
    - Aneurysms usually result from arterial wall weakness, from either trauma or disease.
    - **Trauma** is the most common cause.
      - An aneurysm in the hand can result from a single episode of blunt trauma or from repetitive trauma, such as using a jackhammer.
      - Repetitive trauma can result in **hypothenar hammer syndrome.**
        - Results from thrombosis of ulnar artery in the area of Guyon's canal from **repeated blunt trauma** to base of hypothenar eminence (occurs in upholsterers, carpet layers, ball players)
        - Results in media damage followed by aneurysm formation and eventual thrombosis
        - If intima damaged first, then thrombosis occurs first
        - Syndrome associated with cold intolerance, pain, and sometimes ulceration of ring and small fingers

- **False aneurysms**
  - Much **more common than true aneurysms** in the hand
  - Result from arterial perforation
  - Blood leaks into surrounding tissue
  - Hematoma resolves and cavity replaced by scar tissue (usually takes weeks)
  - Does **not** involve all three layers of the arterial wall

**TIP:** *True* aneurysms are usually *fusiform shaped,* and *false* aneurysms are *saccular shaped.*

- **Diagnosis**
  - Perform a physical examination; frequently, a **pulsatile painful mass** is felt.
  - If aneurysm is deep or small, patient may have pain in the digits from emboli and show pallor of digits.
  - Allen's test should be performed, and any of the imaging studies in Table 86-1 can be used, although an arteriogram is rarely needed.
- **Treatment**
  - Resection and primary repair or vein graft is used.
  - If collateral flow is sufficient, an aneurysm involving the arch can be resected and ligated.

### Ulnar Artery and Other Local Artery Thromboses[3,7]

Thrombosis of the ulnar artery in Guyon's canal can occur from direct trauma.

- Patients with ulnar artery thrombosis at the wrist may present with **pain at night or with repetitive activity** and **cold intolerance.**
- **Exquisite tenderness** is present at the site of thrombosis.
- Eventually, patients may have **dependent rubor** or **ulceration** at the tips of the ring and little fingers.
- Excitation of the sympathetic fibers of the ulnar proper digital nerves is frequently noted.
- Diagnosis is confirmed with **Allen's test.**
- **Arteriography** is often helpful before a definitive treatment is determined.
- The standard treatment is **ligation and resection of the thrombosed segment.**
- Reconstruction of the artery with a vein graft is necessary only when backflow from the radial side of the arch is insufficient.

## Ischemia

### Emboli[9,10]

Emboli to the arm and hand are unusual; approximately **15%** of all emboli go to the upper extremity.

- **Source:** The **heart is the most common source.** Emboli result from arterial fibrillation or a recent myocardial infarction (MI). Other sources include:
  - Thoracic outlet syndrome
  - Atherosclerotic plaques
  - Subclavian and axillary artery aneurysm (traumatic or atherosclerotic)
  - Takayasu's disease and giant cell arteritis
  - Mechanical problems in a graft, usually an arteriovenous fistula graft for dialysis or an axillofemoral bypass graft
  - Penetrating trauma
  - Catheter related
  - Supracondylar humeral fractures

- **Clinical presentation**
  - Emboli from the heart are *macroemboli* and produce immediate symptoms of acute arterial obstruction (**the five Ps: P**ain, **p**allor, **p**ulselessness, **p**aresthesia, **p**oikilothermia).
  - Emboli from an artery are either *atheroemboli* or *thromboemboli* and result in multiple *microemboli* showering the distal end arteries of the hand. This can lead to Raynaud's phenomenon (see later).
- **Diagnosis is made by arteriography.** The groin should always be accessed so that the subclavian and distal arteries can be entirely evaluated.
- **Treatment**
  - Emboli in the arteries need **aggressive treatment.**
  - **Proximal arteriotomy with embolectomy using a Fogarty catheter** (small enough to pass through the superficial and deep arches in the hand) is the treatment of choice.
  - **Percutaneous intraarterial thrombolysis of the distal upper extremity** is controversial but has been shown to be effective in select cases. Local delivery of thrombolytic agent provides more precise action while minimizing risk of systemic side effects.
    - In contrast to lower limb vessels, upper extremity arteries are extremely sensitive to stimuli and respond with significant vasospasm. Thus both a thrombolytic and vasodilatory agent are given for acute thrombolysis.[11] In one study, urokinase was combined with a calcium channel blocker to obtain the desired result.
    - A comparison of percutaneous access via upper extremity or groin suggests greater ease with groin access; however, it may not be feasible because of the need for a long catheter.[11] Direct percutaneous access to the distal upper extremity is via the brachial artery.
  - Acute, severe pain that is not alleviated by the following treatment plans may be relieved with a **stellate ganglion block.**
  - A **cervicodorsal sympathectomy** can provide long-term relief for chronic pain caused by distal small-vessel occlusion.
  - **Emboli from the heart**
    - **Immediate intravenous heparin therapy** and embolectomy are needed.
    - Arterial embolization recurs in up to 33% of patients who do not receive long-term anticoagulative therapy.[9]
    - After an embolectomy, all patients must receive maintenance therapy with intravenous heparin to maintain activated partial thromboplastin time at 1.5-2.5 times the control values.
    - Patients should also receive **outpatient anticoagulation therapy** with oral warfarin or low-molecular-weight heparin. Treatment duration depends on the cause of the emboli (e.g., chronic atrial fibrillation, acute MI). Treatment is 95% effective.[9]
  - **Emboli from sources other than the heart**
    - **Trauma**
      - **Penetrating and catheter related**[5]
        - Although embolectomy alone is effective in treating 95% of patients with emboli of cardiac origin, thrombectomy alone is successful in restoring circulation in only **20%** of patients with catheter-related brachial artery occlusions.
        - Underlying pathology includes arterial stenosis at the site of arteriotomy closure, and intimal disruption from catheter manipulation.
        - In one series of arterial traumas, 80% of patients required arterial repair as well as clot retrieval. Treatment included primary resection and repair, vein patch angioplasty, and interposition vein grafting.

- Level of arterial injury is often localized to **the site of arterial cannulation,** and perioperative arteriography is rarely warranted.
- **Heparin** is used preoperatively to prevent propagation of distal thrombus but is discontinued once the operative repair is complete. Long-term anticoagulation therapy is **not** required.

♦ **Supracondylar humeral fractures**
  - These fractures are usually seen in **children.**
  - **Noninvasive Doppler studies** may be helpful in documenting abnormal perfusion in the injured extremity.
  - Persistent abnormal Doppler pressures after fracture reduction warrant operative exploration.
  - Arteriography may occasionally be helpful, but judicious use is required because of risk of iatrogenic catheter injury in children.
  - Brachial artery injury repairs are indicated in virtually all pediatric patients.
  - Thrombectomy and adjunctive arterial repairs are usually required.

▸ **Subclavian and axillary arteries**
  ♦ Regardless of underlying pathology, exclude the diseased proximal artery, restore circulation, and for patients with macroembolization, retrieve distal clot.
  ♦ Carotid-subclavian, axillary-axillary, and carotid-axillary bypass grafts have been used to reconstruct proximal arterial circulation with excellent long-term patency.
  ♦ Because early intervention is crucial for limb salvage, **brachiocephalic arteriography** is strongly encouraged for all unexplained cases of upper extremity ischemia.

▸ **Takayasu's disease and giant cell arteritis**
  ♦ Both conditions often respond to **nonoperative therapy** with corticosteroids.
  ♦ Surgery is the mainstay of treatment for severely symptomatic, chronic, upper extremity ischemia.
  ♦ Treatment of subclavian artery lesions includes carotid-subclavian, axillary-axillary, or carotid-axillary bypass grafts.
  ♦ Excellent results and low morbidity can be expected with either surgical procedure.
  ♦ Autogenous vein bypass is the treatment of choice for diseases of axillary and brachial arteries.

▸ **Thrombosed grafts**
  ♦ **Intravenous heparin** therapy should be started as soon as the clinical problem is recognized.
  ♦ **Embolectomy** should be performed in conjunction with revision of the thrombosed graft if possible.
  ♦ Multiple graft configurations can be used depending on the vascular anatomy.
  ♦ Three common polytetrafluoroethylene (PTFE) graft configurations include **forearm loop, upper arm straight,** and **brachial–internal jugular vein graft.**
  ♦ Optimally, a new graft may remain patent for an **average of 8-19 months.**
  ♦ Traditionally, surgical thrombectomy and revision of the venous end of the graft have been used to restore function to a thrombosed graft.
  ♦ With each successful revision, the subsequent period of patency decreases.
  ♦ Percutaneous endovascular thrombectomy and angioplasty of the venous anastomosis have been used to restore perfusion with improved secondary patency rates.[12]

## Raynaud's Phenomenon and Related Disorders[9,13-15]

*Raynaud's phenomenon* refers to reversible ischemia of peripheral arterioles. This can occur in response to a variety of stimuli, but it is most commonly caused by exposure to cold or stress.

- Raynaud's phenomenon is related to *Raynaud's disease.* They are **distinct disorders** that share a similar name.
- **Raynaud's disease** is *vasospasm alone,* with no other associated illness.
- **Raynaud's phenomenon** is a *vasospasm associated with another illness,* most commonly an autoimmune disease.
- Other terms used for this distinction are **primary Raynaud's** phenomenon (the disease) and **secondary Raynaud's** phenomenon (the phenomenon).
  - Patients who have had Raynaud's phenomenon for >2 years and have not developed additional manifestations are at low risk for developing an autoimmune disease. Most of these patients are considered to have primary Raynaud's phenomenon.
  - Although Raynaud's phenomenon has been described with a variety of autoimmune diseases, the **most common association is with progressive systemic sclerosis** *(scleroderma).* It is an almost universal association.
  - Raynaud's phenomenon has also been described with such diseases as systemic lupus erythematosus and other disorders not classified as autoimmune, including frostbite, vibration injury, polyvinyl chloride exposure, and cryoglobulinemia.
- **Pathophysiology**
  - One or more body parts have intense vasospasm with associated pallor and often cyanosis.
  - This is often followed by a hyperemic phase with associated erythema.
  - The affected body parts are usually those **most susceptible to cold injury.**
    - It most commonly affects fingers but may affect toes, nose, and ears.
  - A clear line of demarcation exists between the ischemic areas and unaffected areas.

**TIP:** These effects are *reversible* and need to be distinguished from irreversible causes of ischemia such as vasculitis or thrombosis. Rarely, tissue necrosis occurs distal to the affected vessel, usually in the periphery of the vasculature.

- **Incidence**[9,15]
  - **In the United States:** One survey reported a 5%-10% incidence of primary Raynaud's phenomenon in nonsmokers. However, the more accepted figure is **3%-4%.**
    - The frequency of secondary Raynaud's phenomenon depends on the underlying disorder. For example, it is **almost universal in patients with scleroderma** (progressive systemic sclerosis).
  - **Internationally:** The prevalence of primary Raynaud's phenomenon varies among populations, ranging from 4.9%-20.1% in women to 3.8%-13.5% in men. The commonly accepted rate is 3%-4%.
    - As in the United States, the prevalence of secondary Raynaud's phenomenon depends on the underlying disorder.
- **Race**
  - Primary Raynaud's phenomenon shows **no racial predilection.**
  - Secondary Raynaud's phenomenon approximates the **racial prevalence of the underlying disease.**
- **Age**
  - Primary Raynaud's phenomenon usually occurs in the second or third decade of life.
  - Secondary Raynaud's phenomenon begins simultaneously with the underlying disorder.

- **History**
  - **Numbness and pain** may be present in the affected areas.
  - **Affected areas** show at least **two** color changes: White (pallor), blue (cyanosis), and red (hyperemia).
    - The color changes are usually in the order noted, but not always.
    - The affected body part usually changes colors at least twice during the episode.
    - These changes should be completely reversible.
  - Any history of associated symptoms should raise a suspicion of an underlying disorder.
  - **Obtain an occupational history.**
    - **Secondary Raynaud's** phenomenon has been associated with the **frequent use of vibrating tools** such as jackhammers and sanders.
    - Industrial exposure to **polyvinyl chloride** has been implicated.
    - History of **injury or frostbite** may leave the involved limb vulnerable to vasospasm.
  - Syndromes associated with Raynaud's phenomenon are listed in Box 86-1.[15]

**Box 86-1** *SYNDROMES ASSOCIATED WITH RAYNAUD'S PHENOMENON*

**Autoimmune Disorders**

Progressive systemic sclerosis (scleroderma), including diffuse and localized (formerly called CREST syndrome)
Systemic lupus erythematosus
Mixed connective tissue disease (and other overlap syndromes)
Dermatomyositis and polymyositis
Rheumatoid arthritis
Sjögren's syndrome
Vasculitis
Primary pulmonary hypertension

**Infectious Syndromes**

Hepatitis B and C (especially associated with mixed or type 3 cryoglobulinemia)
Mycoplasma infections (with cold agglutinins)

**Neoplastic Syndromes**

Lymphoma
Leukemia
Myeloma
Waldenström's macroglobulinemia
Polycythemia
Monoclonal or type 1 cryoglobulinemia
Lung adenocarcinoma
Other paraneoplastic disorders

**Environmental Associations**

Vibration injury
Vinyl chloride exposure
Frostbite
Lead exposure
Arsenic exposure

**Metabolic and Endocrine Syndromes**

Acromegaly
Myxedema
Diabetes mellitus
Pheochromocytoma
Fabry's disease

**Hematologic Syndromes**

Paroxysmal nocturnal hemoglobinuria

**Drug-Related Associations**

Oral contraceptives
Ergot alkaloids
Bromocriptine
Beta-adrenergic–blocking drugs
Antineoplastics (e.g., vinca alkaloids, bleomycin, cisplatin)
Cyclosporine
Alpha-interferon

- **Differential diagnosis**

Some syndromes can be confused with Raynaud's phenomenon.

- **Anatomic syndromes**
  - Carpal tunnel syndrome
  - Reflex sympathetic dystrophy syndromes
  - Thoracic outlet syndrome
- **Miscellaneous circulatory syndromes**
  - Atherosclerosis
  - Thromboangiitis obliterans
  - Vasculitis
  - Thromboembolic disease
- **Vasospastic syndromes**
  - Livedo reticularis
  - Acrocyanosis
  - Chilblains
- **Laboratory studies**
  - Complete blood cell count: To evaluate polycythemia disorders, underlying malignancies, or autoimmune disorders
  - Blood urea nitrogen: To evaluate possible renal impairment or dehydration
  - Creatinine: To evaluate possible renal impairment
  - Prothrombin time: To detect evidence of hepatic dysfunction
  - Activated partial thromboplastin time: To detect evidence of antiphospholipid antibody syndrome or hepatic dysfunction
  - Serum glucose: To evaluate for diabetic disease
  - Thyroid-stimulating hormone: To detect thyroid disorders
- **Optional laboratory tests**
  - Antinuclear antibody: May be positive in autoimmune disorders and should be ordered for patients with features of these disorders
  - Serum viscosity: Elevated with hyperviscosity syndromes such as paraproteinemia
  - Serum creatine kinase: Elevated with muscle damage such as polymyositis and dermatomyositis
  - Rheumatoid factor: May be elevated with rheumatoid arthritis, other autoimmune disorders, and some forms of cryoglobulinemia (monoclonal proteins in multiple myeloma and Waldenström's macroglobulinemia have an increased frequency of rheumatoid factor activity)
  - Hepatitis panel: Positive for B or C infection in many patients with cryoglobulinemia
  - Cold agglutinins: Present with *Mycoplasma* infections and lymphomas
  - Heavy metal screen: To detect patients with neuropathic pain resulting from poisoning
  - Growth hormone: To evaluate patients for acromegaly
  - Serum vanillylmandelic acid: To evaluate for pheochromocytoma
  - Metanephrine: To detect pheochromocytoma in appropriate patients
  - Catecholamines: To detect pheochromocytoma
  - Leukocyte alkaline phosphatase: To evaluate for leukemias in appropriate patients

- **Imaging studies**[16] (Fig. 86-1)
  - **Thermography** and **arteriography** both have been used, but neither has proved superior to clinical assessment.
  - A fixed, nonreversible, cyanotic lesion is **not** Raynaud's phenomenon and may require further evaluation of the vasculature.

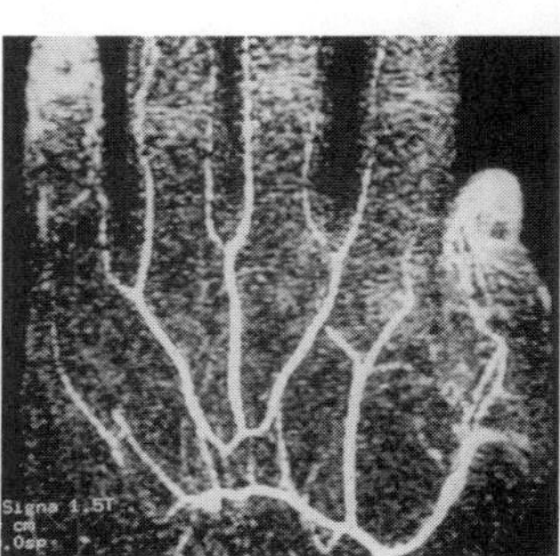

**Fig. 86-1** Contrast-enhanced MR angiogram of Raynaud's with cold-induced vasospasm.

- **Medical treatment**[13-15]
  - **Primary Raynaud's phenomenon**
    - Use **calcium channel blockers,** especially those that cause vasodilation.
    - **The most commonly used drug is nifedipine.**
      - Use the lowest dose of a long-acting preparation, and titrate up as tolerated.
      - If adverse effects occur, decrease dosage or use another agent such as nicardipine, amlodipine, or diltiazem.
    - The following have been advocated, but they are still experimental.
      - Angiotensin-converting enzyme inhibitors
      - Angiotensin receptor antagonists
      - Intravenous prostaglandins
    - Therapy with antiplatelet agents has been tried but has not proved effective.
    - Anticoagulation is **not** indicated.
    - Dziadzio et al[14] showed that losartan at 50 mg/day was effective in patients with primary Raynaud's phenomenon and scleroderma.
  - **Secondary Raynaud's phenomenon**
    - Therapy must be **tailored to the underlying disorder.**
    - If disease is associated with occupational or toxic exposure, patient should avoid inciting environment.
    - Patients with hyperviscosity syndromes and cryoglobulinemia improve with treatments that decrease viscosity and improve the rheologic properties of their blood (e.g., plasmapheresis).
    - Patients with autoimmune disorders and associated Raynaud's phenomenon do **not** usually respond well to therapy.
    - Treat the following:
      - Hepatitis B
      - Hepatitis C
      - *Mycoplasma* infections
    - In older patients with new-onset Raynaud's phenomenon and no obvious underlying cause, consider **malignancy.**
- **Botulinum neurotoxin A (BoNT-A)** effectively treats Raynaud's symptoms, including ulcers and pregangrene. (Disclosure: BoNT-A is not FDA approved for this use.)[17]
  - Mechanism: Cleaves SNAP-25 to prevent vesicle fusion and thus neurotransmitter release into synaptic cleft
  - BoNT-A is injected on the volar aspect under the dermis into the interstitial fluid surrounding the neurovascular bundles of the hand/fingers.
  - A typical treatment involves 100 U dissolved in 10 ml of normal saline. The hand is injected in 10 places with 1 ml aliquots of the solution.[17]

- Injections take effect within several days and may be repeated every 4-6 months.
- Studies show that BoNT-A injections help with pain relief, increase blood flow to fingers, and improve function.
- Potential side effects include anhydrosis and hand/grip weakness.
- Long-term effects and toxicity are unknown.

- **Surgical treatment**
  - **Cervical sympathectomy** still is considered controversial and may offer only temporary relief.
  - **Digital sympathectomy** has been gaining support for patients with severe or tissue-threatening disease.
    - May be used for patients with either primary or secondary disease
    - More commonly necessary with the secondary forms
  - Flatt[18] described an alternative approach to digital sympathectomy.
    - He stripped a 3-4 mm length of the adventitia (without compromising the vessel).
    - Eight treated patients had relief of symptoms and an increase of skin hand temperature for 1-12 years.
    - Only one patient had a relapse.
  - In a later 1999 report, seven patients underwent digital artery sympathectomy as a salvage procedure to prevent amputation. In six patients the digital ulcers healed, and amputation was avoided.
- **Complications**
  - Rarely, digital ulceration and tissue loss result from primary Raynaud's phenomenon.
  - The complications associated with secondary Raynaud's phenomenon are usually related to the underlying disease. The worst are loss of tissue pulp in the distal phalanx, ulceration, and digital gangrene.
- **Prognosis**
  - **Primary Raynaud's: Very good,** with no mortality and little morbidity
  - **Secondary Raynaud's: Related to the underlying disease**
    - Prognosis for the involved digit is related to the severity of ischemia and effectiveness of maneuvers to restore blood flow.
- **Mortality and morbidity**
  - **Primary Raynaud's:** Does not usually cause death or serious morbidity. However, ischemia of the affected body part can result in necrosis; this is very rare.
  - **Secondary Raynaud's: Possible marker for other diseases** that may lead to morbidity and mortality, such as:
    - Scleroderma (progressive systemic sclerosis)
    - Systemic lupus erythematosus
    - Hyperviscosity syndromes

## OTHER VASOSPASTIC DISEASES[9]

- Buerger's disease *(thromboangiitis obliterans)*
  - Usually **not** seen in the upper extremities
  - Inflammatory thrombosis mostly in **young men who smoke**
  - Characterized by **progressive ischemic changes**
  - The only practical treatment is **smoking cessation;** lesions are treated symptomatically as local condition dictates.

- Giant cell arteritis
- Wegner's granulomatosis
- Polyarteritis nodosa
- Takayasu's arteritis
- Hyperparathyroidism
- Iron overload in dialysis patients
- Vinyl chloride exposure

### ATHEROSCLEROTIC DISEASE

- Incidence of below-elbow ischemia from chronic vascular disease is likely underreported.
- Comorbidities are common: Diabetes, end-stage renal disease on dialysis, or systemic atherosclerosis.[19]
- About 5% of all patients with chronic ischemia have upper extremity involvement.[20]
  - When ischemia reaches a critical level, soft tissue necrosis begins.
- **History/physical:** Thorough routine history with complete vascular examination, including noninvasive tests[20]
- **Screening lab tests** for clotting disorder or collagen vascular disease
- **Arteriography:** Imaging modality of choice
- **Goals of treatment**[20]
  - Improve distal blood flow.
  - Promote healing of chronic wounds.
  - Decrease pain.
  - Maintain/improve function.
- **Treatment options**
  - **Arterial vascular bypass:** Best choice for isolated occlusion and patent distal vessels[20]
  - **Arterialization of venous system:** Salvage procedure for atherosclerotic disease when no patent distal vessels exist[20]
    - An in situ vein is stripped of its valves and anastomosed to an artery to provide retrograde flow through the vein to the distal hand and fingers.
  - **Percutaneous transluminal angioplasty:** Prospective study showed a technical success rate of 82% and hand-healing rate of 65%.[19] There is a risk of restenosis and need for repeat procedures.
    - Endoscopic balloon angioplasty can be performed as distally as the volar arch.
    - Stenting is typically reserved for more proximal lesions (i.e., proximal subclavian artery) because of poor or inconsistent patency rates when stenting more distal occlusions.

## THORACIC OUTLET SYNDROME[9,21-23]

Refers to compression of the neurovascular structures at the superior aperture of the thorax

- It involves a constellation of symptoms.
- Cause, diagnosis, and treatment are controversial.
- Affected structures include the brachial plexus (95%), subclavian vein (4%), and subclavian artery (1%).
- Most presentations are nonemergent and require only symptomatic treatment and referral.
- **Incidence**
  - **3-8:1000**

- **Sex**
  - Varies depending on the type of thoracic outlet syndrome
  - **Three times more common in women than in men, overall**
    - **Neurologic:** Female/male ratio approximately 3.5:1
    - **Venous:** More common in males than in females
    - **Arterial:** No sexual predilection
- **Age**
  - Usually **20 to 50 years old**
  - *Never* occurs before puberty and *rarely* after age 50 years
- **History**
  - **Ache or dull pain** and **swelling** in the affected arm
  - **Engorged veins** on hands and arms
  - Patients with arterial compression have "ischemic-like" pain or pain brought on when exercising an arm **(upper extremity claudication).**
- **Causes**
  - **Three major causes:**
    1. **Anatomy**
       - **Scalene triangle:** Anterior scalene muscle anteriorly, middle scalene muscle posteriorly, and upper border of the first rib inferiorly account for most neurologic and arterial thoracic outlet syndrome cases.
       - **Cervical ribs** are involved in most **arterial** cases (rarely in venous and neurologic cases).
       - **Congenital fibromuscular bands** occur in up to 80% of patients with neurologic thoracic outlet syndrome.
       - The transverse process of C7 is elongated.
    2. **Traumatic or repetitive activities**
       - **Motor vehicle accident:** Hyperextension injury with subsequent fibrosis and scarring
       - **Effort vein thrombosis:** Spontaneous thrombosis of the axillary veins after vigorous arm exertion
       - **Playing a musical instrument:** Musicians particularly susceptible because of need to maintain the shoulder in abduction or extension for long periods
    3. **Neurovascular entrapment** at the costoclavicular space
       - Occurs in the costoclavicular space between first rib and head of clavicle
- **Physical examination**

**NOTE: In most cases, physical examination findings are completely normal.**[22,23]

- **Provocative tests** such as Adson's maneuver or the costoclavicular and hyperabduction maneuvers are unreliable.
  - With interscalene compression of the subclavian artery, Adson's test is positive if radial pulse is lost when the affected arm is held in extension and dependent while the patient looks toward the ipsilateral shoulder.
  - *Approximately 92% of asymptomatic patients have variation in strength of the radial pulse during positional changes.*

- The **elevated arm stress test (EAST)** is of debatable use, but it may be the most reliable screening test. It evaluates **all three types** of thoracic outlet syndrome.
  - The patient sits with arms abducted 90 degrees from the thorax and elbows flexed 90 degrees, then opens and closes hands for 3 minutes.
  - Patients with thoracic outlet syndrome cannot continue this for 3 minutes, because symptoms soon appear. Patients with carpal tunnel syndrome have dysesthesia in fingers, but no shoulder or arm pain.
- **Venous**
  - Edema
  - Cyanosis
  - Distended superficial veins of the shoulder and chest
- **Arterial**
  - Pallor and pulselessness
  - Coolness on the affected side
  - Lower blood pressure in affected arm (a reliable indicator of arterial involvement)
  - Multiple small infarcts on hand and fingers (embolization)

■ **Imaging**

- **Cervical radiographs:** May demonstrate skeletal abnormality
- **Chest radiographs**
  - Cervical or first rib
  - Clavicle deformity
  - Pulmonary disease
  - Pancoast's tumor
- **Color-flow duplex scanning** for suspected vascular thoracic outlet syndrome
- **Arteriogram indications**
  - Evidence of peripheral emboli in the upper extremity
  - Suspected subclavian stenosis or aneurysm (e.g., bruit or abnormal supraclavicular pulsation)
  - Blood pressure differential >20 mm Hg
  - Obliteration of radial pulse during EAST
- **Venography indications**
  - Persistent or intermittent edema of the hand or arm
  - Peripheral unilateral cyanosis
  - Prominent venous pattern over the arm, shoulder, or chest

■ **Treatment**

- **Offending structure** (first rib, cervical rib, and middle third of the clavicle, scalenus muscle, or fibrous band) should be surgically removed.
- If arterial obstruction is present, **thromboendarterectomy** or an **interposition graft** may be performed. If symptoms persist, a **cervicodorsal sympathectomy** may help to alleviate hand pain and ischemia.
- Rarely, an arterial bypass graft may be needed.
- Venous obstruction can require the additional step of thrombectomy.
- Nonoperative treatment can be tried, but it should not be continued for >4 months if it fails. Options include:
  - Postural reeducation
  - Activity modification
  - Weight loss

## THORACIC OUTLET SYNDROME TREATMENT ALGORITHM[24] (Fig. 86-2)

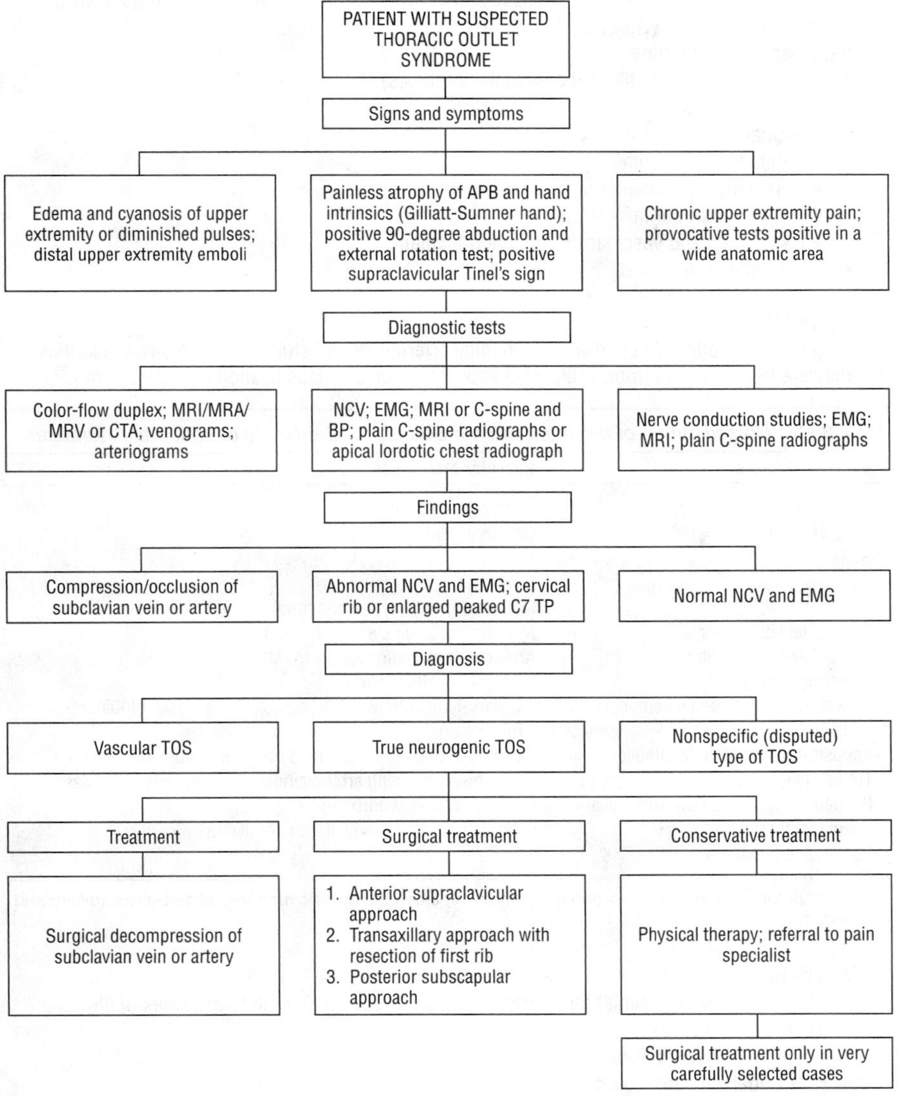


**Fig. 86-2** Treatment algorithm for thoracic outlet syndrome. (*APB,* Abductor pollicis brevis; *BP,* blood pressure; *CTA,* computed tomographic angiography; *EMG,* electromyography; *MRA,* magnetic resonance angiography; *MRI,* magnetic resonance imaging; *MRV,* magnetic resonance venography; *NCV,* nerve conduction velocity; *TOS,* thoracic outlet syndrome; *TP,* transverse process.)

## VASCULAR TUMORS[2,9,25-28]

- Vascular tumors in the hand are **not common.**
  - Two studies show the incidence of vascular tumors at 5%-8% of all hand tumors, with hemangiomas making up 50%-70% of these.
- **Vascular tumors include:**
  - Hemangiomas (infantile and congenital subtypes)
  - Glomus tumors
  - Malignant vascular tumors
    - Hemangiosarcoma
    - Hemangioendothelioma
    - Kaposi's sarcoma
    - <1% of hand vascular tumors are malignant.
  - Lymphangioma

### HEMANGIOMAS

Hemangiomas are often grouped with congenital arteriovenous fistulas (share many similarities), but they are technically a tumor. Table 86-3 shows the current classification schema of both.[25]

**Table 86-3** *Classification of the International Society for the Study of Vascular Anomalies*

| Vascular Tumors | Vascular Malformations |
|---|---|
| Hemangioma of infancy* (GLUT1-positive) | Simple malformation |
| Superficial | Capillary (port-wine stain) |
| Deep | Venous |
| Mixed | Lymphatic |
| Congenital hemangioma | Microcystic (e.g., lymphangioma) |
| Rapidly involuting congenital hemangioma (RICH) | Macrocystic (e.g., cystic hygroma) |
| Noninvoluting congenital hemangioma (NICH) | Arteriovenous malformation (AVM) |
| Kaposiform hemangioendothelioma | Combined malformation |
| Tufted angioma | Capillary-lymphatic-venous (includes most cases of Klippel-Trénaunay) |
| Pyogenic granuloma (lobular capillary hemangioma) | Capillary-venous (includes mild cases of Klippel-Trénaunay) |
| Hemangiopericytoma | Capillary-venous with arteriovenous shunting and/or fistulas (Parkes Weber syndrome) |
| | Cutis marmorata telangiectatica congenita |

*The descriptors *superficial, deep,* and *mixed* have replaced the archaic modifiers *strawberry, capillary,* and *cavernous.*

- **Description**
  - Although 30% are seen at birth, 70%-90% are discovered by the fourth week of life.
  - There are two types:
    - Infantile hemangioma
    - Congenital hemangioma
- **Natural history**
  - Classic infantile hemangiomas undergo **three phases of growth.**[9,25,26]
    1. It appears as a vascular stain or a small vascular papule at birth or during the first few weeks of life.

2. The rapid growth phase starts in the first month and lasts approximately 10-14 months. During this time, the mass may develop from a reddish-purple lesion to a large, bright red or bright blue mass.
3. During the last phase, the lesion involutes over many months or years. **By the age of 7 years, 70% of lesions have involuted.**

- **Congenital hemangiomas**
  - Growth phase is in utero, reaching peak size before birth.[2,25] Lesions are mature at birth.
  - The appearance can be different from a classic infantile hemangioma. Congenital hemangiomas may be purplish or have telangiectasias or peripheral blanching.
  - Based on differences in natural history, congenital hemangiomas are divided into two subtypes.
    - Rapidly involuting congenital hemangioma **(RICH)**
    - Noninvoluting congenital hemangioma **(NICH)**
    - RICH and NICH are both glucose transporter isoform 1 (GLUT1) negative, compared with hemangiomas of infancy, which are GLUT1 positive.
- **Imaging**
  - On plain radiographs, hemangiomas have a soft tissue shadow and may contain calcifications.
  - Typically, hemangiomas have well-defined borders on CT.
  - With the increased use of MRI, the reliance on angiography has diminished.
- **Treatment**[2,27]
  - Traditional management has been based on assumption that the birthmark will **involute spontaneously** by age 3-7 years.
    - With our current understanding and the known history that the RICH subtype quickly involutes, this remains sound practice.
  - **Surgical intervention** is indicated for **symptomatic problems** such as ulceration, infection, bleeding, obstruction of orifices, or psychosocial factors.
    - Hemangiomas on palm of the hand and some on face are usually aggressively treated early, without a "wait and see" period.

**NOTE: It is difficult to attribute efficacy to any of these modalities, because many hemangiomas involute spontaneously without any intervention.**

> **TIP:** Future treatment protocols will need to differentiate infantile from congenital hemangiomas (by GLUT1 testing) and RICH from NICH congenital hemangiomas.

- Cryotherapy with carbon dioxide snow and liquid nitrogen
- Radiotherapy
- Steroid therapy has been advocated for palliation of symptomatic hemangiomas.
- Interferon-alpha2-alpha has been given in cases of rapidly expanding, life-threatening hemangiomas that have failed an initial trial of steroids and require early intervention.
- Compression therapy
- Injection of sodium tetradecyl sulfate (Sotradecol 3%) alone or with surgery
- Laser therapy: Nd:YAG lasers are used for intralesional laser photocoagulation.

> **TIP:** *Maffucci's syndrome* is a rare disorder characterized by multiple hamartomas, including enchondromas and subcutaneous hemangiomas. It is frequently included on written examinations.

## Arteriovenous Malformations and Fistulas[2,9,27,28]

*Arteriovenous malformation* (AVM) is an abnormal communication between an artery and a vein.

- **Congenital AVMs** occur at any point in vascular system, and vary in size, length, location, and number.
- **Arteriovenous fistula (AVF)** is a **single communication** between an artery and a vein that usually has an acquired cause.
- Table 86-4 summarizes the differences between AVM and AVF.[2]

**Table 86-4** *Differences Between Arteriovenous Malformation and Arteriovenous Fistula*

| | AVM | AVF |
|---|---|---|
| **History** | | |
| Discovered early in life | Often | |
| Discovered after trivial injury | Often | |
| Seen after penetrating injury | No | Only mechanism |
| **Symptoms** | | |
| Mass, fullness, discomfort | Often | Often |
| **Signs** | | |
| Mass | Yes | Yes |
| Warm limb | Yes | Yes |
| Limb longer | Often | No |
| Distal ischemia | Sometimes | Sometimes |
| Bruit and thrill | Sometimes | Usually |
| Scar of trauma | No | Yes |
| **Arteriogram** | | |
| Large, single feeder | Sometimes | Yes |
| Rapid shunting | Sometimes | Yes |
| **Treatment** | | |
| Conservative often best | Yes | No |
| May need multiple stages | Yes | No |
| May require amputation | Yes | No |
| Single stage, straightforward | Rarely | Usually |

*AVF,* Arteriovenous fistula; *AVM,* arteriovenous malformation.

- **Pathophysiology**
  - Congenital vascular malformations are inborn errors in embryologic development.
  - Most AVMs are developmental errors that occur between **weeks 4 and 10** of embryogenesis.
  - The causes of these errors are **unknown.**
  - Potential exogenous causes such as viral infections, toxins, and drugs have been implicated but not proven.
  - Almost all AVMs are sporadic and nonfamilial, although a few syndromes such as Sturge-Weber and Klippel-Trénaunay include inherited vascular abnormalities.
  - Although the pathogenetic mechanisms of AVMs are not understood yet, hemodynamic alterations that lead to clinical manifestations of AVMs have been described.

- An abnormal communication causes shunting of blood from the high-pressure arterial side to the low-pressure venous side. This creates an abnormal low-resistance circuit that steals from the high-resistance, normal capillary bed.
- Blood follows the path of least resistance. Flow in the afferent artery and efferent vein increases, causing dilation, thickening, and tortuosity of the vessels.
- If resistance in the fistula is low enough, the fistulous tract will steal from the distal arterial supply, causing a reversal of arterial flow in the segment distal to the AVM. This is known as a *parasitic circulation,* which causes decreased arterial pressures in distal capillary beds and can cause tissue ischemia.
- Increased flow into the venous circulation does not necessarily cause higher venous pressures. However, it can cause vessel wall abnormalities such as thickening of the media and fibrosis of the wall. These changes are known as *arterialization.*
- Blood flow into the venous circulation causes turbulence, which is responsible for the **palpable thrill.** The thrill depends on the geometry of the fistula and does not represent volume of flow accurately.
- In addition to the decreased distal arterial pressures, peripheral venous pressures are increased, leading to tissue ischemia and its sequelae.
- The heart responds to decreased peripheral vascular resistance by increasing stroke volume and cardiac output. This leads to tachycardia, left ventricular dilation, and eventually heart failure.

- **Sex**
  - AVMs occur with **equal frequency** in males and females.
- **Age**
  - All AVMs are present at birth, but they are not always evident clinically.
  - A triggering stimulus during puberty or pregnancy or after minor trauma can precipitate clinical features of the malformation.
- **Symptoms**
  - Mass, pink stain, dilated veins, unequal limb length and girth, or skin ulceration.
  - Limb heaviness that is aggravated with dependency and relieved with elevation.
  - 50% of patients report having pain, which can be caused by tissue ischemia or mass effect on local nerves.
- **Physical findings**
  - The lesion can be **pulsatile.**
  - **Branham's sign** (slowing of the heart rate during compression proximal to AVM) may be present.
  - Patients can develop hyperhidrosis, hypertrichosis, hyperthermia, or a palpable thrill or bruit over the lesion.
  - Patients may have functional impairment of limbs or joints from mass effect or gangrene from prolonged tissue ischemia.
  - Visceral AVMs can present with hematuria, hematemesis, hemoptysis, or melena.
  - Rarely, patients present with signs of congestive heart failure (e.g., dyspnea, leg edema).
- **Laboratory studies**
  - Blood gas analysis in an AVM case reveals a higher oxygen partial pressure in the venous blood immediately distal to the fistula, compared with normal venous blood.
- **Imaging studies**
  - Plain films can show soft tissue masses or abnormalities within bony structures.
  - **Duplex ultrasonography** can be used to characterize **direction and velocity of blood flow.** Doppler scan can be used preoperatively and intraoperatively. However, ultrasound has no therapeutic use.

- **Contrast-enhanced CT scans** are useful to locate abnormality, evaluate for aneurysm formation, and identify bony involvement.
- **Contrast angiography is the most important method for investigating AVMs.**
  - Delineates the number, location, and extent of arteriovenous connections
  - Angiographic signs include early filling of veins, hypertrophied and tortuous arteries proximal to malformation, and varicose and dilated veins distal to fistula.
- **MRI** has become the new standard in preoperative evaluation of patients with AVMs.
  - Generates multiplanar views and can be used to accurately define tissue planes and identify critical flow characteristics
  - Best modality to define local soft tissue and adjacent organ involvement, which helps with preintervention planning
  - MR sequences can be postprocessed into **MR angiogram images,** which help define malformation more clearly.
- **Radiolabeled studies** can determine the shunt fraction, which is the proportion of blood being shunted through the fistulous tract.

■ **Other tests**
- Invasive and noninvasive cardiac evaluation may be indicated in patients with congestive heart failure, because cardiac output can be markedly elevated in patients with large proximal AVMs.

CAUTION: **Percutaneous biopsy is never indicated! Biopsy can be helpful if a lesion is suspected to be sarcomatous or if the clinical impression is unclear.**

■ **Medical treatment**
- Most can be managed and controlled **medically.**
- Only a few demonstrate progressive growth and require surgical intervention.
- Most symptoms are caused by venous hypertension (pain, heaviness, and swelling).
- The cornerstone approach in managing lower extremity symptoms is **elastic support hose.**
  - An elastic support stocking that provides **30-40 mm Hg** of compression usually is sufficient to relieve leg symptoms.
- Arm and some hand lesions can also be managed with compressive garments.
- **Alcohol sclerotherapy** may shrink the size of the AVM, but it places patient at risk for peripheral nerve injury.
  - Treatment of large AVMs with alcohol needs to be performed by an experienced interventional radiologist. Risks must be explained to patients before therapy.

■ **Surgical treatment**
- **Indications for surgical intervention of AVMs:**
  - Hemorrhage
  - Painful ischemia
  - Congestive heart failure
  - Nonhealing ulcers
  - Functional impairment
  - Limb-length inequality
- **Embolization** is an option for treatment and should be considered when conservative measures have failed or when vascularity of the malformation needs to be reduced before surgical resection.
  - Procedure involves the injection of particulate matter into the malformation.
  - Common adverse effects are pain and tenderness near malformation, transient fever, and leukocytosis.
  - Excision should be performed **48-72 hours** after embolization.[29]

- Most AVMs are not amenable to complete surgical excision, and it is not required.
  - A lesion must be well localized for a chance of complete resection.
  - Resectability depends on the degree of extension into adjacent structures.
- Patients severely afflicted with malformations, who are not candidates for local extirpation, may be candidates for amputation and rehabilitation with a limb prosthesis.

■ **Prognosis**
- Lee et al[2] reported their results with **nonsurgical management of AVMs.**
  - 32 patients with surgically inaccessible lesions were treated with embolism and sclerotherapy alone.
  - There were nine failures from a total of 171 sessions.
  - There were 31 complications, mostly minor (27 of 31), and four major.
    - Facial nerve palsy
    - Pulmonary embolism
    - Deep venous thrombosis
    - Massive necrosis of an ear cartilage
- Sofocleous et al[26] reported their results of **embolization** of hand and forearm AVMs.
  - In a 15-year period, 39 patients (22 men, mean age 22.5 years) had symptomatic vascular lesions diagnosed in the forearm and hand.
    - 21 AVMs
    - 17 primary venous malformations (PVMs)
    - One complex lesion with both AVM and PVM
  - Lesions were treated in 34 cases (87%), with immediate technical success achieved in 31 (91%); lesions were not amenable to percutaneous treatment in 5 (13%).
  - There were no major complications, but three embolized AVMs had significant residual flow (81.6% technical success on intention-to-treat basis).
  - Long-term follow-up of up to 5 years in 26/34 treated patients; mean symptom-free period was 30 months for AVM patients and 30.5 months for PVM group (average 1.5 and 1.2 embolization procedures, respectively).

## GLOMUS TUMORS[2,9,30]

*Glomus tumors* are **benign lesions** containing cells from the **glomus apparatus.**

■ The **glomus body** lies in the reticular layer and is responsible for **thermoregulatory control.**

■ The **glomus apparatus** contains an afferent vessel, a Sucquet-Hoyer canal (an arteriovenous shunt in the dermis that contributes to temperature regulation), and multiple shunts in the glabrous skin of the hand and beneath the nail beds.

■ Numerous nonmyelinated nerve fibers are seen histologically.

■ Up to **75%** of glomus tumors are found in the **hand;** up to **65%** of these are found in the **fingertip.**

■ **Classification:** Glomus tumors are classified into three groups:
1. Solitary lesions
2. Multiple painful lesions
3. Multiple painless lesions

■ **Symptoms:** A **classic triad** is observed with glomus tumors.
- Cold hypersensitivity
- Paroxysmal pain
- Pinpoint tenderness

**TIP:** This triad of symptoms for glomus tumors is frequently seen on written examinations.

- Pain caused by glomus tumors is **not primarily nocturnal,** has a paroxysmal pattern, and is **not usually relieved with salicylates.** Tumor is located by applying pressure to the suspected area with the head of a pin, which elicits intense pain **(Love's sign).** If a blood pressure cuff is inflated proximally, the pain is abolished **(Hildreth's sign).**[30]

- **Physical findings**
  - Painful subcutaneous nodules subungually
  - Bluish discoloration in the nail beds, with or without nail plate ridges
- **Imaging**
  - Includes **MRI,** which reveals a dark, well-defined lesion on T1-weighted images and a bright lesion on T2-weighted images[31,32] (Figs. 86-3 and 86-4)
  - Doppler ultrasound studies useful to help detect the **high blood flow** in glomus tumors
- **Treatment:** Excision
  - After nail is removed, the nail bed is exposed.
  - Careful examination of the matrix is necessary, because recurrence rates reportedly are as high as **20%.**
  - Persistence of symptoms after exploration may require reexploration, secondary to the likelihood of **multiple lesions.**
  - Vasisht et al[30] describe an alternative technique that uses a lateral incision and raises a subperiosteal flap to gain full access to the subungual region in 19 patients with only a 15.4% recurrence rate.

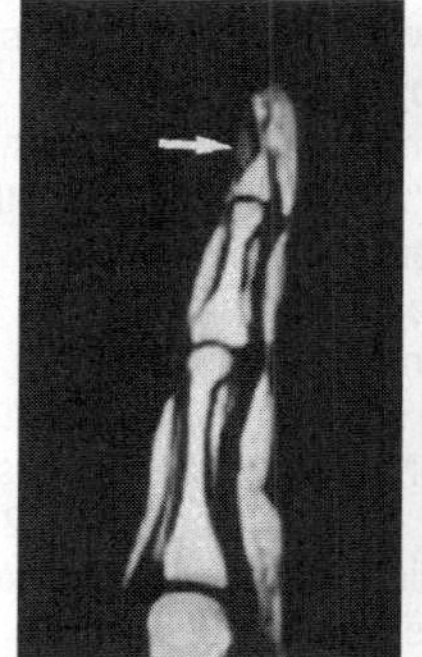
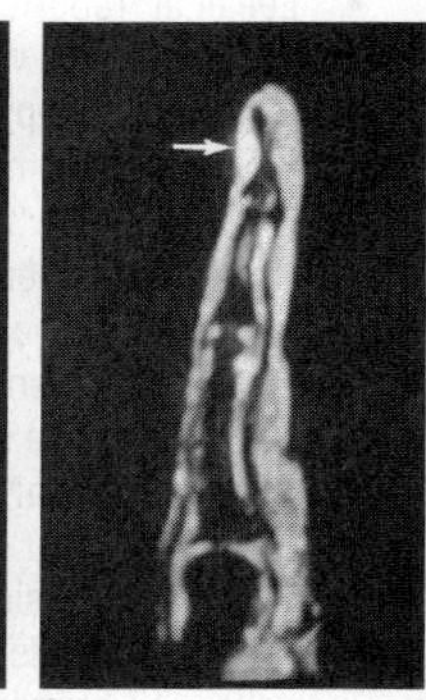

**Fig. 86-3** MRI of subungual glomus tumor.

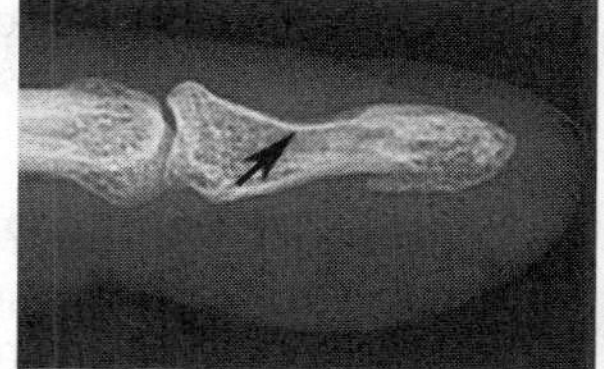

**Fig. 86-4** Radiograph of subungual glomus tumor.

## Malignant Tumors[9,33]

**Angiosarcoma** and **Kaposi's sarcoma (KS)** are most common in adult white men and are seen in the extremities.

- **Angiosarcomas** are red vascular tumors and can metastasize; their behavior is variable. Wide excision is usually curative.
- **KS** shows small bluish-red to dark brown plaques and nodules.
  - Clinical course variable—rapidly fatal or indolent for many years
  - Usually starts on the extremities and spreads to other cutaneous sites or to bowel viscera
  - Has become much more common since **AIDS** became prevalent and can be found in young men
  - Treated by highly active antiretroviral therapy (HAART) treatment for AIDS. In lesions not treated with HAART, variety of systemic and sometimes topical therapies used with variable results.
  - **Surgical treatment** on the hand or extremities **rarely indicated,** except for symptomatic complications. (KS-associated aneurysm of the ulnar artery has been reported.)

## LYMPHANGIOMAS

- Very rare subgroup of malignant hemangiomas; subtypes and treatment options summarized in Table 86-5[26]

**Table 86-5** *Subtypes of Lymphangiomas*

| Subtype | Description | Treatment |
|---|---|---|
| Simple lymphangiomas | Lesions are small and well circumscribed with a wartlike appearance and little tendency to grow | Local excision |
| Cavernous lymphangiomas | Most common variety<br>Appear within the first month of life<br>Can grow to become massive<br>Consist of dilated lymphatic sinuses | Usually excision or amputation is needed<br>Radiation treatments are helpful for common recurrences |
| Cystic hygromas | Occur in the neck or rarely axilla<br>Originate from primitive jugular sacs<br>Present at birth and grow rapidly | Excision |

## KEY POINTS

- ✓ MRA and CTA are useful imaging studies for vascular disorders. CTA is particularly useful for evaluation of vascular trauma.
- ✓ Injuries to arteries of the hand (the arch) and forearm usually can be safely managed with ligation when backbleeding is sufficient. An injured blood vessel should be repaired if there is an accompanying nerve injury, regardless of whether there is adequate bleeding.
- ✓ Emboli have traditionally been treated surgically with embolectomy; however, localized endovascular administration of thrombolytic agent is being recognized as a viable option in some scenarios. Always, the source of the emboli needs to be addressed.
- ✓ Raynaud's phenomenon is vasospasm that is associated with another illness (usually autoimmune), whereas Raynaud's disease is vasospasm that is not associated with other illnesses.
- ✓ Management of Raynaud's phenomenon and disease is difficult; medical therapy helps to manage the symptoms. Surgical therapy is used for failed medical therapy and includes cervical sympathectomy, which only offers temporary relief; digital sympathectomy; and BoNT-A injection, which has shown promise with severely symptomatic disease.
- ✓ Diagnosis of vascular compression at the neck (thoracic outlet syndrome) is difficult, and physical examination findings are usually normal. Most provocative tests are unreliable; only the EAST test has some debatable usefulness.
- ✓ There are two types of hemangiomas. **Classic infantile hemangiomas** have three growth phases, are GLUT1 positive, and undergo 70% involution by the age of 7 years. **Congenital hemangiomas** are GLUT1 negative and have two subtypes: RICH and NICH. RICH rapidly involutes by age 6-10 months, but NICH never involutes.
- ✓ Most AVMs can be successfully treated with embolization and sclerotherapy. Lesions that require surgical excision (symptomatic or psychologically symptomatic facial lesions) should be embolized preoperatively, and the lesion should be excised within 48-72 hours.
- ✓ A glomus tumor is characterized by the classic triad of cold hypersensitivity, paroxysmal pain, and pinpoint pain. Treatment is excision.

## REFERENCES

1. Craig PS, Murphy MS. Vascular problems of the upper extremity: a primer for the orthopedic surgeon. J Am Acad Orthop Surg 10:401-408, 2002.
2. Lee BB, Do YS, Yakes W, et al. Management of arteriovenous malformations: a multidisciplinary approach. J Vasc Surg 39:590-600, 2004.
3. Menzoian JO, Doyle JE, LoGerfo FW, et al. Evaluation and management of vascular injuries of the extremities. Arch Surg 118:93-95, 1983.
4. Gelberman RH, Blasingame JP, Fronek A, et al. Forearm arterial injuries. J Hand Surg Am 4:401-408, 1979.
5. Scheer B, Perel A, Pfeiffer UJ. Clinical review: complications and risk factors of peripheral arterial catheters used for haemodynamic monitoring in anaesthesia and intensive care medicine. Crit Care 6:199-204, 2002.
6. Brzezinski M, Luisetti T, London M. Radial artery cannulation: a comprehensive review of recent anatomic and physiologic investigations. Anesth Analg 109:1763-1781, 2009.
7. Perry MO, Thal ER, Shires GT. Management of arterial injuries. Ann Surg 173:403-408, 1971.
8. Leclercq DC, Carlier AJ, Khuc T, et al. Improvement in the results in sixty-four ulnar nerve sections associated with arterial repair. J Hand Surg Am 10:997-999, 1985.
9. Koman LA, Smith BP, Smith TL, et al. Vascular disorders. In Wolfe SW, Pederson WC, Hotchkiss RN, et al, eds. Operative Hand Surgery, 6th ed. Philadelphia: Churchill Livingstone, 2011.
10. Hood DB, Kuehne J, Yellin AE, et al. Vascular complications of thoracic outlet syndrome. Am Surg 63:913-917, 1997.
11. Barbiero G, Cognolato D, Casarin A, et al. Intra-arterial thrombolysis of acute hand ischaemia with or without microcatheter: preliminary experience and comparison with the literature. Radiol Med 116: 919-931, 2011.
12. Savader SJ, Lund GB, Scheel PJ. Forearm loop, upper arm straight, and brachial-internal jugular vein dialysis grafts: a comparison study of graft survival utilizing a combined percutaneous endovascular and surgical maintenance approach. J Vasc Interv Radiol 10:537-545, 1999.
13. McCall TE, Petersen DP, Wong LB. The use of digital artery sympathectomy as a salvage procedure for severe ischemia of Raynaud's disease and phenomenon. J Hand Surg Am 24:173-177, 1999.
14. Dziadzio M, Denton CP, Smith R, et al. Losartan therapy for Raynaud's phenomenon and scleroderma: clinical and biochemical findings in a fifteen-week, randomized, parallel-group, controlled trial. Arthritis Rheum 42:2646-2655, 1999.
15. Wigley FM, Flavahan NA. Raynaud's phenomenon. Rheum Dis Clin North Am 22:765-781, 1996.
16. Connell D, Koulouris G, Thorn D, et al. Contrast-enhanced MR angiography of the hand. Radiographics 22:583-599, 2002.
17. Mannava S, Plate JF, Stone AV, et al. Recent advances for the management of Raynaud phenomenon using botulinum neurotoxin A. J Hand Surg Am 36:1708-1710, 2011.
18. Flatt AE. Digital artery sympathectomy. J Hand Surg Am 5:550-556, 1980.
19. Ferraresi R, Palloshi A, Aprigliano G, et al. Angioplasty of below-the-elbow arteries in critical hand ischaemia. Eur J Vasc Endovasc Surg 43:73-80, 2012.
20. Matarrese MR, Hammert WC. Revascularization of the ischemic hand with arterialization of the venous system. J Hand Surg Am 36:2047-2051, 2011.
21. Franklin GM, Fulton-Kehoe D, Bradley C, et al. Outcome of surgery for thoracic outlet syndrome in Washington state workers' compensation. Neurology 54:1252-1257, 2000.

22. Plewa MC, Delinger M. The false-positive rate of thoracic outlet syndrome shoulder maneuvers in healthy subjects. Acad Emerg Med 5:337-342, 1998.
23. Oates SD, Daley RA. Thoracic outlet syndrome. Hand Clin 12:705-718, 1996.
24. Huang J, Zager E. Thoracic outlet syndrome. Neurosurgery 55:897-903, 2004.
25. Chang MW. Updated classification of hemangiomas and other vascular anomalies. Lymphat Res Biol 1:259-265, 2003.
26. Sofocleous CT, Rosen RJ, Raskin K, et al. Congenital vascular malformations in the hand and forearm. J Endovasc Ther 8:484-494, 2001.
27. Achauer BM, Chang CJ, Vander Kam VM. Management of hemangioma of infancy: review of 245 patients. Plast Reconstr Surg 99:1301-1308, 1997.
28. Mulliken JB, Glowacki J. Hemangiomas and vascular malformations in infants and children: a classification based on endothelial characteristics. Plast Reconstr Surg 69:412-422, 1982.
29. Weinzweig N, Chin G, Polley J, et al. Arteriovenous malformation of the forehead, anterior scalp, and nasal dorsum. Plast Reconstr Surg 105:2433-2439, 2000.
30. Vasisht B, Watson HK, Joseph E, et al. Digital glomus tumors: a 29-year experience with a lateral subperiosteal approach. Plast Reconstr Surg 114:1486-1489, 2004.
31. Al-Qattan M, Al-Namla A, Al-Thunayan A. Magnetic resonance imaging in the diagnosis of glomus tumours of the hand. J Hand Surg Br 30:535-540, 2005.
32. Drapé J. Imaging of tumors of the nail unit. Clin Podiatr Med Surg 21:493-511, 2004.
33. Noy A. Update in Kaposi sarcoma. Curr Opin Oncol 15:379-381, 2003.

# Part VII

# Aesthetic Surgery

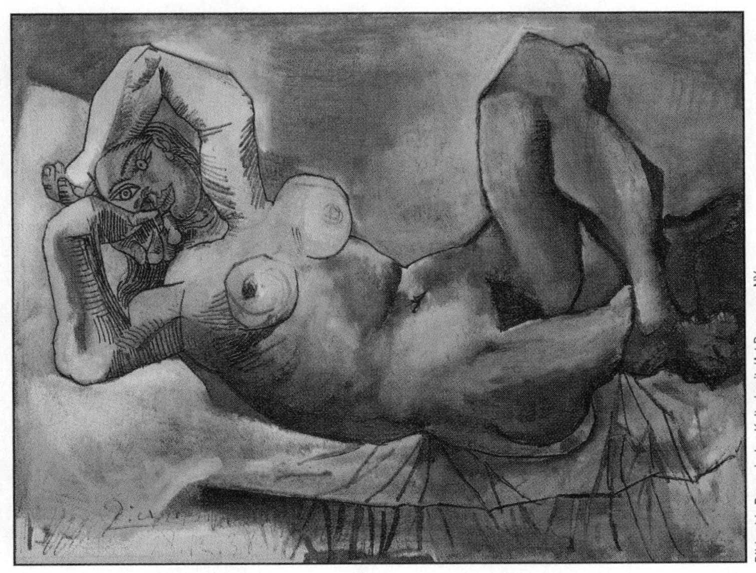

Part VII opening art: Picasso, Pablo (1881-1973) © Artist Rights Society (ARS), NY. Reclining Female Nude. 1938. Black ink, pastel and gouache on paper, 26 × 34 cm. Photo: Jens Ziehe, Nationalgalerie, Museum Berggruen, Staatliche Museen zu Berlin, Berlin, Germany. Photo Credit: Bildarchiv Preussischer Kulturbesitz/Art Resource, NY. © 2006 Estate of Pablo Picasso/ARS, New York.

# 87. Facial Analysis

Janae L. Maher, Raman C. Mahabir

## SKIN QUALITY[1,2]

- **Skin type and complexion**
  - **Fitzpatrick classification:** Ranks the skin's tendency to tan or burn after actinic exposure (Table 87-1)
- **Skin texture and thickness**
  - Total dermal thickness decreases approximately 6% per decade.
  - Actinic exposure and smoking increase the rate of dermal deterioration.
- **Photoaging**
  - **Glogau classification**: Ranks the degree of skin wrinkling and severity of photoaging (Table 87-2)
- **Severity of facial rhytids**
  - **Classification of rhytids**
    - Grade I: No rhytids at rest or on animation
    - Grade II: Superficial rhytids on animation only
    - Grade III: Deep rhytids on animation only
    - Grade IV: Superficial rhytids at rest, deep on animation
    - Grade V: Deep rhytids at rest, deeper on animation

**Table 87-1** *Fitzpatrick Skin Type Classification*

| Skin Type | Sun Exposure History/Skin Color |
|---|---|
| I | Never tans; burns easily and severely; extremely fair skin |
| II | Usually burns; tans minimally |
| III | Burns moderately; tans moderately |
| IV | Tans moderately and easily; burns minimally |
| V | Rarely burns; dark brown skin |
| VI | Never burns; dark brown or black skin |

**Table 87-2** *Glogau Classification*

| Photoaging Group | | Degree of Skin Wrinkling and Photoaging |
|---|---|---|
| I | Mild (age 28-35) | Little wrinkling or scarring; no keratosis; requires little or no makeup |
| II | Moderate (age 35-50) | Early wrinkling, mild scarring; sallow color with early actinic keratosis; requires little makeup |
| III | Advanced (age 50-65) | Persistent wrinkling; discoloration with telangiectasias and actinic keratosis; wears makeup always |
| IV | Severe (age 60-75) | Wrinkling; photoaging: gravitational, dynamic; actinic keratosis with or without skin cancer; wears makeup with poor coverage |

## FACIAL CANONS OF DIVINE PROPORTION[3]

Classical Greek canons of proportion were formulated and documented by the Renaissance artists. These neoclassical canons are as follows (Fig. 87-1):

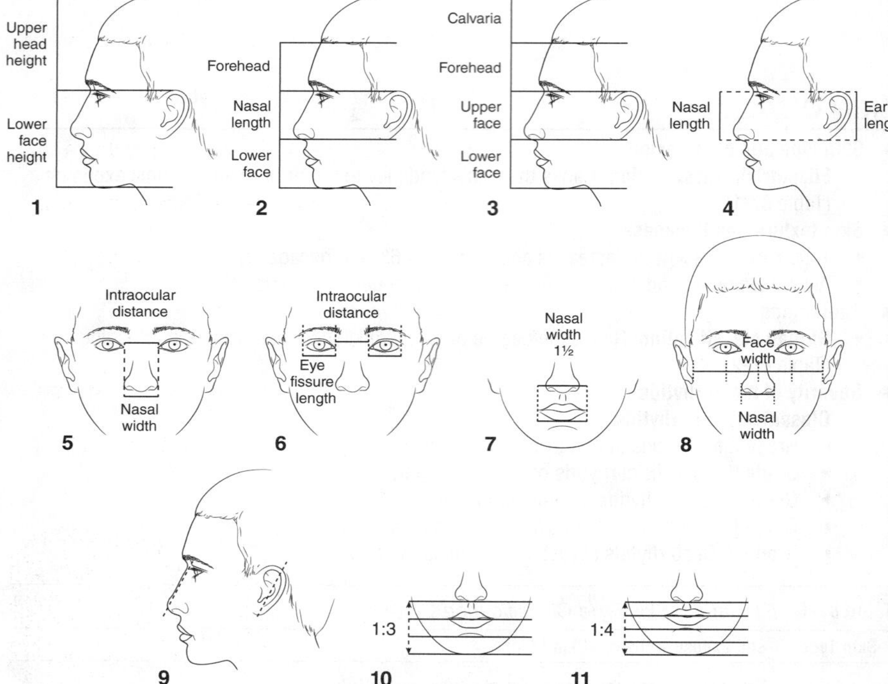


**Fig. 87-1** Neoclassical canons. **1,** The head can be divided into equal halves at a horizontal line through the eyes. **2,** The face can be divided into equal thirds, with the nose occupying the middle third. **3,** The head can be divided into equal quarters, with the middle quarters being the forehead and nose. **4,** The length of the ear is equal to the length of the nose. **5,** The distance between the eyes is equal to the width of the nose. **6,** The distance between the eyes is equal to the width of each eye (the face width can be divided into equal fifths). **7,** The width of the mouth is 1½ times the width of the nose. **8,** The width of the nose is one fourth the width of the face. **9,** The nasal bridge inclination is the same as the ear inclination. **10,** The lower face can be divided into equal thirds. **11,** The lower face can be divided into equal quarters.

- The head can be divided into equal halves by a horizontal line through the eyes.
- The face can be divided into equal thirds, with the nose occupying the middle third.
- The head can be divided into equal quarters, with the middle quarters being the forehead and nose.
- The length of the ear is equal to the length of the nose.
- The distance between the eyes is equal to the width of the nose.
- The distance between the eyes is equal to the width of each eye. (The face width can be divided into equal fifths.)
- The width of the mouth is 1½ times the width of the nose.
- The width of the nose is a fourth the width of the face.
- The nasal bridge inclination is the same as the ear inclination.
- The lower face can be divided into equal thirds.
- The lower face can be divided into equal quarters.

**TIP:** The golden ratio of Fibonacci (1:1.618) is a common theme seen throughout facial aesthetics.

## FRONTAL VIEW[4]

- Vertical fifths: Lines drawn adjacent to the most lateral projection of the head, the lateral canthi, and the medial canthi (Fig. 87-2, *A*)
- Horizontal thirds: Lines drawn adjacent to the menton, nasal base, brows at the supraorbital notch level, and hairline
  - The lower third can be divided into an upper third and lower two thirds by a line drawn through the oral commissures (Fig. 87-2, *B*).
  - The lower third can be divided into halves by a horizontal line adjacent to the lowest point of the lower lip vermilion (Fig. 87-2, *C*).
- Horizontal line through the labiomental groove divides the stomion-to-menton distance into a 1:2 ratio (Fig. 87-2, *D*).
- Width of the mouth and the stomion-to-menton distance are equal (Fig. 87-2, *E*).
- Width of the mouth approximates the distance between the medial limbi of the corneas (Fig. 87-2, *F*).
- The width of the face at the malar level is equal to the distance from the brows to the menton (Fig. 87-2, *G*).
- The distance from the infraorbital rim to the base of the nose equals the nasal base length, which is equal to half of the length of the middle third of the face (Fig. 87-2, *H*).

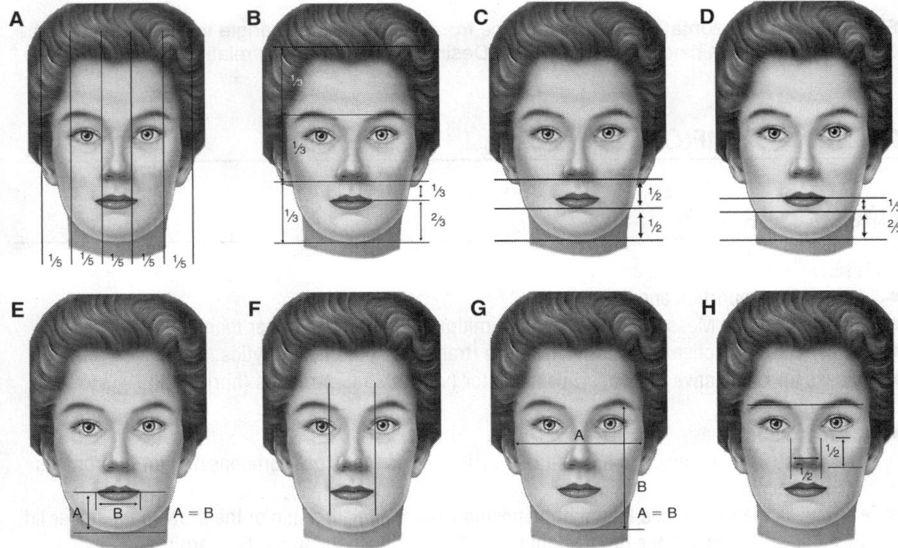


**Fig. 87-2** **A,** Vertical fifths. **B,** Horizontal thirds. **C,** Division of the lower third. **D,** 1:2 ratio of the lower third. **E,** Stomion to menton *(A)* and the width of the mouth *(B)* are equidistant. **F,** Distance between the medial limbi approximates the width of the mouth. **G,** Width of the face at the malar level *(A)* is equal to the distance from the brow to the menton *(B).* **H,** Infraorbital rim to base of nose distance is equal to the nasal base distance, which is equal to half the length of the middle third of the face.

## Lateral View[4]

- The face profile can be divided into horizontal thirds.
  - The lower third can be divided into an upper third and two lower thirds by a line drawn through the oral commissure (Fig. 87-3, *A*).
- The distance from the mandibular angle to the menton is half the distance from the hairline to the menton (Fig. 87-3, *B*).
- The desired lip-chin complex relationship is an upper lip that projects ~2 mm more than the lower lip (Fig. 87-3, *C*).
  - In women the chin lies slightly posterior to the lower lip.
  - In men the chin is slightly stronger.

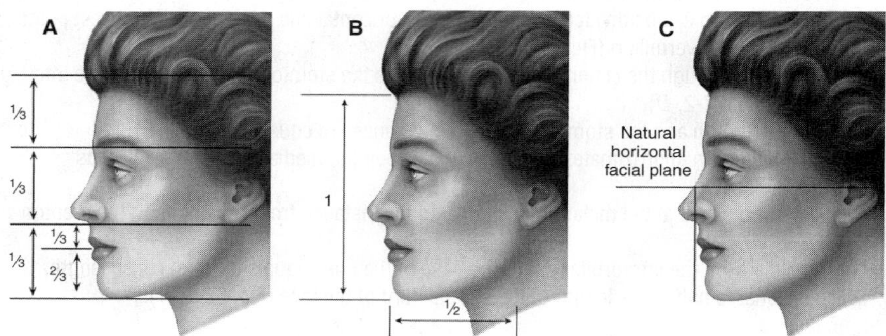


**Fig. 87-3 A,** Horizontal thirds. **B,** Distance from the mandibular angle to menton is half the distance from the hairline to the menton. **C,** Desired lip-chin complex relationship.

# REGION-SPECIFIC ANALYSIS

## UPPER THIRD

### Forehead[1]

- Assess for proportion and contour.
- Forehead height: Measure from hairline to midpupil (fixed point rather than hairline to brow).
- Assess for both active and passive frontalis (transverse) forehead rhytids.
- Assess for both active and passive corrugator (vertical) and procerus (horizontal) rhytids at the glabella.
- Brow position
  - Assess for compensated brow ptosis. (The brow is ptotic but compensated for by frontalis hyperactivity.)
  - Assess the medial and lateral brow position and the relationship of the brow to the upper lid.
    - With lid closed, the brow should be 2-2.5 cm above the upper lid margin.
    - At midpupil, the ratio of the aperture of the eye (1) to the distance from brow to lash line (1.618) is consistent with the golden ratio.
    - Highest portion should be at (or just lateral to) the lateral third point corresponding to lateral edge of the limbus in straight gaze.
    - The medial portion of brow should be caudal to the lateral portion.
    - Greatest degree of brow descent often occurs at the lateral orbit (lateral brow hooding).

## UPPER EYELID[1]

- Assess for redundant skin, skin quality, fat herniation, and soft tissue excess (subcutaneous fat, preseptal fat, lacrimal gland ptosis).
- Intercanthal distance is 31-33 mm; however, 33-36 mm can be considered attractive.
- Intercanthal axis is normally tilted slightly upward from medial to lateral. (Lateral canthus is 2 degrees higher.)
- Vertical opening is ~10 mm.
- Lid position
  - Upper lid extends down at least 1.5 mm below the upper limbus but no more than 3 mm.
  - Pretarsal skin is visualized on relaxed forward gaze: 3-6 mm (varies with ethnicity).
  - The ratio of distance from the lower edge of eyebrow to the open lid center margin to visualized pretarsal skin should never be less than 3:1, preferably more.
- Supratarsal fold
  - 7-11 mm from lash line
  - Indicator of levator dehiscence: Elevation of supratarsal fold; accentuated supratarsal hollow[5] (Fig. 87-4)

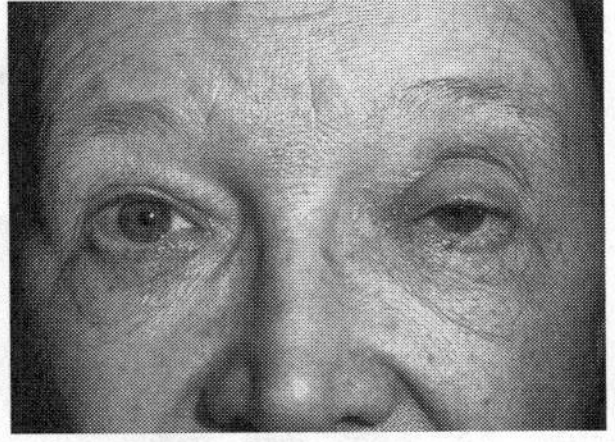

**Fig. 87-4** This woman shows classic signs of left levator dehiscence with ptosis, a high lid crease, and thinning of the lid above the tarsal plate.

## LOWER EYELID

- Assess for redundant skin, skin quality, rhytids (crow's feet), tarsal laxity, skin pigmentation (blepharomelasma), festoons, fat herniation, tear trough deformity, and scleral show.
- The lower lid ideally covers 0.5 mm of the lower limbus but no more than 1.5 mm.

> **TIP:** The lid-cheek junction must also be assessed and factored into the analysis, because it is one of the more complex areas of the face.

## GLOBE

- Determine whether positive, neutral, or negative vector relationship exists.
- Assess for globe prominence/proptosis, enophthalmos/exophthalmos, dystopia, visual acuity, and Bell's phenomenon.

# MIDDLE THIRD

## NOSE[4,6]

- First evaluate skin type and texture.
  - Thick and sebaceous skin does not drape as well, and edema takes longer to subside.
  - Thin skin may drape too well and can show small deformities underneath the skin.
- Evaluate for deviation: A line drawn from midglabella to menton should bisect the nasal bridge, nasal tip, and cupid's bow (Fig. 87-5, *A*).
- The width of the body of the nose at the nasal-cheek junction should equal 80% of the alar base width (Fig. 87-15, *B*).
- The alar base width should be about the same as the intercanthal distance, which should be the same as the width of an eye (Fig. 87-5, *C*).
  - If interalar width is wider than intercanthal width, determine whether it is caused by increased interalar width or alar flaring.

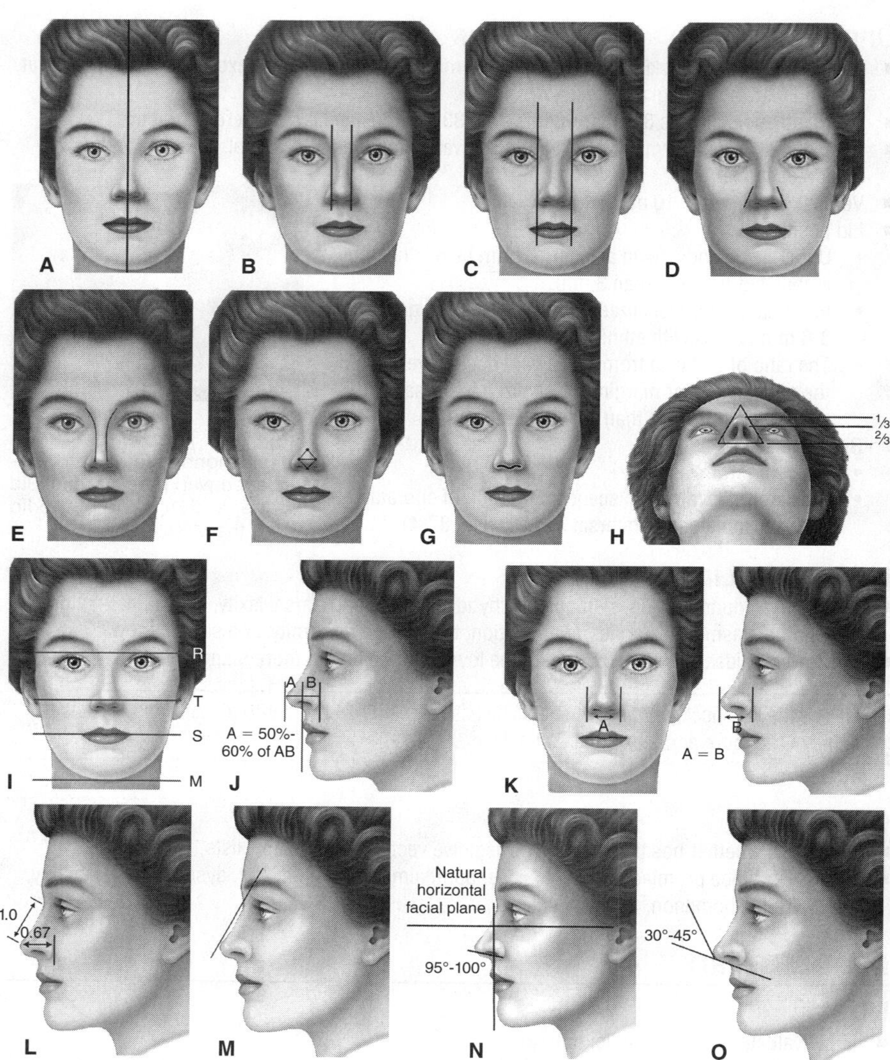


**Fig. 87-5** **A,** Deviation of the nose is evaluated by drawing a line from the midglabella to the menton. **B,** The body of the nose at the nasal-cheek junction should equal 80% of the alar base width. **C,** Alar base width should equal the intercanthal distance. **D,** Alar rims flare slightly outward inferiorly. **E,** Slightly curved divergent lines should extend from the medial supraciliary ridges to the tip-defining points on the dorsum. **F,** The tip-defining points bilaterally, the supratip break above, and the columellar-lobular angle below should form two equilateral triangles. **G,** Gull-wing appearance of the columella. **H,** Basal view. **I,** Nasal length evaluation; RT = 1.6 × TS. (*M,* Menton; *R,* radix, *S,* stomion; *T,* tip.) **J,** Evaluation of the nasal tip projection. **K,** Alar base width *(A)* equals tip projection *(B).* **L,** Tip projection equals 0.67RT (nasal length). (*R,* Radix; *T,* tip.) **M,** Nasal dorsum evaluation. **N,** Nasolabial angle. **O,** Columellar-lobular angle.

- Normal alar flaring in Caucasian females is 2 mm wider than alar base; if it is greater than this, alar base resection should be considered.
- If interalar width is increased, then nostril resection may be indicated.

- The alar rims should flare slightly outward in an inferior direction (Fig. 87-5, *D*).
- Two slightly curved divergent lines should extend from the medial supraciliary ridges to the tip-defining points on the dorsum (Fig. 87-5, *E*).
- Nasal tip evaluation: Locate the tip-defining points bilaterally, supratip break above, and the columellar-lobular angle below; these should form two equilateral triangles (Fig. 87-5, *F*).
- Columella evaluation: It should hang just inferior to the alar rims, giving a gentle gull-wing appearance (Fig. 87-5, *G*).
- Basal view: An equilateral triangle is visualized with a 2:1 ratio of columella to lobular portion; the nostrils should be teardrop shaped (Fig. 87-5, *H*).
- Nasal length evaluation
  - Ideal nasal length (RT) should equal the distance from the stomion to the menton (SM), which equals 1.6 × distance from tip to stomion (TS) (Fig. 87-5, *I*).
  - Nasal length should be approximately two thirds of midfacial (middle third) height.
- Nasal tip projection evaluation
  - A line drawn from the alar-cheek junction to the tip of the nose, when bisected by a vertical line drawn adjacent to the most projecting portion of the upper lip, should have 50%-60% of the horizontal line anterior to the vertical line (Fig. 87-5, *J*).
    - If >60% of the tip is anterior to the vertical line, the tip is overprojected and should be reduced.
    - If <50% of the line lies anterior to it, projection is inadequate and should be augmented.

**TIP:** This relationship only holds true if the upper lip projection is normal.

- Tip projection equals the alar base width (Fig. 87-5, *K*).
- Tip projection should be approximately 0.67RT (Fig. 87-5, *L*).

**TIP:** This relationship only holds true if the nasal length is correct.

- Nasal dorsum evaluation
  - In women it lies 2 mm behind and parallel to a line connecting the nasofrontal angle with the desired tip projection; a slight supratip break is preferred (Fig. 87-5, *M*).
  - In men it lies slightly more anteriorly.
  - If it is too far posterior to this line, augmentation will be required.
  - If it is too far anterior to this line, reduction is indicated.
- Tip rotation
  - This is determined by the degree of the nasolabial angle.
  - Draw a straight line through the most anterior and posterior points of the nostrils on lateral view. Where this bisects with a perpendicular line to the natural horizontal facial plane is the nasolabial angle (Fig. 87-5, *N*).
    - In women 95- to 100-degree angle is preferred.
    - In men 90- to 95-degree angle is preferred.

**TIP:** A nose with a high dorsum without a supratip break will appear less rotated than one with a low dorsum and supratip break, even though the degree of rotation is the same.

- Columellar-lobular angle: Formed by the junction of the columella with the infratip lobule (Fig. 87-5, *O*)

- It is usually 30-45 degrees.
- Increased fullness in this area (usually caused by prominent caudal septum) will give the appearance of increased tip rotation even though the angle of rotation (nasolabial angle) is within normal limits.

■ Intranasal examination
- Inspect airways, nasal valve, septum, and turbinates.

■ Ethnic variations in nasal structure
- Compared with nasal ideals for whites, the nose of black patients and those of Middle Eastern descent have the following characteristics.
  - Blacks (Fig. 87-6)
    - Wide, low nasal dorsum
    - Decreased nasal length and tip projection
    - Poor nasal tip definition
    - Acute columellar-labial angle
    - Alar flaring
  - Middle Eastern (Fig. 87-7)
    - Wide nasal bones
    - Thick, sebaceous skin
    - Ill-defined bulbous tip
    - High dorsum and over projecting radix
    - Acute columellar-labial angle
    - Slight alar flaring

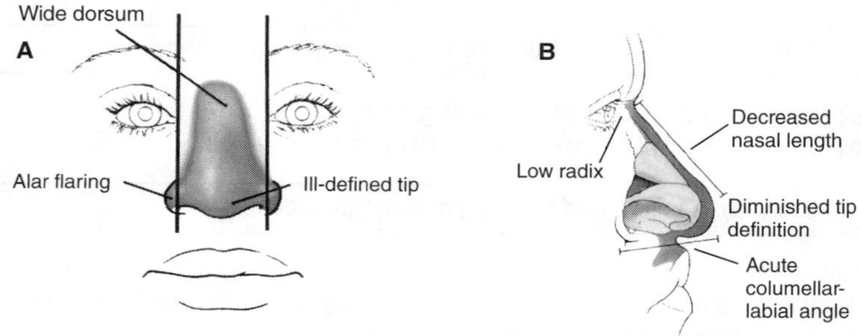


**Fig. 87-6** Typical characteristics of the noses of black patients.

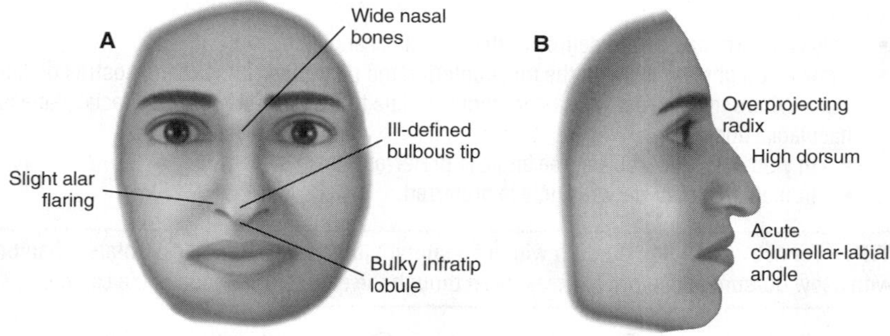


**Fig. 87-7** Typical characteristics of the noses of patients of Middle Eastern descent.

## Cheek

- Assess rhytids, lid-cheek junction, volume of facial fat, descent of the malar fat pad, and skeletal proportions.
- A youthful face has high cheekbones with concavity in the buccal area.

## Ears[7,8] (Fig. 87-8)

- Normal ear aesthetics
  - It is positioned approximately one ear length posterior to the lateral orbital rim and centered in middle third horizontal plane.
  - Long axis inclines posteriorly ~20 degrees from the vertical plane.
  - Width is ~50%-60% of length.
  - Anterolateral aspect of helix protrudes 21-30 degrees (1.5-2 cm) from scalp.
  - Helix should project 2-5 mm more laterally than antihelix in frontal view.

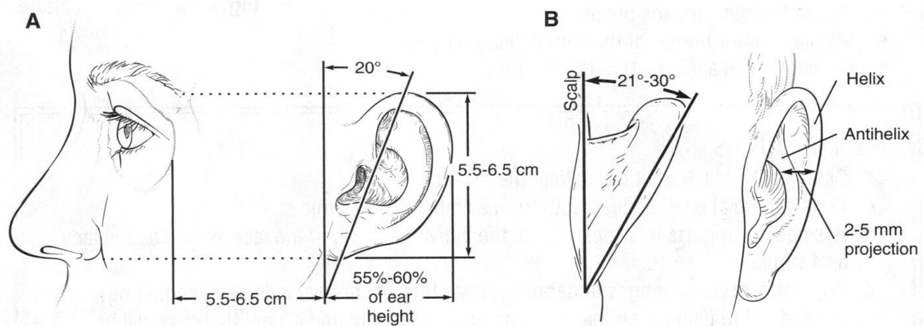


**Fig. 87-8** Normal ear aesthetics.

# LOWER THIRD

## Mouth

- Assess dental occlusion.
- Lips
  - Examine key landmarks, including vermilion-cutaneous junction, cupid's bow, and philtral columns.
  - Assess for presence of perioral rhytids.
  - Assess for volume loss.
  - Assess lateral angles of the mouth; aging lowers this, causing downward slant.
  - Upper lip length: At rest with the lips slightly separated, the upper lip should expose approximately one half of the incisor teeth.
- Nasolabial grooves and marionette lines (lines from the corner of the mouth to the mandibular border): Assess depth at rest and during animation.

## Chin

- Assess projection in relation to other facial proportions; pogonion should be 3 mm posterior to the nose-lip-chin plane.
- Nasal length (RT) = Vertical chin length (SM).

- Reidel's plane: Line touching projected lips should touch pogonion (Fig. 87-9).
- Assess labiomental groove definition, which should be approximately 4 mm deep.

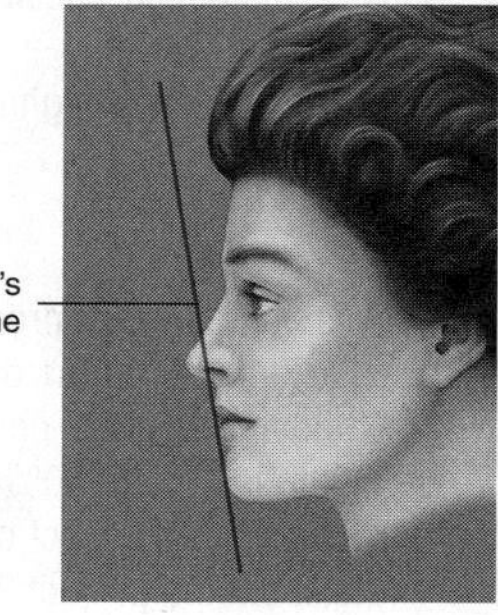


**Fig. 87-9** Reidel's plane.

## Neck[9]

- Assess skin for quality, tone, excess, and rhytids.
- Evaluate for subcutaneous and preplatysmal fat.
- Assess for static or dynamic platysmal banding.
- Look for submandibular gland ptosis.
- Mandibulocutaneous ligament: Tethering of the descending facial tissues at this ligament produces the appearance of jowls.
- Qualities of a youthful neck
  - Distinct inferior mandibular border
  - Subhyoid depression
  - Visible thyroid cartilage bulge
  - Visible anterior border of the sternocleidomastoid
  - Cervicomental angle of 105-120 degrees

## Key Points

- ✓ Skin quality will dramatically affect the results.
- ✓ Consider facial relationships both from a static and dynamic standpoint.
- ✓ It is equally important to look at both the individual parts of the face as well as the face as a whole.
- ✓ Preoperative counseling is imperative. Areas that will not be addressed should be pointed out to patients so that they can recognize them and accept that they will be present postoperatively.
- ✓ These are only guidelines. Many aesthetically pleasing faces do not have these proportions. These assessments are useful in determining factors that are responsible for individual appearances.
- ✓ Ensure that what a patient wants is congruent with what you, the surgeon, can do. It is acceptable to say NO.

## References

1. Barton FE Jr, ed. Facial Rejuvenation. St Louis: Quality Medical Publishing, 2008.
2. Nahai F, ed. The Art of Aesthetic Surgery: Principles & Techniques. St Louis: Quality Medical Publishing, 2005.
3. Bashour M. History and current concepts in the analysis of facial attractiveness. Plast Reconstr Surg 118:741-756, 2006.
4. Gunter JP, Rohrich RJ, Adams WP Jr, eds. Dallas Rhinoplasty Nasal Surgery by the Masters. St Louis: Quality Medical Publishing, 2002.
5. McCord CD Jr, Codner MA, eds. Eyelid & Periorbital Surgery. St Louis: Quality Medical Publishing, 2008.
6. Byrd HS, Hobar PC. Rhinoplasty: a practical guide for surgical planning. Plast Reconstr Surg 91:642-654, 1993.
7. Janis JE, Rohrich RJ, Gutowski KA. Otoplasty. Plast Reconstr Surg 115:60e-72e, 2005.
8. Ha RY, Trovato MJ. Plastic surgery of the ear. Sel Read Plast Surg 11(R3):1-46, 2011.
9. Ellenbogen R, Karlin JV. Visual criteria for success in restoring the youthful neck. Plast Reconstr Surg 66:826-837, 1980.

# 88. Nonoperative Facial Rejuvenation

Daniel O. Beck, Sacha I. Obaid, John L. Burns, Jr.

## CAUSES AND CLASSIFICATION OF FACIAL AGING[1-3]

### ACTINIC DAMAGE

- **Chronic sun exposure** causes changes in the skin.
  - Elastic fibers accumulate in abnormal arrangements.
  - Tissue collagenases and matrix metalloproteinases increase.
  - The number of collagen fibers decreases, and the remaining fibers become increasingly disorganized.
  - A thin layer of dermis called the *grenz zone,* or *border zone,* forms between the abnormal dermis and the epidermis.
- **The net result of these changes causes several conditions to develop:**
  - Fine rhytids
  - Skin laxity
  - Dyschromia
  - Cutaneous malignancies
- Glogau[4] developed a classification system to describe the degree of actinic damage in a patient (Table 88-1).

**Table 88-1** *Glogau Classification of Photoaging*

| Group | Severity | Age (years) | Findings |
|---|---|---|---|
| I | Mild | 28-35 | Minimal wrinkles; no keratosis; minimal acne scarring; little or no makeup |
| II | Moderate | 35-50 | Dynamic wrinkling/smile lines; early keratosis; mild scarring; some makeup |
| III | Advanced | 50-65 | Actinic keratosis; telangiectasia; wrinkling present at rest; moderate scarring; always wears makeup |
| IV | Severe | 60-75 | Actinic keratoses and skin cancers; severe wrinkling (static and dynamic); severe acne scarring; makeup cakes on |

### CHRONOLOGIC AGING

- **Skin changes occur with age.**
  - Thinning of the dermis and epidermis
  - Stratum corneum less organized
  - Fewer fibroblasts, mast cells, and blood vessels
  - Decreased number and organization of collagen and elastin fibers
    - Decreased ratio of type I/type III collagen
- Dynamic forces from underlying mimetic muscles cause rhytids in the overlying skin.
- Gravitational forces cause deep wrinkles, because facial fat descends.

- Fitzpatrick et al[5] developed a classification of facial wrinkling (Table 88-2).

**Table 88-2** *Fitzpatrick's Classification of Facial Wrinkling (Perioral and Periorbital)*

| Class | Score | Wrinkling | Degree of Elastosis |
|---|---|---|---|
| I | 1-3 | Fine wrinkles | Mild (fine textural changes with subtly accentuated skin lines) |
| II | 4-6 | Fine to moderate | Moderate (distinct papular elastosis, individual papules with yellow translucency under direct lighting, dyschromia); intermediate number of lines |
| III | 7-9 | Fine to deep | Severe (multipapular and confluent elastosis, thickened yellow and pallid wrinkles, cutis rhomboidalis); numerous lines with or without redundant skin |

## CHOICE OF PROCEDURE

- Complete physical examination
  - Static versus dynamic rhytids
  - Associated skin conditions
  - Skin thickness
  - Fitzpatrick skin type classification: Scale of a patient's ability to tan (Table 88-3)

**Table 88-3** *Fitzpatrick Skin Type Classification*

| Skin Type | Sun Exposure History/Skin Color |
|---|---|
| I | Never tans; burns easily and severely; extremely fair skin |
| II | Usually burns; tans minimally |
| III | Burns moderately; tans moderately |
| IV | Tans moderately and easily; burns minimally |
| V | Rarely burns; dark brown skin |
| VI | Never burns; dark brown or black skin |

  - Hypopigmented or hyperpigmented skin
  - Extent of photodamage (Glogau classification)
- The surgeon and patient must decide together:
  - Which aspects of facial appearance are most distressing
  - Realistic treatment goals
  - Acceptable downtime
- Patients must understand:
  - Nonoperative facial rejuvenation can restore a more youthful appearance.
  - Nonoperative facial rejuvenation is not as powerful nor as long lasting as operative techniques.
- Resurfacing techniques
  - Cause dermal collagen reorganization and new collagen deposition
    - Reduce actinic damage
    - Improve dyschromias
    - Restore a more youthful appearance
- Fillers
  - Augment depressions in the soft tissue
  - Mask the appearance of fine lines and wrinkles

**TIP:** In general, deeper and more aggressive resurfacing techniques create longer downtime, erythema, edema, and time to reepithelialization, but more dramatic results. The patient and surgeon need to be willing to accept multiple treatments or less dramatic results if faster recovery is desired.

## METHODS OF NONOPERATIVE TREATMENT

- **Lasers**
- **Pulsed light**
- **Dermabrasion**
- **Chemical peels**
- **Radiofrequency**
- **Ultrasound**
- **Botulinum toxin**
- **Soft tissue fillers**

## LASERS

### METHOD OF ACTION

- Lasers produce **heat** in target tissue that rapidly dissipates by conduction.
- The **energy wavelength** and the **exposure duration** determine the amount of heat transferred and the extent of induced tissue damage.
- Selective tissue injury is produced by the selection of a wavelength of energy that is specifically targeted to a **chromophore** in the skin.
- Common chromophore targets (Fig. 88-1)
  - Hemoglobin/oxyhemoglobin (vasculature)
  - Melanin (skin pigment, hair follicles)
  - Water (epidermis, dermis)
- To prevent collateral damage and protect surrounding tissue, the duration of exposure of the laser must be **equal to or shorter than the thermal relaxation time** of the chromophore target.
- Both **ablative** and **nonablative** lasers can be used for facial rejuvenation.
- See Chapter 11 for a comprehensive review of lasers and their use in plastic surgery.

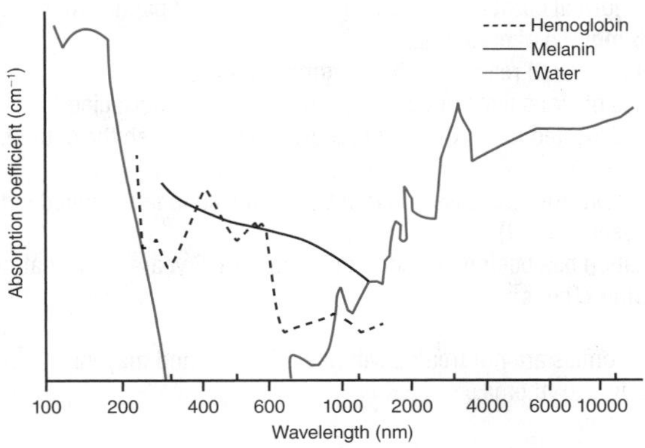


**Fig. 88-1** Common chromophores and their absorption spectrums.

## ABLATIVE LASERS

- The goal is to vaporize superficial epidermal tissues and coagulate deeper tissues without causing scarring.
- Thermal damage induces collagen remodeling, with the goal of tightening the skin and reversing actinic and chronologic changes seen with age.
- Laser treatment has various effects on skin.
  - The area of direct contact is vaporized.
  - A surrounding area of thermal damage is produced.
  - Areas of irreversible and reversible damage are produced, both of which produce inflammation and wound healing.
- **Two most common types of ablative lasers**
  - $CO_2$ laser
  - Erbium:YAG laser

### $CO_2$ LASER

- This is one of the first and longest-used laser types in facial rejuvenation.
- It can be used for treatment of fine or deep rhytids.
- The wavelength is **10,600 nm.**
- The target chromophore is **water.**
- **Depth of ablation** depends on the **number of passes** and **amount of cooling time** allowed between passes.
  - 20-60 μm of vaporization can be produced with the first pass, and 20-150 μm of additional thermal injury can be produced, depending on the settings.[6-10]
  - **$CO_2$ lasers** have a higher ablation threshold than erbium lasers, resulting in **deeper thermal heating.**

**CAUTION: If cooling time is insufficient, less ablation and increased thermal damage will result.**

- With each additional pass, vaporization decreases and thermal injury increases because of the reduced water content (target chromophore) after the initial pass.
- The **clinical endpoint** is a pale yellow color of the skin surface (midreticular dermis).
- Ablated epidermis is replaced with normal, healthy epidermal cells from adnexal structures.
  - The mean time for reepithelialization is **8½ days.**
- **The greatest effect is in the papillary dermis,** where disorganized damaged collagen masses are replaced with normal compact collagen bundles arranged parallel to the skin's surface.
- Patients have **3-6 months** of erythema.
- The most common adverse reaction is **hypopigmentation.**
  - This can lead to obvious lines of demarcation if regional resurfacing is performed.
  - Stuzin et al[11] advocated using $CO_2$ laser resurfacing only when the entire face will be treated rather than just one area.
  - Hypopigmentation from $CO_2$ lasers is most pronounced in fair-skinned individuals (i.e., Fitzpatrick classes I and II).
  - Hypopigmentation has been reported to occur up to 1-2 years after treatment.
- **Other potential side effects**[12-16]
  - Erythema
    - Skin dyschromias are not treated with the $CO_2$ laser and may initially be accentuated by postprocedure erythema.
  - Hyperpigmentation
    - Schwartz et al[17] reported that the incidence of hyperpigmentation was reduced from 43% to 6% by adding hydroquinone, kojic acid, and sunscreen to the postoperative regimen.

- Milia formation
- Acne exacerbation
- Contact allergies with soaps and moisturizers
- Superficial infection
- Stimulation of herpes simplex flare-ups
- Hypertrophic scarring
- Ectropion

■ **Absolute contraindications**
- Active viral, bacterial, or fungal infection
- **Isotretinoin use** within the previous 6-12 months (because of its suppressive effects on adnexal structures)

## Fractionated $CO_2$ Laser[18]

■ Combines **fractional photothermolysis** with an ablative **10,600 nm** wavelength

■ Pulse delivered in an evenly spaced "pixilated" pattern known as ***microthermal zones*** **(MTZ)**
- Supplies dermal coagulative energy without confluent epidermal damage
- Rapid reepithelialization and dermal reconstruction occurs from unaffected cells within punctate zones of injury.

■ Indicated for treatment of facial rhytids, actinic damage, and scarring
- Coverage density typically ranges from 20%-60% per pass, depending on the area treated.

■ Multiple treatments over large areas can be performed without concern for alterations in pigment.

■ Therapy is guided by proper selection of coverage density and energy settings, not clinical endpoints as with the $CO_2$ laser.

■ Handpieces with larger spot sizes targeting pigmentary disorders have demonstrated promising early results.

## Erbium:YAG Laser[19-29]

■ The wavelength is **2940 nm.**

■ The target chromophore is **water.**

■ Energy is absorbed by water 12-18 times more efficiently than with $CO_2$ lasers.

■ There is **less thermal diffusion** to the surrounding tissues than with $CO_2$ lasers.

■ The ablated, desiccated tissue is ejected when hit by the laser, producing a popping sound.

> **TIP:** The combination of less thermal diffusion and ejection of tissues may give a more consistent result with each pass, compared with the $CO_2$ laser.

■ Because of the consistent penetration depth with each pass, treatment can be administered in multiple passes at lower fluences (5 J/cm$^2$) or fewer passes at higher fluences (e.g., 10-25 J/cm$^2$) to effect a deeper peel.[19]
- Provides 3-5 $\mu$m of ablation per pass
- Generates 20-50 $\mu$m of thermal damage[19-24]

■ The **clinical endpoint** can be recognized by a punctate bleeding pattern and a fragmented appearance of the dermis.

■ It does not stimulate continued collagen remodeling as a $CO_2$ laser does. Consequently, it does not function well as a tightening device.

> **TIP:** Because the depth of penetration is much less than with a $CO_2$ laser, erbium:YAG lasers are reserved for more superficial problems such as epidermal or dermal lesions, mildly atrophic acne scars, mild actinic damage, and subtle dyspigmentation.

- The primary advantage of an erbium:YAG laser over a $CO_2$ laser is a shorter recovery time.
  - 5½ days for reepithelialization
  - 3-4 weeks of erythema[21-23]
  - Controversy exists about the shorter recovery time.
    - It may result from **decreased thermal diffusion** in the surrounding tissue.
    - It may result from **lower depth of penetration.**
    - Adrian[25,26] found that when the $CO_2$ laser and erbium:YAG laser were adjusted to the same depth of penetration, there was **no difference in the duration of clinical erythema.**
    - Because a decrease in penetration depth results in less inflammation and collagen remodeling, the result is less dramatic. If the decreased erythema seen with erbium:YAG lasers is the result of decreased penetration depth, the use of erbium over $CO_2$ means accepting a less dramatic result in exchange for less downtime.
- The incidence of transient hyperpigmentation is 3.4%-24%.[19]
- The incidence of hypopigmentation is 0%-12%.[19,27-29]
- The potential side effects are similar to those seen with $CO_2$ lasers.

**CAUTION: $CO_2$ and erbium:YAG laser resurfacing have been safely performed at the same time as rhytidectomy. However, surgeons must consider the dual insult to the skin flaps with such a procedure.[30]**

## NONABLATIVE LASERS

- Epidermal vaporization is **not** produced. Consequently, **recovery is much easier** with nonablative lasers than with ablative lasers.
- Heat is generated in the dermis and causes inflammation, collagen reorganization, and new collagen generation, thus tightening and rejuvenating the skin.
  - Dermal coagulation is not as significant as with ablative devices; clinical results are comparatively modest.
- Nonablative lasers can treat dyschromia.

### FRACTIONAL RESURFACING

- Fractional photothermolysis uses a light with a **1.5 μm** wavelength.[31]
- Light penetrates **300 μm** into skin.
- **Blue dye** is laid down on the skin in a "pixilated" pattern and **functions as the target chromophore** for the laser.
- The blue dye pattern is confined to small areas known as *microscopic thermal zones.* When the laser strikes the skin, it heats only these microscopic thermal zones and leaves the surrounding skin untreated.
- The distance between microscopic thermal zones can be as little as **250 μm.**
  - The blue dye can be laid down to treat various portions of the skin. Traditionally **13%-17%** of the skin is targeted at each application.
  - Patients receive repeat treatments once a week, with four or five treatments total.
  - The net result is treatment of the entire face, with no more than 17% of the skin experiencing the inflammatory response at one time.
- Fractional resurfacing represents a compromise.
  - Downtime is minimized; typically 24 hours.
  - Results are less dramatic with each treatment.
  - Multiple treatments are needed to achieve the desired results.

- The treatment is excellent for dyschromia.
- Fine wrinkles of the neck, chest, hands, and face can be treated safely.

## Nd:YAG Laser

- It is also known as a *neodymium:yttrium-aluminum-garnet laser.*
- The **wavelength** is **1064 nm.**
- Energy is **nonspecifically absorbed** by target tissue.
  - Various proteins appear to be the main target.
  - Blood vessels, red blood cells, collagen, and melanin are the most sensitive.
  - Water is a secondary target.
  - Because of the nonspecific target, there is **nonspecific heating of the tissue.**
- The scattering of laser energy by the tissues at the 1064 nm wavelength causes the area of greatest photon density to be 1-2 mm below the surface of the skin, in the dermis.[32-35]
- All Fitzpatrick skin types can be safely treated.
- Transmission of energy causes photo damage and inflammation in the dermis, leading to collagen reorganization and neocollagenesis, which in turn may have a mild tightening effect on the skin.
- The epidermis is not ablated, because the energy is concentrated on the dermis.

**TIP:** Although overall collagen remodeling and neocollagenesis is less than with ablative lasers, the Nd:YAG laser is attractive because the crusting, edema, and prolonged erythema of ablative lasers do not occur.

- A **1320 nm Nd:YAG** laser has been developed and marketed specifically for nonablative facial rejuvenation.
  - The **1320 nm** wavelength targets **dermal water.**
- The greater water absorption and nonspecific dermal scatter of the 1320 nm laser increases dermal heating and requires a cooling agent to be placed on the epidermis to prevent blistering.
- Like the 1064 nm version, the 1320 nm laser produces much less dramatic results than ablative lasers. Patients must have realistic expectations before treatment.[36,37]

## Posttreatment Care

Posttreatment care is critical to prevent complications, especially with ablative laser resurfacing.

- Patients will often be concerned.
- Moist wound healing is best.
- Prescribe valacyclovir (Valtrex) or acyclovir (Zovirax) for 1 week to prevent herpes simplex flare-up.
- Cephalexin (Keflex) or other antibiotics aimed at skin flora should be given for 1 week to prevent superficial infections.
- Fluconazole (Diflucan) may be given for 1 week to prevent fungal infections.
- A steroid dose pack may decrease inflammation or swelling.
- A 10% topical vitamin C cream can be used.

**CAUTION: Do not use topical growth factors, because they may promote hypertrophic scarring.**

- Use lipid-based ointments to provide a moist environment.
  - **Occlusive** and **nonocclusive** dressings are acceptable alternatives.
- Hydroquinone, kojic acid, and sunscreen can help prevent hyperpigmentation.

## INTENSE PULSED LIGHT (IPL)

- IPL is **not** a laser technique.
- IPL emits a spectrum of photons in the **500-1300 nm** range.
- **The chromophore is water and hemoglobin at 550-580 nm, superficial pigment at 550-570 nm, and deeper pigment at 590-755 nm.**
- Filters can be used to include or exclude particular wavelengths.
  - If filters are used that limit transmission to shorter wavelengths, such as 550-800 nm, superficial chromophores such as melanin and dermal oxyhemoglobin are treated.
  - If a filter is used that allows transmission of higher wavelengths, dermal water will be nonspecifically targeted. This results in dermal heating and inflammation, which then can lead to collagen deposition and reorganization to provide a mild tightening effect.
- **Indications**
  - Signs of hypervascularity (flushing, telangiectasias, or rosacea)
  - Signs of hyperpigmentation (solar lentigines, melasma [chloasma], or freckling)
  - Improvement of skin texture
  - Decrease pore size
- **Contraindications**
  - Unrealistic expectations
  - Tanned skin
  - Hypersensitivity to sunlight
  - Photosensitizing medications
  - Active isotretinoin (Accutane) treatment
  - Therapeutic anticoagulation medications
  - Pregnancy
  - Active lupus
  - History of wound-healing problems
  - Skin cancer
  - Fitzpatrick VI skin type (Fitzpatrick V is a relative contraindication.)
- **Potential side effects** include prolonged redness, transient speckling of pigmentation, scabbing, edema, hair loss, purpura, hyperpigmentation, hypopigmentation, herpes eruption, infection, and scarring.
- A series of treatments, usually 4-7, is needed to provide a long-lasting effect.
- The interval between treatments should be 2-3 weeks.
- **Realistic expectations are essential.** Reasonably, IPL can be expected to improve facial flushing or rosacea by **50%-75%** and dyschromia by **40%-60%.**[38-40]
- Pretreatment of the skin is **not** necessary.
- Patients should **not** be tanned when undergoing treatment.
- Topical anesthesia can be placed before treatment.
- Patients should expect **24 hours** of slight redness and dermal edema.
- **Sunblock** should be used between treatments.
- If the goal is to treat superficial dyschromia, supplement IPL treatments with topical retinoids and/or bleaching creams such as hydroquinone.

## MECHANICAL RESURFACING

### DERMABRASION

*Dermabrasion uses a handheld rotary device to remove superficial layers of the skin to promote reepithelialization with new collagen deposition.*

- It can be used to treat fine rhytids in the perioral region with good results.
- It is also very effective for reducing superficial acne scarring and scarring from other surgical procedures.
- It can be used for minor skin tightening when larger areas are treated.
- Brush strokes are made opposite burr rotation to maintain control and prevent damage to normal tissue.
- The **depth of resurfacing** can be controlled by the **amount of pressure** the device applies to the skin, **speed** of rotation, **coarseness** of the tip, **length** of treatment, and patient's **skin type and texture.**
  - Manual control of the depth of resurfacing is an advantage over other resurfacing methods that offer less precise control.
- Postoperative results are **highly technique and operator dependent.**
  - If resurfacing is performed too deeply, scarring occurs. If resurfacing is too superficial, minimal or no results are seen.

**CAUTION: When treating deeper rhytids, avoid the upper lip, malar prominence, chin, and mandible, because these areas are prone to hypertrophic scarring.**

- **Paprika bleeding indicates penetration into the superficial papillary dermis and is a safe endpoint for treatment.**
  - Yellow globules of sebaceous glands should be avoided when treating deeply.

**TIP:** As resurfacing proceeds deeper into the reticular dermis, the bleeding vessels become larger, and white parallel lines of frayed collagen may be seen if loupe magnification is used.

- Mechanical factors limit the ability to treat periorbital wrinkling and wrinkles between the lower lip and chin.
- Cryoanesthetic sprays can provide anesthesia, maintain rigid tissue, and reduce bleeding.

**TIP:** When resurfacing a large area, two things can be done to produce a more consistent result. First, plan the operative sequence based on the knowledge that dermabraded areas bleed, and the blood will flow downward, potentially obscuring your vision in untreated areas. Second, apply topical gentian violet to the target areas. The pigment is removed as areas are treated, leaving a guide of what is left to treat.

- **Reepithelialization time** depends on the depth of resurfacing but is generally **7-10 days.**
- Typically, treated skin is red for 1-2 weeks and pink for up to 2-3 months.[41,42]
- Intradermal postoperative swelling improves over 3 months.
- Collagen remodeling takes 3-6 months.
- Milia formation may occur for several weeks postoperatively.
- Acne outbreaks may occur.
- Hypopigmentation can occur in **10%-20%** of patients.[43,44]
- Hyperpigmentation may complicate recovery, but it is almost always reversible with hydroquinone and sun avoidance.
- Antibacterial ointments, especially those with neomycin, can cause contact dermatitis and should be used with caution postoperatively.

## Microdermabrasion

*Microdermabrasion uses a handheld, particle-containing device applied to the skin to produce a superficial injury.*

- A microdermabrator uses mild suction to pull skin into the handpiece, then removes dirt, oil, surface debris, and dead skin by sending a stream of particles toward the skin.
- The particles can be **aluminum oxide** or **sodium chloride.**
- After microtrauma to the skin, the crystals are aspirated into a container within the machine.
- The **particle flow rate** and **strength of the suction** control the **depth of penetration.**
- **Repetitive intraepidermal injury is the result,** which may cause gradual improvement in damaged skin by stimulating fibroblast proliferation and generation of new collagen.
- Microdermabrasion can improve rough skin, texture irregularities, acne scarring, and mottled pigmentation resulting from photoaging. Its ability to treat fine rhytids is inconsistent.[45]
- Because it penetrates only the epidermis, microdermabrasion can be repeated frequently with minimal erythema and does not require anesthesia.
- 4-12 weekly or bimonthly treatments should be performed.[46-48]
- Patients should avoid the sun for 1 week before the procedure.
- Patients should refrain from using retinoids and glycolic acid creams for a few days.
- Patients with darker color skin types should be treated with a less aggressive power setting.
- After the treatment, clean the skin and apply protective moisturizer and sunscreen.
- Skin recovery takes 7-10 days.
- Potential complications include excessive bleeding, infection, scarring, hypopigmentation, and infection.
- **Relative** contraindications include **rosacea** and **telangiectasias,** both of which may be exacerbated by treatment.[48-50]
- **Absolute** contraindications include **impetigo, flat warts,** and **active herpes simplex virus infection.**

**CAUTION: To prevent hypertrophic scarring, wait 1 year after isotretinoin (Accutane) treatment before considering microdermabrasion.**

# OTHER NONABLATIVE SKIN-TIGHTENING MODALITIES

## Monopolar Radiofrequency Dermal Remodeling (Thermage)

*Thermage is used to remodel the dermis using radiofrequency.*

- Thermage is used to tightens and contours mild laxity of the skin on the lower face or neck for patients without underlying structural ptosis.
- **Radiofrequency** is applied to the skin with **simultaneous cryogenic cooling.**
- The radiofrequency changes polarity on the skin 6 million times per second.
- **Capacitive coupling** causes **uniform distribution of heat.**
- The **geometry** and **size** of the tip affect the **depth** of injury.
- The treatment energy is typically **85-135 J/cm$^2$**, and it is usually titrated to the patient's tolerance for pain.
- Typically, erythema occurs for 24-36 hours after the procedure.
- Treated skin shows preservation of epidermis with alteration in underlying collagen.
- Collagen deposition is increased in the grenz zone and is thought to be the mechanism of skin tightening.
- Patients typically have mild edema and mild-to-moderate erythema immediately after treatment.
- Rare dysesthesias are reported.

- Results are variable and not as dramatic as with a face lift or ablative resurfacing techniques.
- Disadvantages include potential pain, less dramatic results, or rare indentations.
- **Fat atrophy** is possible.[51]

### Focused Ultrasound Dermal Remodeling (Ultherapy)

**Ultherapy** seeks to remodel the dermis and SMAS/platysma using focused **ultrasound.**

- **Ultherapy** is FDA approved for treatment of contour deformities in the head, neck, and submental regions.
- Device incorporates ultrasound imaging capability for visualizing target tissue and an **ultrasound** module configured to create multiple linear sites of localized thermal injury.
- Depth and volume of the thermally induced lesions are determined by the chosen ultrasound probe.
- Source energy range is typically **0.5-1.2 J** and can be titrated based on patient tolerance.
- Pulses are delivered with progression along a parallel treatment plane.
- Patients usually feel minor discomfort with treatment over bony prominences (e.g., angle of mandible).
- Histologic studies show preservation of the epidermis with focal zones of collagen disruption.
- Treatment depths of up to 4.5 mm are reported.
- Immediate skin flushing with up to 24 hours of erythema is typical.
- Other less common side effects include mild edema, tingling, tenderness, numbness, and bruising.
- Like Thermage, the results are variable and not as dramatic as with a face lift or ablative resurfacing techniques.

> **TIP:** Though noticeable results after a single treatment are reported, patients may require multiple treatments to obtain noticeable results with Thermage and Ultherapy. Patients must be educated before treatment about the possibility of obtaining moderate results at best.
>
> These modalities are probably best reserved for patients who desire nonsurgical alternatives to rejuvenation and are willing to accept modest results with minimal downtime.

## CHEMICAL PEELS

### Purpose

- Chemical peels involve the application of a chemical exfoliant to initiate a controlled wound of the epidermis and/or dermis to correct contour irregularities and stimulate cellular activity for regeneration.

### Indications

- **Superficial peels**
  - Upper epidermal defects
  - Mild dyschromia
  - Melasma
- **Medium-depth peels**
  - Superficial dermal defects
  - Mild dermatoheliosis
  - Superficial rhytids
- **Deep peels**
  - Deeper dermal defects
  - Severe dyschromia
  - Deep rhytids

## Types of Peels

- **Superficial peeling agents**
  - Alpha hydroxy acid (AHA) peels
  - Jessner's solution
  - Salicylic acid
  - Dry ice
- **Medium-depth peels**
  - Trichloroacetic acid (TCA) peels
  - Combination peels
- **Deep peels**
  - Phenol
    - Baker-Gordon formula
    - Hetter's formula

## Factors Affecting the Depth of Penetration

- Peeling formula used
- Concentration of acid
- Skin preparation before peeling
- Skin degreasing
- Skin cleansing
- Abrasion or topical retinoic acid
- Sebaceous gland density
- Cutaneous anatomy
- Occlusion
- Method of application
- Time of contact
- Acid neutralization (for AHAs)
- Repetition and frequency of peel
- Storage and age of peeling solution

## Comparison With Laser Resurfacing

- Less dermal thinning
- Cheaper
- More effective in treating deep rhytids
- Redness lasts longer
- More swelling in first 5 days
- Can perform light peels—repeatable without scarring and with minimal erythema
- Deep peels: Take longer to heal with prolonged erythema, higher risk of hypopigmentation and dermal scarring[41,52,53]

## Patient Evaluation

An accurate assessment of a patient's skin type is essential to optimize rejuvenation and prevent complications.

- As with other types of nonsurgical rejuvenation, **preoperative evaluation** and **patient selection** are essential.
- **Step 1:** Assess the patient's ability to tan (see Table 88-3).

**TIP:** In general, the absence of tanning ability is closely related to a patient's sensitivity to a peel.

- **Step 2:** Assess the **amount of actinic damage.**
  - In general, the worse the actinic damage, the thicker the skin, and the more aggressive the peel should be.
- **Step 3:** Evaluate previous or current skin care regimen.

## Pretreatment Regimen

- **Pretreatment is critical for preventing complications, optimizing the effect of the peel, and ensuring the most dramatic results.**
- Pretreatment begins with **avoidance of sun and cigarette smoke** and the **initiation of a daily skin care regimen** that consists of a buffing grain cleanser, an AHA toner, and a vitamin A conditioning lotion.
  - Buffing grains strip off dead skin cells.
  - AHA toners strip off the upper layer of epidermal cells, forcing the skin to proliferate rapidly.
  - Vitamin A conditioning lotions are thought to help regenerate the skin.
- The net result of this skin care regimen is to **increase the cell turnover** from the normal 28 days to 10-12 days.
  - Ideally, a rosy red hue should be produced, indicating rapid skin turnover.
  - This skin care regimen can be adjusted as needed.
- For patients who will eventually need more aggressive treatments, this regimen is used as the **first-line pretreatment** of the skin for several weeks or months before deeper peels or resurfacing is performed.
  - Patients who have more significant photoaging should have either microdermabrasion or a glycolic acid peel monthly, in addition to this skin care regimen.
  - IPL therapy can be used for patients with moderate to severe actinic damage. Intermediate to deep resurfacing with a laser, dermabrasion, and TCA or phenol peels also can be used.
- **Sunscreen** should be used daily.
- **Tretinoin** (Vesanoid), a synthetic retinoic acid, should be prescribed.
  - Stimulates papillary dermal collagen synthesis and angiogenesis
  - Increases glycosaminoglycan (GAG) deposition
  - Exfoliates the stratum corneum, which makes the skin more sensitive to the peel
  - Especially beneficial in patients with thick or oily skin

**CAUTION: Users should be aware of increased photosensitivity during tretinoin use. Sunscreen should be worn during use.**

- **Tyrosinase inhibitors** such as **hydroquinone** should be used in patients with Fitzpatrick types III-VI skin or with pigment dyschromias.
  - Used to block tyrosinase, a key enzyme in the production of melanin
  - Prevents new melanosome formation but does not lighten existing pigment
  - Helps prevent postpeel hyperpigmentation

**NOTE: Significant controversy exists about the optimal duration of the prepeel regimen. As little as 2 weeks and as much as 3 months have been recommended.**

## Superficial Peeling Agents

- **Alpha hydroxy acid (AHA) peels**
  - AHA occurs naturally in many fruits including apples, grapes, and citrus fruits.
  - Lactic acid, glycolic acid, tartaric acid, and malic acid can be used.
  - Concentrations range from 10%-70%, with 50% or 70% being the most common.
    - At **lower** concentrations, AHAs **decrease keratinocyte cohesion** above the stratum granulosum, causing desquamation.
    - At **higher** concentrations, AHAs can cause **epidermolysis.**
  - The primary use of AHA is as an **exfoliant.**
  - Exfoliation occurs over a few days.
  - The **pH** of the solution controls the effect.

**CAUTION: A pH of $<2$ causes epithelial necrosis instead of exfoliation.**

  - The FDA has approved AHAs for consumer sale if the pH is $>3.5$ and the acid concentration is $\leq 10\%$.
  - The FDA has approved AHAs for use by cosmetologists, as long as the pH is $>3.0$ and the concentration is $\leq 30\%$.
  - Physicians can use higher concentrations of AHAs with a lower pH.
  - Moy et al[54] have developed different concentrations and treatment times for various skin conditions (Table 88-4).

**Table 88-4** *Recommended Duration of Glycolic Acid Peels for Different Skin Conditions*

| Condition | Glycolic Acid (%) | Time (minutes) |
|---|---|---|
| Melasma | 50 | 2-4 |
| Acne | 50 | 1-3 |
| Actinic keratosis | 70 | 5-7 |
| Wrinkles | 70 | 4-8 |
| Solar lentigines | 70 | 4-6 |

**TIP:** Pretreatment with tretinoin (Retin-A) increases the depth of penetration and accelerates wound healing.[55-57]

- **Jessner's solution**
  - Can be used as another superficial peel or as an intermediate peel
  - Like AHAs, functions as a **keratolytic**
  - **Solution consists of:**
    - Resorcinol: 14 g
    - Salicylic acid: 14 g
    - Lactic acid: 14 ml
    - qs ethanol: 1000 ml
  - Can be used to perform a **superficial peel** or as a **keratolytic** to prepare the skin for a TCA peel
    - Produces keratolysis that allows subsequent use of a TCA peel to have a deeper and more profound effect.
  - **Depth of penetration determined by number of coats**
  - Can be applied in six or seven coats for an intermediate peel
    - The skin will slough, starting with the central face area in 3 days, progressing to the midcheek in 5 days, and toward the ears in 7 days.
  - Peel repeatable every 2-3 months

**TIP:** Jessner's solution is easy to use, with no timing necessary. Neutralize with water after creating a light frost.

- **Salicylic acid**
  - Use at concentrations of **20%-30%.**
  - It is lipid soluble, and therefore good for comedonal acne.
  - Antiinflammatory and anesthetic effects result in decreased erythema and pain.
- **Carbon dioxide ice (dry ice)**
  - Apply with an alcohol-acetone mixture.
  - Apply for 5-15 seconds, depending on the desired depth.
  - Dry ice is applied at –78° C versus –196° C for liquid nitrogen.

## MEDIUM-DEPTH PEELS

- **Trichloroacetic acid**
  - TCA is a derivative of acetic acid and can be used for **intermediate to deep peels.**
  - TCA is commonly used at concentrations of 15%-50%.
    - At concentrations of **20%-35%,** it functions as an **intermediate** peel.
    - At concentrations of **45%-55%,** it can penetrate the skin irregularly and cause **scarring.**
  - TCA causes **coagulation necrosis** of cells through extensive protein denaturation and cell death.
  - Over 5-7 days, the epidermis and superficial dermis slough.[58-61]
  - Skin slough usually begins centrally and proceeds laterally.

**TIP:** If the TCA peel is performed at midweek, most of the skin sloughing will occur over the weekend.

- **Depth of penetration** is directly related to **strength of the solution** and to **pretreatment of the skin.**

**TIP:** Retin-A can be used to pretreat the skin, causing dekeratinization and allowing greater depth of penetration. It also can accelerate the postoperative healing process.

- **Penetration can be improved** and made more uniform by using the following procedure immediately before the TCA peel.
  - **Wash** and **degrease** the skin to remove oil.
  - **Mechanically remove** surface debris.
  - **Chemically disrupt the skin barrier** with mild acid solutions such as **Jessner's solution.**
- When using Jessner's solution before the TCA peel, apply 3-4 coats. Then follow with a 20%-35% TCA peel.
- The **endpoint** for an intermediate-depth peel, using Jessner's solution and TCA, is the production of Obagi's level 1 frost, which is a **foggy white frost on an erythematous base.**
- A **second endpoint** is an epidermal slide, which is produced if a cotton tip applicator is applied to the surface of the skin.
  - This has also been given the name *accordion sign.*
  - The epidermal slide disappears as the peel penetrates deeper.
- As a peel is made deeper, an intense white to yellow blanch is produced, indicating a peel at Obagi's level 2 or 3.[53,62]
- The wounds are healed by **secondary intention,** during which the epidermis is repopulated and the disorganized, damaged collagen of the superficial dermis is replaced by orderly, newly formed collagen.

**CAUTION: Dingman et al[63] have shown that TCA peels can be used safely in conjunction with a deep-plane face lift. Peeling in the setting of undermined skin in face-lift patients is nevertheless worrisome because of the potential development of postoperative skin slough.**

## Deep Peels

- **Indicated for Glogau level III and IV photodamage**
- **Phenol peel**
  - **Phenol** is a derivative of **coal tar** that causes rapid denaturation and coagulation of surface keratin.
  - Phenol produces a new zone of collagen.
  - Phenol is effective for wrinkles and severe dyschromia.
  - Phenol penetrates to the **middle reticular dermis.**
  - Similar to TCA peels, the **depth of penetration** can be greatly affected by preparing the skin with **washing** and **degreasing** before peel application.

**CAUTION: Cardiac monitoring is required, because phenol can cause arrhythmias. Avoid use in patients with a history of cardioarrhythmia, hepatic or renal compromise, and those on medications with potential cardiac side effects.**

  - Occluding methods (e.g., waterproof zinc oxide tape) prevent evaporation, resulting in deeper penetration.
  - Significant controversy exists about the concentration required for optimal results.
    - Mackee and Karp[64] used 88% phenol to produce superficial peels that were repeatable every month for 4-6 months.
    - Spira et al[65] found that 50% concentrations of phenol were as effective as stronger concentrations, with fewer complications.
  - Today the most common formulation is the **Baker-Gordon peel.**[66-68]
    - **Phenol:** 3 ml
    - **Tap water:** 2 ml
    - **Liquid soap:** 8 drops
      - Soap acts as a surfactant to lower surface tension. It also emulsifies and aids in penetration.
    - **Croton oil:** 3 drops
      - **Croton oil** is a skin irritant that causes inflammation, vesication, and secondary collagen formation.
- **Hetter's croton oil peel**
  - Hetter[69-72] believes that the true active ingredient in phenol peels is the **croton oil, not the phenol,** and that minute changes in concentration of croton oil can cause very different results.
  - Hetter[69] has published the **"heresy phenol formulas,"** which give the concentrations of ingredients needed for different levels of peeling in different anatomic regions (Table 88-5).

**Table 88-5** *Formulas With Varying Concentrations of Phenol and Croton Oil*

**35% Phenol Vehicle***

| | Croton Oil (%) | | | |
|---|---|---|---|---|
| | **0.4** | **0.8** | **1.2** | **1.6** |
| Water | 5.5 | 5.5 | 5.5 | 5.5 |
| USP phenol 88% | 3.0 | 2.0 | 1.0 | 0.0 |
| Stock solution containing croton oil | 1.0 | 2.0 | 3.0 | 4.0 |
| Septisol | 0.5 | 0.5 | 0.5 | 0.5 |
| TOTAL | 10 | 10 | 10 | 10 |

**48.5% Phenol Vehicle†**

| | Croton Oil (%) | | | | |
|---|---|---|---|---|---|
| | **0.4** | **0.8** | **1.2** | **1.6** | **2.0** |
| Water | 4.0 | 4.0 | 4.0 | 4.0 | 3.5 |
| USP phenol 88% | 4.5 | 3.5 | 2.5 | 1.5 | 1.0 |
| Stock solution containing croton oil | 1.0 | 2.0 | 3.0 | 4.0 | 5.0 |
| Septisol | 0.5 | 0.5 | 0.5 | 0.5 | 0.5 |
| TOTAL | 10 | 10 | 10 | 10 | 10 |

*For eyelids and neck, mix 1 ml of 0.4% solution with 1.2 ml of USP phenol 88% and 1.8 ml of water for a 0.1% solution of croton oil in 35% phenol.
†For eyelids and neck, mix 1 ml of 0.4% solution with 1.7 ml of USP phenol 88% and 1.3 ml of water for a 0.1% solution of croton oil in 50% phenol.

- **Hetter has suggested the following order for mixing the solution:**
  1. Croton oil is added to undiluted phenol.
  2. After this mixture dissolves completely, water is added.
  3. Finally, Septisol soap is added.
- Truppman and Ellenby[73] found a significant incidence of cardiac arrhythmias when 50% of the face was treated with a phenol–croton oil peel in <30 minutes. If this treatment was spread out over 60 minutes, no arrhythmias were seen.

**TIP:** Cardiac monitoring should be employed whenever phenol peels are used. Giving supplemental $O_2$ during the procedure may be helpful in preventing arrhythmic complications.

- To prevent arrhythmias, Binstock[74] advises peeling the face by small sections 15-20 minutes apart, preparing the skin with washing, and degreasing the skin before peel application.

- **Comparison of TCA peel with phenol–croton oil peel**
  - Phenol–croton oil peels produce **less hypertrophic scarring** than TCA peels for every layer of wrinkle depth.
  - All deep phenol peels cause some degree of hypopigmentation.
  - Phenol–croton oil peels tend to produce less hypopigmentation than TCA peels.

## COMPLICATIONS OF RESURFACING

- **Infection:** Bacterial, viral, or fungal
  - Antiviral prophylaxis is indicated for those with a history of herpes simplex.
- **Prolonged erythema**
  - Topical hydrocortisone can improve erythema.
- **Acne:** Possible between days 3 and 9
- **Scarring**
  - Avoid resurfacing for patients with a history of keloid scars.
- **Pigmentary change**
  - Hyperpigmentation usually resolves.
  - Hypopigmentation can be permanent.
- **Milia:** Sometimes appear 2-3 weeks after reepithelialization
  - May be aggravated by ointments because of occluded sebaceous glands

## BOTULINUM TOXIN

- Botulinum toxin is derived from the bacterium *Clostridium botulinum.*[75]
  - Varying strains of *C. botulinum* produce seven distinct neurotoxins: serotypes A through G.
  - Produces **chemodenervation** of muscle by targeting the SNAP/SNARE docking protein complex thus **preventing binding and release of acetylcholine** at the neuromuscular endplate
    - Botulinum toxins A, C, and E target the SNAP-25 protein within the SNARE complex.
    - Botulinum toxins B, D, F, and G target synaptobrevin within the SNARE complex.
- Botulinum toxins A and B are commercially available.
  - Type A was initially FDA approved for treatment of glabellar frown lines in patients 65 years or younger.
    - Approval has expanded to include hyperhidrosis, blepharoptosis, and cervical dystonia.
  - Type B is FDA approved for treatment of cervical dystonia.
- Three preparations of botulinum toxin A are currently available with on-label and off-label indications for facial aesthetics.
  - **Botox: Onabotulinumtoxin A** (Allergan, Santa Barbara, CA)[76]
    - FDA approved in 2002 for treatment of glabellar rhytids
    - Available in 50- or 100-unit vials; typically diluted to a final concentration of **2.5-4 U/0.1 ml**
    - Stored at 2°-8° C before use
  - **Dysport: Abobotulinumtoxin A** (Medicis Aesthetics, Scottsdale, AZ)[77-79]
    - FDA approved in 2009 for treatment of glabellar rhytids and cervical dystonia
      - Used for nearly two decades outside of the United States before approval
    - Available in 300-unit vials; typically diluted to a final concentration of **10-30 U/0.1 ml**
    - Stored at 2°-8° C before use
  - **Xeomin: Incobotulinumtoxin A** (Merz Pharmaceuticals, Greensboro, NC)[80,81]
    - FDA approved in 2010 for treatment of cervical dystonia and blepharoptosis, 2011 for glabellar rhytids
      - Used in Europe since 2005
    - Available in 50- and 100-unit vials; typically diluted to a final concentration of **2.5-4 U/0.1 ml**
    - Lyophilized preparation; does **not** require refrigeration before use

## Pretreatment Preparation and Considerations

- When reconstituted, botulinum toxin should be clear, colorless, and free from particulate matter.
- Preserved or nonpreserved normal saline solution may be used for reconstitution.
  - Preserved saline may be associated with decreased pain from injections.[82,83]
- Manufacturer guidelines promote one-time use within 4 hours of reconstitution.
  - These products do not contain an antimicrobial agent; prolonged storage is outside FDA guidelines.
  - Consensus reports support safe and effective use of botulinum toxin A up to 6 weeks after reconstituting and storage at 4° C.[82,83]
- Bruising can be decreased by stopping medications that inhibit clotting 10-14 days before treatment. These include aspirin, nonsteroidal anti-inflammatory drugs (NSAIDs), and vitamin E.
- Botulinum toxin is contraindicated by active infection at the proposed treatment sites and by hypersensitivity to any of the ingredients contained within the diluent, including albumin (all three toxin A products) or lactose (Dysport).
- **Use botulinum toxin cautiously with:**
  - Patients who have a peripheral motor neuropathic disease such as **myasthenia gravis** or **Eaton-Lambert syndrome**
  - **Coadministration of aminoglycoside antibiotics** or other agents that interfere with neuromuscular transmission
  - **Inflammatory skin disorders** at the injection site
  - **Pregnancy:** Category C drug
  - **Lactation**[82]

## Immunogenicity

- Botulinum toxin A is expressed as a 150 KDa core toxin within a larger 900 KDa protein complex.
  - The immune system may recognize any component of this complex and trigger an immune reaction.
  - The amount of neurotoxin and complexing protein injected defines the foreign protein load.
  - High or repeat protein loads may trigger toxin A antibody production and secondary nonresponse.
  - Current commercial preparations seek to minimize delivered protein load by eliminating complexing proteins.
    - Xeomin has effectively eliminated complexing proteins during preparation, which may suggest the lowest immunogenicity of the available preparations.
- Primary nonresponders to botulinum toxin A are rare and may be caused by **underdosing, genetics,** or **preformed antibodies.**
- Botulinum toxin B can be used off-label in primary or secondary nonresponders if underdosing is eliminated as the cause.

## Administration and Efficacy

- Units of botulinum toxin A are not directly interchangeable between brands. Activity on a per-unit basis depends on the bacteria strain, manufacturing process, and resulting toxin complex size.
  - The **calculated median lethal dose (LD50)** of onabotulinum toxin A is **2700 U** for a **70 kg** human.[84]
- Similar results can be achieved with different preparations using **normalized clinical dosing.**[77-79]
  - Consensus recommendations suggest
    - **1:1** dosing ratio between Botox and Xeomin
    - **2:1 or 2.5:1** dosing ratio between Dysport and Botox or Xeomin

- Spread of toxin occurs immediately and depends on injection **volume** and **injection technique.**
  - Diffusion from the injection site occurs over days and follows a concentration gradient (**toxin-dose** dependent).
- Onset of effect is typically 1-3 days.
- Complications include injection site pain, injection site reaction, headache, brow/eyelid ptosis, respiratory tract infection, and acne.
- Reassess the patient at 14 days and consider any touch-ups at that time.
- The typical interval for treatment is 3-4 months.
  - Avoid boosting the immune system by administering toxin more frequently than every 3 months.

**TIP:** No universal dosage is applicable to all patients at a given anatomic location. Treatment must be individualized to address severity of rhytids, muscle bulk, choice of neurotoxin, and response to any previous treatments.

**NOTE: All doses given are for administration of Botox or Xeomin. The suggested 2:1 or 2.5:1 ratio pertains to Dysport.**

## Glabellar Complex and Vertical Forehead Lines[82,83]

- The targeted muscles include the **corrugator supercilii, procerus,** and **orbicularis oculi.**
- The starting dose is 20-30 U for women and 30-40 U for men.
- 4-6 injection points are recommended[82] (Fig. 88-2).
- Avoid injecting too low around the orbit—all injections should be directed outside the orbital rim.

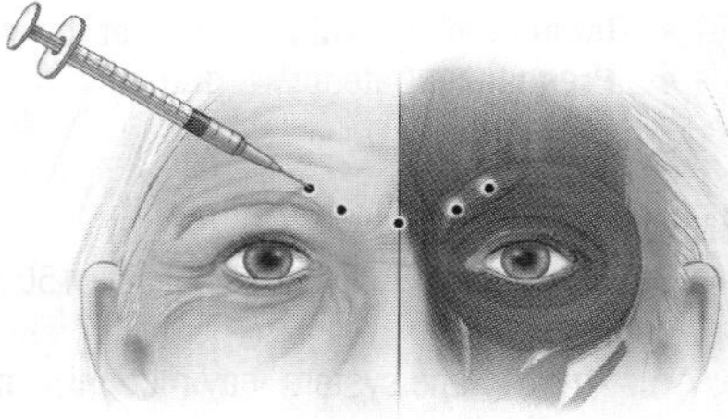

**Fig. 88-2** Injection points for glabellar complex and vertical forehead lines.

**TIP:** Stay well above the superior orbital rim with the lateral injections.

## Horizontal Forehead Lines[82,83]

- The target muscle is the **frontalis.**
- The starting dose is 10-20 U for women and 20-30 U for men.
- 4-8 injection points may be used.
- Stay at least **2 cm** above the brow to reduce the risk of brow ptosis.
- Look for brow asymmetry before injecting. This may be partially corrected by additional injections on the side where the brow is the most depressed.

**CAUTION: If injections are too centralized, a "quizzical" eyebrow appearance results, with lateral brow elevation and central depression.**

- Avoid low, lateral brow injections. A high, lateral brow injection results in a significant alteration of the lateral brow.

## Crow's Feet (Lateral Orbital Wrinkles)[82,83]

- The target is the **lateral portion of the orbicularis oculi muscle.**
- The total starting dose is 12-30 U.
- Use 2-4 injection points per side, 1 cm lateral to the bony orbit[82] (Fig. 88-3).
- Before injecting this area, perform a snap test to the lower lids. If they are lax, there is significant risk for postinjection ectropion, and low injections must be avoided.
- Use caution around the lower third of the canthal area.
- **Do not inject below the zygomatic arch** or in the region of the **zygomaticus muscle,** because this can cause lip and cheek ptosis.

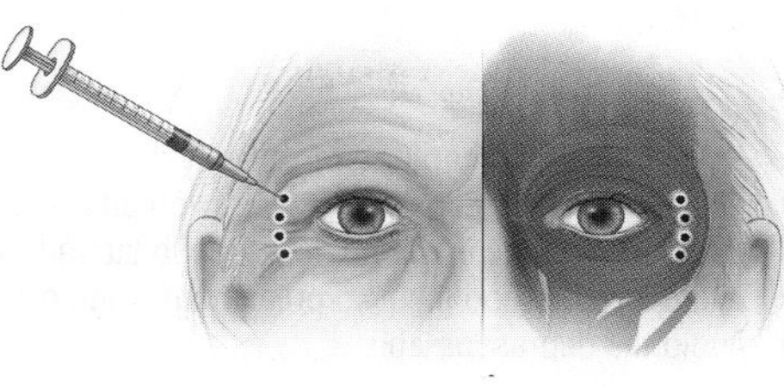

**Fig. 88-3** Injection points for crow's feet.

**CAUTION: To prevent postoperative bruising, take care to search for veins and do not injure them.**

- Use caution with patients who have a history of dry eyes, recent blepharoplasty, or LASIK surgery.

## Bunny Lines[82,83]

*Bunny lines appear on the sides of the nose and radiate downward.*

- Targets include the **nasalis** and **procerus** muscles.
- The typical starting dose is 3-6 U.
- Usually, three injection points are used, one in the midline and one on each side[82] (Fig. 88-4).
- Keep injections in this area superficial to prevent bruising.
- To prevent drooping of the upper lip, take care **not to inject the levator labii superioris alaeque nasi** and **levator labii superioris.** To prevent botulinum toxin from diffusing into these muscles, do not massage too vigorously or in a downward direction.

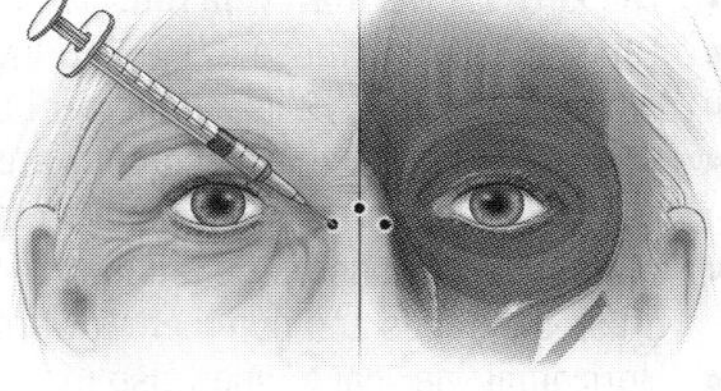

**Fig. 88-4** Injection points for bunny lines.

## Perioral Wrinkles[82,83]

- Use to decrease the appearance of fine vertical wrinkles of the upper lip.
- Use to produce a fuller upper lip by relaxing the orbicularis, causing slight eversion of the upper lip.
- The target is the **orbicularis oris** muscle.
- The usual starting dose is 4-10 U, evenly divided between the two sides.
- 2-7 injection points can be used[82] (Fig. 88-5).
- Do **not** use in patients who use their lips for their professions, such as musicians, singers, or public speakers.
- Always inject symmetrically.
- Avoid the corners of the lips (to prevent drooling).
- Avoid the midline (to prevent flattening of the lip).

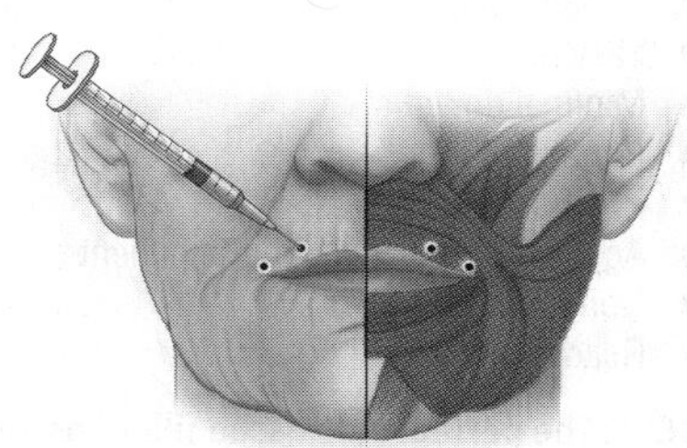

**Fig. 88-5** Injection points for perioral wrinkles.

- Stay within 5 mm of the vermilion border.
- *Lower lip injections have a more significant effect on muscle function and should be limited or avoided.*

### Dimpled Chin[82,83]

- The target is the **mentalis** muscle.
- The usual starting dose is 2-6 U in women and 2-8 U in men.
- One injection site in the midline, or two laterally, are recommended.
- Avoid injecting too high (to prevent affecting orbicularis function in the lower lip).
- Avoid the depressor labii.

### Marionette Lines[83]

- The target is the **depressor anguli oris** muscle.
- The total starting dose is 5 U per side.
- Inject symmetrically, 1 point per side.
- Inject superficially 1 cm lateral and inferior to oral commissures.

### Platysmal Bands[82,83]

- Treatment with botulinum toxin may be effective for patients with platysmal banding who have retained their skin elasticity or for those with banding and previously had skin tightening from a rhytidectomy.
- The target is the **platysma** muscle.
- The usual starting dose is 10-30 U in women and 10-40 U in men.
- Women receive 2-12 injections per band, and men receive 3-12 injections.
- Patient selection and expectations are critical. Botulinum toxin is **not** an alternative to surgery, and it **will not correct skin laxity or fat deposits.**
- **Strap muscles should be avoided.** To ensure that the treatment is limited to the platysma, grasp the bands and pull them toward the injecting hand, and then inject.
- Horizontal "necklace" lines also may be treated.

## SOFT TISSUE FILLERS

### Ideal Soft Tissue Filler[85,86]

- Safe and nontoxic
- Nonallergenic
- Easy to use
- Minimal downtime
- Predictable
- Potentially reversible
- Ages appropriately with the patient
- Nonpalpable
- Readily available

**NOTE: The perfect soft tissue filler has yet to be created. The fillers that we have now incorporate many, but not all, of the ideal characteristics.**

## Classes of Soft Tissue Fillers

- Autologous materials
- Biologic materials
- Synthetic materials
- Off-label materials

## Autologous Materials

- **Safety** is perhaps the biggest advantage of using autologous materials.
- Toxicity, allergic reactions, immunogenicity, carcinogenicity, and teratogenicity are not concerns.
- **Potential pitfalls** with autologous materials include infection, migration, inflammatory reactions, impermanence, technique dependence, and lack of reproducibility and reliability.
- Examples include fat, dermis, fascia, cartilage, subcutaneous musculoaponeurotic system (SMAS), and laViv (tissue-culture–derived fibroblasts from a patient's own fibroblasts; Fibrocell Science, Exton, PA).

## Biologic Materials

- Biologic materials are derived from **organic sources.**
- Primary **advantages** include ready, off-the-shelf availability and ease of use.
- **Disadvantages** include sensitization to foreign animal or human proteins, transmission of disease, and immunogenicity.
- Longevity is limited.
- Collagen products and hyaluronic acid products are the two major types.

## Synthetic Materials

- **Advantages** include potential permanence, reduced concerns of disease transmission, and sensitization to foreign animal or human proteins.
- **Disadvantages** include potential for granuloma formation, acute and delayed infections, migration or displacement, and deformities that can result from complications or removal of the material.
- Calcium hydroxyapatite (Radiesse, Merz Aesthetics, San Mateo, CA) and poly-L-lactic acid (Sculptra, Valeant Aesthetics, Bridgewater, NJ) are FDA approved as **semipermanent** fillers for facial augmentation.
- Polytetrafluoroethylene (PTFE) and polymethylmethacrylate (Artefill, Suneva Medical, San Diego, CA) are FDA approved for **permanent** facial augmentation.
- The FDA approval process limits the availability of synthetic materials for use as a soft tissue filler. Many more products are available outside the United States.

## Off-Label Materials

- Many synthetic fillers are FDA approved for use with conditions unrelated to plastic surgery.
- The FDA limits and prevents manufacturers from marketing these products for other uses; however, plastic surgeons have found alternative off-label uses for some of these products.
    - Calcium hydroxyapatite (Radiesse) was initially FDA approved for vocal cord injections but was used by plastic surgeons for soft tissue augmentation.
- Liability is a concern if complications arise.

## CHARACTERISTICS OF SPECIFIC COMMON SOFT TISSUE FILLERS

### Autologous Fat

- Autologous fat can be injected for soft tissue augmentation.
- It does not act as a dermal filler, but subcutaneous volume is enhanced.
- Common areas of use in facial rejuvenation include the infraorbital hollow, malar region, angle of the mandible, anterior or posterior jaw line, chin, nasolabial fold, supraorbital and temporal region.
  - It is also used to fill iatrogenic deformities after liposuction.
- Discrete fat compartments of the face have been identified and characterized by their age-related changes. Knowledge of this anatomy can guide placement of fat injections to restore youthful appearance.[87-90]
- Current literature does not support a standardized procedure for harvest, preparation, and injection.[91]
- Coleman[92] demonstrated long-term survival of fat with his *structural fat grafting* technique and provided the following principles and guidelines for structural fat grafting:
  - Fatty tissue is more fragile than most other human tissues and is damaged easily outside the body by mechanical insults.
  - To survive harvesting, transport, and implantation with cannulas and syringes, fat must be harvested in intact parcels, small enough to be inserted through a small cannula but large enough so that the tissue architecture is maintained.
  - Fat is living tissue that must be in close proximity to a nutritional and respiratory source to survive.
  - Placement by keeping the fat parcels separate from one another promotes longevity and stability.
  - It is essential to maximize the contact surface area of each fatty tissue parcel with the surrounding host tissues for successful integration and anchoring of newly placed tissue.
  - Whenever possible, incisions are placed in wrinkle lines, folds, or hair-bearing areas to facilitate placement of the fat grafts in at least two directions when indicated.
  - To strengthen bony or underlying support, the fat can be layered against bone or cartilage in the deeper levels.
  - To support the skin, fat is layered immediately under the skin.
  - For filling and plumping or restoring fullness, tissues are placed in the intermediate layers between skin and the appropriate underlying layers.
- **Technique**
  - Harvest with a Coleman 14-gauge harvesting cannula or a Lambros 3 mm cannula.[93-95]
  - Harvesting should be done with a 10-20 cc syringe held at 1-2 cc of negative pressure to minimize trauma to the fat.
  - **The site of fat harvest does not alter success or longevity.**[96]
  - Spin the harvested fat for 1 minute at 1500 RPM to remove blood, oil, and local anesthetic.
  - Inject fat in the facial region using a 1 cc syringe, with 0.1 cc of fat placed during each pass.[95]
  - The fat that survives transfer can be permanent, and it gains and loses volume with fluctuations in the weight of the patient.
  - **Great care must be taken when injecting fat into the eyelids.**
    - Small injection amounts should be used with each pass to prevent fat emboli to the eye or brain.
    - If the fat is injected too superficially, such as just below the thin eyelid skin or at the junction of the muscle and subcutaneous tissue, palpability or irregularities may occur.

## Hyaluronic Acid (HA) Derivatives

- HA was approved by the FDA in 2003. Its use has supplanted collagen as the biologic filler of choice.
- HA is a normal component of the ground substance responsible for dermal hydration.
- HA is a linear polysaccharide composed of repeating disaccharide units of N-acetyl-glucosamine and N-acetyl-glucuronic acid. It belongs to a larger class of molecules called **glycosaminoglycans.**
- It is a polysaccharide with no species specificity, so there is **no immunologic activity** and **no need for a skin test.**
- HA absorbs water and **expands after injection.**
- HA products include Restylane and Restylane-L (Medicis Aesthetics), Perlane and Perlane-L (Medicis Aesthetics), Juvederm Ultra(XC) and Ultra Plus(XC) (Allergan), Belotero Balance (Merz Aesthetics), and Hydrelle (Anika Therapeutics, Bedford, MA).
  - Some formulations of HA injectables are now available with lidocaine infused into the filler material for improved comfort during treatment.
- The distinct properties of various HA products should be considered when deciding on the appropriate filler for use[97] (Box 88-1).

**Box 88-1** *Factors to Consider When Choosing a Hyaluronic Acid Filler*

- Concentration of hyaluronic acid
- Cost
- Cross-linking
  - Degree of cross-linking
  - Quantity of hyaluronic acid cross-linked versus non-cross-linked
  - Type of cross-linking technology used
- Duration of correction
- G′ (elastic modulus)
- Hydration level of product in the syringe
- Presence of lidocaine
- Required needle size for injection
- Sizing technology
- Syringe design and size

- **Perlane, Juvederm Ultra Plus(XC)** are the **largest HA** particles and should be injected into the **deepest layer of the dermis.**
- **Restylane, Juvederm Ultra(XC)** are **midsized particles** and should be injected at the **middle dermis level.**
- **Restylane Fine Lines** contains the **smallest particles,** and should be injected at the **dermal-epidermal junction.**
- **Belotero Balance** contains **midsize particles** formulated to create a **low-viscosity** product that can be injected at the **middle dermis** or **dermal-epidermal junction.**

**TIP:** Combining different particle sizes allows tailoring of the therapy to treat a range of conditions, from deeper folds such as the nasolabial folds to finer lines.

- **Injections can be painful.** Topical and/or injectable anesthesia should be used for comfort.
- Inject with an even flow to prevent lumps or irregularities.
- If lumps are noted at the time of injection, **massage** immediately.
- **Inject to the final desired volume.**

**CAUTION: Injection of HA too superficially can lead to a bluish discoloration (Tyndall effect).**

- After injection, patients should cool the area with ice packs for the first 24 hours and take oral antihistamines.
- Patients should expect 3-5 days of swelling, which can cause worry of overcorrection.
  - Bruising may last up to 1½ weeks.
  - Intermittent swelling may occur for the first 2-6 weeks in rare cases.
    - If massive swelling occurs, consider using a steroid dose pack.
- HA lasts approximately **6-9 months.**
- With repeated injections of HA, the product lasts longer, and less volume is required.
- **Potential complications** include erythema, edema, ecchymosis, and acneiform dermatitis.
  - Telangiectasias may form, especially in response to larger injections or in patients with either preexisting telangiectasias in the injection region, or rosacea.
  - Rarely, patients may develop erythema of the overlying skin, which can be treated with a light topical steroid.
  - With larger injection volumes, abscesses may occur, which can be drained with an 18-gauge needle.
- Intralesional **hyaluronidase** injection is used for reversal in overcorrection, asymmetries, nodules, and compressive vascular compromise.
- **Lip augmentation**
  - Use midsized HA products such as Juvederm Ultra(XC), Restylane-L, or a combination of a midsized HA and another filler.
  - Use infraorbital and mental nerve blocks or a topical anesthetic.
  - Lidocaine with epinephrine can be used to decrease bruising and can be used with fillers. Some fillers come with lidocaine already mixed.
  - If lip shape is good initially, then augmenting the vermilion border alone may be enough to produce a good result.
  - Note preexisting asymmetries between the right and left sides of the lips before injecting.
  - Long, thin lips tend to have a higher resting tension and less dramatic results.
  - In patients with lips that are tight to the dentition or with an Angle class II occlusion, augmentation should be conservative to prevent irregularities of the dentition to be reflected in the lips and to prevent the lips from appearing too prominent.
  - Use viral prophylaxis in patients with a history of herpes to prevent herpetic outbreak and scarring.
  - Begin with augmentation of the vermilion border.
  - If desired, proceed to augmentation of the philtral columns.
  - Injection within the lip itself should be performed in the substance of the orbicularis oris.
  - Limit injection of the skin above the upper lip vermilion border, because augmentation of this region lengthens the upper lip skin.
  - HA can be combined with botulinum toxin to limit pinching of the lip and the formation of vertical lines.
    - 2 U of Botox/Xeomin or 6 U of Dysport is used per side in the upper lip.
    - Take care to avoid the midline.
    - Botulinum toxin should be placed within 5 mm of the vermilion border. The closer it is placed to the vermilion border, the greater the resulting lip projection.

- **Effacement of nasolabial folds**
  - A reasonable goal is **50% correction** of the depth of the nasolabial fold.
  - Place HA at angles to the fold, and layer to enhance longevity.
  - If the fold has a superficial line etched into it, use small-sized HA particles to address the condition.
  - Taping the fold for a few days after injection can prevent lateral displacement of the product when the patient smiles.
  - **Do not completely correct the fold,** because this will give the patient an odd appearance.
  - Too much filler in the areas over the dentition can appear as a bump.
- **Scar correction**
  - More than one treatment may be required to achieve full correction.
  - Using an 18-gauge needle to release the scar before injection improves results.
- **Glabellar folds**
  - Treat in combination with botulinum toxin.
  - Use either a small or midsize HA product.
    - A low-viscosity product such as Belotero can minimize compression of delicate vessels in this area.
  - Use a cross-radial tunneling injection technique.
- Restylane and Perlane are ideal for correcting lipoatrophy from antiretroviral therapy for HIV.
  - The areas most frequently treated are the inframalar hollow, concavities adjacent to the zygomatic temporal bone, and the zygomatic arch.
  - In the temple and adjacent to the arch, place the filler deep within or under the periosteum.
- The goal of lipoatrophy correction should be to soften the contours but not totally correct them.[85]

## Calcium Hydroxyapatite (CaHA)

- CaHA (Radiesse) is a pure synthetic made primarily of calcium and phosphate ions.
- The particles are identical to the mineral portion of human bone.
- CaHA particles have a consistent, uniform, smooth, spherical shape with a narrow size range of 25-45 mm.
- CaHA particles are suspended in an aqueous gel composed of sodium carboxymethyl cellulose, glycerin, and sterile water.
- The carrier gel is replaced with the patient's own connective tissue over 3-6 months.
- The carrier gel is 70% of the product's volume.
- Fibrous tissue grows on the spheres and holds them in place. The manufacturer reports no evidence of fibroblastic encapsulation or particle migration.
- **No sensitivity testing** is required.
- Originally used for oral or maxillofacial defects and vocal cord insufficiency.
- Now FDA approved for the correction of moderate to severe facial rhytids.
  - CaHA is best used for nasolabial folds, lips, radial lip lines, white rolls, glabellar lines, acne scars, facial lipoatrophy, posttraumatic or poststeroid atrophy, and cheek, chin, or mandibular border augmentation.[85]
- The average longevity of soft tissue augmentation is 9-18 months.
- Place CaHA in the **deep dermis.**
- Place the material as the needle is withdrawn with a linear injection technique.
- Layer the product for deep folds.
- Postinjection massage is important to smooth any irregularities.
- The maximum volume occurs at 4-6 weeks.
- There is an 8%-10% incidence of lumps.[98-100]

- Treat irregularities monthly with dilute triamcinolone (Kenalog) until resolved.
- Use intermittent icing for 24 hours and avoid blood thinners before injecting.

## Poly-L-Lactic Acid (PLLA)

- **Sculptra** (Valeant Aesthetics, Bridgewater, NJ) is injectable PLLA.
- Sculptra is a synthetic polymer that is biodegradable, biocompatible, and immunologically inert.
- Because it is neither human nor animal derived, **no skin test is required.**
- The initial tissue reaction is inflammatory, involving mononuclear macrophages and proliferating fibroblasts with capsule formation around the microspheres.
- Microparticles are broken down by nonenzymatic hydrolysis into lactic acid monomers, which are then metabolized into $CO_2$ or incorporated into glucose.
- **PLLA eventually degrades and is replaced with collagen.**
- PLLA is currently FDA approved for midfacial to deep facial rhytids and folds, and volume restoration of HIV lipoatrophy.
- Because it must be injected **deeply,** Sculptra is **not** indicated for correction of perioral, periorbital, and facial lines requiring superficial deposition.
- **Reconstitute at least 2 hours before injection, preferably overnight.**
- Once reconstituted, it may be stored at room temperature for 72 hours.
- Before use, the vial must be rolled or agitated to ensure a uniform translucent suspension.
- Reconstitute each vial with 5 ml or more of sterile water.
  - The more water that is used for reconstitution, the less dense and viscous the injection product will be.
  - 1%-2% lidocaine (Xylocaine) may be added to solution to reduce pain.[101]
  - A final volume of 8-9 ml is commonly used.
- Injection requires a relatively large needle. **(A 26-gauge needle is the smallest that can be used.)**
- Inject into deep dermal, subcutaneous tissues, or directly over the periosteum.[101]
- Multiple injections in a crisscross pattern produce the best results.
- If the product is injected over bone, place the needle on the periosteum and inject an aliquot. Then use fingers to massage and spread the filler over the bone.
- After injection, place moisturizer on the area, massage the area for at least 5 minutes, and then place ice packs.
- The patient should massage the injected area at home every day.
- Edema will give the initial appearance of a full correction, but it will resolve over several hours to several days, causing the contour defect to reappear.
- If patients require significant volume correction, multiple conservative sessions are preferred over filling it all at once.
  - In severe facial fat loss, 3-6 treatments may be required.
- The final effect may last up to **2 years.**[101-104]
- **Side effects** include delayed occurrence of subcutaneous papules, bleeding from the injection site, discomfort, erythema or inflammation, ecchymosis, granulation formation, and edema.[85,101]

## Polymethylmethacrylate (PMMA)

- Artefill is composed of collagen-covered PMMA beads.
- The collagen is a transport vehicle and is absorbed over a 4- to 6-week period.
- The volume of the tissue is increased by the body making connective tissue around the PMMA beads.
- PMMA is a **permanent filler.**

- The safest areas of injection are the nasolabial folds and deep marionette lines.
- PMMA works well for deep soft acne scars.

**CAUTION: Rhytids in the glabellar and periorbital region can thin with age, eventually causing the permanent filler to become visible.**

- Do **not** use PMMA for superficial rhytids.
- Use caution and **preinjection testing** for patients with known collagen allergies.
- Use a 26-gauge needle for injection.
- Inject as the needle is withdrawn from the deep dermal plane.
- After injection, massage the area to ensure that there are no lumps.
- Immediately after injection into mobile areas, such as the lips or nasolabial folds, place tape on them to limit movement and filler migration.
- If filling depressed scars, release the scar before injecting the PMMA. In the case of scars, serial injections every 8 weeks should be used for complete correction.
- Although Artefill is considered a permanent filler, more volume may be required after approximately 1½ years.[105-107]
- Inform patients that initial results are not seen for 6-8 weeks, because collagen is absorbed during this time and replaced with tissue growth into the PMMA beads.[106,107]
- Irregularities discovered soon after injection should be treated with injection of a dilute dose of a steroid (Kenalog 0.2 mg/ml) to soften the irregularity. If this is unsuccessful, surgical excision of the irregularity may be required.
- Rare granulomas may form in response to PMMA beads.[85,108,109]

## Key Points

- ✓ Successful rejuvenation of an aging face requires thorough analysis of both actinic and chronologic damage.
- ✓ A variety of nonsurgical options are available to treat an aging face. These include resurfacing, paralysis of underlying musculature, and soft tissue augmentation.
- ✓ When considering resurfacing, patients and physicians must balance the desire for dramatic results with the desire for minimal recovery.
- ✓ Botulinum toxin injections require a thorough understanding of the anatomy of the facial muscles. Successful injections can provide dramatic results, but poorly located injections can cause deformities.
- ✓ A variety of soft tissue fillers exist, each with its own profile of sensitivity and longevity. Patients and physicians must understand the limitations and potential benefits of each filler.

## References


1. Glogau RG. Aesthetic and anatomic analysis of the aging skin. Semin Cutan Med Surg 15:134-138, 1996.
2. Sauermann K, Clemans S, Jaspers S, et al. Age related changes of human skin investigated with histometric measurements by confocal laser scanning microscopy in vivo. Skin Res Technol 8:52-56, 2002.
3. West MD. The cellular and molecular biology of skin aging. Arch Dermatol 130:87-95, 1994.
4. Glogau RG. Chemical peeling and aging skin. J Geriatr Dermatol 2:30-35, 1994.
5. Fitzpatrick RE, Goldman MP, Satur NM, et al. Pulsed carbon dioxide laser resurfacing of photo-aged facial skin. Arch Dermatol 132:395-402, 1996.

6. Burkhardt BR, Maw R. Are more passes better? Safety versus efficacy with the pulsed $CO_2$ laser. Plast Reconstr Surg 100:1531-1534, 1997.
7. Walsh JT Jr, Deutsch TF. Pulsed $CO_2$ laser tissue ablation: measurement of the ablation rate. Lasers Surg Med 8:264-275, 1988.
8. Stuzin JM, Baker TJ, Baker TM, et al. Histologic effects of the high-energy pulsed $CO_2$ laser on photoaged facial skin. Plast Reconstr Surg 99:2036-2050, 1997.
9. Smith KJ, Skelton HG, Graham JS, et al. Depth of morphologic skin damage and viability after one, two, and three passes of a high-energy, short-pulse $CO_2$ laser (Tru-Pulse) in pig skin. J Am Acad Dermatol 37:204-210, 1997.
10. Grossman AR, Majidian AM, Grossman PH. Thermal injuries as a result of $CO_2$ laser resurfacing. Plast Reconstr Surg 102:1247-1252, 1998.
11. Stuzin JM, Baker TJ, Baker TM. $CO_2$ and erbium:YAG laser resurfacing: current status and personal perspective. Plast Reconstr Surg 103:588-591, 1999.
12. Weinstein C, Ramirez OM, Pozner JN. Postoperative care following $CO_2$ laser resurfacing: avoiding pitfalls. Plast Reconstr Surg 100:1855-1866, 1997.
13. Williams EF III, Dahiya R. Review of nonablative laser resurfacing modalities. Facial Plast Surg Clin North Am 12:305-310, 2004.
14. Jacobson D, Bass LS, VanderKam V, et al. Carbon dioxide and ER:YAG laser resurfacing. Results. Clin Plast Surg 27:241-250, 2000.
15. Chajchir A, Benzaquen I. Carbon dioxide laser resurfacing with fast recovery. Aesthetic Plast Surg 29:107-112, 2005.
16. Brunner E, Adamson PA, Harlock JN, et al. Laser facial resurfacing: patient survey of recovery and results. J Otolaryngol 29:377-381, 2000.
17. Schwartz RJ, Burns AJ, Rohrich RJ, et al. Long-term assessment of $CO_2$ facial laser resurfacing: aesthetic results and complications. Plast Reconstr Surg 103:592-601, 1999.
18. Hunzeker CM, Weiss ET, Geronemus RG. Fractionated $CO_2$ laser resurfacing: our experience with more than 2000 treatments. Aesthet Surg J 29:317-322, 2009.
19. Bass S. Erbium:YAG laser skin resurfacing: preliminary clinical evaluation. Ann Plast Surg 40:328-334, 1998.
20. Pozner JM, Goldberg DJ. Histologic effect of a variable pulsed Er:YAG laser. Dermatol Surg 26:733-736, 2000.
21. Goldman MP, Marchell N, Fitzpatrick RE. Laser skin resurfacing of the face with a combined $CO_2$/Er:YAG laser. Dermatol Surg 26:102-104, 2000.
22. Zachary CB. Modulating the Er:YAG laser. Lasers Surg Med 26:223-226, 2000.
23. Weinstein C. Erbium laser resurfacing: current concepts. Plast Reconstr Surg 103:602-616, 1999.
24. Perez MI, Bank DE, Silvers D. Skin resurfacing of the face with the Erbium:YAG laser. Dermatol Surg 24:653-658, 1998.
25. Adrian RM. Pulsed carbon dioxide and erbium-YAG laser resurfacing: a comparative clinical and histologic study. J Cutan Laser Ther 1:29-35, 1999.
26. Adrian RM. Pulsed carbon dioxide and long pulse 10-ms erbium-YAG laser resurfacing: a comparative clinical and histologic study. J Cutan Laser Ther 1:197-202, 1999.
27. Tanzi EL, Alster TS. Side effects and complications of variable-pulsed erbium:yttrium-aluminum-garnet laser skin resurfacing: extended experience with 50 patients. Plast Reconstr Surg 111:1524-1529, 2003.
28. Ross EV, Miller C, Meehan K, et al. One-pass $CO_2$ versus multiple-pass Er:YAG laser resurfacing in the treatment of rhytids: a comparison side-by-side study of pulsed $CO_2$ and Er:YAG lasers. Dermatol Surg 27:709-715, 2001.

29. Jimenez G, Spencer JM. Erbium:YAG laser resurfacing of the hands, arms, and neck. Dermatol Surg 25:831-834, 1999.
30. Alster TS, Doshi SN, Hopping SB. Combination surgical lifting with ablative laser skin resurfacing of facial skin: a retrospective analysis. Dermatol Surg 30:1191-1195, 2004.
31. Manstein D, Herron GS, Sink RK, et al. Fractional photothermolysis: a new concept for cutaneous remodeling using microscopic patterns of thermal injury. Lasers Surg Med 34:426-438, 2004.
32. Trelles MA, Alvarez X, Martin-Vasquez MJ, et al. Assessment of the efficacy of nonablative long-pulsed 1064-nm Nd:YAG laser treatment of wrinkles compared at 2, 4, and 6 months. Facial Plast Surg 21:145-153, 2005.
33. Carniol PJ, Farley S, Friedman A. Long-pulse 532-nm diode laser for nonablative facial skin rejuvenation. Arch Facial Plast Surg 5:511-513, 2003.
34. Papadavid E, Katsambas A. Lasers for facial rejuvenation: a review. Int J Dermatol 42:480-487, 2003.
35. Friedman P, Skover GR, Payonk G, et al. Quantitative evaluation of nonablative laser technology. Semin Cutan Med Surg 21:266-273, 2002.
36. Trelles MA. Short and long-term follow-up of nonablative 1320 nm Nd:YAG laser facial rejuvenation. Dermatol Surg 27:781-782, 2001.
37. Trelles MA, Allones I, Luna R. Facial rejuvenation with a nonablative 1320 nm Nd:YAG laser: a preliminary clinical and histologic evaluation. Dermatol Surg 27:111-116, 2001.
38. Mark KA, Sparacio RM, Voigt A, et al. Objective and quantitative improvement of rosacea-associated erythema after intense pulsed light treatment. Dermatol Surg 29:600-604, 2003.
39. Huang L, Liao YL, Lee SH, et al. Intense pulsed light for the treatment of facial freckles in Asian skin. Dermatol Surg 28:1007-1012, 2002.
40. Raulin C, Greve B, Grema H. IPL technology: a review. Lasers Surg Med 32:78-87, 2003.
41. Fulton JE Jr. Dermabrasion, chemabrasion, and laserabrasion. Historical perspectives, modern dermabrasion techniques, and future trends. Dermatol Surg 22:619-628, 1996.
42. Branham GH, Thomas JR. Rejuvenation of the skin surface: chemical peel and dermabrasion. Facial Plast Surg 12:125-133, 1996.
43. Fulton JE Jr, Rahimi AD, Mansoor S, et al. The treatment of hypopigmentation after skin resurfacing. Dermatol Surg 30:95-101, 2004.
44. Kunachak S, Leelaudomlipi P, Wongwaisayawan S. Dermabrasion: a curative treatment for melasma. Aesthetic Plast Surg 25:114-117, 2001.
45. Karimipour DJ, Karimipour G, Orringer JS. Microdermabrasion: an evidence based review. Plast Reconstr Surg 125:372-377, 2010.
46. Grimes PE. Microdermabrasion. Dermatol Surg 3:1160-1165, 2005.
47. Spencer JM. Microdermabrasion. Am J Clin Dermatol 6:89-92, 2005.
48. Shpall R, Bedingfield FC III, Watson D, et al. Microdermabrasion: a review. Facial Plast Surg 20:47-50, 2004.
49. Koch RJ, Hanasono MM. Microdermabrasion. Facial Plast Surg Clin North Am 9:377-382, 2001.
50. Shim EK, Barnette D, Hughes K, et al. Microdermabrasion: a clinical and histopathologic study. Dermatol Surg 27:524-530, 2001.
51. Abraham MT, Vic Ross E. Current concepts in nonablative radiofrequency rejuvenation of the lower face and neck. Facial Plast Surg 21:65-73, 2005.
52. Kauvar AN, Dover JS. Facial skin rejuvenation: laser resurfacing or chemical peel: choose your weapon. Dermatol Surg 27:209-212, 2001.
53. Fulton JE, Porumb S. Chemical peels: their place within the range of resurfacing techniques. Am J Clin Dermatol 5:179-187, 2004.

54. Moy LS, Murad H, Moy RL. Glycolic acid peels for the treatment of wrinkles and photoaging. J Dermatol Surg Oncol 19:243-246, 1993.
55. Kim IH, Kim HK, Kye YC. Effects of tretinoin pretreatment on TCA chemical peel in guinea pig skin. J Korean Med Sci 11:335-341, 1996.
56. Vagotis FL, Brundage SR. Histologic study of dermabrasion and chemical peel in an animal model after pretreatment with Retin-A. Aesthetic Plast Surg 19:243-246, 1995.
57. Hevia O, Nemeth AJ, Taylor JR. Tretinoin accelerates healing after trichloroacetic acid chemical peel. Arch Dermatol 12:678-682, 1991.
58. Monheit GD. The Jessner's 1 TCA peel: a medium-depth chemical peel. J Dermatol Surg Oncol 15:945-950, 1989.
59. El-Domyati MB, Attia SK, Saleh FY, et al. Trichloroacetic acid peeling versus dermabrasion: a histometric, immunohistochemical, and ultrastructural comparison. Dermatol Surg 30:179-188, 2004.
60. Chiarello SE, Resnik BI, Resnik SS. The TCA masque. A new cream formulation used alone and in combination with Jessner's solution. Dermatol Surg 22:687-690, 1996.
61. Glogau RG, Beeson WH, Brody HG, et al. Re: Obagi's modified trichloroacetic acid (TCA)–controlled variable depth peel: a study of clinical signs correlating with histological findings. Ann Plast Surg 38:298-302, 1997.
62. Tse Y, Ostad A, Lee HS, et al. A clinical and histologic evaluation of two medium-depth peels. Glycolic acid versus Jessner's trichloroacetic acid. Dermatol Surg 22:781-786, 1996.
63. Dingman DL, Hartog J, Siemionow M. Simultaneous deep-plane face lift and trichloroacetic acid peel. Plast Reconstr Surg 93:86-93, 1994.
64. Mackee GM, Karp FL. The treatment of postacne scars with phenol. Br J Dermatol 64:456-459, 1952.
65. Spira M, Gerow FJ, Hardy SB. Complications of chemical face peeling. Plast Reconstr Surg 54:397-403, 1974.
66. Butler PE, Gonzalez S, Randolph MA, et al. Quantitative and qualitative effects of chemical peeling on photo-aged skin: an experimental study. Plast Reconstr Surg 107:222-228, 2001.
67. Stuzin JM, Baker TJ, Gordon HL. Chemical peel: a change in the routine. Ann Plast Surg 23:166-169, 1989.
68. Kligman AM, Baker TJ, Gordon HL. Long-term histologic follow-up of phenol face peels. Plast Reconstr Surg 75:652-659, 1985.
69. Hetter GP. An examination of the phenol-croton oil peel. Part 4. Face peel results with different concentrations of phenol and croton oil. Plast Reconstr Surg 105:1061-1083, 2000.
70. Hetter GP. An examination of the phenol-croton oil peel. Part 3. The plastic surgeons' role. Plast Reconstr Surg 105:752-763, 2000.
71. Hetter GP. An examination of the phenol-croton oil peel. Part 2. The lay peelers and their croton oil formulas. Plast Reconstr Surg 105:240-248, 2000.
72. Hetter GP. An examination of the phenol-croton oil peel. Part 1. Dissecting the formula. Plast Reconstr Surg 105:227-239, 2000.
73. Truppman ES, Ellenby JD. Major electrocardiographic changes during chemical face peeling. Plast Reconstr Surg 63:44-48, 1979.
74. Binstock JH. Safety of chemical face peels. J Am Acad Dermatol 7:137-138, 1982.
75. Carruthers J, Stubbs HA. Botulinum toxin for benign essential blepharospasm, hemifacial spasm and age-related lower eyelid entropion. Can J Neurol Sci 14:42-45, 1987.
76. Lorenc ZP, Kenkel JM, Fagien S, et al. A review of onabotulinumtoxinA (Botox). Aesthet Surg J 33 (1 Suppl):S9-S12, 2013.
77. Lorenc ZP, Kenkel JM, Fagien S, et al. A review of abobotulinumtoxinA (Dysport). Aesthet Surg J 33 (1 Suppl):S13-S17, 2013.

78. Matarasso A, Shafer D. Botulinum toxin neurotoxin type A-ABO (Dysport): clinical indications and practice guide. Aesthet Surg J 29(6 Suppl):S72-S79, 2009.
79. Maas C, Kane MA, Bucay VW, et al. Current aesthetic use of abobotulinumtoxin a in clinical practice: an evidence based consensus review. Aesthet Surg J 32(1 Suppl):S8-S29, 2009.
80. Lorenc ZP, Kenkel JM, Fagien S, et al. IncobotulinumtoxinA (Xeomin): background, mechanism of action and manufacturing. Aesthet Surg J 33(1 Suppl):S18-S22, 2013.
81. Lorenc ZP, Kenkel JM, Fagien S, et al. IncobotulinumtoxinA in clinical literature. Aesthet Surg J 33 (1 Suppl):S23-S34, 2013.
82. Carruthers J, Fagien S, Matarasso SL; Botox Consensus Group. Consensus recommendations on the use of botulinum toxin type a in facial aesthetics. Plast Reconstr Surg 114(Suppl 6):S1-S22, 2004.
83. Lorenc ZP, Kenkel JM, Fagien S, et al. Consensus panel's assessment and recommendations on the use of 3 botulinum toxin type A products in facial aesthetics. Aesthet Surg J 33(1 Suppl):S9-S12, 2013.
84. Gill DM. Bacterial toxins: a table of lethal amounts. Microbiol Rev 46:86-94, 1982.
85. Nahai F, ed. The Art of Aesthetic Surgery: Principles & Techniques, 2nd ed. St Louis: Quality Medical Publishing, 2011.
86. Homicz MR, Watson D. Review of injectable materials for soft tissue augmentation. Facial Plast Surg 20:21-29, 2004.
87. Rohrich RJ, Pessa JE. The fat compartments of the face: anatomy and clinical implications for cosmetic surgery. Plast Reconstr Surg 119:2219-2227, 2007.
88. Rohrich RJ, Pessa JE. The retaining system of the face: histologic evaluation of the septal boundaries of the subcutaneous fat compartments. Plast Reconstr Surg 121:1804-1809, 2008.
89. Rohrich RJ, Pessa JE, Ristow B. The youthful cheek and the deep medial fat compartment. Plast Reconstr Surg 121:2107-2112, 2008.
90. Rohrich RJ, Arbique GM, Wong C, et al. The anatomy of suborbicularis fat: implications for perioral rejuvenation. Plast Reconstr Surg 124:946-951, 2009.
91. Gir P, Brown SA, Oni G, et al. Fat grafting: evidence based review on autologous fat harvesting, processing, reinjecting and storage. Plast Reconstr Surg 130:249-258, 2012.
92. Coleman SR, ed. Structural Fat Grafting. St Louis: Quality Medical Publishing, 2005.
93. Coleman WP III. Autologous fat transplantation. Plast Reconstr Surg 88:736, 1991.
94. Coleman SR. Long-term survival of fat transplants: controlled demonstrations. Aesthetic Plast Surg 19:421-425, 1995.
95. Coleman WP III. Fat transplantation. Dermatol Clin 17:891-898, 1999.
96. Rohrich RJ, Sorokin ES, Brown SA. In search of improved fat transfer viability: a quantitative analysis of the role of centrifugation and harvest site. Plast Reconstr Surg 113:391-395; discussion 396-397, 2004.
97. Baumann L, Blyumin M, Saghari S. Dermal fillers. In Baumann L, ed. Cosmetic Dermatology: Principals and Practice, 2nd ed. New York: McGraw-Hill, 2009.
98. Sklar JA, White SM. Radiance FN: a new soft tissue filler. Dermatol Surg 30:764-768, 2004.
99. Flaharty P. Radiance. Facial Plast Surg 20:165-169, 2004.
100. Tzikas TL. Evaluation of the Radiance FN soft tissue filler for facial soft tissue augmentation. Arch Facial Plast Surg 6:234-239, 2004.
101. Fitzgerald R, Vleggaar D. Facial volume restoration of the aging face with poly-L-lactic acid. Dermatol Ther 24:2-27, 2011.
102. Woerle B, Hanke CW, Sattler G. Poly-L-lactic acid: a temporary filler for soft tissue augmentation. J Drugs Dermatol 3:385-389, 2004.
103. Sterling JB, Hanke CW. Poly-L-lactic acid as a facial filler. Skin Therapy Lett 10:9-11, 2005.

104. Borelli C, Kunte C, Weisenseel P, et al. Deep subcutaneous application of poly-L-lactic acid as a filler for facial lipoatrophy in HIV-infected patients. Skin Pharmacol Physiol 18:273-278, 2005.
105. Lemperle G, Romano JJ, Busso M. Soft tissue augmentation with Artecoll: 10-year history, indications, techniques, and complications. Dermatol Surg 29:573-587, 2003.
106. Lemperle G, Sadick NS, Knapp TR, et al. Artefill permanent injectable for soft tissue augmentation. Part I. Mechanism of action and injection techniques. Aesthetic Plast Surg 34:264-272, 2010.
107. Lemperle G, Sadick NS, Knapp TR, et al. Artefill permanent injectable for soft tissue augmentation. Part II. Indications and applications. Aesthetic Plast Surg 34:273-286, 2010.
108. Alcalay J, Alkalay R, Gat A, et al. Late-onset granulomatous reaction to Artecoll. Dermatol Surg 29:859-862, 2003.
109. Lombardi T, Samson J, Plantier F, et al. Orofacial granulomas after injection of cosmetic fillers. Histopathologic and clinical study of 11 cases. J Oral Pathol Med 33:115-120, 2004.

# 89. Fat Grafting

**Phillip B. Dauwe**

## GENERAL PRINCIPLES

- Fat grafting is the free nonvascularized transfer of adipose tissue.
- It is used to correct soft tissue contour deformities.
- Successful long-term volume maintenance is the goal.
- The main drawback is **unpredictable long-term results** from graft volume loss over time.
- Current efforts investigate methods to minimize graft resorption and provide more long-term predictability.

> **TIP:** Peer's "cell survival theory": The number of viable adipocytes at the time of transplantation correlates with ultimate fat graft survival volume.[1]

## FAT CHARACTERISTICS

- Fat grafting transfers adipocytes, preadipocytes, and surrounding stroma
- Adipocytes: Mature fat cells
- Preadipocytes:
  - Adipogenic precursor cells (stem cells)
  - Tolerate ischemia better than mature adipocytes[2]
  - Have the potential to differentiate into adipocytes and proliferate after grafting[2]

## INDICATIONS[3]

### BREAST[4] (Fig. 89-1)

- Contour irregularity after reconstruction or augmentation
- Primary breast augmentation with or without external tissue expansion[3]
- Micromastia, tuberous breast, or other congenital breast deformity
- Poland's syndrome

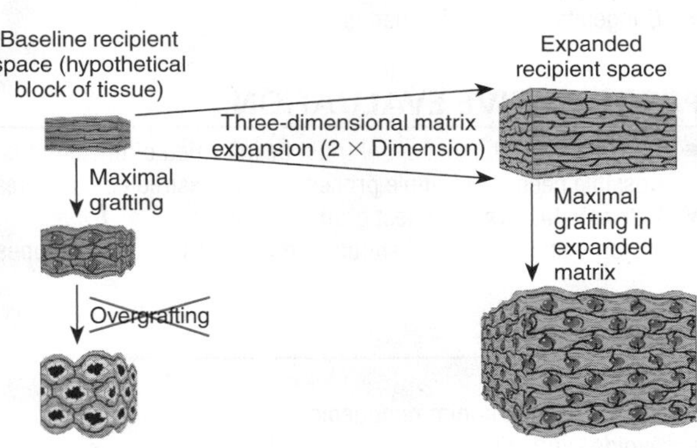


**Fig. 89-1** Megavolume grafting after expansion. The block of tissue is maximally filled with fat grafts, and then overfilled to crowding *(left)*. The block is three-dimensionally stretched to show how many more grafts can be placed in the expanded and hypervascular space *(right)*.

- Deformity following partial mastectomy
- Damaged skin resulting from radiotherapy[5]
  - Decreases collagen deposition
  - Attenuates thickened epidermis
  - Improves hyperpigmentation
- Nipple reconstruction

### FACE

- Lipoatrophy (HIV, drug-related, facial aging)
- Posttraumatic contour deformity
- Lip augmentation
- Malar augmentation
- Periorbital rejuvenation
- Nasolabial fold augmentation
- Depressed acne scars

### TRUNK

- Iatrogenic liposuction deformities

### GLUTEAL REGION

- Gluteal crease augmentation
- Buttock augmentation

### HAND REJUVENATION

- Dorsal hand rejuvenation[6]
- Dupuytren's contracture release[7]

### OTHER INSTRUCTIONS

- Penile enlargement
- Burn scar contractures
- Radiation damage[8,9]
- Congenital constriction bands

## PREOPERATIVE EVALUATION

- Patient expectations: Patient must be informed of the tenuous nature of fat grafting and the possible need for multiple procedures for desired cosmetic result.[10]
- **Extrinsic factors** can affect graft viability.
  - Smoking, nutritional status, sympathomimetic drugs, obesity, diabetes, COPD

## ADVANTAGES

- Safe
- Biocompatible, nonimmunogenic
- Avoids synthetic fillers
- Abundant, readily available
- Natural appearance

- Inexpensive
- Soft tissue contouring at donor site
- Low donor site morbidity

## DISADVANTAGES

- No uniform technique has proved superior for maximizing long-term results.[11]
- Amount of graft resorption is unpredictable.
  - A result of acute graft ischemia and failure of graft nutrition
- Results are highly technique dependent.
- Graft volume fluctuates with weight change.

## FAT HARVEST

- Atraumatic harvesting, handling, and transplantation correlates with higher long-term volume maintenance.
- Manual harvest (Coleman technique) results in higher percentage of viable adipocytes compared with conventional liposuction.
- Graft viability increases with the use of large-bore harvest cannulas and low pressure.
- **Coleman technique: Harvest**[6,12]
  - Small incision (~5 mm) placed strategically for broad access to donor site (Fig. 89-2)
  - Infiltration of donor site with 1:1 wetting solution (if under local anesthesia, 0.5% lidocaine with 1:200,000 epinephrine; if under general anesthesia, 1:400,000 epinephrine in lactated Ringer's solution)
  - Harvesting cannula[12] (Fig. 89-3): 3 mm diameter, 17-gauge lumen, 15 or 23 cm length, blunt tip; connected to a 10 cc Luer-Lok syringe
  - Cannula is introduced through the same incision made for infiltration.
  - Gentle back-pressure on the 10 cc syringe plunger creates a light negative pressure.
  - Cannula is advanced and retracted in long, even radial strokes through subcutaneous tissue.
  - After syringe is filled with subcutaneous tissue, cannula is removed from syringe, and a Luer-Lok plug is placed to prevent leakage.

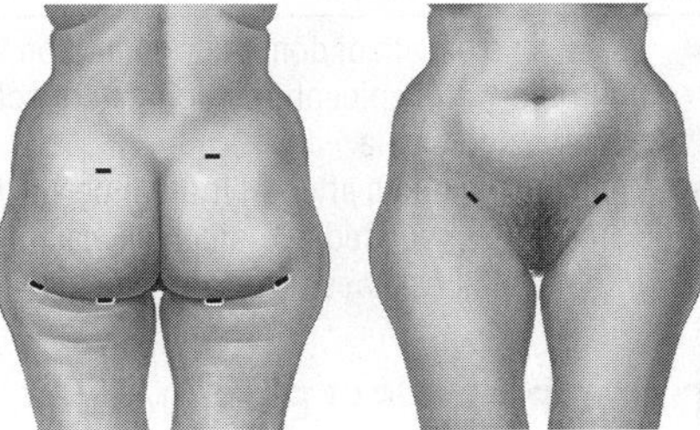

**Fig. 89-2**

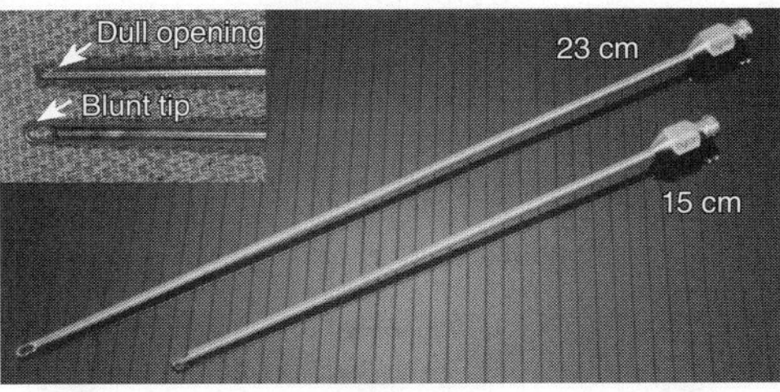


**Fig. 89-3** The harvesting cannula is usually 15 cm long. A longer cannula increases torque on the Luer-Lok aperture and can break the syringe tip during extraction.

- Suction-assisted fat harvest[13,14]
  - Fat harvest with liposuction has been reported as successful.[4]
  - A larger oil layer is often observed after suction-assisted fat harvest, indicating fat cell rupture.[13]
  - Fat cell viability correlates with amount of shear trauma, but does not correlate with pressure amount used to harvest.[15]
    - Therefore fat cell rupture is likely caused by mechanical shear trauma from travel through the suction circuit.
  - Suction provides a more efficient method of fat harvest in large-volume fat grafting, and larger lipoaspirate volumes can be harvested.

**TIP:** Maintain continuous negative pressure in the harvest syringe, with the plunger pulled back to the 2 or 3 cc mark.

## INFILTRATION TECHNIQUE BEFORE FAT HARVEST

- There is no benefit of donor site infiltration with epinephrine or local anesthetic on fat cell viability.[16]
- Infiltration with epinephrine-containing solution reduces blood loss and reduces blood fraction of harvested tissue.
- Wait 7-10 minutes after infiltration before harvest to allow maximal epinephrine effect.
- Some report reduced preadipocyte viability and impaired differentiation into mature adipocytes with use of local anesthetics.[17,18]

## DONOR SITE SELECTION

- Adipocyte viability not affected by choice of donor site.[19]
- Consider convenience of access and patient positioning.
- Consider possible need to enhance body contour at donor site.
- Consider patient request.
- Be aware of **zones of adherence** (Fig. 89-4).
  - Distal iliotibial tract
  - Gluteal crease
  - Lateral gluteal depression
  - Middle medial thigh
  - Distal posterior thigh

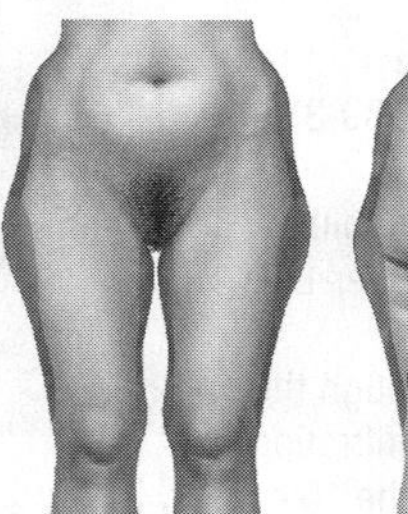
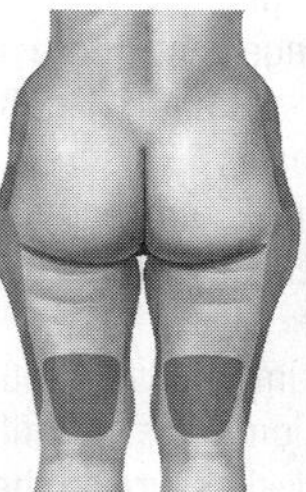
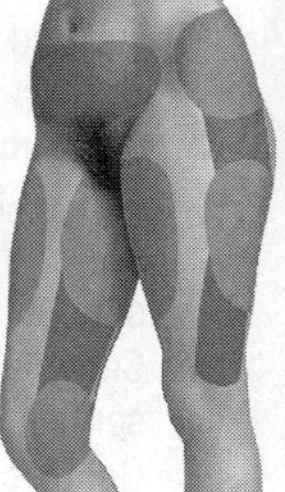

**Fig. 89-4**

**TIP:** Donor site selection depends mostly on positioning.

- Supine: Abdomen and medial thigh
- Prone: Back, flank, and buttock

## FAT PROCESSING

*Refinement of the harvested subcutaneous tissue into pure fat is crucial for predictable fat grafting.*

- **Three methods:** Centrifugation, washing, or sedimentation
  - All three techniques have shown equivalent results.[20]

### CENTRIFUGATION

- Ideal centrifugation is approximately 1500-3000 rpm for 2-3 minutes, but significantly lower G force centrifugation (15-20 G) has been reported as successful.[6,20,21]
- After 2-3 minutes no further separation occurs, and fat cell destruction takes place.[22]
- **Coleman technique: Refinement**[8]
  - The plunger is removed from capped 10 cc syringe, and syringe is placed in central-rotor centrifuge.
  - Syringe is centrifuged at approximately 3000 rpm for 3 minutes.
  - The harvested material is now separated into three layers (Fig. 89-5).
    1. **Upper layer:** Oil from ruptured fat cells
    2. **Middle layer:** Parcels of adipose tissue
       - Most viable adipose cells are consistently found at bottom of the fat layer.[22]
    3. **Lower layer:** Blood, water, lidocaine
  - The upper (oil) layer is decanted using a cotton pledget.
  - The lower (aqueous) layer is drained through bottom of the syringe.
  - Exposure to air is minimized to prevent dessication and fat cell lysis.

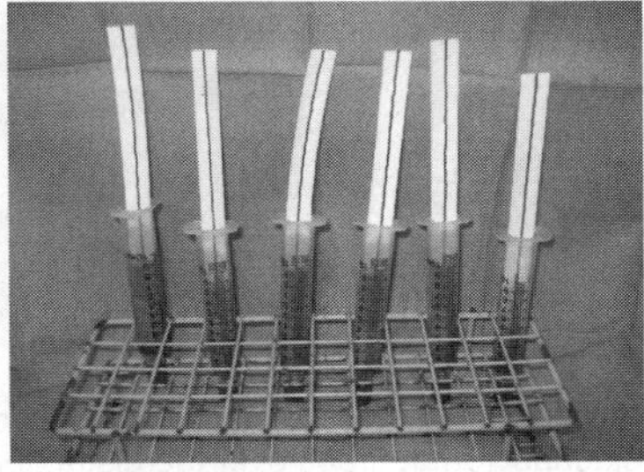

**Fig. 89-5** Harvested graft is separated into three layers by centrifugation.

### WASHING[23]

- Cleansing of the harvested graft removes cellular debris that invokes inflammatory response.
- Washing solution options are normal saline, 5% glucose, lactated Ringer's, or sterile water.
- Fat aspirate is mixed with washing solution in washing syringes.
- Syringes are placed upright until the fat layer separates from the aqueous layer, which contains blood and debris.
- Aqueous layer is removed, and procedure is repeated until supernatant is clear.
- Osmotic gradient created by the washing solution may affect adipocyte viability.[24]

### SEDIMENTATION, DECANTATION, AND STRAINING[24]

- Least traumatic method
- Harvested tissue allowed to sediment in the harvest syringe
- Can take up to 1 hour
- Can be combined with decanting of harvested tissue on an absorbent surface
- Aspirate can be strained through a cotton towel or finely meshed wire basket.

### COTTON-GAUZE ROLLING[25]

- Low trauma method of fat processing.
- Lipoaspirate is poured from the harvest syringe onto a nonstick, absorbent gauze.
- The fat is gently rolled and kneaded along the gauze with an instrument handle for 5 minutes.
- Aqueous and oil layers are removed nearly completely, but the stromal component is largely retained with this method.
- Reported as having the highest graft retention in vivo.

## FAT INJECTION

- **Cannula selection**[4,13] (Fig. 89-6)
  - 7 or 9 cm injection cannula
  - 17-gauge lumen
  - 1 cc or 3 cc Luer-Lok syringe
  - Tip types:
    - Blunt
    - Sharp: "Pickle fork"
      - Used to break up fibrous tissue

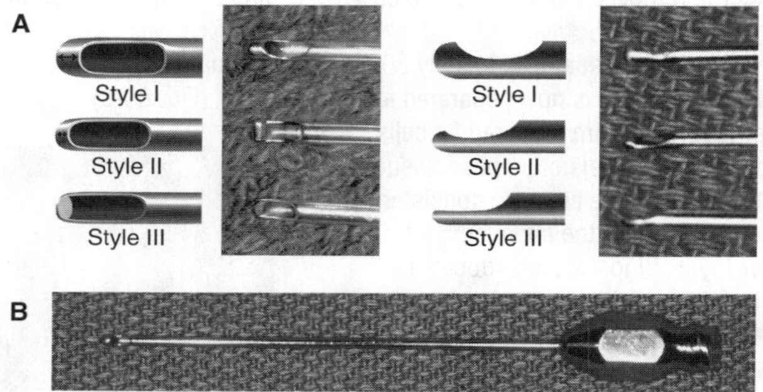


**Fig. 89-6 A,** The Coleman style I cannula is completely capped on the tip and has a lip that extends 180 degrees over the distal aperture. The Coleman style II cannula is similar, with a lip that extends 130 to 150 degrees over the distal aperture. The Coleman style III cannula is flat on the end to allow dissection of tissues in specific situations, for example, when pushing through scars or fibrous tissue. **B,** Structural fat placement is usually achieved using a blunt 17-gauge cannula with one distal aperture just proximal to the tip.

- **Injection technique**
  - **"Structural" fat placement**[12]
    - Transfer refined fat tissue from the 10 cc harvest syringes into 1 cc (face) or 3 cc (body) syringe by injection into open barrel of injection syringe.
    - Place incisions for wide access to recipient site.
    - Advance cannula and inject on withdrawal.
    - Deposit in 0.1 cc aliquots to maximize surface area of contact with surrounding tissue.
    - Place fat in cross-hatched pattern using long radial passes from multiple directions.
    - Use digital manipulation to flatten clumps and minor irregularities.
- **Large-volume fat injection**[4,26]
  - Up to 4-6 L of regional fat grafting can be performed safely, but more commonly performed volumes include 200-300 cc per site.
  - 10 cc and 60 cc syringes are used for large-volume injections to increase efficiency.
  - Multiplanar radially oriented passes performed, but larger aliquots are deposited.
  - Large aliquot fat injections have better survival when injected intramuscularly.
  - Volumetric studies using Vectra imaging have shown better long-term fat retention when a larger volume of fat is injected.[27]
  - Survival of large-volume fat grafts is higher when combined with external tissue expansion.[3]

## GRAFT VIABILITY

- Grafted fat relies initially on plasmatic imbibition from surrounding tissue before neovascularization takes place.
- If graft aliquots are too large, central necrosis will occur.
- Maximum viable percentage of graft at 1.5 mm from vascularized margin is 40%.[28]
- Ideal fat graft aliquot is 3 mm diameter.
- Histologic zones of grafted fat[16]
  - **Peripheral zone:** Viable adipocytes
  - **Intermediate zone:** Inflammatory cells
  - **Central zone:** Necrosis
- **Graft success may correlate with the number of viable preadipocytes transferred with the graft.**
- Infusion of platelet-rich plasma (PRP) improves fat graft survival and neovascularization.[29,30]
- PRP reduces inflammatory reaction and reduces rate of oil cyst formation.[31]

## FAT STORAGE

- Tissue viability drops significantly with cryopreservation.[32]
- At room temperature, aspirated fat should be transplanted as quickly as possible.
- Fat cells begin to degenerate rapidly at 4 hours after harvest.[33]
- Controlled rate of freezing reduces cell destruction.
- Addition of a cryopreservative agent to improve adipocyte viability is controversial.
  - Most agents are cytotoxic.
  - Effect on metabolic activity is variable.
  - Adipose-derived stem cell yield is significantly less in cryopreserved fat than that obtained from fresh fat.[33]

## CLINICAL TECHNIQUES

- **The Coleman technique** (see pp. 1103-1104)
  - Popular method of atraumatic fat harvest, processing, and injection
  - Goal of this technique is to maximize graft take
- Breast augmentation with external tissue expansion[3,26]
  - The Brava system is an external tissue expansion system used in conjunction with fat grafting for primary breast augmentation.
    - External tissue expanders worn for 4 weeks preoperatively
    - Brava worn for 7 days postoperatively
    - Breasts are infiltrated with lipoaspirate through 10-14 needle puncture sites and fanned over a 3D pattern
    - Brava worn for 7 days postoperatively
    - Breast volumes increased by 233 cc per breast
    - Graft survival substantially higher when external tissue expander used (82% vs. 55%)
- **Facial fat grafting**[34]
  - Useful for rejuvenation of the aging face and correction of craniofacial disorders such as hemifacial atrophy
  - Facial volume loss is primarily due to loss of facial fat, therefore fat represents the ideal filler for the aging face
  - When combined with other facial rejuvenation procedures, superior cosmetic outcomes can be obtained

  - Atraumatic manual fat harvest is performed with a 10 cc syringe and blunt cannula
  - Purification is performed by rolling fat on absorbent nonstick gauze to minimize injury to adipocytes.
  - Injection is performed using the Coleman technique.
- Percutaneous aponeurotomy and lipofilling (PALF)[21]
  - Used for subdermal scar release, congenital constriction band, radiation scarring, Dupuytren's contracture[7]
  - Percutaneous "Rigottomies" (4-5 nicks/$cm^2$) with 18g needle releases the scar in a scaffold manner and the 3D matrix interstices are filled with lipoaspirate in microliter aliquots.
  - Open, broad fasciotomies should be avoided to avoid large cavities where fat may collect and fail to revascularize
  - Multiple stages required
- Gluteal augmentation[4]
  - Gluteal augmentation with fat grafting
  - Harvest lipoaspirate with 4-5 mm liposuction cannula
  - Strain fat through large metal strainer
  - Large aliquot fat injections do better when injected intramuscularly than subcutaneous
  - Inject fat with 2.4 mm cannula on a 10 cc syringe in subcutaneous space and a 3 mm cannula on a 60 cc syringe for intramuscular injection
  - Total fat graft amount = up to 6-8 L
  - Compression garment for 4-6 weeks, no sitting for 10 days, no pressure on buttock for 6 weeks
  - 75%-80% fat survival

## APPLICATIONS IN IRRADIATED TISSUE

- Fat grafting can alleviate the sequelae of radiation damage to skin and soft tissue.
- Although not fully elucidated, the most likely mechanism is the effect of adipose-derived stem cells present within the stromal vascular fraction of the graft.[9]
- After fat grafting, irradiated skin becomes softer and more pliable, with resolution of ulceration and improvement in scar index.[8]
- Histologic and electron micrographic evaluation reveals progressive regeneration of tissue ultrastructure.[8,9,35]
  - Reduction of epidermal thickening
  - Decrease in vascular density
  - Down-regulation of fibrotic response to radiation
  - Restoration of collagen organization

## APPLICATIONS IN REGENERATIVE MEDICINE

- Adipose tissue is a rich source of multipotent stromal cells that can be applied towards regenerative cellular therapy.
- Two cell fractions containing multipotent cell lines can be derived from lipoaspirate[36]:
  1. **Stromal vascular fraction (SVF)**
     - Heterogeneous mesenchymal cell population that includes adipose stromal cells, hematopoietic stem cells, endothelial cells, fibroblasts, macrophages, and pericytes

2. **Adipose tissue-derived stem cells (ASCs)**
   - ASCs have been shown to contain cell lines that can differentiate into adipocytes, chondrocytes, osteoblasts, myocytes, and cardiomyocytes.[37,38]
   - When compared with conventional lipotransfer, fat containing supraphysiologic concentrations of ASCs (cell-enriched lipotransfer) have a higher survival rate and more prominent microvasculature on histologic evaluation.[39-41]
   - The potential applications of cell-enriched lipotransfer are extensive. In addition to soft tissue augmentation, these include involutional disorders, radiation damage, and chronic wound-healing problems.[8]
   - Applications in other fields of medicine include treatment of inflammatory disorders, diabetes, neurologic disorders, and cardiovascular disease.
   - The ASAPS/ASPS joint position on cell-enriched lipotransfer is that scientific evidence on both safety and efficacy is limited.[42]

## POSTOPERATIVE CARE

- Compression garment at all times for 2 weeks, then at night for 2 weeks
- Edema minimized to prevent fat migration and resorption
  - Elevation and application of cold packs
- Swelling and bruising possible up to 4-5 months[6]
- Permanent results not seen until 6 months postoperatively
- Activity limitation
  - Massage or manipulation of grafted area is minimized for at least 1 week to prevent graft migration.
  - Full activity is resumed 3 weeks after procedure.

## COMPLICATIONS[43]

- **Fat resorption**
  - Reports of varying amounts of volume resorption over time
  - Six months needed to determine permanent results before repeating fat grafting
- **Aesthetic deformity**
  - Recipient or donor site
- **Graft size fluctuation with weight changes**
- **Fat necrosis and formation of calcifications**
  - Fat grafting to the breast may result in microcalcifications, which can be misinterpreted as sign of malignancy on subsequent mammogram.
  - This does not interfere with detection of malignancy if evaluated by an experienced radiologist.[44]
- **Pseudocyst formation**
- **Fat emboli**
- **Lipoid meningitis**
- Arterial **occlusion** leading to blindness, stroke, and skin necrosis[45,46]
  - Incidence is 7% of partial- or full-thickness skin loss.
  - Do not use sharp cannulas and needles when injecting the face.
  - Inject face with epinephrine to vasoconstrict surrounding arteries.
  - Limit volume of each injection to 0.1 cc per pass.

## Key Points

- ✓ Counsel patients regarding long-term unpredictability of fat grafting and the need for multiple procedures to obtain the desired cosmetic result.
- ✓ Graft success correlates with the number of viable adipocytes and preadipocytes transferred.
- ✓ Use an atraumatic fat harvest technique with a large-bore cannula and low-pressure system.
- ✓ Graft must be injected in small aliquots (0.1 cc) to maximize surface area contact with surrounding tissue.
- ✓ Avoid manipulation of grafted site postoperatively to minimize graft migration.
- ✓ Compression garments are essential to prevent graft migration, contour deformity, and seroma.
- ✓ Fat grafting to the breast does not interfere with malignancy detection if subsequent mammograms are evaluated by an experienced radiologist.

## References


1. Peer LA. Cell survival theory versus replacement theory (1946). Plast Reconstr Surg 16:161-168, 1955.
2. von Heimburg D, Zacharia S, Heschel I, et al. Human preadipocytes seeded on freeze-dried collagen scaffolds investigated in vitro and in vivo. Biomaterials 22:429-438, 2001.
3. Khouri RK, Eisenmann-Klein M, Cardoso E, et al. Brava and autologous fat transfer is a safe and effective breast augmentation alternative: results of a 6-year, 81-patient, prospective multicenter study. Plast Reconstr Surg 129:1173-1187, 2012.
4. Coleman SR, Mazzola RF. Fat Injection: From Filling to Rejuvenation. St Louis: Quality Medical Publishing, 2009.
5. Mendieta CG. Gluteal reshaping. Aesthet Surg J 27:641-655, 2007.
6. Coleman SR. Hand rejuvenation with structural fat grafting. Plast Reconstr Surg 110:1731-1744; discussion 1745-1747, 2002.
7. Hovius SE, Kan HJ, Smit X, Selles RW, Cardoso E, Khouri RK. Extensive percutaneous aponeurotomy and lipografting: a new treatment for Dupuytren disease. Plast Reconstr Surg 128:221-228, 2011.
8. Phulpin B, Gangloff P, Tran N, et al. Rehabilitation of irradiated head and neck tissues by autologous fat transplantation. Plast Reconstr Surg 123:1187-1197, 2009.
9. Rigotti G, Marchi A, Galiè M, et al. Clinical treatment of radiotherapy tissue damage by lipoaspirate transplant: a healing process mediated by adipose-derived adult stem cells. Plast Reconstr Surg 119:1409-1422; discussion 1423-1424, 2007.
10. Ersek RA. Transplantation of purified autologous fat: a 3-year follow-up is disappointing. Plast Reconstr Surg 87:219-227; discussion 228, 1991.
11. Gir P, Brown SA, Oni G, Kashefi N, Mojallal A, Rohrich RJ. Fat grafting: evidence-based review on autologous fat harvesting processing reinjection and storage. Plast Reconstr Surg 130:249-258, 2012.
12. Coleman SR. Structural fat grafts: the ideal filler? Clin Plast Surg 28:111-119, 2001.
13. Coleman SR. Structural Fat Grafting. St Louis: Quality Medical Publishing, 2004.
14. Gonzalez AM, Lobocki C, Kelly CP, Jackson IT. An alternative method for harvest and processing fat grafts: an in vitro study of cell viability and survival. Plast Reconstr Surg 120:285-294, 2007.
15. Lee JH, Kirkham JC, McCormack MC. The effect of pressure and shear on autologous fat grafting. Plast Reconstr Surg 131:1125-1136, 2013.

16. Moore JH Jr, Kolaczynski JW, Morales LM, et al. Viability of fat obtained by syringe suction lipectomy: effects of local anesthesia with lidocaine. Aesthetic Plast Surg 19:335-339, 1995.
17. Keck M, Zeyda M, Gollinger K, et al. Local anesthetics have a major impact on viability of preadipocytes and their differentiation into adipocytes. Plast Reconstr Surg 126:1500-1505, 2010.
18. Keck M, Janke J, Ueberreiter K. Viability of preadipocytes in vitro: the influence of local anesthetics and pH. Dermatol Surg 35:1251-1257, 2009.
19. Rohrich RJ, Sorokin ES, Brown SA. In search of improved fat transfer viability: a quantitative analysis of the role of centrifugation and harvest site. Plast Reconstr Surg 113:391-395; discussion 396-397, 2004.
20. Botti G, Pascali M, Botti C, et al. A clinical trial in facial fat grafting: filtered and washed versus centrifuged fat. Plast Reconstr Surg 127:2464-2473, 2011.
21. Khouri RK, Smit JM, Cardoso E, Pallua N, Lantieri L, Mathijssen IM, Khouri RK Jr, Rigotti G. Percutaneous aponeurotomy and lipo-filling (PALF)—a regenerative alternative to flap reconstruction? Plast Reconstr Surg 2013 Aug 6. [Epub ahead of print]
22. Boschert MT, Beckert BW, Puckett CL, et al. Analysis of lipocyte viability after liposuction. Plast Reconstr Surg 109:761-765; discussion 766-767, 2002.
23. Ersek RA, Chang P, Salisbury MA. Lipo layering of autologous fat: an improved technique with promising results. Plast Reconstr Surg 101:820-826, 1998.
24. Rose JG Jr, Lucarelli MJ, Lemke BN, et al. Histologic comparison of autologous fat processing methods. Ophthal Plast Reconstr Surg 22:195-200, 2006.
25. Fisher C, Grahovac TL, Schafer ME, et al. Comparison of harvest and processing techniques for fat grafting and adipose stem cell isolation. Plast Reconstr Surg 132:351-361, 2013.
26. Del Vecchio DA, Bucky LP. Breast augmentation using preexpansion and autologous fat transplantation: a clinical radiographic study. Plast Reconstr Surg 127:2441-2450, 2011.
27. Choi M, Small K, Levovitz C, et al. The volumetric analysis of fat graft survival in breast reconstruction. Plast Reconstr Surg 131:185-191, 2013.
28. Carpaneda CA, Ribeiro MT. Percentage of graft viability versus injected volume in adipose autotransplants. Aesthetic Plast Surg 18:17-19, 1994.
29. Jin R, Zhang L, Zhang YG. Does platelet-rich plasma enhance the survival of grafted fat? An update review. Int J Clin Exp Med 6:252-258, 2013.
30. Liao HT, Marra K, Rubin PJ. Application of Platelet-Rich Plasma and Platelet-Rich Fibrin in Fat Grafting: Basic Science and Literature Review. Tissue Eng Part B Rev 2013.
31. Rodríguez-Flores J, Palomar-Gallego MA, Enguita-Valls AB, et al. Influence of platelet-rich plasma on the histologic characteristics of the autologous fat graft to the upper lip of rabbits. Aesthetic Plast Surg 35:480-486, 2011.
32. Lidagoster MI, Cinelli PB, Leveé EM, et al. Comparison of autologous fat transfer in fresh refrigerated and frozen specimens: an animal model. Ann Plast Surg 44:512-515, 2000.
33. Matsumoto D, Shigeura T, Sato K, et al. Influences of preservation at various temperatures on liposuction aspirates. Plast Reconstr Surg 120:1510-1517, 2007.
34. Bucky LP, Kanchwala SK. The role of autologous fat and alternative fillers in the aging face. Plast Reconstr Surg 120(6 Suppl):89S-97S, 2007.
35. Sultan SM, Stern CS, Allen RJ Jr, et al. Human fat grafting alleviates radiation skin damage in a murine model. Plast Reconstr Surg 128:363-372, 2011.
36. Bourin P, Bunnell BA, Casteilla L, et al. Stromal cells from the adipose tissue-derived stromal vascular fraction and culture expanded adipose tissue-derived stromal/stem cells: a joint statement of the International Federation for Adipose Therapeutics and Science (IFATS) and the International Society for Cellular Therapy (ISCT). Cytotherapy 15:641-648, 2013.

37. Zuk PA, Zhu M, Ashjian P, et al. Human adipose tissue is a source of multipotent stem cells. Mol Biol Cell 13:4279-4295, 2002.
38. Choi YS, Vincent LG, Lee AR, et al. Mechanical derivation of functional myotubes from adipose-derived stem cells. Biomaterials 33:2482-2491, 2012.
39. Matsumoto D, Sato K, Gonda K, et al. Cell-assisted lipotransfer: supportive use of human adipose-derived cells for soft tissue augmentation with lipoinjection. Tissue Eng 12:3375-3382, 2006.
40. Brayfield C, Marra K, Rubin JP. Adipose stem cells for soft tissue regeneration. Handchir Mikrochir Plast Chir 42:124-128, 2010.
41. Sterodimas A, de Faria J, Nicaretta B, et al. Autologous fat transplantation versus adipose-derived stem cell-enriched lipografts: a study. Aesthet Surg J 31:682-693, 2011.
42. ASAPS/ASPS position statement on stem cells and fat grafting. Aesthet Surg J 31:716-717, 2011.
43. Gutowski KA. Current applications and safety of autologous fat grafts: a report of the ASPS fat graft task force. Plast Reconstr Surg 124:272-280, 2009.
44. Delay E, Garson S, Tousson G, et al. Fat injection to the breast: technique results and indications based on 880 procedures over 10 years. Aesthet Surg J 29:360-376, 2009.
45. Kling RE, Mehrara BJ, Pusic AL, et al. Trends in autologous fat grafting to the breast: a national survey of the american society of plastic surgeons. Plast Reconstr Surg 132:35-46, 2013.
46. Coleman SR. Avoidance of arterial occlusion from injection of soft tissue fillers. Aesthet Surg J 22:555-557, 2002.

# 90. Hair Transplantation

Jeffrey E. Janis, Daniel O. Beck

## HAIR[1,2]

### EMBRYOLOGY

- Hair follicles originate from **ectoderm** and **mesoderm.**
  - Arise in the **third gestational month.**

### ANATOMY (Fig. 90-1)

- Hair shaft made of **keratinized protein**
  - Several layers, including melanocytes
  - Hair bulb
  - Papilla
- Sebaceous glands
- Sweat glands
- Erector pili muscle
- **Follicular unit**
  - One to four terminal hairs
  - One vellus hair
  - Nine sebaceous glands
  - Insertions of erector pili muscles
  - Perifollicular vascular plexus
  - Perifollicular neural net
  - Perifolliculum
- Average human scalp has approximately **100,000-150,000 hairs.**
  - **Blondes,** on average, have slightly **more** hair.
  - **Redheads,** on average, have slightly **less** hair.

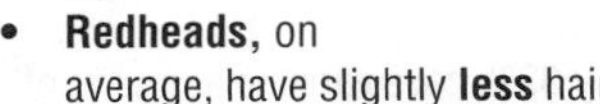

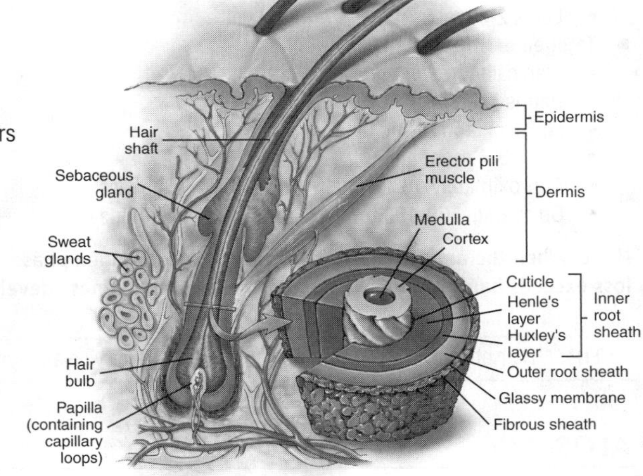


**Fig. 90-1** Anatomy.

- There are as many hair follicles in a bald scalp as a nonbald scalp (histologically).

## PHYSIOLOGY OF HAIR GROWTH[2,3]

### THREE PHASES (Fig. 90-2)

- **Anagen**
  - **Active growth**
  - Follicular cells actively multiplying and becoming keratinized
  - **90%** of hairs normally in this phase
  - Lasts approximately **1000 days in men** and **2-5 years longer in women**
- **Catagen**
  - Also called *degradation phase*
  - Keratinization of hair base (i.e., forms a club)
  - Separation of base from dermal papilla
  - Moves toward the surface
  - Lasts **2-3 weeks**
- **Telogen**
  - Also called *resting phase*
  - Hair is shed.
  - Follicle **inactive** and hair growth stops
  - Lasts **3-4 months**
  - Approximately **10%** of hairs normally in this phase
  - On average, **50-100 telogen hairs** fall out every day

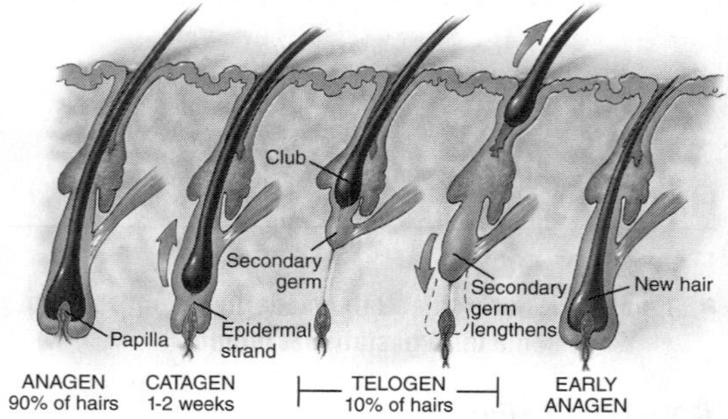

**Fig. 90-2** Three phases of hair growth.

**NOTE: When the anagen phase shortens and the telogen phase is prolonged (i.e., rate of hair loss exceeds hair growth), thinning and eventual baldness develop.**

**TIP:** Hair physiology is frequently covered on in-service and written board examinations.

## ALOPECIA

### INCIDENCE[4,5]

- It is estimated that 35,000,000 men and 21,000,000 women in the United States have hair loss.
- It is so common in men that it is actually accepted as **normal.**
  - Of men seeking hair replacement surgery, approximately **33%** have variable amounts of alopecia by their **mid-30s.**
  - **50%** have variable amounts of alopecia by age 50 years.
  - **66%** have variable amounts of alopecia by their mid-60s.
- Highest incidence is in whites, followed by Asians and blacks, and the lowest is in American Indians.

### Etiologic Factors[2,4,5]

- **Androgenic alopecia**
  - Male pattern baldness is the conversion of healthy, thick terminal hairs to clear, microscopic vellus hairs.
  - It is an **X-linked, dominant condition.**
  - **5α-reductase,** which is in the cells of susceptible hair follicles and the skin, is responsible for converting testosterone to dihydrotestosterone (DHT).
  - Normal circulating amounts of testosterone may be excessively converted to DHT, or the hair follicle may be abnormally sensitive to DHT, which creates androgenic alopecia.
- Donor follicles from **occipital regions** have decreased or absent DHT and thus are **not** influenced by hormonal factors, making them attractive for use as donor grafts.

NOTE: **In general, the earlier the onset of alopecia, the more severe it will be.**

- **Discoid lupus erythematosus**
- **Lichen planopilaris**
  - Lichen planus of skin and hair follicles
- **Alopecia areata**
- **Cicatricial alopecia**
- **Traumatic alopecia**

## HAIR TRANSPLANTATION

### Indications

- Androgenic alopecia
- Cicatricial alopecia
- Traumatic alopecia
- Traction alopecia

### Contraindications

- Diffuse female pattern baldness
- Non-donor-dominant alopecia
- Alopecia areata
- Active scarring alopecias (discoid lupus erythematosus, lichen planopilaris, and other cicatricial alopecia)

## PATIENT EVALUATION

### Male Classification[5] (Fig. 90-3)

- **Hamilton**[6] described **seven major types** of male pattern baldness.
- The **Norwood modification** is most commonly used.[4,5,7]
  - **Type I:** Minimal or no hairline recession at the frontotemporal areas
  - **Type II:** Symmetrical triangular frontotemporal recessions extend posteriorly, no more than 2 cm anterior to the coronal plane drawn between the external auditory canals
  - **Type III:** Symmetrical triangular frontotemporal recessions extend posteriorly more than 2 cm
  - **Type $III_{vertex}$:** Primarily vertex hair loss; may be accompanied by frontotemporal recession that conforms to type III guidelines
  - **Type IV:** Sparse or absent vertex hair with more severe frontotemporal recession; areas separated by a band of moderately dense hair that extends across the top of the head

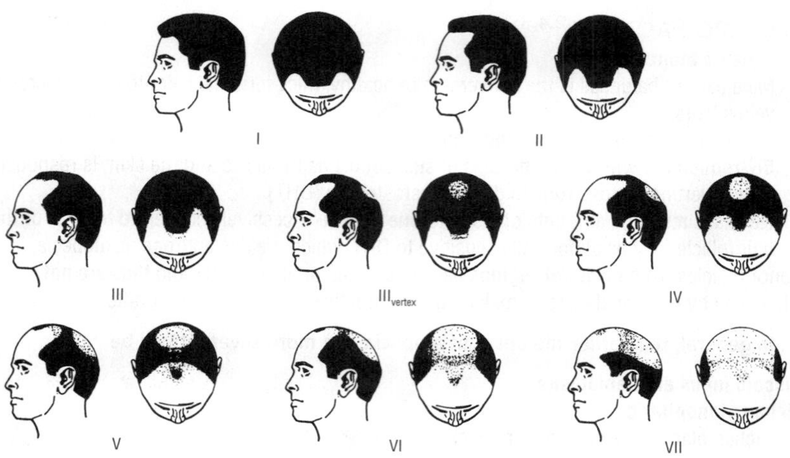


**Fig. 90-3** Norwood male classification of alopecia.

- **Type V:** Same as type IV, but more severe hair loss; band of hair narrower and more sparse
- **Type VI:** Band is absent and two areas interconnect.
- **Type VII:** Most severe form; only a narrow horseshoe-shaped band of fine, sparse hair

## Female Classification[8] (Fig. 90-4)

- The **Ludwig classification**[8] is most commonly used.
- The following patient characteristics must be taken into account.
  - **Hair density:** A natural result is more difficult to achieve with poor density.
  - **Thickness of hair follicles:** Fine, thin hair is harder to disguise than curly, thicker hair.
  - **Straight versus curly hair:** Natural curl produces a better result.
  - **Hair color:** Light-colored, gray, or salt-and-pepper hair is more natural than thin, straight, black hair.

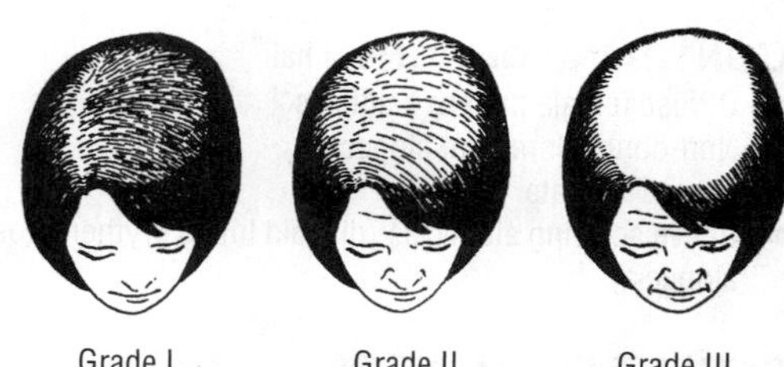


**Fig. 90-4** Ludwig female classification of alopecia.

# Treatment[2,9]

## Medical Therapy

- Frequently used in conjunction with hair restoration surgery
- **Minoxidil (Rogaine)**
  - Available in 2% and 5% topical solutions
  - Used on scalp twice daily
  - Cosmetically useful hair obtained only in about **one third** of cases
  - *Must be used indefinitely to maintain a response*

- **Finasteride (Propecia)**
  - **5α-reductase inhibitor**
  - Promotes conversion of hair follicles to the anagen phase
  - Available in 1 mg tablets and given once daily
  - Lowers DHT on the scalp and in serum of treated patients
  - Effective in **preventing further hair loss** and **increasing hair counts** to the point of cosmetically appreciable results
  - Hair loss on temples is **not** improved (although vertex and frontal hair counts are increased).
  - Side effects rare (<1%)
  - Must be used indefinitely to maintain a response

## Laser Therapy

- Promoted as a preventive measure against androgenic alopecia; thickens and induces growth of existing follicles.
- FDA-permitted devices are approved for safety not efficacy.
- Large-scale, placebo-controlled trials are lacking.
  - **Low-level laser (light) therapy** (LLLT)[10,11]
    - Uses wavelengths within the red/infrared spectrum **(600-900 nm)** to induce hair growth
    - Mester et al[12] (1967) first noted faster hair regrowth in shaved mice while attempting to induce skin cancer using a 694 nm ruby laser.
    - Interest in LLLT maintained by literature reports of paradoxical hair growth after laser treatment for hair removal
    - Mechanism of action for LLLT commonly referred to as *photobiomodulation,* although exact mechanism not known
    - **Theories for mechanism of action include:**
      - Increased blood flow at dermal papilla
      - Direct stimulation of dermal follicles
      - Synchronization of hair growth cycles
      - Upregulation of mitochondria and ATP production
    - **Side effects**
      - Pain
      - Pruritis
      - Mild paresthesia
      - Erythema
      - Dry scalp and dandruff
      - Transient shedding after treatment
    - **Outcome studies**
      - Avram and Rogers[13]
        - 7 patients; 20-minute treatments of superior scalp using a 650 nm laser twice weekly for 3-6 months
        - Nonspecific trend toward decrease in vellus hairs, increased terminal hairs, and increased hair shaft diameter
        - However, blinded subjective clinical evaluation noted improvement in only 2/7 patients and no change in 4/7 patients.
      - Shukla et al[14]
        - Evaluated the effect of helium-neon (He-Ne) laser (632.8 nm) irradiation on the hair follicle growth cycle of testosterone-treated and untreated mice
        - Found significant increase in percentage anagen, indicating stimulation of hair growth

- Leavitt et al[15]
  - Evaluated HairMax LaserComb (HairMax, Boca Raton, FL)
  - FDA-approved device using a 655 nm source for promotion of hair growth
  - Randomized, blinded, sham device-controlled, multi-center trial
  - 110 male patients, treated three times/week for 26 weeks over scalp vertex
  - Increase in terminal hair density >5 hairs/cm$^2$ seen in 86.1% of treatment group versus 5% in control group
  - Subjective patient assessment reported minimal to moderate growth in 62% of treated versus 46% of control group
- **Fractional photothermolysis**
  - Use of a **1550 nm** erbium-glass laser to create controlled microscopic zones of thermal injury
  - Exact mechanism of action not known; theories include:
    - Direct stimulation of the dermal papilla
    - Direct stimulation of stem cells
    - Induction of increased blood flow
    - Upregulation of cytokines and growth factors involved in the hair cycle
  - Side effects similar to those of LLLT
  - **Outcome studies**
    - Kim et al[16]
      - Two study arms: Androgenic alopecia mouse model and human trial
      - Significant increase in hair density and growth rate up to 1 month after treatment
      - Histologic studies demonstrated an increased anagen/telogen ratio
      - Improvement primarily from increase in vellus hair
      - No significant change in hair caliber
      - All parameters returned to pretreatment baseline level by 4-month follow-up
    - Lee et al[17]
      - 27 females treated biweekly for 5 months
      - 24/27 patients judged as responders based on hair density and thickness
        - 3 significant improvement, 21 moderate improvement, 3 stabilized state
      - Most notable improvement was seen at frontal hair recesses in all responding patients.
      - 26/27 patients noted improvement or stabilization of hair loss on self-assessment.
      - There was no long-term follow-up to determine maintenance of effects.

## SURGICAL THERAPY[2,14,15,18,19]

### PRINCIPLES

- Provide a natural look.
- Reconstitute a normal anterior hairline with normal hair growth patterns.
- Minimize scalp scars in both the donor and recipient sites.

### PREOPERATIVE CARE

- Ensure that the patient has discontinued medications that may result in excessive bleeding (e.g., NSAIDs, anticoagulants, herbal medications).
- Assess for allergies to medications, including local anesthetics, anxiolytics, and narcotic pain medication.

## Preoperative Planning

- Average scalp measures **500 cm**$^2$ (50,000 mm$^2$)
- Average **200 hairs/cm**
- **One follicular unit/mm**$^2$ for normal nonbalding scalp
  - Each follicular unit (FU) contains two **hairs** (therefore two hairs/mm$^2$)
- Approximately **12.5%** of scalp available for hair transplantation in type V or type VI male pattern baldness
  - Equivalent to 12,500 hairs or 6250 FU (two hairs each)
  - Can be transplanted in two megasessions of 3000-4000 micrografts or minigrafts (see later)
  - A good visual result is apparent with densities of 25-40 FU/cm$^2$
- Donor site location
  - **Occipital** and **temporal** areas best donor sites
  - Optimal donor site varies with **age**
    - **In patients older than 40 years:** Donor site is half the vertical distance from the posterior upper healthy fringe to the lower hairline (Fig. 90-5, *A*).
    - **In patients younger than 40 years:** Donor site is at the junction of the middle and caudal thirds of the same vertical distance described previously (Fig. 90-5, *B*).

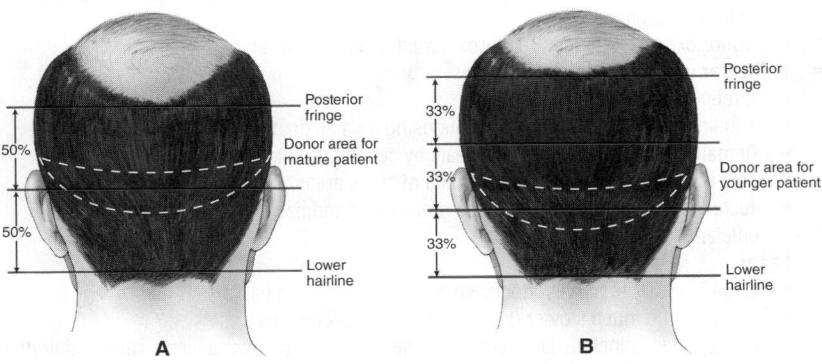


**Fig. 90-5** Donor site locations.

## Minigrafts and Micrografts (Fig. 90-6)

- **Micrografts** contain one or two hairs per graft.
- **Minigrafts** contain three to eight hairs per graft.
- When properly placed, smaller grafts provide a more natural, less abrupt hairline than punch grafts (usually 4 mm).
- It is best to place grafts into incision sites, called *slits,* which are arranged in horizontal rows along the frontal hairline.
  - Slit techniques represent a simpler method for placing hair grafts.

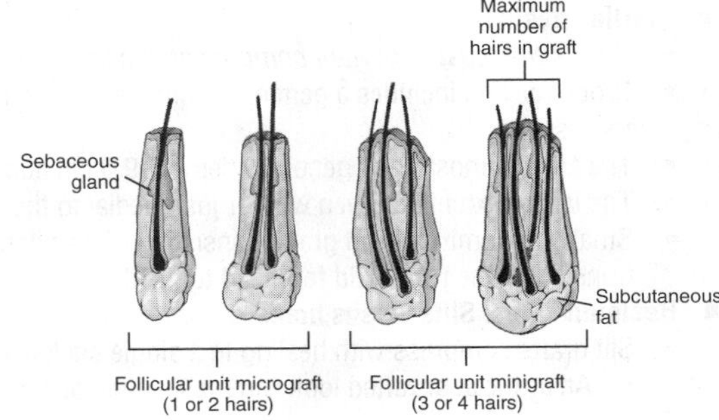


**Fig. 90-6** Minigrafts and micrografts.

- Large numbers of one- to three-hair micrografts are placed in slit incisions without using recipient punches to remove bald scalp.
- Fine micrograft hairs are placed in the front line and are backed up by larger micrografts and minigrafts.
- Slits can be used for younger patients with thinning hair without sacrificing existing hair follicles in the recipient area.
- Slits may require more than one session to complete.

## TECHNIQUE

- **Harvesting the grafts**
  - **Strip excision (elliptical excision)**
    - Can be subdivided into minigrafts or micrografts
    - Less follicular loss
    - Knife blade angulation **parallel to hair shafts** reduces follicle transection.
  - **Triple- or quadruple-blade knives**
    - Used to make 2 mm parallel excisions across the scalp
    - Easier and more precise
    - Allow surgeons to accurately trim 1 mm and 2 mm grafts with no waste and little follicular damage
    - Donor excision site then reapproximated by sutures or staples
  - **Follicular unit extraction**
    - A refined micropunch graft
    - 1 follicular unit is removed at a time using a small diameter (0.8-1.5 mm) punch.
    - Remaining puncture donor site heals by secondary intention.
    - This is a good technique for coverage of small areas.
    - Technique is gaining popularity as motorized handpieces make harvest time more efficient.
  - **Laser**
    - Er:YAG or $CO_2$ to harvest donor strip
    - Harvest time much slower than with blade dissection
    - Disadvantages include laser cost, less yield, longer postoperative crusting and erythema, telogen precipitation.

**TIP:** It is extremely helpful to have an assistant trained in harvesting and processing to drastically shorten the procedure time.

- **Hairline design**
  - *This is the most important component to achieving a natural appearance.*
  - Proper design includes a gentle, curving hairline with maintenance of frontotemporal recessions.
  - The anteriormost point generally lies 7.5-9.0 cm above the glabella (Fig. 90-7).
  - The lateral extent lies even with or just medial to the lateral canthus.
  - Small, randomly spaced grafts consisting of less course hairs are used to re-create the soft transition zone from bald forehead to the dense posterior hairline.
- **Recipient sites: Slits versus holes**
  - Slit grafts compress with healing to a single stalk from which 2-5 hairs grow.
    - An artificial or tufted look can result when only slit minigrafts are used.

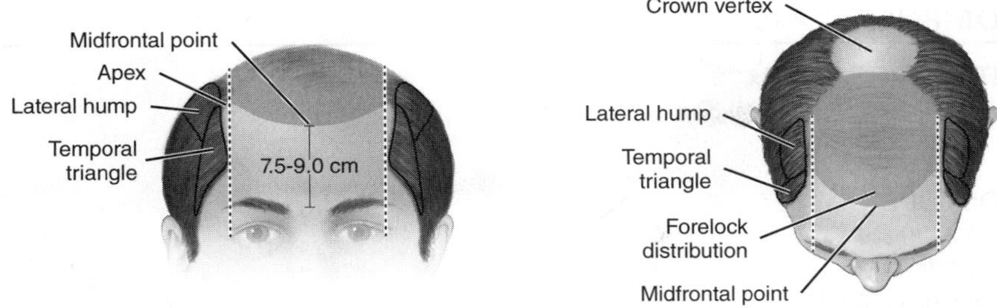


**Fig. 90-7** Anatomic subunits in hair transplantation.

- Similar minigrafts placed in holes seem to remain spread out and do not have a compressed, artificial appearance.
- Some doctors mix slits with holes and varying graft size to obtain a more natural result.

- **Proper orientation**
  - **Natural angles** (Fig. 90-8)
    - **Frontal hairline:** 45-60 degrees
    - **Posterior to hairline:** 75-80 degrees
    - **Crown/vertex:** 90 degrees (i.e., perpendicular to scalp)
    - **Posterior to crown:** 45-60 degrees downward
    - **Lateral fringes:** Follow direction of existing hair

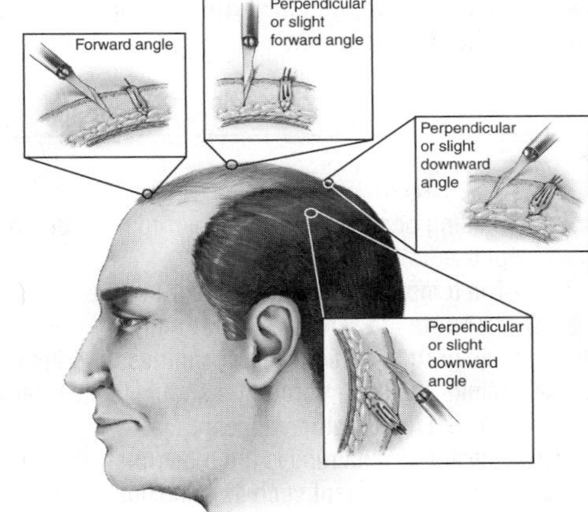


**Fig. 90-8** Natural angles in hairline design.

**TIP:** It is helpful to wear loupes during harvest and transplantation.

## POSTOPERATIVE CARE

- Cover the donor grafts with a nonstick dressing (Telfa), and wrap patient's head in a turban.
- Keep the patient for approximately 1 hour after surgery, and give oral fluids and a light snack.
- The patient should be accompanied home.
- The patient should not engage in strenuous exercise or heavy lifting for 2 weeks.
- The patient should avoid direct sunlight.
- The patient should wash hair using the "pour method" (i.e., mix light shampoo with warm water and pour over the scalp without massaging).
- The patient may resume normal hair washing at postoperative day 14.
- The patient should follow up in the clinic 1 week after surgery.

## COMPLICATIONS

### INTRAOPERATIVE

- Hemorrhage
- Lidocaine toxicity

### POSTOPERATIVE

- Hemorrhage
- Infection
- Scarring (including keloids)
- Poor hair growth
- Unnatural hairline
- Doll's head appearance

**CAUTION: Be sure to plan for future hair loss when designing the donor incisions and recipient sites. Further hair loss may eventually expose donor site incisions or result in unnatural tufts of hair.**

### KEY POINTS

✓ Balding occurs when more hair follicles are in the telogen phase than in the anagen phase.
✓ The temporal and occipital hair follicles are usually resistant to the effects of DHT; therefore they are excellent donors.
✓ Minigraft and micrograft techniques produce more natural results than punch grafts.
✓ Minigrafts and micrografts should be inserted at the proper angle and orientation to prevent an unnatural appearance.
✓ The anterior hairline is the most important location to reconstruct.
✓ Medical treatment such as minoxidil and finasteride are useful adjuncts to surgical treatment and have minimal side effects.
✓ Complete restoration may require more than one procedure.

### REFERENCES


1. Orentreich N, Durr NP. Biology of scalp hair growth. Clin Plast Surg 9:197-205, 1982.
2. Barrera A. Hair Transplantation. The Art of Micrografting and Minigrafting. St Louis: Quality Medical Publishing, 2002.
3. Orentreich N. Scalp hair replacement in man. In Oregon Regional Primate Research Center, Montagna W, Dobson RL, eds. Advances on Biology of Skin, vol 9. Proceedings of the University of Oregon Medical School Symposium on the Biology of Skin. New York: Pergamon Press, 1969.
4. Norwood OT. Male pattern baldness: classification and incidence. South Med J 68:1359-1365, 1975.
5. Norwood OT, Shiell RC, eds. Hair Transplant Surgery, 2nd ed. Springfield, IL: Charles C Thomas, 1984.
6. Hamilton JB. Patterned loss of hair in man: types and incidence. Ann N Y Acad Sci 53:708-728, 1951.
7. Norwood OT. Patient selection, hair transplant design, and hairstyle. J Dermatol Surg Oncol 18:386-394, 1992.
8. Ludwig E. Classification of the types of androgenetic alopecia (common baldness) occurring in the female sex. Br J Dermatol 97:247-254, 1977.
9. Beran S. Hair restoration. Sel Read Plast Surg 9:29, 2001.

10. Willey A, Torrontegui J, Azpiazu J, et al. Hair stimulation following laser and intense pulsed light photoepilation: review of 543 cases and ways to manage it. Lasers Surg Med 39:297-301, 2007.
11. Avram MR, Leonard RT Jr, Epstein ES, et al. The current role of laser/light sources in the treatment of male and female pattern hair loss. J Cosmet Laser Ther 9:27-28, 2007.
12. Mester E, Szende B, Tota JG. [Effect of laser on hair growth of mice] Kiserl Orvostud 19:628-631, 1967.
13. Avram MR, Rogers NE. The use of low-level light for hair growth: part I. J Cosmet Laser Ther 12:116, 2010.
14. Shukla S, Sahu K, Verma Y, et al. Effect of helium-neon laser irradiation on hair follicle growth cycle of Swiss albino mice. Skin Pharmacol Physiol 23:79-85, 2010.
15. Leavitt M, Charles G, Heyman E, et al. HairMax LaserComb laser phototherapy device in the treatment of male androgenetic alopecia: a randomized, double-blind, sham device-controlled, multicentre trial. Clin Drug Investig 29:283-292, 2009.
16. Kim W, Lee H, Lee JW, et al. Fractional photothermolysis laser treatment of male pattern hair loss. Dermatol Surg 37:41-51, 2011.
17. Lee GY, Lee SJ, Kim WS. The effect of a 1550 nm fractional erbium-glass laser in female pattern hair loss. J Eur Acad Dermatol Venereol 25:1450-1454, 2011.
18. Vogel JE, Jimenez F, Cole J, et al. Hair restoration surgery: the state of the art. Aesthet Surg J 33:128-151, 2013.
19. Bunagan MJ, Banka N, Shapiro J. Hair transplantation update: procedural techniques, innovations and applications. Dermatol Clin 31:141-153, 2013.

# 91. Brow Lift

Jonathan Bank, Jason E. Leedy

## ANATOMY

### MUSCULATURE[1] (Fig. 91-1)

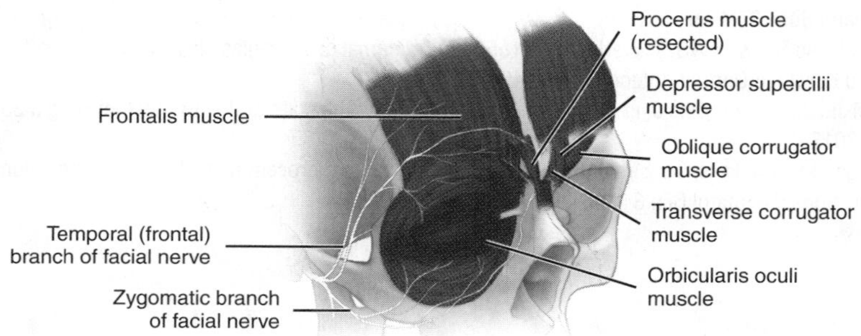


**Fig. 91-1** Periorbital motor nerves and the muscles they activate.

- **Frontalis muscle**
  - Origin: Galea aponeurosis
  - Insertion: Supraorbital dermis by interdigitating with orbicularis oculi
    - Loose connective tissue under muscle allows movement, but muscular and periosteal adhesions limit brow movement (important in surgical releases).
  - Innervation: Temporal (frontal) branch of facial nerve
  - Action: Brow elevator; creates transverse forehead rhytids
  - **Galea aponeurosis:** Splits into two sheaths that encapsulate the frontalis
    - Posterior sheath extends to the periosteum at the superior orbital rim.
- **Corrugator supercilii muscle**
  - **Lies deep to frontalis muscle**
  - Origin begins 3 mm lateral to the vertical midline drawn through the nasion.
  - Extends 85% of distance between the nasion and lateral orbital rim[2]
  - **Oblique head**
    - Origin: Superior-medial orbital rim
    - Insertion: Dermis at medial eyebrow
    - Innervation: Zygomatic branches
    - Action: Depresses brow; creates oblique glabellar lines

- **Transverse head**
  - Origin: Superomedial orbital rim
  - Insertion: Dermis just superior to the middle third of the eyebrow
  - Innervation: Frontal branch
  - Action: Moves the brow medially; creates oblique and vertical glabellar lines
- **Depressor supercilii muscle**
  - Origin: Superior-medial orbital rim
  - Insertion: Medial brow dermis
  - Innervation: Zygomatic branches
  - Action: Depresses brow; creates oblique glabellar lines
- **Procerus muscle**
  - Origin: Superior-medial orbital rim
  - Insertion: Dermis of medial brow
  - Innervation: Superior portion by frontal branch, inferior portion by zygomatic branches
  - Action: Depresses brow; creates oblique glabellar and transverse nasal root lines
- **Orbicularis oculi**
  - **Medial orbital portion** can cause medial brow depression.
    - Insignificant contributor to glabellar rhytids
  - **Lateral orbital portion** can cause lateral brow depression.
    - Creates lateral orbital rhytids (i.e., crow's-feet)
  - Innervated by zygomatic branch of facial nerve

## SENSATION

- **Supratrochlear nerve**[3]
  - Exits orbit **medially** (1.5 cm from midline) and usually arborizes
  - Enters corrugator then frontalis to supply the forehead[3]
  - Partial injury during corrugator resection inevitable but of low consequence
- **Supraorbital nerve**[4-6]
  - Exits through foramen or notch **lateral to supratrochlear nerve** (3-4 cm from midline, or midpupillary line)
  - Divides into **superficial** and **deep** branches
  - **Superficial branch** enters frontalis 2-3 cm above rim, and supplies forehead.
  - **Deep branch** supplies scalp posterior to the hairline.
  - Runs laterally up to 0.5-1.5 cm medial to the superior temporal line (temporal crest)

> **TIP:** Transection of the deep branch with subgaleal dissection and coronal incisions is believed to be responsible for postoperative scalp paresthesias.[4]

## SENTINEL VEIN

- Medial of two zygomaticotemporal communicating veins (between superficial and deep systems)[7] (Fig. 91-2)
- 1.5 cm above and lateral to lateral canthus
- Lowest branch of **frontal branch of facial nerve** is 1 cm above the vein.

## BROW-RETAINING LIGAMENTS

- **Orbital ligament:** Fibrous band connecting the orbital rim and the superficial temporal fascia deep to the lateral eyebrow[8]

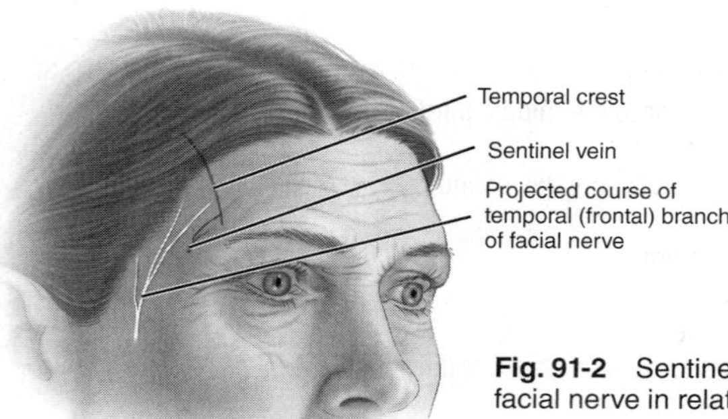


**Fig. 91-2** Sentinel vein and frontal branch of facial nerve in relation to the temporal crest.

- **Temporal and supraorbital ligamentous adhesions and lateral brow and lateral orbital thickening of the periorbital septum (Fig. 91-3):** Periorbital attachments released for brow elevation[9]
- **Brow-retaining ligament and upper lid-retaining ligament:** Zones of attachment from bone to overlying skin that require release for brow elevation[10]

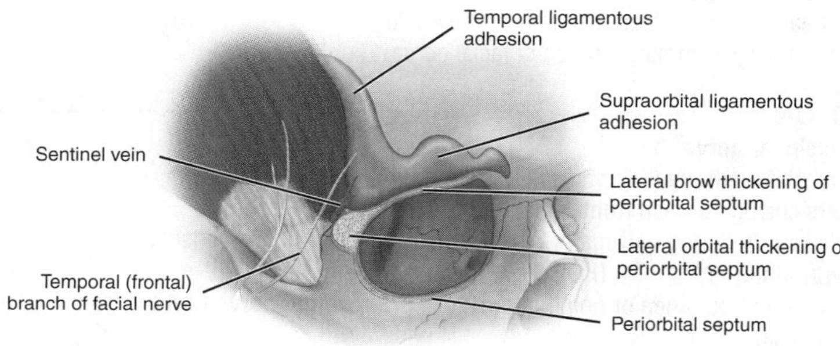


**Fig. 91-3** Temporal and supraorbital adhesions.

## AESTHETICS

### YOUTHFUL APPEARANCE

- Absence of forehead and glabellar rhytids
- Absence of dyschromia
- Appropriately positioned hairline
- Pleasing eyebrow shape and position

### AESTHETIC MEASUREMENT GUIDELINES[11,12] (Fig. 91-4)

- **Anterior hairline to brow:** 5 cm in women; 6 cm in men
- **Eyebrow position at lateral limbus:** On orbital rim in men; 1 cm above orbital rim in women
- **Medial brow** club shaped and **lateral brow** tapers; ends lie at approximately same level, but lateral end may be slightly elevated
- **Gentle arch:** Peak at junction of the medial two thirds and lateral one third, lying halfway between lateral limbus and lateral canthus

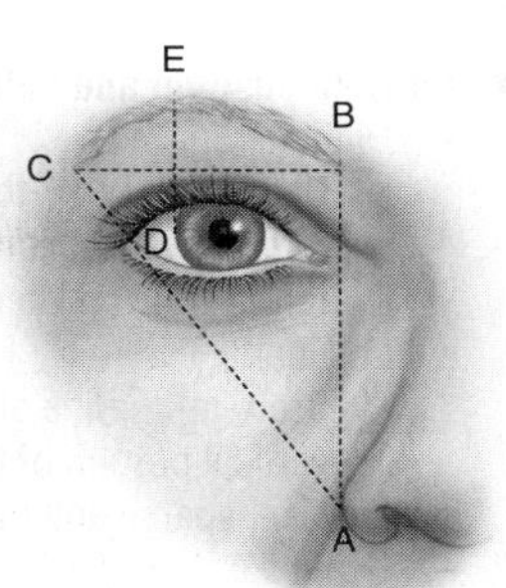


**Fig. 91-4** Standard configuration and spacing of the brow in women. (*A,* Nasal alar base; *B,* medial eyebrow; *C,* lateral eyebrow; *D,* lateral limbus.)

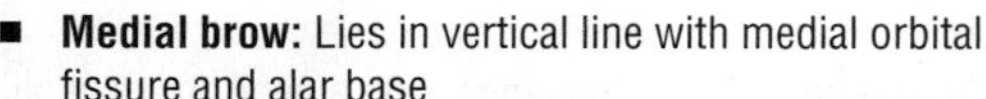

- **Medial brow:** Lies in vertical line with medial orbital fissure and alar base
- **Lateral brow:** Lies on oblique line from alar base through lateral orbital fissure
- **In midpupillary line**
    - Anterior hairline to brow: 5-6 cm
    - Brow to superior orbital rim: 1 cm
    - Brow to supratarsal crease: 1.6 cm
    - Brow to midpupil: 2.5 cm

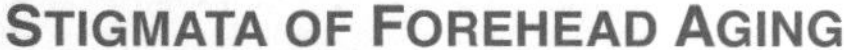

### STIGMATA OF FOREHEAD AGING

- Transverse forehead rhytids
- Glabellar rhytids
- Brow ptosis
- Skin dyschromia

## PREOPERATIVE EVALUATION

### ASSESSMENT OF ANATOMIC FEATURES

- Degree of frontal bone convexity
- Prominence of supraorbital rim
- Forehead height
- Amount of retroorbicularis fat (ROOF)
- Hairline and hair thickness

### ASSESSMENT OF AGING CHANGES

- **Brow position and shape (medial and lateral)**
    - As per previously mentioned aesthetic guidelines
    - May be artificially elevated from plucking and makeup
- **Rhytids (transverse, vertical) at rest and on animation**
    - Dynamic rhytids
        - **Present only during animation**
        - Amenable to botulinum toxin
        - Surgical improvement with weakening of the involved muscles
    - Static rhytids
        - **Present at rest;** result of sustained muscle hyperactivity
        - In general, partially improved with surgical muscle weakening but require redraping of soft tissue
        - **Superficial rhytids:** Amenable to fillers and resurfacing procedures
        - **Deep rhytids:** Require extensive soft tissue redraping (e.g., subcutaneous dissection)
    - Note periorbital features such as crow's-feet and lateral orbital crowding.
- **Skin quality and color**
    - Improvement in dyschromia and skin texture dramatically improves surgical result.
    - Adjunctive skin care should be considered.

- **Hairline position and anterior hair**
  - High hairline
    - Defined as brow-to-hairline distance >5 cm in women and >6 cm in men
    - Alternatively considered when the anterior hairline lies on more oblique aspect of forehead from lateral view
  - Low hairline
    - Brow-to-hairline distance <5 cm in women and <6 cm in men, with anterior hairline on vertical portion of forehead from lateral view
    - Fine, sparse anterior hair less likely to conceal a coronal incision than thicker, dark hair

## SURGICAL TECHNIQUE

### SURGICAL APPROACHES[13]

- **Typically, brow lifts are combined with other procedures that involve periorbital rejuvenation (upper, lower blepharoplasty).**
- **Coronal**
  - Universal option, fallen out of favor because of extent of dissection and ability to achieve similar results with less-invasive techniques
  - Incision can be beveled to allow hair to grow through scar
  - Coronal, modified coronal, or anterior hairline incision
  - Incision placed at least **3 cm posterior to hairline** for better scar camouflage
  - **Useful for low hairline:** 1.5 mm of anterior hairline retrodisplacement required for every 1 mm of eyebrow elevation
- **Anterior hairline incision**
  - Useful if hairline is high (hairline on oblique portion of forehead from lateral view)
  - Incision 1-2 mm posterior to hairline
  - Risk of scar visibility

> **TIP:** In bald men, place the incision farther posteriorly to make it less visible from the frontal view.

  - Greater scalp excision (up to 3-4 cm) performed laterally (versus medially) to preferentially correct lateral brow descent
- **Endoscopic**
  - Usually small central incision with two temporal incisions (can add two paramedian incisions)
  - Arguably limits morbidity of coronal and hairline incision
  - **Adequate release of periorbital septa and adhesions essential**
  - Multiple fixation options (see below)
- **Temporal**[5] (Fig. 91-5)
  - Keep incision over temporalis muscle. (More medial location places supraorbital nerve at risk.)
  - Dissect plane just above deep temporal fascia to prevent frontal nerve injury.
  - Technique is otherwise similar to coronal but spares vertex incision.

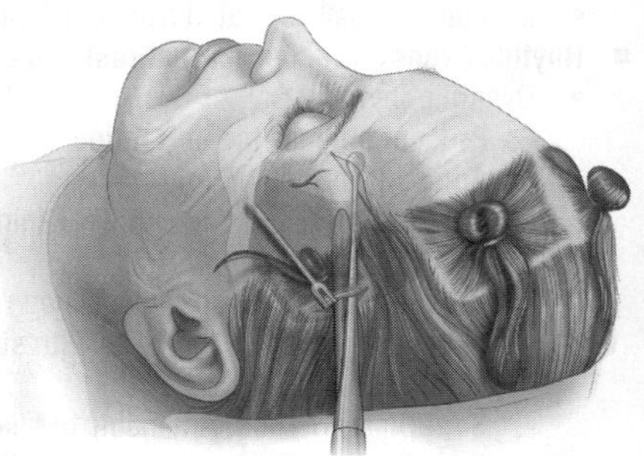

**Fig. 91-5** Temporal approach.

- **Transblepharoplasty**
  - Involves tacking lateral brow to periosteum or deep temporal fascia to obtain mild lateral lift
  - Adequate undermining critical to avoid overhang
  - Can also perform simultaneous corrugator and procerus excision for glabellar rhytids[7,14] (Fig. 91-6)
- **Combined**
  - Temporal with transpalpebral incisions (Knize[8])
  - Can achieve results similar to those of coronal approach

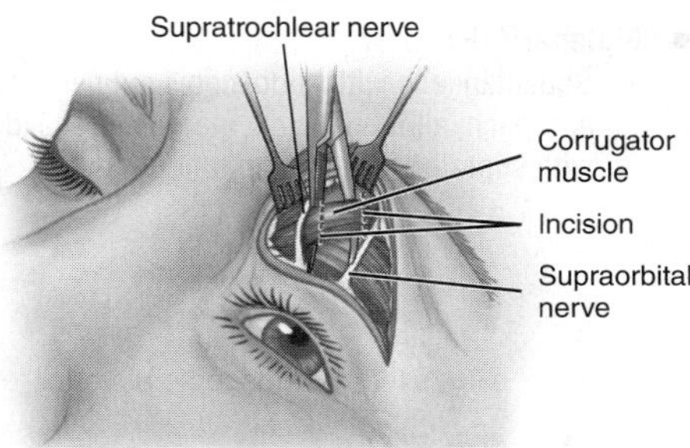


**Fig. 91-6** Transblepharoplasty approach.

- **Direct**
  - **Supraciliary**
    - Removal of ellipse of skin and subcutaneous tissue only at supraorbital rim to conceal scar above eyebrow
    - **Useful in men with thick skin, deep rhytids (hide scar), and alopecia** (coronal and temporal incisions less favorable)
  - **Midbrow**
    - Removal of midforehead skin strip to conceal incision in transverse rhytid
    - **Useful in men with thick skin, deep rhytids, and alopecia,** thereby making coronal or temporal incisions less favorable
    - Advances hairline downward

## Plane of Dissection

- **Subcutaneous**
  - Preserves posterior scalp sensation
  - Useful for improving deep transverse rhytids by disconnecting dermal adhesions
  - Decreases flap vascularity and *can be associated with increased wound complications*
  - Tedious dissection
  - Difficult to perform medial brow depressor muscle excision
- **Subgaleal**
  - Rapid, easy dissection
  - Allows direct excision or scoring of muscle

**TIP:** Some surgeons argue that fixation of galea to periosteum is quicker than periosteum to bone, which may improve durability of the lift.[15]

- **Subperiosteal**
  - Some surgeons believe that lifting the pericranium provides more sustained lift.[16]
  - Requires release of arcus marginalis for effective lift
  - Should be avoided in the medial brow area if medial brow elevation is not desired

- **Biplanar**[12] (Fig. 91-7)
  - Subcutaneous with endoscopic subperiosteal approach; allows improvement in forehead rhytids with suprabrow muscle excision[17]

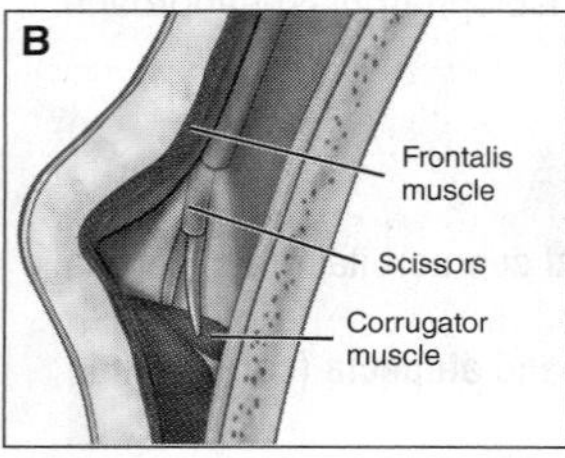


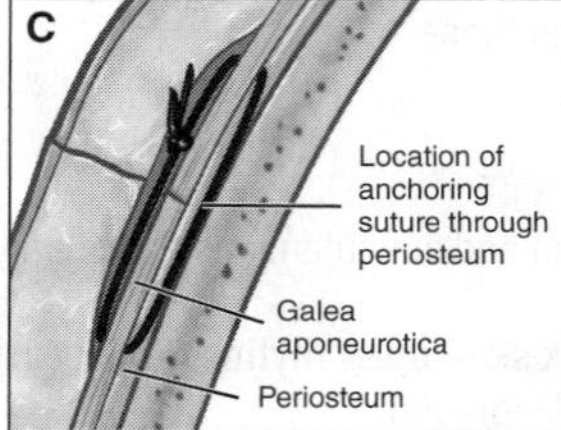


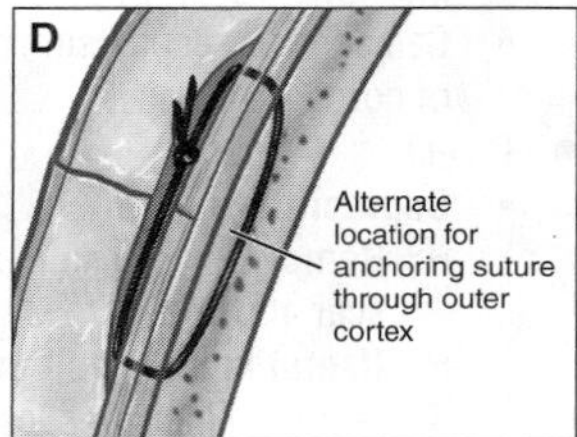


**Fig. 91-7** Endoscopic biplanar forehead lift.

## Muscle Weakening

- **Direct muscle excision**
  - Can remove corrugators and portions of frontalis
    - ▸ Preserve suprabrow frontalis (at least 2 cm) to maintain brow animation
  - Can graft glabella with fat after removal of corrugators to correct depression deformities after resection of muscle bulk[18]
- **Muscle scoring**
  - Frontalis, corrugators (decreases rhytids), and lateral orbicularis (can assist with brow fixation by minimizing downward pull)
- **Chemical paralysis**
  - Botulinum toxin

## Securing Brow Elevation

Elastic band principle: *The farther away the suspension point is from the brow, the less effective the lift.*[15]

- **Skin excision:** Open technique
  - Skin excision/brow elevation ratio is 2:1 (3:1 if frontalis removed for brow elevation).[19]
  - Some authors recommend up to 5:1 ratio to achieve longer-lasting results.
- **Suture techniques**
  - **Endoscopic techniques**
    - ▸ Cortical tunnel: Suture secured to tunnel made in outer table of calvarium
    - ▸ Lateral spanning suspension sutures

- **Devices**
  - **Percutaneous or internal screw placement with attached suture:** Screws removed at later follow-up
  - **K-wire placement:** Can be left permanently or removed
  - **Endotine** (Coapt Systems, Palo Alto, CA): Dissolvable, fan-shaped anchoring device
  - **DePuy Mitek** (Raynham, MA): Bone anchor with attached suture
  - **Lactosorb suspension screws** (Biomet Microfixation, Jacksonville, FL): Resorbable screws with hole in screw head for suture threading

## PROCEDURE SELECTION[7,20] (Table 91-1)

**Table 91-1** *Choosing the Best Option*

| Morphology | Coronal | Endoscopic | Temporal | Transpalpebral | Temporal + Transpalpebral | Direct | Brow Pexy |
|---|---|---|---|---|---|---|---|
| **Forehead** | | | | | | | |
| High | + | | + | + | + | + | |
| Low | + | + | + | + | + | + | |
| Flat | + | + | + | + | + | + | |
| Convex | + | | + | + | + | + | |
| **Hairline** | | | | | | | |
| High | | | + | + | + | + | |
| Low | + | + | + | + | + | + | |
| Receding | | | + | + | + | + | |
| **Skin Excess** | | | | | | | |
| Lateral | + | + | + | | + | + | + |
| Medial | + | + | | | | + | |
| **Skin** | | | | | | | |
| Thick | + | + | + | + | + | | |
| Normal | + | + | + | + | + | | |
| Deep rhytids | + | + | | + | + | | |
| Superficial rhytids | + | + | | + | + | | |
| **Brow Position** | | | | | | | |
| Lateral | | | | | | | |
| Normal | | | | | | | |
| Low | + | + | + | | + | | + |
| Medial | | | | | | | |
| Normal | + | + | | + | + | | |
| Low | + | + | | | | | |

## COMPLICATIONS

- **Sensory nerve deficit:** Results from injury to supraorbital or supratrochlear nerves; requires careful preservation during corrugator excision
- **Posterior scalp dysesthesias:** Results from transection of deep branch of supraorbital nerve
- **Frontalis muscle paralysis:** Results from frontal branch injury in temporal dissection
- **Skin necrosis:** Results from excessive tension
- **Alopecia:** Results from excessive tension or thermal injury; keep anterior hairline incision 1-2 mm posterior to hairline to prevent damage to anterior hair follicles
- **Infection**
- **Hematoma and bleeding**
- **Abnormal hair part or visible scar:** Excessive tension
- **Chronic pain:** Supraorbital nerve dysesthesias; more likely if history of migraines
- **Permanent overcorrection:** Limit traction and scalp excision
- **Abnormal soft tissue contour:** Can occur with muscle excision
- **Asymmetry, poor cosmesis, or lateral displacement of brow:** Results from excessive corrugator excision
- **Dimpling:** In transpalpebral brow pexy, prevented by keeping sutures in deep dermis

### KEY POINTS

- ✓ Frontalis muscle action is antagonized by the corrugator, procerus, depressor supercilii, and orbicularis oculi muscles.
- ✓ A high hairline occurs when hairline is on the superior, oblique portion of the frontal bone.
- ✓ Coronal incisions cause posterior scalp paresthesias, which may be troublesome for patients postoperatively.
- ✓ Endoscopic approaches require fixation techniques.

## REFERENCES


1. Nahai F, Saltz R, eds. Endoscopic Plastic Surgery, 2nd ed. St Louis: Quality Medical Publishing, 2008.
2. Janis JE, Ghavami A, Lemmon JA, et al. The anatomy of the corrugator supercilii muscle revisited. I. Corrugator topography. Plast Reconstr Surg 120:1647-1653, 2007.
3. Janis JE, Hatef DA, Hagan R, et al. Anatomy of the supratrochlear nerve: implications for the surgical treatment of migraine headaches. Plast Reconstr Surg 131:743-750, 2013.
4. Knize DM. Reassessment of the coronal incision and subgaleal dissection for foreheadplasty. Plast Reconstr Surg 102:478-489, 1998.
5. Janis JE, Ghavami A, Lemmon JA, et al. The anatomy of the corrugator supercilii muscle: part II. Supraorbital nerve branching patterns. Plast Reconstr Surg 121:233-240, 2008.
6. Fallucco M, Janis JE, Hagan RR. The anatomical morphology of the supraorbital notch: clinical relevance to the surgical treatment of migraine headaches. Plast Reconstr Surg 130:1227-1233, 2012.
7. Nahai F, ed. The Art of Aesthetic Surgery: Principles & Techniques, 2nd ed. St Louis: Quality Medical Publishing, 2011.
8. Knize DM. Limited-incision forehead lift for eyebrow elevation to enhance upper blepharoplasty. Plast Reconstr Surg 97:1334-1342, 1996.

9. Moss CJ, Mendelson BC, Taylor GI. Surgical anatomy of the ligamentous attachments in the temple and periorbital regions. Plast Reconstr Surg 105:1475-1490, 2000.
10. Byrd HS, Burt JD. Achieving aesthetic balance in the brow, eyelids, and midface. Plast Reconstr Surg 110:926-933, 2002.
11. Ellenbogen R. Transcoronal eyebrow lift with concomitant upper blepharoplasty. Plast Reconstr Surg 71:490-499, 1983.
12. McCord CD, Codner MA, eds. Eyelid & Periorbital Surgery. St Louis: Quality Medical Publishing, 2008.
13. Janis JE, Potter JK, Rohrich RJ. Brow lift techniques. In Fahien S, ed. Putterman's Cosmetic Oculoplastic Surgery, 4th ed. Philadelphia: Saunders Elsevier, 2008.
14. Paul MD. Subperiosteal transblepharoplasty forehead lift. Plast Reconstr Surg 99:605, 1997.
15. Flowers FS, Caputy GC, Flowers SS. The biomechanics of brow and frontalis function and its effect on blepharoplasty. Clin Plast Surg 20:255-268, 2003.
16. Troilius C. A comparison between subgaleal and subperiosteal brow lifts. Plast Reconstr Surg 104:1079-1090, 1999.
17. Ramirez OM. Endoscopically assisted biplanar forehead lift. Plast Reconstr Surg 96:323-333, 1995.
18. Guyuron B. Corrugator supercilii resection through blepharoplasty incision. Plast Reconstr Surg 107:606-607, 2001.
19. Ortiz Monasterio F. Aesthetic surgery of the facial skeleton: the forehead. Clin Plast Surg 18:19-27, 1991.
20. Nahai F. Clinical decision-making in brow lift. In Nahai F, ed. The Art of Aesthetic Surgery: Principles & Techniques, 2nd ed. St Louis: Quality Medical Publishing, 2011.

# 92. Blepharoplasty

Kailash Narasimhan, Jason E. Leedy

## DEFINITIONS AND EPIDEMIOLOGY[1]

- Blepharoplasty: Excision of excessive eyelid skin, with or without orbital fat, for either functional or cosmetic indications
- Most common aesthetic facial procedure
- More common in younger women than men
- Most commonly performed in fifth decade of life

## ANATOMY[2-4] (Fig. 92-1)

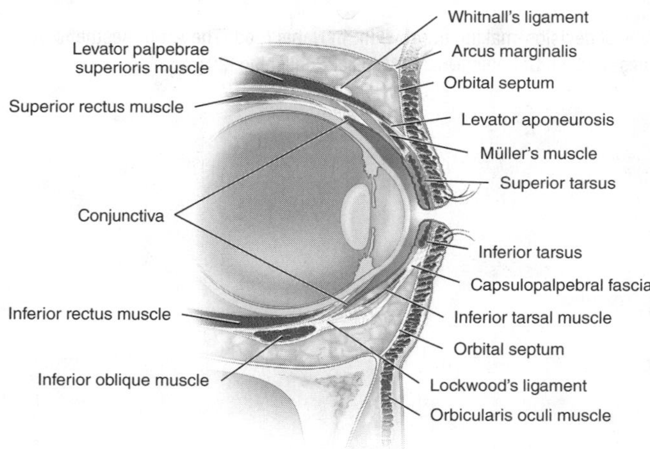


**Fig. 92-1** Cross-section of the upper and lower eyelids.

### EYELID: LAMELLAR STRUCTURE

- **Anterior lamella:** Skin and orbicularis muscle
- **Posterior lamella:** Tarsus and conjunctiva

**NOTE: Many also consider the septum to be the "middle lamella."**

## ORBICULARIS MUSCLE[4] (Fig. 92-2)

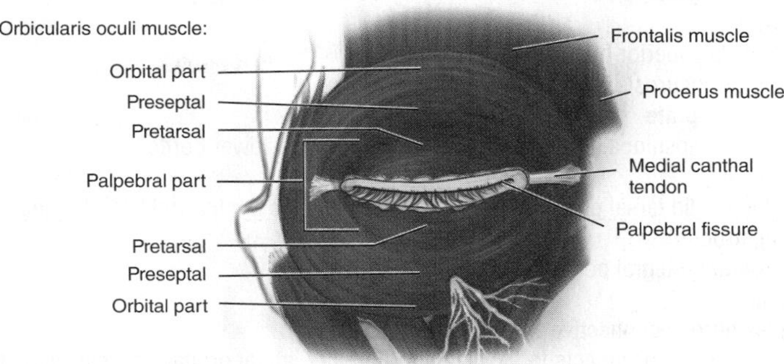


**Fig. 92-2** Orbicularis oculi.

- **Three portions**
  1. **Orbital**
     - Outermost portion
     - Superficial to corrugators and procerus
     - Voluntary
     - Allows tight closure of eye; protecting globe
     - Allows medial brow depression
  2. **Preseptal**
     - Overlies septum
     - Both voluntary and involuntary
     - Assists with blinking
  3. **Pretarsal**
     - Adherent to tarsus
     - Involuntary
     - Assists with blinking
     - Innervation primarily from the zygomatic branch, inferolateral on the deep surface

## TARSOLIGAMENTOUS COMPLEX

- Makes up posterior lamella (Fig. 92-3)

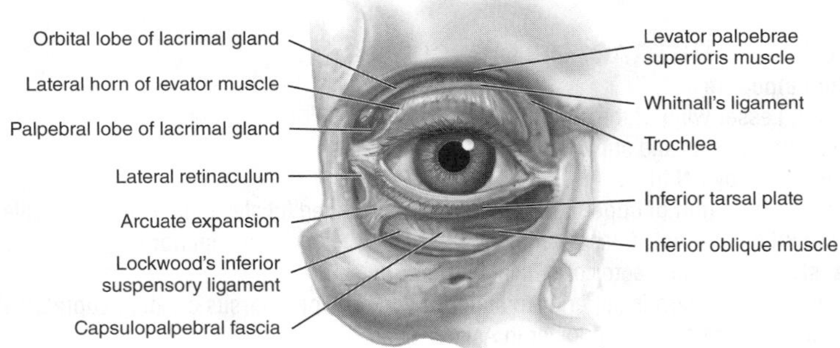


**Fig. 92-3** Tarsoligamentous anatomy of the orbit.

- Constitutes connective tissue framework of upper and lower lids
- **Upper lid tarsal plate** is 30 mm horizontally by 10 mm vertically
  - 7-10 mm wide
  - Inserts onto superior border of Müller's muscle
  - Levator apроneurosis inserts onto superior border
- **Lower lid tarsal plate**
  - Made up of capsulopalpebral fascia, which inserts onto lower border
  - 4-5 mm wide
- Upper and lower lid tarsal plates attach to orbital rim by the medial and lateral retinacular supporting structures.
- **Lateral canthus:** Integral point of fixation for the lower lid
  - 5 mm long
  - Complex fibrous connective tissue network formed by:
    - Fibrous crura: Connects tarsal plate to Whitnall's lateral orbital tubercle within the lateral orbital rim
    - Lateral retinaculum
    - Fibrous condensation consisting of:
      - Lateral horn of levator aponeurosis
      - Lateral rectus check ligaments
      - Whitnall's suspensory ligaments
      - Lockwood's inferior suspensor ligament

## Preseptal Fat

- Located between septum and orbicularis muscle
- Can be a significant factor in upper lid hooding and puffiness
- **Upper lid:** Retroorbicularis oculi fat **(ROOF)**
- **Lower lid:** Suborbicularis oculi fat **(SOOF)**

## Orbital Septum

- Septum is an extension of orbital periosteum.
- Upper septum extends from superior orbital rim to insertion on levator aponeurosis at varying levels (10-15 mm above superior tarsal border).
- Lower septum extends from inferior orbital rim to the capsulopalpebral fascia (5 mm below lower tarsal border).

**TIP:** Attenuation of the septum results in pseudoherniation of intraorbital fat.

## Levator and Retractor Muscles

- **Levator palpebrae**
  - Origin: Lesser wing of the sphenoid
  - Insertion: Dermis and superior edge of upper tarsus
  - Innervation by CN III
  - Action: 10-15 mm of upper lid excursion and sustained lid elevation from contractile tone
  - **Whitnall's ligament:** A fascial condensation 14-20 mm from superior edge of tarsus; translates posterior vector of pull into superior vector
    - Inserts into dermis superior to superior edge of upper tarsus creating supratarsal crease; insertion much lower in Asians

- **Müller's muscle**
  - Origin: Levator muscle
  - Insertion: Superior edge of tarsus
  - Innervation: Sympathetics
  - Action: 2-3 mm of upper lid lift

**TIP:** At the fornix the levator muscle splits into superficial and deep layers. The superficial layer continues as the levator aponeurosis, but the deep layer is Müller's muscle.

- **Capsulopalpebral fascia**
  - *Lower lid equivalent of levator muscle*
  - Origin: Inferior oblique muscle fascia
  - Insertion: Septum 5 mm below tarsus
  - Action: 1-2 mm of downward lower lid migration with downward gaze

## Orbital Fat

- **Physiologically different from normal body fat**
  - Smaller cells
  - Fat more saturated
  - Less lipoprotein lipase
  - Less metabolically active
  - Minimally affected by diet
- **Distinct compartments** (Fig. 92-4)
  - **Two** in **upper** lid (medial and middle)
  - **Three** in **lower** lid (medial, central, and lateral)

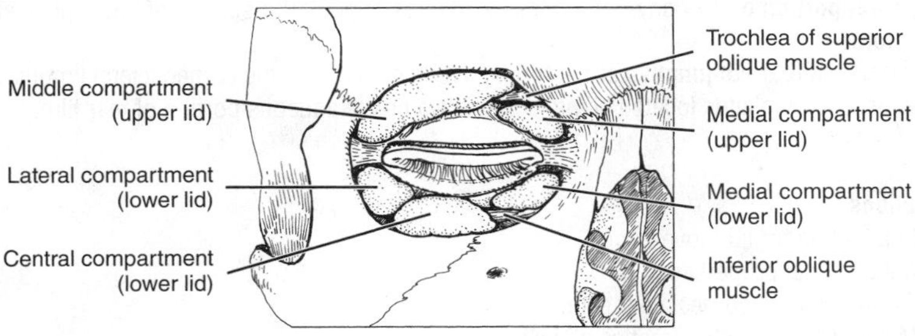


**Fig. 92-4** Orbital fat pads.

**TIP:** The medial compartment fat of the upper lid is more vascular than the others and pale with smaller lobules and more fibrous tissue. The trochlea of the superior oblique muscle separates the medial and middle compartments in the upper lid. The inferior oblique muscle separates the medial and central compartments in the lower lid.

## Anatomy of Midface and Lid-Cheek Junction[2]

- Prezygomatic space includes skin and subcutaneous fat that cover orbicularis oculi fat (SOOF).
- Preperiosteal fat is found deep to the origins of the lip elevator muscles.
- Upper border of prezygomatic space is the orbitomalar ligament, which connects periosteum to SMAS and skin.
- **Tear-trough** consists of orbitomalar ligament, levator labii superioris, and levator alaeque nasi.
- Lower border of prezygomatic space is formed by the zygomatic ligaments.
- Zygomatic ligaments are osteocutaneous ligaments that radiate outward to attach to dermis of cheek.
- **Malar fat pad** is a triangular fat pad over the malar eminence.

## Lacrimal Apparatus

- Comprises **palpebral** and **orbital** portions, separated by **levator aponeurosis.**
- Located beneath and behind lateral portion of superior orbital rim, it is normally not visible externally.
- **Lacrimal drainage system**
  - Punctum drains to canaliculus, which drains to lacrimal sac, which drains to the nasolacrimal duct.
  - **Active pump mechanism**
    - Blinking creates negative pressure in lacrimal sac, allowing tears to pass through the punctum and canaliculus into the sac.
    - Eye opening increases sac pressure and passes tears into nasolacrimal duct.

## Conjunctiva[2]

- Most posterior layer of the eyelid
- Continues over Tenon's capsule
- **Palpebral portion** of the conjunctiva closely adheres to posterior surface of tarsal plate and lid retractors.
- It becomes **bulbar conjunctiva** at the fornix, overlying globe to the corneoscleral limbus.
- Small accessory glands located within conjunctiva create aqueous portion of tear film.

## Tears

- **Functions**
  - Lubrication for lid movement
  - Antibacterial properties
  - Oxygenation of corneal epithelium
  - Maintains a smooth refractive globe surface
- **Three layers**
  1. **Lipid layer:** Superficial, thin; reduces evaporative losses; secreted by meibomian glands and accessory sebaceous glands of Zeiss and Moll
  2. **Aqueous layer:** Thick; from main lacrimal gland as well as accessory glands of Wolfring and Krause within the conjunctival tissue
  3. **Mucoid layer:** Maintains contact with the globe; hydrophilic; produced by mucin goblet cells
- **Basic secretion:** Accessory lacrimal glands of Wolfring and Krause, mucin goblet cells, and meibomian glands
- **Reflex secretion:** Main lacrimal gland, parasympathetic innervation

## AESTHETIC MEASUREMENTS[5] (Fig. 92-5)

- **Palpebral fissure:** 12-14 mm vertically, 28-30 mm horizontally
- **Upper lid:** At level of upper limbus, highest point just medial to pupil
- **Lower lid:** At level of lower limbus, lowest point slightly temporal, forms "lazy-S"
- **Visible pretarsal skin:** 3-6 mm
- **Lash line to supratarsal crease:** 8-10 mm
- **Lateral canthus:** 1-2 mm above medial canthus
- **In midpupillary line**
  - **Anterior hairline to brow:** 5-6 cm
  - **Brow to orbital rim:** 1 cm
  - **Brow to supratarsal crease:** 16 mm, minimum 12 mm
  - **Brow to midpupil:** 2.5 cm

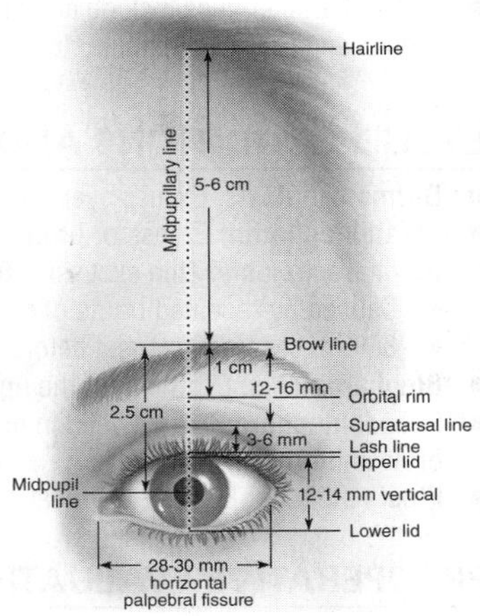


**Fig. 92-5** Aesthetic measurements.

## AESTHETIC PERIORBITAL CHARACTERISTICS[6,7]

- **Aesthetically positioned brow** (see Chapter 91)
- **Full superior orbital sulcus**
  - Aging and trauma can give hollowed appearance.
  - Excessive volumes are unattractive and can cause blepharoptosis.
- **Crisp, precise supratarsal crease with pretarsal show**
  - Formed by levator muscle insertion into dermis above tarsus
  - 3-6 mm of pretarsal show favorable
- **Appropriate lid position:** No ptosis or ectropion
- **Lower lid pretarsal bulge often present in attractive eyes**
  - Results from pretarsal orbicularis muscle fullness
- **Smooth lid-cheek junction**
  - Stigmata of aging: Excess skin, pseudoherniation of intraorbital fat, malar pad descent, nasojugal groove, visible inferior orbital rim
  - Hollowed appearance from paucity of intraorbital fat

## ASIAN EYELID ANATOMY[8] (Fig. 92-6)

- Asians have aesthetic eyelid features distinct from those of individuals of other ethnicities.
- Main anatomic features of the Asian lower eyelid include: (1) an absent or short supratarsal crease, (2) a shorter tarsus, (3) descending preaponeurotic fat, and (4) minimal to absent connections between the levator aponeurosis to the upper lid dermis.

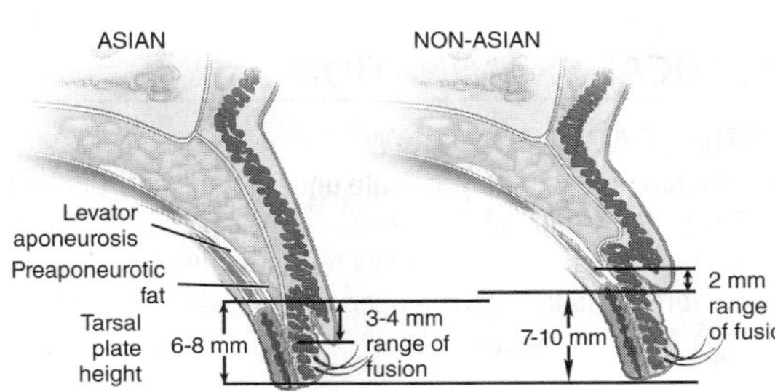


**Fig. 92-6** Asian eyelid anatomy demonstrates absent supratarsal crease, shorter tarsus, and absent connection from levator to upper lid dermis.

- Outer characteristics include an almond-shaped fissure with a varying degree of slant, lash ptosis, and medial epicanthal fold.

## EYELID CONDITIONS AND DEFORMITIES

- **Dermatochalasis:** Excess eyelid skin
- **Steatoblepharon:** Excess or protruding fat through a lax septum
- **Blepharochalasis:** Thin excessive upper and lower lid skin
  - Caused by repeated bouts of painless edema
  - 80% of cases have onset before age 20 years; edema refractory to antihistamines and steroids
- **Blepharoptosis:** Drooping of the upper eyelid; disorder of eyelid levator mechanism
- **Pseudoblepharoptosis:** Eyelid in normal position but appearance of ptosis as a result of a ptotic brow and brow skin
- **Ptosis adiposa:** Extreme attenuation of the canthus and septum

## PREOPERATIVE EVALUATION[9]

### HISTORY

- **Patient expectations**
  - Functional versus aesthetic
  - Mirror examination
  - Assessment of potentially unrealistic expectations
- **Inquire about**[10]
  - Coagulopathies
  - Thyroid dysfunction
  - Hypertension
  - Renal or cardiac abnormalities that may predispose to edema
  - Anticoagulant or antiplatelet medications
    - Vision
    - Corrective lenses
    - Trauma
    - Glaucoma
    - Allergies
    - Excess tearing
    - Dry eyes

> **TIP:** History of vision correction or refractive surgery should be obtained, because they predispose to dry-eye symptoms postoperatively. These patients should wait 6 months before blepharoplasty.

## PHYSICAL EXAMINATION

### FOREHEAD AND BROW

- **Frontalis crease:** May indicate unconscious effort to keep brows elevated
- **Brow ptosis** (Fig. 92-7)
  - With eyes closed and brow relaxed, immobilize frontalis function with gentle pressure on forehead; have patient open eyes.

- If the brow position is lower than when the patient is looking straight forward, **compensated brow ptosis** is diagnosed (i.e., the brow is ptotic but is compensated by frontalis hyperactivity).

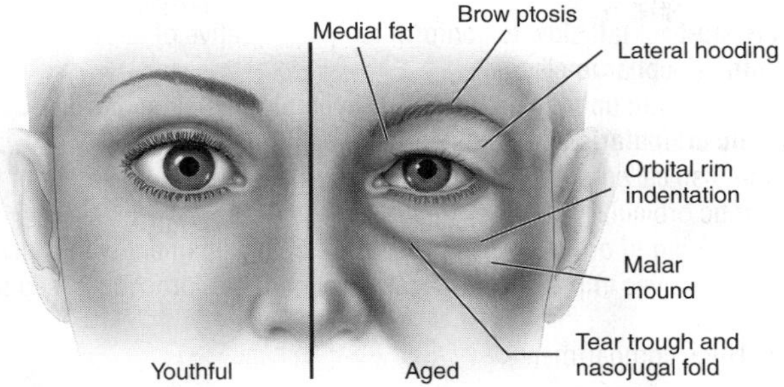


**Fig. 92-7** Characteristics of aging periorbital region.

> **TIP:** Identify compensated brow ptosis preoperatively, because upper blepharoplasty alone may exacerbate brow ptosis and failure to identify brow ptosis in artificially positioned brows before blepharoplasty may result in excessive skin resection.

- **Glabellar frown lines:** Indicate corrugator hyperactivity

## Upper Lid

- **Redundant skin:** Lateral hooding
- **Position of supratarsal fold**
  - 7-11 mm from lash line
  - Examine during downward gaze
  - High supratarsal fold indicative of **levator dehiscence** (see Chapter 93)
- **Fat herniation** (pseudohernia)
- **Soft tissue excess**
  - Subcutaneous fat
  - Preseptal fat
  - Lacrimal gland ptosis
- **Lid position:** Should be at the superior border of the limbus

> **TIP:** If upper lid ptosis is acquired, consider myasthenia gravis as a potential underlying etiologic factor.

- Canthal tilt[11] (Fig. 92-8)
  - Determined by the angle of the intercanthal line
  - Patients can have positive canthal tilt or negative tilt.

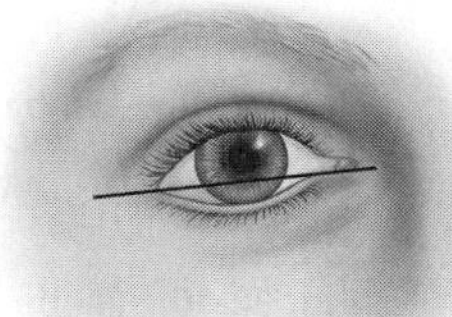


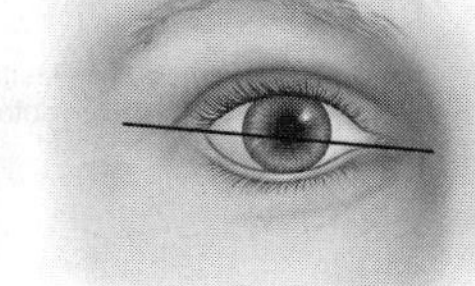


**Fig. 92-8** Canthal tilt is measured by the angle between the medial and lateral canthi and as a measurement of the orbital vector.

## Lower Lid

- **Redundant skin**
  - Rhytids: Fine and deep (crow's feet)
- **Tarsal laxity**
  - **Pinch test** (snap-back): If slow to conform to eye, indicative of tarsal laxity
- **Skin pigmentation** (blepharomelasma)
  - Possibly thin skin with underlying muscle or hyperpigmentation of skin
- **Redundant, ptotic orbicularis oculi muscle** (festoons)
  - **Squinch test** (also called *squint test;* forcible eye closure): Improvement of festoon if caused by ptotic orbicularis muscle
  - **Malar bag:** Shelving of orbicularis over orbital retaining ligament with excess intraorbital fat
    - Correction involves improving lid-cheek junction (Loeb procedure, septal reset, midface lift).
- **Fat herniation:** Three compartments
- **Tear trough**
  - According to Barton,[25] created by herniation of orbital fat, tight attachment of the orbicularis along the arcus marginalis, and malar retrusion (Fig. 92-9)
  - According to Codner et al,[11] created by herniation of fat over the orbitomalar ligament, which arises from periosteum and attaches to skin
    - According to this definition, the tear trough arises over a triangular space defined by the orbitomalar ligament, levator labii superioris, and levator alaeque nasi.

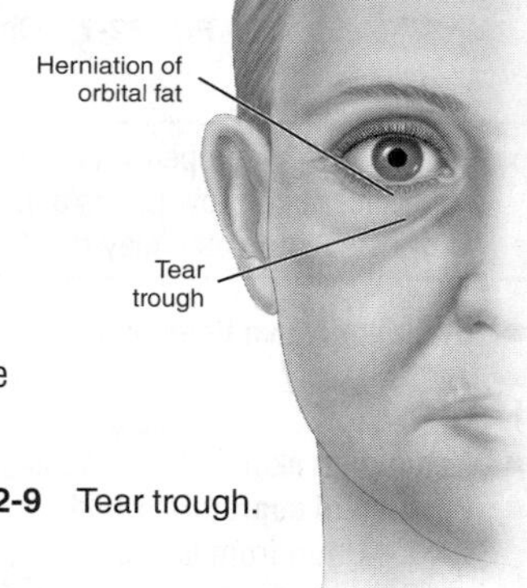


**Fig. 92-9** Tear trough.

- **Scleral show**
  - Lower lid should be up to 2 mm below inferior limbus.
  - Tarsal laxity, negative vector orbit, exophthalmos, or middle lamellar contracture of lower lid can be present.

## Globe Position (Fig. 92-10)

- **Proptosis:** Thyroid disease
- **Enophthalmos:** Posttraumatic
- **Negative vector:** If anterior portion of globe is anterior to most projecting portion of the zygoma

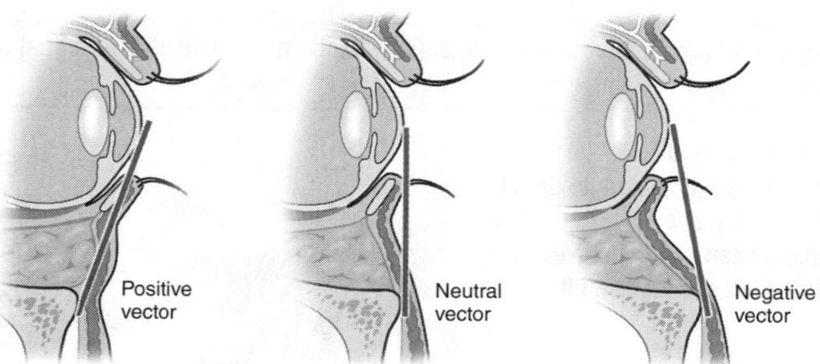


**Fig. 92-10** Globe vectors.

**TIP:** A patient undergoing lower lid procedures is at risk of scleral show and ectropion, because tightening of the lower lid can cause downward migration of the lower lid on a prominent globe.

## Ocular Examination

- Record the best corrected visual acuity for each eye. Use a Snellen eye chart.
- If there is a visual field defect, refer to ophthalmologist or optometrist.
- **Bell's phenomenon:** If lids are forcibly held open while patient attempts to close them, the globe rotates upward.
  - When condition is **not** present, patient may be **more susceptible** to dry-eye symptoms with postoperative lagophthalmos.
- Evaluate for eyelid ptosis.

**TIP:** Suspect ptosis if supratarsal fold is high or asymmetrical.

## Lacrimal Function Test

- Useful for **elderly patients** and all patients with **dry-eye symptoms;** consider ophthalmologic consultation
- **Schirmer's test I:** Basic and reflexive secretion
  - Whatman filter paper (Whatman Inc., Florham Park, NJ) (5 by 35 mm, distal 5 mm folded) placed on lateral sclera: >10 mm of wetting after 5 minutes is normal
- **Schirmer's test II:** Basic secretion
  - Perform after topical anesthetic applied; usually <40% of Schirmer's I
- **Advanced tests:** Tear film breakup, rose bengal staining, tear lysozyme electrophoresis

# UPPER BLEPHAROPLASTY PRINCIPLES AND TECHNIQUES[6,12]

**Objective:** To create a well-defined supratarsal fold, exposing smooth pretarsal skin, while refining volume of the supratarsal lid

## Markings

- **Lower line**
  - Mark in upright position with upper lid under "closing tension" (i.e., mark while applying gentle upward traction on upper lid to smooth the pretarsal skin as desired postoperatively)
  - Usually made 9-11 mm above the lash line. Be meticulous about making symmetrical bilateral lower marks.
- **Upper line**
  - Mark varies depending on the amount and location of redundancy.
  - Extend the lateral excision by canting upward from lower line to upper line so that closure will lie within a rhytid. Avoid medial extension (Fig. 92-11).

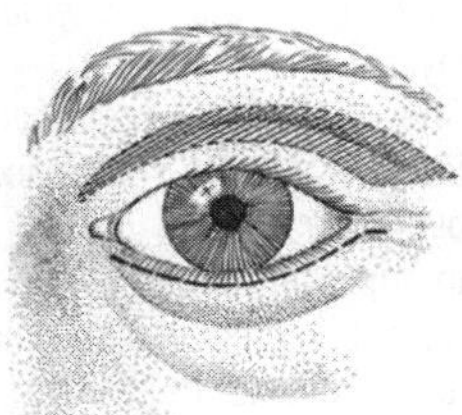

**Fig. 92-11** Blepharoplasty markings.

## TECHNIQUE

**NOTE: Anesthetic choice depends on surgeon's preference, length of procedure, and whether concomitant procedures are to be performed.**

- Excise skin (can use knife or $CO_2$ laser).
- Open/excise orbicularis muscle (if desired). Pretarsal orbicularis must be maintained to preserve blink. Excision is usually performed concurrently with skin excision.
  - Excision of muscle can decrease bulk of upper lid and allow adherence of skin to septum, thereby creating supratarsal fold.
  - Preservation of muscle maintains upper lid fullness. The literature varies on treatment of the muscle.
- Incise orbital septum high to prevent injury to levator palpebrae.
  - Use separate stab incisions rather than opening widely.
- Excise redundant intraorbital fat, if indicated.
  - Medial fat has more compact, dense fat lobules that are more pale than in central compartment. It is also more vascular.
  - Central compartment has more loosely organized yellow fat lobules.

**CAUTION: Avoid overresection of intraorbital fat to prevent a hollowed appearance with advancing age. Conservative resection involves removal of only the excess fat that comes easily through the septal perforation.**

- Excise the retroorbicularis fat, if indicated. This fat lies anterior to the septum but posterior to the orbicularis and creates lateral fullness.[13]
- Assess the lacrimal gland. If lacrimal gland ptosis is contributing to lateral fullness, consider glandulopexy rather than resection to prevent dry-eye symptoms.
- Recognize a prominent superolateral bony orbit preoperatively. Bony reduction can be performed.
- Close skin. Multiple techniques and suture types are practiced (subcuticular Prolene pull-out sutures to running fast-absorbing gut). In general, single-layer closure is all that is needed. Permanent sutures should be removed early (4 days) to help prevent inclusion cyst.

## TARSAL FIXATION TECHNIQUES

- Techniques designed to help create a **high supratarsal fold**
- **Indicated in:**
  - Asian eyelids
  - Preoperative lid fold $<$4-7 mm from lid margin
  - Secondary blepharoplasty
  - Men with brow ptosis
- **Principles**
  - Flowers[14]: *"Anchor blepharoplasty"* uses a permanent suture from skin to tarsus and then levator.
  - Sheen[15]: Sutures pretarsal orbicularis to levator
  - Baker et al[16]: No suture, excise at least 5 mm of orbicularis, and allow skin to scar to septum overlying levator
- Asian upper lid surgery[8]
  - Operation creates a supratarsal that is more aesthetically pleasing.
  - Ideal look "opens the eye" and brings out its inherent shape and beauty.
  - Open and closed techniques involve some element of suspending the levator and/or tarsus to the dermis.
  - Closed technique uses two sutures to anchor tarsus to deep dermis.

## LOWER BLEPHAROPLASTY PRINCIPLES AND TECHNIQUES

**Objective:** Restore youthful appearance with lower lid just touching inferior edge of limbus and lateral canthus being elevated approximately 1-2 mm above the medial canthus; recontour or excise redundant fat, tighten skin, and smooth lid-cheek interface

### APPROACHES TO LOWER LID

- **Skin flap**[17]
  - Subciliary incision to create a skin flap over preseptal orbicularis
  - Removal of excess skin possible without disturbing the orbicularis
  - Useful for removing a large amount of skin
  - Tedious dissection with risk of skin perforation
  - Can result in scarring of skin with muscle
- **Skin-muscle flap**[18]
  - Subciliary incision with skin-muscle flap; pretarsal muscle left undisturbed
  - Allows resection of skin and muscle together, up to 3-5 mm
  - Easier dissection
- **Transconjunctival**[19]
  - Incision made in palpebral conjunctiva, just above fornix, through capsulopalpebral fascia, thereby giving access to intraorbital fat
- **Fat resection**
  - Can be removed through transcutaneous and transconjunctival preseptal and postseptal approaches
- **Fat manipulation**
  - **Loeb procedure:** Medial fat slid out of compartment into tear trough, sutured to angular muscles[20]
  - **Arcus marginalis release:** Lower compartment fat redraped over rim[21,22]
  - **Septal reset:** Lower compartment fat redraped over rim with repositioning of orbital septum by suturing it to periosteum[23-26] (Fig. 92-12)
- **Fat augmentation**
  - Malar injection of fat can help smooth the lid-cheek junction when used in conjunction with transconjunctival blepharoplasty.
  - Five-step lower blepharoplasty involves fat augmentation in the deep medial fat pad, transconjunctival fat removal, release of orbital retaining ligament, lateral retinacular suspension, and removal of skin.[26]

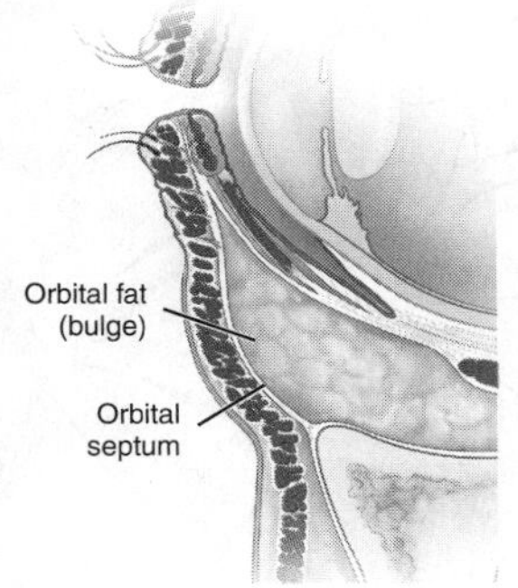


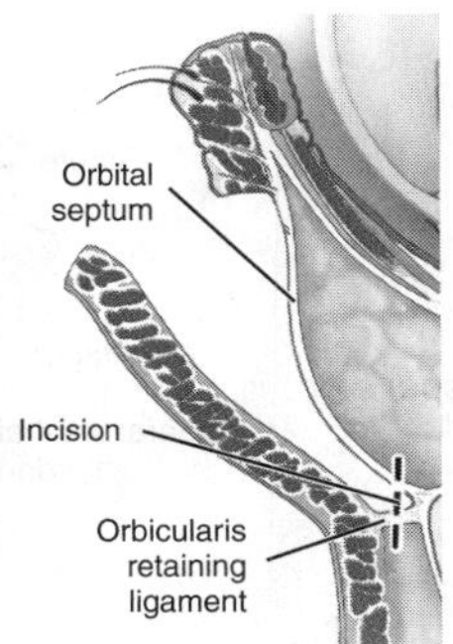


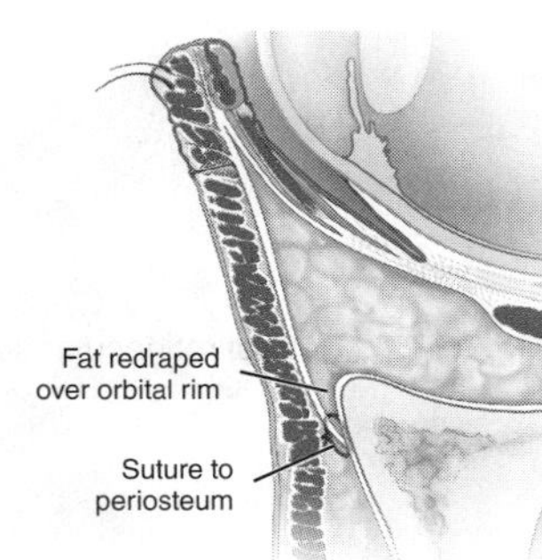


**Fig. 92-12** Septal reset.

## Lower Lid Laxity

- **Tarsal shortening**
  - **Kuhnt-Szymanowski procedure:** Pentagonal excision lateral to lateral limbus to avoid visible notching
    - Useful for patients with **true lower lid tarsal excess**
- **Lateral canthoplasty**
  - Involves division of commissure with repositioning of lower canthal tendon (tarsal strip procedure) and lateral canthus
  - Can correct more lower lid laxity than tarsal wedge excision because of repositioning the lateral canthus[27] (Fig. 92-13)
  - Synechia of upper and lower lid can occur at commissure.

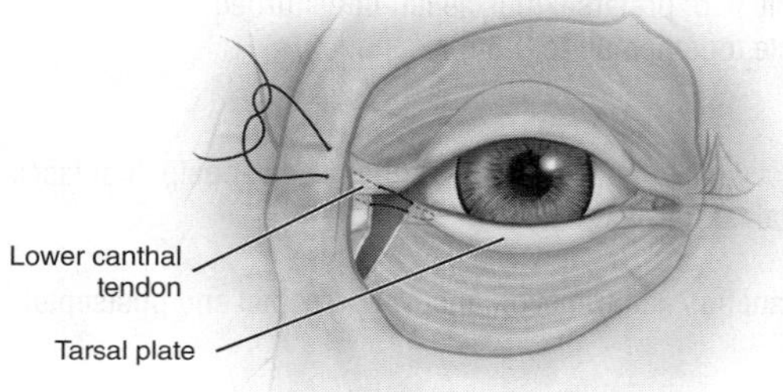


**Fig. 92-13** Canthoplasty.

- **Canthopexy/retinacular suspension: Suture suspension to orbital rim**[27]
  - Involves tightening the lateral canthus or lateral retinaculum to periosteum using sutures
  - Does not involve disinsertion of the lateral canthus
  - Provides mild lid tightening and canthal elevation, mainly to counteract downward scar forces during healing from lower lid procedures (Fig. 92-14)
    - In patients with prominent eyes, the position of the canthopexy should be adjusted slightly superiorly to prevent malposition of the lower lid below the globe and scleral show.[11]

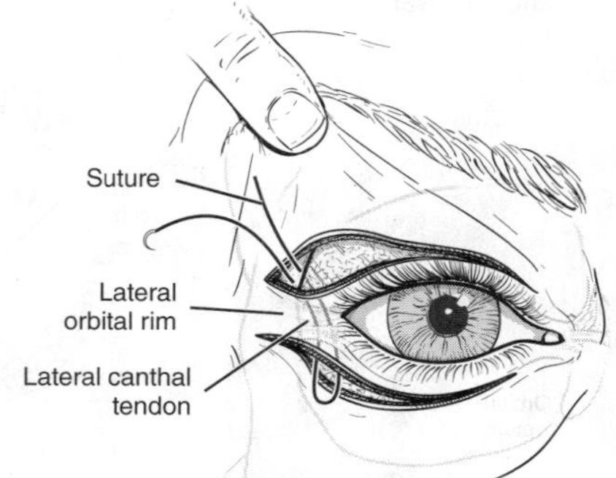


**Fig. 92-14** Lateral retinacular suspension.

## COMPLICATIONS[28]

### Asymmetry

- **Most common complication,** may require corrective surgery

### Retrobulbar Hematoma

- Related to fat excision
- **Signs/symptoms**
  - Pain
  - Proptosis
  - Lid ecchymosis
  - Decreased vision and extraocular movements
  - Dilated pupils
  - Scotomas
  - Increased intraocular pressure
- **Treatment**
  - Elevate head of bed
  - Release surgical incisions
  - Lateral cantholysis
  - Mannitol (12.5 g IV bolus over 3-5 minutes)
  - Acetazolamide (Diamox) (500 mg IV bolus)
  - Steroids (Solu-Medrol) (100 mg IV)
  - Rebreathe in bag (elevates $CO_2$)
  - Topical beta-blockers (Betopic)
  - Emergent ophthalmologic consultation
  - Reoperation

### Blindness

- 0.04% incidence, usually only occurs if there is bleeding after fat removal
- **Pathophysiology**
  - Retrobulbar hematoma leading to central retinal artery occlusion or optic nerve ischemia
  - Considered irreversible after 100 minutes

### Ectropion

- **Causes**
  - Excessive skin resection
  - Scar contracture
  - Cicatricial adhesion to orbital septum
  - Dystonia of the orbicularis
  - Contraction of the capsulopalpebral fascia
  - Disinsertion of lateral canthus
  - Midfacial descent
- **Predisposing factors**
  - Lower lid laxity
  - Proptosis
  - Unilateral high myopia (increase anteroposterior eye dimension)
  - Thyroid disease

- **Early treatment**
  - Taping
  - Frost sutures
  - Massage (Carraway exercises)[29]
  - Steroid injection
- **Late treatment**
  - **Skin loss:** Midface lift or skin graft
  - **Hypotonic lid:** Wedge resection or canthoplasty
  - **Posterior/middle lamella scarring:** Release and spacer graft (AlloDerm [LifeCell Corp, Branchburg, NJ], palatal mucosa)

## Lagophthalmos

- Usually temporary, but if not may require skin grafting

## Keratoconjunctivitis Sicca (Dry-Eye Syndrome)

- If identified preoperatively, should approach very conservatively, if at all
- Postoperatively treat with topical moisturizers
  - Can also be avoided by preserving lacrimal gland during dissection

## Corneal Injury

- Confirm with **fluorescein testing**
  - Superficial injury treated with **topical antibiotics** and **eye patching**
  - Should resolve in 24-48 hours

## Diplopia

- **Inferior oblique muscle most commonly injured** followed by superior oblique muscle
- Usually resolves spontaneously but may require corrective muscle surgery

## Ptosis

- Often present preoperatively but not identified by surgeon and patient until postoperatively
- Can occur from direct injury to levator
- A-frame deformity[2]
  - Peaked arch deformity over supratarsal crease caused by overresection of central and nasal fat pads over the area of the interpad septum

## Key Points

✓ The pretarsal muscle is the most important for blink.
✓ The upper eyelid has two fat compartments; the lower lid has three.
✓ Avoid aggressive fat resection in upper and lower lid blepharoplasty.
✓ Lower lid blepharoplasty techniques should limit orbicularis denervation and cicatricial adhesions between lamellae.
✓ Retrobulbar hematoma is a surgical emergency.

## REFERENCES


1. Wolfort FG, Kanter WR. History of blepharoplasty. In Wolfort FG, Kanter WR, eds. Aesthetic Blepharoplasty. Boston: Little Brown, 1995.
2. Codner MA, Ford DT. Blepharoplasty. In Aston SJ, Beasley RW, Thorne HM, et al, eds. Grabb and Smith's Plastic Surgery, 6th ed. Philadelphia:Lippincott Williams and Wilkins, 2007.
3. Carraway JH. Surgical anatomy of the eyelids. Clin Plast Surg 14:693-701, 1987.
4. Furnas DW. The orbicularis oculi muscle. Clin Plast Surg 8:687-715, 1981.
5. Muzaffar AR, Mendelson BC, Adams WP Jr. Surgical anatomy of the ligamentous attachments of the lower lid and lateral canthus. Plast Reconstr Surg 110:873-884, 2002.
6. Flowers RS, DuVal C. Blepharoplasty and periorbital aesthetic surgery. In Aston SJ, Beasley RW, Thorne HM, et al, eds. Grabb and Smith's Plastic Surgery, 6th ed. Philadelphia: Lippincott and Wilkins, 2007.
7. Guyuron B. Blepharoplasty and ancillary procedures. In Achauer BH, Eriksson E, Guyuron B, et al, eds. Plastic Surgery: Indications, Operations, and Outcomes. St Louis: Mosby–Year Book, 2000.
8. Lee CK, Ahn ST, Kim N. Asian upper lid blepharoplasty surgery. Clin Plast Surg 40:167-178, 2013.
9. Jelks GW, Jelks EB. Preoperative evaluation of the blepharoplasty patient: bypassing the pitfalls. Clin Plast Surg 20:213-223, 1993.
10. Trussler AP, Rohrich RJ. MOC-PSSM CME article: Blepharoplasty. Plast Reconstr Surg 121(Suppl 1):1-10, 2008.
11. Codner MA, Kikkawa DO, Korn BS, et al. Blepharoplasty and brow lift. Plast Reconstr Surg 126:1e-17e, 2010.
12. Rohrich RJ, Coberly DM, Fagien S, et al. Current concepts in aesthetic upper blepharoplasty. Plast Reconstr Surg 113:32-42, 2004.
13. May JW, Feron J, Zingarelli P. Retro-orbicularis oculi fat (ROOF) resection in aesthetic blepharoplasty: a 6 year study in 63 patients. Plast Reconstr Surg 86:682-689, 1990.
14. Flowers RS. Upper blepharoplasty by eyelid invagination: anchor blepharoplasty. Clin Plast Surg 20:193-207, 1993.
15. Sheen JH. A change in the technique of supratarsal fixation in upper blepharoplasty. Plast Reconstr Surg 59:831-834, 1977.
16. Baker TJ, Gordon HL, Mosienko P. Upper lid blepharoplasty. Plast Reconstr Surg 60:692-698, 1977.
17. Casson P, Siebert J. Lower lid blepharoplasty with skin flap and muscle split. Clin Plast Surg 15:299-304, 1988.
18. Aston SJ. Skin-muscle flap lower lid blepharoplasty. Clin Plast Surg 15:305-308, 1988.
19. Tomlinson F, Hovey L. Transconjunctival lower lid blepharoplasty for removal of fat. Plast Reconstr Surg 56:314-318, 1978.
20. Loeb R. Fat pad sliding and fat grafting for leveling lid depressions. Clin Plast Surg 8:757-776, 1981.
21. Hamra ST. Arcus marginalis release and orbital fat preservation in midface rejuvenation. Plast Reconstr Surg 96:354-362, 1995.
22. McCord CD Jr, Codner MA, Hester TR. Redraping the inferior orbicularis arc. Plast Reconstr Surg 102:2471-2479, 1998.
23. Hamra ST. The role of orbital fat preservation in facial aesthetic surgery. Plast Reconstr Surg 23:17-28, 1996.
24. Hamra ST. The role of the septal reset in creating a youthful eyelid-cheek complex in facial rejuvenation. Plast Reconstr Surg 113:2124-2142, 2004.

25. Barton FE, Ha R, Awada M. Fat extrusion and septal reset in patients with the tear trough triad: a critical appraisal. Plast Reconstr Surg 13:2115-2121, 2004.
26. Rohrich RJ, Ghavami A, Mojallal A. The five-step lower blepharoplasty: blending the eyelid-cheek junction. Plast Reconstr Surg 128:775-783, 2011.
27. Fagien S. Algorithm for canthoplasty: the lateral retinacular suspension: a simplified suture canthopexy. Plast Reconstr Surg 103:2042-2053, 1999.
28. Lisman RD, Hyde K, Smith B. Complications of blepharoplasty. Clin Plast Surg 15:309-335, 1988.
29. Carraway JH, Mellow CG. The prevention and treatment of lower lid ectropion following blepharoplasty. Plast Reconstr Surg 85:971-981, 1990.

# 93. Blepharoptosis

Jason E. Leedy, Jordan P. Farkas

## DEFINITION

*Blepharoptosis* is drooping of the upper lid margin to a position that is lower than normal. (Normal upper lid position is at the level of the upper limbus.)

## ANATOMY[1] (Fig. 93-1)

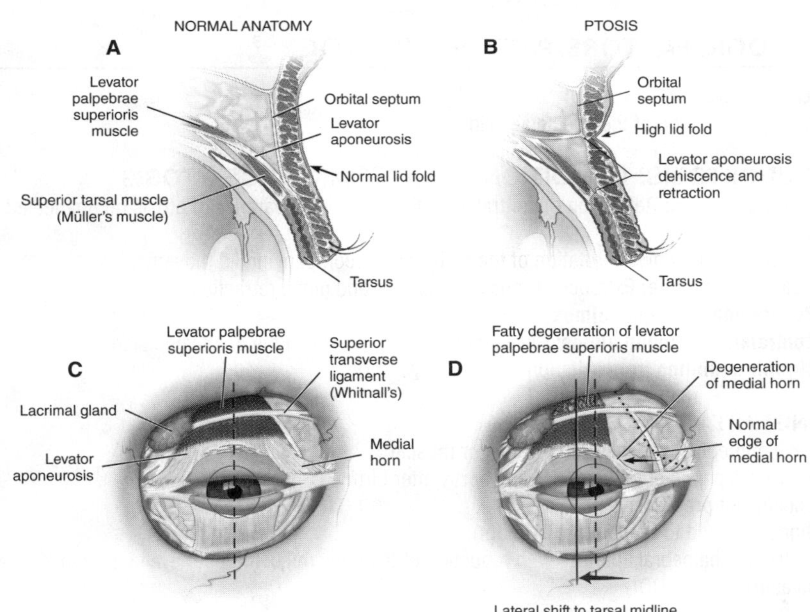


**Fig. 93-1** Differences between normal and ptotic upper eyelid anatomy.

### LEVATOR APONEUROSIS

- **Origin:** Lesser wing of the sphenoid
- **Insertion:** Orbicularis oculi, dermis, tarsus
- **Innervation:** Superior division of oculomotor nerve (CN III)
- **Action:** Provides 10-12 mm of eyelid elevation
- **Embryology:** Develops in the third gestational month from the superior rectus muscle
- Anterior lamella of the levator muscle forms aponeurosis

- Posterior lamella of the levator muscle forms Müller's muscle
- Approximately 2-5 mm above the tarsus the anterior portion of the levator aponeurosis joins the orbital septum.

### Müller's Muscle

- **Origin:** Posterior lamella of levator muscle
- **Insertion:** Superior border of tarsus
- **Innervation:** Sympathetics
- **Action:** Provides 2-3 mm of eyelid elevation

### Frontalis Muscle

- **Origin:** Galeal aponeurosis
- **Insertion:** Suprabrow dermis
- **Innervation:** Frontal branch of facial nerve
- **Action:** Elevates brow and upper eyelid skin

## ETIOLOGIC FACTORS/PATHOPHYSIOLOGY[2,3]

### True Ptosis

- Intrinsic drooping of the affected eyelid

### Pseudoptosis: Conditions That Mimic True Ptosis

- **Grave's disease:** Retraction of contralateral lid can give appearance of ptosis on unaffected side
- **Hypotropia:** Downward rotation of the globe with accompanying lid movement
- **Duane's syndrome:** Extraocular muscular fibrosis and globe retraction
- **Posttraumatic enophthalmos**
- **Contralateral exophthalmos:** Gives impression of ptosis on the unaffected side
- **Chronic squinting** from irritation

### Congenital Ptosis[2,3]

- Developmental dysgenesis in the levator muscle
- Idiopathic persistent ptosis noticed shortly after birth
- Usually not progressive
- Signs confined to the affected eyelid(s)
- Decreased palpebral aperture with reduction of the pupil reflex to upper eyelid margin measurement (MRDI)
- Decreased levator excursion
  - Poor or absent levator function reflected in the absence of the supratarsal crease
- Ptotic eyelid generally higher than the normal eyelid during downgaze
- Inheritance pattern unclear
- Levator biopsies in congenital ptosis show absence of striated muscle fibers with fibrosis.

> **TIP:** History alone usually can distinguish congenital from acquired ptosis, but if there is a question, lagophthalmos on downward gaze is characteristic of congenital ptosis, because levator fibrosis prevents downward lid migration.

- **Associated ocular abnormalities**
  - **Coexistent strabismus and amblyopia**
    - Caused by pupil occlusion
  - **Marcus Gunn's jaw-winking syndrome**
    - Synkinesis of upper lid with chewing
    - Seen in 2%-6% of congenital ptosis
    - Caused by aberrant innervation from fifth cranial nerve
  - **Blepharophimosis syndrome**
    - Triad of **ptosis, telecanthus,** and **phimosis** of lid fissure
  - **Congenital anophthalmos or microphthalmos**
    - Hypoplasia of the lids, globe, and orbital bones
  - **Coexistent eyelid hamartoma**
    - Neurofibromas
    - Hemangiomas
    - Lymphangiomas

## ACQUIRED PTOSIS[2,3]

- **Myogenic**
  - **Involutional myopathic (senile ptosis)**
    - *Most common type*
    - Stretching of the levator aponeurosis attachments to the anterior tarsus
    - Dermal attachments are maintained and therefore the *supratarsal crease rises.*
    - Levator function is usually good.
  - **Chronic progressive external ophthalmoplegia**
    - Progressive muscular dystrophy affects the extraocular muscles and levator.
    - 5% of cases involve the facial and oropharyngeal muscles.
- **Traumatic**
  - *Second most common type*
  - Allow recovery of myoneural dysfunction, resolution of edema, and softening of scar (approximately 6 months).
  - This can occur after cataract surgery from dehiscence of levator aponeurosis.
- **Neurogenic**
  - **Third nerve palsy:** Paralyzes levator muscle
  - **Horner's syndrome:** Paralyzes Müller's muscle
  - **Myasthenia gravis**
    - Primarily, young women and old men are affected.
    - Ptosis worsens with fatigue, at the end of the day.
    - Improvement with neostigmine or edrophonium is characteristic.
- **Mechanical**
  - Upper lid tumors
  - Severe dermatochalasis (excessive upper lid skin), brow ptosis

## EVALUATION[2,3]

### Determination of Cause

- Congenital or acquired

**TIP:** Evaluate for lagophthalmos during downward gaze. This indicates levator fibrosis, which is more commonly seen with congenital cases.

### Degree of Ptosis (Table 93-1)

- Always compare with contralateral side.
- Measure amount of descent over upper limbus.
  - 1-2 mm: Mild
  - 3 mm: Moderate
  - 4 mm or more: Severe
- Record palpebral fissure height.

**Table 93-1** *Degree of Ptosis*

| Degree of Ptosis | Mild | Moderate | Severe |
|---|---|---|---|
| Lid descent over upper limbus | 1-2 mm | 3 mm | >4 mm |

### Levator Function (Table 93-2)

- Measure from extreme downward gaze to extreme upward gaze while immobilizing the brow.
- >10 mm: Good
- 5-10 mm: Fair
- <5 mm: Poor

**Table 93-2** *Levator Function*

| Levator Function | Good | Fair | Poor |
|---|---|---|---|
| Levator excursion | >10 mm | 5-10 mm | 0-5 mm |

### Preoperative Evaluation for Dry-Eye Symptoms

- **Schirmer's tests I and II** (see Chapter 92)
- **Bell's phenomenon:** Upward rotation of globe when eyes forcibly opened, corneal protective mechanism during sleep
- **Tear film breakup and tear lysozyme electrophoresis:** Advanced ophthalmologic tests useful to further characterize causes of dry-eye symptoms

**TIP:** General rule: If contact lenses can be worn, then tear production is adequate.

- **Assess lower lid position:** Scleral show or lower lid laxity—patient more prone to postoperative dry-eye symptoms and may benefit from lower lid procedure to improve position or tone in conjunction with ptosis correction

**TIP:** All ptosis procedures cause lagophthalmos; therefore dry-eye symptoms must be evaluated preoperatively.

### Contralateral Eye

- **Hering's law**[4]
  - Levator muscles receive equal innervation bilaterally.
  - Severe ptosis on one side creates impulse for bilateral lid retraction. Therefore, if the severely affected side is corrected, innervation impulse for lid retraction diminishes, which may reveal ptosis of the contralateral side.
- **Hering's test**
  - Attempt to reveal contralateral ptosis.
  - With brow immobilized in straightforward gaze, elevate affected lid with cotton-tipped applicator to alleviate ptosis; then examine for contralateral ptosis.

### Lid Contour and Lid Crease

- Evaluate contralateral lid contour and lid crease to determine proper postoperative lid crease on affected side.

### Ocular Examination

- Assess general ocular visual function and consider ophthalmologic consultation for formal examination.
- Consult with ophthalmologist preoperatively for baseline visual field testing.

### Complicating Issues[5,6]

- **Dry eyes**
  - Postoperative lagophthalmos with corneal exposure may threaten vision.
- **Hypoplastic tarsus**
  - This is seen in congenital cases. Ptosis repair can cause lid eversion.
- **Floppy upper lid**
  - Medial horn of levator aponeurosis is commonly dehisced and creates temporal shift of tarsus. Ptosis repair must recenter tarsus.
- **Asymmetrical ptosis**
  - Correction of ptosis in the severe eye can unmask ptosis in the contralateral eye.
- **Widened intercanthal distance**
  - Ptosis gives illusion of narrower intercanthal distance; if widened preoperatively, patient should be informed about possible appearance of telecanthus postoperatively.

## ANESTHESIA FOR PTOSIS REPAIR

- IV sedation with local anesthetic
- Useful for mild to moderate degrees of ptosis correction in cooperative patients
- Most amenable to anterior-approach levator surgery
- Allows active patient participation with eye opening and closure so that precise correction can be achieved

### Technique

- Inject local anesthetic (use sparingly).
- Expose aponeurosis.

- Place key sutures.
- Have patient sit upright and focus on premarked spot on distant wall.
- Adjust key sutures until ptosis is corrected at appropriate level.

**TIP:** Excess local anesthetic may impair levator function, which can markedly affect results.

## CHOICE OF SURGICAL PROCEDURE[7] (Fig. 93-2)

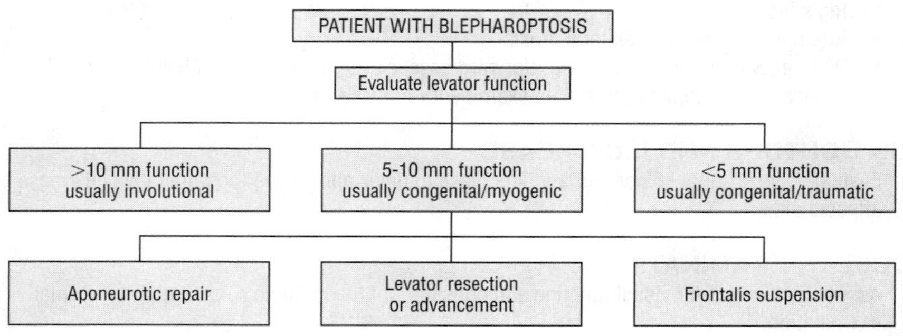


**Fig. 93-2** Algorithm for ptosis repair.

- If >**10 mm** of levator excursion (excellent), then **aponeurotic surgery** or **müllerectomy**
- If **5-10 mm** of excursion (moderate), then **levator resection** or advancement
- If **0-5 mm** of excursion (poor), then **frontalis suspension** required

**TIP:** In patients with mechanical ptosis, treat contributing factor(s) (e.g., brow ptosis, upper lid tumor).

- **The most important factor is the amount of levator excursion.**
  - Limit use of epinephrine in local anesthetic, because it stimulates Müller's muscle, which gives 0.5-1 mm of temporary lid elevation. If using epinephrine with monitored anesthesia care, the operated side should be slightly overcorrected to compensate for postoperative relaxation of Müller's muscle.

### FASANELLA-SERVAT PROCEDURE[8] (Fig. 93-3)

- Conjunctival approach to excise tarsus, Müller's muscle, and conjunctiva
- Should be considered only when levator function is excellent with minimal ptosis
- Avoids external incision—therefore cannot alter supratarsal crease
- Somewhat less predictable than external approaches
- Resection of tarsus can result in postoperative floppy lid with lid peaking and eversion.

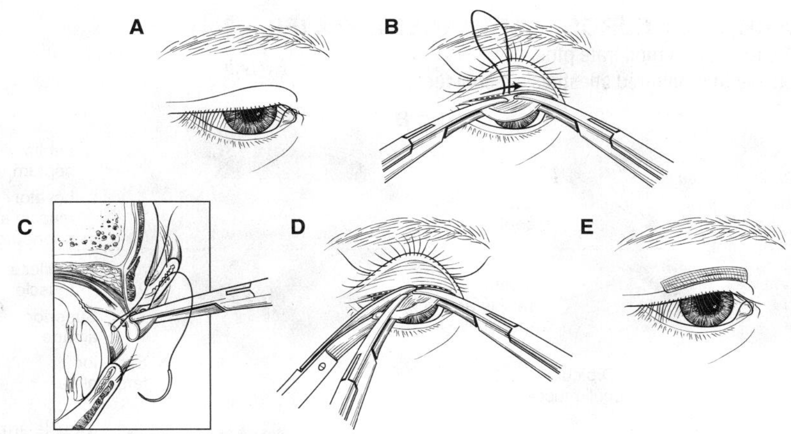


**Fig. 93-3** The Fasanella-Servat (tarsal-conjunctival müllerectomy) procedure is indicated for patients with good levator excursion and mild ptosis.

## MÜLLER'S MUSCLE–CONJUNCTIVAL RESECTION (PUTTERMAN PROCEDURE)[9,10]

- Appropriate candidates for surgery were tested with instillation of 2.5% phenylephrine hydrochloride drops into the conjunctival sac.
- Phenylephrine-stimulated contraction of the sympathetically-innervated Müller's muscle provided an excellent guide to the results of Müller's muscle–conjunctival resection[10] (Table 93-3).
- 3.5-4.5 mm of folded Müller's muscle conjunctiva complex is resected using a noncrushing vascular clamp. This corresponds to the 7-9 mm resection length determined by the phenylephrine evaluation.
- Double-armed catgut is placed in a running horizontal mattress fashion and then inserted from the conjunctiva through the external lid and tied loosely over the tarsal plate.

**Table 93-3** *Phenylephrine Response Guideline*

| Ptosis Response to Phenylephrine | Length of Müller's Muscle–Conjunctiva to Resect (mm) |
|---|---|
| Excessive lid elevation | 7-7.5 |
| Perfect height | 8 |
| Inadequate lid elevation | 9 |
| No response | Müller's muscle–conjunctival resection not indicated |

## Levator Aponeurosis Advancement[11] (Fig. 93-4)

- Useful for mild to moderate ptosis
- Amenable to monitored anesthesia technique

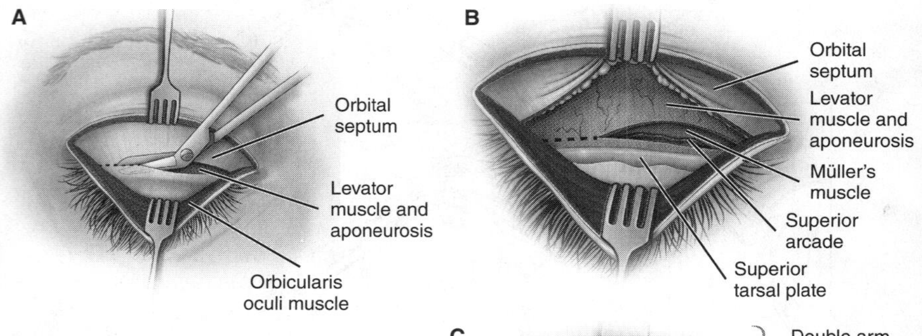


**Fig. 93-4** Dissection of the levator aponeurosis.

- **Technique**[7] (Fig. 93-5)
  - Incise skin at desired supratarsal fold.
  - Expose orbital septum and distal levator aponeurosis beneath orbicularis fibers.
  - Incise septum and retract preaponeurotic fat to expose the aponeurosis, which can be identified by the vertically oriented vessels on its superior surface.
  - Incise distal aponeurosis at the superior tarsal border, and dissect it free from Müller's muscle.
  - Place a central-lifting suture: Double-arm 6-0 suture passed into superior tarsus and levator aponeurosis. Tarsus will need to be recentered in cases of temporal displacement.

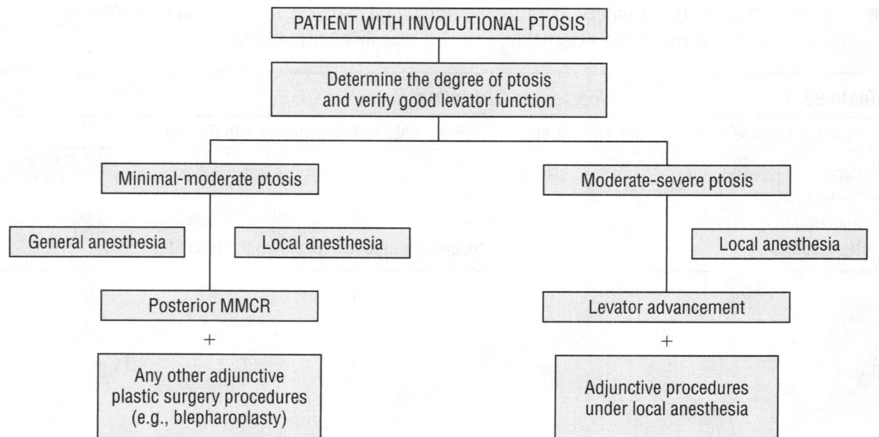


**Fig. 93-5** Algorithm for treatment of involutional ptosis. (*MMCR,* Müller's muscle–conjunctival resection.)

**TIP:** In general, 4 mm of levator advancement is needed for every 1 mm of ptosis correction.

**TIP:** If this patient is under general anesthesia, a gapping method can be applied, in which an advancement is performed until upper and lower eyelids are separated by an amount corresponding to preoperative levator excursion.

- If levator excursion is 8-10 mm, upper lid should be slightly lower than the upper limbus after advancement; if it is 6-8 mm, it should be at the limbus; if it is 4-6 mm, it should be slightly higher than the limbus.
- Additional medial and lateral sutures are placed.
- Perform supratarsal crease fixation—"anchor blepharoplasty" or resection of orbicularis.

- Alternatively, levator aponeurosis advancement can be performed by exposing levator muscle above Whitnall's ligament and resecting muscle in ratio of 4:1 for desired correction.[11]
- Levator plication has also been described using a 3:1 ratio without incision of aponeurosis, performed concurrently with aesthetic facial procedures under general anesthesia.[12]

## External Levator Resection[1,13] (Fig. 93-6)

- Best used when levator function is fair
- Sacrifices the viable levator muscle

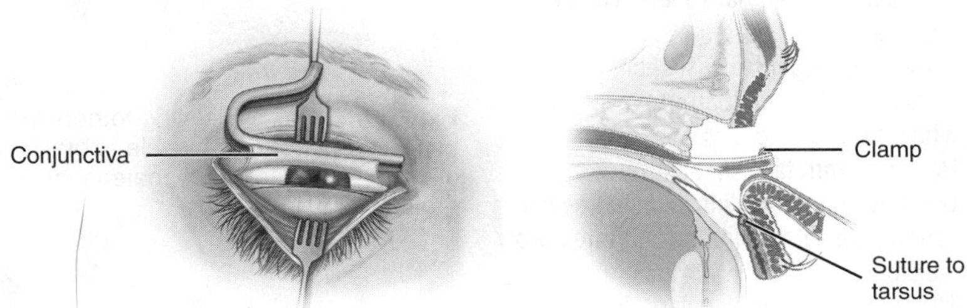


**Fig. 93-6** Müller's muscle–conjunctiva complex. The flap is everted exposing the conjunctiva. Conjunctiva is then dissected free from the overlying levator complex. It should be dissected in the fornix and reattached to the superior edge of the tarsus with absorbable sutures. This is then resected.

**TIP:** Carraway and Vincent[11] espouse levator advancement over external levator resection because of improved results with less morbidity.

- **Technique**
  1. Incise skin and orbicularis muscle at the desired supratarsal crease.
  2. Expose superior border of the tarsus.
  3. Incise full thickness through superior tarsal attachments and place ptosis clamp.
  4. Dissect levator and Müller's muscle complex from conjunctiva and orbital septum/preaponeurotic fat; cut medial and lateral horns as necessary.
  5. Remove full thickness of levator aponeurosis/muscle and Müller's muscle.

6. **Beard method:** If there are 1-2 mm of ptosis with 8-10 mm of levator function, resect 10-12 mm; if there are 2 mm of ptosis with 5-7 mm of levator function, resect 18 mm.
7. **Berke method:** Use the gapping method (see previous description).

### Levator Reinsertion

- Only useful in true levator dehiscence, which is likely only after trauma
- Involves resuturing the dehisced end to the tarsus
- Uncommon procedure because of uncommon indication

### Frontalis Suspension[8] (Fig. 93-7)

- Required if levator function **poor** (<5 mm) (congenital cases, neurogenic cases)
- Can provide 1 cm of excursion; good result in straightforward gaze; may produce lagophthalmos while asleep, which requires ointment or nighttime patching
- Incorporates a sling (fascia lata, temporalis fascia, homograft fascia, silicone strips, Gore-Tex) from frontalis to lid
  - If eyes are dry preoperatively proceed with caution. Consider use of biologic or alloplastic material so level can be adjusted.
- For unilateral congenital cases, bilateral suspension performed to improve symmetry
- **Crawford's technique**
  - Harvest 3 mm fascia lata strip.
  - Use three supralash incisions at medial, central, and lateral limbus and three brow incisions.
  - Thread fascia submuscularly from upper lid to brow.
- **Direct tarsal suturing with lid crease formation**
  - Creates supratarsal crease and fixation of sling material to tarsus to prevent late entropion seen with Crawford's procedure

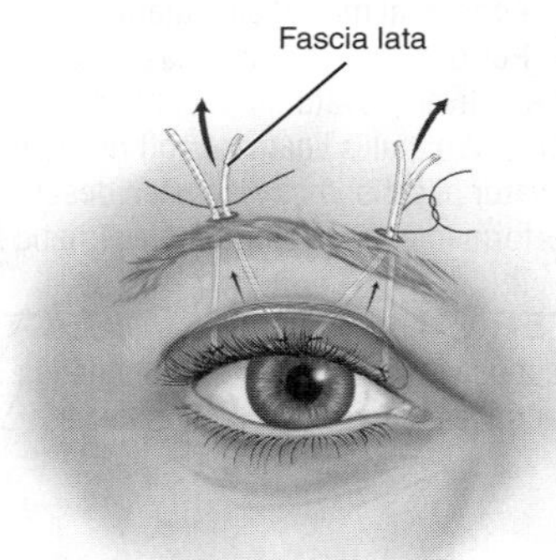


**Fig. 93-7** A frontalis sling tethers the upper eyelid to the frontalis muscle above by way of alloplastic or autologous material beneath the orbicularis oculi muscle.

## COMPLICATIONS[12]

- Undercorrection
- Overcorrection
- Excessive lagophthalmos
- Corneal exposure or keratitis, dry-eye syndrome
- Eyelid contour abnormality, temporal overcorrection
- Eyelid crease asymmetry
- Eyelash ptosis or lash abnormalities
- Entropion or ectropion/eversion of the upper lid
- Extraocular muscle imbalance
- Conjunctival prolapse

## Key Points

- ✓ Congenital ptosis usually requires frontalis suspension.
- ✓ Acquired ptosis is most often involutional.
- ✓ For correction of involutional ptosis, use levator advancement with monitored anesthesia and advance approximately 4 mm for every 1 mm of desired lid elevation.

## References

1. McCord CD Jr, Codner MA, eds. Eyelid & Periorbital Surgery. St Louis: Quality Medical Publishing, 2008.
2. McCord CD. The evaluation and management of the patient with ptosis. Clin Plast Surg 15:169-184, 1988.
3. McCord CD. Evaluation of the ptosis patient. In McCord CD Jr, Codner MA, Hester TR, eds. Eyelid Surgery: Principles and Techniques, 2nd ed. New York: Lippincott Williams & Wilkins, 2006.
4. Parsa FD, Wolff DR, Parsa MM, et al. Upper eyelid ptosis repair after cataract extraction and the importance of Hering's test. Plast Reconstr Surg 108:1527-1536, 2001.
5. Carraway J. Correction of blepharoptosis. In Achauer BM, Eriksson E, Guyuron B, et al, eds. Plastic Surgery: Indications, Operations, and Outcomes, St Louis: Mosby–Year Book, 2000.
6. Carraway JH. Cosmetic and function considerations in ptosis surgery: the elusive "perfect" result. Clin Plast Surg 15:185-193, 1988.
7. Chang S, Lehrman C, Itani K, et al. A systematic review of comparison of upper eyelid involutional ptosis repair techniques: efficacy and complication rates. Plast Reconstr Surg 129:149-157, 2012.
8. Bentz ML, Bauer BS, Zuker RM, eds. Principles & Practice of Pediatric Plastic Surgery. St Louis: Quality Medical Publishing, 2008.
9. Guyuron B, Davies B. Experience with the modified Putterman procedure. Plast Reconstr Surg 82:775-780, 1988.
10. Liu MT, Totonchi A, Katira K, et al. Outcomes of mild to moderate upper eyelid ptosis correction using Müller's muscle-conjunctival resection. Plast Reconstr Surg 130:799e-809e, 2012.
11. Carraway JH, Vincent MP. Levator advancement technique for eyelid ptosis. Plast Reconstr Surg 77:394-402, 1986.
12. de la Torre JI, Martin SA, De Cordier BC, et al. Aesthetic eyelid ptosis correction: a review of technique and cases. Plast Reconstr Surg 112:655-660, 2003.
13. McCord CD Jr. Complications of ptosis surgery and their management. In McCord CD Jr, Codner MA, Hester TR, eds. Eyelid Surgery: Principles and Techniques. New York: Lippincott-Raven, 1995.

# 94. Face Lift

Jason Roostaeian, Sumeet S. Teotia, Scott W. Mosser

## ANATOMY

A thorough grounding in facial anatomy is crucial when attempting to deliver consistent, safe, and reproducible results in rhytidectomy.

### SOFT TISSUE LAYERS OF THE FACE[1] (Fig. 94-1)

- **The layers of the facial soft tissues can be conceptualized as a series of concentric layers from superficial to deep.**
- **Retaining ligaments and fascial septa will span across these layers to support the soft tissue.**
  - Skin
  - Subcutaneous tissue/superficial fat compartments
  - Superficial musculoaponeurotic system (SMAS), temporoparietal fascia (above), platysma (below)
  - Facial mimetic muscles (NOTE: The SMAS attaches to the fascia around the **zygomatic muscles anteriorly.**)
  - Deep facial fascia (parotidomasseteric fascia)/deep fat compartments
  - Neurovascular structures
  - Bone
- **The neurovascular plane contains the following:**
  - Facial nerve
  - Parotid duct
  - Buccal fat pad
  - Facial vessels

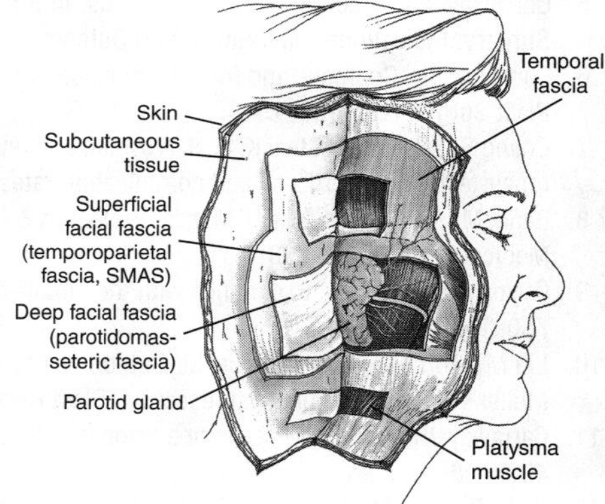


**Fig. 94-1** Facial soft tissue layers.

- **SMAS**[1-3]
  - The SMAS is a well-defined portion of the superficial facial fascia.
  - SMAS thickness varies by patient and region of the face. It is thickest over the parotid and becomes thinner medially.
  - The superficial facial fascia is a discrete fascial layer.
    - Forms a continuous sheath through the face and neck
    - Extends into malar region, lip, and nose, covering the mimetic muscles
  - The SMAS is an upward extension of the superficial cervical fascia into the face.
  - The fascia of the platysma muscle is part of the superficial cervical fascia and is continuous with the SMAS below.
  - The temporoparietal fascia (superficial temporal fascia) is an extension of the SMAS over the temporal region above.

- There are **four fascial layers** in the temporal region[1,4,5] (Fig. 94-2).
  1. Temporoparietal fascia
  2. Parotidotemporal fascia
  3. Superficial layer of the deep temporal fascia
  4. Deep layer of the deep temporal fascia
- From the level of the superior orbital margin to the zygomatic arch, the superficial and deep layers of the deep temporal fascia are separated from each other by the **superficial temporal fat pad.**
- The facial nerve runs just deep to the parotidotemporal fascia.

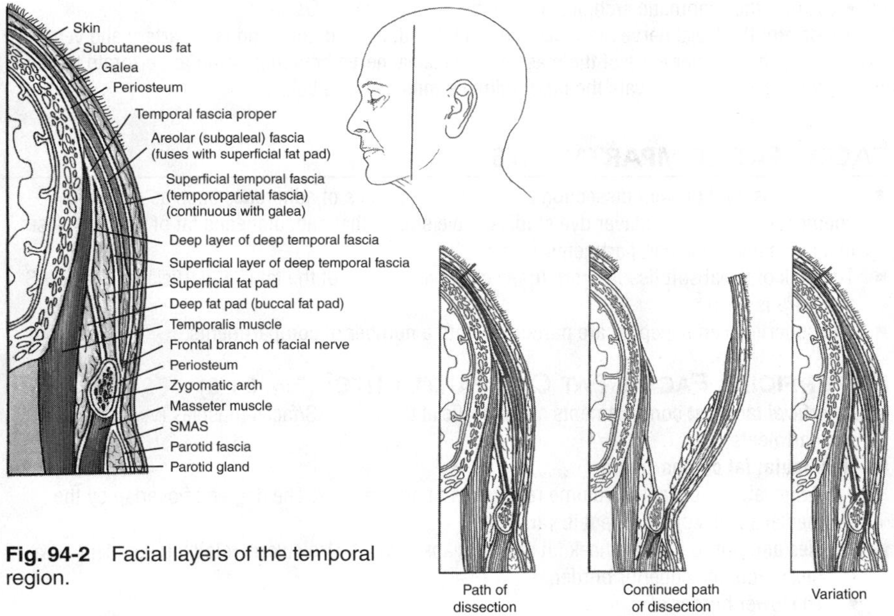


**Fig. 94-2** Facial layers of the temporal region.

> **TIP:** The superficial layer of the deep temporal fascia is often used as a landmark to protect the frontal branch, which runs superficial to it.

- The galea runs over the scalp and is continuous with the SMAS, frontalis, and temporoparietal fascia.
- **Fixed SMAS**
  - Adheres to and lies over the parotid
  - Thicker portion of the SMAS allowing greater protection of the facial nerve
- **Mobile SMAS**
  - Lies beyond the parotid gland, directly over the mimetic muscles, facial nerves, and parotid duct

    - Not adherent, tends to be relatively thin, and relatively mobile
    - At its most anterior extent, the mobile SMAS forms the fascia around the zygomaticus major, which can be a tethering point.
  - Traction and mobilization of the mobile SMAS allow movement of the midface and lower face during rhytidectomy.
    - Allow proper elevation, repositioning, and rotation for optimal outcome
- **Deep facial fascia (parotidomasseteric fascia)**[4]
  - A continuation of the superficial layer of the deep cervical fascia on the face
  - Over the parotid, it is called the *investing fascia of the parotid.*
  - Over the masseter, it is called the *masseteric fascia.*
  - Above the zygomatic arch, it is called the *deep temporal fascia.*
  - Covers the facial nerve branches, buccal fat pad, parotid duct, and facial artery and vein
  - Over the anterior edge of the masseter, the facial nerve branches begin to perforate the deep facial fascia to innervate the facial mimetic muscles (see below).

## FACIAL FAT COMPARTMENTS

- Clinical observation with dissection across discrete zones of adherence such as retaining ligaments, as well as cadaver dye studies, have shown that subcutaneous fat of the face exists in distinct anatomic compartments.
- The bulk of facial soft tissue is fat. In the cheek area, 56% of the fat is superficial to the SMAS and 44% is deep.[6]
- The superficial and deep fat are partitioned into a number of compartments.

### SUPERFICIAL FACIAL FAT COMPARTMENTS[7] (Fig. 94-3)

All superficial facial fat compartments are superficial to the SMAS/facial muscles (versus the deep fat compartments).

- **Nasolabial fat compartment**
  - Relatively consistent in volume regardless of age and sex. The degree of overlap by the medial cheek compartment is variable.
  - Lies anterior to medial cheek fat and overlaps jowl fat. Orbicularis retaining ligament represents the superior border.
  - The lower border of the zygomaticus major muscle is adherent to this compartment.
- **Cheek fat compartments**
  - Medial cheek fat
    - Bordered superiorly by the orbicularis retaining ligament/lateral orbital compartment, inferiorly by jowl fat, medially by nasolabial fat, and laterally by middle cheek fat

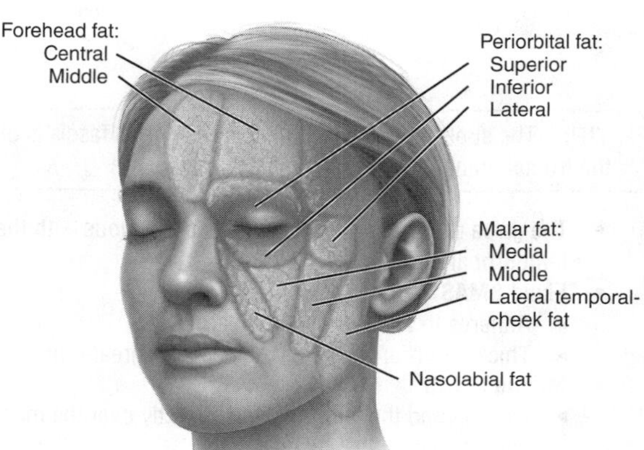


**Fig. 94-3** Superficial facial fat compartments.

- Middle cheek fat
  - Anterior and superficial to the parotid gland
  - At its superior portion, the zygomaticus major muscle is adherent. A confluence of septa is present at this location, where the zygomatic ligament has been described.[8]
  - Location of the parotidomasseteric ligaments corresponds to where the medial fat abuts the middle cheek fat.[4]
- Lateral temporal-cheek compartment
  - Most of the lateral cheek compartment lies immediately superficial to the parotid gland, connecting the temporal fat to cervical subcutaneous fat.
  - A true septum, referred to as the *lateral cheek septum,* can be located anterior to this compartment and is the first septal boundary encountered during a face lift.

- **Forehead and temporal fat compartments**
  - Composed of three compartments
    1. Central
    2. Middle temporal fat compartments on either side of it (superior temporal septum forms the lateral border)
    3. Lateral temporal-cheek compartment (described above)
- **Orbital fat compartments**
  - Composed of three compartments
    1. Superior compartment, bounded by orbital retaining ligament (ORL) above and the canthi medially and laterally
    2. Inferior compartment, bounded by ORL inferiorly and the canthi medially and laterally
    3. Lateral compartment, bounded superiorly by the inferior temporal septum, inferiorly by the superior cheek septum, where the zygomaticus major muscle is adherent
- **Jowl fat compartment**
  - Adheres to the depressor anguli oris muscle
  - Bounded medially by the depressor labii, superiorly and laterally by the cheek compartments, and inferiorly by the membranous fusion of the platysma muscle. This occurs at the region of the mandibular retaining ligament.[8]

## Malar Fat Pad[1,9,10]

- A commonly used term introduced by Owsley,[10] referring to the region of the superficial fat compartments that is thought to play an important role in the youthful cheek.
- The two primary components of the malar fat pad are the nasolabial and medial cheek fat compartments. The inferior orbital fat compartment can also be considered as part of the "malar fat pad."
- Triangular in shape, overlies the zygomaticus major, the zygomaticus minor, and the lower orbicularis oculi.
- Its base is along the nasolabial sulcus, and its apex is toward the zygomatic prominence.
- With age the fat pad descends and loses volume, which creates fullness and deepening of the nasolabial sulcus.

## Deep Facial Fat Compartments[9]

- Deep medial fat compartment
- Suborbicularis oculi fat (SOOF) compartment
- Retroorbicularis oculi fat (ROOF) compartment
- Loss of volume in the deep medial fat may be responsible for the loss of fullness seen in the aging midface.[10,11]

## Buccal Fat Pad[11]

The buccal fat pad is an important structure that contributes to cheek and facial contour.

- It consists of a **central body and three extensions:** Temporal, pterygoid, and buccal.
- The central body and buccal extensions contribute to cheek contour.
- The buccal fat pad is similar to an egg yolk in color, size, and consistency.
- The zygomatic and buccal branches of the facial nerve lie superficial to the buccal extension, with the parotid duct passing through it.
- In select cases, the buccal extension can be removed using an intraoral approach with a longitudinal incision in the buccal sulcus to reduce cheek fullness and enhance the malar eminence.

# LIGAMENTS AND ADHESIONS OF THE FACE[1,14-17] (Fig. 94-4)

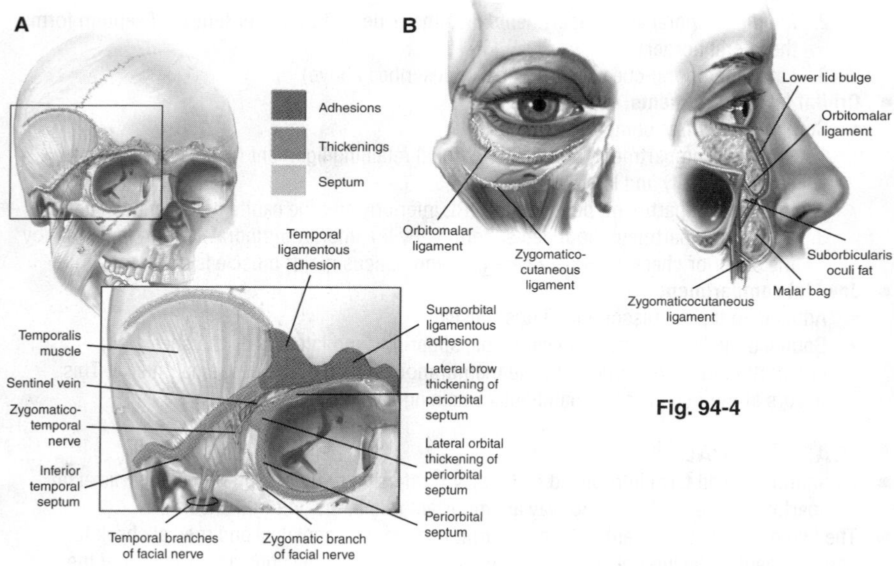


Fig. 94-4

## Retaining Ligaments

- The **retaining ligaments** of the face anchor the relatively fixed deep structures such as bone or muscular fascia to the overlying soft tissue, thereby supporting the facial skin and preventing displacement.
- Originally described by Bosse and Papillon,[12] as well as Furnas,[8] and later further characterized by Stuzin et al.[4]
- Various names given to these anatomic structures have created some confusion.
- They are present throughout the face, and some also represent the fascial boundary of the fat compartments (see above).[13]

- It is important to be familiar with the main retaining ligaments that may require division for adequate moblization of the face during a face-lift procedure.
- These must be released for mobilization of the brow and periorbital tissues as part of upper facial rejuvenation procedures such as brow lift and blepharoplasty.
- The orbitomalar ligament and zygomaticocutaneous ligament have been referred to as the *orbital retaining ligament* and *malar membrane,* respectively. Both structures are important in development of the tear trough deformity and malar bags.[15]

## Ligaments and Adhesions of the Middle and Lower Face[1,8]

- **Two types** of retaining ligaments have been described.
  1. **Osteocutaneous ligaments**
     - **Zygomatic osteocutaneous ligament**
       - Extends from the zygomatic arch and body, through the malar fat pad, to the overlying dermis
       - **McGregor's patch:** Part of the ligament over the zygomatic body
     - **Mandibular osteocutaneous ligament**
       - Extends from the parasymphyseal mandibular region to the overlying dermis
  2. **Parotid and masseteric cutaneous ligaments** (Fig. 94-5)
     - Formed by coalescence of the superficial and deep facial fascia
     - Fixes these facial layers to the parotid and masseter, and attaches to the overlying dermis by fibrous septa
- The functional significance of these ligaments is important for understanding the pathophysiology of the aging face.[1]
  - These ligaments attenuate and relax with age, causing creases by pivoting facial tissue.
  - The characteristics of facial aging are the result of these ligaments relaxing, along with loss of skin elasticity and atrophy of soft tissues.
    - Weakening of the zygomatic ligaments, which suspend the malar soft tissues and fat pad
      - Causes downward migration of the malar soft tissues
      - Creates redundant skin that hangs over the fixed nasolabial fold (not deepening of the nasolabial fold)

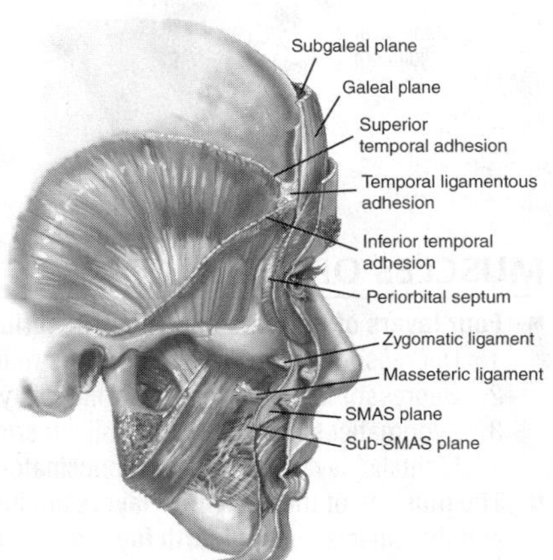


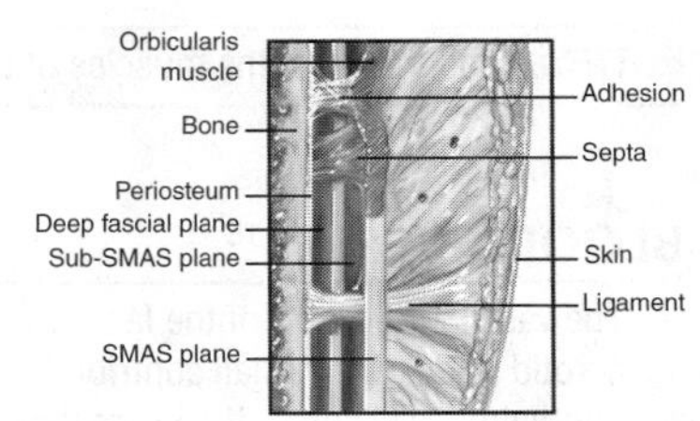


**Fig. 94-5**

- Weakening of the masseteric ligaments
  - Causes downward migration of the cheek tissue, thereby creating **marionette lines** and **jowls** (descent below the mandibular margin)
  - **Jowls** formed from tethering by the **mandibular ligament** (Fig. 94-6)

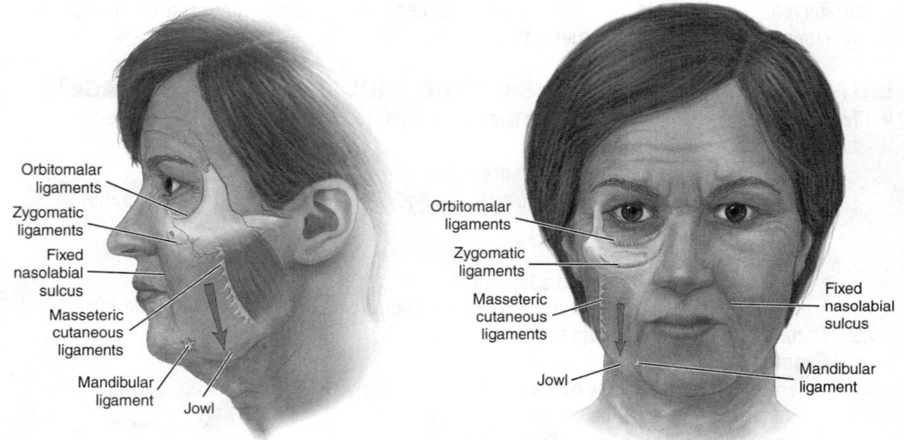


**Fig. 94-6**

## MUSCLES OF THE FACE

- **Four layers of muscles have been described (from superficial to deep).**[1,18]
  1. Depressor anguli oris, zygomaticus minor, orbicularis oris
  2. Depressor labii inferioris, risorius, platysma
  3. Zygomaticus major, levator labii superioris alaeque nasi
  4. Mentalis, levator anguli oris, buccinator
- The muscles of the **first three layers** are innervated by the facial nerve on their **deep** surfaces, and the muscles of the **fourth layer** are innervated by the facial nerve on their **superficial** surfaces.

**TIP:** Innervation of the muscles of the face is a common test question.

## BLOOD SUPPLY[1,18]

- The vascular territory of the face and scalp is supplied primarily by the branches of the external carotid artery, with small contributions to the eyelid, brow, forehead, and scalp through ophthalmic division of the internal carotid artery.
  - **Anterior face arteries:** Facial, superior and inferior labial, supratrochlear, and supraorbital
  - **Lateral face arteries:** Transverse, submental, zygomaticoorbital, anterior auricular
  - **Scalp and forehead:** Superficial temporal, frontal and temporal branches of the superficial temporal, posterior auricular, occipital

- Facial vessels lie in the deepest plane with the parotid duct and buccal and zygomatic branches of the facial nerve.
- Blood supply of the facial skin is through a network of myocutaneous perforators located along the oral commissures and nasolabial folds.
  - The **anterior region** of the face is supplied by a dense network of **myocutaneous** perforators.
  - The **lateral face** is supplied by a network of sparsely populated **fasciocutaneous** perforators.
- Skin undermining during face lift divides the fasciocutaneous perforators located laterally; thus the blood supply of the facial flap is dependent on the medially based myocutaneous perforators.

**NOTE: Many of the blood vessels that supply the face tend to travel in proximity to the retaining ligament. For example, in the area of the zygomatic ligament, McGregor's patch is known to contain a density of blood vessels that often bleed during dissection in that area.**

## SENSORY NERVES[1]

- The sensory supply of the face is supplied by branches of the trigeminal nerve ($V_{1\text{-}3}$) and cervical spinal nerves, with a small contribution to the auditory canal through CN VIII and CN X.
- The sensory nerves run from their respective deep foramina as a main branch, becoming superficial while branching multiple times to supply sensation to an area of skin. Therefore these small superficial branches are frequently disrupted during a face lift. However, at that level, they will regenerate.

**CAUTION: Disruption at the main trunk should be avoided, because regeneration may not occur and neuromas can form.**

- **Great auricular nerve** (C2-C3)
  - *Most common nerve injured during face lifts (symptomatic)*
  - It is at greatest risk in its superficial location, which begins along the posterior border of the sternocleidomastoid (SCM) muscle, 6.5 cm inferior to the tragus, *McKinney's point.*
  - It then runs parallel and just posterior to the external jugular vein. The nerve is technically deep to the superficial cervical fascia as it runs up the posterior border of the SCM muscle; however, the platysma is absent here placing the nerve at risk.
  - Division of the nerve leads to numbness of the lower half of the ear on both the cranial and lateral surfaces.
- **Auriculotemporal nerve**
  - Courses with the superficial temporal artery
  - Can be divided during a face lift
  - **Frey's syndrome:** Sympathetic reinnervation of facial skin flap after division of auriculotemporal nerve fibers causing gustatory sweating
- **Lesser occipital nerve**
  - Travels mostly over the SCM muscle, running between the muscle fascia and superficial facial fascia
  - Innervates the superior third of the ear and mastoid region in about 60% of cases
  - Occasionally supplies two thirds of the superior ear
- **Skin of midface supplied by branches of the maxillary division**
  - Zygomaticotemporal, zygomaticofacial, and infraorbital nerves
  - Knowing the locations of the main nerve trunks helps to prevent division during face lifts.

## MOTOR NERVES

### FACIAL NERVE[19] (Fig. 94-7)

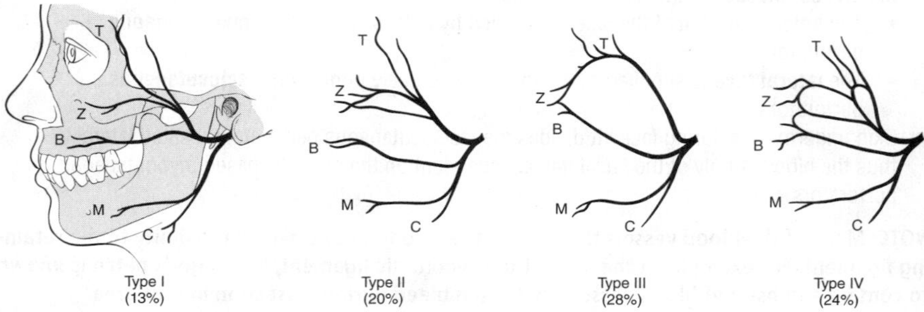


**Fig. 94-7** Variations in the branching pattern of the facial nerve. (*B,* Buccal branch; *C,* cervical branch; *M,* mandibular branch; *T,* temporal branch; *Z,* zygomatic branch.)

- Emerges through the stylomastoid foramen and is immediately protected by the parotid gland
- Divides into an upper and lower portion within the parotid gland, and then divides into **five major branches** with variable branching patterns:
  1. Temporal (frontal)
  2. Zygomatic
  3. Buccal
  4. Marginal mandibular
  5. Cervical

**CAUTION: The temporal (frontal) and marginal mandibular branches are most at risk for permanent deficit during rhytidectomy, because they are considered terminal branches with minimal to no interconnections with other branches.[5,20,21]**

- **Frontal branch**[19] (Fig. 94-8)
  - Courses more superficially after crossing the zygomatic arch (at midpoint between the tragus and lateral canthus) within the sub-SMAS fat just deep to the temporoparietal fascia
  - Travels superiorly, approximately along a trajectory from the tragus to a point 1.5 cm above the lateral brow, *Pitanguy's line.*[22]
  - Protected by an additional layer of fascia deep to the SMAS called the *parotidotemporal fascia*[5]

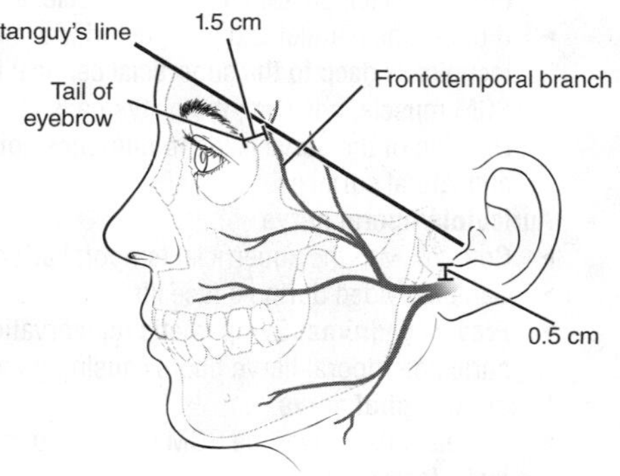


**Fig. 94-8** Frontal branch course.

- **Buccal and zygomatic branches**
  - Emerge from the anterior parotid
  - Lie in the loose areolar tissue and fat superficial to the masseter and deep to the SMAS and parotidomasseteric fascia
  - Injury to one or more branches typically yields only a temporarily noticeable deficit.

**NOTE: Permanent injuries are rare as a result of their multiple interconnections.**

- **Marginal mandibular branch**
  - Protected by the deep cervical fascia layer after exiting the anteroinferior border of the parotid at the angle of the mandible
  - Courses forward deep to the anterior facial vein in contact with the superolateral portion of the submandibular gland near the mandibular midbody in the region of the facial vessels; swings superiorly and perforates the deep fascia to run between the fibroareolar plane between the deep cervical fascia and the platysma
  - Follows the mandibular border, and before crossing the facial vessels may extend 3 cm below the mandibular border[23]
  - Runs above the mandibular border after crossing the facial vessels
  - Runs deep to platysma throughout its course

**CAUTION: The vulnerable point for injury is after it exits the deep cervical fascia and courses up and over the anterior mandible in the region of the facial artery.**

  - Dissection above platysma laterally, and inferior to the mandibular border centrally, prevents injury to the nerve.
- **Cervical branch**
  - Located roughly half the distance from the mentum to the mastoid and approximately 1 cm below this line at the level of the angle of the mandible[24]
  - Exits the inferior portion of the parotid slightly anterior to the angle of the mandible
  - Immediately perforates the deep cervical fascia and then runs in the fibroareolar tissue that attaches to the platysma at its superolateral border
  - Platysma should be dissected at this superolateral border from the deep fascia bluntly to prevent injury.
  - Injury to the cervical branch leads to "pseudoparalysis of the mandibular branch," with an asymmetrical full denture smile. This is distinguished from marginal mandibular nerve injury by the ability to evert and purse the lower lip.[25,26]
  - Cervical branch injury is generally associated with complete recovery within 3-4 weeks on average.[26]

## Facial Danger Zones[27]

- Figs. 94-9 and 94-10 and Table 94-1 outline the zones of the face where motor branches of the facial nerves and sensory nerves are at greatest risk during face lift.[27]

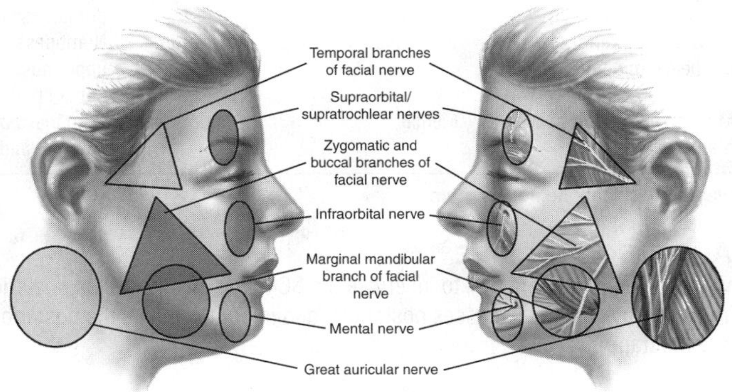


**Fig. 94-9** Facial danger zones: Motor and sensory nerves.

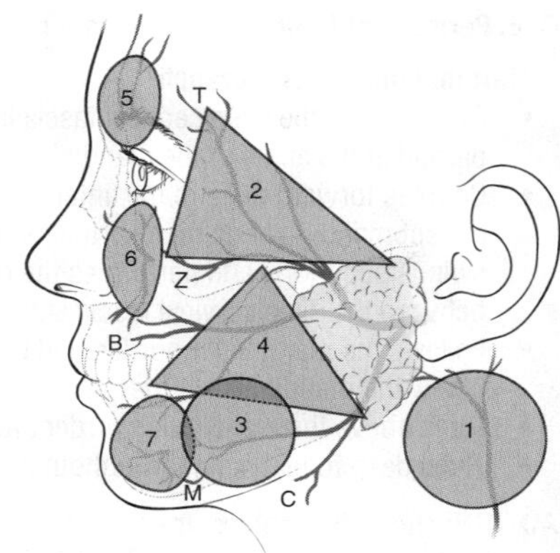


**Fig. 94-10** Underlying nerves running through each facial danger zone after the skin and SMAS layer have been removed. (*B,* Buccal branch; *C,* cervical branch; *M,* mandibular branch; *T,* temporal branch; *Z,* zygomatic branch.)

**Table 94-1** *Seckel's Facial Danger Zones*

| Facial Danger Zone | Location | Nerve | Relationship to SMAS | Sign of Zonal Injury |
|---|---|---|---|---|
| 1 | 6.5 cm below external auditory canal | Great auricular | Posterior to | Numbness of inferior two thirds of ear, adjacent cheek and neck |
| 2 | Below a line drawn from 0.5 cm below tragus to 2 cm above lateral eyebrow and above zygoma | Temporal branch of facial | Beneath | Paralysis of forehead |
| 3 | Midmandible 2 cm posterior to oral commissure | Marginal mandibular branch of facial | Beneath | Paralysis of lower lip |
| 4 | Triangle formed by connecting dots on malar eminence, posterior border of mandibular angle, and oral commissure | Zygomatic and buccal branches of facial | Beneath | Paralysis of upper lip and cheek |
| 5 | Superior orbital rim above midpupil | Supraorbital and supratrochlear | Anterior to | Numbness of forehead, upper eyelid, nasal dorsum, scalp |
| 6 | 1 cm below inferior orbital rim below midpupil | Infraorbital | Anterior to | Numbness of side of upper nose, cheek, upper lip, lower eyelid |
| 7 | Midmandible below second premolar | Mental | Anterior to | Numbness of half of lower lip and chin |

*SMAS,* Superficial musculoaponeurotic system.

## Spinal Accessory Nerve[28,29]

- This nerve exits the jugular foramen to innervate the SCM and then leaves its posterior border 7-9 cm from the clavicle. It then passes posteriorly and inferiorly across the posterior triangle to innervate the trapezius.

**CAUTION: The spinal accessory nerve is vulnerable to injury as it leaves the posterior border of the SCM. It stays deep to the investing layer of the deep cervical fascia on the levator scapulae but is separated from the muscle by the prevertebral layer of deep cervical fascia and adipose tissue.**

- It is relatively superficial in this position, especially more proximally, and can be injured during elevation of neck skin.

## CHANGES IN THE AGING FACE

### SKIN[30]

- **Intrinsic processes**
  - Epidermis becomes thinner, with flattening of the dermal-epidermal junction.
  - Cell turnover decreases, which may account for slower wound healing.
  - Dermis becomes atrophic with reduced numbers of fibroblasts.
  - Subdermal adipose tissue decreases.
  - Number and diameter of collagen fibers decrease, and the ratio of type III to type I collagen increases.
- **Extrinsic processes:** Photoaging[31]
  - It is primarily caused by sun exposure. Other causes are smoking and weight fluctuation.
  - Characteristics include dryness, rhytids, irregular pigmentation, loss of elasticity, telangiectasias, and areas of purpura.
  - Histologically this process is also called *basophilic degeneration* or *elastosis.*
    - Epidermis atrophies.
    - Elastic fibers thicken in the dermis.
    - Ground substance increases.

### WRINKLES

Wrinkling occurs as a result of aging, actinic damage, or genetic disorders. Normal aging is a process of atrophy.

- **Three types of creases occur in the skin.**[31]
  1. Animation creases from mimetic muscle insertions
  2. Fine, shallow wrinkles (caused by disruption of skin elastic structures)
  3. Coarse, deep wrinkles resulting from solar elastosis and epidermal atrophy
- **Histologic changes**[31]
  - Loss of dermoepidermal papillae
  - Fewer melanocytes and Langerhans cells
  - Less dermal collagen, leading to thinning of the skin
  - Loss of reticular dermis with reduced dermal organization
  - Decreases in ground substance (elastic fibers, collagen, glycosaminoglycan gel)
  - Larger sebaceous glands

### SOFT TISSUE

- Aging in the soft tissue appears to have four main mechanisms:
  1. Descent from gravitational forces
  2. Deflation/volume loss
     - There is a loss of soft tissue volume in the middle and upper thirds of the aging face.[32-34]
     - Tissue along the inferior orbital rim does not become ptotic but instead appears to do so because of volume loss.[35]
  3. Fat accumulation in the lower third, especially the neck and jowl area[36,37]

4. Radial expansion: Repeated animation stretches retaining ligaments and allows the soft tissue to expand away from the face.
   - This is perhaps most apparent with the nasolabial fold with smiling, because the skin of the lip is forced beneath the subcutaneous fat of the cheek, allowing that soft tissue to prolapse outward from the skeleton, thereby deepening the fold.[38]

### BONE[39]

- The infraorbital rim and anterior maxilla gradually retrude, contributing in part to development of the **tear trough deformity.**
- The orbit expands inferolaterally and superomedially.
- The adult facial skeleton continues to grow unless there is bone demineralization or dentition is lost, then there is a reduction in overall facial height because of loss of alveolar bone in the mandible and maxilla.
- Facial structures rotate downward and inward with respect to the cranial base.

## PREOPERATIVE FACIAL ANALYSIS

- The entire face should be evaluated and treated to prevent a patchwork appearance, with an algorithm developed to correct aspects of aging.
- History is obtained to exclude high-risk patients: Smokers, patients with poorly controlled hypertension, diabetics, chronic NSAID users, and those with other medical conditions.
- Treatment of aged skin with resurfacing techniques such as laser or chemical peel should be considered.
- Divide the face into zones during examination, and develop a checklist. Use a consistent approach, such as top to bottom, to ensure a complete analysis.

### PERIORBITAL ZONE (FOREHEAD, BROW, AND MIDFACE)[1]

- **Brow position:** Assess the medial and lateral brow position and the relationship of the brow to the upper lid.
- **Forehead height:** Note the distance from the hairline to the brow. The brow is not an exact point, but measurement between fixed points such as hairline to pupil is exact and therefore a better gauge.
- **Glabellar creases:** Assess for corrugator (vertical) wrinkling, procerus (horizontal) wrinkling, and depth of rhytids.
- **Temporal region:** Evaluate the presence of crow's feet, excess skin, and temporal atrophy.
- **Upper eyelid:** Assess the skin, the effect of brow ptosis (pseudoptosis), lid ptosis (congenital or senile), and fat (mostly medial).
- **Lower eyelid:** Observe the lower lid–cheek junction; assess lid tone; look for festoons and tear-trough deformity with orbital fat herniation.
- **Lateral canthal position:** Note the canthal relationship and lid tone.
- Assess the lid-cheek junction for **tear-trough deformity**.
- Assess malar projection and for negative or positive vector orbit (less versus greater malar projection relative to cornea, respectively).[40]
- Assess for malar descent and/or atrophy.

### PERIORAL ZONE: MIDDLE THIRD (LOWER FACE)[1]

- **Nasolabial folds and marionette grooves:** Assess depth at rest and animation.
- **Angle of the mouth:** Aging lowers the angle of the mouth.

- **Upper lip:** Note presence of perioral rhytids, length of upper lip, and volume loss with increased distance from nose to vermilion border of upper lip, leading to loss of definition of philtral columns.
- **Lower lip:** Assess volume loss.
- **Chin:** Assess the depth of labiomental fold, chin ptosis (witch's chin), and jowls.
- **Nose:** Assess the aging, ptotic nose.
- **Ear position:** Assess for lobular ptosis and elongation; observe increased vertical height of the ear.

### Neck Zone: Lower Third of Face/Neck[1]

- The neck is discussed in detail in Chapter 95.
- Examine for excess skin, platysmal bands causing transverse cervical creases, and subcutaneous and subplatysmal fat.
- Generally the neck skin should be elevated past the inferior extent of the platysmal band and ideally past the last transverse rhytid.
- Assess the jawline and the submandibular gland.

### Facial Proportions[41]

- Overall width, length, and fullness can help determine an individualized approach to face lift.
- Both the vector of pull on the SMAS (horizontal versus vertical) and whether to excise excess fullness (SMASectomy versus stacking or plication) can be determined with this approach.
- Analysis focuses on three basic facial parameters:
  1. *Midface width:* Determined by a horizontal line through the infraorbital rims
  2. *Facial length:* Vertical height from the malar projection point to the inferior jowl point
  3. *Facial fullness:* Overall distribution of soft tissue fullness

## VARIATIONS IN TECHNIQUE

### Incision Placement[1]

- Scar location depends on location of hairline and sideburns, Fitzpatrick skin classification, and ear topography.
- **Temple incision** (Fig. 94-11)
  - Widening the distance between the lateral canthus and the anterior part of the temporal hairline creates an unnatural appearance.
  - **Prehairline:** Ideal with short sideburns, secondary face lifts, and when excision of excess skin would widen the distance from the lateral canthus
  - **Posthairline:** Often used in continuation with an open-coronal brow-lift procedure, and when minimal excess temporal skin is recruited; often possible when differential vectors between skin and SMAS are used, allowing more of a pure posterior vector for the skin

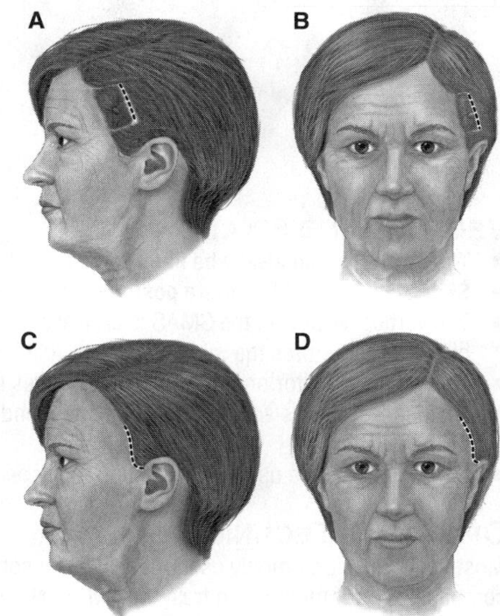


**Fig. 94-11** **A** and **B,** Posthairline temporal incision. **C** and **D,** Prehairline temporal incision.

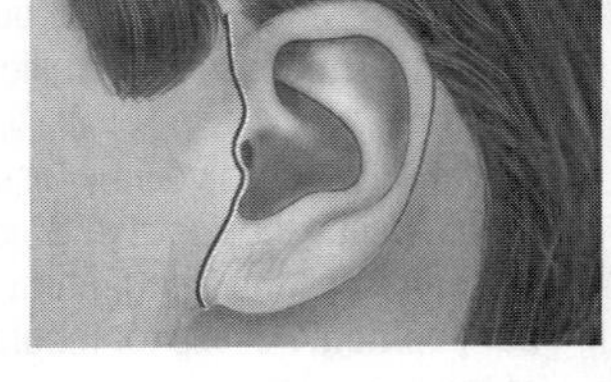

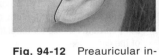

Fig. 94-12 Preauricular intertragal incision.

- **Preauricular incision** (Fig. 94-12)
  - Incision is made between the anatomic margin of the face and ear, taking notice of the width of the root of the helix.
  - The incision is curved along the anterior border of the helix to the upper tragus.
  - An intratragal incision along its posterior border is best suited to hide the scar.
  - Pretragal incision should be considered in men, given the possibility of hair follicles moving to the area of the tragus otherwise.
  - Some surgeons prefer pretragal incision if cheek skin is dramatically different from tragal skin.
- **Postauricular incision** (Fig. 94-13)
  - The incision is best placed at the retroauricular sulcus.
  - A consistent landmark should be used, such as the posterior auricularis muscle or top of the tragus, to place incision at the same height on both sides.
  - **Occipital incision can also be prehairline or posthairline into the scalp. With a prehairline incision, the surgeon need not worry about aligning the hairline after skin excision; however, the scar may become hypertrophic and visible.**

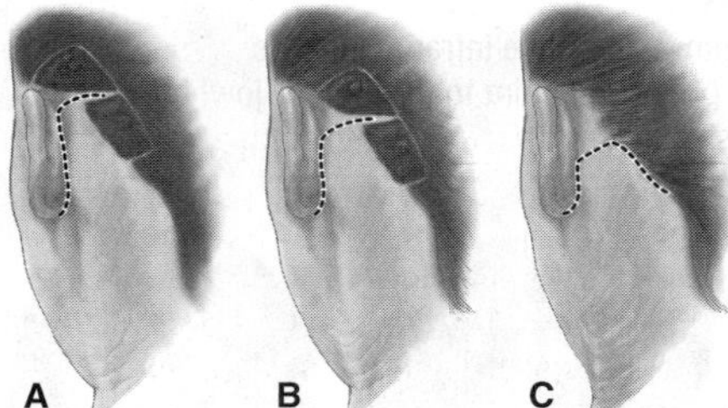


**Fig. 94-13 A,** A high retroauricular crossing to the hairline is best suited to patients with modest redundancy of neck skin. **B,** A lower retroauricular crossing to the hairline is best suited to patients with modest to excessive redundancy of neck skin. **C,** An occipital hairline incision is best suited to those with excessive or massive skin redundancy, especially in the lower neck.

## Vectors and Fixation[1]

- The **SMAS** should ideally be fixed and elevated in a more **vertical** or **diagonally vertical** vector.
- **Skin** fixation should be more **posterior** and vertical.
- The vertical vector on the SMAS is critical and improves the jawline and perioral areas, and the high SMAS restores the midface.
- The diagonal vector on the platysma improves the neck and submental areas.
- Permanent sutures are mostly used to suspend the SMAS, and absorbable sutures are used for the skin.
- Some propose the use of Vicryl mesh to suspend the SMAS for added support and fixation.[17]

## Operative Techniques

Most techniques commonly used today involve some degree of subcutaneous dissection in combination with methods to treat the SMAS. No study has demonstrated a clear advantage of one technique over another.

- **Subcutaneous face lift**[31]
  - The standard subcutaneous face lift with variable skin undermining

- The SMAS and deeper fat compartments are not addressed.
- **Advantages:** Safe, relatively easy to perform, rapid recovery; ideal for thin patients with a lot of excess skin and minimal ptosis of deep structures.
- **Disadvantages:** Persistence is shortened, because tension is provided by skin, a relatively elastic structure compared with the SMAS, which has a fascial component.

■ **Deep subcutaneous face lift**
- A thicker flap may be developed, as with the "extended supraplatysmal plane" technique, in which skin and superficial fat compartments are dissected as a unit and redraped.[42]
- **Advantages:** Flap is robust, SMAS is not penetrated, and superficial fat compartments are captured, allowing defatting and/or mobilization into desired location.
- **Disadvantages:** Flap is unidirectional (skin and fat must move together), and fixation depends on suture tension on fat and skin, neither of which is ideal.

■ **Subcutaneous face lift with plication and/or imbrication**
- **SMAS plication** (suture infolding) is the elevation of a subcutaneous flap and placement of direct sutures to tighten the SMAS without elevating it as a discrete layer.
- **SMAS imbrication** involves incision, advancement, and overlapping with suture fixation.
- The fatty tissues of the cheek and neck are suspended upward and laterally without SMAS undermining.
- **Advantages:** Technique is relatively safe and rapid compared with sub-SMAS dissection, relatively easy to perform, and can treat and reshape deeper structures and take tension off of the skin closure. Proponents claim long-lasting results.
- **Disadvantages:** A branch of the facial nerve can theoretically be caught with the suture. Some believe the lack of a raw surface edge prevents adequate scar formation for long-term benefit (although the superficial surface is dissected with skin elevation).
- **Minimal access cranial suspension (MACS) short-scar face lift** of Tonnard and Verpaele[43]
  - ▸ A variation of the plication method
  - ▸ Subcutaneous tissues are dissected from the underlying SMAS-platysma layer and then suspended from the deep temporal fascia.
  - ▸ Long looping sutures with multiple bites (microimbrication) are used to elevate the deep tissues in a vertical vector[43] (Fig. 94-14, *A*). One loop is placed for the neck, another for the jowl, and an optional third suture (extended MACS-lift) for midface elevation[43] (Fig. 94-14, *B*).
- **Suture placement for lateral SMASectomy** (with or without short scar)[44]:
  - ▸ A variation of the imbrication method.
  - ▸ Strip of SMAS is excised in the region overlying the anterior edge of the parotid gland parallel to the nasolabial fold.

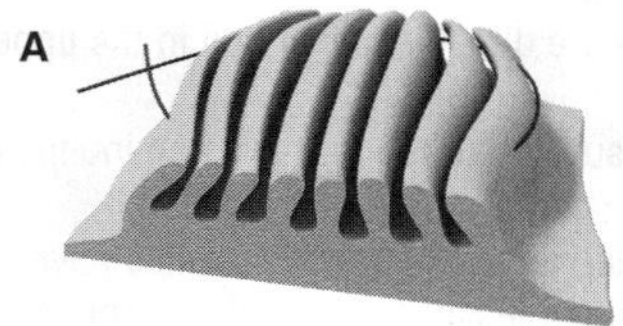


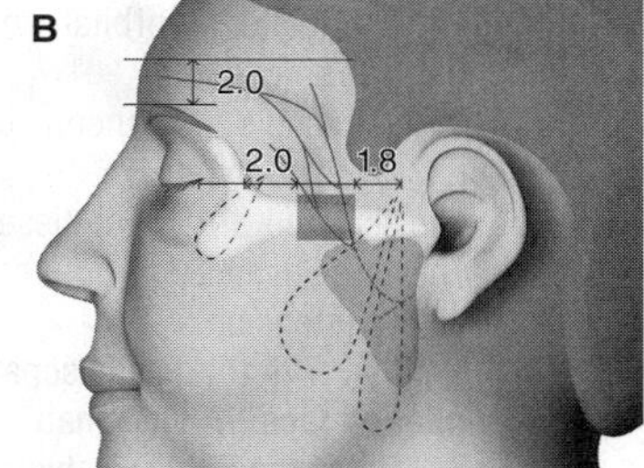


**Fig. 94-14 A,** A purse-string suture technique, as advocated in the MACS-lift, is a facial sculpturing technique that involves multiple microimbrications of the SMAS. **B,** Extended MACS-lift.

- The vector of elevation is perpendicular to the nasolabial fold.
- SMAS is not undermined. Tissue is excised at the junction of the mobile and immobile SMAS, allowing the mobile SMAS to be advanced.
- Ideal in a patients with a full face in place of a plication to remove some of the deep tissue excess.
- Gives more complete raw surface of the SMAS, which some believe helps with its longevity.

• **SMAS stacking**[41]
  - Ideal in patients who could benefit from increased fullness
  - SMAS is incised on two sides, leaving a strip of SMAS variable in width, oriented in the chosen vector of pull.
  - SMAS anterior and posterior to the strip is then brought together over the strip, "stacking" one layer of SMAS over the SMAS strip.

■ **Skoog face lift**[45]
- In 1974 Skoog described skin and SMAS elevation as a single unit, advancing the entire skin-SMAS unit posteriorly onto the cheek and neck.
- Identified the relatively stretch-resistant SMAS as a discrete layer that could be used to augment skin suspension
- Fails to improve nasolabial folds and anterior neck pull caused by tethering of the SMAS to lip elevators[46]
- Modified further by Barton[47] and by Hamra[48] to treat the nasolabial fold (Fig. 94-15)
- **Advantages:** Flap is thick with robust blood supply. A longer-lasting result is possible, given the inelasticity of the SMAS, which holds the tension of the mobilized skin and soft tissues.
- **Disadvantages:** Dissection is at a deeper, more dangerous level that can lead to facial nerve injury. SMAS can be tethered without adequate release of retaining ligaments and attachment to facial muscles, compromising the result. The skin and deep tissues move as a unit in one direction.

■ **Subcutaneous and sub-SMAS dissection with several variations**[19] (see Fig. 94-15)
- The term *deep plane* or *sub-SMAS* or *deep SMAS* refers to dissection that lifts the SMAS layer.
- A **low SMAS** technique (inferior to the zygomatic arch) treats the lower face only and has no effect on tissues of the midface or perioral and infraorbital regions.
- A **high SMAS** technique (superior to the zygomatic arch) treats the midface and periorbital area in combination with the lower face.
  - Refined, perfected, and popularized by Barton[47]
- **Composite face lift** of Hamra[48-51]
  - Carries not only the platysma and subcutaneous fat but also the lower lid orbicularis muscle as a single dissected unit
  - The malar and periorbital areas are directly suspended in the upper face with this rhytidectomy.
  - The skin and subcutaneous tissues are not elevated as an independent layer.
- **Lamellar SMAS face lift**[52]
  - The skin and SMAS are dissected as two separate lamellae (layers).
  - They are advanced to different degrees along separate vectors and suspended under different tension.
  - Each layer is addressed separately.
- **Foundation face lift** of Pitman[53]
  - Separates the SMAS-platysma only from the underlying tissues while simultaneously raising a composite flap of SMAS-platysma, subcutaneous fat, and skin.

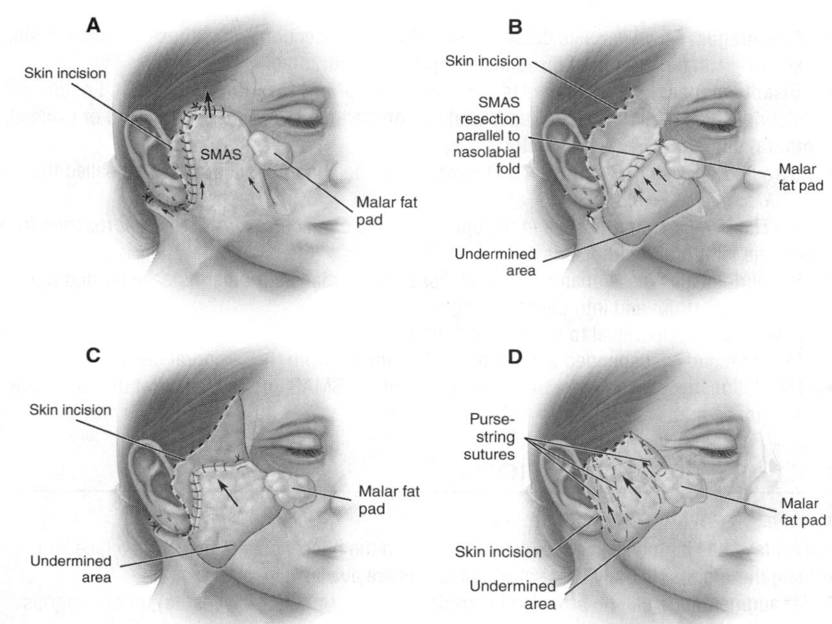


**Fig. 94-15** **A,** Barton: High SMAS lift. **B,** Baker: Short-scar lift. **C,** Stuzin: Extended SMAS lift. **D,** Tonnard and Verpaele: Extended MACS-lift.

- **Advantages of these types:** Same as Skoog procedure with the additional advantage of greater release of the SMAS, allowing improved mobilization and greater effect on the anterior face.
- **Disadvantages of these types:** Deeper more dangerous level of dissection and more extensive dissection can lead to facial nerve injury. SMAS skin and deep tissues will move as a unit unless two planes of dissection above and below the SMAS are performed. (This, however, can compromise the integrity of the SMAS layer, which gets very thin past the parotid anteriorly.)

■ **Subperiosteal face lift**[31]

- First introduced by Tessier,[54] who applied craniofacial principles to lifting the facial soft tissues
- Does not dissect the SMAS or skin as an independent layer
- Midface periosteum is elevated as a single unit and then redraped and affixed to achieve tissue repositioning.
- Little[36] advocated a combined **temporal and perioral subperiosteal midface release,** which stacks the entire cheek–soft tissue unit to further accentuate the malar eminence.
- The superiosteal technique allows adequate redraping of the forehead and malar areas.
  - ▸ The perioral and neck region requires an additional procedure for suspension.
  - ▸ Additional procedure may involve skin, SMAS, or a combination.
- Patients with great skin redundancy of the nasolabial folds, jawline, and neck are not candidates for the isolated subperiosteal face lift.

- **Advantages:** Facial nerve is deeper to this plane of dissection and is thus protected. Visible scarring can be minimized through a temporal and intraoral approach.
- **Disadvantages:** Learning curve is steep. Skin and SMAS must move as a unit. Endoscopic technology is often required. Superficial fat compartments cannot be reshaped or excised.

- **Temporal supraperiosteal dissection**
  - Byrd and Andochick[55] and Hunt and Byrd[56] described an **endoscopic method** called the *endoscopic brow midface lift.*
    - The bony and soft tissues in the upper face are treated as a single unit approached from the temporal region.
  - Subperiosteal plane is abandoned, and dissection is made supraperiosteally around the lateral orbital rim and into the malar region.
  - Dissection is superficial to origin of zygomaticus major.
  - Malar fat pad is suspended independently by sutures from the temporal fascia.
  - Dissection involves an avascular plane between the SMAS and the periosteum around the zygomatic arch.

## ANCILLARY CONSIDERATIONS

### MALAR ENHANCEMENT[31]

A youthful face has high cheekbones, with concavity in the buccal area. The goal of a face lift is to accentuate the zygomatic body, and several methods are available.

- Malar augmentation can be provided by implants, fillers (fat, hydroxyapatite), or autologous tissues (SMAS).
- The goal is to resuspend or reposition the ptotic malar fat pad.
- Malar prominence can be enhanced by folding redundant, dissected SMAS onto itself and suturing it to the zygomatic body.
- The cheek mass can be anchored to the lateral orbital rim using materials such as permanent suture, tendon, fascia, or Gore-Tex.
- Transblepharoplasty techniques have been described that suspend the cheek mass to the temporal fascia at its insertion near the lateral orbital rim.[39,41]
- Temporal supraperiosteal approaches for elevating the cheek flap also exist (see previous discussion).[56,57]
- Methods exist that treat the ptotic orbicularis oculi muscle.
- The **malar septum** is the basis of malar mounds and malar edema. Adequate release of this septum may be necessary to smooth the lower orbital and malar soft tissues.[58,59]

### NASOLABIAL FOLDS[10,46,47,58,60]

- The lower and middle thirds of the nasolabial fold generally show better correction than the upper third with most face-lift techniques.
- Deep nasolabial folds have been treated by various techniques.
  - A sub-SMAS face lift that goes through the SMAS to the subcutaneous plane at the level of the belly of the zygomaticus major muscle can stretch the nasolabial fold if sufficient tension is placed on the anterior cheek skin.
  - Dermal attachments of the fold can be released and filled with fat or dermal fat grafts.
  - Soft tissue fillers can be used to smooth the fold but have variable longevity and are not appropriate for all patients.
  - Adjunctive suction can be applied to thick folds, but success is variable.
- No single ideal method has been identified.

## The Aging Lip[31]

- **Signs**
  - Longer distance between the columellar base and upper vermilion border
  - Less exposed vermilion (thin lips)
  - Loss of volume in the vermilion (pout)
- **Vermilion advancement technique**
  - Directly and precisely positions the Cupid's bow.
  - A visible scar is left on the lip margin.
- **Skin removal along the alar and columellar bases**
  - Can shorten the aging upper lip
  - Hidden scar along the base of the nose
- **Volume enhancement**
  - Can add bulk to vermilion volume using fat injections, fillers, AlloDerm (LifeCell, Branchburg, NJ), dermal/fascial grafts (using redundant SMAS), and tendon grafts (Palmaris).

## Jawline[31]

- Slings and sutures may be placed along the mandibular border in an attempt to smooth the jawline, but caution must be exercised.
- **Submandibular gland** and **digastric muscle excision** has been advocated by some surgeons but is not widely accepted.
- Suction may be applied with caution along the submandibular border, but only after a face lift has been performed to prevent contour hollowing.

## Chin Ptosis[31]

- Occasionally, an aging lower face may have a "witch's chin" (prominent submental crease and a hanging soft tissue mass below the lower mandibular border).
- Most effective correction is by resuspension of chin mass and insertion of a chin implant.
- Cutaneous dissection to release the mental crease and retaining ligaments is important when redraping.

## Fat Injections[1]

- The purpose of fat injections is to restore age-associated volume loss and tissue atrophy (see Chapter 89).
- Fat can be placed in the lips, nasolabial folds, chin, jawline, tear trough and periorbicular deformities, zygomatic prominence, and labiomandibular folds.
- Aim for slight overcorrection with much expected loss over time.
- Repeat injections are almost always necessary.
- Dermal fat grafts can also be used adjunctively.
- Injections must be deep and contour irregularities corrected by massaging.
- Generally aim for about 3 cc in the upper lip and 2 cc in the lower lip; expect a 50% loss over several months.
- The injected fat can be filtered first using a sieve (a double-overlap gauze) and can also be centrifuged.
- The viability of fat injections is highly variable.

## PERIOPERATIVE MANAGEMENT AND ASSESSMENT

### Preoperative Assessment Management

- All NSAIDs must be discontinued at least 2 weeks before surgery.
- Supplements such as fish oils, garlic, ginkgo, and ginger should not be taken for at least 2 weeks before surgery.
- If the patient is on other anticoagulants such as Plavix or Coumadin, then a face lift is high risk and not medically advisable.
- As with any cosmetic procedure, unrealistic expectations should be assessed; do not operate if they are present.
- Evaluate psychological and social issues of the patient, and learn why a face lift is wanted; if reason is unusual, do not operate.
- Contraindications for a face lift include smoking, obesity, skin disorders (such as Ehlers-Danlos), systemic medical problems such as diabetes, uncontrolled hypertension, history of angina.

### Intraoperative Considerations

- Have an exact plan of execution, with a sequence that makes sense for a given operative plan.
  - When to treat the neck and perform ancillary procedures such as fat grafting, blepharoplasty, and/or brow lift should be planned preoperatively.
- Time injection of local anesthetic with epinephrine to at least 10 minutes before incision so that you will not have to wait for effect.
- Careful management of blood pressure is important to keep a clean, relatively bloodless operative field.
  - Have strict guidelines on how to manage intraoperative hypertension, and discuss expectations with the person administering anesthesia.
- The face should not be dependent during surgery to prevent venous pooling.
- The patient's body should remain warm and covered.
- Hair should be washed, braided, or clustered with rubber bands before an incision is made.
- Face lift is performed with the patient in a recumbent position; the final vectors will have gravitational effects not realized in the operating room.

### Postoperative Management

- **Hematoma prevention** is the most important factor immediately after a face lift.
- The head of the bed must be elevated at all times to minimize swelling and edema.
- Strict **blood pressure control** is necessary (see below).
- All incisions, skin flap viability, and the presence of a hematoma must be evaluated on postoperative day 1.
- **Drains:** Neck drains should be used to collect large hematomas and prevent airway compromise and are usually removed on postoperative day 1 or 2, based on drainage.
- **Dressings:** Dressing should not be too tight, especially over the forehead and on undermined skin flaps. Not placing a dressing under the chin can allow monitoring for fluid collection in the neck.
- Small fluid collections can be aspirated with an 18- or 20-gauge needle.
- Hematomas and continued bleeding are treated by returning the patient to the operating room for an immediate evacuation procedure.
- Small hematomas or fluid collections beyond 3 or 4 days can also be treated with needle aspiration after the hematoma has liquefied.

## Hypertension Management[31]

- Systolic blood pressure control is maintained perioperatively to prevent hematoma.
- The goal of blood pressure maintenance is to keep systolic pressure <139 mm Hg.
- Chlorpromazine (Thorazine) (25 mg) 1 hour and 3 hours postoperatively can be very effective for rebound hypertension. This dose can be repeated at 4-hour intervals for up to 24 hours to keep systolic blood pressure <150 mm Hg.
- A clonidine (Catapres) patch (0.2 mg) can be placed for sustained intraoperative or postoperative hypertension.
- Clonidine 0.1-0.3 mg can be given before surgery to patients who are prone to hypertension.
- Alternatively, labetalol (Normodyne, Trandate) (5 mg/ml IV) can be given in 1-2 ml boluses, which will lower blood pressure for 1-2 hours.
- A calcium channel blocker (Hydralazine) can be given when heart rate is low (<65 beats/min).

# COMPLICATIONS

## Hematoma

- *Most common complication*
- Meticulous intraoperative hemostasis and adequate perioperative blood pressure control are the most important factors of prevention.
- The reported rate is about **2%-3% in female patients.**[61]
- **Males** have a higher reported rate of about **8%.**
- Incidence in men can be reduced to ~4% with careful attention to postoperative blood pressure control.[62]
- Increased incidence with:
  - Simultaneous open neck surgery
  - Patients taking platelet inhibitors such as NSAIDs
  - Hypertension in the postoperative period
  - The rebound effect of epinephrine wearing off postoperatively[63]
- Most likely to occur in the first 24 hours postoperatively.
- A randomized prospective trial and a meta-analysis review showed no statistically significant benefit to the use of tissue sealants such as fibrin glue.[64] There was, however, a strong trend toward reduction in postoperative drainage at 24 hours and ecchymosis.
- Drains do not prevent hematoma; however, they reduced the incidence of bruising in a prospective randomized trial.[65]
- Tumescent infiltration (200 ml per facial side) with no epinephrine reduced postoperative hematomas without significantly increasing wound bleeding or facial edema.[63]
- Dilutions as low as 1:800,000 have been shown to provide adequate hemostasis.[66]

## Sensory Nerve Injury[67]

- Sensory innervation of the face-lift skin flap is always damaged, and there is no attempt to preserve these small branches. The sensory disruption of the skin flap, however, is self-limited, usually resolving in 12 months.
- The great auricular nerve, is the *"most often recognized nerve injury"* after a face lift, with an incidence of up to 7%.

**NOTE: If the nerve is inadvertently cut during dissection, it is repaired primarily using magnification and fine sutures.**

- With unrecognized injury a painful neuroma may form, but this sequela is rare.

## Motor Nerve Injury[20]

- Nerve dysfunction in the first few hours after surgery is common and is attributable to the lingering effects of local anesthetic.
- The buccal branch is *most often injured* during a face lift, although long-term sequelae are rare because the buccal and zygomatic branches are multiple and interconnected.
- The reported incidence varies but is likely <1%.
- Paralysis from the marginal mandibular branch results in an inability to evert the lower lip, indicating mentalis paralysis.
- Platysma "pseudoparalysis" is an asymmetrical lower lip with a "full denture smile." It results from injury to the cervical branches innervating the platysma. Patients typically recover completely from this injury within 6 months.
- Very few permanent facial nerve injuries have been reported with sub-SMAS dissections.[19]

## Skin Slough and Necrosis[31]

- Subcutaneous dissection has higher rates of skin slough (4%) than sub-SMAS dissections (1%).
- Skin slough is often preceded by hematoma or infection and most commonly occurs in the **retroauricular region.**
- The incidence is significantly higher in patients with vascular occlusive disorders, particularly smokers.[68]
- Prevention: Avoid surgery on active smokers and do not place undue tension on the skin flap.

> **TIP:** If skin perfusion is questionable postoperatively, then release of skin sutures may be indicated to prevent loss of skin flaps. It is more practical to return to the operating room at a later date for scar revision than to lose a potentially devastating area of the facial skin flap.

- All areas of compromised skin perfusion should be kept moist with triple antibiotic ointment and impregnated gauze such as Xeroform.

## Infection[16]

- Infection is rare after face-lift surgery, reported to be <1%.[67]
- Infection after a face lift is most commonly associated with erythema in the neck, likely related to the less robust blood supply.
- Preauricular infections are often a result of otic canal *Pseudomonas aeruginosa* carriers.[69]
- Methicillin-resistant *Staphylococcus aureus* (MRSA) from nasal colonization is another source of infection.
  - Random testing has shown nasal carrier rates of 21.5% for methicillin-sensitive *S. aureus* (MSSA) and 5.6% for MRSA strains.[70]
- MRSA can be eradicated in nasal carriers by administration of topical mupirocin ointment for 7-10 days and chlorhexidine soap body washes for 5 days.[71]
- If infection is present, empiric antibiotic coverage should be initiated and cultures should be obtained with incision and drainage as necessary. Culture-specific antibiotics are then continued for 1-2 weeks.

## Hypertrophic Scars[39]

- Postauricular scar is most common, where the tension is often greatest.
- Intralesional steroids can be injected directly into scar tissue to reduce redness, itching, and discomfort.
- In general, it is preferable to wait at least 6 months and often a year after surgery to perform scar revision.

## Other Complications

- Prolonged edema, ecchymosis, and contour irregularities are relatively common complications but have been difficult to quantify.
- Parotid fistulas rarely occur and usually respond to aspiration, which can be repeated.
- Prolonged chronic pain, salivary cysts, and pigment changes have been reported but are rare.
- Postoperative thrombosis/pulmonary embolism: In a retrospective study of 126 patients, low-molecular-weight heparin prophylaxis resulted in a higher rate of postoperative bleeding at 16.2% versus 1.1% in the control group. No symptomatic thrombosis or pulmonary embolism was observed in the 89 control patients with the use of compression stockings and mobilization on the day of surgery only.[72]

## The 10 Most Frequent Complications After Rhytidectomy[67]

1. Hematoma (70% of all rhytidectomy complications)
2. Postoperative edema
3. Ecchymosis
4. Nerve injury
5. Unacceptable scarring (hypertrophic)
6. Skin slough
7. Seromas
8. Contour irregularities
9. Infection
10. Patient dissatisfaction

## STIGMATA OF FACE LIFTS AND THEIR PREVENTION[73]

- **An unnatural or "pulled" appearance**
  - Usually results from excessive tension on the skin layer or improper vectors of tension on the SMAS layer
  - Stigmata of face lift can include:
    - **Lateral sweep**
    - **Commissural distortion**
    - **Joker's lines**
    - **Smile blocks**
    - **Flattening of facial contours**
  - Most of these deformities are caused by the orientation, magnitude, and vector of pull.
  - Hamra[74] introduced the term "lateral sweep," caused by strong lateral pull in the lower face without treatment of the midface. This allows natural descent from aging over time to sag over the lateral pleat in the lower face.
  - Lambros and Stuzin[75] described "joker's line," which results from submalar hollowing that becomes accentuated by the rhytidectomy procedure. Prevention is by a more limited release of SMAS and skin, along with less vertical pull. Fat grafting to the area can also help.
  - Smile blocks have been described as hypodynamic cheek mounds that do not move appropriately with animation. Soft tissue augmentation has been suggested as a means of correction over the immobile area to create a smoother appearance.
  - Tension on the SMAS layer, not on the skin, helps prevent the pulled appearance.
  - Skin should be seen as providing a covering function, not a supporting one. It is inherently elastic but should not be expected to provide a sustained support for sagging, deeper facial tissues.
  - Tension on the SMAS should be uniform to prevent an abnormal facial appearance during animation.

- **Visible scars**
  - Visible scars are often too far anterior because of improper planning of incision placement.
  - Widened unfavorable scars are commonly caused by excessive tension on skin flaps.

> **TIP:** To best conceal scars they should (1) follow anatomic contours and (2) be free of tension.

- **Hairline distortion**
  - The sideburn, temporal hairline, and occipital hairline can be distorted with aggressive excision and/or poor incision planning.
  - The temporal hair should ideally be no more than 4-5 cm from the lateral orbit.
  - If preoperative assessment indicates that significant superolateral movement of the midfacial skin is expected, then a sideburn component of the incision should be planned.
  - Prevent significant step-offs in the occipital hairline. One option is a prehairline incision down the occipital scalp; however, this can become visible.
- **Alopecia**
  - Primarily caused by injury to the hair follicles either from cautery or excessive tension that inhibits blood supply.
  - Focal hair transplantation can be performed for persistent deformities.
- **Tragal deformities**
  - Characterized as blunting of the pretragal depression, anterior displacement, excessive fullness, and/or hair growth of the tragus.
  - Blunting and anterior displacement can occur from excessive tension on skin closure, or because the incision was not placed precisely at the tragal border.
  - Prevent excessive fullness and retained cheek skin hair by defatting the thicker cheek skin and disrupting the hair follicles before redraping.
- **"Pixie ear" deformity**
  - Characterized by **inferior migration and axis distortion of the lobule.**
  - To best prevent this deformity, do not place tension on the lobule, and transfer caudal forces to postauricular fascia and skin.
    - Divide excess portion of SMAS flap, transpose it posteriorly, and attach it to mastoid fascia to brace the ear.
- **Contour irregularities**
  - Irregularity in skin flap thickness, buccal fat pseudoherniation, submandibular gland ptosis, or digastric muscle hypertrophy can lead to a contour irregularity.

## SECONDARY FACE LIFTS[73]

- Patients may seek secondary face lifts to treat the natural aging process, an unfavorable result (as listed above), or a combination of the two.
- The average duration between the primary and secondary face lift in a large series was 9 years.[76]
- A significant number of patients will have developed new medical conditions and/or started new medications between their first and second face lift; therefore a thorough preoperative medical evaluation is imperative.
- Preexisting deficits in sensation and facial animation must be identified and documented thoroughly.
- Though it is prudent to obtain the surgical report from the patient's previous operation, it often is not available.

- The SMAS layer has been found to be thinner in secondary face lift.
- Typically less skin can be excised.
- Scarring of the tissue planes increases complexity and concern for facial nerve injury.
- The skin flap may be more robust in terms of blood supply because of the delay phenomenon from previous elevation.
- Pay particular attention to the stigmata of face lifts (listed above) so that they can be treated and prevented during the secondary procedure.

## KEY POINTS

- ✓ No single technique has been proven to provide a consistently superior result or treat all varieties of facial aging.
- ✓ Aging is characterized by soft tissue descent, volumetric redistribution, and skin changes.
- ✓ Resurfacing techniques such as laser or chemical peel should be considered for the treatment of aging skin.
- ✓ Prevent facial nerve injury by always being exceedingly cautious in facial danger zones and in depth of dissection plane.
- ✓ Pitanguy's line is from 0.5 cm below the tragus to 1.5 cm above the lateral brow; it traces the route of the frontal branch.
- ✓ To test the marginal mandibular branch and distinguish it from the cervical branch of the facial nerve, ask the patient to evert the lower lip.
- ✓ The platsyma and its innervation (cervical branch) are responsible for lowering the lower lip in full denture smile.
- ✓ Systolic blood pressure control is important to maintain perioperatively to minimize the risk for hematoma.
- ✓ The upper portion of the nasolabial fold is one of the hardest structures to recontour and is nearly impossible to obliterate.
- ✓ Fat grafting into the facial fat compartments should be considered to help restore a youthful shape in areas that have lost volume.
- ✓ The average duration between the primary and secondary face lift in a large series was 9 years.[75]

## REFERENCES


1. Nahai F, ed. The Art of Aesthetic Surgery: Principles & Techniques. St Louis: Quality Medical Publishing, 2005.
2. Gosain AK, Yousif NJ, Madiego G, et al. Surgical anatomy of the SMAS: a reinvestigation. Plast Reconstr Surg 92:1254-1263; discussion 1264-1265, 1993.
3. Mitz V, Peyronie M. The superficial musculo-aponeurotic system (SMAS) in the parotid and cheek area. Plast Reconstr Surg 58:80-88, 1976.
4. Stuzin JM, Baker TJ, Gordon HL. The relationship of the superficial and deep facial fascias: relevance to rhytidectomy and aging. Plast Reconstr Surg 89:441-449; discussion 450-451, 1992.
5. Trussler AP, Stephan P, Hatef D, et al. The frontal branch of the facial nerve across the zygomatic arch: anatomical relevance of the high-SMAS technique. Plast Reconstr Surg 125:1221-1229, 2010.
6. Raskin E, Latrenta GS. Why do we age in our cheeks? Aesthet Surg J 27:19-28, 2007.
7. Rohrich RJ, Pessa JE. The fat compartments of the face: anatomy and clinical implications for cosmetic surgery. Plast Reconstr Surg 119:2219-2227, 2007.
8. Furnas DW. The retaining ligaments of the cheek. Plast Reconstr Surg 83:11-16, 1989.

9. Rohrich RJ, Arbique GM, Wong C, et al. The anatomy of suborbicularis fat: implications for periorbital rejuvenation. Plast Reconstr Surg 124:946-951, 2009.
10. Owsley JQ. Lifting the malar fat pad for correction of prominent nasolabial folds. Plast Reconstr Surg 91:463-474; discussion 475-476, 1993.
11. Dubin B, Jackson IT, Halim A, et al. Anatomy of the buccal fat pad and its clinical significance. Plast Reconstr Surg 83:257-264, 1989.
12. Bosse JP, Papillon J. Surgical anatomy of the SMAS and the malar region. In Transactions of the Ninth International Congress of Plastic Reconstructive Surgery. New York: McGraw-Hill, 1987.
13. Rohrich RJ, Pessa JE. The retaining system of the face: histologic evaluation of the septal boundaries of the subcutaneous fat compartments. Plast Reconstr Surg 121:1804-1809, 2008.
14. Knize DM. An anatomically based study of the mechanism of eyebrow ptosis. Plast Reconstr Surg 97:1321-1333, 1996.
15. Mendelson BC, Muzaffar AR, Adams WP Jr. Surgical anatomy of the midcheek and malar mounds. Plast Reconstr Surg 110:885-896; discussion 897-911, 2002.
16. Moss JC, Mendelson BC, Taylor GI. Surgical anatomy of the ligamentous attachments in the temple and periorbital regions. Plast Reconstr Surg 105:1475-1490, 2000.
17. Muzaffar AR, Mendelson BC, Adams WP Jr. Surgical anatomy of the ligamentous attachments of the lower lid and lateral canthus. Plast Reconstr Surg 110:873-884; discussion 897-911, 2002.
18. Owsley JQ Jr. Platysma-fascial rhytidectomy: a preliminary report. Plast Reconstr Surg 60:843-850, 1977.
19. Barton FE Jr. Aesthetic surgery of the face and neck. Aesthet Surg J 29:449-463, 2009.
20. Baker DC, Conley J. Avoiding facial nerve injuries in rhytidectomy. Anatomical variations and pitfalls. Plast Reconstr Surg 64:781-795, 1979.
21. Stuzin JM, Wagstrom L, Kawamoto HK, et al. Anatomy of the frontal branch of the facial nerve: the significance of the temporal fat pad. Plast Reconstr Surg 83:265-271, 1989.
22. Pitanguy I, Ramos AS. The frontal branch of the facial nerve: the importance of its variations in face lifting. Plast Reconstr Surg 38:352-356, 1966.
23. Conley J, Baker DC, Selfe RW. Paralysis of the mandibular branch of the facial nerve. Plast Reconstr Surg 70:569-577, 1982.
24. Chowdhry S, Yoder EM, Cooperman RD, et al. Locating the cervical motor branch of the facial nerve: anatomy and clinical application. Plast Reconstr Surg 126:875-879, 2010.
25. Ellenbogen R. Pseudo-paralysis of the mandibular branch of the facial nerve after platysmal face-lift operation. Plast Reconstr Surg 63:364-368, 1979.
26. Daane SP, Owsley JQ. Incidence of cervical branch injury with "marginal mandibular nerve pseudo-paralysis" in patients undergoing face lift. Plast Reconstr Surg 111:2414-2418, 2003.
27. Seckel BR, ed. Facial Danger Zones: Avoiding Nerve Injury in Facial Plastic Surgery. St Louis: Quality Medical Publishing, 1994.
28. Blackwell KE, Landman MD, Calcaterra TC. Spinal accessory nerve palsy: an unusual complication of rhytidectomy. Head Neck 16:181-185, 1994.
29. Millett PJ, Romero A, Braun S. Spinal accessory nerve injury after rhytidectomy (face lift): a case report. J Shoulder Elbow Surg 18:e15-e17, 2009.
30. Khavkin J, Ellis DA. Aging skin: histology, physiology, and pathology. Facial Plast Surg Clin North Am 19:229-234, 2011.
31. Gonyon DL Jr, Barton FE Jr. The aging face: rhytidectomy and adjunctive procedures. Sel Read Plast Surg 11, 2012.
32. Coleman SR. Facial recontouring with lipostructure. Clin Plast Surg 24:347-367, 1997.
33. Lambros V. Observations on periorbital and midface aging. Plast Reconstr Surg 120:1367-1376, 2007.
34. Lambros V. Models of facial aging and implications for treatment. Clin Plast Surg 35:319-327; discussion 317, 2008.

35. Rohrich RJ, Pessa JE, Ristow B. The youthful cheek and the deep medial fat compartment. Plast Reconstr Surg 121:2107-2112, 2008.
36. Little JW. Three-dimensional rejuvenation of the midface: volumetric resculpture by malar imbrication. Plast Reconstr Surg 105:267-285; discussion 286-289, 2000.
37. Little JW. Volumetric perceptions in midfacial aging with altered priorities for rejuvenation. Plast Reconstr Surg 105:252-266; discussion 286-289, 2000.
38. Stuzin JM. Restoring facial shape in face lifting: the role of skeletal support in facial analysis and midface soft-tissue repositioning. Plast Reconstr Surg 119:362-376; discussion 377-378, 2007.
39. Warren RJ, Aston SJ, Mendelson BC. Face lift. Plast Reconstr Surg 128:747e-764e, 2011.
40. Jelks GW, Glat PM, Jelks EB, et al. The inferior retinacular lateral canthoplasty: a new technique. Plast Reconstr Surg 100:1262-1270; discussion 1271-1275, 1997.
41. Rohrich RJ, Ghavami A, Lemmon JA, et al. The individualized component face lift: developing a systematic approach to facial rejuvenation. Plast Reconstr Surg 123:1050-1063, 2009.
42. Hoefflin SM. The extended supraplatysmal plane (ESP) face lift. Plast Reconstr Surg 101:494-503, 1998.
43. Tonnard PL, Verpaele AM, eds. The MACS-Lift: Short-Scar Rhytidectomy. St Louis: Quality Medical Publishing, 2004.
44. Baker DC. Minimal incision rhytidectomy (short scar face lift) with lateral SMASectomy. Aesthet Surg J 21:68-79, 2001.
45. Skoog T, ed. Plastic Surgery: New Methods and Refinements. Philadelphia: WB Saunders, 1974.
46. Barton FE Jr. The SMAS and the nasolabial fold. Plast Reconstr Surg 89:1054-1057; discussion 1058-1059, 1992.
47. Barton FE Jr. Rhytidectomy and the nasolabial fold. Plast Reconstr Surg 90:601-607, 1992.
48. Hamra ST. Composite rhytidectomy. Plast Reconstr Surg 90:1-13, 1992.
49. Hamra ST. Repositioning the orbicularis oculi muscle in the composite rhytidectomy. Plast Reconstr Surg 90:14-22, 1992.
50. Hamra ST. Arcus marginalis release and orbital fat preservation in midface rejuvenation. Plast Reconstr Surg 96:354-362, 1995.
51. Hamra ST. Prevention and correction of the "face-lifted" appearance. Facial Plast Surg 16:215-229, 2000.
52. Stuzin JM, Baker TJ, Baker TM. Refinements in face lifting: enhanced facial contour using vicryl mesh incorporated into SMAS fixation. Plast Reconstr Surg 105:290-301, 2000.
53. Pitman GH. Foundation face lift. In Nahai F, ed. The Art of Aesthetic Surgery: Principles & Techniques. St Louis: Quality Medical Publishing, 2005.
54. Tessier P. [Subperiosteal face-lift] Ann Chir Plast Esthet 34:193-197, 1989.
55. Byrd HS, Andochick SE. The deep temporal lift: a multiplanar, lateral brow, temporal, and upper face lift. Plast Reconstr Surg 97:928-937, 1996.
56. Hunt JA, Byrd HS. The deep temporal lift: a multiplanar lateral brow, temporal, and upper face lift. Plast Reconstr Surg 110:1793-1796, 2002.
57. Seify H, Jones G, Bostwick J, et al. Endoscopic-assisted face lift: review of 200 cases. Ann Plast Surg 52:234-239, 2004.
58. Pessa JE, Brown F. Independent effect of various facial mimetic muscles on the nasolabial fold. Aesthetic Plast Surg 16:167-171, 1992.
59. Pessa JE, Garza JR. The malar septum: the anatomic basis of malar mounds and malar edema. Aesthet Surg J 17:11-17, 1997.
60. Yousif NJ, Gosain A, Matloub HS, et al. The nasolabial fold: an anatomic and histologic reappraisal. Plast Reconstr Surg 93:60-69, 1994.
61. Baker DC, Aston SJ, Guy CL, et al. The male rhytidectomy. Plast Reconstr Surg 60:514-522, 1977.

62. Baker DC, Stefani WA, Chiu ES. Reducing the incidence of hematoma requiring surgical evacuation following male rhytidectomy: a 30-year review of 985 cases. Plast Reconstr Surg 116:1973-1985; discussion 1986-1987, 2005.
63. Jones BM, Grover R. Avoiding hematoma in cervicofacial rhytidectomy: a personal 8-year quest. Reviewing 910 patients. Plast Reconstr Surg 113:381-387; discussion 388-390, 2004.
64. Por YC, Shi L, Samuel M, et al. Use of tissue sealants in face-lifts: a metaanalysis. Aesthetic Plast Surg 33:336-339, 2009.
65. Jones BM, Grover R, Hamilton S. The efficacy of surgical drainage in cervicofacial rhytidectomy: a prospective, randomized, controlled trial. Plast Reconstr Surg 120:263-270, 2007.
66. Siegel RJ, Vistnes LM, Iverson RE. Effective hemostasis with less epinephrine. An experimental and clinical study. Plast Reconstr Surg 51:129-133, 1973.
67. Stuzin JM. MOC-PSSM CME article: face lifting. Plast Reconstr Surg 121:1-19, 2008.
68. Riefkohl R, Wolfe JA, Cox EB, et al. Association between cutaneous occlusive vascular disease, cigarette smoking, and skin slough after rhytidectomy. Plast Reconstr Surg 77:592-595, 1986.
69. Roland PS, Stroman DW. Microbiology of acute otitis externa. Laryngoscope 112:1166-1177, 2002.
70. Lindeque B, Rutigliano J, Williams A, et al. Prevalence of methicillin-resistant Staphylococcus aureus among orthopedic patients at a large academic hospital. Orthopedics 31:363, 2008.
71. Ammerlaan HS, Kluytmans JA, Wertheim HF, et al. Eradication of methicillin-resistant Staphylococcus aureus carriage: a systematic review. Clin Infect Dis 48:922-930, 2009.
72. Durnig P, Jungwirth W. Low-molecular-weight heparin and postoperative bleeding in rhytidectomy. Plast Reconstr Surg 118:502-507; discussion 508-509, 2006.
73. Rasko YM, Beale E, Rohrich RJ. Secondary rhytidectomy: comprehensive review and current concepts. Plast Reconstr Surg 130:1370-1378, 2012.
74. Hamra ST. Frequent facelift sequelae: hollow eyes and the lateral sweep: cause and repair. Plast Reconstr Surg 102:1658-1665, 1998.
75. Lambros V, Stuzin JM. The cross-cheek depression: surgical cause and effect in the development of the "joker line" and its treatment. Plast Reconstr Surg 122:1543-1552, 2008.
76. Beale EW, Rasko Y, Rohrich RJ. A 20-year experience with secondary rhytidectomy: a review of technique, longevity and outcomes. Plast Reconstr Surg 131:625-634, 2012.

# 95. Neck Lift

**Ricardo A. Meade, Trang Q. Nguyen, Deana S. Shenaq**

## ANATOMY[1]

### SKIN

- Evaluate the neck for cervical rhytids and skin excess.
- Amount of fat in the subcutaneous layer varies between the skin and the platysma muscle (Fig. 95-1).
- Additional fatty tissue may be found in the interplatysmal submental region.
- Although a fatty layer maintains the soft appearance of the neck, it may be molded to help address contours.
- The **anterior jugular veins** course within the fatty layer and should be respected when working in the deep interplatysmal area. Other veins of significant caliber can present difficulties if dissection is made in the wrong plane (Fig. 95-2).

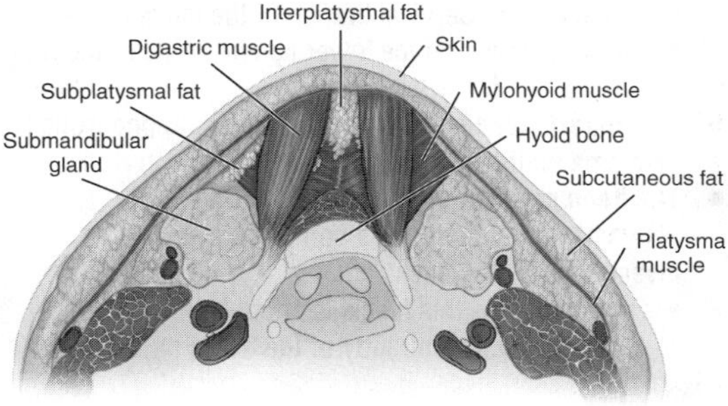

**Fig. 95-1** Practical anatomy of the neck.

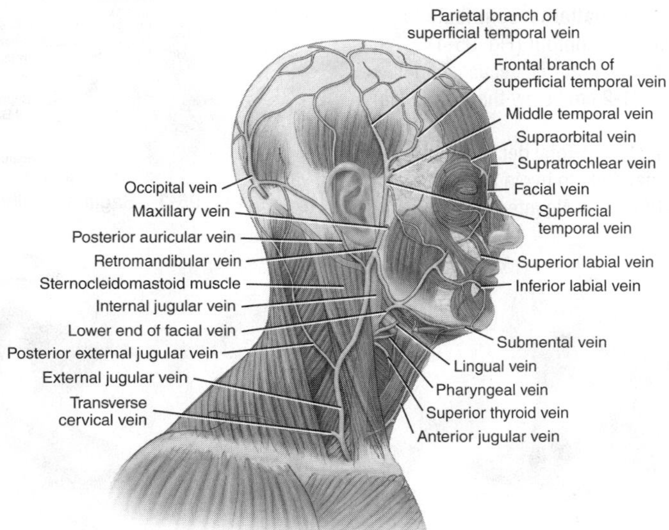


**Fig. 95-2** Venous anatomy.

## MUSCLE

- The **platysma** is a broad, thin muscle that spans the neck and is a key instrument for controlling neck contour.
  - **Origin:** Pectoralis and deltoid muscle fascia
  - **Insertion**
    - **Anterior fibers:** Symphysis of the mandible and slightly laterally
    - **Posterior fibers:** Cross the mandible and insert into the superficial musculoaponeurotic system (SMAS)
  - **Blood supply**
    - Major: Branch of the submental artery
    - Minor: Branch of the suprasternal artery
  - **Innervation:** Cervical branch of the facial nerve
  - **Action:** Draws on the lower lip and angle of the mouth causing oblique wrinkling of the skin of the neck[2]
- The **superficial cervical fascia** is a thin, aponeurotic lamina that immediately covers the platysma on its surface.
- The **deep cervical fascia** lies under the platysma and constitutes a complete investment for the neck.
  - In the midline this fascia is attached to the symphysis and body of the hyoid bone.
  - It divides laterally to enclose the sternocleidomastoid (SCM) muscle, and the investing portion is attached to the ligamentum nuchae and to C7[3] (Fig. 95-3).
- Three classic platysmal **decussation and interdigitation patterns**[4] contribute to submental neck contour (Fig. 95-4).
  - **Type I** (75%): Partial decussation in midline (1-2 cm below the mandibular symphysis)
  - **Type II** (15%): Total decussation from mandible to hyoid bone
  - **Type III** (10%): No interdigitation

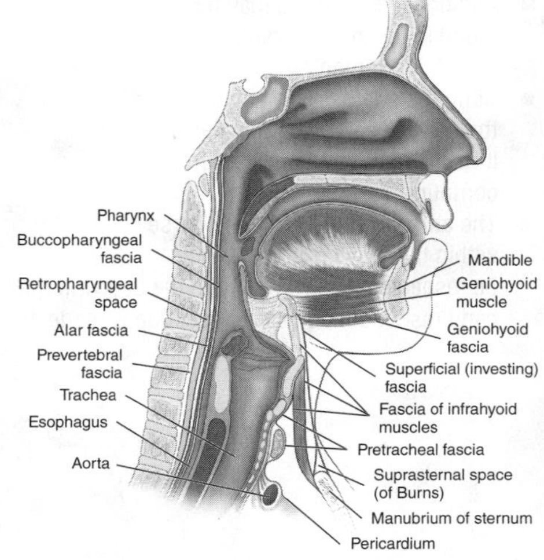


**Fig. 95-3** Sagittal section.

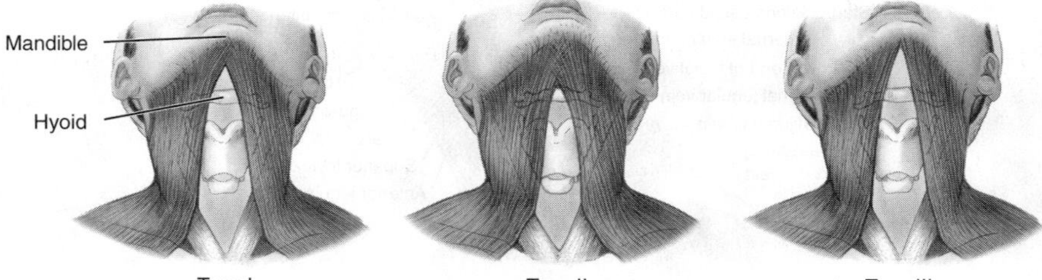


**Fig. 95-4**

**NOTE: Midline decussation creates a supportive sling. When decussation is absent, free medial muscle edges fall away, creating vertical bands.**

## NERVES

- **Inframaxillary** or **cervical nerve branches**
  - Run beneath the platysma across the side of the neck over the suprahyoid region
- **Marginal mandibular nerve**
  - Located at the tail of the parotid in a subplatysmal plane.
  - Posterior to the facial artery, it runs above the inferior border of the mandible (81%) or up to 1 cm below it (19%).[5]
  - Anterior to the facial artery, all of the branches are above the inferior border of the mandible.
  - It innervates the **depressor anguli oris, depressor labii inferioris, mentalis,** part of the **orbicularis oris,** and **risorius.**[3,6]
  - Danger zone is usually a 2 cm radius circle located 2 cm posterior to the oral commissure[7] (Fig. 95-5).

**TIP:** Exercise caution with electrocautery in this zone, because current can be conducted to the nerve.

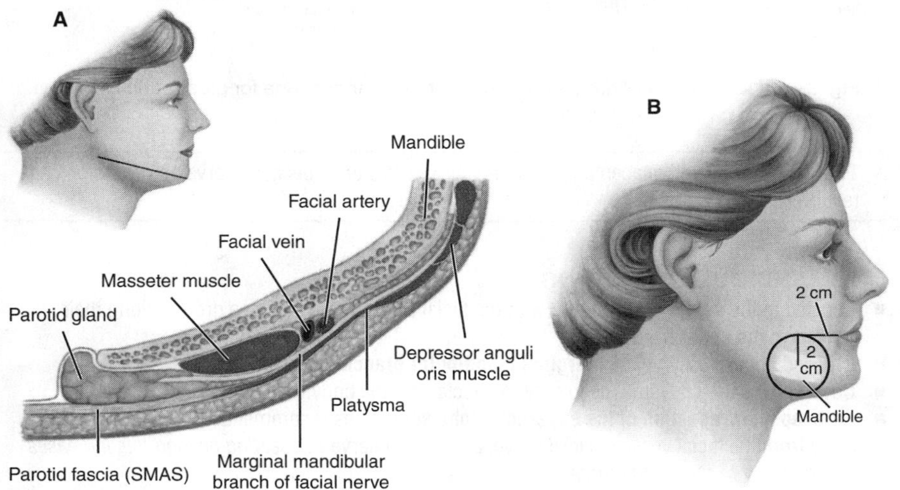


**Fig. 95-5** **A,** Anatomy of the marginal mandibular nerve. **B,** Danger zone for marginal mandibular nerve is a 2 cm radius circle located 2 cm posterior to the oral commissure.

- Great auricular nerve (GAN) (Fig. 95-6)[7]
  - Danger zone is located in 3 cm radius circle dropped 6.5 cm inferior to external auditory canal (EAC) on midpoint of SCM.
  - Emergence of GAN is beneath SCM, 9 cm below EAC.
  - Injury can result in paresthesia/anesthesia of lower 2/3 of ear and adjacent neck/cheek skin.

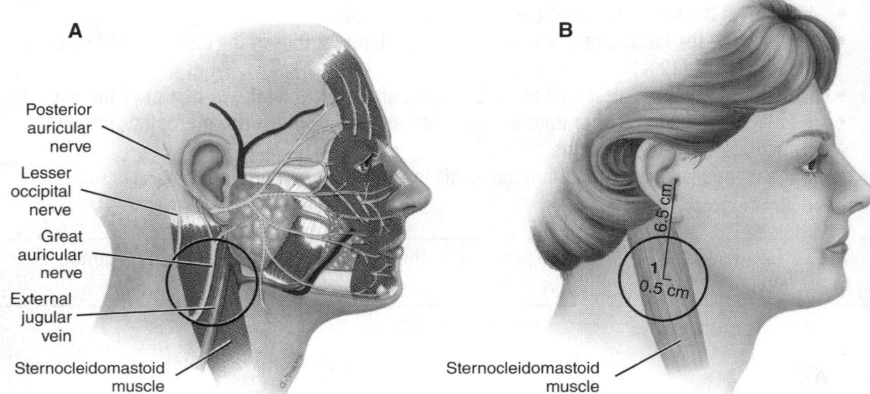


**Fig. 95-6** **A,** Anatomy of great auricular nerve. **B,** Danger zone for great auricular nerve.

**TIP:** Be careful with placement of sutures in/over this area, because nerve compression can result.

## Submandibular Glands

- Located in the **submental triangle** with the facial artery embedded in a groove along their posterior and upper border
- Crossed superficially by the **marginal mandibular branch** of the facial nerve
- Covered by skin, platysma, deep cervical fascia, and the body of the lower jaw
- **Intracapsular resection of the superficial lobe** sometimes recommended, because it is well away from the facial vessels, facial nerve, and lingual nerve *(dissecting beyond this increases risk of injury to these structures).*

## Digastric Muscles

- Each muscle consists of **two muscles** joined by a tendon, forming the **submental triangle.**
  - The **posterior muscle,** the longer of the two, courses from the mastoid process on the temporal bone downward, forward, and medially.
    - **Innervation:** CN VII
  - The **anterior muscle** courses near the symphysis, down and posteriorly.
    - **Innervation:** CN V
  - Both bellies terminate in the **central tendon.**[6]

## RETAINING LIGAMENTS (Fig. 95-7)

- Fascial condensations create adherences between the SMAS, platysma, and overlying dermis to underlying muscular and osseous structures.
- They help support facial soft tissues in their normal location. As these attenuate, the stigmata of aging appear.
- Four ligaments: **Zygomatic, mandibular, masseteric-cutaneous, platysma-auricular**
- **Zygomatic** and **mandibular** ligaments are examples of true osteocutaneous ligaments. (They extend from bone to overlying skin.)
- Mandibular ligaments lie in the parasymphyseal region of the mandible, lateral to the chin pad, and delineate the anterior border of the jowl.
- **Platysma-auricular** ligaments serve as a surgical guide to the posterosuperior platysmal border, an anchoring location in many suspension techniques.

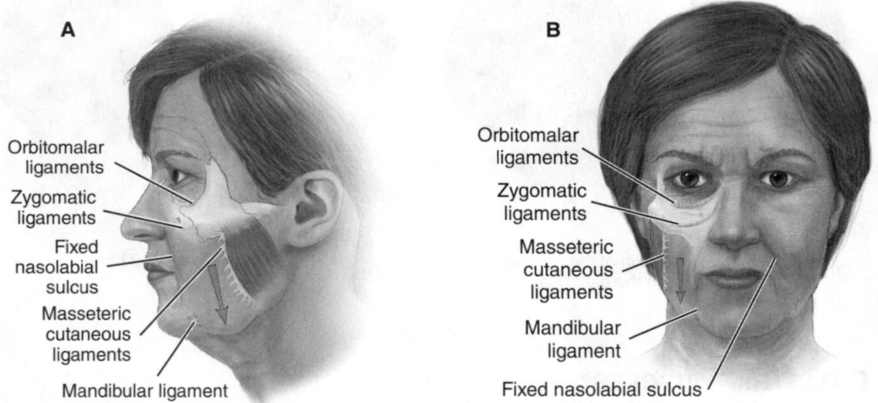


**Fig. 95-7 A,** Lateral and **B,** AP views of retaining ligaments of the face.

# PREOPERATIVE ASSESSMENT

## SKIN

- Skin quality, with rhytids **at rest** and **during animation,** must be evaluated in detail.
- Skin excess may suggest elasticity of the skin, or lack thereof.
- The quality of skin elasticity is inversely related to the length of incision required.
  - Normal skin elasticity is essential for all short-scar procedures.
  - Skin damage and actinic changes alone require a full-length retroauricular incision because of the increased need to redrape.
- Evaluation of skin excess can help determine which direction to redrape the skin flap. Hairline distortion is unacceptable after rhytidectomy.
  - The direction of pull is slightly cephalad and mostly lateral. This vector is parallel to the cervical creases.
- **Apparent** skin excess redrapes after neck contouring. **Real** skin excess usually extends below the thyroid cartilage and posteriorly beyond the SCM.

## FAT

- Evaluate for **subcutaneous** and **preplatysmal** fat.
- Differentiate this from **subplatysmal** fatty excess by pinching the submental area at rest and then after contraction of the platysma muscles.
- Displaced facial fat can contribute to ptotic jowls and loss of definition of inferior mandibular border, which results from platysmal laxity and mandibular ligament attenuation.

## PLATYSMA[8] (Fig. 95-8)

- Look for static or dynamic banding of the platysma.
- Evaluate imperfections in the neck and jaw shadows.
- Assess the neck-face interface to determine how facial soft tissue ptosis affects the jawline.

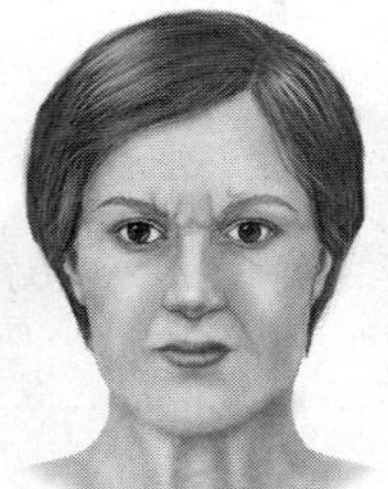
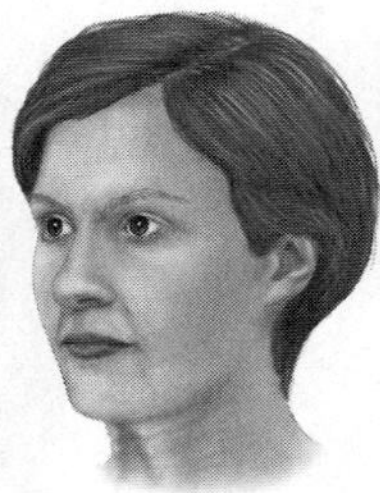

Evaluation of excess skin of the neck and platysmal bands with the patient at rest

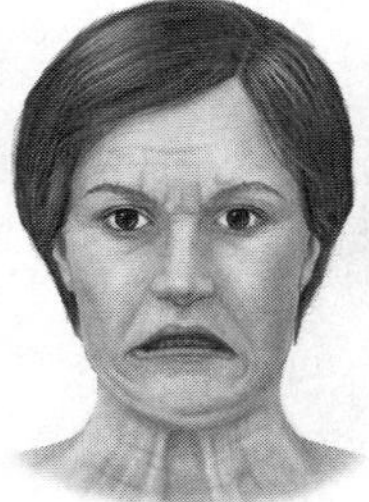
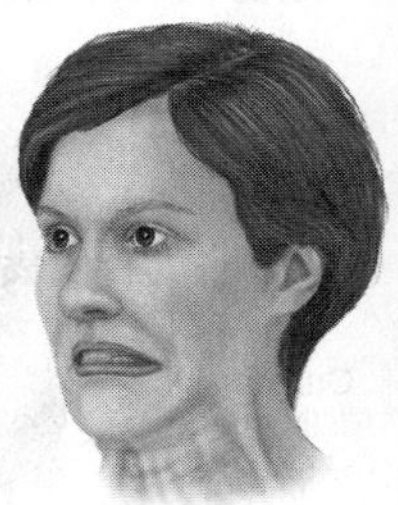

Evaluation of platysmal bands on animation

**Fig. 95-8**

## DIGASTRIC MUSCLES[9]

- These bulge below the inferior border of the mandible.

> **TIP:** Persistent bulging after fat removal from the neck is often caused by prominence of the digastric muscles.

## SUBMANDIBULAR GLAND

- Evaluate for submandibular gland ptosis. Prominent glands should be brought to the patient's attention preoperatively.
- Look for a bulge below the mandibular rim within the submandibular triangle.

> **TIP:** It can be helpful to accentuate this deformity by having the patient flex his or her neck.

## MANDIBULOCUTANEOUS LIGAMENT

- Tethering of the relaxing facial tissues at this ligament produces the appearance of **jowls.**
- Feel the volume of jowling tissue with the patient in a supine position to evaluate the need for liposuction of the fat pad or simple tightening of the SMAS-platysma laterally.

## CHIN

- Assess the projection of the chin relative to all facial proportions.

**TIP:** An alloplastic chin implant or osseous genioplasty may complement neck contours.

## VISUAL CRITERIA OF A YOUTHFUL NECK[10,11] (Fig. 95-9)

- Distinct inferior mandibular border
- Visible subhyoid depression
- Visible thyroid cartilage bulge
- Visible anterior border of the SCM muscle
- Cervicomental angle of 105-120 degrees

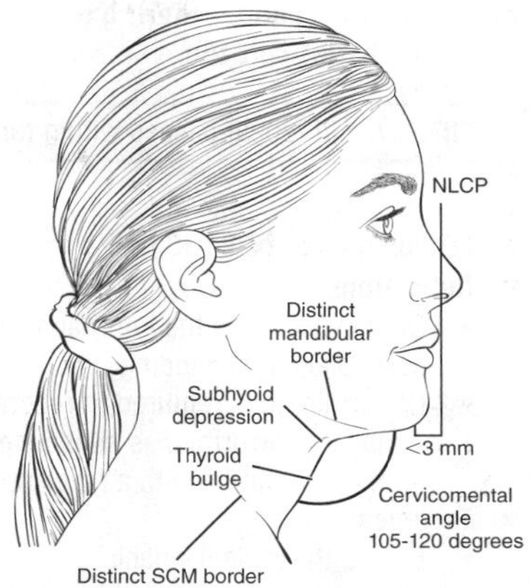


**Fig. 95-9** Visual criteria for a youthful neck. (*NLCP,* Nose-lip-chin plane; *SCM,* sternocleidomastoid.)

## OPTIONS FOR NECK REJUVENATION

### PROCEDURES

- **Options to address superficial, intermediate, and deep tissues**
  - **Superficial tissues:** Skin and subcutaneous fat
  - **Intermediate tissues:** Platysma, fat lying between the two muscles, lymph nodes
  - **Deep tissues:** Subplatysmal fat, digastric muscles, submandibular glands, suprahyoid fascia
- **Surgical approaches**
  - Suction lipectomy only
  - Submental cervicoplasty
  - Short-scar face lift without submental incision (lateral pull)
  - Short-scar face lift with submental incision (direct view)
  - Full-scar face lift without submental incision (lateral pull)
  - Full-scar face lift with submental incision (direct view)

### LIPOSUCTION ALONE

- **Indications**
  - Young patients
  - Good dermal quality
  - Localized fat
- **Technical tips**
  - Incision is made in submental neck area and/or behind earlobes.
  - 2-3 mm single-hole cannula is recommended for suction-assisted liposuction (SAL).
  - 50% energy ultrasound-assisted lipectomy (UAL) with a 2 mm solid probe for no longer than 2-3 minutes is recommended, if using UAL.
  - No drains are required if it is the sole procedure.
  - A compression garment is used.

**TIP:** Small quantities of aspirate can create big differences.

**NOTE: After suctioning the neck, platysmal banding that may have been present only on animation or other underlying irregularities may become evident.**

**CAUTION: Avoid oversuctioning. Leave 3-5 mm of fat on the skin to give it a soft contour and prevent scarring and tethering to the underlying platysma. Excessive fat removal is a common error that is difficult to reverse.**

**TIP:** Avoid repeat passes within tunnels. Make crisscross strokes.

## Submental Neck Lift[12]

- **Indications**
  - Direct viewing of the internal neck anatomy is indicated by findings from neck examination (e.g., platysmal banding).
  - Undermining is required to recontour the neck.
  - It may be performed as an isolated procedure for recontouring the submental area and neck or in combination with a face lift.
- **Technical tips**
  - Extend the patient's neck.
  - Make incision just posterior to the submental crease to prevent scarring that may deepen crease.
  - Release the crease anteriorly from underlying tissues.
  - **Interplatysmal or subplatysmal fat excision** may be performed in addition to subcutaneous defatting. If a lymph node is seen in this fatty layer, include it in the resection. Leave adequate subcutaneous fat to prevent a submental depression.
  - The mandibular ligaments can be released as the dissection is continued forward and laterally.
  - Tangential (partial) resection of the anterior belly of the digastric muscles can be performed through this incision.[9] Use a hemostat to partially divide it halfway through the thickness of the muscle.
  - Piecemeal intracapsular submandibular gland resection can be considered with this approach.

**CAUTION: Be sure to discuss complications with the patient (i.e., increased risk of bleeding, nerve injury, dry mouth, or salivary fistula).**

- ▸ If the submandibular gland is removed partially, a drain is usually placed deep to the platysma after layered closure.

**NOTE: Necessity of digastric muscle or submandibular gland resection has not achieved general acceptance among surgeons because of risks and complications. Some have advocated for more conservative maneuvers such as suspension sutures or platysmal suturing to support the ptotic submandibular gland[13-15]**

## Short-Scar Face and Neck Lift[16] (see Chapter 94)

- **Indications**
  - No excess neck skin
  - Presence of jowling
  - Aged neck-face interface
- **Technical tips**
  - Technique involves prehairline incision below the sideburn and a preauricular intratragal incision around the earlobe.

- Neck recontouring through a submental approach or liposuction may be performed at the same time.
- Skin flap is elevated, extending to the posterior border of SCM.
- An SMAS-platysma flap is then dissected and pulled up in the face and posteriorly in the neck.
- Lateral plication is performed to further define the neck.

### Full-Scar Face and Neck Lift

- **Indications**
  - Patients with aging changes in the face and neck, with inelastic and excess lower and posterior neck skin
- **Technical tips**
  - Incision is retroauricular around the earlobe up to the level of the tragus or higher and across into the occipital hairline, which allows more skin excision in patients with significant excess.
  - First align the hairline, then remove the excess skin.
  - Close the retroauricular sulcus with three-point suture technique, incorporating the deep fascia to prevent migration of the scar.

## NONOPERATIVE TECHNIQUES

- **Injection with botulinum toxin**[17,18]
  - This is a good nonsurgical intervention for patients with prominent platysmal bands but little or no skin excess, patients who are not surgical candidates, or patients with recurrent platysmal bands after prior neck rejuvenation.
  - 5-100 units of neurotoxin is injected per band.
  - Grasp platysma between fingers and inject toxin at 1 cm intervals.
  - Complications include dysphagia at high doses, edema, ecchymosis, neck discomfort, and weakness.

## OPERATIVE TECHNIQUES

### Skin Flap Procedures

- In general, a **vertical vector** of pull is required for a youthful, harmonious lift of the neck.
- A **posterior and diagonal vector** is required when using a **retroauricular approach.**
- Management of neck skin differs from management of facial skin. Often, neck skin need not be excised, because it will redrape and redistribute to provide excellent results.
  - If excision is necessary, consider retroauricular incision or hairline incision according to the amount to be removed.
- Cronin and Biggs[19] excised excess skin in the severe "turkey gobbler" neck deformity using a **T-Z incision,** restoring a youthful contour to the cervical angle.
  - The scarring that results is only occasionally acceptable in men who present with a generous redundancy of skin.
  - It may be appropriate for older patients willing to accept scar trade-off for a less involved operation and faster recovery.[20]

**TIP:** This has become a particularly popular option for patients who have experienced massive weight loss.

## Platysmal Procedures

- The platysma may be imbricated, plicated, incised, lengthened, or suspended.[9,21]
  - Once platysmal diastasis is plicated, surrounding skin is recruited toward midline. Tethered areas must be released from their attachments to platysmal fascia.
- **Platysmal flap cervical rhytidoplasty**[21]
  - Sectional myotomy of the medial edge of platysma allows lateral rotation and advancement of flap edges.
  - Suture flaps to mastoid fascia laterally to avoid recurrence of vertical banding.
  - Consider thyroid cartilage's capability for masculinization of the neck when performing a myotomy. Some describe controlling the effect by performing platysmal transection above or below the cartilage to camouflage or accentuate it.
- **Suspension sutures** (Fig. 95-10)
  - Suspension sutures running along the inferior border of the mandible over superficial fascia on platysma can help define jawline.
  - Sutures are interlocked at midline and tacked to mastoid fascia, as described by Guerrero-Santos[22] and later popularized by Giampapa and Di Bernardo.[23]
  - Suspension sutures can be used to define the jaw line, support enlarged or prolapsed submandibular glands, and enhance neck-jaw angle, though long-term results may not be maintained.[23,24]
  - Modification of suspension suture includes horizontal plication of platysma below the submandibular gland to further correct contour deformity caused by the gland.[23]

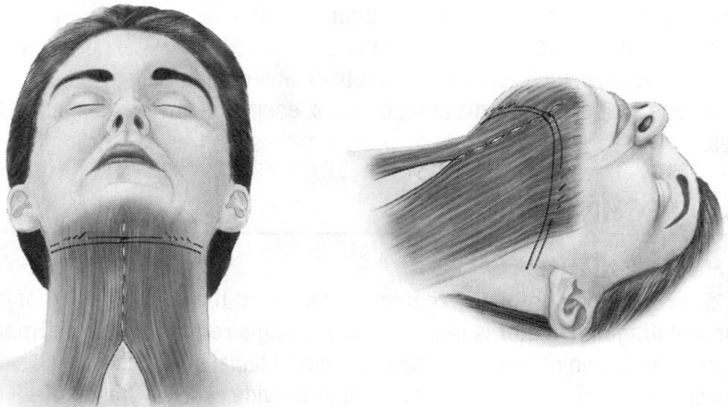

**Fig. 95-10** Suspension sutures, interlocked at midline, run along the inferior mandibular border.

- **Platysma muscle sling**[9] (Fig. 95-11)
  - A sling is made by dividing the platysma horizontally across the entire width.
  - A wide gap is created that is potentially visible.
  - Retraction of the platysma superiorly results in the *window-shading* effect, which has diminished the popularity of this method of treating vertical banding.[14]

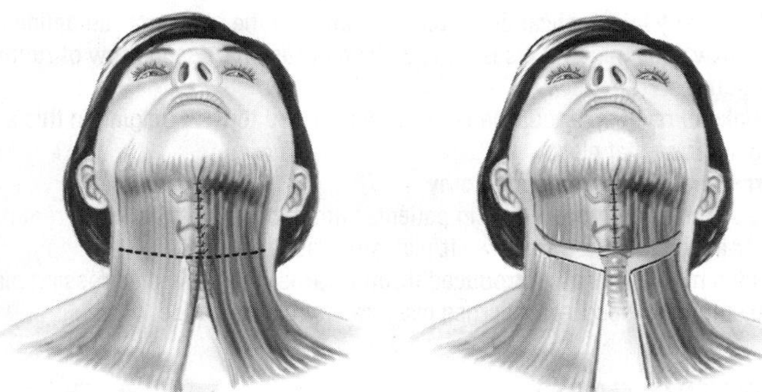

**Fig. 95-11** Full transection of the platysma creates a wide gap and window-shading effect.

- **Corset platysmaplasty**[25,26] (Fig. 95-12)
  - Its use has multiple purposes: to eliminate static paramedian muscle bands, shape the waistline of the neck, and flatten the submental plane.
  - The neck skin is shifted posteriorly, but the platysma pull is forward toward the anterior midline.
  - No muscle is resected. Redundant muscle is folded inward to form a flat midline seam.
  - The procedure is performed through a 4 cm submental incision.
  - A multilayered seam approximates the full height of the midline platysma edges, creating a "waistline" to the neck from an anterior platysmal shift.
  - Plication continues to 3 fingerbreadths above the suprasternal notch.
  - Crisscrossing and backtracking are advocated to keep the seam tight.

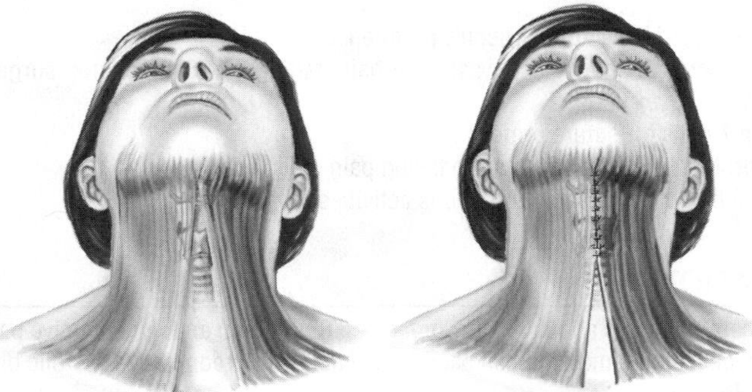

**Fig. 95-12** Coaptation of decussated platysmal fibers in the midline creates a corset-type effect.

**TIP:** This technique is highly effective in recontouring the submental area.

- If combined with lateral plication, midline plication of the platysma can define the jawline and neck-jaw angle nicely. This is done with an occasional second row of running vertical oblique sutures.
- Additional submandibular suturing may be performed to treat bulging in this area by creating a strong, flat pleat.

- **Closed percutaneous platysma myotomy**[27]
  - Use this as an isolated procedure in patients with minor skin laxity, recurrent platymsal bands, or in conjunction with face lift/platysmaplasty.
  - 3-0 braided nylon suture is introduced through large-gauge needle crossing platysma muscle; suture is used to saw across platysma to release bands.

## POSTOPERATIVE CARE[1]

- Monitor postoperative blood pressure closely; consider a beta-blocker such as metoprolol or the alpha-agonist clonidine to maintain normotensive systolic blood pressure and prevent hematomas.
- Provide oral analgesics and antiemetics, with specific instructions for their use.
- Instruct patients to avoid pillows that flex the neck to keep the cervicomental angle open.
- Avoid folding the neck skin flaps, because this contributes to edema by obstructing neck lymphatics.
- Drains are surgeon's preference; they help eliminate serum and small amounts of blood oozing, potentially reducing postoperative edema.
- Remove drains on the first postoperative day after examining patient.
- Without applying pressure, place cotton dressings or foam tape and an elastic garment on the wound overnight to absorb wept fluids.
- On the first postoperative day, remove operative dressing and replace it with a neck strap for no longer than 4 weeks.
- Instruct patients to maintain an open neck angle, similar to angle created when elbows are on knees while sitting.
- Antibiotics are used based on surgeon's preference.
- Encourage patients to shower and wash their hair starting 24-48 hours after surgery to keep suture lines clean.
- Follow up in 7 days for suture removal.
- Alcohol is prohibited until patients stop taking pain medications.
- Recommend that patients avoid strenuous activities for 6 weeks.

## COMPLICATIONS[28]

- Overall hematoma rate is about 3% in women and 8% in men and hypertensive patients.[29]
- A higher incidence of hematoma has been associated with preoperative systolic blood pressure >150 mm Hg.
- Marginal mandibular nerve injury is most common in neck-lift procedures; however, injury to the cervical branch can also occur that may mimic marginal mandibular injury. Cervical branch injury can be distinguished from the former, because patient is able to evert lower lip (mentalis muscle is still functioning).
- Idiopathic trauma to the GAN may cause temporary loss of sensation of a portion of the ear, scalp, or face.
- Skin slough often preceded by hematoma or infection is most common in the retroauricular area.

- Underestimating submental fat removal is often caused by fatty deposits deep to the platysma.
- Overresection of fat is an error that is difficult to correct and leaves a hollowed out appearance especially in the submental region.

## Key Points

- ✓ When evaluating a neck for cervicoplasty, evaluate the midface for an ideal combined result.
- ✓ Patients rarely need cervicoplasty only. Diligently examine facial proportions, including chin projection.
- ✓ If the skin is sun damaged and inelastic, a full periauricular incision is required.
- ✓ Submental approach to neck lift will improve a patient's profile, cervicomental angle, and jawline but does not address neck-face aging above mandibular border or angle.
- ✓ Do not overresect fat; leave 3-5 mm of a subcutaneous cushion on the flap.
- ✓ Look and gently pinch the neck to consider the need for fat removal.
- ✓ Evaluate muscles and banding.
- ✓ With an anterior platysmaplasty the neck is better consolidated, but this does not suffice to treat banding. A myotomy must be performed on the platysma to solve the problem.
- ✓ The height of the myotomy is usually at the level of the cricoid cartilage.
- ✓ The best result provides harmony of all facial proportions.
- ✓ Discuss the risks of procedures thoroughly with patients, and set realistic goals and expectations.

## References

1. Nahai F, ed. The Art of Aesthetic Surgery: Principles & Techniques, 2nd ed. St Louis: Quality Medical Publishing, 2011.
2. Gray H, Pick TP, Howden R, eds. Gray's Anatomy: Descriptive and Surgical. 1901 Edition. Philadelphia: Running Press, 1974.
3. Netter FH, ed. Atlas of Human Anatomy, 5th ed. Summit, NJ: CIBA-GEIGY, 2010.
4. Fedok FG, Sedgh J. Managing the neck in the era of the short scar face-lift. Facial Plast Surg 28:60, 2012.
5. Dingman RO, Grabb WC. Surgical anatomy of the mandibular ramus of the facial nerve based on the dissection of 100 facial halves. Plast Reconstr Surg 29:266, 1962.
6. Cardoso de Castro C. The anatomy of the platysma muscle. Plast Reconstr Surg 66:680, 1980.
7. Seckel BR, ed. Facial Danger Zones: Avoiding Nerve Injury in Facial Plastic Surgery, 2nd ed. St Louis: Quality Medical Publishing, 2010.
8. Connell BF. Contouring the neck in rhytidectomy by lipectomy and a muscle sling. Plast Reconstr Surg 61:376, 1978.
9. Connell BF, Shamoun JM. The significance of digastric muscle contouring for rejuvenation of the submental area of the face. Plast Reconstr Surg 99:1586, 1997.
10. Ellenbogen R, Karlin JV. Visual criteria for success in restoring the youthful neck. Plast Reconstr Surg 66:826, 1980.
11. Rohrich RJ, Rios JL, Smith PD, et al. Neck rejuvenation revisited. Plast Reconstr Surg 118:1251, 2006.
12. Knize DM. Limited incision submental lipectomy and platysmaplasty. Plast Reconstr Surg 101:473, 1998.
13. Baker DC. Face lift with submandibular gland and digastric muscle resection: radical neck rhytidectomy. Aesthetic Surg J 26:85, 2006.

14. Barton FE. Aesthetic surgery of the face and neck. Aesthet Surg J 29:449, 2009.
15. de Castro CC, Aboudib JH, Roxo AC. Updating the concepts on neck lift and lower third of the face. Plast Reconstr Surg 130:199-205, 2012.
16. Baker DC. Lateral SMASectomy. Plast Reconstr Surg 100:509, 1997.
17. Matarasso A, Matarasso SL, Brandt FS, et al. Botulinum A exotoxin for the management of platsyma bands. Plast Reconstr Surg 103:645, 1999.
18. Kane MA. Nonsurgical treatment of platysmal bands with injection of botulinum toxin A. Plast Reconstr Surg 103:656, 1999.
19. Cronin TD, Biggs TM. The T-Z-plasty for the male "turkey gobbler" neck. Plast Reconstr Surg 47:534, 1971.
20. Zins JE, Fardo D. The "anterior-only" approach to neck rejuvenation: an alternative to face lift surgery. Plast Reconstr Surg 115:1761, 2005.
21. Fuente del Campo A. Midline platysma muscular overlap for neck restoration. Plast Reconstr Surg 102:1710, 1998.
22. Guerrero-Santos J. Neck lift: simplified surgical techniques, refinements, and clinical classification. Clin Plast Surg 10:379, 1983.
23. Giampapa VC, Di Bernardo BE. Neck recontouring with suture suspension and liposuction: an alternative for the early rhytidectomy candidate. Aesthetic Plast Surg 19:217, 1995.
24. Nahai F. Reconsidering neck suspension sutures. Aesthet Surg J 24:365, 2004.
25. Feldman JJ. Corset platysmaplasty. Plast Reconstr Surg 85:333, 1990.
26. Feldman JJ. Neck Lift. St Louis: Quality Medical Publishing, 2006.
27. Gonzalez R. Composite platysmaplasty and closed percutaneous platysma myotomy: a simple way to treat deformities of the neck caused by aging. Aesthet Surg J 29:344, 2009.
28. Gonyon DL, Barton FE. The aging face: rhytidectomy and adjunctive procedures. Sel Read Plast Surg 10:21, 2005.
29. Baker DC, Stefani WA, Chiu ES. Reducing the incidence of hematoma requiring surgical evacuation following male rhytidectomy: a 30 year-review of 985 cases. Plast Reconstr Surg 116:1973, 2005.

# 96. Rhinoplasty

Michael R. Lee

Jacques Joseph, a surgeon from Berlin, is known as *the father of modern rhinoplasty.*[1]

## NASAL ANATOMY

### Skin

Upper two thirds of the skin envelope is thinner and more mobile than the lower third.

### Muscles

- Three clinically significant muscles:
  - **Levator labii superioris alaeque nasi:** Assists in patency of external nasal valve
  - **Nasalis:** Assists in nasal airway patency
  - **Depressor septi:** When hyperactive, may shorten the upper lip and decrease tip projection on animation. Division of the muscle during rhinoplasty can alleviate this problem.

> **TIP:** Patients with facial paralysis may have nasal obstruction from a nonfunctional levator labii superioris alaeque nasi muscle.

### Blood Supply (Fig. 96-1)

- Arterial supply to nose is located superficial to the nasal musculature in the subcutaneous plane.
- Ophthalmic and facial arteries create a rich vascular cascade that supplies the nasal envelope.
- **Ophthalmic artery**
  - Supplies the superior portion of nasal envelope
  - **Branches:** Anterior ethmoidal artery, dorsal nasal artery, and external nasal artery
- **Facial artery**
  - Supplies most of nasal envelope and responsible for nasal tip blood supply
  - **Branches:** Superior labial artery and angular artery
  - Superior labial artery branches to create columellar artery (present 68.2% of cases).[2,3]

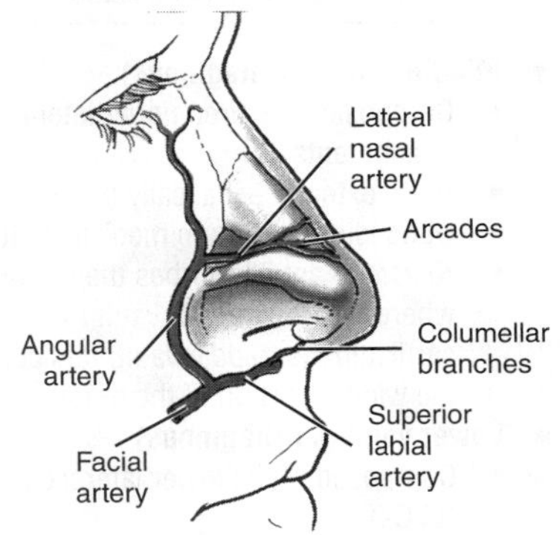


**Fig. 96-1** Blood supply.

  - Angular artery branches to create lateral nasal artery (unilateral or bilateral 100% of cases).
    - Lateral nasal artery is found 2-3 mm above alar groove.[2,3]
      - Primary blood supply to tip in open rhinoplasty, because the columellar arteries are sacrificed.[4]

**TIP:** Understanding the nasal tip blood supply is crucial to prevent vascular embarrassment. Inadvertent sacrifice of the lateral nasal artery during alar base resection may lead to soft tissue necrosis.

## INNERVATION

- Maxillary and ophthalmic branches of CN V provide sensation to nose.
- Supraorbital and supratrochlear branches of ophthalmic nerve supply cephalic portion.
- External nasal branch of anterior ethmoid innervates middle vault and nasal tip.

## NASAL VAULTS (Fig. 96-2)

- The nose can be divided into three vaults.
- **Upper vault (bony)**
  - Composed of paired nasal bones and ascending frontal processes of maxilla.
  - Nasal bones average 2.5 cm in length.
  - Nasal bones have greater thickness and density above the medial canthus and gradually become thinner toward the tip.
  - Nasal bones are widest at the nasofrontal suture and then become narrowest at the nasofrontal angle, before widening again inferior to the radix and then narrowing again at the inferior margin.

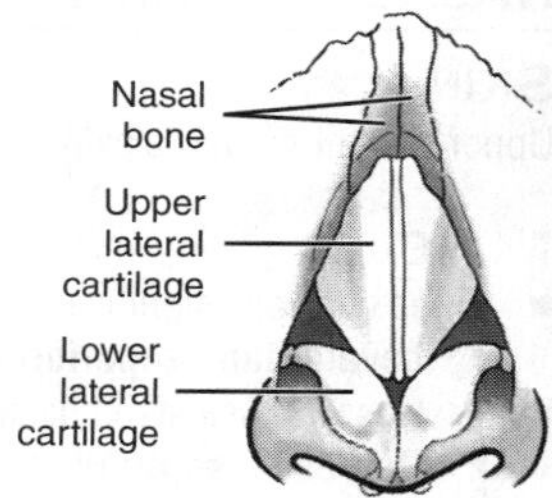


**Fig. 96-2** Nasal vaults.

**TIP:** Osteotomies that extend into the thick nasal bone above the level of the medial canthus may lead to fragment lateralization known as a *rocker deformity.*

- **Middle vault (cartilaginous)**
  - Composed of paired upper lateral cartilages (ULCs), dorsal septum, and soft tissue attachments.
  - ULCs extend cephalically underneath the nasal bones for 6-8 mm.
  - ULCs join the septum medially to form a "T" in cross-section, creating the internal nasal valve.
  - *Keystone area* describes the region where the bony upper vault meets the cartilaginous middle vault. It is commonly the widest portion of the dorsum.
- **Lower vault (cartilaginous)**
  - Composed of the lower lateral cartilages (LLCs).
  - *Scroll area* describes the region of abutment between the ULCs and LLCs.
  - Each LLC may be divided into three crura: **medial, middle,** and **lateral** (Fig. 96-3).
  - Lateral crus attaches laterally to accessory cartilages, which then connect to the piriform aperture.
  - The lateral crus shares a common perichondrium with the accessory cartilage.
  - Lateral crus and accessory cartilage function as a single unit called *lateral crura complex.*
  - LLCs are intimately related to tip projection, rotation, and definition.

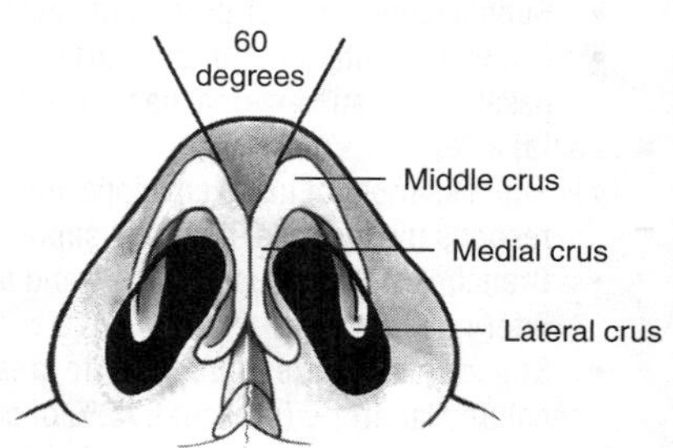


**Fig. 96-3** Each lower lateral cartilage may be divided into three crura: Medial, middle, and lateral.

- **The lateral crural complex is supported by three structures:**
  - Suspensory ligaments of the tip
  - Fibrous connections to the ULC
  - Abutment with the piriform aperture

## Nasal Tip

- **Support and projection of the nasal tip are provided by the following[5]:**
  - LLC and attachment to the piriform aperture
  - Domal suspensory ligament
  - Fibrous intercartilaginous connections between ULC and LLC
  - Medial crural ligaments
  - Anterior septal angle

## Septum

- Composed of quadrangular septal cartilage and bone of ethmoid and vomer (Fig. 96-4).
- Variations in anatomy of the osteocartilaginous junction are common.[6]
- Evaluate septum for deviation, perforation, or bone spurs.
- Fractures from prior trauma occur in patterns based on underlying biomechanics.[6]

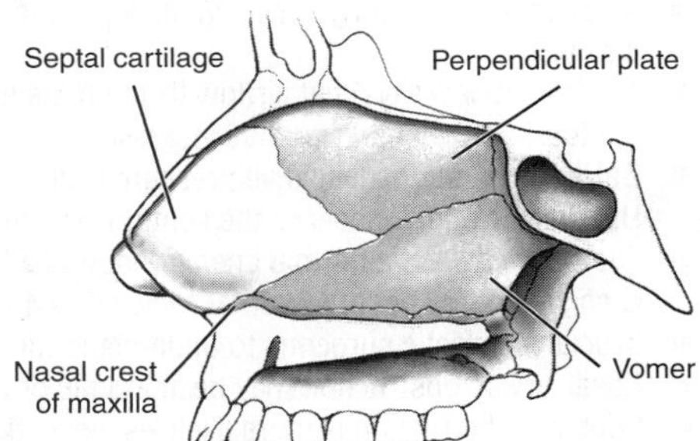


**Fig. 96-4** Nasal tip.

## Turbinates

- Paired bony structures regulate and humidify inspired air.
- Superior, middle, and inferior turbinates are extensions of the lateral nasal wall.
- Superior and middle turbinates are components of the ethmoid bone.
- The inferior turbinate is a separate bone and the primary turbinate treated in rhinoplasty.
- A severely deviated septum may induce the contralateral inferior turbinate to hypertrophy to balance nasal resistance of bilateral nasal cavities.
- A hypertrophied inferior turbinate may be responsible for up to two thirds of total airway resistance.[7]
- Complete removal of the inferior turbinate may cause nasal obstruction with *empty nose syndrome.*

## Internal Nasal Valve

- Originally described in 1920 by Mink.[8]
- Narrowest portion of the nasal airway thus regulating airflow resistance.
- Typically provides half of total airway resistance.[9]
- Created by junction of caudal border of the ULC and nasal septum.
- Normal angle is **10-15 degrees,** with a more acute angle leading to nasal obstruction.[10]
- *Cottle maneuver:* The cheek is pulled laterally to displace the lateral nasal wall to identify internal valve collapse. The specificity of the Cottle maneuver is not well defined.

> **TIP:** Spreader grafts are placed between the ULC and nasal septum to widen the internal nasal valve.

### External Nasal Valve

- Created primarily by caudal edge of lateral crus and nasal septum.
- Contributions from soft tissue of ala and nasal sill.
- The nasal ala is void of cartilage.
- External valve collapse may be seen with nostril collapse on inspiration.
- Assess alar rims for notching or eversion on inspiration, which may be a compensatory response for external valve collapse.

## NASAL PHYSIOLOGY

- The nasal airway contributes 50% of the overall airway resistance.
- Nasal mucosal engorgement significantly decreases lumen from a relatively fixed-volume nasal cavity.
- *Poiseuille's law* says that airflow through the nose, similar to fluid through a tube, increases to the fourth power as the radius increases.
- During inspiration a negative pressure is generated, and the internal nasal valve narrows as the ULCs are brought closer to the septum. The nostrils enlarge.
- The *nasal cycle* is a normal phenomenon of alternating mucosal constriction and dilation on each side of the nose. A normal cycle takes 4 hours to complete.
- Crucial for plastic surgeons to understand functional implications of aesthetic techniques.
- Nasal airway obstruction may be anatomic or the result of a physiologic response.
- Constant obstruction is more likely associated with a fixed structural abnormality such as septal deviation.
- Gradual worsening of nasal obstruction, particularly with epistaxis in smokers, should raise concern for neoplasm.
- Nasal obstruction is a frequent complaint of patients seeking cosmetic rhinoplasty.
- Seasonal obstruction or obstruction related to dust, mold, pollen, or other allergens may suggest allergic rhinitis.
- Presence of *allergic shiners* (dark circles under eyes) may suggest *allergic rhinitis.*
- Bilateral obstruction that changes in severity suggests mucosal disease.
- The nose should be examined before and after application of a vasocontrictive agent. This allows the surgeon to quantify the extent of mucosal disease.
- Trial medical management for nasal airway obstruction may be used to clarify the clinical presentation.
- Allergic rhinitis treated with avoidance of specific allergens, environmental control, antihistamines, and topical intranasal corticosteroids (e.g., Nasonex or Flonase).
- Crusting, ulceration, or polypoid changes should prompt a medical workup for a systemic condition before surgical intervention. Lesions potentially suspected of neoplasia should prompt appropriate referral and tissue biopsy.
- Viral rhinitis (common cold) is self-limited but may progress to bacterial superinfection (antibiotics and nasal toilet).
- *Rhinitis medicamentosus:* Rebound vasodilatation and engorgement of the nasal mucosa in response to overuse of topical nasal decongestants such as Neo-Synephrine or Afrin. Treatment includes stopping use of the offending agent, patient education, a combination of oral antihistamines and decongestants, topical nasal steroid sprays, and possibly a steroid taper.
- *Ozena:* Primary atrophic rhinitis associated with aggressive submucosal septal resection and complete turbinectomy.

- Factors important in identifying cause:
  - Time of onset
  - Duration of obstruction
  - Precipitation or relieving factors
  - Rhinorrhea
  - Epistaxis
  - Prior trauma or surgery
  - Headaches, visual disturbances, otologic symptoms
  - Medication use, in particular vasoactive nasal sprays
  - Use of tobacco, alcohol, or drugs
  - Seasonal obstruction

**TIP:** Before surgical treatment, identify and perform nasal swab culture for patients at risk for MRSA colonization.

## NASAL ANALYSIS

- Successful rhinoplasty begins with understanding the patient's objectives.
- Cultural differences exist, and surgeons should be aware of these (see Chapter 87 for additional information).
- The patient should be educated regarding achievable results.
- Software imaging systems allow improved communication between surgeon and patient.
- Preoperative assessment involves evaluating the nose on frontal, lateral, and basilar views.
- A systematic method is crucial for comprehensive facial and nasal evaluation.
- After surgical goals are established, a focused plan is developed.

### Frontal View

- **Assess overall facial proportions and their relationship to the nose.**
- **Determine thickness and quality of nasal skin envelope.**
- **Determine if nose is straight or crooked.**
  - Imaginary vertical line from midglabella to menton helps establish midline.
  - Determine if deviation involves bone and/or cartilage.
  - Cartilaginous deviation is often related to underlying septal deviation.
- **Analyze the dorsal aesthetic lines.**
  - These should appear as two slightly curved, divergent lines that extend from the medial superciliary ridge to the tip-defining points.
- **Evaluate width of upper vault.**
  - The bony vault should be 75%-80% of the ideal alar base.
- **Evaluate middle vault.**
  - Determine whether an inverted-V deformity is present at the middle vault origin.
  - Assess for lateral nasal wall collapse or contour deformity.
- **Evaluate width of alar base.**
  - The ideal alar base should be equivocal to the intercanthal distance.
  - If the width is greater than ideal norms, then degree of alar flaring should be determined.
    - Compare the maximum alar width with the width of ala at the alar base.
    - If difference between these two is >2 mm, problem is excessive flaring.
    - If difference is <2 mm, problem is primarily excessively wide alar base.

- Alar rims should be symmetrical with a slight outward flare in the inferior and lateral direction.
- The outline of the alar rims and columella should resemble a gull in flight (Fig. 96-5).

■ **Assess nasal tip definition.**
- Nasal tip should receive the distal end of the dorsal aesthetic lines.
- Two tip-defining points should exist, with each providing individual but symmetrical light reflexes.
- A diamond can be created in the ideal tip by connecting four points.

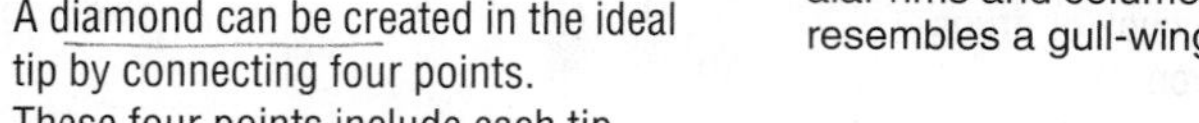

- These four points include each tip-defining point, the supratip point, and columellar-lobular angle point.

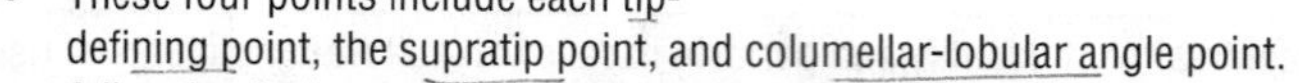

Fig. 96-5 Outline of alar rims and columella resembles a gull-wing.

- A line that is drawn to connect each tip-defining point inside of the diamond should yield two equilateral triangles.
- Determine if the tip appears bulbous or boxy, and assess the likelihood of lateral and/or middle crural malposition.
- Evaluate the infratip lobule for excess fullness or asymmetry.
- The *infratip lobule* is bordered by the tip-defining points superiorly and columellar base inferiorly. A line drawn through the nostril apex should bisect it into equal divisions.[11]

## Lateral View

■ **Evaluate nasal dorsum and tip.**
- Radix should be at a level between upper lash line and supratarsal fold.
- Low radix may give appearance of overprojected nose.
- Evaluate the slope of the nasal dorsum (line drawn from radix to nasal tip).
  - ▸ Males should have a smooth, straight line with no supratip break.
  - ▸ Females should have a smooth, slightly concave dorsum 2 mm inferior to the line and contain supratip break.
- A *tension nose* is defined as a high nasal dorsum from excess of quadrangular cartilage with inferior displacement of the nasal tip cartilages.

■ **Assess nasal tip projection.**
- *Tip projection* is defined as distance from alar-cheek junction to nasal tip.
- Nasal length is measured from the radix to the nasal tip.
- Tip projection should equal 67% of the nasal length.
- Tip projection should approximately equal alar base width.
- Line is drawn from the alar-cheek junction to the nasal tip. 50%-60% of the nasal tip should lie anterior to a vertical line tangent to the most projecting part of the upper lip vermilion.

■ **Assess nasal tip rotation.**
- Determination of the nasolabial angle helps to assess tip rotation (Fig. 96-6).
  - ▸ Should be 95-110 degrees in females and 90-95 degrees in males.

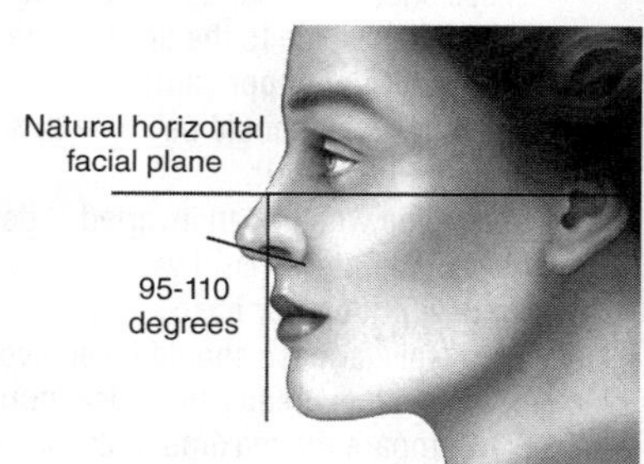


**Fig. 96-6** Nasolabial angle.

- **Evaluate nasal ala.**
  - The alar rim should also have a smooth oval contour from the lateral view.
  - Normal columellar show is 2-3 mm.
  - The greatest distance from the long axis of the nostril to either the columella or alar rim should be 1-2 mm.
  - Nasal tip/columella ratio should be 1:2.
- **Assess infratip lobule.**
  - The columellar-labial angle is created by the junction of the columella with the upper lip.
  - Fullness in this area is typically the result of a prominent caudal septum.
  - The ideal columellar-labial angle is 30-45 degrees (Fig. 96-7).

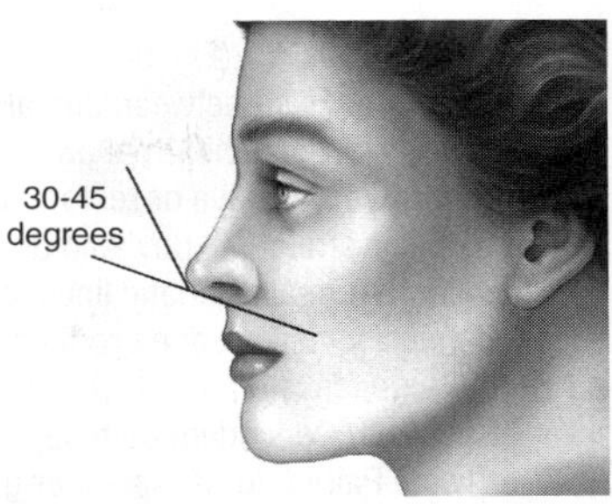


**Fig. 96-7** Columellar-labial angle.

## Basal View

- The alar rims and nasal tip should form an equilateral triangle.
- Nasal tip/columella (nostril) ratio should be 1:2.
- The nostril should have a slight teardrop shape with the apex slightly medial to the base.
- The lateral border of the columella (medial nostril) should be smooth in contour.
- Septal deviation or excess, premature flaring of the medial crura, or soft tissue fullness may distort columella.

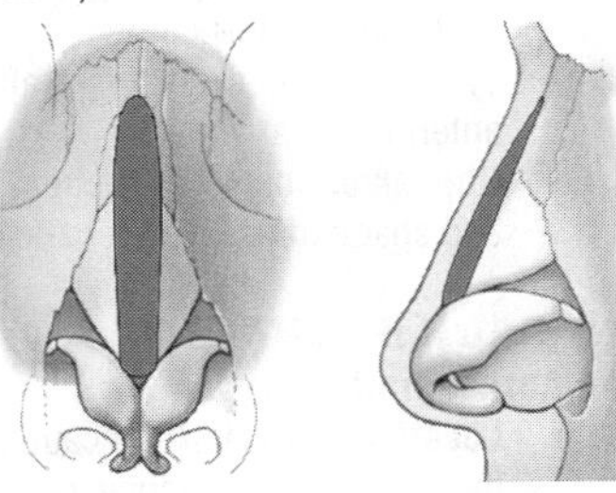

**Fig. 96-8** Dorsal onlay graft.

# GRAFT NOMENCLATURE[12]

## Nasal Dorsum Grafts

- **Dorsal onlay graft**[12] (Fig. 96-8)
  - **Location:** Longitudinal graft placed directly on the nasal dorsum
  - **Objective:** Augmentation and/or contour improvement

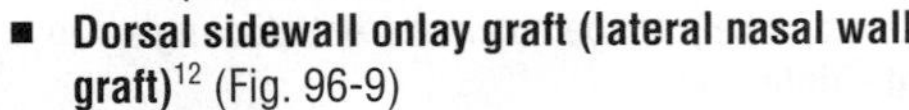

- **Dorsal sidewall onlay graft (lateral nasal wall graft)**[12] (Fig. 96-9)
  - **Location:** Lateral nasal wall
  - **Objective:** Correct depressions or irregularities, improve contour of depressed ULCs
- **Radix graft**[12] (Fig. 96-10)
  - **Location:** Upper dorsum usually in a customized soft tissue pocket
  - **Objective:** Augment inadequate nasofrontal angle or redefine radix further cephalad. Provides appearance of lengthened nose.

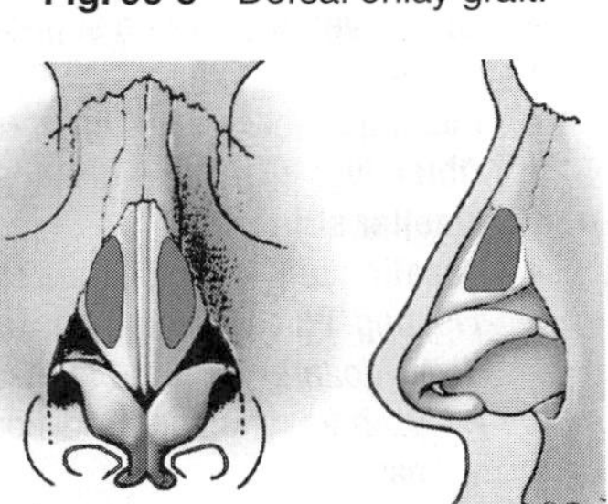

**Fig. 96-9** Dorsal sidewall onlay graft (lateral nasal wall graft).

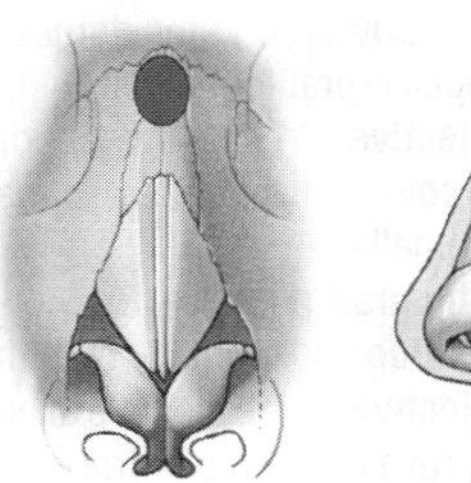

**Fig. 96-10** Radix graft.

- **Spreader grafts**[13,14] (Fig. 96-11)
  - **Location:** Fixed between dorsal septum and ULC in submucoperichondrial pocket
  - **Objective:** Improve or restore nasal valve patency, straighten deviated dorsal septum, smooth dorsal aesthetic lines, correct inverted-V deformity, correct open roof deformity
- **Septal extension grafts**[13,15] (Fig. 96-12)
  - **Location:** Dependent on type of graft
  - *Type I:* Paired dorsal spreader grafts that extend beyond anterior septal angle into the interdomal space
  - *Type II:* Paired batten grafts that extend diagonally across the septal L-strut into the tip-lobule complex
  - *Type III:* Direct extension graft affixed to anterior septal angle
  - **Objective:** Control projection, rotation, support, and shape of nasal tip; create supratip break

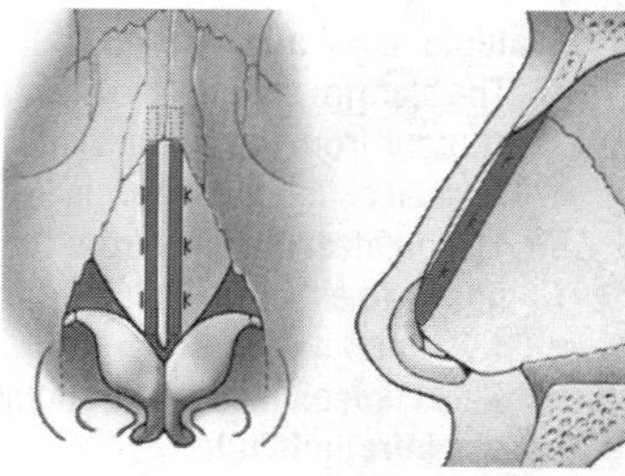

**Fig. 96-11** Spreader grafts.

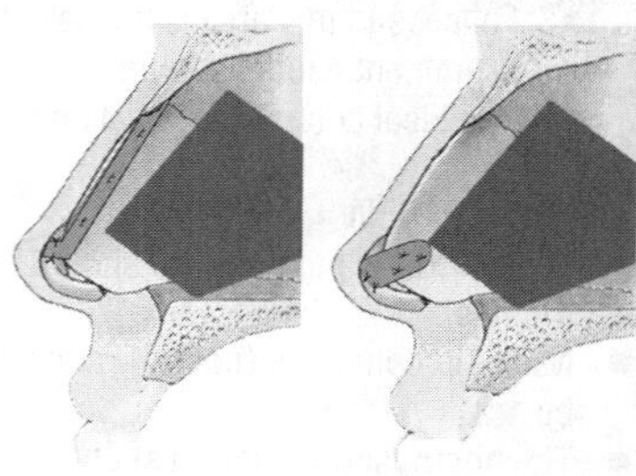

Type I Type II

**Fig. 96-12** Septal extension grafts.

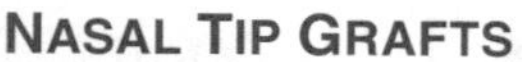

## NASAL TIP GRAFTS

- **Anchor graft**
  - **Location:** Shaft fixed to caudal margin of medial crura, and transverse limbs to lateral crura
  - **Objective:** Improve tip support and projection and correct deformity of lateral crura
- **Cap graft**
  - **Location:** Space between tip-defining points and medial crura
  - **Objective:** Increase projection or refine nasal tip, refine infratip lobule
- **Columellar strut**
  - **Location:** Between the medial crura
  - *Floating:* Placed in tight pocket via closed approach
  - *Fixed-floating:* Secured to medial crura via open approach
    - Both floating and fixed-floating have 2-3 mm of soft tissue between base of graft and nasal spine.
  - *Fixed:* Secured directly to nasal spine or premaxilla
  - **Objective:** Maintain or increase tip projection and help shape columellar-lobular angle
- **Extended columellar strut-tip graft (extended shield graft)**
  - **Location:** Caudal to or between the medial crura, extending anteriorly beyond the domes and posteriorly toward the medial crural footplates
  - **Objective:** Provide tip support, projection, and definition; improve volume caudal to medial crura and shape columella
- **Onlay tip graft** (Fig. 96-13)
  - **Location:** Horizontally over the alar domes
  - **Objective:** Increase tip projection and definition, improve contour of infratip-lobule

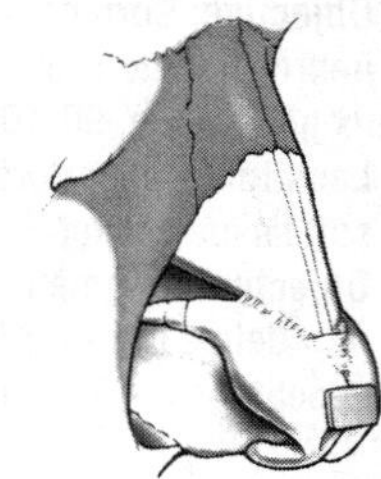

**Fig. 96-13** Onlay (Peck) graft.

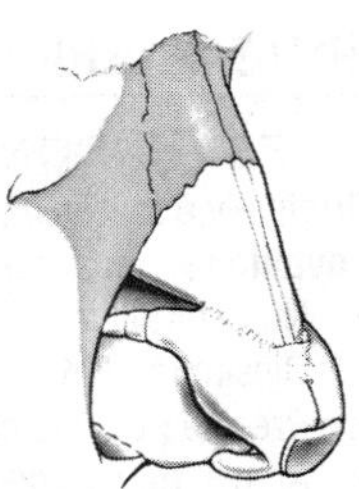

Fig. 96-14 Infralobular graft.

- **Shield graft (Sheen or infralobular graft)** (Fig. 96-14)
  - **Location:** Rests on anterior middle crura and extends to nasal tip
  - **Objective:** Improve tip projection and definition, improve infraftip-lobule contour
- **Subdomal graft**
  - **Location:** Bar-shaped graft placed in pocket under the domes
  - **Objective:** Improve domal symmetry and crural orientation, correct pinched nasal tip deformity
- **Umbrella graft**
  - **Location:** Vertical columella strut between medial crura with addition of horizontal tip onlay graft
  - **Objective:** Increase tip projection and support

## Nasal Alar Grafts

- **Alar batten graft**
  - **Location:** Pocket from the piriform aperture to paramedian position in alar sidewall
  - **Objective:** Improve internal or external valve collapse
- **Alar contour graft (alar rim graft)**
  - **Location:** Subcutaneous pocket immediately above and parallel to alar rim
  - **Objective:** Correct or avert alar retraction or collapse
- **Alar spreader graft (lateral crural spanning graft)**
  - **Location:** Bridges the intercrural space in pocket, lateral crura, and vestibular skin
  - **Objective:** Correct pinched nasal tip deformity and improve nasal valve function
- **Composite alar rim graft**
  - **Location:** Intranasal alar rim
  - **Objective:** Correct severe alar retraction or notching
- **Lateral crural onlay graft**
  - **Location:** Anterior surface of lateral crura
  - **Objective:** Improve contour, strength, and shape of nasal ala; improve external valve function
- **Lateral crural strut graft**
  - **Location:** Underneath lateral crura, extending laterally to or onto piriform aperture, inferior to alar groove
  - **Objective:** Correct alar retraction, rim collapse, and malpositioned lateral crura
- **Lateral crural turnover graft**[16]
  - **Location:** Cephalic portion of lateral crura turned over onto the remaining caudal lateral crura
  - **Objective:** Improve strength and position/shape of lateral crura

## Alar Base Grafts

- **Alar base graft**
  - **Location:** Placed along lateral piriform aperture
  - **Objective:** Augment recessed lip–alar base junction
- **Columellar plumping graft**
  - **Location:** Space between the medial crura and nasal spine
  - **Objective:** Augment inadequate columellar-labial angle, correct columellar contour deformities
- **Premaxillary graft**
  - **Location:** Caudal portion of piriform aperture
  - **Objective:** Correct premaxillary recession

## SURGICAL APPROACH

### CLOSED (ENDONASAL)

- Originally described by Roe[17] in 1887
- **Advantages** (according to Sheen[18])
  - No external scar
  - Dissection limited to areas of interest
  - Precise pockets can be created for insertion of graft material without fixation.
  - Allows percutaneous fixation when large pockets are made
  - Minimizes postsurgical edema
  - Decreased operative time
  - Faster recovery
  - Creates an intact tip graft pocket
  - Allows composite grafting to the alar rim
- **Disadvantages**
  - Need for experience and great reliance on preoperative diagnosis
  - Does not allow simultaneous viewing of surgical fields by surgeons and students
  - Does not allow direct viewing of nasal anatomy
  - Difficult dissection of alar cartilages, especially if they are malpositioned
- **Surgical incisions**
  - Approach is usually through combination of incisions needed to access areas of concern.
  - **Alar incisions** (Fig. 96-15)
    - **Intercartilaginous:** Located between upper and lower lateral cartilages, with LLCs delivered through incision using retrograde or eversion approach
    - **Transcartilaginous:** Located at the level of the LLC, with LLC accessed using cartilage-splitting approach
    - **Marginal:** Located in alar rim and in conjunction with intercartilaginous incision to deliver LLC

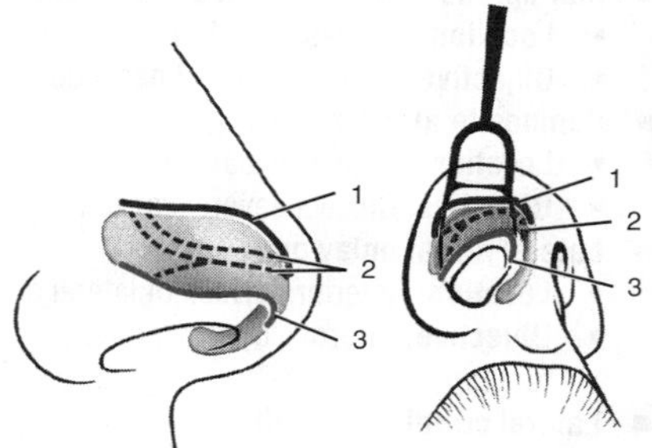


**Fig. 96-15** Preferred incisional approaches: *1,* Intercartilaginous; *2,* transcartilaginous; *3,* marginal.

  - **Septal incisions**
    - **Complete (full) transfixion:** Entire septum incised at membranous and caudal cartilaginous junction, releases tip completely, exposes nasal spine and depressor septi muscle
    - **Limited partial transfixion:** Less tip access but allows preservation of attachments between medial crural footplates and caudal septum
    - **Partial transfixion:** Begins caudal to anterior septal angle and ends just short of medial crural attachments to the caudal septum
    - **Hemitransfixion:** Created unilaterally at junction of caudal septum and columella
    - **High septal transfixion** (Fig. 96-16): Does not violate the junction of the caudal septum and the medial crura or membranous septum

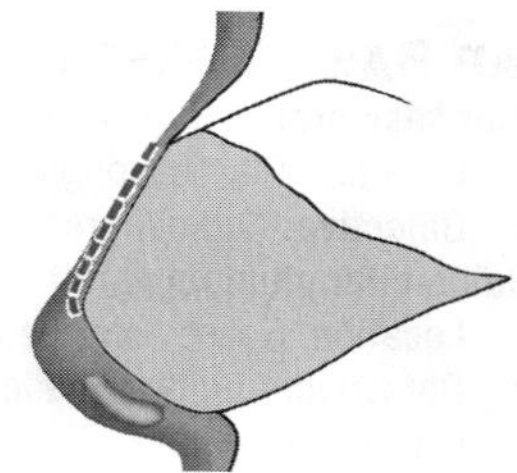

**Fig. 96-16** High septal transfixion.

> **TIP:** A complete transfixion incision disrupts the attachments of the medial crural footplate to the caudal septum. This results in significant loss of tip support and potential loss of tip projection.

## Open (External)

- Originally described by Vogt[19] in 1983
- **Advantages** [20]
  - Binocular vision
  - Evaluation of the complete deformity without disruption
  - Precise diagnosis and correction of deformities
  - Use of both hands
  - Increased options with original tissues and cartilage grafts
  - Direct control of bleeding with electrocautery
- **Disadvantages**
  - External nasal incision
  - Prolonged operative time
  - Increased tip edema
  - Columellar incision separation and delayed wound healing
  - May require suture stabilization of grafts

# SURGICAL TECHNIQUE

## Nasal Tip

A graduated approach is optimal, with reassessment after each maneuver implemented.

- **Tip projection: Influenced by several factors** (Fig. 96-17):
  - **Cartilaginous**
    - Anterior septal angle
    - LLCs (length and strength)
  - **Soft tissue**
    - Suspensory ligaments spanning the LLCs
    - Fibrous connections between the upper and lower lateral cartilages
    - Fibrous connections of lateral crura with piriform aperture
- **Increasing tip projection**
  - **Suture techniques**[21]
    - Used to increase tip projection 1-2 mm
    - Refine the tip and improve definition

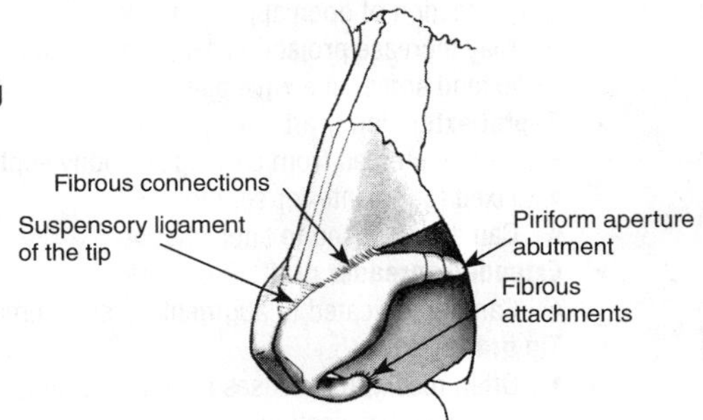


**Fig. 96-17** Support structures of the nasal tip.

- **Medial crural sutures** (Fig. 96-18)
  - Horizontal mattress sutures placed between the medial crura
  - Unify the LLCs and can stabilize the columellar strut either in front of or between the medial crura
  - Can correct premature flaring of the medial crura
- **Interdomal sutures** (Fig. 96-19)
  - Placed between the domes of the two LLCs
  - Increase infratip columellar projection and refine the nasal tip
- **Transdomal sutures** (Fig. 96-20)
  - Placed between the medial and lateral portions of a single LLC
  - Allow correction of domal asymmetry and provide tip projection and definition

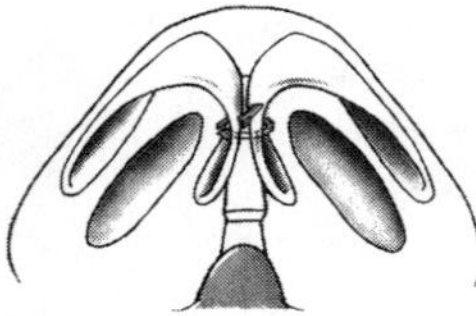

**Fig. 96-18** Medial crural sutures.

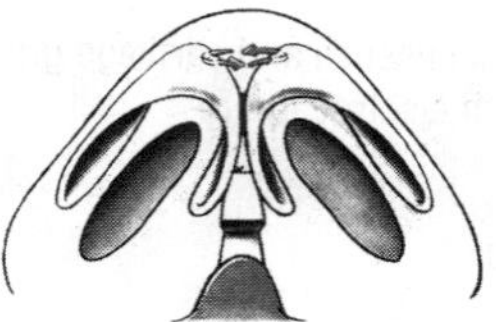

**Fig. 96-19** Interdomal sutures.

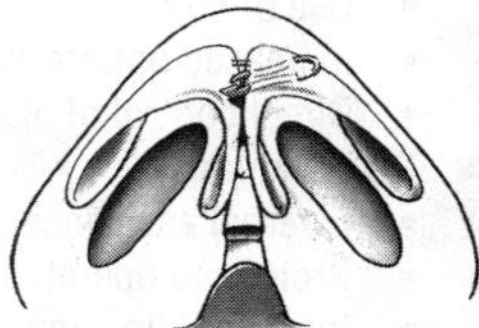

**Fig. 96-20** Transdomal sutures.

- **Medial crural septal sutures** (Fig. 96-21)
  - Placed between the medial crura and the septum
  - Cause rotation of the nasal tip, which increases tip projection and corrects rotation from a drooping nasal tip or aging nose

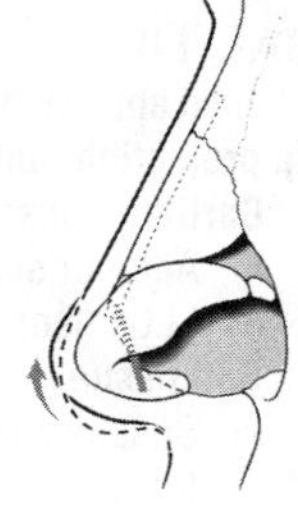

**Fig. 96-21** Medial crural septal sutures.

- **Cartilage grafting techniques**
  - **Columellar strut graft**
    - Used commonly to maintain projection lost through dissection of open approach
    - May increase projection 1-2 mm if graft long enough to extend soft tissue envelope
  - **Septal extension graft**
    - Can be created from cartilage or bony septum
    - Fixed to the anterior septum
    - Can also be used to alter rotation
  - **Extended spreader graft**
    - Can be fabricated to augment dorsum, create supratip break and definition
  - **Tip grafts**
    - Often reserved for cases in which other graft and suture techniques are insufficient for needed projection
    - Includes anchor graft, cap graft, onlay tip graft, shield graft, subdomal graft, and umbrella grafts

- **Decreasing tip projection**[22] (Fig. 96-22)
  - **Soft tissue**
    - Release of the ligamentous and fibroelastic attachments of the lower lateral crura
  - **Cartilage techniques**
    - Transection of **lateral** crura of LLC. Remaining cartilage may be spliced or sewn end to end.
    - Transection of **medial** crura of LLC. Remaining cartilage may be spliced or sewn end to end.

- Transection of **both lateral and medial crura** of LLC. Remaining cartilage may be spliced or sewn end to end.

**TIP:** Tripod model is useful to understand relationship between projection and rotation. When the lateral crura are shortened, the tip will be rotated as projection is decreased, whereas shortening of the medial crura will derotate and deproject the tip. If equivalent portions of both medial and lateral crura are resected, the projection is decreased while the rotation should remain the same.

**TIP:** Alar base flaring commonly occurs after a 2 mm setback of the nasal tip.

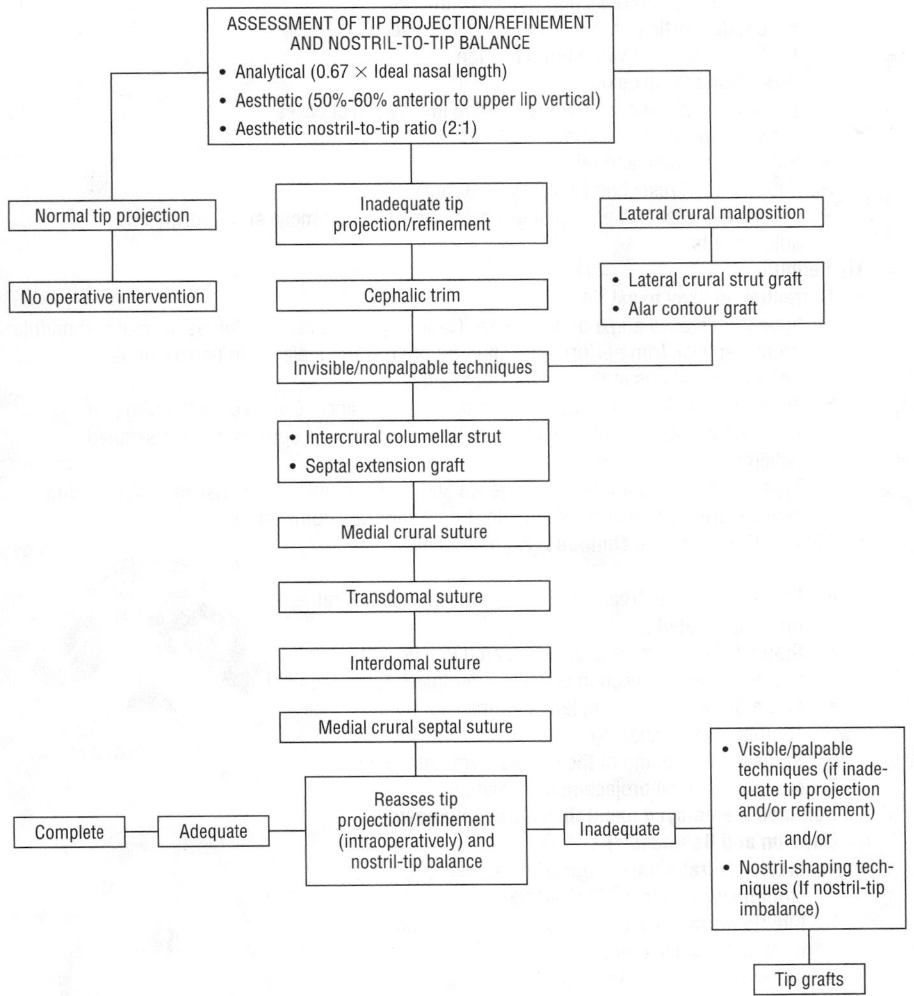


**Fig. 96-22** Algorithm for achieving adequate tip projection and refinement.

- **Tip rotation**
  - Tip grafts may also be used to improve the appearance of tip rotation.
  - Redundant mucosal resection is often necessary.
  - If increased projection is needed with rotation, *lateral crural steal* can be performed.
  - **Increasing tip rotation (cephalad rotation)**
    - **Suture techniques**
      - Multiple suspension suture techniques have been described.
      - Most techniques use suture to suspend LLC to either dorsal septum or osteocartilaginous junction.
    - **Cartilage techniques**
      - Cephalic trim of LLC
      - Caudal septum resection (typically anterior)
      - Caudal portion of medial crura of LLC resection
      - Columella strut with suture fixation
    - **Resection of radix skin**
      - Transverse resection of excess skin in very select cases
  - **Decreasing tip rotation (caudal rotation)**
    - Skin undermining and release of LLC
    - Caudal septal resection (typically posterior)
    - Cartilage grafts such as septal extension grafts or columella struts fortify tip adjustments.
- **Tip definition**
  - **Correction of boxy nasal tip**[23]
    - **Type I:** Increased angle of divergence (>30 degrees) between domes. Domal and middle crural cephalic trim performed with interdomal sutures placed to narrow angle. Consider intradomal sutures in thick-skinned patients.
    - **Type II:** Wide dome arc but normal angle of divergence. Domal cephalic trim and transdomal sutures with possible addition of intradomal sutures in thick-skinned patients
    - **Type III:** Increased angle of divergence and a wide dome arc. Domal and middle crural cephalic trim with placement of interdomal and transdomal sutures
  - **Modern tip-suturing techniques (suggested by Tebbetts**[24]**)**
    - **Stage 1:** Open approach and symmetrical lateral crural rim strip created
    - **Stage 2:** Medial crura positioned, arch unified and secured, dome projection equalized, footplate corrected
    - **Stage 3:** Columella strut, lateral crural spanning sutures, and tip shaping
    - **Stage 4:** Positioning of the unified, symmetrical tip complex for final projection and rotation
  - **Commonly employed nasal tip sutures (suggested by Guyuron and Behmand**[25]**)**
    1. **Medial crural suture:** Approximates medial crura and strengthens support[13] (Fig. 96-23)
    2. **Middle crural suture:** Approximates most anterior portion of medial crura
    3. **Interdomal suture:** Approximates domes and equalizes asymmetrical domes[13] (Fig. 96-24)

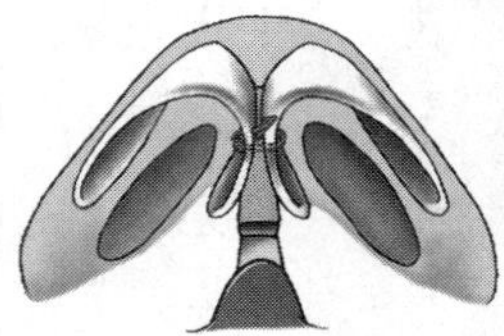

**Fig. 96-23** Medial crural suture.

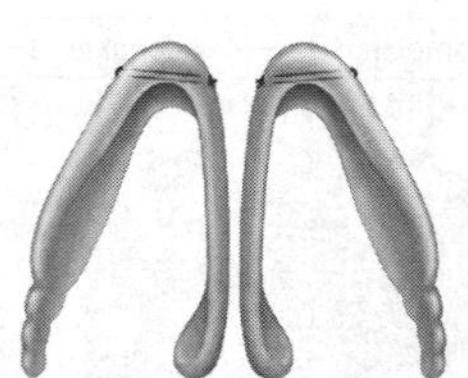

**Fig. 96-24** Interdomal suture.

4. **Transdomal sutures:** Narrows domal arch and medializes lateral crura[13] (Fig. 96-25)
5. **Lateral crural suture:** Increases concavity of lateral crura, reduces interdomal distance, retracts alar rims[13] (Fig. 96-26)
6. **Medial crural septal suture:** Increases tip projection and retracts columella (Fig. 96-27)
7. **Tip rotation suture:** Shifts tip cephalad while retracting columellar base, and improves notril shape[13] (Fig. 96-28)

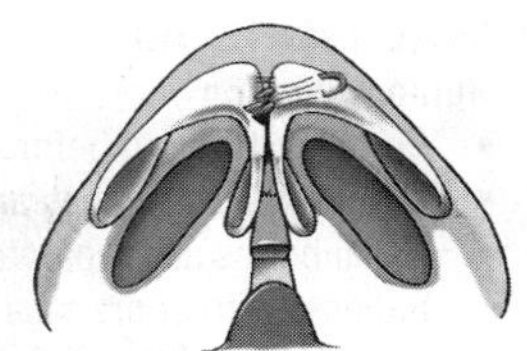

**Fig. 96-25** Transdomal suture.

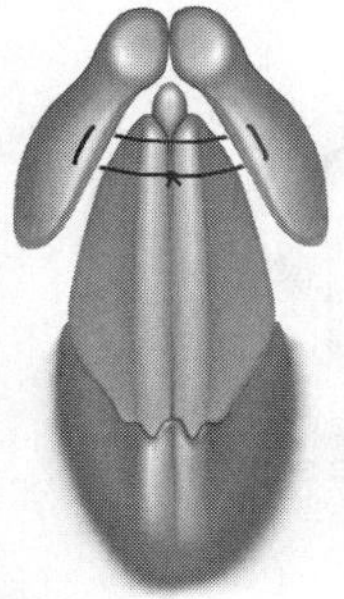

**Fig. 96-26** Lateral crural suture.

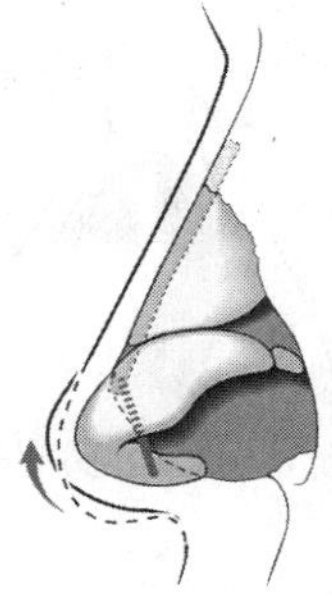

**Fig. 96-27** Medial crural septal suture.

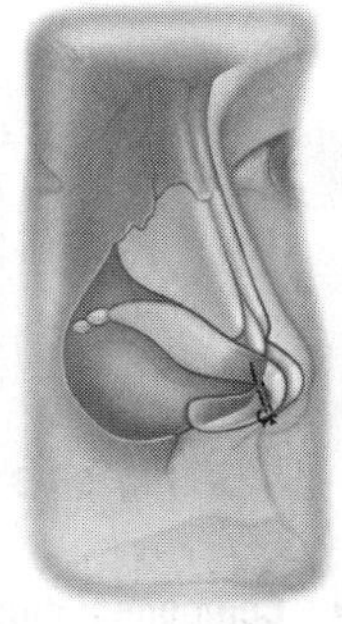

**Fig. 96-28** Tip rotation suture.

8. **Medial crural footplate suture:** Approximates footplates, narrows columellar base, improves nostril shape[13] (Fig. 96-29)
9. **Lateral crural convexity-control mattress suture:** Alters degree of convexity of lateral crura[13] (Fig. 96-30)

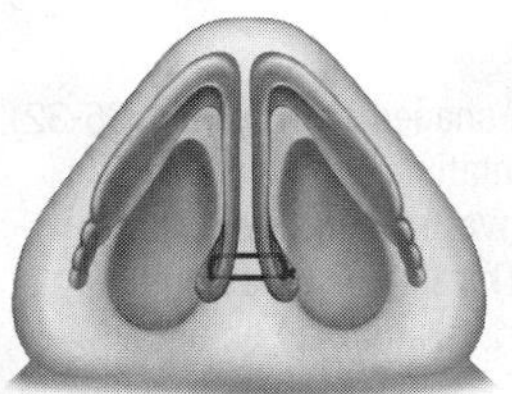

**Fig. 96-29** Medial crural footplate suture.

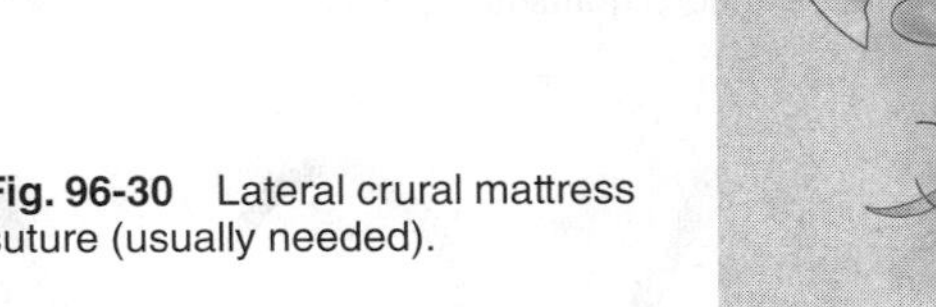

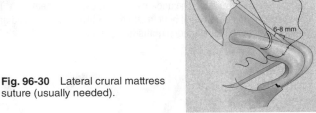


**Fig. 96-30** Lateral crural mattress suture (usually needed).

## Nasal Dorsum

- **Hump reduction**
  - Perform this step before septal cartilage harvest and tip refinement.
  - Numerous techniques are described, with osteotome and rasp being the most common.
  - Nasal bones are separated from the ULCs, resulting in an inverted-V deformity.
  - Patients with short nasal bones are at increased risk of an inverted-V deformity.
  - Restoration of the ULC position is crucial to maintain the nasal valve (Fig. 96-31).
  - Reduction of a dorsal hump often results in an *open roof deformity,* which requires either osteotomies or grafting to close.

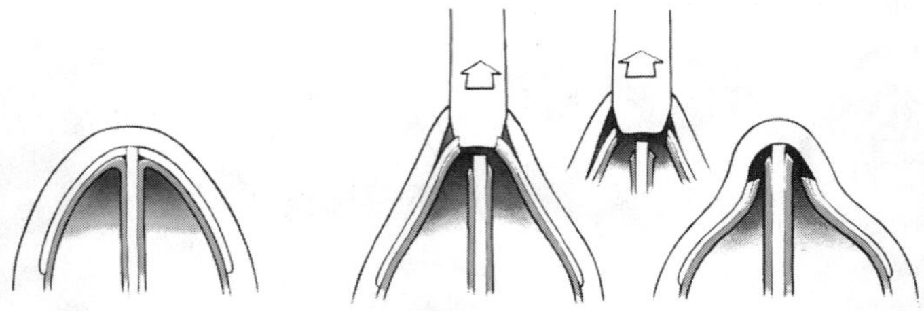

**Fig. 96-31** Preservation of the ULCs during reduction of the septum.

  - **Component dorsal hump reduction**[26]
    1. Separation of the ULC from the septum
    2. Incremental reduction of the septum proper
    3. Incremental dorsal bony reduction with rasp
    4. Verification by palpation
    5. Final modifications (spreader grafts, suturing techniques, osteotomies)
    6. Placement of ULC tension-spanning suture when needed
- **Dorsal augmentation**

Multiple options exist for augmentation, though cartilage is most commonly employed.[27]

  - **Septal cartilage**
    - Obviates morbidity of additional donor site
    - May not be option in secondary rhinoplasty
    - Partial-thickness incisions may be used to create V-, U-, or A-shaped grafts[28] (Fig. 96-32).
    - An inverted-V–shaped graft provides minimal dorsal augmentation but fits well with arched contour of dorsum. A-shaped grafts are essentially inverted-V grafts with a crossbar of cartilage underneath for greater augmentation. Thin-skinned patients may develop graft visibility of inverted-V or inverted-A–shaped grafts and may be better served with inverted-U grafts for contour.

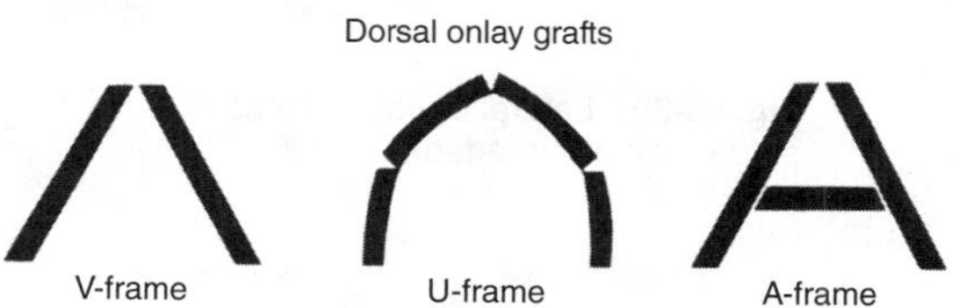


**Fig. 96-32** Partial-thickness incisions may be used to create V-, U-, or A-shaped grafts.

- **Auricular cartilage**
  - Lacks rigidity and volume of other sites
  - Must preserve crucial landmarks to prevent secondary defects of ear[29]
- **Costal cartilage**
  - Offers ample volume and strong support
  - Main drawback is propensity for warping
  - Balanced cross-sectional carving described by Gibson and Davis[30] may limit warping.
  - Lopez et al[31] suggested placing the concave side down, thus limiting effect of warping.
  - Gunter et al[32] suggested use of percutaneous K-wire to limit warping.
- **Irradiated costal cartilage**
  - Offers benefits of costal cartilage, obviating morbidity of donor site
  - Adams et al[33] showed that warping exists despite irradiation.
- **Diced or morselized cartilage**
  - Erol[34] described the Turkish delight (diced cartilage wrapped in Surgicel [Ethicon, Somerville, NJ]).
  - Daniel[35] suggested wrapping diced cartilage in fascia for less resorption.
- **Synthetic implants**[27]
  - **Silicone**
  - **Expanded polytetrafluoroethylene** (Gore-Tex)
  - **High-density polyethylene** (Medpor; Porex Surgical, Newnan, GA)
  - **Polyethylene terephthalate** (Dacron)
  - **AlloDerm** (LifeCell, Branchburg, NJ).
  - More commonly used in Asian countries

## OSTEOTOMIES

- *Control* is critical to successful osteotomies.
- May be percutaneous or endonasal.
- May be continuous or discontinuous (postage stamped).
- **Medial osteotomies**
  - The two most common medial osteotomies are the **medial oblique** and the **paramedian** (Fig. 96-33).
  - Typically used to narrow the bony vault
  - May also be used to widen the bony vault with lateral displacement of nasal bones
  - Involve a separation of the nasal bones and nasal septum
    - Should be performed *before* lateral osteotomies if medial osteotomies are to be successful
  - Separation provides stable upper vault bones on which the medial osteotomies can be performed
  - If lateral osteotomies are performed first, the bones will have little support, making them a moving target during the medial osteotomies.

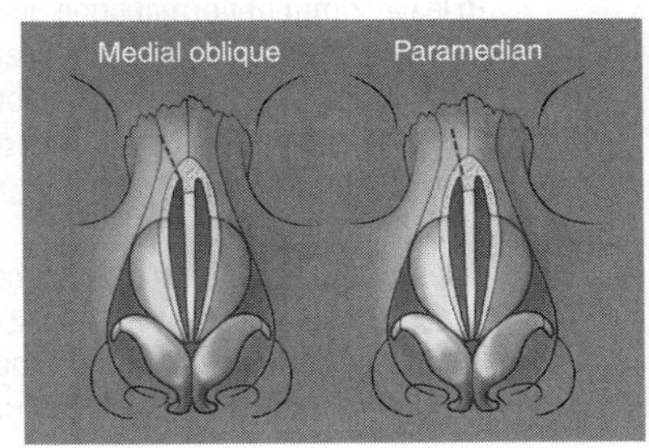


**Fig. 96-33** The two most common medial osteotomies.

- **Lateral osteotomies**
  - Serve to narrow wide bony dorsum, reposition asymmetrical nasal bones, or close open-roof deformity
  - Can be used to create complete fracture or to weaken the vault (with subsequent greenstick fracture to mobilize)

- **Three main types of lateral osteotomies**[36] (Fig. 96-34)
  - Classification nomenclature: *References height relative to face of maxilla*
    - **Low-high:** Begins low (lateral) at piriform aperture and extends cephalad to intercanthal line, ending high (medial) on the dorsum; used to mobilize a medium-wide nasal base or small open-roof deformity
    - **Low-low:** Begins low (lateral) at the piriform aperture and continues low (lateral), ending near the intercanthal line; used to mobilize bony roof and correct an excessively wide nasal base or a large open-roof deformity
    - **Double-level:** Lateral osteotomy performed first along nasal sidewall, approximating the nasomaxillary suture, and combined with low-low osteotomy; used for excessive lateral wall convexity and symmetrical or asymmetrical lateral nasal deformities

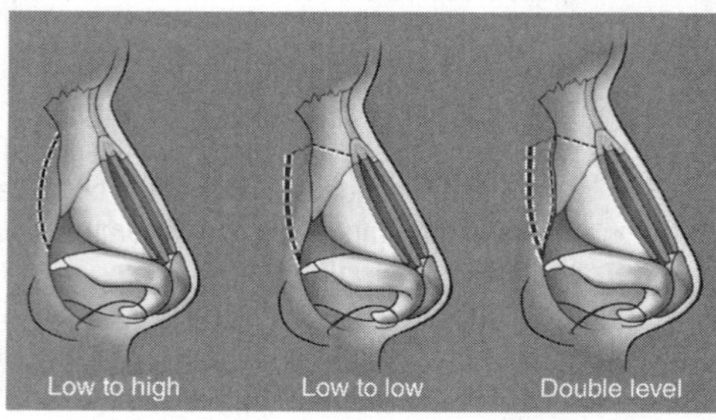


**Fig. 96-34** Types of lateral osteotomies.

- **Technique**[36]
  1. Lidocaine is infiltrated with epinephrine.
  2. A 2 mm osteotome is introduced at level of inferior orbital rim and nasofrontal junction.
  3. Osteotome should be parallel to surface of maxilla and positioned at the midportion of the bony vault.
  4. Nondominant hand is placed on nose while dominant hand holds osteotome.
  5. Gentle pressure is exerted on the nasal bones with the osteotome, and the osteotome is swept down the lateral nasal wall and laterally along the frontal process of the maxilla in a subperiosteal plane to the site of the first osteotomy. This effectively displaces the angular artery, thus minimizing bleeding.
  6. Multiple 2 mm osteotomies are carried out in the paths described previously, taking care to leave 2 mm of normal bone between each osteotomy. When moving the osteotome from one position to the next, keep osteotome against the maxilla to prevent the angular artery from returning to its previous position and potentially being injured.
  7. Once the osteotomies have been made, the thumb and index finger are used to gently reposition the bones.
- **Relative contraindications**
  - Elderly patients with thin nasal bones
  - Patients who wear heavy eyeglasses
  - Ethnic noses that are low and broad
  - Short nasal bones with a distal border <1 cm below the intercanthal line

**TIP:** The nasal bones are thickest at anatomic suture lines. Osteotomies in these areas would require increased force, which would lead to less control. Therefore they should be designed where cutting will be through thinner transition zones.

**TIP:** Angle the osteotome so that only one edge contacts the bone, thereby increasing force per square centimeter and maximizing control.

## Nasal Alae

- **Alar Rim Deformities**
  - May be congenital or acquired
  - Acquired deformities are usually the result of prior overzealous lateral crus resection.
  - Nonanatomic alar grafts lend structural support to the alar rim.
  - These include alar contour or rim grafts, alar batten grafts, and alar spreader grafts.
  - The most commonly used grafts are alar contour and lateral crural strut grafts.
  - **Alar contour grafts**
    - **Indications for placement of nonanatomic alar contour grafts**[37]
      - Secondary rhinoplasty patients with minimal vestibular lining loss and at least 3 mm of residual LLC
      - Primary rhinoplasty patients with congruent alar rim notching
      - Primary or secondary rhinoplasty patients with malpositioning of the LLCs
    - **Nonanatomic alar contour grafts are not effective for:**
      - Patients with alar rim retraction secondary to significant vestibular lining loss
      - Severe alar scarring
      - No LLC remnant
    - **Principles for nonanatomic alar contour graft placement**[37]
      - A 6 by 2 mm cartilage graft is fashioned; septal cartilage is preferred for this technique.
      - Use long, sharp Stevens scissors to create a pocket immediately above the alar rim.
      - Place cartilage graft in this pocket, and confirm that alar notching is corrected and that the graft is not visible.
      - A wider or second additional graft may be necessary for patients with severe scarring from previous rhinoplasty.
  - **Lateral crural strut grafts**
    - **Indications for placement of a lateral crural strut graft** [38]
      - Correction of the boxy nasal tip
      - Malpositioned lateral crura
      - Alar retraction
      - Alar rim collapse
      - Concave lateral crura
    - **Principles of lateral crural strut graft placement**[38]
      - Perform cephalic trim of lateral crura using an open rhinoplasty approach.
      - Undermine the vestibular skin off the lateral crura.
      - Carve a cartilage graft 3-4 by 15-25 mm, preferably of septal cartilage.
      - Place the lateral crural strut graft on the deep surface of the lateral crus in the undermined pocket.
      - Secure cartilage graft with two or three 5-0 Vicryl sutures.
      - Place the lateral end of the graft caudal to the alar groove to prevent visibility.

- Lateral crural strut grafts will be thicker and longer than the LLCs, and the lateral crura will assume the shape of the grafts.
- If alar rim is severely deformed, the LLCs may need to be separated from the accessory chain of cartilages to allow the lateral crural strut graft to extend further laterally (Fig. 96-35).

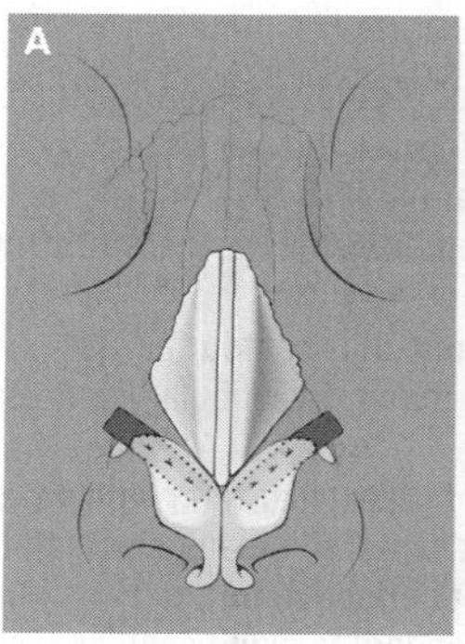


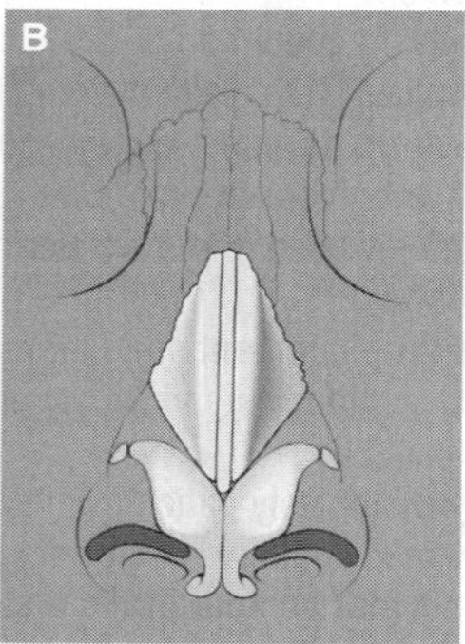


**Fig. 96-35** **A,** Lateral crural strut graft. **B,** Nonanatomic alar contour graft.

> **TIP:** It is essential to closely examine the basal view at conclusion of surgery. Any hint of alar notching should prompt the surgeon to place alar contour grafts.

- **Wide alae**
  - **Alar flaring**
    - Alar flare should be wedge excised with preservation of the alar base.
    - Inferior portion of wedge should preserve 1-2 mm of alar base to prevent alar notching.
    - The incision should not be carried into the nasal vestibule (Fig. 96-36).
  - **Excessively wide alar base**
    - A complete wedge is excised, with excision extending into the nasal vestibule 2 mm above the alar groove (Fig. 96-37).

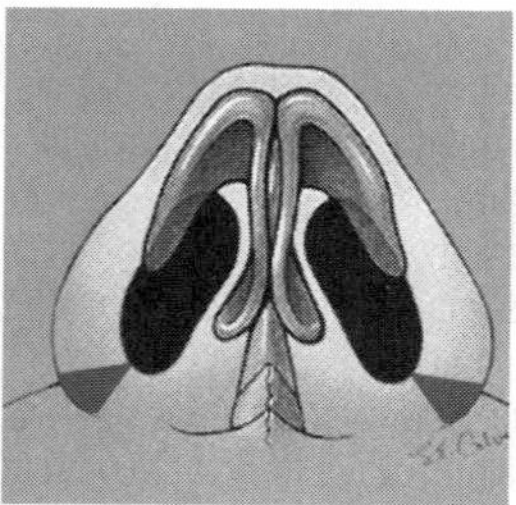

**Fig. 96-36** Correction of alar flaring.

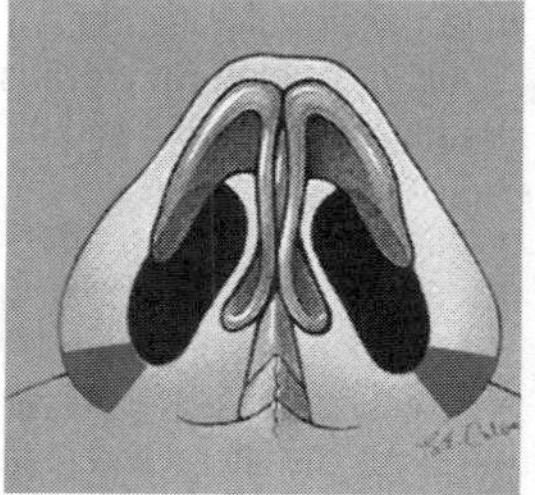

**Fig. 96-37** Correction of excessively wide alar bases.

  - A No. 11 blade is used to make the medial incision at the sill.
  - The blade is angled 30 degrees laterally. This results in a small flap medially, which is important to prevent notching postoperatively.

**TIP:** When correcting alar flare by wedge excision, the alar groove incision is longer than the incision on the alar surface. To ensure optimal approximation, the wound is closed using the halving principle.

**TIP:** Alar base resection alters the alar-cheek junction, affecting the overall appearance of nasal projection.[39]

## Nasal Airway

- **Deviated septum**
  - Deviated portion may be resected by open or closed technique.
  - Open rhinoplasty allows dissection to be centered on the anterior septal angle to expose the septum.
  - Closed rhinoplasty or septoplasty alone is approached through two main incisions.
    - **Hemitransfixion incision:** Incision is made at junction of cartilaginous and membranous septum, providing optimal access to caudal septum.
    - **Killian incision:** Incision is made posterior to the cartilaginous and membranous septal junction, allowing a more focused approach to the deviation at the expense of limited caudal septum access.
    - In either approach the mucoperichondrium and mucoperiosteum are separated from the underyling cartilage.
  - Deviated cartilage is treated either through resection or a combination of scoring, suture, or strut to straighten.
  - A minimum of 1 cm septal *L strut* (dorsal and caudal septum) must be preserved to prevent *saddle-nose deformity.*
  - Placement of mattress sutures in weakened cartilage is an effective way to preserve tissue while straightening.[40]
  - Bony spurs or deviation is cautiously removed without disturbing the skull base.
  - Skull base (cribriform plate) disruption may lead to cerebrospinal fluid leakage.
  - The end result should be a midline septum secured to the nasal spine.
  - Doyle splints, transseptal suture, or nasal packing is used to appose mucosal flaps back to the remaining septum.
  - If bilateral mucosal tears occur at the same position, a septal perforation may result.
    - If none exist, a small stab incision should be made to serve as a drainage hole to deter hematoma formation.
- **Turbinate hypertrophy**
  - Beekhuis[41] reviewed 1000 rhinoplasty patients and found that 10% had nasal obstruction postoperatively, most resulting from turbinate hypertrophy.
  - After correction of septal deviation, surgeons should determine whether hypertrophied turbinate will lead to obstruction.
  - Turbinate hypertrophy can correct over time, with medication relief in interim.

- Two common methods of surgical correction:
  - **Outfracture:** Performed using a Boise elevator or a Vienna speculum (Fig. 96-38). The turbinates are fractured and displaced laterally. Crucial to be aware of orbit and skull base in relation to any instrument introduced into the nasal cavity.
  - **Submucosal resection:** Mucosa preserved with removal of underlying anterior bone. Excessive resection of the inferior turbinate decreases its ability to regulate airflow.

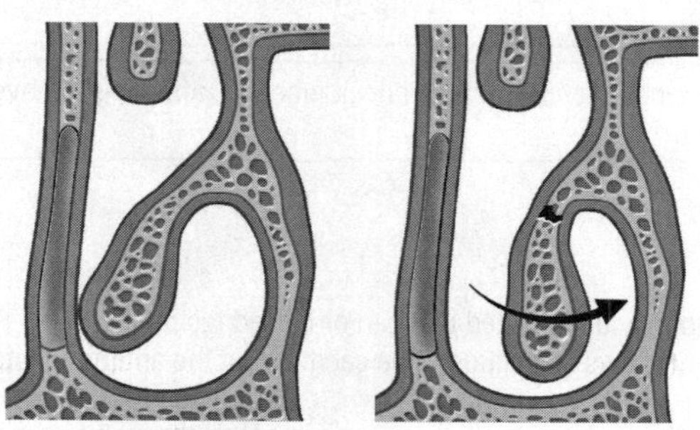

**Fig. 96-38** Outfracture of the inferior turbinate.

- **Nasal valve**
  - Treatment of the internal nasal valve centers on increasing the angle between the caudal ULC and dorsal septum.
  - Suture techniques have been described, but spreader grafts are the most popular method presently used.[42]
  - Use of a lateral nasal wall graft may add support and fortify the nasal valve.
  - Correction of external valve deformity centers on fortification of the LLC and nasal ala, and removal of obstruction.
  - **Alar position and support**
    - Cartilage grafts (e.g., alar contour grafts, lateral crural strut grafts, batten grafts)
    - Suture techniques
  - **Obstruction**
    - Correction of deviated caudal septum
    - Correction of abnormal flaring of the medial crura
    - Reduction of soft tissue excess
    - Combination of above
  - **Five-step medial crural footplate modification**[43]
    1. Location and extent of splayed footplates are marked by two symmetrical lines that parallel the columella along the inferior medial portion of the nasal sill.
    2. Minimal mucosa (1-2 mm) is excised overlying the marked area of the medial crural footplates.
    3. A 5-0 PDS horizontal mattress spanning suture is passed across the columella to secure the medial crural footplates.

4. A second 4-0 chromic gut horizontal mattress suture is used to capture the soft tissue mass at the columellar base.
5. Mucosa is closed with 5-0 chromic gut.

## Deviated Nose

- Causes are deviated septum, ULC-deforming forces, or asymmetrical nasal bones.
- Obtain wide exposure of the deviated structures.
- Release all of the mucoperichondrial attachments of the deviated septum.
- Release deforming forces, including the LLCs and ULCs from each other, and the ULCs from the septum.
- If deviation is caused by asymmetry of the ULCs, the septal deviation can be corrected by the release of the ULCs from the LLCs.
- If the deviation is result of septal deviation, the septum must be straightened.
- The caudal septum must be anatomically reduced onto the nasal spine.
  - May require a vertical sectioning to create a "swinging door"
    - If this is insufficient, small wedges of cartilage can be excised from the convex side of the deviation, with cartilage scoring on the concave side to destroy the cartilage memory and straighten the septum.
- The caudal septum is sutured to the periosteum of the nasal spine and held reduced with a graft of septal cartilage.
- If septal deviation occurs higher in the nose, correction should first be attempted by shaving the convex side of the deviation with addition of cartilage dorsal spreader grafts to the concave side of the dorsum to camouflage the deformity.
  - If this is unsuccessful in correcting the deformity, cartilage-scoring techniques such as those described for caudal defects can be attempted.
- If high dorsal deviation persists after these maneuvers, a series of full-thickness cuts can be made through the deviated portion of the dorsal septum.
  - These full-thickness cuts must be made only through 50% of the dorsal L-strut.
  - If the cuts are thicker than this, the L-strut will not be able to support the dorsum and collapse will occur.
- If full-thickness cuts need to be made, then bilateral cartilage spreader grafts should be placed for support and better definition of the dorsal aesthetic lines.
- Straightening of the septum narrows the nasal airway in patients with preexisting inferior turbinate hypertrophy.
- Submucous resection of the hypertrophied inferior turbinate must be performed to prevent postoperative airway obstruction.
- Asymmetrical nasal bones are treated next.
- Correction begins with asymmetrical oblique rasping of the nasal bones.
- If this fails to correct the deviation or asymmetry, osteotomies are performed to correct the deviation.
- If the nasal bones are symmetrical, lateral osteotomies alone will be sufficient.
- If the nasal bones are asymmetrical, then medial osteotomies may be required[44] (Fig. 96-39).

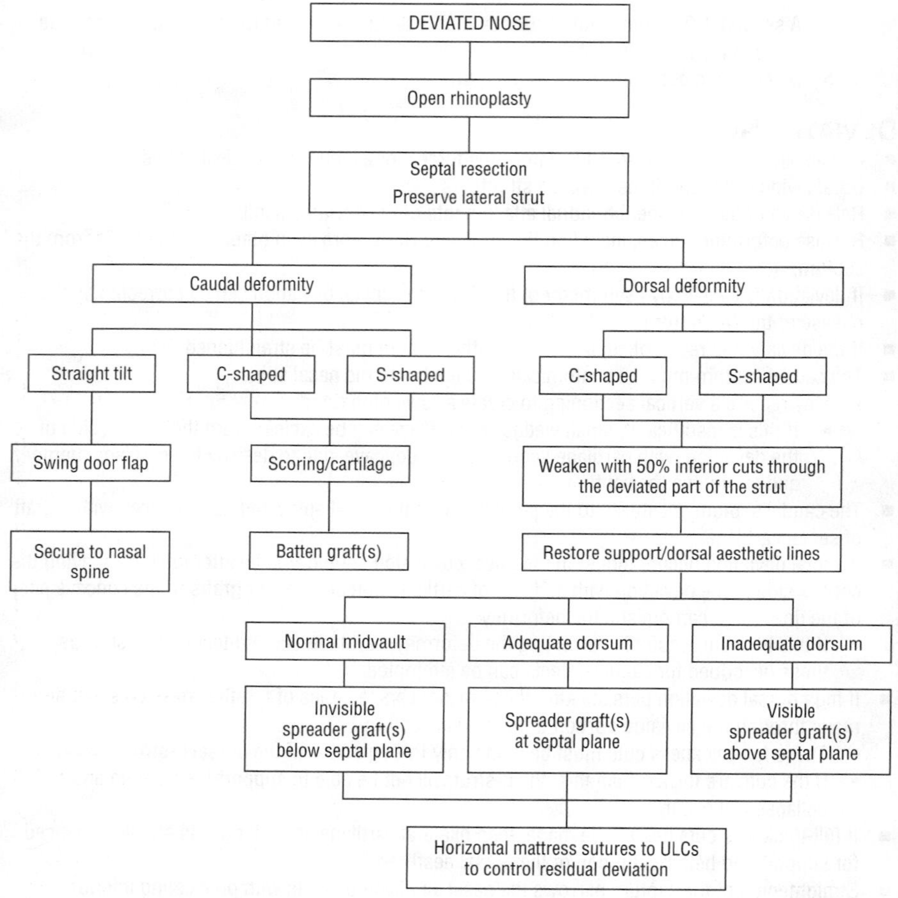


**Fig. 96-39** Algorithm for correction of a deviated nose. (*ULCs,* Upper lateral cartilages.)

## SECONDARY RHINOPLASTY

- More challenging operation than primary rhinoplasty.
- Scar formation, prior grafts, cartilage deficiency are responsible for complexity.
- Gunter and Rohrich[20] published the classic article in 1987 for open approach rationale.
- Common problems seen in secondary rhinoplasty[45]:
  - Residual bony deviation
  - Middle vault collapse
  - Graft visibility/palpability
  - Underresected or overresected dorsum
  - Damaged LLC and subsequent tip deformities
  - Pinched tip
  - Alar notching or retraction

- The amount of LLC reconstruction is related to the existing deformity.[46,47]
- Tip grafts are more commonly reserved for secondary rhinoplasty tip alteration.

## Key Points

- ✓ A thorough understanding of nasal anatomy and nasal aesthetics is essential for successful rhinoplasty.
- ✓ Planning begins with comprehensive analysis using AP, lateral, and basilar views.
- ✓ The open and closed approaches have advantages and disadvantages.
- ✓ Rhinoplasty has evolved from a cartilage-destructive operation to a more cartilage preserving/manipulating operation.
- ✓ Nasal airway obstruction may be caused by reversible medical conditions or by surgically correctible conditions such as internal or external nasal valve collapse, septal deviation, or inferior turbinate hypertrophy.
- ✓ A graduated approach to nasal tip projection is recommended; columellar strut followed by tip suturing with tip grafts is reserved for patients in whom the prior methods are inadequate.
- ✓ The tripod model helps in understanding tip projection and rotation.
- ✓ Reduction of the dorsum should be completed using the component method to preserve the middle vault.
- ✓ Regardless of the osteotomy method, maximizing control is crucial for success.
- ✓ Choosing the correct approach to alar base surgery requires determining the degree of alar flaring.
- ✓ Secondary rhinoplasty is a more difficult operation than primary rhinoplasty, underscoring the importance of getting it right the first time.

## References


1. Joseph J. Nasenplastick und Sonstige Gesichtsplastik Nebsteinen Anhang Ueber Mammaplastik. Leipzig: Verlag von Curt Kabitzsch, 1931.
2. Rohrich RJ, Huynh B, Muzaffar AR, et al. Importance of the depressor septi nasi muscle in rhinoplasty: anatomic study and clinical application. Plast Reconstr Surg 105:376-383; discussion 384-388, 2000.
3. Rohrich RJ, Gunter JP, Friedman RM. Nasal tip blood supply: an anatomic study validating the safety of the transcolumellar incision in rhinoplasty. Plast Reconstr Surg 95:795-799; discussion 800-801, 1995.
4. Rohrich RJ, Muzaffar AR, Gunter JP. Nasal tip blood supply: confirming the safety of the transcolumellar incision in rhinoplasty. Plast Reconstr Surg 106:1640-1641, 2000.
5. Adams WP Jr, Rohrich RJ, Hollier LH, et al. Anatomic basis and clinical implications for nasal tip support in open versus closed rhinoplasty. Plast Reconstr Surg 103:255-261; discussion 262-264, 1999.
6. Lee MR, Inman J, Callahan S, et al. Fracture patterns of the nasal septum. Otolaryngol Head Neck Surg 143:784-788, 2010.
7. Rohrich RJ, Krueger JK, Adams WP Jr, et al. Rationale for submucous resection of hypertrophied inferior turbinates in rhinoplasty: an evolution. Plast Reconstr Surg 108:536-544; discussion 545-546, 2001.

8. Mink PJ. Physiologie der Obern Luftwege. Leipzig: Vogel, 1920.
9. Toriumi DM, Josen J, Weinberger M, et al. Use of alar batten grafts for correction of nasal valve collapse. Arch Otolaryngol Head Neck Surg 123:802-808, 1997.
10. Rohrich RJ, Hollier LH. Use of spreader grafts in the external approach to rhinoplasty. Clin Plast Surg 23:255-262, 1996.
11. Rohrich RJ, Liu JH. Defining the infratip lobule in rhinoplasty. Anatomy, pathogenesis of abnormalities and correction using an algorithmic approach. Plast Reconstr Surg 130:1148-1158, 2012.
12. Gunter JP, Landecker A, Cochran CS. Frequently used grafts in rhinoplasty: nomenclature and analysis. Plast Reconstr Surg 118:14e-29e, 2006.
13. Gunter JP, Rohrich RJ, Adams WP. Dallas Rhinoplasty: Nasal Surgery by the Masters, 2nd ed. St Louis: Quality Medical Publishing, 2007.
14. Sheen JH, Sheen AP. Aesthetic Rhinoplasty, 2nd ed. St Louis: Quality Medical Publishing, 1998.
15. Byrd JS, Burt JD, Andochick S, et al. Septal extension grafts: a method for controlling tip projection and shape. Plast Reconstr Surg 100:999-1010, 1997.
16. Janis J, Trussler A, Ghavami A. Lower lateral crural turnover flap in open rhinoplasty. Plast Reconstr Surg 123:1830-1841, 2009.
17. Roe JO. The deformity of the pug nose and its correction by a simple operation. Med Rec 31:621, 1887.
18. Sheen JH. Closed versus open rhinoplasty—and the debate goes on. Plast Reconstr Surg 99:859-862, 1997.
19. Vogt T. Tip rhinoplastic operations using a transverse columellar incision. Aesthetic Plast Surg 7:13-19, 1983.
20. Gunter JP, Rohrich RJ. External approach for secondary rhinoplasty. Plast Reconstr Surg 80:161-174, 1987.
21. Rohrich RJ, Griffin JR. Correction of intrinsic nasal tip asymmetries in primary rhinoplasty. Plast Reconstr Surg 112:1699-1712; discussion 1713-1715, 2003.
22. Ghavami A, Janis JE, Acikel C, et al. Tip shaping in primary rhinoplasty: an algorithmic approach. Plast Reconstr Surg 122:1229-1241, 2008.
23. Rohrich RJ, Adams WP Jr. The boxy nasal tip: classification and management based on alar cartilage suturing techniques. Plast Reconstr Surg 107:1849-1863; discussion 1864-1868, 2001.
24. Tebbetts JB. Shaping and positioning the nasal tip without structural disruption: a new, systematic approach. Plast Reconstr Surg 94:61-77, 1994.
25 Guyuron B, Behmand RA. Nasal tip sutures. II. The interplays. Plast Reconstr Surg 112:1130-1145, 2003.
26. Rohrich RJ, Muzaffar AR, Janis JE. Component dorsal hump reduction: the importance of maintaining dorsal aesthetic lines in rhinoplasty. Plast Reconstr Surg 114:1298-1308; discussion 1309-1312, 2004.
27. Lee MR, Unger JG, Rohrich RJ. Management of the nasal dorsum in rhinoplasty: a systematic review of the literature regarding technique, outcomes, and complications. Plast Reconstr Surg 128:538e-550e, 2011.
28. Gunter JP, Rohrich RJ. Augmentation rhinoplasty: dorsal onlay grafting using shaped autogenous septal cartilage. Plast Reconstr Surg 86:39-45, 1990.
29. Lee MR, Callahan S, Cochran S. Auricular cartilage: harvest and versatility in rhinoplasty. Am J Otolaryn 32:547-552, 2011.
30. Gibson T, Davis WB. The distortion of autologous cartilage grafts: its cause and prevention. Br J Plast Surg 10:257, 1958.
31. Lopez MA, Shah AR, Westine JG, et al. Analysis of the physical properties of costal cartilage in a porcine model. Arch Facial Plast Surg 9:35-39, 2007.

32. Gunter JP, Rohrich RJ, Adams WP. Dallas Rhinoplasty: Nasal Surgery by the Masters. St Louis: Quality Medical Publishing, 2002.
33. Adams WP, Rohrich RJ, Gunter JP, et al. The rate of warping in irradiated and nonirradiated homograft rib cartilage: a controlled comparison and clinical implications. Plast Reconstr Surg 103:265-270, 1999.
34. Erol O. Tip rhinoplasty in broad noses in a Turkish population: Eurasian noses. Plast Reconstr Surg 130:185-197, 2012.
35. Daniel RK. Diced cartilage grafts in rhinoplasty surgery: current techniques and applications. Plast Reconstr Surg 122:1883-1891, 2008.
36. Rohrich RJ, Krueger JK, Adams WP Jr, et al. Achieving consistency in the lateral nasal osteotomy during rhinoplasty: an external perforated technique. Plast Reconstr Surg 108:2122-2130; discussion 2131-2132, 2001.
37. Rohrich RJ, Raniere J Jr, Ha RY. The alar contour graft: correction and prevention of alar rim deformities in rhinoplasty. Plast Reconstr Surg 109:2495-2505; discussion 2506-2508, 2002.
38. Gunter JP, Friedman RM. Lateral crural strut graft: technique and clinical applications in rhinoplasty. Plast Reconstr Surg 99:943-952; discussion 953-955, 1997.
39. Unger JG, Lee MR, Kwon RK, et al. A multivariate analysis of nasal tip projection. Plast Reconstr Surg 129:1163-1167, 2012.
40. Gruber RP. Suture correction of nasal tip cartilage concavities. Plast Reconstr Surg 100:1616-1617, 1997.
41. Beekhuis GJ. Nasal obstruction after rhinoplasty: etiology, and techniques for correction. Laryngoscope 86:540-548, 1976.
42. Lee MR, Unger JG, Gryskiewicz J, Rohrich RJ. Current clinical practices of the rhinoplasty society members. Ann Plast Surg 71:453-455, 2013.
43. Geissler PJ, Lee MR, Roostaeian J, Unger JG, Rohrich RJ. Reshaping the medial nostril and columellar base: five-step medial crural footplate approximation. Plast Reconstr Surg 132:553-557, 2013.
44. Rohrich RJ, Gunter JP, Deuber MA, et al. The deviated nose: optimizing results using a simplified classification and algorithmic approach. Plast Reconstr Surg 110:1509-1523, 2002.
45. Rohrich RJ, Lee MR. External approach for secondary rhinoplasty: advances over the past 25 years. Plast Reconstr Surg 131:404-415, 2013.
46. Gunter JP, Yu YL. The tripod concept for correcting nasal-tip cartilages. Aesthet Surg J 24:257-260, 2004.
47. Menick FJ. Anatomic reconstruction of the nasal tip cartilages in secondary and reconstructive rhinoplasty. Plast Reconstr Surg 104:2187-2198, 1999.

# 97. Genioplasty

Lee W.T. Alkureishi, Matthew R. Greives, Ashkan Ghavami

## ANATOMY

### Relevant Muscles[1] (Fig. 97-1)

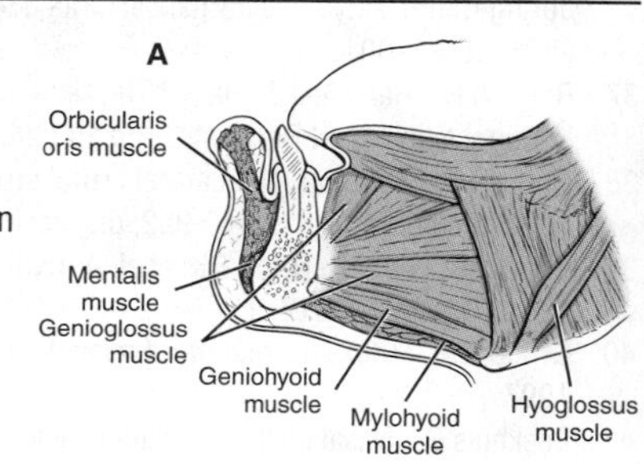


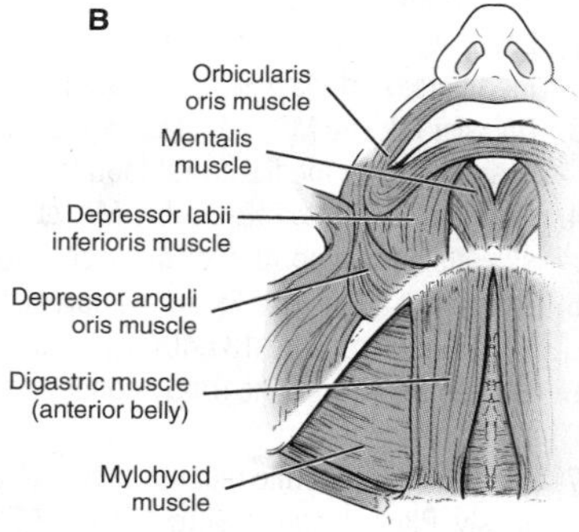


Fig. 97-1

- Mentalis: Most important muscle, encountered via intraoral approach
  - Conelike geometry
  - Vertical fibers from incisor fossa to overlying skin
    - Can cause wrinkling
    - If hyperdynamic, may be visible under lower lip
    - Midline void between fibers seen when chin dimple is present
  - Intraoral incisions transect mentalis: Must be reattached to prevent chin ptosis *(witch's chin deformity)*
- Orbicularis oris (lower fibers)
- Depressor anguli oris
- Quadratus (depressor) labii inferioris
- Geniohyoid, genioglossus, mylohyoid, and anterior belly of digastric
  - Attach to lingual (posterior) aspect of chin

### Bony Landmarks

- Mental foramen: In line with pupil, infraorbital foramen, and second premolar; may be multiple
- Digastric fossa: Origin of anterior belly of digastric
- Mental protuberance: Triangular bony prominence of lower anterior aspect of the mandible
- Mental spines: Muscular attachments for geniohyoid, suprahyoid muscles, and genioglossus
- Submandibular fossa: Impression on medial surface of mandible below the mylohyoid line

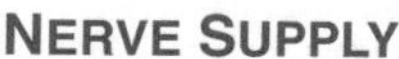

### Nerve Supply

- Inferior alveolar nerve (from mandibular nerve): Enters mandibular foramen and travels within mandibular canal
- Mental nerve is terminal branch: Exits at mental foramen. Path of nerve is below level of foramen.
  - Genioplasty procedures carry risk of injury.

**CAUTION: Osteotomies should be 5-6 mm below mental foramen to prevent injury to nerve branches or tooth apices.**

- Nerve can be absent or distorted in patients with hemifacial microsomia or other facial deformities.

## Blood Supply

- Labial branches of facial artery
- Inferior alveolar artery: Runs with inferior alveolar nerve in mandibular canal. Mental branch exits with mental nerve.

## Significant Cephalometric Points (Fig. 97-2)

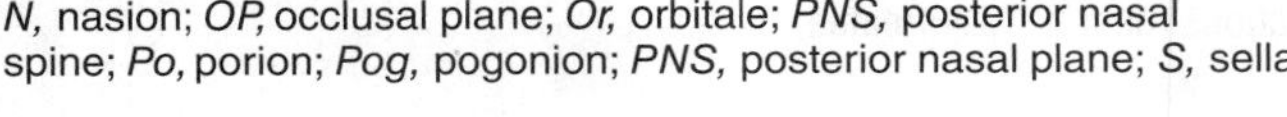


**Fig. 97-2** Significant cephalometric points. (*A,* A-point; *ANS,* anterior nasal spine; *Ar,* articulaire; *B,* B-point; *Ba,* basion; *FH,* Frankfort horizontal plane; *GN,* gnathion; *Go,* gonion; *Me,* menton; *MP,* mandibular plane; *N,* nasion; *OP,* occlusal plane; *Or,* orbitale; *PNS,* posterior nasal spine; *Po,* porion; *Pog,* pogonion; *PNS,* posterior nasal plane; *S,* sella.)

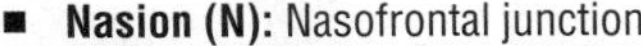

- **Nasion (N):** Nasofrontal junction
- **Subspinale (A):** Columella-labial junction
- **Supramentale (B):** Deepest point between pogonion and incisor
- **Pogonion (Pog):** Most projecting portion of mandible. Indicates chin excess or deficiency in relation to other structures (e.g., nasion and lip position)
- **Menton (Me):** Lowest (most caudal) portion of chin

# CLASSIFICATION OF CHIN DEFORMITIES (Table 97-1)

- **Microgenia:** Small chin
- **Macrogenia:** Large chin
- **Combined deformities:** Short or long macrogenia/microgenia
  - Horizontal (off center) asymmetries can also exist.
- Classification system proposed by Guyuron et al[2] can guide surgical planning (see Table 97-1).

**Table 97-1** *Classification System*

| Type | Deformity | Vector and Surgical Treatment |
|---|---|---|
| Class I | Macrogenia | Horizontal: Osteotomy with setback or ostectomy<br>Vertical: Osteotomy and resection<br>Both horizontal and vertical: Osteotomy, resection, and setback |
| Class II | Microgenia | Horizontal: Osteotomy with advancement, autogenous or alloplastic augmentation<br>Vertical: Osteotomy and lengthening, with or without graft<br>Both horizontal and vertical: Osteotomy, lengthening, and advancement, with or without graft |
| Class III | Combined | Horizontal macrogenia with vertical microgenia: Osteotomy with lengthening and setback<br>Horizontal microgenia with vertical macrogenia: Osteotomy with resection of horizontal segment and advancement |
| Class IV | Asymmetrical | Short anterior lower face: Addition of wedge of bone to short side<br>Normal lower facial height: Removal of wedge of bone from long side; add to short side<br>Long anterior facial height: Removal of wedge of bone based on long side |
| Class V | Witch's chin | Soft tissue correction |
| Class VI | Pseudomacrogenia | Soft tissue adjustment (not predictable) |
| Class VII | Pseudomicrogenia | Maxillary osteotomy |

## PREOPERATIVE EVALUATION

### Complete History and Physical Examination

- Diabetes mellitus: Poor candidates for implantation; at risk for infection and wound-healing problems
- Poorly controlled hypertension: Increased risk for ecchymosis/hematoma
- Smoking history: Healing problems and infection risk, especially with implantation or grafts
- **Dental history**
  - Before dentition is fully erupted (~age 15), risk of injury to teeth with osteotomies is greater.
  - Alloplastic augmentation may be most appropriate in elderly/edentulous patients with poor bone stock.
  - Dental/intraoral infections must be fully treated.

### Occlusion Type (Fig. 97-3)

- **Angle class I**
  - Mesiobuccal cusp of maxillary first molar rests in the buccal groove of mandibular first molar (see Fig. 97-3, *A*).
- **Angle class II (retrognathia, overjet)**
  - Mesiobuccal cusp of maxillary first molar rests **mesial (anterior)** to buccal groove (see Fig. 97-3, *B*).
  - *Most common malocclusion in North American white individuals.*
  - Orthognathic surgery with maxillary and mandibular osteotomies may be necessary.
- **Angle class III (prognathism, negative overjet)**
  - Mesiobuccal cusp of the maxillary first molar rests **distal (posterior)** to buccal groove of mandibular first molar (see Fig. 97-3, *C*).

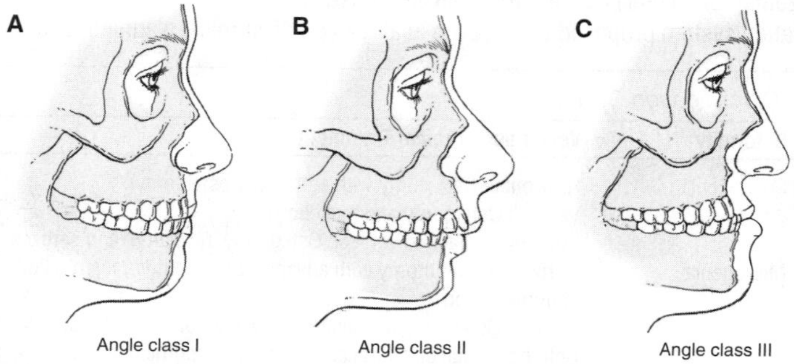


**Fig. 97-3** Occlusion types. **A,** Angle class I. **B,** Angle class II. **C,** Angle class III.

> **TIP:** Obtaining previous orthodontic history is important, because occlusion may have been corrected without adjusting for maxillary and mandibular disharmonies (deformity is masked). These patients frequently seek genioplasty, but wish to avoid "undoing" their previous orthodontia. The limits of this approach should be discussed in detail.[3]

## IMAGING: EVALUATION OF SOFT TISSUES[4]

- Standardized frontal view, bilateral oblique (three-quarter) views, and bilateral sagittal (lateral) views
- **Assess symmetry.**
  - Identification of preexisting asymmetries is crucial.
  - Subtle nerve palsies (idiopathic or iatrogenic) may only be evident on animation.
  - Bony asymmetries may be corrected with offset osteotomies.
- **Determine lower facial height.**
  - Divide the face horizontally into thirds.[5]
  - Glabella to subnasale distance should equal subnasale to menton distance.[6]
    - Decreased facial height may be caused by vertical maxillary deficiency, decreased vertical chin height, or both.
    - Elongation via osteotomy may be required.[7]
  - Vertical maxillary excess is best seen by maxillary incisal show of >3 mm.
    - Lip strain is a puckered appearance caused by compensatory contraction of mentalis to achieve lip closure.
    - Patients are better served with formal orthognathic correction.
- **Assess for lip incompetence.**
  - If it is present, osseous genioplasty may be most appropriate.[8]
- **Upper lip–lower lip relationship and chin projection**
  - Riedel's line (Fig. 97-4): Connects most prominent point of upper and lower lips
    - Pogonion ideally touches this line (variations with horizontal microgenia versus macrogenia, or excess soft tissue of the chin).
  - Porion-orbitale-subnasale (P-O) line: Perpendicular to the Frankfort horizontal plane[9]
    - Upper lip vermilion ($0 \pm 2$ mm from P-O line)
    - Lower lip vermilion ($-2 \pm +2$ mm from P-O line)
    - Soft tissue pogonion ($-4 \pm 2$ mm from P-O line)
- **Labiomental crease**
  - Fold aesthetics dependent on **vertical proportion of mandible and facial length**[2,10] (Fig. 97-5)

**TIP:** A deep fold may look good on longer faces.[11]

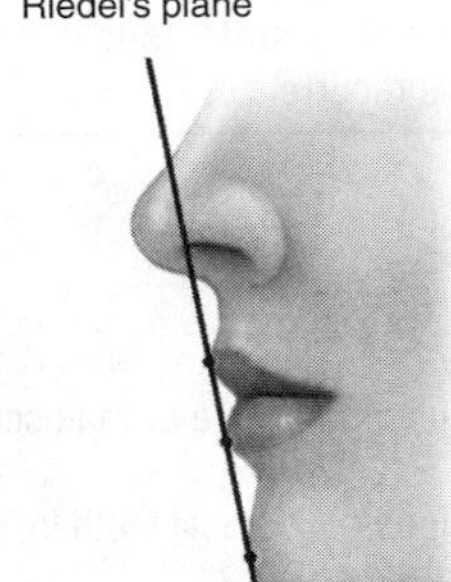


**Fig. 97-4** Riedel's plane is a simple line that connects the most prominent portion of the upper and lower lip, which on a balanced face should touch the pogonion.

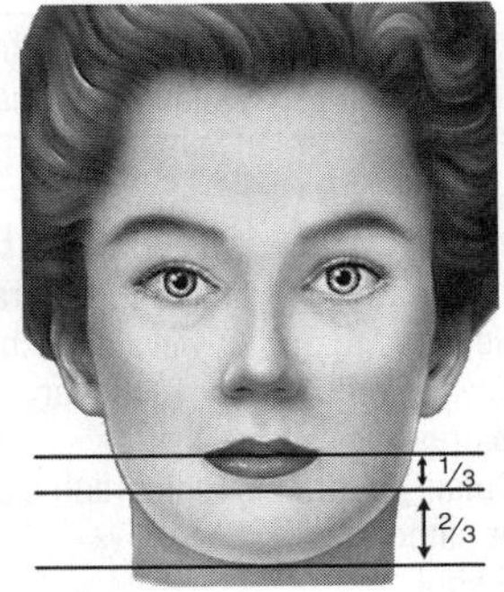


**Fig. 97-5** A horizontal line through the labiomental groove is a third of the distance from the stomion to the menton.

- Evaluate for **height** (if dividing stomion to menton into thirds, fold often falls at junction of upper and middle thirds).
  - If fold is too low, augmentation may only treat chin pad.[4]
- **Depth** should be 4 mm in women, 6 mm in men.
  - Deep crease may be caused by excessive chin projection or prominent/flared lower incisors. Horizontal vector chin augmentation can lead to exaggerated deep fold and overprojected chin.
  - Shallow crease can result from horizontal microgenia or lingually inclined teeth and can be further effaced by vertical augmentation.
  - Shape and depth of fold can be influenced by both alloplastic and osseous genioplasty.

- **Soft tissue pad:** Normally 9-11 mm thick
  - Palpate at pogonion and off midline with patient in repose and when smiling.
  - Soft tissue contribution can predict effects of augmentation.
- **Lower lip**
  - Length: Subnasale-stomion distance should be half the stomion-menton distance.
  - Lower lip eversion from deep bite, excess lip bulk, or excess overjet may deepen labiomental fold.[12]
- **Witch's chin deformity**
  - Soft tissue ptosis caudal to menton exaggerates submental crease.
  - Correction requires elliptical skin and soft tissue and muscle resection/repositioning.
  - Augmentation can exaggerate the deformity.
- **Cervicomental angle: Angle between chin and neck in sagittal view**
  - Normal angle is 105-120 degrees.
  - Submental lipectomy, platysmaplasty, or resection of anterior digastric/submandibular gland can be used as adjuncts to genioplasty.

## Dynamic and Static Chin Pad Analysis[4]

- A **thin** chin pad when smiling can increase pad effacement with increased bony prominence (can be native or caused by augmentation).
  - Burr reduction or osteotomy setback may be required.
- A **thick** pad may increase submental soft tissue fullness and worsen the cervicomental angle if bony setback is performed.

> **TIP:** Mentalis muscle fixation superiorly is essential for preventing soft tissue descent. Secondary cases may require soft tissue fixation to prevent ptosis recurrence.[13]

## Imaging: Evaluation of Bony Deformities

- **Cephalograms and/or panoramic radiographs (Panorex)**
  - Required to properly evaluate chin deficiency or excess
  - Always indicated for secondary cases or if maxillary/mandibular imbalance or malocclusion is present
  - Obtain panoramic radiograph if any concern about nerve malposition, apical teeth location, or pathology
- **Occlusion**
  - Angle class I occlusion can usually be managed with genioplasty.
  - Angle class II/III occlusion may require mandibular/maxillary osteotomies, with or without genioplasty.[7]

- **Steiner analysis:** Provides information on the relationship between the skull base, maxilla, and mandible (see Fig. 97-2).
  - S-N-A (sella-nasion-subspinale) angle: Relationship of midface to skull base
  - S-N-B (sella-nasion-supramentale) angle: Relationship of mandible to skull base
  - A-N-B (A point-nasion-B point) angle: Relationship of midface to mandible

## OSSEOUS GENIOPLASTY[1] (Fig. 97-6)

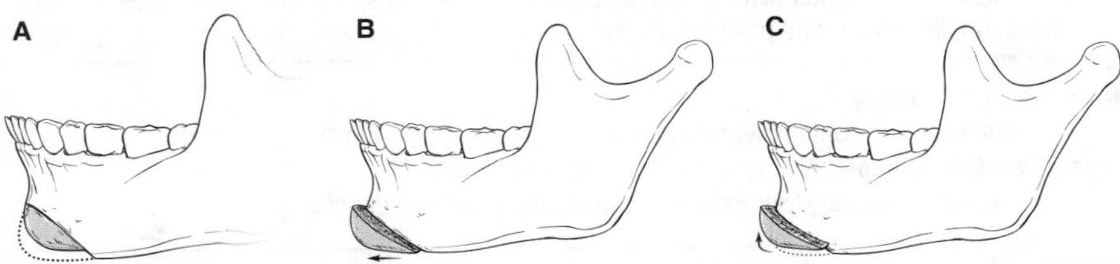


**Fig. 97-6** Types of genioplasty. **A,** Reduction genioplasty. **B,** Sliding genioplasty. **C,** Jumping genioplasty.

- **More versatile** than alloplastic augmentation
  - Sliding genioplasty is well suited to treatment of more complex deformities.
  - Careful planning of osteotomies allows correction in three dimensions.
- **Indications**
  - Horizontal asymmetries of any magnitude
  - Deficiency or excess in both vertical and sagittal planes
    - Moderate-to-severe microgenia
  - Direct reduction of inferior cortex with saw or burr
  - Secondary cases (especially after implant-related complications)[14]
  - As an adjunct to formal orthognathic surgery
- **Contraindications**
  - Inadequate bone stock (e.g., elderly patient)
  - Abnormal dentition or intraoral infections: Require treatment before genioplasty
  - Patient preference against osteotomies

Malocclusion requires consideration of orthognathic surgery and a more extensive workup, including cephalometric analysis and occlusion models.

### Soft Tissue Response/Osseous Movement Ratio

- **Osteotomy and alloplastic augmentation:** Approximately 0.8-0.9:1
- **Ostectomy:** Approximately 0.25-0.50:1

### Patient Selection

- Increased vertical height or sagittal excess
- Can be used in conjunction with orthognathic surgery

## Types of Osteotomies

- **Reduction genioplasty**
  - **Indication:** Increased vertical height or sagittal excess
  - Osteotomy angled inferiorly to produce vertical reduction

**NOTE: Excess vertical height of the mandible requires formal orthognathic procedures, commonly with a simultaneous genioplasty.**

> **TIP:** Genioplasty results can be enhanced with submental soft tissue procedures such as liposuction, lipectomy, and platysmaplasty.

- **Sliding genioplasty**
  - **Indication:** Horizontal (sagittal) deficiency (standard operation)
  - **Two-tier genioplasty:** Two segments advanced anteriorly
    - Rarely necessary: For extreme sagittal and/or vertical deficiency

> **TIP:** Dissection carried in an oblique anterior direction or at right angle to the bone provides a small cuff of intact mentalis muscle to facilitate soft tissue approximation when closing.

- **Jumping genioplasty**
  - **Indication:** Very minor chin height excess
  - Inferior fragment "jumped" over superior segment as an onlay
  - Augment anterior projection with small reduction in vertical height.

> **TIP:** Excess inferior/posterior stripping may devascularize the lower bone segment after osteotomy is performed. Only lateral exposure is required to view the mental nerves.

- **Ostectomy**
  - **Indication:** Significant height reduction
- **Interpositional bone grafts (or hydroxyapatite)**
  - **Indication:** To add more vertical length
  - Added to osteotomy segment that has been angled superiorly
- **Centralizing genioplasty**
  - **Indication:** To correct horizontal asymmetries
  - Wedges of autogenous bone graft or hydroxyapatite often needed
- **Approaches**
  - Intraoral: allows easy access for osteotomy and fixation
- **Fixation**
  - Plates/screws
  - Wires
  - Sutures

## IMPLANT GENIOPLASTY[1]

- Technically straightforward
- Low complication rate
- **Indications**
  - Mild isolated sagittal (horizontal) deficiencies
  - Shallow labiomental fold

- Relative: Concomitant neck lift/face lift
  - Cosmetic surgery patients tend to favor implants over osteotomy.
  - Face-lift/neck-lift procedures often include a submental incision that can easily be used for placing a chin implant.
- **Contraindications**
  - Excess horizontal deficiency
  - Vertical mandibular deficiency of any severity
  - Mandibular asymmetry
  - Secondary cases with bony erosion
  - Significant microgenia
  - Relative contraindication: Smokers, diabetics
  - Malocclusion: May require orthognathic surgery

## Implant Types[15]

- **Synthetic**
  - **Silicone** (smooth or textured)
  - **Porous polyethylene (Medpor; Porex Surgical, Newnan, GA):** Pores allow tissue ingrowth and incorporation of implant rather than encapsulation (as with silicone and nonporous implants).
    - Infection rate may be lower for porous implants, but removal is much more challenging.
  - Custom-made implants based on three-dimensional modeling (perhaps more useful if multiple facial implants required)
  - Comprehensive approach: Large implants for lateral augmentation combined with mandibular angle implants or other facial implants[1]

## Approach

- **Extraoral**
  - **Advantages**
    - **Submental exposure** allows more precise placement.
    - Possibly fewer cases of malposition and mental nerve injury.
    - Soft tissue/muscle closure should be strong to prevent soft tissue ptosis.
  - **Disadvantage:** Visible scar
- **Intraoral**
  - **Advantages**
    - No visible scars
    - Similar infection rate
  - **Disadvantages**
    - Can lead to improper implant position (often too superior): No direct view of pocket

> **TIP:** In general, alloplastic augmentation should be used only for patients with mild-to-moderate chin deficiency in the sagittal plane and a shallow labiomental fold.[1,4,11,12]

## Fixation

- **Methods**
  - Screws[16]
  - Sutures[12,13,17]
  - Mitek

- Wires
- Tissue-adhering implant ± tabs
- If no fixation: Precise pocket dissection and soft tissue approximation becomes even more important.

### Implant Position

- **Proper position:** Directly over pogonion
- **Superior positioning**
  - Can cause increased bone and/or tooth root resorption/erosion, movement, and asymmetries
- **Superficial placement**
  - Implant can be visible, palpable, and show irregularities.

**TIP:** A pocket that is too large can increase malposition rates.

### Implant Removal/Secondary Cases

- **Often requires:**
  - Replacement with a smaller implant and fixation
  - Osseous genioplasty to fill the soft tissue void
  - Soft tissue/muscle manipulations (resection, repositioning) to prevent:
    - Soft tissue pad balling
    - Chin pad ptosis
    - Fasciculations: Not preventable, but can be treated with botulinum toxin type A injections[13]

## COMPLICATIONS

### Poor Aesthetic Results

- **Most common complication;** however, dissatisfaction rate very low
- **Satisfaction rates**[18]
  - **Osseous genioplasty:** 90%-95%
  - **Alloplastic augmentation:** 85%-90%
- **Overcorrection**
  - More common in women
  - May result in overprojection and masculinization
- **Implant versus osseous genioplasty aesthetics**
  - Very controversial with limited reports
  - One study showed slightly higher satisfaction and self-esteem improvement rates with osseous genioplasty.[18]
- **Asymmetries**
  - Related to technique of improper soft tissue/muscle (mentalis) dissection and fixation/reapproximation
  - Bony asymmetries with osseous genioplasty: Increased chance if osteotomy is not posterior enough

## Hematoma

- Rare[19]
- Commonly at lateral osteotomy site
- Responds to simple aspiration

## Infection

- Uncommon (5% for implants [Proplast; Vitek, Houston, TX], approximately 3% for osseous genioplasty)[1,17]
- Prophylactic antibiotics should cover for oral flora
- More likely with hematomas in osseous techniques
- Presents with tissue swelling, pain, or draining fistula/sinus
- May be treated with local wound care, antibiotics, or incision/drainage of abscess
- Overall may be more common in **alloplastic implantation** (may require implant removal)
- Some surgeons report no infections.[16]
- Implant extrusion: Very rare—most series report 0%; may be related to infection or inappropriate placement of incision with inadequate gingival tissue for closure[20]

## Muscular Complications

- Must resuspend mentalis muscle: Prevents **witch's chin**
- **Ball phenomenon:** Removal of implant causes capsule to contract and "ball up" mentalis muscle.
  - Treated with capsulectomy and larger implant versus osseous genioplasty
- **Fasciculations:** Treated with lifelong botulinum toxin[13]

## Malposition

- Perhaps more common with **intraoral** implant placement
- Leads to increased bone resorption rates

## Nerve Injury

- **Neurapraxia**
  - Often a retraction injury and resolves in 2-6 weeks

**TIP:** Limit retraction and manipulation of mental nerves as much as possible.

- **Lower lip paresthesias**
  - Transient lower lip numbness in almost all patients
  - $<1\%$ persistent numbness at 1 year[21,22]
    - 15%-29% in patients undergoing combined genioplasty with orthognathic surgery[22,23]
  - Possible temporary drooling
    - If it lasts longer than 6 weeks, consider removal, trimming of implant.
    - Permanent deficits may be related to improper osteotomy technique and damage of inferior alveolar nerve as it courses caudally.

## Bone Erosion

- As high as 0.1 mm/month
- Higher if placed over alveolar bone rather than lower mandible
- Larger implant associated with more bony erosion

## Key Points

- ✓ The chin should never project beyond a vertical line drawn from the anterior upper and lower lips (Riedel's line).
- ✓ The lower lip, chin pad (dynamic and static), nose-lip-chin relationship, and labiomental fold (depth and height) should be incorporated into preoperative analysis.
- ✓ Malocclusion and/or midface deficiency or excess warrants workup for orthognathic surgery.
- ✓ Osteotomy must be at least 5 mm below the mental foramen to prevent inferior alveolar nerve injury.
- ✓ Soft tissue/bone response ratio to osseous and alloplastic genioplasty is approximately 0.8:1.
- ✓ Alloplastic augmentation genioplasty is the most common genioplasty technique used today.
- ✓ The position of a chin implant is critical; it should rest directly over the pogonion.
- ✓ Alloplastic genioplasty cannot correct vertical deficiencies or asymmetry.

## References


1. Cohen SR. Genioplasty. In Achauer BH, Eriksson E, Guyuron B, et al, eds. Plastic Surgery: Indications, Operations, and Outcomes, vol 5. St Louis: Mosby–Year Book, 2000.
2. Guyuron B, Michelow BJ, Willis L. Practical classification of chin deformities. Aesthetic Plast Surg 19:257-264, 1995.
3. Rosen HM. Aesthetic guidelines in genioplasty: the role of facial disproportion. Plast Reconstr Surg 95:463-469, 1995.
4. Guyuron B, ed. Genioplasty. Boston: Little Brown, 1993.
5. Powell N, Humphries B, eds. Proportions of the Aesthetic Face. New York: Thieme-Stratton, 1984.
6. Rosen HM. Surgical correction of the vertically deficient chin. Plast Reconstr Surg 82:247-256, 1988.
7. Guyuron B. Genioplasty. Plast Reconstr Surg 121(4 Suppl):S1-S7, 2008.
8. Schendel SA. Cephalometrics and orthognathic surgery. In Bell WH, ed. Modern Practice in Orthognathic Surgery. Philadelphia: WB Saunders, 1992.
9. Jones BM, Vesely MJ. Osseous genioplasty in facial aesthetic surgery: a personal perspective reviewing 54 patients. J Plast Reconstr Aesthet Surg 59:1177-1187, 2006.
10. Gunter JP, Rohrich RJ, Adams WP, eds. Dallas Rhinoplasty: Nasal Surgery by the Masters, 2nd ed. St Louis: Quality Medical Publishing, 2007.
11. Rosen HM. Osseous genioplasty. In Aston SJ, Beasley RW, Thorne HM, et al, eds. Grabb and Smith's Plastic Surgery, 5th ed. Philadelphia: Lippincott, 1997.
12. Zide BM, Pfeifer TM, Longaker MT. Chin surgery. I. Augmentation—the allures and the alerts. Plast Reconstr Surg 104:1843-1853, 1999.
13. Zide BM, Boutros S. Chin surgery. III. Revelations. Plast Reconstr Surg 111:1542-1550; discussion 1551-1552, 2003.
14. Wolfe SA, Rivas-Torres MT, Marshall D. The genioplasty and beyond: an end-game strategy for the multiply operated chin. Plast Reconstr Surg 117:1435-1446, 2006.
15. Terino EO. Alloplastic facial contouring by zonal principles of skeletal anatomy. Clin Plast Surg 19:487-510, 1992.
16. Yaremchuk MJ. Improving aesthetic outcomes after alloplastic chin augmentation. Plast Reconstr Surg 112:1422-1432, 2003.
17. Zide BM, Longaker MT. Chin surgery. II. Submental ostectomy and soft-tissue excision. Plast Reconstr Surg 104:1854-1860; discussion 1861-1862, 1999.

18. Guyuron B, Raszewski RL. A critical comparison of osteoplastic and alloplastic augmentation genioplasty. Aesthetic Plast Surg 14:199-206, 1990.
19. White JB, Dufresne CR. Management and avoidance of complications in chin augmentation. Aesthet Surg J 31:634-642, 2011.
20. Guyuron B, Kadi JS. Problems following genioplasty: diagnosis and treatment. Clin Plast Surg 24:507-514, 1997.
21. Gui L, Huang L, Zhang Z. Genioplasty and chin augmentation with Medpor implants: a report of 650 cases. Aesthetic Plast Surg 32:220-226, 2008.
22. Hoenig JF. Sliding osteotomy genioplasty for facial aesthetic balance: 10 years of experience. Aesthetic Plast Surg 31:384-391, 2007.
23. Lindquist C, Obeid G. Complications of genioplasty done alone or in combination with sagittal split-ramus osteotomy. Oral Surg Oral Med Oral Pathol 66:13-16, 1988.

# 98. Liposuction

**Fadi C. Constantine, José L. Rios**

## HISTORY

- First description traced to Dujarrier in 1920s[1]
  - Used a uterine curette to remove fat from the knees of a ballerina
    - Resulted in eventual amputation from damage to femoral artery
- Popularized in Europe in the 1970s by Drs. Yves-Gerard Illouz, Pierre Fournier, and Francis Otteni
  - They first presented their experience at the 1982 ASPS meeting in Hawaii.
    - Key advancements were the introduction of blunt cannulas and evacuation using negative pressure.

## ANATOMY

### SUBCUTANEOUS LAYERS[2] (Fig. 98-1)

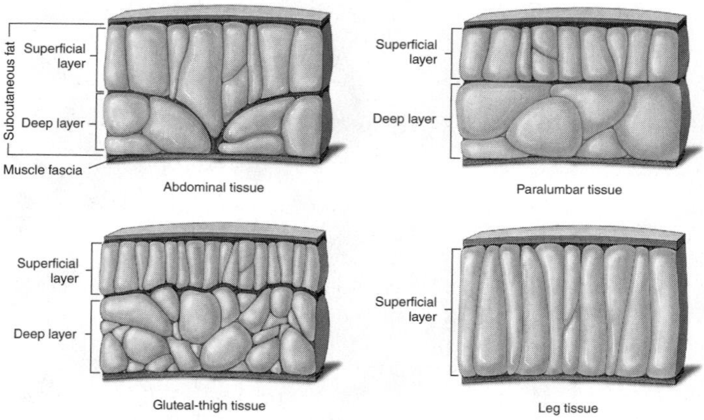


**Fig. 98-1** Differences in subcutaneous tissues in various areas of the body.

- **Superficial**
  - Fat is dense and adherent to overlying skin.
  - **Suction with caution to prevent surface irregularities.**
- **Intermediate**
  - **Safest** layer
  - Most commonly suctioned layer
- **Deep**
  - Loose and less compact
  - Can be removed safely in most areas except the buttocks

- **Cellulite** (gynoid lipodystrophy)
  - **Illouz**[3]
    - Caused by hypertrophy of superficial fat within septa that connect the superficial fascial system and the epidermis
  - **Lockwood**[4] (two types of cellulite)
    - First is similar to Illouz's theory.
    - Second is related to skin laxity that more commonly is seen in women >35 years of age as a result of age, sun damage, massive weight loss, and/or liposuction.
    - Treated with skin-tightening procedures.

## Zones of Adherence[5] (Fig. 98-2)

- Distal iliotibial tract
- Gluteal crease
- Lateral gluteal depression
- Middle medial thigh
- Distal posterior thigh

**CAUTION: Do not violate the zones of adherence during liposuction. This will result in contour deformities.**

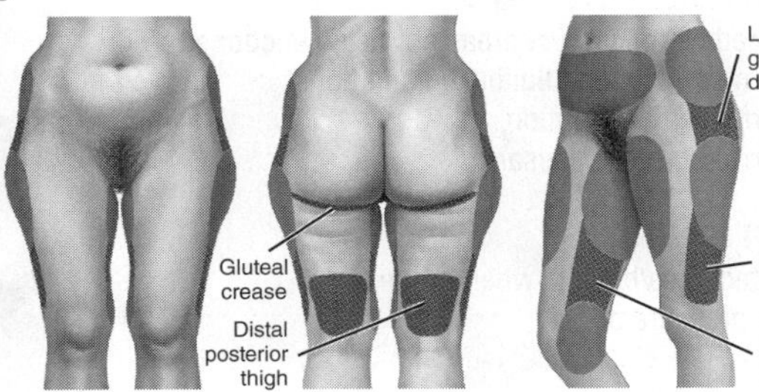


**Fig. 98-2** Zones of adherence.

# PHYSICS OF LIPOSUCTION[6]

- The typical unit of measure of the vacuum pump is the ***torr.*** 1 atm = 760 torr or 760 mm Hg.
  - One torr is the pressure necessary to support a column of mercury 1 mm high at 0° C and standard gravity.
  - A pump that produces 30 torr used at sea level will show 730 mm Hg on the gauge and will have 30 mm inside the vacuum. (The pump will remove all but 30 mm of pressure from within the system.)
  - Cannulas are designed with blunt tips to lessen the chance of tearing fascia, veins, arteries, and nerves.
  - The smaller the diameter of the cannula, the more even the fat removal.
  - The shorter the shaft of the cannula, the better the surgeon's control of the instrument.
  - $R = r^4(l)K$, where *R* is the resistance, *r* is the radius of the tube, *l* is the length, and *K* is a constant factor.
  - Resistance increases dramatically as the radius of the cannula decreases.

# PREOPERATIVE EVALUATION

## Physical Examination

- Check for deviation from the ideal contour.
- **Note any of the following:**
  - Asymmetries
  - Dimpling/cellulite
  - Location of fat deposits
  - Areas of adherence
- Examine spine for **scoliosis** (may cause asymmetry).
- Check **laxity** of skin.
- Assess for **hernias/diastasis.**

### PHOTOGRAPHS

- Standard photographs of areas to be treated should be obtained (see Chapter 13).

## PREOPERATIVE CONSIDERATIONS

### GENERAL

- Complete blood count if expecting to perform **large-volume** procedure
- IV antibiotics
- Deep venous thrombosis prophylaxis

### HYPOTHERMIA

- Forced warm air over areas not being suctioned
- Warm intravenous fluid (IVF) solutions
- Warm wetting solution
- Warm room if necessary

### POSITIONING

- Protect face/breasts when prone
- Pad pressure points

## MARKINGS (Fig. 98-3)

- Use indelible marker to outline areas to be treated.
- Use circled *X's* over areas of maximal prominence.
- Mark parallel lines over zones of adherence and other areas to be avoided.

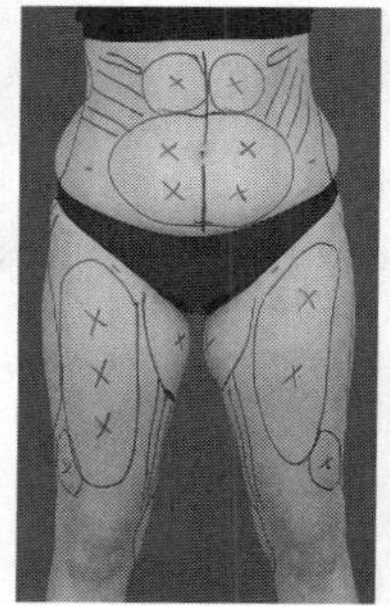
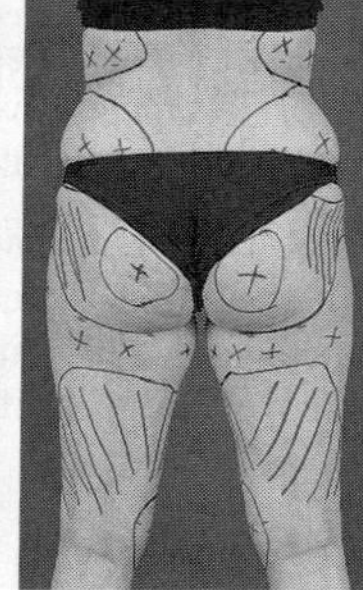

**Fig. 98-3** Markings. Circled *X's* are over zones of prominence and lines are over zones of adherence.

## WETTING SOLUTIONS[7-13] (Tables 98-1 and 98-2)

**Table 98-1** *Volume of Infiltrate By Technique*

| Technique | Infiltrate |
|---|---|
| Dry | No infiltrate |
| Wet | 200-300 ml/area* |
| Superwet | 1 ml infiltrate:1 ml aspirate* |
| Tumescent | Infiltrate to skin turgor<br>2-3 ml infiltrate:1 ml aspirate |

*Infiltrate may contain lidocaine, epinephrine, and/or sodium bicarbonate, depending on surgeon's preference.

**Table 98-2** *Estimated Blood Loss By Technique*

| Technique | Estimate of Blood Loss (as % of volume) |
|---|---|
| Dry | 20-40 |
| Wet | 4-30 |
| Superwet | 1 |
| Tumescent | 1 |

## PURPOSES OF WETTING SOLUTION

- Volume replacement
- Provide hemostasis
- Provide pain control
- Enhance cavitation (ultrasound-assisted liposuction [UAL])
- Dissipate heat (UAL)
- **Can vary in constituents. One example:**
  - 1000 ml of lactated Ringer's solution at 21° C
  - 30 ml of 1% lidocaine (15 ml if large volume)
  - 1 ml of 1:1000 epinephrine
- **Klein[8]:**
  - 1000 ml normal saline solution
  - 50 ml 1% lidocaine
  - 1 ml 1:1000 epinephrine
  - 12.5 ml of 8.4% sodium bicarbonate (alkalization may decrease pain with infiltration but not needed with general anesthesia)

**NOTE: Regardless of the anesthetic route, large-volume liposuction (>5000 ml total aspirate) should be performed in an acute care hospital or in a facility that is either accredited or licensed. Vital signs and urinary output should be monitored postoperatively, and patients should be monitored overnight in an appropriate facility by qualified and competent staff familiar with the perioperative care of liposuction patients.**

## LIDOCAINE IN WETTING SOLUTION

- Analgesia is provided for up to 18 hours postoperatively.
- Recommended maximum is **7 mg/kg.**
- Klein[8] used up to 35 mg/kg, resulting in peak levels (12 hours) less than the toxic threshold (3 μg/ml).
- **Use of such high quantities of lidocaine is possible because of:**
  - Diluted solution
  - Slow infiltration
  - Vasoconstriction of epinephrine
  - Relative avascularity of fatty layer
  - High lipid solubility of lidocaine
  - Compression of vessels by infiltrate

**NOTE: After 20-30 minutes, wet environment may be lost.**

# INCISIONS (Figs. 98-4 and 98-5)

- Longer for UAL than suction-assisted lipoplasty (SAL) (6-8 mm vs. 2-3 mm)
- **Locations**
  - **Breast (male):** Lateral inframammary fold (IMF) or periareolar
  - **Lateral back:** Lateral bra line
  - **Vertical back:** Midline
  - **Flank/hip:** Lateral gluteal fold/lateral lower hip/flank in bikini line/posteriorly may use paraspinous locations
  - **Abdomen:** Lateral lower abdomen/suprapubic/umbilical
  - **Buttock:** Lateral gluteal fold

- **Lateral thigh:** Lateral gluteal fold
- **Posterior thigh:** Lateral gluteal fold
- **Medial thigh:** Medial gluteal crease (posterior)
- **Anterior thigh:** Inguinal crease
- **Upper arm:** Posterior radial proximal humerus (prone), distal radial humerus (supine)

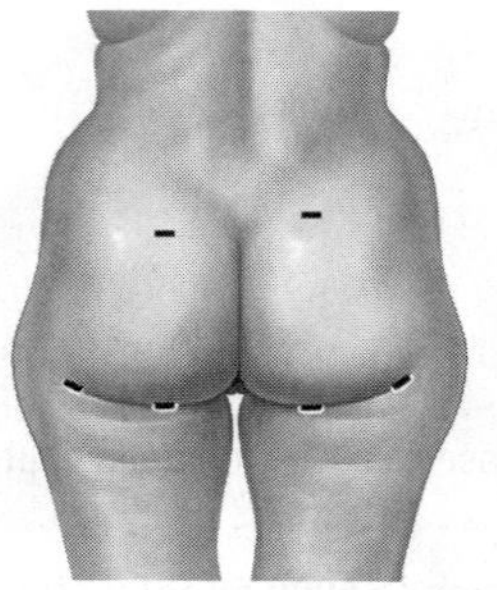
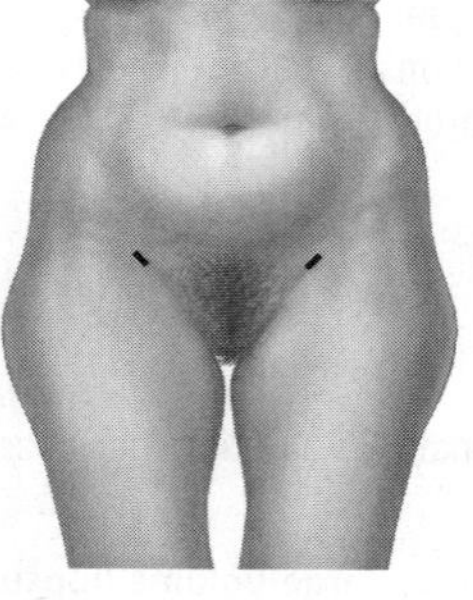

**Fig. 98-4** Incisions for buttocks and medial thighs.

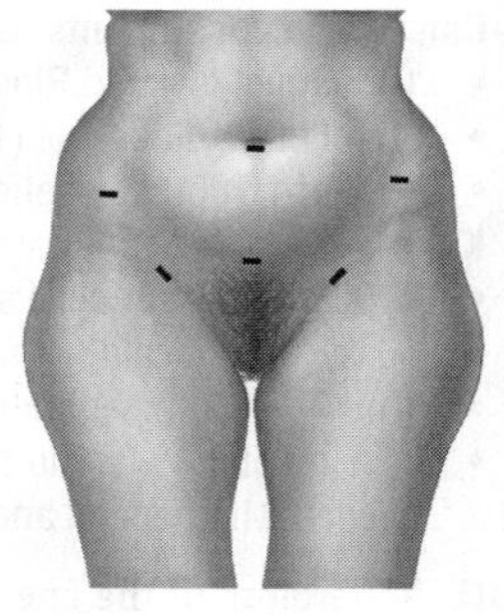

**Fig. 98-5** Abdominal incisions.

## UAL[14,16]

- First described by Zocchi in Italy in 1993
- A result of alternating currents that cause piezoelectric crystals to expand and contract, releasing ultrasonic waves
- UAL typically more advantageous over SAL for **fibrous areas** or **moderately lax skin**
  - Radiographic dye studies of postperfusion vasculature in treated areas showed significantly less vascular disruption with UAL than with traditional techniques.
- Ultrasonic energy emulsifies subcutaneous fat by three processes:
  1. **Micromechanical**
     - Direct tissue trauma by the ultrasonic wave
     - "Jackhammer effect"
  2. **Thermal**
     - Tissues absorb the sound waves, producing heat.
     - Friction
     - Internal heating (electric → mechanical energy)
  3. **Cavitation**
     - Tissue fragmentation by means of formation and collapse of intracellular microbubbles
     - Less dense tissue more susceptible to cavitation
- SAL is then used for evacuation.
- UAL has three stages:
  - *Stage I:* Subcutaneous infiltration of fluids to decrease blood loss and tissue density
  - *Stage II:* Ultrasound treatment to emulsify subcutaneous fat
  - *Stage III:* Evacuation of emulsified fat and final contouring
- Complications of UAL[17]
  - Thermal injury
  - Seroma
  - Hyperpigmentation

## POWER-ASSISTED LIPOSUCTION[18]

- Externally powered cannula oscillating in a 2 mm reciprocating motion at rates of 4000-6000 cycles/minute.
- Faster and less labor intensive
  - **Advantages**
    - Large volumes
    - Fibrous areas
    - Revision liposuction
  - **Disadvantages**
    - Significant noise generation
    - Mechanical vibration transmitted to operating surgeon
    - Bulky and somewhat cumbersome
    - Difficult to perform fine contouring changes

## LASER-ASSISTED LIPOSUCTION[18]

- Treatment involves insertion of a laser fiber through a small skin incision.
  - Fiber is either housed within the cannula or is stand-alone device.
- Acts by disrupting fat cell membranes and emulsifying fat.
- Most common wavelengths in United States are 924/975 nm, 1064 nm, 1319/1320 nm, and 1450 nm.
- **Four-stage technique is employed.**
  1. Infiltration
  2. Application of energy to subcutaneous tissue
  3. Evacuation through traditional techniques
     - Some suggest skipping this stage in smaller regions (neck) and allowing the body to absorb liquefied contents.
  - Subdermal skin stimulation
- **Mechanism of action:** Heating of the subdermal tissue is thought to be the contributing factor for possible skin-tightening effect.
  - Anecdotal: No large prospective trials to show difference between laser-assisted liposuction and conventional techniques.
    - Prado et al[19] showed no difference in smaller study.
    - DiBernardo and Reyes[20] showed some efficacy in five patients.

## FLUID RESUSCITATION

- 1 L of isotonic fluid is absorbed from the interstitium in 167 minutes.
- **25%-30%** of the infiltrate is removed during suctioning.
  - Rest is reabsorbed over 6-12 hours postoperatively.
- **IVF (using superwet infiltration):**
  - Crystalloid at maintenance (adjust to urine output and vital signs)
  - Replacement IVF of 0.25 ml per cubic centimeter of aspirate over 5 L
    - The use of superwet over tumescent technique results in equivalent blood loss, but with decreased chances of fluid overload and congestive heart failure.[21]
  - Continue maintenance IVF until oral intake is adequate.

## LIPOSUCTION STAGES

### Stage I: Infiltration[11]

- Infiltrate **intermediate plane** with superwet technique.
- Record delivered amount to each area.
- Endpoint is uniform blanching and skin turgor.
- Allow 7-10 minutes for maximal vasoconstriction from epinephrine.

### Stage II: UAL Treatment (Omit if Performing SAL Only)

- Place access incisions asymmetrically.
- Use port protector and wet towels.
- Treat posterior areas first **(can treat 70%-80% of the circumference from this position).**
- Move cannula at all times.
- Withdraw to within 3 cm of incision to redirect and minimize torque.
- Move from **superficial to deep. (SAL goes from deep to superficial.)**
- **Endpoints** (Table 98-3):
  - **Primary:** Loss of resistance, blood in aspirate
  - **Secondary:** Final contour, treatment time

**Table 98-3** *Surgical Endpoints for UAL and SAL/PAL*

| Endpoint | UAL | SAL/PAL |
|---|---|---|
| Primary | Loss of tissue resistance<br>Blood aspirate | Final contour<br>Symmetrical pinch test results |
| Secondary | Treatment time<br>Treatment volume | Treatment time<br>Treatment volume |

*PAL,* Power-assisted liposuction; *SAL,* suction-assisted liposuction; *UAL,* ultrasound-assisted liposuction.

### Stage III: Evacuation and Final Contouring[15]

- Set aspirator at 60%-70% of usual suction.
- Begin with deep layer and move superficially.

## LIPOSUCTION BY AREA

### Hips and Flanks

- **Flank (males)**
  - Begins in paraspinous area
  - Widest just above iliac crest
  - Anteriorly blends with lower abdominal adiposity of lateral rectus sheath
  - Begins at convexity below flare of rib cage; becomes convex and full over the iliac crests
  - Inferiorly defined by zone of adherence lying along the iliac crest
- **Hips (females)**
  - Similar area as the flank, only more inferior so that its bulk is centered **over the crests**
  - Ends lower than the flank

- **Gluteal depression**
  - Convexity between the hips above and the lateral thigh below
  - Also known as the *saddlebag*
- **Technical details**
  - Jackknife when prone
  - Average infiltration volumes: 500-800 ml in the hip

## Thighs

- Thigh should be a shallow convex arc on both anterior and posterior surfaces.
- Lateral thigh extends from the gluteal depression to the knee.
- Buttock extends from sacrum to inferior gluteal fold.
- *Banana roll* is the fullness from inferior gluteal fold to posterior upper thigh zone of adherence.
- There should be an unbroken curve from the iliac crest to the distal thigh.
- Medially there should be a slight convexity of the upper third of the medial thigh; middle to distal third is flat or slightly concave.
- **Ideal buttock**
  - Slightly convex
  - Nonptotic
  - Firm with a slight lateral gluteal depression
- In **women** the buttocks are **rounded** and flow into the lateral thigh.
- **Male** buttocks are more **angular** and almost **squared laterally** (more muscle, less fat, more firm).

## Abdomen

- **Borders**
  - Xiphoid superiorly
  - Pubic ramus inferiorly
  - Laterally extends to the anterior iliac crest along the inguinal ligament
- Clearly delineated linea alba depression from top to bottom
- **Anteriorly**
  - Slight supraumbilical concavity
  - Infraumbilical convexity
- **Women**
  - Highlighted by bilateral concavities, as defined by the flank from the rib to the iliac crest
- **Men**
  - Do **not** have a bilateral convexity (hourglass shape)
  - No flare at the iliac crest
  - Infraumbilical region should be flat

## Arms

- Ideal arm is lean and has an anterior convexity of the deltoid merging with a convexity of the biceps.
- Posterior surface of the arm should be slightly convex from axilla to elbow.
- Patients with at least 1.5 cm of fat by the pinch test are good candidates.

- **Technical details**
  - When prone: Incision placed in posterior axillary fold, and SAL incision at radial elbow
  - Long radial strokes to prevent waviness/contour deformity
  - Use full-length contoured TopiFoam

**CAUTION: Perform UAL from a radial incision-only to prevent ulnar nerve problems.**

## DRAINS

- Not routinely used
- Consider for liposuction procedures combined with resection

## INCISION CLOSURE

- Massage out excess fluid.
- Close with suture of choice.
- Place antibiotic ointment, 2 × 2 gauze, and paper tape.
- Place compression garment with TopiFoam (Byron Medical, Tucson, AZ), except on buttocks, posterior flank, or back.

## POSTOPERATIVE CARE

- Change dressing after 3-4 days.
  - Tell patient to sit at bedside for 5 minutes after removing the garment before standing.
- No tub baths are allowed for the first week.
- Compression garment worn at all times for 2 weeks, then at night for 2 weeks.
- Foam is worn under garments for first 7 days.

**CAUTION: Make sure foam padding is flat against the patient's body to prevent potential contour deformities from rippling.**

- Patients return to work in 3-5 days, after small-volume procedures.
- Large-volume procedures may require 7-10 days before return to work.
- Full activities are resumed in 3-4 weeks as tolerated.

## HEALING COURSE

- **1-3 days:** Access incisions drain
- **3-5 days:** Edema maximizes, drainage slows
- **7-10 days:** Ecchymosis resolves
- **4-6 weeks:** Edema resolves
- **8-10 weeks:** Induration in large-volume areas[16]
- **3-4 months:** Final contour

## COMPLICATION, PREVENTION, AND TREATMENT[21] (Boxes 98-1 and 98-2)

**Box 98-1** *SAFETY GUIDELINES IN LIPOSUCTION*

- Appropriate patient selection (ASA class I, within 30% of ideal body weight)
- Use of superwet techniques of infiltration
- Meticulous monitoring of volume status (urinary catheterization, noninvasive hemodynamic monitoring, communication with anesthesiologist)
- Judicious fluid resuscitation*
  - For aspirate <5 liters: Maintenance fluid plus subcutaneous infiltrate
  - For aspirate >5 liters: Maintenance fluid plus subcutaneous infiltrate plus 0.25 ml of intravenous crystalloid per milliliter of aspirate >5 liters
- Overnight monitoring of large-volume (>5 liters of total aspirate) liposuction patients in an appropriate health care facility
- Use of pneumatic compression devices in cases performed under general anesthesia or lasting >1 hour
- Maintaining total lidocaine doses <35 mg/kg (wetting solution)

*Individualized based on patient's urine output and hemodynamics.

**Box 98-2** *LOCAL ANESTHETIC SYSTEM TOXICITY (LAST) TREATMENT*[22]

- **Infuse** 20% lipid emulsion. (Values in parentheses are for a 70 kg patient.)
  1. Bolus 1.5 ml/kg (lean body mass) intravenously over 1 minute (~100 ml).
  2. Provide continuous infusion at 0.25 ml/kg/minute (~18 ml/minute; adjust by roller clamp).
  3. Repeat bolus once or twice for persistent cardiovascular collapse.
  4. Double the infusion rate to 0.5 ml/kg/minute if blood pressure remains low.
  5. Continue infusion for at least 10 minutes after circulatory stability is achieved.
- Recommended upper limit is approximately 10-12 ml/kg lipid emulsion over the first 30 minutes.

### KEY POINTS

- ✓ Consider whether you have chosen the correct procedure: liposuction versus skin resection.
- ✓ Mark patients while they are awake; allow them to provide guidance in choosing the areas to be treated.
- ✓ Allow 7-10 minutes after infiltration and before suction for maximal epinephrine effect. (Consider infiltration before preparation and draping to save time.)
- ✓ Perform repeated assessments of progress to prevent contour deformities.
- ✓ Underresection is preferable to a difficult-to-correct contour deformity.
- ✓ Strict garment use is essential to prevent contour deformity and chronic seroma formation.

## References


1. Grazer FM. Suction-assisted lipectomy, suction lipectomy, lipolysis, and lipexeresis [discussion]. Plast Reconstr Surg 72:620, 1983.
2. Markman B, Barton FE Jr. Anatomy of the subcutaneous tissue of the trunk and lower extremity. Plast Reconstr Surg 80:248, 1987.
3. Illouz YG. Study of subcutaneous fat. Aesthetic Plast Surg 14:165, 1990.
4. Lockwood TE. Superficial fascial system (SFS) of the trunk and extremities: a new concept. Plast Reconstr Surg 86:1009, 1991.
5. Rohrich RJ, Smith PD, Marcantonio DR, et al. The zones of adherence: role in minimizing and preventing contour deformities in liposuction. Plast Reconstr Surg 107:1562, 2001.
6. Hetter GP. Lipoplasty: The Theory and Practice of Blunt Suction Lipectomy. Boston: Little Brown, 1984.
7. Rohrich RJ, Beran SJ, Fodor PB. The role of subcutaneous infiltration in suction-assisted lipoplasty: a review. Plast Reconstr Surg 99:514, 1997.
8. Klein JA. The tumescent technique for local anesthesia improves safety in large-volume liposuction. Plast Reconstr Surg 92:1085, 1993.
9. Goodpasture JC, Bunkis J. Quantitative analysis of blood and fat in suction lipectomy aspirates. Plast Reconstr Surg 78:765, 1986.
10. Courtiss EH, Choucair RJ, Donelan MB. Large-volume suction lipectomy: an analysis of 108 patients. Plast Reconstr Surg 89:1068, 1992.
11. Klein JA. The tumescent technique: anesthesia and modified liposuction technique. Dermatol Clin 8:425, 1990.
12. American Society of Plastic Surgeons. Practice Advisory on Liposuction: Executive Summary, 2003. Available at *http://www.plasticsurgery.org/Documents/medical-professionals/health-policy/key-issues/Executive-Summary-on-Liposuction.pdf.*
13. Rohrich RJ, Kenkel JM, Janis JE, et al. An update on the role of subcutaneous infiltration in suction-assisted lipoplasty. Plast Reconstr Surg 111:926-927, 2003.
14. Kenkel JM, Janis JE, Rohrich RJ, Beran SJ. Aesthetic body contouring: ultrasound-assisted liposuction. In Matarasso A, ed. Operative Techniques in Plastic and Reconstructive Surgery. Philadelphia: Saunders-Elsevier, 2003.
15. Zocchi ML. Ultrasonic assisted lipoplasty. Technical refinements and clinical evaluations. Clin Plast Surg 23:575, 1996.
16. Rohrich RJ, Kenkel JM, Beran SJ. Ultrasound-Assisted Liposuction. St Louis: Quality Medical Publishing, 1998.
17. Illouz YG. Complications of liposuction. Clin Plast Surg 33:129, 2006.
18. Farkas JP, Stephan PJ, Kenkel JM. Liposuction: basic techniques and safety considerations. In Nahai F, ed. The Art of Aesthetic Surgery: Principles & Techniques, 2nd ed. St Louis: Quality Medical Publishing, 2011.
19. Prado A, Andrades P, Danilla S, et al. A prospective, randomized, double-blind, controlled clinical trial comparing laser-assisted lipoplasty with suction-assisted lipoplasty. Plast Reconstr Surg 118:1032, 2006.
20. DiBernardo BE, Reyes J. Evaluation of skin tightening after laser-assisted liposuction. Aesthet Surg J 29:400, 2009.
21. Rohrich RJ, Grazer FM, de Jong RH. Fatal outcomes from liposuction: census survey of cosmetic surgeons [discussion]. Plast Reconstr Surg 105:447, 2000.
22. Weinberg GL. Lipid emulsion infusion: resuscitation for local anesthetic and other drug overdose. Anesthesiology 117:180, 2012.

# 99. Brachioplasty

Sacha I. Obaid, Jeffrey E. Janis, Jacob G. Unger, Jason E. Leedy

## ANATOMY (Fig. 99-1)

- Subcutaneous fat in the arms tends to collect **posteriorly** and **inferiorly;** very little subcutaneous fat is found medially.
- The fat and skin of the upper arm are supported by **two fascial systems.**
  - **Superficial fascial system**
    - Encases the fat of the upper arm circumferentially from axilla to elbow
  - **Longitudinal fascial system**[1]
    - Begins at the clavicle as the clavipectoral fascia
    - Extends to the axillary fascia
    - Connects to the superficial fascial system
- With age and weight gain, the superficial fascial system and axillary fascia loosen.
  - Creates a "loose hammocklike" effect
  - Results in significant ptosis of the posteromedial arm
- There is also a deep fascial system, which should not be violated during brachioplasty.
- Arm musculature is enveloped by the deep investing fascia.
- *All major neurovascular bundles lie deep to the deep investing fascia.*

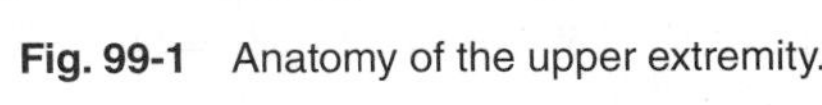

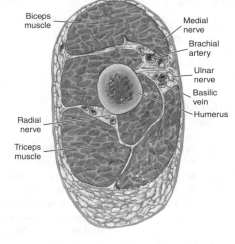


**Fig. 99-1** Anatomy of the upper extremity.

**NOTE: The only nerves located superficial to the deep investing fascia are the medial brachial cutaneous and medial antebrachial cutaneous (MABC) nerves. The most commonly referenced nerve is the MABC, which runs with the basilic vein and pierces the deep fascia an average of 14 cm proximal to the medial epicondyle.**[2]

> **TIP:** The entire dissection in excisional or liposuction brachioplasty should remain superficial to the deep investing fascia. If this plane is not violated, then all important neurovascular structures in the upper extremity are preserved. The only at-risk structure is the MABC nerve, which can still cause a painful neuroma if injured!

## PATIENT EVALUATION

### ASSESSMENT

- A complete history is obtained, including weight loss/gain, tobacco use, nutritional status (especially if massive-weight-loss [MWL] patient) and all medical problems.
- A physical examination is performed.
  - Evaluate the arms, including ROM at shoulder/elbow/hand and grip strength.
  - Assess for excess fat, excess skin, particular areas of excess, and overall skin quality and tone.
- **Upper arm rejuvenation** patients can be divided into **three types** (Table 99-1).[3]

**Table 99-1** *Classification of Upper Arm Contouring*

| Type | Skin Excess | Fat Excess | Location of Skin Excess |
|---|---|---|---|
| I | Minimal | Moderate | N/A |
| IIA | Moderate | Minimal | Proximal |
| IIB | Moderate | Minimal | Entire arm |
| IIC | Moderate | Minimal | Arm and chest |
| IIIA | Moderate | Moderate | Proximal |
| IIIB | Moderate | Moderate | Entire arm |
| IIIC | Moderate | Moderate | Arm and chest |

- **Type I:** Relative excess of fat in the upper arm with good skin tone and minimal laxity
  - Best treated with liposuction alone
- **Type II:** Skin laxity can be **horizontal, vertical,** or **both.**
  - **Type IIA:** Only **proximal** arm redundancy
    - If redundancy is strictly **horizontal,** a vertically oriented wedge or an elliptical excision of skin is made, isolated to the axillary fold (Fig. 99-2).
    - If laxity is **vertical and horizontal,** a **T-shaped resection** along the proximal upper arm is required (Fig. 99-3).

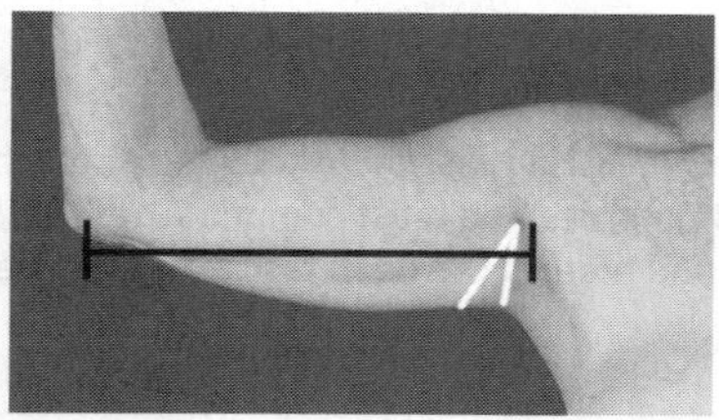

**Fig. 99-2** Type IIA: Horizontal redundancy is treated by a vertically oriented wedge or elliptical skin excision in the axilla.

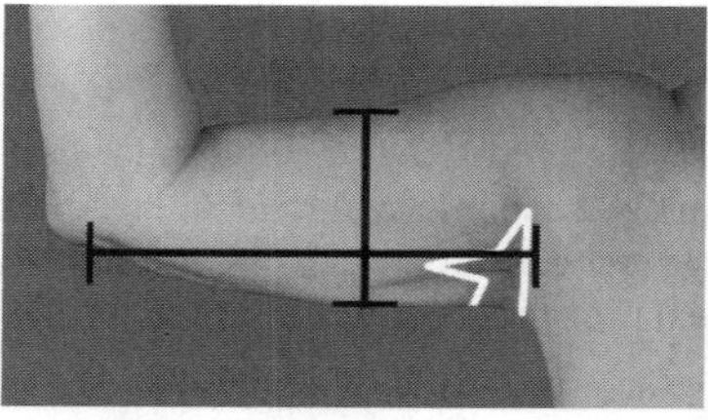

**Fig. 99-3** Type IIA: Vertical and horizontal laxity is treated by a T-shaped resection along the proximal upper arm.

- **Type IIB:** Skin redundancy of the **entire upper arm** from elbow to chest wall
  - For isolated **vertical** skin redundancy, a **horizontal excision** can be performed along the brachial groove (Fig. 99-4).
  - If excess is **horizontal and vertical,** an **L-shaped excision** is made in the axilla (Fig. 99-5).

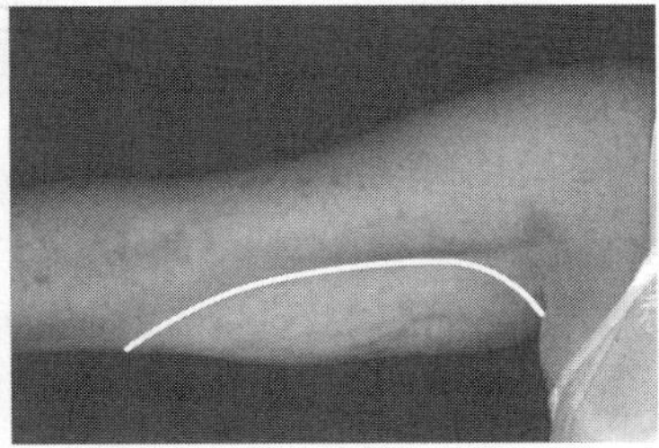

**Fig. 99-4** Type IIB: Isolated vertical skin redundancy is treated with a horizontal excision along the brachial groove.

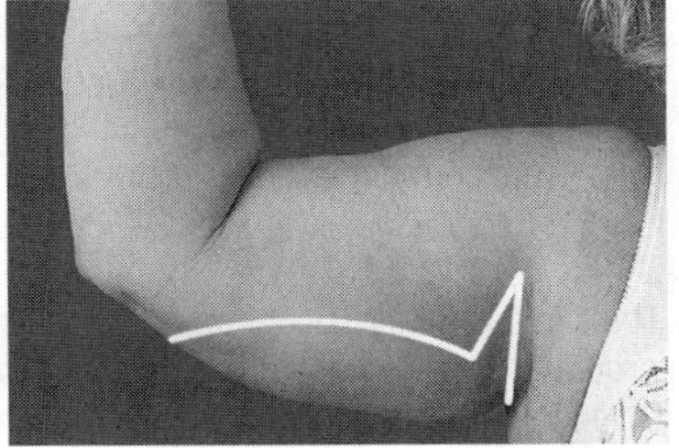

**Fig. 99-5** Type IIB: Horizontal and vertical excess is treated with an L-shaped excision in the axilla.

    - Excision extends into the arm as far as the excess skin in the arm does.
    - The L may extend all the way to the elbow if necessary. (This is commonly the case.)
- **Type IIC:** Laxity extends **onto the lateral chest wall** (Fig. 99-6).
  - An **extended brachioplasty** is needed that extends onto the chest wall.
  - *These are typically MWL patients.*
- **Type III:** Both **significant excess fat** and **redundant skin** in the arm; several options:
  - Further weight loss before surgery
  - Staged treatment with liposuction first, followed by subsequent excisional brachioplasty
  - Combined single-stage liposuction and excisional brachioplasty
  - Subtypes **A, B,** and **C:** Specific locations of the skin excess
    - A: Proximal
    - B: Entire arm
    - C: Arm and chest

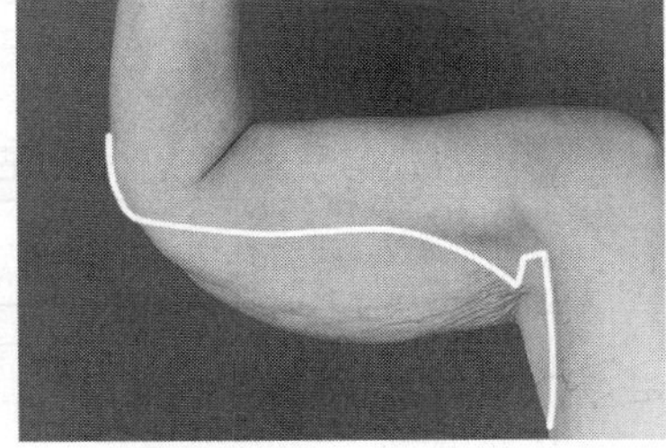

**Fig. 99-6** Type IIC: Laxity extends onto the lateral chest wall and requires extended brachioplasty.

- Patients with isolated **vertical** skin redundancy and some lipodystrophy distally along the entire upper arm with **good** skin quality may be candidates for limited incision medial brachioplasty.[4]
- For type IIIB and IIIC arms, newer techniques such as the liposuction-assisted posterior brachioplasty have achieved effective results in one stage.[5]

**TIP:** When considering treatment for excess tissue, remember that the resection is performed in the "opposite" vector from the direction of the excess (i.e., vertical excess is removed via a horizontal excision, and horizontal excess is removed via a vertical excision).

## Contraindications

- **Absolute**
  - Neurologic or vascular disorders of the upper extremity such as reflex sympathetic dystrophy
  - Lymphedema of the arms secondary to previous axillary lymph node dissection
  - Unrealistic patient expectations
- **Relative**[6]
  - Symptomatic Raynaud's disease
  - Connective tissue disorders
  - Advanced rheumatoid arthritis

## Patient Education

- The scars from excisional brachioplasty are frequently exposed by everyday clothing and *are probably the most noticeable aesthetic surgery scars.*
- Given the prominence of the scars, this **must** be discussed with patients preoperatively.

> **TIP:** It is often helpful to draw the scars on the patient's arm during the preoperative consultation and to document this in the medical record. At the same time, the proposed effect of an excisional brachioplasty can be demonstrated.

- Patients must also be warned of temporary areas of numbness in the upper arm secondary to transection of branches of MABC nerves, as well as the risk for painful neuroma.

> **TIP:** If the MABC nerve is injured while performing brachioplasty, it should be crushed, cauterized, and neurotized into muscle to help prevent a painful neuroma.

# ALGORITHM FOR TREATMENT[3] (Fig. 99-7)

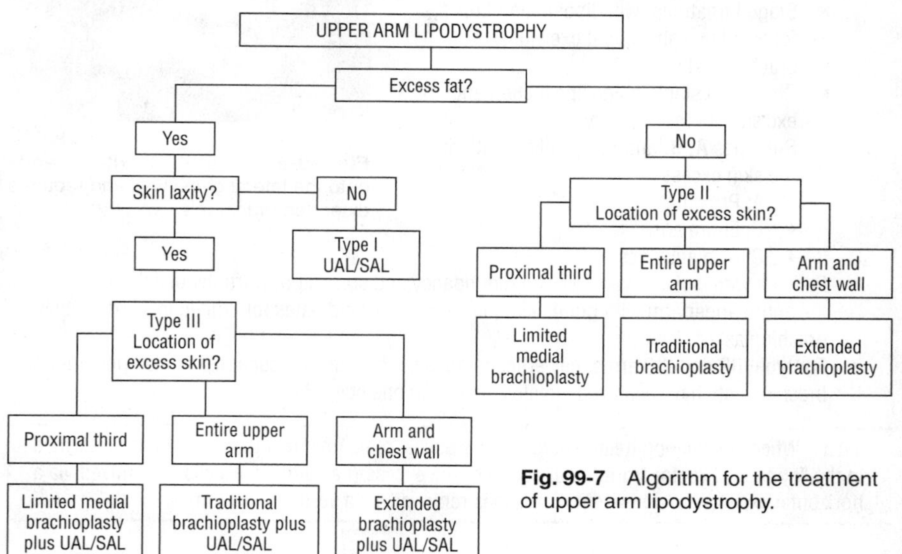


**Fig. 99-7** Algorithm for the treatment of upper arm lipodystrophy.

## PATIENT MARKINGS AND OPERATIVE TECHNIQUE

### LIPOSUCTION

- Liposuction can be performed as a stand-alone procedure for arm rejuvenation.
- It can also be performed as the first step in excisional brachioplasty, because it:
  - Decreases arm bulk
  - Increases the amount of skin that can be successfully resected
- Suction is concentrated in the medial and posterior quadrants of the proximal half of the upper arm.
- Incisions are made in posterior lateral elbow region and in superior portion of axilla anteriorly for infiltration of wetting solution and liposuction.

**CAUTION: Care must be taken to keep the cannula away from the axilla and the posteromedial elbow to prevent damage to the nerves of the brachial plexus or the ulnar nerve. Special caution should also be taken when using ultrasound-assisted liposuction (UAL).**

- Liposuction should be performed at an intermediate depth.
- Approximately 0.5 cm of subcutaneous fat is left on the skin to prevent contour irregularities.[6]

**TIP:** Do not use UAL near the medial epicondyle to prevent damage to the ulnar nerve.

### MINIBRACHIOPLASTY/LIMITED MEDIAL INCISION BRACHIOPLASTY[6] (Fig. 99-8)

- For patients with **mild skin laxity** and **mild-to-moderate excess fat** in the upper arm, a **minibrachioplasty** can be performed.
  - Combines removal of excess fat through liposuction with removal of skin laxity through an incision limited to the axilla ± the proximal portion of the upper arm.

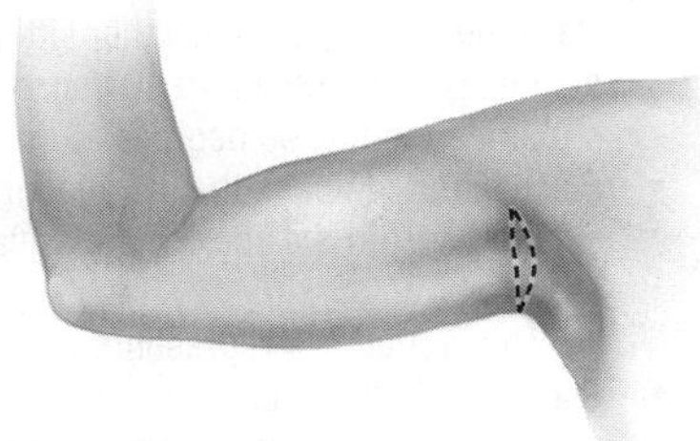

**Fig. 99-8** Minibrachioplasty of axillary brachioplasty incision.

- **Preoperative markings**
  - Liposuction should concentrate on the excess fat found in the **posteromedial** region of the upper arm.
  - After being marked, the patient abducts the arm 90 degrees at the shoulder and flexes 90 degrees at the elbow.
  - A **pinch test** is used to mark an ellipse of skin in the axilla that can be resected to help restore an aesthetic contour of the upper arm. This usually will be limited to 3-5 cm at its widest point.
  - If the proposed elliptical resection does not appear to correct skin laxity, or if there is focal horizontal excess as well, then a vertical dart can be added to create a T-shaped incision that is confined to the upper third of the arm.
- **Principles**
  - The first step is **liposuction** of excess upper arm fat, concentrated in the posteromedial regions, as described earlier.

- After liposuction, an elliptical skin excision is performed transversely in the axilla.
  - **High potential for scar widening or dehiscence**
    - Lockwood's technique[1] uses permanent sutures to anchor the superficial fascial system of the arm to longitudinal fascia (dense axillary fascia and clavipectoral fascia), which is a strength layer affixed to the clavicular periosteum.
      - Helps correct the laxity of the longitudinal fascial sling that develops with age

**TIP:** The most important step to successful minibrachioplasty or limited-incision medial brachioplasty is patient selection. A minibrachioplasty with superficial fascial suspension to the axillary and clavipectoral fascia can be a highly effective operation for patients with mild-to-moderate skin excess in addition to excess fat; however, for moderate-to-severe skin excess with or without excess fat, a standard brachioplasty should be performed to achieve the desirable contour. Patients MUST have good skin quality to have a good response to this type of repair.

## Standard Brachioplasty[6] (Fig. 99-9)

- A standard brachioplasty should be used for patients with moderate-to-severe excess skin with or without excess fat.
- If there is a significant amount of excess fat in addition to excess skin, then the procedure should begin with liposuction.
- **Preoperative markings for standard brachioplasty are as follows[6]:**
  - Have the patient (who is either sitting or standing) abduct the arm 90 degrees at the shoulder and flex 90 degrees at the elbow.
  - Place a dotted line in the bicipital groove, extending from the apex of the axilla down to the elbow.
    - This dotted line represents the proposed scar location.
  - Place a solid line 1 cm above and parallel to the line in the bicipital groove.
    - This line marks the proposed upper incision for the brachioplasty.
  - The surgeon places an index and long finger along the proposed upper-line incision and uses the thumb to pinch the inferomedial skin upward toward the upper incision.
    - This pinch test signals how much skin can be excised; marks are placed inferiorly to delineate the proposed lower incision.
  - Draw three to five vertical lines perpendicular to the longitudinal lines.
    - This divides the proposed resection into thirds or fifths.
    - These lines assist in aligning the closure (see later).

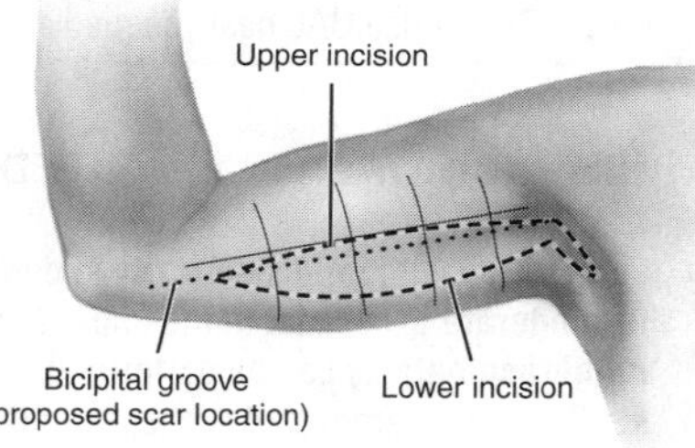


**Fig. 99-9** Standard brachioplasty incision.

## Two-Ellipse Technique[7] (Fig. 99-10)

- **Outer Ellipse** based on tissue redundancy
- **Inner Ellipse** adjusted to allow for closure
  - Avoids potential issues with overaggressive resection, vascular compromise
- Steps
  - Patient is marked seated with arm abducted and elbow at 90 degrees.
  - Amount of redundancy marked using pinch test on medial and lateral arm from the axillary crease to the elbow (Fig. 99-11, *A*).
  - Inner ellipse is designed by cheating in one half *X*, where *X* is pinch thickness (Fig. 99-11, *B*).
  - Orientation marks made for guidance of closure techniques (Fig. 99-11, *C*).

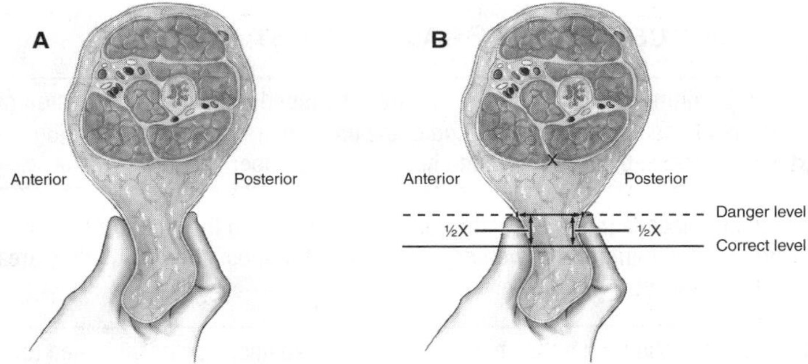


**Fig. 99-10 A,** Amount of tissue resection based on pinch thickness does not take into account the distance between the surgeon's fingers. **B,** To account for this discrepancy, the amount of resection is reduced by one half *X* on each side.

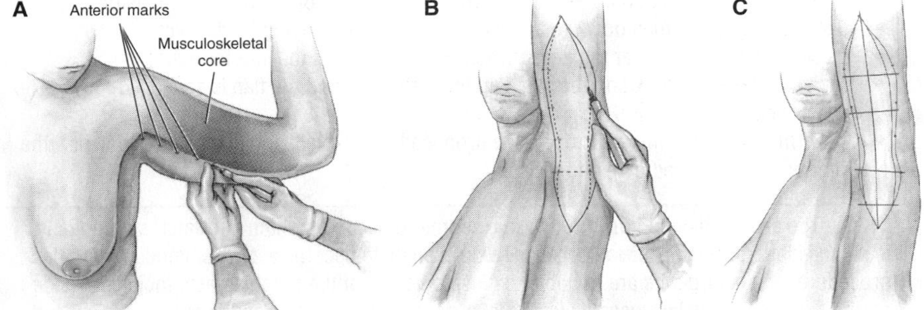


**Fig. 99-11 A,** Tissue is pinched below the underlying muscle mass, and anterior and posterior marks are made. Marks can continue to the distal end of the upper arm to eliminate excess tissue. **B,** Marks continue around the upper arm to the axillary crease. These marks are used to create the inner ellipse but serve as the actual resection line. **C,** A line through the midline is marked to orient the resection and allow placement of retraction clamps. Crosshatched marks guide alignment at closure.

**NOTE: There is a commonly debated concept regarding scar placement posteriorly versus medially. A medial scar lies in a less visible area (only seen when the arm is externally rotated and abducted); however, the poor dermal quality of the skin here creates an often wider scar. A posteriorly placed scar can be a fine-line scar because of better dermal quality, but this will be visible from behind when the patient wears sleeveless clothing.**

**NOTE: In a newer concept, the scar is placed at a happy medium between the true posterior and true medial (bicipital groove) area at the posteromedial aspect of the arm. This allows better dermal alignment without the high visibility of a posterior scar. It requires slight variation in determining possible resection. Conservative resection is advised when learning this technique to prevent overly tight closures (Kenkel JM, personal communication, 2012).**

## Operative Sequence for Brachioplasty

**TIP:** To help minimize edema, concerns are discussed with the anesthesiologist preoperatively. The IV line should not be placed in the upper extremity. An external jugular line or lower extremity line can be used instead to help minimize upper extremity edema.

- Incisions are made in the posterolateral elbow region and in the superior portion of the axilla anteriorly for the infiltration of wetting solution and for liposuction (within the area to be resected if possible).

**TIP:** Even if liposuction will not be performed, wetting solution can be infiltrated to decrease blood loss and assist with dissection.

To prevent ulnar nerve injury, do not place liposuction access incisions medially at the elbow.

- Liposuction is performed; a **minimum of 0.5 cm of fat** is left on the skin.
- A No. 10 blade is used to incise through the proximal portion of the upper incision.
- Dissection is performed down to the deep investing fascia using Bovie electrocautery.
- Dissection continues over the deep investing fascia toward the inferior mark.
- Towel clips are placed along the skin flap to be excised, and the flap is advanced toward the upper incision.
- Confirm that the wound will close if the proposed inferior incision is made; if it will not, the inferior incision is redrawn and incised.

**TIP:** The arm is divided into three to five segments, each of which is treated sequentially, including closure. This is critical, because the arm tends to become very edematous during this procedure. Often surgeons are not able to close portions of the brachioplasty incision. These portions can generally be closed if closure is performed immediately and progressively instead of after the entire wound is dissected.

- Closure begins with reapproximation of the superficial fascial system, followed by deep dermal and subcuticular layers.
  - ▶ The superficial fascial system is closed with long-lasting absorbable suture to help relieve tension.

**TIP:** To prevent postoperative numbness, leave some fat on the deep investing fascia at the junction between the middle and lower third of the upper arm. This helps to protect the MABC nerve, which exits the deep investing fascia here, often with the basilic vein.[6]

- **If the wound crosses the axilla, a Z-plasty** can be performed to try to decrease scar retraction and axillary banding.
  - The necessity of Z-plasty is debated. Many surgeons find increased risk of wound dehiscence with these flaps and prefer to treat banding with a delayed Z-plasty only if necessary.
- Drains are placed to prevent seroma formation.
- The wound is dressed and wrapped with an Ace bandage, beginning distally at the hands and continuing proximally to the axilla to assist with edema.

## BRACHIOPLASTY IN MASSIVE-WEIGHT-LOSS PATIENTS

- MWL patients often develop a "bat-wing" appearance to their arms, with severe skin laxity that extends from the olecranon across the axilla to the chest wall (Fig. 99-12).[8]
- A standard brachioplasty treats skin laxity from the olecranon to the axilla.
  - This does not significantly affect excess skin of the axilla or the lateral chest wall.
  - To treat skin in this zone, brachioplasty must extend across the axilla and onto the chest wall.
- Patient is marked with the arms abducted 90 degrees and the elbow flexed 90 degrees.

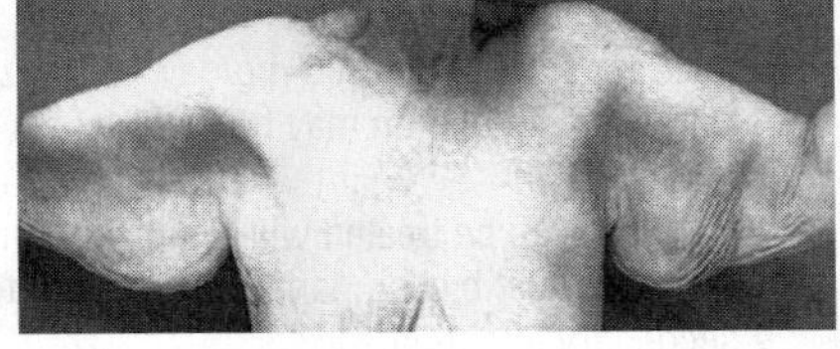

**Fig. 99-12** Bat-wing appearance of a massive-weight-loss patient.

- An elliptical incision is planned as in a standard upper arm brachioplasty.
  - However, instead of terminating the incision in the axillary dome, the incision is carried further into the axilla and down on to the chest wall as necessary.
  - The incision is continued as far as the skin laxity continues.
- To help make the scar less noticeable, a sinusoidal variation can be added to the proposed excision so that the final scar does not lie in a straight line.
- An axillary Z-plasty can be added to the proposed skin excision to prevent contracture across the axilla and to restore the appearance of the axillary dome (Fig. 99-13).
  - This should be designed with 60-degree angles to the longitudinal incision.
  - Central transverse limb of the Z should lie in transverse axis of axillary dome.
  - Pros/Cons of immediate versus delayed Z-plasty previously discussed.
- The intraoperative technique is similar to the standard brachioplasty described previously.
- **Minimal undermining of the skin flaps** should be necessary given the already lax nature of the skin.

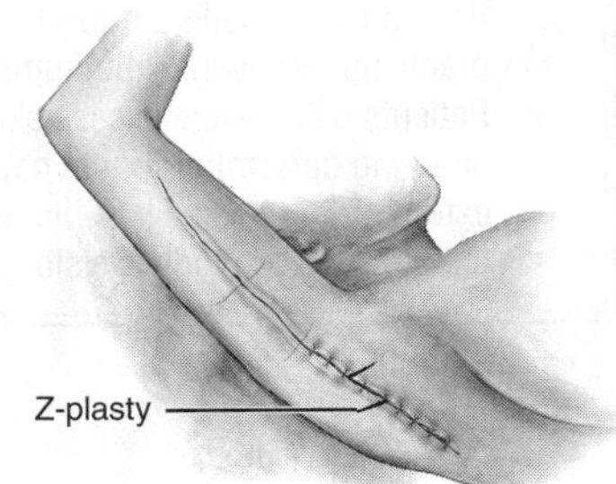


**Fig. 99-13** Axillary Z-plasty.

- It is critical to divide the incision into thirds, fourths, or fifths.
  - Perform the operation segmentally to ensure that edema will not prevent closure of appropriately designed skin flaps.
  - Conversely, the L brachioplasty described by Hurwitz and Holland[9] treats chest wall laxity without use of a Z.
    - A standard ellipse is drawn along the arm into the deltopectoral groove, and a second ellipse is created at a 90-degree angle within the axilla to elevate the posterior axillary fold and create a smoother contour.
    - Results were good with a low incidence of delayed wound healing.

## POSTOPERATIVE CONSIDERATIONS

- Postoperative complications include seroma, hematoma, infection, lymphocele, numbness, peripheral nerve pain, and wound dehiscence, especially in the axilla.
  - Postoperative complication rates were as high as 40% in many studies.[2,9-11]
  - Wound-healing complications were especially high in the MWL population and in those undergoing concomitant procedures with brachioplasty.[11]
    - Ace wraps should be worn for at least 2 days postoperatively to help minimize edema.
    - After 2 days, patients can continue to use Ace wrap or switch to surgical sleeve or long-sleeved surgical vest.
    - Gabapentin, 100-300 mg/day, can be used to treat peripheral nerve pain if needed.[6]
  - Surgical intervention may be required if a painful neuroma forms from injury to the MABC nerve.
  - Seromas can be treated with multiple aspirations and will usually resolve.
  - Lymphoceles, by comparison, may need to be marsupialized and allowed to heal via secondary intention.

### KEY POINTS

✓ Successful rejuvenation of the arm requires accurate assessment of the deformity and appropriate treatment selection.

✓ Patients with mild-to-moderate excess fat but good skin quality should have traditional, CAST, or ultrasound-assisted liposuction.

✓ Patients with mild-to-moderate amounts of excess skin and fat should have a minibrachioplasty or limited medial brachioplasty, with skin excision confined to the axilla.

✓ Patients with moderate-to-severe amounts of excess skin should have a traditional brachioplasty, with a longitudinal skin excision planned from the axilla to the elbow.

✓ Patients with severe excess skin, such as massive-weight-loss patients and those with bat-wing deformity, should have an extended brachioplasty. The skin excision should extend from the elbow to the axilla and onto the lateral chest wall. This can take many forms, but all include excision of skin within and below the axilla.

## REFERENCES


1. Lockwood T. Brachioplasty with superficial fascial system suspension. Plast Reconstr Surg 96:912-920, 1995.
2. Knoetgen J, Moran S. Long-term outcomes and complications associated with brachioplasty: a retrospective review and cadaveric study. Plast Reconstr Surg 117:2219-2223, 2006.
3. Appelt EA, Janis JE, Rohrich RJ. An algorithmic approach to upper arm contouring. Plast Reconstr Surg 118:237-246, 2006.
4. Trussler A, Rohrich RJ. Limited incision medial brachioplasty: technical refinements in upper arm contouring. Plast Reconstr Surg 121:305-307, 2008.
5. Nguyen A, Rohrich RJ. Liposuction-assisted posterior brachioplasty: technical refinements in upper arm contouring. Plast Reconstr Surg 126:1365-1369, 2010.
6. Nahai F, ed. The Art of Aesthetic Surgery: Principles & Techniques, 2nd ed. St Louis: Quality Medical Publishing, 2011.
7. Aly AS. Body Contouring After Massive Weight Loss. St Louis: Quality Medical Publishing, 2006.
8. Strauch B, Greenspun D, Levine J, et al. A technique of brachioplasty. Plast Reconstr Surg 113:1044-1049, 2004.
9. Hurwitz D, Holland S. The L brachioplasty: an innovative approach to correct excess tissue of the upper arm, axilla, and lateral chest. Plast Reconstr Surg 117:403-411, 2006.
10. Shermak M. Body contouring. Plast Reconstr Surg 129:963e-978e, 2012.
11. Gusenoff JA, Coon D, Rubin JP. Brachioplasty and concomitant procedures after massive weight loss: a statistical analysis from a prospective registry. Plast Reconstr Surg 122:595-603, 2008.

# 100. Abdominoplasty

**Luis M. Rios, Jr., Sacha I. Obaid, Jason E. Leedy**

## ANATOMY

- **The abdominal wall is composed of seven layers:**
  1. Skin
  2. Subcutaneous fat
  3. Scarpa's fascia (the superficial fascial system of the abdomen)
  4. Subscarpal fat
  5. Anterior rectus sheath
  6. Muscle
  7. Posterior rectus sheath

### SKIN

- The skin of the abdominal wall receives a rich vascular supply from multiple muscle and fascial perforating vessels.
- The skin of the abdominal wall can vary in quality depending on a person's genetics, age, previous pregnancies, and history of weight gain and loss.
- The skin of the abdominal wall may feature multiple **striae,** which are evidence of **attenuated or absent dermis.**

### FAT

- The abdominal wall has **two** layers of fat, **superficial and deep,** separated by Scarpa's fascia (Fig. 100-1).

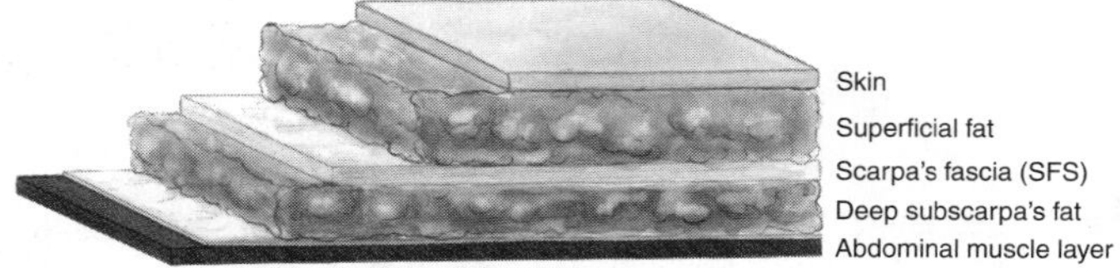


**Fig. 100-1** Layers of fat. (*SFS,* Superficial fascial system.)

- The **superficial layer** of fat is thicker, more dense, more durable, and has a heartier blood supply.
- The **deeper layer** of fat is less dense and receives most of its blood from the subdermal plexus and underlying myocutaneous perforators.

> **TIP:** Because the blood supply to the deeper fat is distinct from the blood supply to the skin, it can be more easily excised when thinning the abdominal wall flap in an abdominoplasty. By contrast, thinning the superficial layer of fat may lead to vascular compromise of the overlying skin.

- There are **four paired muscle groups** of the abdominal wall.
  1. Rectus abdominis
  2. External oblique
  3. Internal oblique
  4. Transversus abdominis
- The aponeurotic portions of the transversus muscle and the two oblique muscles envelop the rectus abdominis muscles, forming the anterior and posterior rectus sheaths and meeting in the midline to form the linea alba.
- The **arcuate line** represents a transition point.
  - **Above the arcuate line,** there are distinct anterior and posterior rectus sheaths.
  - **Below the arcuate line,** contributions from the internal oblique and transversus join contributions from the external and internal obliques to form a single anterior rectus sheath with no posterior rectus sheath.
  - The arcuate line is roughly halfway between the umbilicus and symphysis pubis.

## Vascularity of the Abdominal Wall (Box 100-1)

**Box 100-1** *Vascular Supply to the Abdominal Wall According to Huger*[1]

Zone I: Superior and inferior epigastric systems
Zone II: Circumflex iliac and external pudendal systems
Zone III: Intercostals and external pudendal systems

- **Huger**[1] divided the vascular supply to the abdominal wall into **three zones** (Fig. 100-2).
  - **Zone I**
    - Between the lateral borders of the rectus sheath from the costal margin to a horizontal line drawn between the two anterior superior iliac spines (ASISs)
    - Supplied primarily by superficial branches of the **superior and inferior epigastric systems**
  - **Zone II**
    - Below the horizontal line between the two ASISs to the pubic and inguinal creases
    - Supplied by the superficial branches of the **circumflex iliac** and **external pudendal vessels**

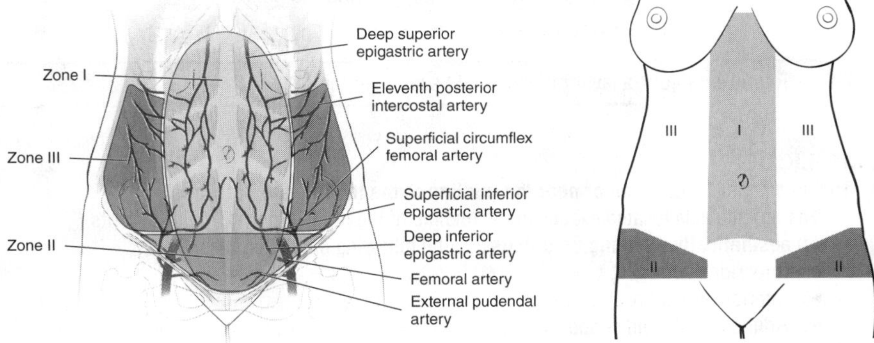


**Fig. 100-2** Huger vascular zones.

- **Zone III**
  - Superior to zone II and lateral to zone I
  - Supplied by **intercostals, subcostals,** and **lumbar** vessels
- Sensation to the abdomen is from **intercostal nerves T7-12.**

## NERVES AND THE ABDOMINAL WALL

- **Lateral cutaneous branches**
  - Perforate the intercostal muscles at the midaxillary line
  - Then travel within the subcutaneous plane
- **Anterior cutaneous branches**
  - Travel between the transversus and internal oblique muscles to penetrate the posterior rectus sheath just lateral to the rectus
  - Eventually enter the rectus muscles and then pass to the overlying fascia and skin
- **Lateral femoral cutaneous nerve** (Fig. 100-3)
  - Innervates the skin in the lateral aspect of the thigh
  - Immerges close to the ASIS

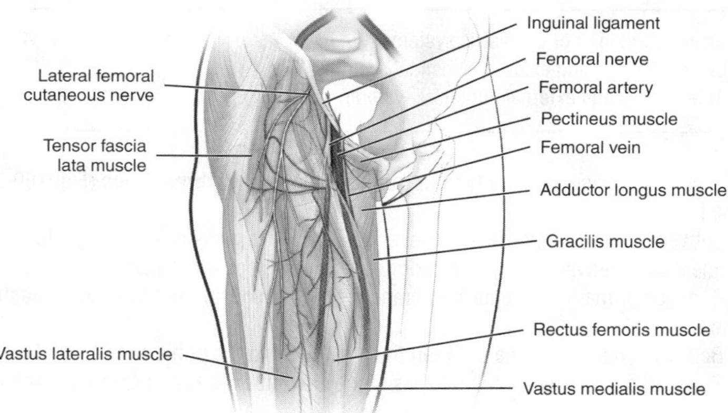


**Fig. 100-3** Lateral femoral cutaneous nerve.

> **TIP:** To prevent injury, a layer of fat should be left over the ASIS.

## UMBILICUS

- The umbilicus is located **on or near the midline at the level of the iliac crest.**
  - The umbilicus is located exactly in the midline of the body in only 1.7% of patients.[2]
  - An **aesthetically pleasing umbilicus** has the following characteristics[3]:
    - Superior hooding
    - Inferior retraction
    - Round or ellipsoid shape
    - Shallow

- **Blood supply to the umbilicus** (Fig. 100-4) **is from:**
  - Subdermal plexus
  - Right and left deep inferior epigastric artery (DIEA)
  - Ligamentum teres
  - Median umbilical ligament

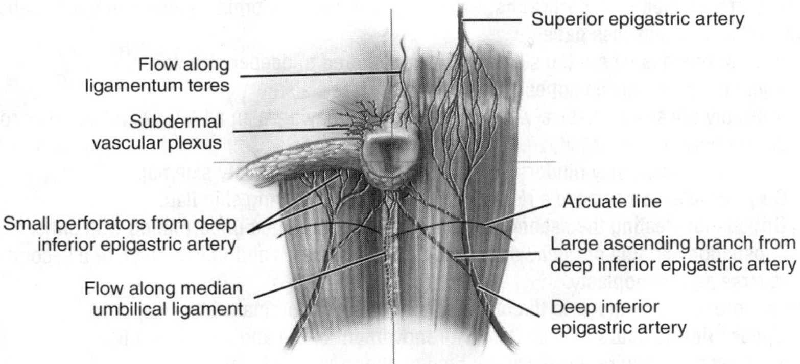


**Fig. 100-4** Blood supply to the umbilicus.

# PREOPERATIVE EVALUATION

## History and Physical Examination

- **Complete history should include**[3]**:**
  - Number of pregnancies and children
  - Previous cesarean section or other abdominal surgery
  - Previous or current hernias
  - Exercise routine
  - Gastrointestinal history, including irritable bowel syndrome or constipation
  - Respiratory history, including asthma, smoking, or sleep apnea
  - History of weight loss and gain, and active diet regimen
  - History of weight loss surgery, including location of ports

**CAUTION: Abdominoplasty is a huge stressor in terms of blood supply to the abdominal wall flap. To minimize complications, surgeons should not operate on active smokers, but instead should insist that these patients quit smoking before abdominoplasty and openly discuss the increased risk of complications. This will not only encourage cessation of smoking but also will help discourage patients from lying about their smoking history. A urine or blood nicotine test may be indicated.**

- Examine the skin of the abdominal wall for **striae,** which represent thinning or absent dermis.
  - Surgeons must explain to patients that:
    - Striae located inferior to the umbilicus may be removed as part of the abdominoplasty.
    - Most striae above the umbilicus will not be removed.
    - Striae above the umbilicus may become more prominent, because the abdominal wall flap is stretched by the abdominoplasty.

- **Excess skin** must be treated.
  - The patient must be examined while standing, supine, and sitting.
  - If the patient is examined only in the standing or supine position, the surgeon may be fooled into thinking there is little or no excess skin.
  - When the patient sits, the surgeon immediately determines whether there is excess abdominal skin.
- Examine for **rashes or excoriations,** especially under the abdominal pannus in obese patients and massive-weight-loss patients.
- Look for **adhesions** where the skin and fat are tethered to deeper structures.
  - There is commonly an adhesion at that level at the waist.
  - Morbidly obese or massive-weight-loss patients may have an additional adhesion or roll of skin superiorly.
  - These adhesions may hinder movement of the abdominoplasty skin flap.
  - Surgical release can pose a risk of ischemia in the overlying skin flap.
  - Options for treating the second adhesion are discontinuous undermining with either a liposuction cannula or Lockwood dissector, a *fleur-de-lis* abdominoplasty, or a second-stage reverse abdominoplasty.
- **Scars** represent alterations to the blood supply of the abdominal wall.
  - **Upper midline scars** may limit inferior movement of the abdominal skin flap.
    - They may require release at the time of abdominoplasty.
    - For some patients *fleur-de-lis* abdominoplasty should be considered.
  - **Subcostal scars** are particularly troubling.
    - They represent an interruption of the superolateral blood supply that the abdominoplasty skin flap relies on for blood supply postoperatively.
    - **Of all those undergoing abdominoplasty, these patients are at the highest risk for postoperative wound-healing complications.**

**CAUTION: To prevent wound-healing complications, the abdominal wall skin flap *must not* be undermined beneath a subcostal incision. The limitations of undermining, limited results, and high risk of complications must be discussed with these patients. Many are not candidates for an abdominoplasty.**

- **Myofascial laxity** must be treated.
  - **A diver's test** can be performed with the patient first standing and then flexing at the waist.
    - Worsening of lower abdominal wall fullness indicates **myofascial laxity** (Fig. 100-5, *A* and *B*).
  - The **pinch test** is an additional test for myofascial laxity (Fig. 100-5, *C*).
    - Abdominal fullness is assessed with the patient both relaxed and actively tensing the abdominal wall.

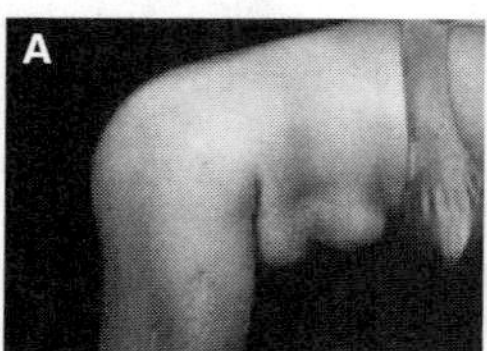


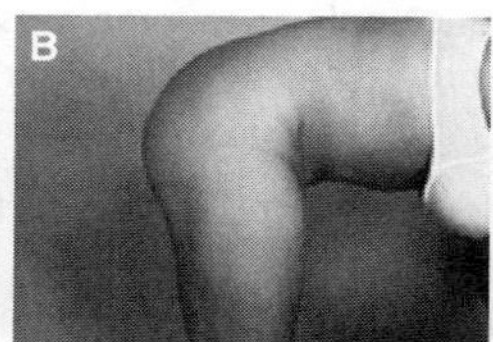


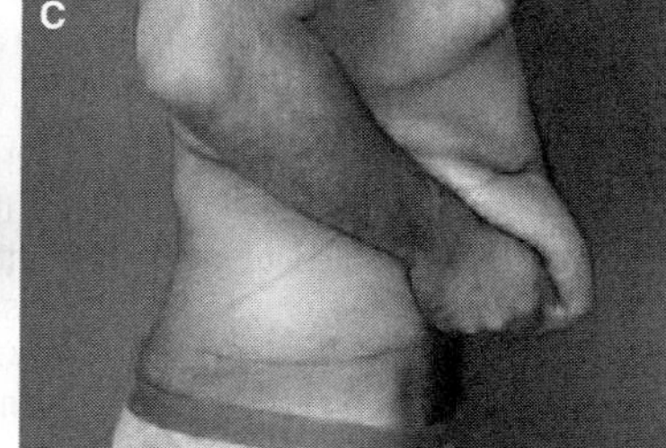


**Fig. 100-5** **A** and **B,** Diver's test. **C,** Pinch test.

    - If the amount of fullness that can be pinched is significantly decreased by tensing the abdominal wall, then the patient has significant myofascial laxity.
- Midline **diastasis recti abdominis** must be examined.
  - If upper abdominal fullness exists, have the patient lie down.
  - If abdomen is scaphoid, plication will work.
  - If fullness is still present, plication will be difficult and the patient should be encouraged to lose weight.

**TIP:** Nearly all patients who have previously been pregnant have some degree of myofascial laxity of the abdominal wall in addition to excess skin.

- Examine and document any **hernias,** including incisional, epigastric, periumbilical, and inguinal hernias, especially in patients who have had previous surgeries and massive-weight-loss patients.

**NOTE: The importance of a thorough hernia examination cannot be overstated. Preoperative knowledge of hernias can help the surgeon prevent injuring the bowel during dissection. In addition, depending on the size of the hernia and the comfort level of the plastic surgeon, preoperative knowledge of a hernia may allow the plastic surgeon to potentially coordinate with a general surgeon to assist with hernia repair at the time of the operation.**

## Informed Consent

- **In location and length of scars.**
  - The standard lower abdominal transverse scar
  - The potential need for a short vertical midline scar
    - This "T scar" may be necessary for patients with smaller amounts of excess abdominal wall skin and fat.
  - Potential for cutaneous deformities ("dog-ears") at the lateral ends of the abdominoplasty incision
    - If these are present, revision surgeries, including excision of this skin or liposuction of the underlying fullness, may be necessary.
  - **Overall complication rate is 20%-34%.**[4]
- **Wound-healing complications.**
  - Both the transverse incision at the waist and the umbilicus itself are at risk for poor wound healing because of poor vascularity.
  - Smokers (49.7%) versus nonsmokers (14.8%)[5]
- **Loss or malposition of the umbilicus.**
  - Patients should be reminded preoperatively that the umbilicus is truly midline in only 1.7% of patients.[2]
- **Seromas** (0%-14% incidence).[4]
  - The need for and purpose of postoperative drains should be explained.
- Potential need for **revision surgeries or procedures** (5%-43%).
- Surgeons need to discuss financial arrangements and patients' responsibilities for these procedures.
- Patients must understand that they will not be able to walk fully erect for several days after the operation.
  - They will need a minimum of 2-3 weeks off from work.
  - They will not be able to do any strenuous exercise or lifting for at least 6 weeks postoperatively.

- Abdominoplasty carries an increased risk of **pulmonary embolism (PE).**
  - Factors that increase PE risk include general anesthesia and longer operative times (>140 minutes).[4]
  - Every patient should be placed in thromboembolism-deterrent (TED) hose, starting with sequential compression devices (SCDs) in the preoperative area, and encouraged to ambulate and maintain hydration.
  - Serious consideration should be given to the use of low-molecular-weight heparin (Lovenox 40 mg SQ) on the evening of surgery and continued for 7 days.
- **Infection:** Risk in the literature is 0%-8%.[4] The Surgical Care Improvement Project (SCIP) identifies areas to reduce risk of infection (Box 100-2).

**Box 100-2** *SCIP PROTOCOL*

Shaving is not required. Do not use razors.
Give IV antibiotics 30-59 minutes before the incision.
Give postoperative antibiotics for 24 hours.
Perform elective surgery with $A_1C < 7$.
Prevent intraoperative hypothermia.

*SCIP,* Surgical Care Improvement Project.

**TIP:** Abdominoplasty carries a moderate complication rate. Therefore patients should be optimal candidates for the procedure.

## PROCEDURE SELECTION (Table 100-1)

**Table 100-1** *Procedure Selection*

| Procedure | Excess Fat | Excess Skin | Skin Tone | Diastasis |
|---|---|---|---|---|
| Liposuction | Mild | None | Good | None |
| Liposuction and endoscopic repair | Mild | None | Good | Present |
| Miniabdominoplasty | Infraumbilical | Infraumbilical | Good | Present |
| Traditional or lipoabdominoplasty | Significant and not confined to infraumbilical region | Significant and not confined to infraumbilical region | Fair to poor | Present |
| Circumferential | Mild to moderate | Extends to back | Fair to poor | Present |
| High-lateral-tension | Mild to moderate | Lateral abdominal area and thigh | Poor | Present |
| Fleur-de-lis | Mild to moderate | Vertical and horizontal | Fair to poor | Present |

- Patients with mild fat excess, no excess skin, and good skin tone are candidates for **liposuction alone.**[6]
- Patients with mild fat excess, no excess skin, good skin tone, and rectus diastasis should have **liposuction combined with endoscopic diastasis repair.**

- Patients with skin and fat excess isolated to the infraumbilical region should have an **infraumbilical miniabdominoplasty** with liposuction and diastasis repair.
- Patients with significant amounts of skin and fat excess that is not limited to the infraumbilical region should have a **traditional abdominoplasty** with or without liposuction of the flank.
- Patients with significant extra skin that may extend far laterally and even around to the back should have **circumferential abdominoplasty.**
  - *This is the procedure of choice for most massive-weight-loss patients.*
- Patients with excess skin at the lateral abdominal area, lateral hip and thigh, pubis, and possibly anteromedial thigh are candidates for **Lockwood's high-lateral-tension abdominoplasty.**
- Patients with excess skin both vertically and horizontally (especially in the upper midline region) are candidates for a **fleur-de-lis abdominoplasty.**

## TRADITIONAL ABDOMINOPLASTY

### Preoperative Markings

- Patients should be encouraged to wear their undergarments of choice the day of surgery.
  - This helps the surgeon plan the lower incision with the goal of hiding as much of it under these garments as possible.
- Preoperative markings begin with identification of the pubic bone and ASIS bilaterally.
- With the patient standing, the lateral aspects of the abdominal fold are marked. This is a guide to the lateral extension of the incision.
- The planned incision is marked beginning transversely at the level of the pubic bone.
  - At least **5-7 cm** must be left between this incision and the top of the vulval commissure to prevent distortion of the vulvar region postoperatively.
- The transverse marks are extended laterally and superiorly toward the hips bilaterally.
  - The lateralmost points of the incision should lie inferior to the ASIS to prevent visibility of the scar postoperatively.
- A pinch test is performed to determine how much skin can be resected from the abdomen comfortably and to design a proposed upper incision.
  - The surgeon should determine whether the skin and fat all the way up to and just past the umbilicus should be excised in the operating room.
  - If there is any question, the surgeon must discuss with the patient the high likelihood of needing a **small vertical component** to the incision with a final "inverted-T"–shaped scar, which is more noticeable than a traditional transverse abdominoplasty scar.
- Areas to be considered for concomitant liposuction are marked preoperatively.

> **TIP:** Most patients who present for abdominoplasty have at least some degree of fat excess in the hips, flanks, and/or thighs. These deposits frequently become more noticeable postoperatively. Both the surgeon and the patient must be aware of this and consider concomitant or staged liposuction with the abdominoplasty procedure for optimal results. Failure to recognize this and discuss it preoperatively may result in an unhappy patient with a compromised final result.

### Principles

- Before the patient enters the operating room, the surgeon and anesthesiologist must **test the bed** to make sure it can flex at the patient's waist to an optimal level.

> **TIP:** Failure to test the bed preoperatively can cause significant intraoperative difficulties.

- After induction of anesthesia, liposuction is performed in all planned areas.
- The patient's temperature must be maintained by warming in the preoperative area and warming the OR and IV fluids. Warm blankets and thermal caps are used throughout the case.
- SCDs and TED hose are started in the preoperative room before the induction of anesthesia.
- To decrease the risk of infection, IV antibiotics for *Staphylococcus aureus* are given 30-59 minutes before the incision. Ancef 1 g or clindamycin 900 mg (patients with penicillin allergies) is given. Ancef is given every 3 hours and clindamycin every 6 hours during the procedure.
- No shaving is performed at the time of surgery or for 2 weeks before surgery. Razors are prohibited. Clippers can be used.
- The umbilicus must be cleaned of all particulate matter. Give the patient surgical soap and cotton-tipped applicators to clean the umbilicus 1 week before surgery.
- Abdominoplasty begins with placement of two traction sutures at 3 o'clock and 9 o'clock positions in the umbilicus.

**TIP:** Before making the circumumbilical incision, take care to orient the umbilicus by placing these sutures with asymmetrical tails, for instance, with one long tail and one short tail on the right and two long tails on the left. This helps to prevent twisting of the umbilical stalk during closure and subsequent poor blood flow.

- The umbilicus is incised circularly, and dissecting scissors are used to separate the umbilicus from the abdominal skin and fat down to the rectus sheath.
  - *Avoid skeletonizing the umbilical stalk, which leads to compromised vascularity of the umbilicus.*
- The inferior incision is made bilaterally.
- Dissection is taken straight down to the fascia overlying the rectus and oblique musculature.
- The skin and fat of the abdominal wall are elevated from the underlying muscular fascia in a loose areolar plane up to the costal margins laterally and to the xiphoid process medially.

**TIP:** Central undermining preserves the blood supply to the abdominal wall. By limiting the central undermining to only what is needed to perform the rectus plication, 80% (versus 30%) of the abdominal blood supply can be preserved.[7]

- Leave a small amount of fat on the muscular fascia in the region of the ASIS to prevent injury to the lateral femoral cutaneous nerve.

**TIP:** The importance of leaving a small amount of fat on the muscular fascia in the region of the ASIS cannot be overemphasized. This prevents injury to the lateral femoral cutaneous nerve, which can cause significant pain, numbness, and dysesthesia in the hip and lateral thigh region postoperatively. van Uchelen et al[8] reported a 10% incidence of injury to this nerve in their review of abdominoplasty procedures.

**CAUTION: As dissection is taken along the muscular fascia centrally, care must be taken to identify and preserve the umbilical stalk. Failure to do so results in transection of the umbilical blood supply and likely umbilical necrosis postoperatively.**

**TIP:** There are a number of periumbilical myocutaneous perforating vessels. These should signal the surgeon to slow the dissection and search for the umbilical stalk to prevent transection.

- The bed is flexed, bringing the patient to a seated position, and the amount of skin and fat that can be resected from the abdominal wall while allowing a tension-free closure is marked.
- This excess skin and fat are resected.
- The wound is copiously irrigated.
- Once the abdominal flap is resected, the rectus diastasis is repaired.
    - A cotton-tipped applicator is used to apply methylene blue to the rectus sheath elliptically as a proposed area to be imbricated.
    - The rectus sheath is imbricated or reinforced by placing interrupted sutures along the marked repair.
    - Rectus plication helps to narrow the waist and correct laxity in the abdominal wall that occurs in all women who have been pregnant.
- After a first row of interrupted permanent sutures is placed, a second reinforcing permanent suture can be run from the xiphoid to the umbilicus, and a separate reinforcing suture can be run infraumbilically to the pubis.
- Horizontal plication sutures can be placed to help narrow the waist (Fig. 100-6).

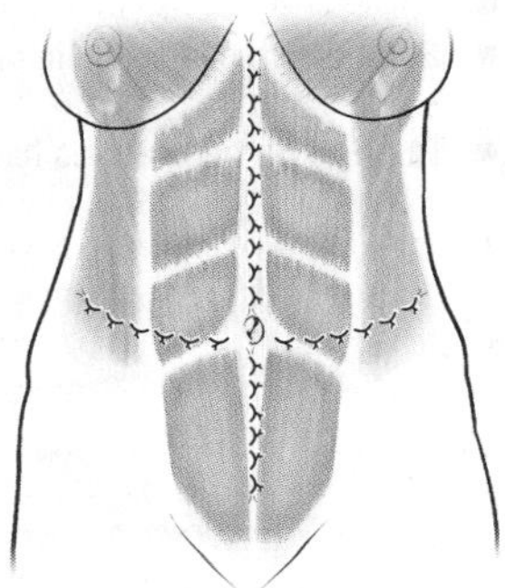

**Fig. 100-6** Plication sutures of abdomen, including horizontal sutures.

> **TIP:** It is essential to begin rectus plication just inferior to the xiphoid process. Failure to do so can result in a postoperative bulge that is fairly distressing to the patient.

- **Rectus plication** must be performed using **permanent sutures.**
    - Using ultrasound imaging, van Uchelen et al[8] revealed a 40% recurrence rate for diastasis in 40 patients at 64 months when plication had been performed using absorbable sutures.
    - Nahas et al[9-11] reported a 0% recurrence rate for diastasis in 12 patients by CT scans at 76-84 months when permanent sutures were used.

> **TIP:** Plication of the rectus fascia tends to be the most painful portion of the operation. Local anesthetic delivered by continuous-infusion catheters to the region of the rectus plication can significantly reduce postoperative pain.

- Progressive tension sutures (PTSs) can be used to attach the flap to the abdominal musculature (see Fig. 100-7).

> **TIP:** PTSs advance the flap and distribute the tension of the closure throughout the abdominal flap instead of the incision. They also reduce the risk of seroma. Pollock and Pollock[12,13] have reported a 0% incidence of seroma with these sutures without drains.

- The level of the umbilicus is transposed with a marking pen to the overlying skin of the abdominal wall.
- The umbilicus is inset.
- If used, Jackson-Pratt drains can be exteriorized through the hair-bearing skin of the pubic region or a separate lateral incision.
- The superficial fascial system is closed, followed by closure of the deep dermal and subcuticular layers.
- An abdominal binder is placed postoperatively.

## PROGRESSIVE TENSION SUTURES[12-14] (Fig. 100-7)

- The abdominal flap is sutured and advanced onto the muscular fascia using interrupted 2-0 Vicryl.
- As the flap is advanced, progressive tension is exerted on each suture and away from the incision.
- Decreased tension on the incision prevents necrosis and hypertrophic scars.
- The dead space is closed, preventing hematoma and seroma formation.
- Sutures can be used in lipoabdominoplasty, other forms of abdominoplasty, and body contour surgery.
- Running barbed sutures have also been effectively used as PTS sutures.[14]

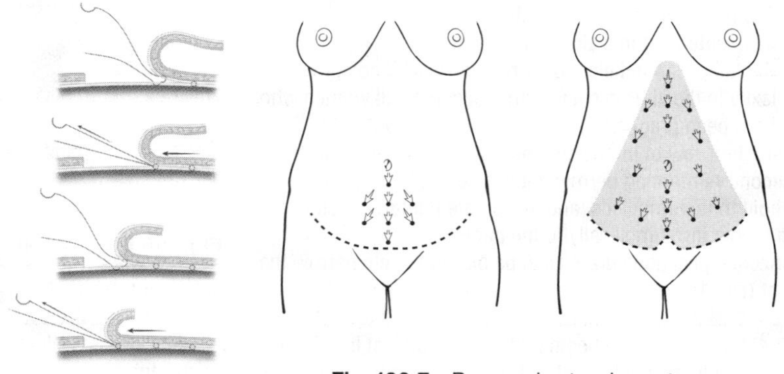

**Fig. 100-7** Progressive tension sutures.

## LIPOABDOMINOPLASTY[7]

- The areas for liposuction are marked.
- Superwet technique is used.
- Ultrasonic or traditional suction-assisted liposuction (SAL) is safe.
- A thin layer of fat is left on the abdominal wall to preserve lymphatic supply.
- Selective undermining of the flap is limited to the central area that will require plication, most commonly to the lateral border of the rectus[15] (Fig. 100-8).

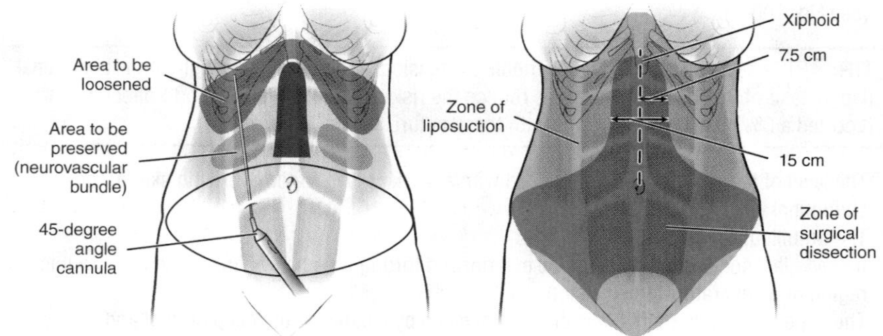


**Fig. 100-8** Central (selective undermining) of abdominoplasty flap.

- The abdominal perforators at the lateral aspect of the rectus muscle are preserved.[7]
- PTSs and drains can be used.
- Saldanha et al[7] theorized that 80% of blood supply, nerves, and lymphatics are preserved with this technique, thus contributing to their low rate of seroma (0.4%), dehiscence, necrosis, and hematoma. The incidence of DVT and PE remain the same.

**TIP:** Lipoabdominoplasty is safe if selective undermining principles are followed. More than 80% of the blood supply to the abdominal wall can be preserved with this technique, compared with 30% in a traditional abdominoplasty.

## MINIABDOMINOPLASTY[3] (Fig. 100-9)

- Miniabdominoplasty is useful for patients with primarily **infraumbilical excess of skin and fat.**
- A **shorter scar (12-16 cm)** is planned than for a traditional abdominoplasty.
- Rather than separate the umbilicus from the abdominal wall flap, it **remains attached.**
- The umbilical stalk is transected at the level of the anterior abdominal wall fascia.
- The resulting umbilical fascial defect is repaired.
- The rectus diastasis is repaired using permanent sutures.
- A more conservative skin and fat resection is performed than for a traditional abdominoplasty.
  - The umbilicus is usually moved approximately 2 cm inferiorly with this procedure.
- Liposuction is frequently included to further improve abdominal contour, especially in the supraumbilical region.

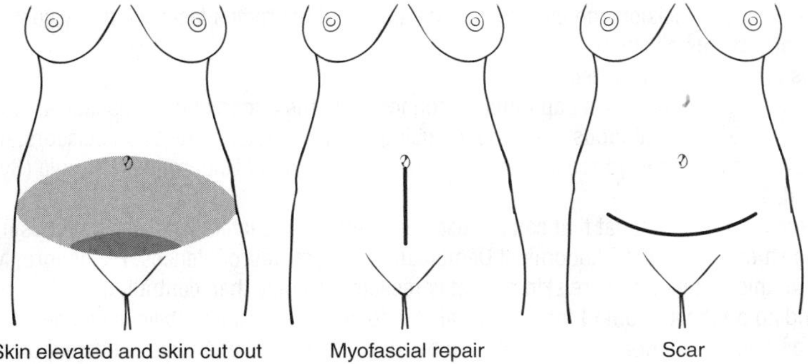


**Fig. 100-9** Miniabdominoplasty.

## HIGH-LATERAL-TENSION ABDOMINOPLASTY[16]

- One basis for this procedure: Although the excess skin infraumbilically is primarily **vertical,** the excess skin in the epigastrium is primarily **horizontal.**
  - Lockwood[16] believed that the skin of the epigastrium develops laxity horizontally because of a strong superficial fascial adherence to the linea alba, which limits vertical descent of skin and fat.
  - Therefore less skin is taken centrally and more is taken laterally.
  - This results in an **oblique vector of pull** that treats both the infraumbilical vertical excess and the epigastric lateral pull.

- Another basis for this procedure: Direct undermining to the costal margins, which is a fundamental part of traditional abdominoplasty, is actually unnecessary.
  - **Direct undermining is performed only centrally** in an area that allows rectus plication.
  - Limited, direct undermining makes liposuction safer throughout a much larger area of the abdominal flap.
  - Liposuction superolaterally creates a discontinuous undermining, allowing advancement of the abdominal flap.[16]
- Other advantages: Performs a lift of the anterior and lateral thigh; allows liposculpture of abdomen, leading to a more contoured result[16]

### Preoperative Markings

- A suprapubic mark is made 6.5-7.0 cm superior to the incisura of the vagina or the base of the penis.[3]
- The ASIS is marked bilaterally, and the three marks are connected.
- The marking pen is then placed centrally at the inferior incision line, and the vertical excess of skin is pulled upward until taut. The skin that is now at the tip of the pen is marked.
- Potential excess skin is tested laterally using a pinch test.
- This excess is marked laterally and connected to the central mark.
- The resultant proposed upper incision should be located infraumbilically and superior to the umbilicus laterally.
- The proposed areas of liposuction are marked both centrally and laterally.

### Principles and Technique

- Create the lower incision and elevate the skin and fat of the rectus fascia centrally, just enough to perform rectus plication.
- Rectus plication is performed.
- Laterally the abdominal skin flap remains connected to the underlying rectus fascia, but it is loosened by discontinuous undermining using vertical spreading or Mayo scissors, the surgeon's finger, an oversized suction cannula, or a Lockwood Underminer Cannula (Byron Medical, Tucson, AZ).[3]
- The amount of skin and fat that can be resected centrally and laterally is confirmed using a pinch test or a Lockwood Abdominal Demarcator (Integra NeuroSciences, Plainsboro, NJ).
  - With this technique, more skin and fat is resected laterally than centrally.
- Depending on the amount of infraumbilical skin to be excised, the umbilicus can be left in place and pulled inferiorly, or the stalk can be transected and the umbilicus floated, or it can be excised and relocated.
- The wound is tacked closed, and liposuction is performed in both a superficial and deep plane.
- Drains are placed.
- The superficial fascial system is repaired, followed by closure of the deep dermis and the skin.

## FLEUR-DE-LIS ABDOMINOPLASTY[17,18]

- The **fleur-de-lis** technique allows excision of the lower abdominal excess skin and fat through a transverse incision.
- It allows simultaneous removal of the supraumbilical horizontal skin excess through a vertical excision.
- The abdominoplasty can be taken as high as the xiphoid in the midline and as low as the mons pubis, depending on the area of skin laxity.

- To maximize vascularity, it is critical that skin flaps are left attached to the underlying fascia, except in the areas contained within the fleur-de-lis excision.[3]
- Although this procedure can completely change abdominal contour, the expected scars must be discussed preoperatively because they can be significant.
- Complication rate for this procedure is 31%, similar to that of traditional abdominoplasty (26%).[18]

## REVERSE ABDOMINOPLASTY

- Baroudi et al[19] first described reverse abdominoplasty in 1979.
- A transverse upper abdominal incision is made roughly at the level of the inframammary fold, and redundant superior abdominal tissue is pulled up to meet this incision and excised.
- The principal indication is for cleanup of residual redundant tissue that remains superiorly after lower abdominoplasty.
- The other indication is the rare patient who presents with excess skin and abdominal protuberance that is primarily in the upper pole of the abdomen.[3]
- This procedure can be combined with a breast procedure (e.g., Wise-pattern reduction or mastopexy), because the inframammary fold incisions can be used for both procedures.

### KEY POINTS

- ✓ Successful rejuvenation of the abdomen requires a thorough understanding of the anatomy of the abdominal wall and the techniques available for rejuvenation.
- ✓ Selection of the optimal procedure is of paramount importance for obtaining a good result.
- ✓ A graduated approach should be taken for liposuction performed in patients with minimal to moderate excess fat and good skin tone or quality with little laxity. Patients with more excess skin and fat are better candidates for traditional abdominoplasty.
- ✓ During abdominoplasty, care must be taken to preserve the lateral femoral cutaneous nerve to prevent painful postoperative neuromas.
- ✓ Permanent sutures must be used during rectus plication to prevent recurrent rectus diastasis.
- ✓ Newer techniques have been developed, including the fleur-de-lis abdominoplasty and the high-lateral-tension abdominoplasty, to treat supraumbilical horizontal abdominal laxity and vertical infraumbilical abdominal laxity.
- ✓ PTSs can reduce or eliminate seromas.
- ✓ Lipoabdominoplasty is safe if the key principles of selective undermining are followed.
- ✓ Infection rates can be reduced by keeping the patient warm, not using razors, optimizing the patient's medical status (glucose), and the proper use of antibiotics.
- ✓ DVT prophylaxis includes assigning a risk assessment score, placing TED hose and SCDs in the preoperative suite, encouraging postoperative ambulation and hydration, and considering the use of anticoagulants in the postoperative period.

## REFERENCES

1. Huger WE Jr. The anatomic rationale for abdominal lipectomy. Am Surg 45:612-617, 1979.
2. Rohrich RJ, Sorokin ES, Brown SA, et al. Is the umbilicus truly midline? Clinical and medicolegal implications. Plast Reconstr Surg 112:259-265, 2003.
3. Nahai F. The Art of Aesthetic Surgery: Principles & Techniques. St Louis: Quality Medical Publishing, 2005.

4. Buck DW, Mustoe TA. An evidence-based approach to abdominoplasty. Plast Reconstr Surg 126:2189-2195, 2010.
5. Manassa EH, Hertl CH, Olbrisch RR. Wound-healing problems in smokers and nonsmokers after 132 abdominoplasties. Plast Reconstr Surg 111:2082-2087; discussion 2088-2089, 2003.
6. Rohrich RJ, Beran SJ, Kenkel JM, et al. Extending the role of liposuction in body contouring with ultrasound-assisted liposuction. Plast Reconstr Surg 101:1090-1102, 1998.
7. Saldanha OR, Federico R, Daher PF, et al. Lipoabdominoplasty. Plast Reconstr Surg 124:934-942, 2009.
8. van Uchelen JH, Kon M, Werker PM. The long-term durability of plication of the anterior rectus sheath assessed by ultrasonography. Plast Reconstr Surg 107:1578-1584, 2001.
9. Nahas FX, Augusto SM, Ghelfond C. Should diastasis recti be corrected? Aesthetic Plast Surg 21:285-289, 1997.
10. Nahas FX, Ferreira LM, Mendes Jde A. An efficient way to correct recurrent rectus diastasis. Aesthetic Plast Surg 28:189-196, 2004.
11. Nahas FX, Ferreira LM, Augusto SM, et al. Long-term follow-up of correction of rectus diastasis. Plast Reconstr Surg 115:1736-1743, 2005.
12. Pollock H, Pollock T. Progressive tension sutures: a technique to reduce local complications in abdominoplasty. Plast Reconstr Surg 105:2583-2586, 2000.
13. Pollock T, Pollock H. Progressive tension sutures in abdominoplasty: a review of 597 consecutive cases. Aesthet Surg J 32:729-742, 2012.
14. Rosen A. Use of absorbable barbed suture and progressive tension technique in abdominoplasty: a novel approach. Plast Reconstr Surg 125:1024-1027, 2010.
15. Heller JB. Outcome analysis of combined lipoabdominoplasty versus conventional abdominoplasty. Plast Reconstr Surg 121:1821-1829, 2008.
16. Lockwood T. High-lateral-tension abdominoplasty with superficial fascial system suspension. Plast Reconstr Surg 96:603-615, 1995.
17. Dellon AL. Fleur-de-lis abdominoplasty. Aesthetic Plast Surg 9:27-32, 1985.
18. Friedman T, O'Brien Coon D, Michaels J, et al. Fleur-de-lis abdominoplasy: a safe alternative to traditional abdominoplasty for the massive weight loss patient. Plast Reconstr Surg 125:525-535, 2010.
19. Baroudi R, Keppke EM, Carvalho CG. Mammary reduction combined with reverse abdominoplasty. Ann Plast Surg 2:368-373, 1979.

# 101. Medial Thigh Lift

Sacha I. Obaid, Jason E. Leedy, Luis M. Rios, Jr.

## ANATOMY

- The medial thigh has a relatively thin outer layer of epidermis and dermis.
- Beneath the dermis are two layers of fat separated by a relatively weak superficial fascial system.
- Deep to the subcutaneous fat lies the strong, thick **Colles' fascia.**[1-4]
  - Attaches to the ischiopubic rami of the bony pelvis, to Scarpa's fascia of the abdominal wall, and to the posterior border of the urogenital diaphragm
  - Has an especially strong area at the **junction of the perineum and the medial thigh**
  - Provides the **anatomic shelf** that defines the perineal thigh crease
  - Best found intraoperatively by dissecting at the origin of the adductor muscles on the ischiopubic ramus and retracting the skin and superficial fat of the vulva medially
  - Lies just at the deepest and most lateral aspect of the vulvar soft tissue[5]
- The **femoral triangle** lies lateral to the Colles' fascia dissection (Fig. 101-1).
  - Midinguinal point between the pubic symphysis and anterior superior iliac spine
  - **Borders**
    - Superior: Inguinal ligament
    - Medial: Adductor longus
    - Lateral: Sartorius
- *Surgeons must be aware of the femoral triangle and avoid entering it to prevent major vascular or nerve injury and to prevent disruption of the lymphatic channels.*[5]

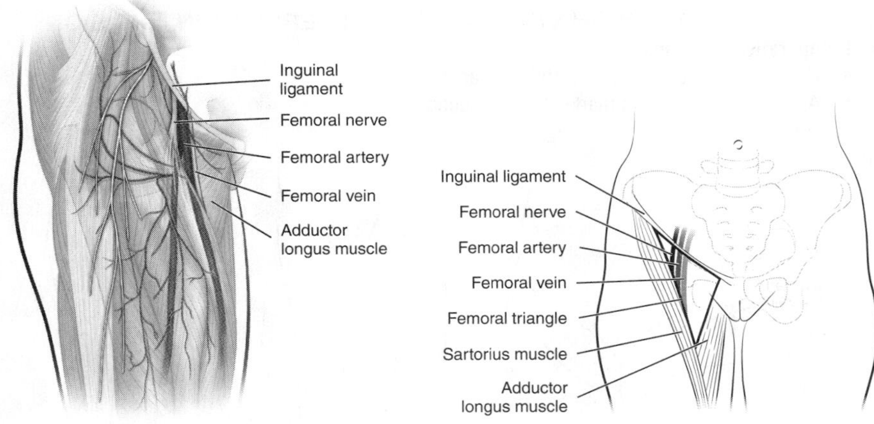


**Fig. 101-1** Femoral triangle.

## PATIENT EVALUATION

- Complete history is taken and physical examination performed.
- The skin quality and tone are assessed, along with the presence, location, and degree of skin ptosis.
- The presence or absence of extra subcutaneous fat in the thighs (medial and lateral) is recorded.
  - Many women have concerns about fat collections in the trochanteric regions. These can be treated with liposuction at the time of medial thigh lift.
  - The lower torso may require liposuction at the time of thigh lift.
- If present, laxity of the abdomen and pubic region are corrected first.
- In massive-weight-loss patients, the lower body lift is performed first, and thigh lift is performed at a second stage.
- If significant lipodystrophy is present, then liposuction is performed at least 3 months before the thigh lift.
- **Classification system** (Table 101-1)

**Table 101-1** *Classification and Surgical Recommendation*

| Classification | Description | Treatment |
|---|---|---|
| **Type I** | Lipodystrophy with no sign of skin laxity | **Liposuction alone** |
| **Type II** | Lipodystrophy and skin laxity confined to the **upper third of the thigh** | Liposuction and a **horizontal skin excision** |
| **Type III** | Lipodystrophy and moderate skin laxity that extends **beyond the upper third of the thigh** | Liposuction, horizontal and vertical excision |
| **Type IV** | Skin laxity that extends the **length of the thigh** | A **longer vertical resection** than for type III |
| **Type V** | Severe medial thigh skin laxity with lipodystrophy | **Two stages:**<br>First stage: Aggressive liposuction<br>Second stage: Excisional medial thigh lift |

## OPERATIVE TECHNIQUE

### Classic Medial Thigh Lift With Transverse Skin Excision[5]

- **Preoperative markings**
  - Patient is marked standing with knees apart (Fig. 101-2).
  - Areas of excess fat are marked for liposuction.

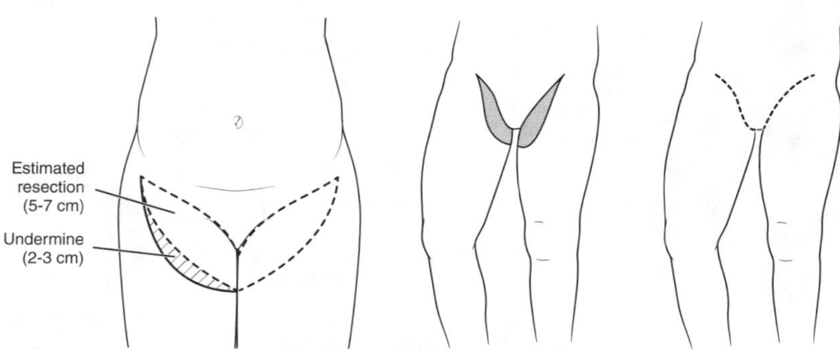


**Fig. 101-2** Preoperative markings.

- The femoral triangle is marked to remind the surgeon to stay away from this region.
- The proposed incision line is marked in the medial thigh crease from the pubic tubercle to the perineal-thigh crease.
  - The posterior incision no longer extends to the buttock crease.
  - Prone position is no longer used.
- A pinch test determines the amount of excess skin that can be removed, and an elliptical excision is marked.
  - 5-7 cm resection is average. Another 3-5 cm is gained with anchoring of the superficial fascial system (SFS) to Colles' fascia.
- For patients with laxity that extends beyond the upper third of the medial thigh skin, a vertical ellipse is added, creating a T-shaped final proposed incision.

■ **Technique**
- Foot and ankle compression devices are placed.
- The patient is placed in the supine position (frog-leg).
- Stirrups are no longer needed, because the incision ends at perineal crease.
  - The anterior incision begins at pubic tubercle and lateral border of mons.
  - Posterior incision stops at perineal-thigh crease and does not extend to buttocks.
  - Inferior flap dissection extends 2-3 cm beyond planned skin excision.
    - Care is taken not to violate the underlying muscular fascia.
    - The wound is closed, including separate closure of the superficial fascial system, deep dermis, and subcuticular areas.
- Colles' fascia is carefully identified near the origin of the adductor muscles on the ischiopubic ramus.
  - The skin and superficial fat of the vulva are retracted medially to aid in identification.

**TIP:** Carefully preserve the soft tissue that lies between the mons pubis and the femoral triangle to prevent lymphedema.

- The superficial fascial system of the medial thigh skin is identified and anchored to Colles' fascia (Fig. 101-3).
- The deep dermal and subcuticular layers are closed after the drain is placed.

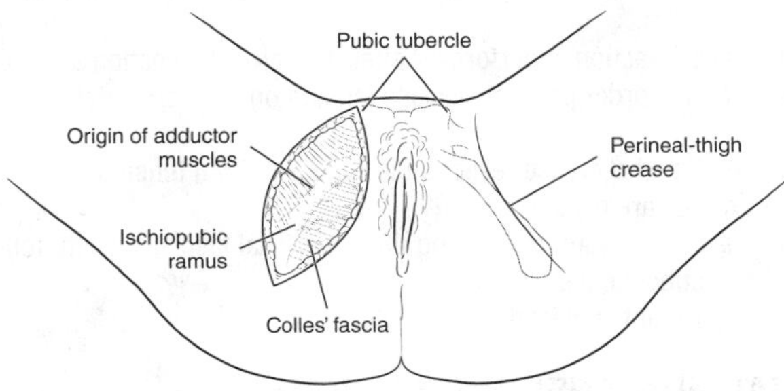


**Fig. 101-3** Colles' fascia.

## Modified Medial Thigh Lift in Massive-Weight-Loss Patients[5]

■ It is best to perform abdominal procedures in conjunction with or before thigh lifts to obtain best contour.

■ These patients often have **severe horizontal skin laxity.**

- This operation focuses on primary correction of horizontal laxity using a **longitudinal medial thigh incision.**
- The transverse medial thigh crease incision is minimized and used primarily for the excision of standing cutaneous deformities (dog-ears).
- There is no need for anchoring to the Colles' fascia.
- **Preoperative markings**
  - The patient is marked standing with the legs apart.
  - The proposed line of closure is determined so that it lies medially in the thigh and is minimally visible.
  - A pinch test determines how much skin and fat can be removed anteriorly and posteriorly.
  - The anterior and posterior incisions are marked.
- **Technique** (Fig. 101-4)
  - Intraoperatively only the supine frog-leg position is used.
  - Liposuction around knees is performed first. Otherwise, perform liposuction 3 months before resection.
  - The anterior incision is made with dissection down to the deep fat.
  - The skin and fat to be excised are elevated as dissection proceeds toward the proposed posterior incision.
  - **Saphenous vein should be preserved.**

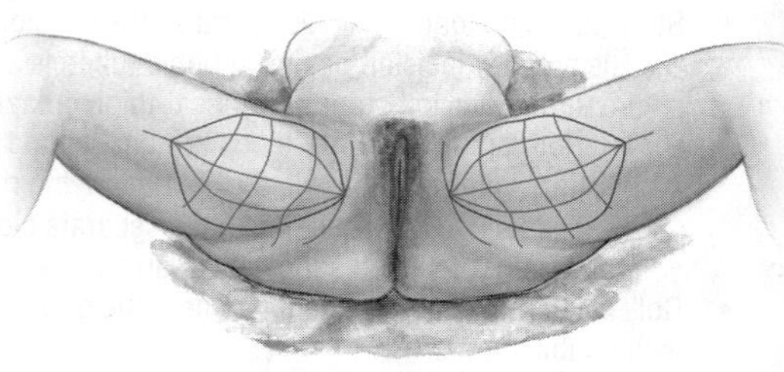

**Fig. 101-4** Anticipated resection. The horizontal incision stops at the posterior perineal crease.

**TIP:** Injury to the saphenous vein can result in prolonged swelling of the lower extremity.

  - The vertical resection is performed first.
  - It is **safest to perform this operation segmentally** to ensure that the wound closes with appropriate tension in each area and to minimize intraoperative edema that could prevent closure of the wounds.
  - The medial crease resection is performed after the vertical resection and closure.
    - Adherence to this order prevents excess tension on the horizontal closure of the medial crease.
    - The horizontal medial crease resection is closed without tension.
  - Jackson-Pratt drains are placed.
  - The wounds are closed by approximating the superficial fascial system, followed by the deep dermal and subcuticular layers.
  - A compression garment is placed.

## Fasciofascial Suspension Technique

- Candiani et al[6] proposed an alternative medial thigh lift that employs a **transverse skin excision with a vertical vector of pull.**
- Instead of relying on anchoring the Colles' fascia, this technique relies on the **strength of overlap between the gracilis and adductor longus fascia.**
- The operation begins with a transverse incision that is made parallel to, but 6-7 cm below, the inguinal crease.

- The skin and fat are undermined down to the fascia of the adductor longus and gracilis muscles.
- This fascia is overlapped and closed by an amount equal to the proposed skin and fat resection.
- The skin and fat are resected and closed under minimal tension, with most of the tension borne by the gracilis and adductor longus fascia.

## POSTOPERATIVE COMPLICATIONS

- Skin irregularities and depressions
- Hypertrophic scars
- Flattening of the buttocks from tension of wound closure
- Distribution of the vulva
- Lymphedema
- Recurrence of thigh ptosis

## POSTOPERATIVE COURSE

- Consider perioperative anticoagulation
- Compression garments for 2-4 weeks
- Encourage ambulation
- Drain removed in 5-7 days
- Daily dressing changes
- Driving restricted for 1-2 weeks
- Exercise restricted for 6 weeks

**TIP:** To prevent recurrence of thigh ptosis, anchor the closures to Colles' fascia or use fasciofascial suspension of the adductor and gracilis muscles.

### KEY POINTS

- ✓ Aesthetic rejuvenation of the thigh begins with a complete history and physical examination to determine the presence, location, and severity of excess skin and fat in the thigh.
- ✓ Based on the degree of excess skin and fat, liposuction alone, a transverse medial thigh incision, or a vertical medial thigh incision is used to correct the deformity.
- ✓ Care must be taken to preserve the soft tissue between the mons pubis and the femoral triangle to prevent postoperative lymphedema.
- ✓ The risk of thigh ptosis recurring is high unless a strong method of fixation is employed. This can be anchoring of Colles' fascia or fasciofascial suspension of the adductor and gracilis muscles.
- ✓ For a moderate amount of lipodystrophy in a massive-weight-loss patient, liposuction is performed in an early stage of contouring. Thigh lift is carried out 3 months later.
- ✓ In vertical excisions, preserve the saphenous vein to avoid prolonged swelling of the lower extremity.
- ✓ In massive-weight-loss patients, abdominal contouring is performed before or in conjunction with the thigh lift.

## REFERENCES


1. Lockwood TE. Fascial anchoring technique in medial thigh lifts. Plast Reconstr Surg 82:299-304, 1988.
2. Lockwood TE. Transverse flank-thigh-buttock lift with superficial fascial suspension. Plast Reconstr Surg 87:1019-1027, 1991.
3. Lockwood TE. Lower body lift with superficial fascial system suspension. Plast Reconstr Surg 92:1112-1122, 1993.
4. Lockwood TE. Maximizing aesthetics in lateral-tension abdominoplasty and body lifts. Clin Plast Surg 31:523-537, 2004.
5. Mathes DW, Kenkel JM. Current concepts in medial thighplasty. Clin Plast Surg 35:151-163, 2008.
6. Candiani P, Campiglio GL, Signorini M. Fascio-fascial suspension technique in medial thigh lifts. Aesthetic Plast Surg 19:137-140, 1995.

# 102. Body Contouring in the Massive-Weight-Loss Patient

**Luis M. Rios, Jr., Rohit K. Khosla**

## CLASSIFICATION OF MORBID OBESITY[1,2]

- **Obesity:** BMI >30 kg/m$^2$
- **Severe obesity:** BMI >35 kg/m$^2$
- **Morbid obesity:** BMI >40 kg/m$^2$
  - Morbidly obese individuals exceed their ideal body weight (IBW) by >100 pounds or are >100% over their IBW.
- **Superobesity:** BMI >50 kg/m$^2$
  - Superobese individuals exceed their IBW by >225%.
- The National Institutes of Health (NIH) also uses this classification (Table 102-1).

**Table 102-1** *NIH Classification by Body Mass Index*

| BMI (kg/m$^2$) | Class |
|---|---|
| 25-29.9 | Overweight |
| 30-34.9 | Class I (low risk) obesity |
| 35-39.9 | Class II (medium risk) obesity |
| ≥40 | Class III (high risk) obesity |

## COMORBIDITIES ASSOCIATED WITH MORBID OBESITY[1,2]

- Osteoarthritis
- Obstructive sleep apnea
- Gastroesophageal reflux
- Lipid abnormalities
- Hypertension
- Diabetes mellitus
- Congestive heart failure
- Asthma
- Coronary artery disease—silent myocardial ischemia

## COMPLICATIONS OF SKIN REDUNDANCY

- Intertriginous infections and rashes
- Musculoskeletal pain
- Functional impairment, especially with ambulation, urination, and sexual activity
- Psychological issues such as depression and low self-esteem

## BARIATRIC SURGERY TECHNIQUES[2-4]

- These techniques are performed through traditional **open** approaches or **laparoscopically.**
- **Laparoscopic techniques** substantially reduce the morbidity from postoperative wound infections, dehiscence, and incisional hernias.
- They result in weight loss and reduce medical comorbities such as type 2 diabetes.

### RESTRICTIVE PROCEDURES[4] (Fig. 102-1)

- Manipulate the **stomach only**
- Reduce caloric intake by decreasing the quantity of food consumed at a single time
  - **Vertical band gastroplasty (VBG)**
    - Not very effective: 50% of patients unable to maintain weight loss
  - **Laparoscopic adjustable gastric band (lap band)**
    - Achieves approximately 50% reduction of excess weight
    - Can be completed by erosion

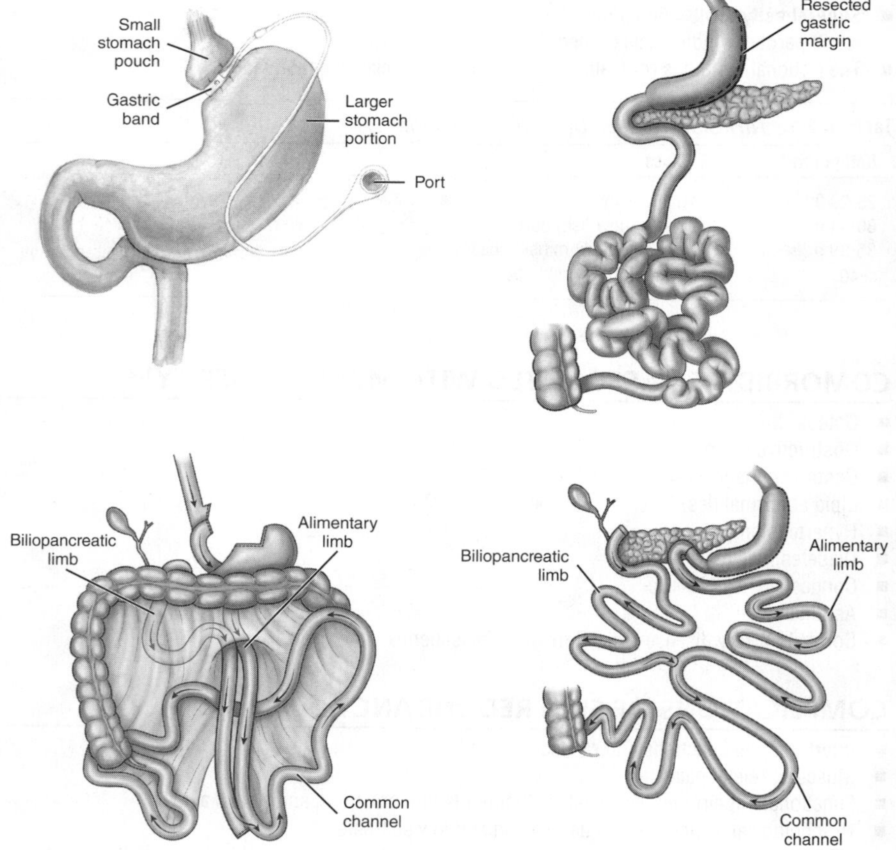


**Fig. 102-1** Restrictive procedures.

- **Gastric sleeve**[4]
  - Gastric tube created by resecting greater curvature of stomach
  - 70% remission of type 2 diabetes, which is less than with gastric bypass[4]
  - Mean excess weight loss 50% at 6 years[4]

### Combination Restrictive and Malabsorptive Procedures

- *Superior for weight reduction*
- **Malabsorptive component**
  - Limits nutrient and calorie absorption from ingested foods by *bypassing the duodenum* and other specific lengths of the small intestine
- **Biliopancreatic diversion (BPD)**
  - Achieves near 75%-80% reduction of excess weight
  - *Produces significant nutritional deficiencies*
- **BPD with duodenal switch**
  - Approximately 73% of excess weight lost
- **Roux-en-Y gastric bypass (RYGB)**
  - **Most common** bariatric procedure performed, and considered the benchmark[3]
  - Achieves excess weight loss of >50%
  - 93% resolution of type 2 diabetes[3]

## FUNDAMENTALS OF BODY CONTOURING AFTER MASSIVE WEIGHT LOSS[1,5,6]

- Bariatric surgery is a life-altering event for patients with morbid obesity; the body contouring that follows has an equally profound impact on the patient's physical and psychological well-being.
- All areas of the body present with varying degrees of skin redundancy that can be treated surgically.
- Deformities of tissue ptosis are typically circumferential.
- Body contouring surgery is not formulaic: Each patient provides distinct challenges of redundant skin distribution and severity.

## LIPOSUCTION

- **Not effective as a sole modality** for massive-weight-loss patients
- Can be used in areas of mild contour irregularities as an adjunct to excisional procedures
- Can be performed after recovery from major excisional procedures for refinement of contour

## SURGICAL STRATEGY

- The goals of surgery are to alleviate functional, aesthetic, and psychological impairments of skin redundancy.
- Determine the priorities of the patient; however, the general sequence should be:
  1. Trunk, abdomen, buttocks, lower thighs
  2. Upper thorax/breasts, arms
  3. Medial thighs
  4. Face
- Attention to intravenous fluid (IVF) resuscitation during the perioperative period is essential for large-volume excisional surgeries (e.g., belt lipectomy).
  - Intraoperative fluid management should consist of **maintenance fluid plus 10 ml/kg/hr.**
  - Monitor urine output closely during the first 24-48 hours postoperatively with continued IVF resuscitation as needed.

> **TIP:** It is best to multistage body contouring surgery in individuals who require several areas of correction to minimize complications, pain, and need for blood transfusions.

## TIMING OF BODY CONTOURING AFTER BARIATRIC SURGERY[1,5-7]

- Delay surgery until patient's weight has stabilized for **at least 6 months,** which corresponds to approximately 12-18 months after gastric bypass.
  - The patient is allowed time to achieve metabolic and nutritional homeostasis.
  - The period of rapid weight loss is detrimental to wound healing.
  - The risk of surgical complications decreases significantly from approximately 80% to 33% as patients approach their IBW.
  - Aesthetic outcomes are better for patients who are near their IBW.
- Most patients settle at a BMI of 30-35 kg/m$^2$ after bariatric surgery (Table 102-2).
  - Consider an initial panniculectomy or breast reduction for motivated patients in this category to improve comfort during exercise.
    - This may facilitate lifestyle changes that result in further weight loss and give better aesthetic outcomes with subsequent surgery.
- **The best candidates for extensive body contouring after massive weight loss have a BMI of 25-30 kg/m$^2$.**

**Table 102-2** *BMI and Operative Recommendations*

| BMI | Recommendation |
|---|---|
| 30-34.9 | Body contouring in appropriate candidates |
| 35-39.9 | Encourage more weight loss |
| 40+ | Do not operate |

## STAGING OF PROCEDURES

- Discuss patient's expectations.
- Remind patients of where they started.
- Ask patients to discuss their priorities.
- Advantages of staging[8,9]
  - Anesthesia time is decreased.
  - Blood loss is decreased.
  - Opposing vectors of pull are minimized.
  - Revisions can be performed at subsequent stages.
  - Complications are not increased in staging procedures.
- Different stages can be performed 3-6 months apart.

## PREOPERATIVE EVALUATION[1,3]

- Record **greatest** and **presenting BMI.**
- Assess stability of medical comorbidities and psychiatric problems.
  - Cardiac evaluation: Consider stress test
  - If there is a history of deep venous thrombosis (DVT), consider hematology consult.
  - **40%** of bariatric patients are treated for psychiatric diagnosis.
- Determine smoking history. *Smoking is a relative contraindication.*
- Common **nutritional deficiencies** include:
  - Iron deficiency anemia
  - Vitamin $B_{12}$
  - Calcium
  - Zinc
  - Fat-soluble vitamins (A, D, E, and K)
  - Protein
- Assess amount of daily protein intake. According to Michaels et al,[9] daily requirement of protein is **70 g.**
- Some patients may require preoperative protein, calcium, iron, and vitamin $B_{12}$ supplementation.
- Preoperative laboratory examinations should include complete blood count (CBC), electrolytes, blood urea nitrogen (BUN), creatinine, urine analysis (UA), liver function (LFTs), glucose, calcium, ferritin, total protein, and albumin.
- Physical examination focuses on regional fat deposition and laxity of the skin envelope. Use pinch test to estimate extent of tissue resection.
- Patients who are highly motivated and have good support are good candidates and may have fewer complications.

## INTRAOPERATIVE STRATEGIES TO MINIMIZE COMPLICATIONS[8,9]

- Proper positioning and padding
- Prevent hypothermia, especially given the amount of exposed area in the surgical field
  - University of Pittsburgh Hypothermia Protocol[9]
    - Preoperative forced-flow air warmer
    - OR temperature at 21° C (70° F)
    - Active warming during surgery
    - Warm preparative solutions and IVFs
- DVT prophylaxis: Massive-weight-loss patients may have a 1% incidence of DVT.
  - Mechanical compression and use of TED hose starts in the preoperative area and continues until patient is ambulating.
  - Low-molecular-weight heparin begins the evening of surgery and continues for 7 days.
- Antibiotics are given 30-59 minutes before the incision and repeated throughout the case.

# TISSUE CHARACTERISTICS AND SURGICAL TECHNIQUES

## TRUNK/ABDOMEN[1,6,10]

- The abdomen usually demonstrates the greatest deformity.
- Most tissue descent is along the lateral axillary lines.
- Truncal tissues have the appearance of an inverted cone (Fig. 102-2).
- The mons pubis has varying degrees of ptosis.
- **Surgical goals**
  - Flatten contour.
  - Tighten abdominal wall with fascial plication.
  - Repair ventral hernia if present.
  - Elevate and widen mons pubis.

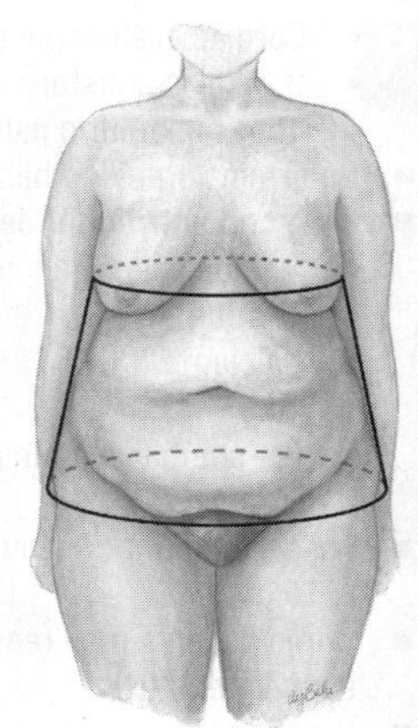

**Fig. 102-2** Truncal body contour after massive weight loss. The trunk takes on the form of an inverted cone. The soft tissue is narrow at the rib cage and wider at the pelvic rim. A belt lipectomy eliminates the inferior aspect of the cone.

- **Surgical approach**
  - *Traditional abdominoplasty* techniques fail to maximally improve body contour, because they do not treat lateral tissue laxity.
  - *Fleur-de-lis abdominoplasty* techniques can be performed for patients who do not have back and lateral thigh ptosis[8,10] (Fig. 102-3).

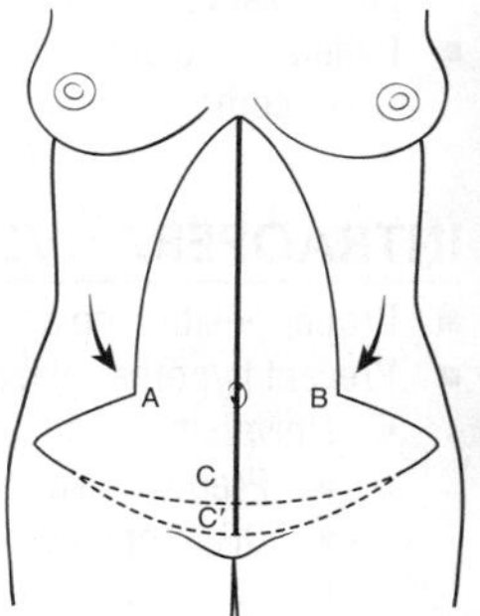


**Fig. 102-3** Markings for fleur-de-lis abdominoplasty. The redundant vertical tissue above the umbilicus is removed as a triangle connected to the redundant skin in the lower abdomen, which is marked as a standard abdominoplasty. Points *A* and *B* will join as an inverted-T closure in the midline at the pubic symphysis *(C)*. In patients with significant mons ptosis, *C′* is marked 4-6 cm below to resect additional inferior redundancy and elevate the mons.

  - *Circumferential belt lipectomy/lower body lift* treats the circumferential nature of tissue ptosis in the trunk[1,6] (Fig. 102-4).
    - Allows resection of the entire lower section of the inverted cone deformity
    - Allows elevation of buttocks and lateral thighs for a comprehensive lower body lift
    - Belt lipectomy improves lower truncal unit with a higher incision.
    - Lower body lift combines truncal and thigh units from the knee and above.
  - Patients with BMI of >35 have a higher risk for complications after belt lipectomy/lower body lift.[1]
  - **Key components of surgical technique**
    - Markings are as shown in Fig. 102-4.
    - Start with the patient in a supine position.
    - Make inferior incision first on the abdomen, similar to traditional abdominoplasty technique.

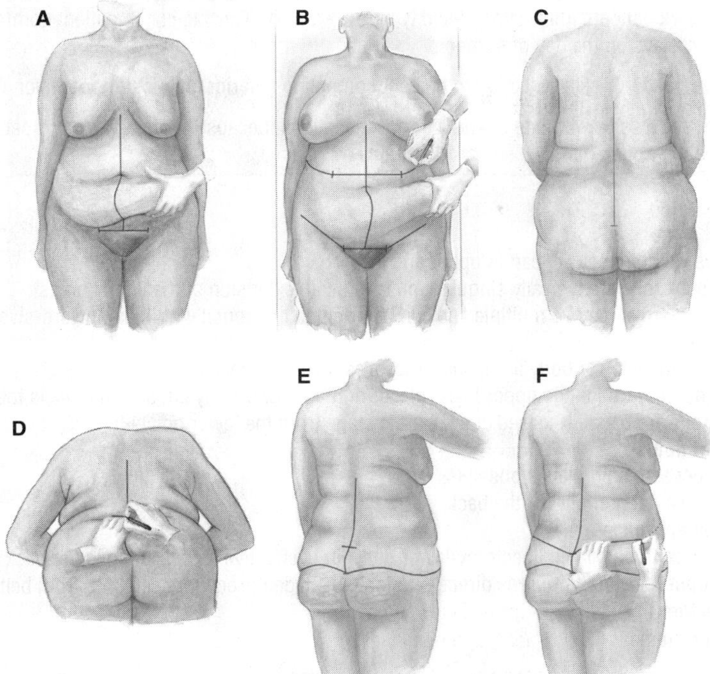


**Fig. 102-4** Markings for belt lipectomy. **A,** The midline is marked initially. The horizontal pubic incision is marked below the natural hairline to allow elevation of the mons. The inferior midline of the closure should be level with the pubic symphysis. The pannus is elevated superiorly and medially to allow marking of the lateral extension of the inferior incision to just below the anterior superior iliac spine. **B,** The superior markings are made anteriorly using the pinch technique to determine the extent of resection. **C,** The midline of the back is marked with the inferior point at the coccyx. **D,** The patient is slightly bent at the waist, and the pinch test is used to estimate the superior extent of resection. **E** and **F,** The superior and inferior back marks are made to meet the abdominal marks laterally.

- An umbilicoplasty is required to shorten the umbilical stalk flush with the newly contoured abdominal skin, regardless of the contouring technique used.
- Perform liposuction on lateral thighs to release zones of adherence, which allows lateral thigh elevation.
- Place patient in right and lateral decubitus positions to perform posterior resection.
- The posterior resection is taken down deep to the superficial fascia to maintain a layer of fat on the deep fascia and to minimize seroma formation.
- Align final scars below pelvic rim (horizontal level across the superior aspect of iliac crests) so that scars will be hidden under most undergarments and bikinis.
- Widely drain anteriorly and posteriorly to prevent seroma formation.

**TIP:** Mark patients in the office the day before surgery. This facilitates patient comfort and prevents delays on the day of surgery.

Minimize posterior skin resection to prevent competing anterior and posterior tension forces.

Be more aggressive with lateral and anterior resections, because these areas are most visible to the patient.

## BACK[1,6-8,11]

- Massive weight loss can lead to upper and lower back rolls.
- Upper back rolls are typically singular and may be an extension of the lateral breast.
- Lower back rolls may be multiple and can be oriented horizontally or in an upward-sweeping direction.
- Circumferential lower body lift usually improves the lower back rolls.
  - Do not undermine the upper back rolls during the lower body lift; seroma rate is too high.
- Upper rolls are usually excised at a separate stage from the lower body lift.
- **Surgical goals**
  - Resect as many rolls as possible.
  - Create a flat contour for the back.
- **Surgical approach**
  - A circumferential belt lipectomy/lower body lift is effective for resecting lower back rolls.
  - An upper back roll requires direct excision in a staged procedure separate from belt lipectomy.
  - Place drains.

**TIP:** Align transverse and posterior scars along the brassiere line in women.

## WAIST AND LATERAL THIGHS[1,6]

- Massive weight loss creates a contour that lacks waist and hip definition.
- Lack of definition is caused by ptosis of the abdomen, lateral thighs, and buttocks.
- Maximal vertical relaxation occurs along lateral body contours.
- Tissue excess spirals down the thigh in an anterior and posterior direction.
- **Surgical goals**
  - Narrow the waist as much as possible.
  - Create a smooth natural curve from the rib cage through the waist and down onto hips.
- **Surgical approach**
  - The lateral thigh is structurally dependent on truncal tissues. It is not possible to effectively elevate the thighs if trunk remains lax.
  - Circumferential belt lipectomy/lower body lift is effective to define the waist and lateral hips in a single-stage procedure.
  - Suture the superficial fascial system (SFS) to the deep fascia with permanent sutures on both skin flaps in a three-point configuration to maintain elevation of the lateral thigh, effectively establishing a new zone of adherence at the level of the final scar.

**TIP:** Use independent leg extensions on the OR table that will allow hip abduction while prone and supine to eliminate tension on the lateral thigh advancement.

## MEDIAL THIGHS[1] (Fig. 102-5)

- Most massive-weight-loss patients have more horizontal skin excess of the thighs relative to the vertical excess.
- A vertical medial thigh lift is more effective than a horizontal medial thigh lift. A combination of both is frequently required.
- To reduce potential for labial spreading **do not place tension on the horizontal scar.**
- Perform abdominal contouring before or in conjunction with the thigh lift to achieve a harmonious result.

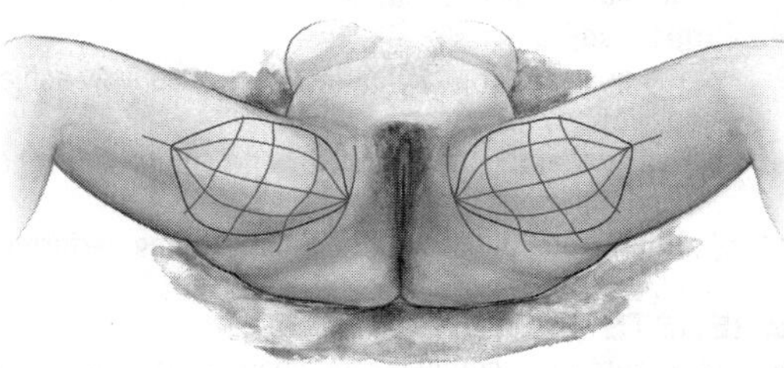

**Fig. 102-5** Medial thighs.

- Medial thigh lift should be performed in a separate staged procedure after the lateral thighs are treated.
  - This can be combined with liposuction of the medial, anterior, and posterior thigh as an adjunct to treat mild contour irregularities.
- **Contraindications**
  - Preexisting lymphedema
  - History of lower extremity DVT
  - Presence of varicose veins
    - Obliterate varicosities before performing medial thigh lipectomy.
- **Surgical goals**
  - Create a flat contour for the medial thigh.
  - Minimize labial spreading.
- **Surgical approach**
  - Mark the perineal crease on the inner thigh as the superior extent of the vertical ellipse.
  - Perform a pinch test in a superior-to-inferior direction to estimate the extent of resection.
  - Preserve the superficial saphenous vein during resection.
  - Avoid dissection anteriorly in the femoral triangle.
  - A superior dog-ear can be worked out along the posterior inferior buttock crease or anterior inguinal crease.

> **TIP:** Wait 3-6 months after lower body lift to minimize tension on the medial thigh.
>
> Resect skin only if incision is taken anteriorly to preserve inguinal lymphatics.
>
> Suture SFS of thigh to Colles' fascia with nonabsorbable sutures if horizontal medial thigh lift is performed.

## BUTTOCKS[1,6,7]

- The back and buttocks tend to blend together, which gives the appearance of a long vertical buttock height.
- The central buttock crease descends, leaving minimal soft tissue coverage over the coccyx.
- The lateral inferior buttock crease lies more horizontally without a shapely curve.
- **Surgical goals**
  - Define the buttocks by creating a line of demarcation from the back to the buttocks. Align the final scar following the superior gluteal curve in a central gull-wing pattern.

- Elevate the buttocks, including the central crease.
- Cover coccyx with additional soft tissue if there is a deficiency.
- Develop an upward curve of the inferior buttock crease.

■ **Surgical approach**
- The goals of buttock definition are effectively achieved with circumferential belt lipectomy/ lower body lift.
- Consider autogenous gluteal augmentation to enhance buttock contour, especially with central buttock projection.
- Autogenous gluteal augmentation can be performed with fat grafting or dermal/fat flaps.

## BREASTS[1,7,12]

■ Breast surgery is complex after changes caused by weight loss.

■ The volume and characteristics of breast tissue are highly variable after massive weight loss.
- Loss of shape
- Loss of elasticity
- Loss of texture
- Loss of support
- Loss of volume

■ **Pittsburgh Rating Scale**[13] (Table 102-3)
- Different from routine ptosis classification

**Table 102-3** *Pittsburgh Rating Scale*

| Grade | Scale |
|---|---|
| 0 | Normal |
| 1 | Ptosis grade I/II or severe macromastia |
| 2 | Ptosis grade III or moderate volume loss or constricted breast |
| 3 | Severe lateral roll and/or severe volume loss with loose skin |

■ Determine the approach.
- Discuss patient's expectations and desires.
- Evaluate breast shape, volume, size, and lateral breast rolls.
- Discuss expectant recurrent ptosis.

■ **Surgical approach**[12] (Tables 102-4 and 102-5)
- Perform augmentation for patients without ptosis and with stable skin envelope.
- Reduction mammaplasty is indicated for persistent macromastia.
  - ▸ *No single reduction technique is superior in this patient population.*
- Mastopexy or augmentation is indicated for patients with grade I/II ptosis.
- Mastopexy with or without augmentation is indicated for patients with grade III ptosis.
- Plication sutures can help support the lower and lateral breast.

**Table 102-4** *Guidelines for Surgical Approach*

| Procedure | Ptosis | Breast Volume | Skin Envelope |
|---|---|---|---|
| Augmentation | None | Minimal | Stable |
| Mastopexy with or without augmentation | Present | Minimal | Unstable (inelastic skin) |
| Mastopexy | Present | Moderate | Unstable |
| Breast reduction | Present | Large | Unstable |

**Table 102-5** *Basic Components Required to Treat Massive-Weight-Loss Breasts*

| Breast Deformity | Suggested Procedure |
|---|---|
| Minimal breast volume<br>No ptosis, stable skin envelope | Implant augmentation |
| Ptosis, unstable skin envelope | Mastopexy with or without augmentation |
| Moderate breast volume with ptosis | Mastopexy |
| Large breasts with ptosis | Breast reduction |

- Dermal suspension techniques can elevate the central mound.
- **Autoaugmentation** from the lateral and inferior breast folds provides more volume.[13]
  - Flap perfusion principles must be followed.
  - Volume will be redistributed with the designed flaps instead of implants.

**TIP:** No one technique works for all massive-weight-loss patients. Depending on each patient's expectations and breast characteristics, a combination of techniques may have to be used to achieve the desired results. Recurrent ptosis is very common[14] (Fig. 102-6).

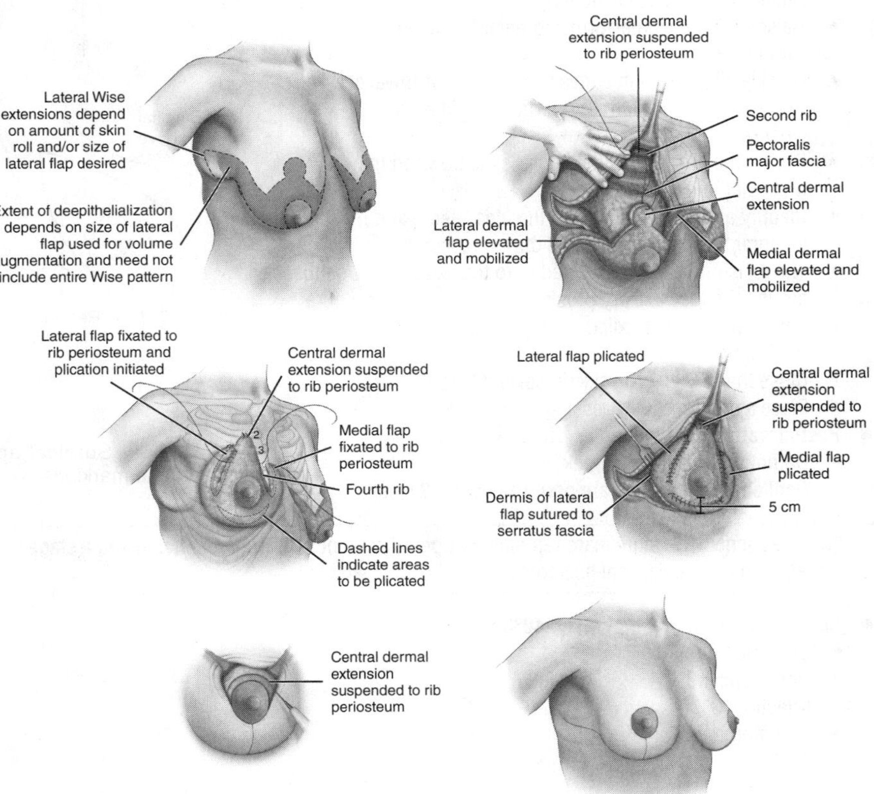


**Fig. 102-6** Breast reconstruction in massive-weight-loss patients.

## UPPER ARMS[1,15,16]

- The upper arms develop severely ptotic skin that extends from the olecranon across the axilla onto the chest wall.
- Excess arm skin is contiguous with the posterior axillary fold on the lateral chest.
- Ideal candidates for brachioplasty have deflated upper arms and a small amount of residual fat.
- Concomitant procedures are safe and performed in 85%-95% of massive-weight-loss patients who have brachioplasty.
- **Surgical goals**
  - Eliminate horizontal upper arm excess.
  - Eliminate lateral thoracic skin excess.
  - Create a smooth transition from the lateral chest onto the upper arm.
  - Minimize scar visibility and contracture.
- **Surgical approach**[1] (Fig. 102-7)
  - Incisions placed posterior to the bicipital groove are less noticeable when viewed from the front.
  - A sinusoidal incision pattern decreases the possibility of linear scar contracture.
  - Z-plasty in the axilla is no longer used.
  - Raise the flap and perform segmental resection using towel clips.
  - Quickly align the skin edges with staples or towel clips to prevent edema from interfering with final wound closure.
  - Resect the entire subcutaneous tissue down to the muscular aponeurosis.
  - Identify and prevent injury to the ulnar nerve and medial antebrachial cutaneous nerve during resection.
  - The incision should be carried onto the axilla with a gentle curve to reduce axillary ptosis and restore a more natural dome shape to the axilla.
  - Place a drain.
  - Close the SFS and the skin in several layers.
  - Place a compressive dressing.
- **Postoperative instructions**
  - Do not raise arm for 1 week.
  - Gentle ROM exercises are performed after 2 weeks.

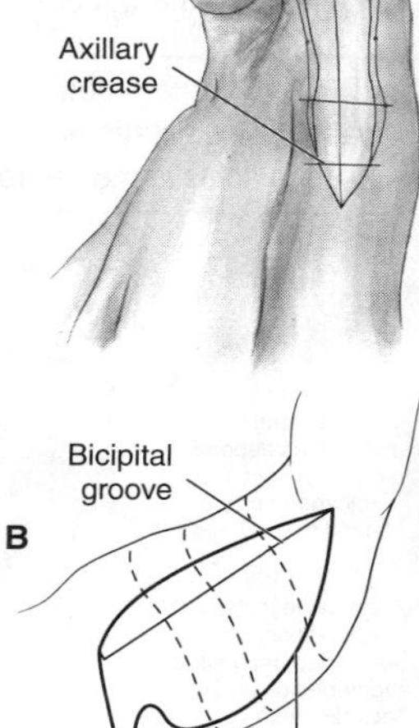


**Fig. 102-7** Surgical approach and markings.

> **TIP:** Patients with significant remaining upper arm fat benefit from liposuction as a staged procedure before excisional lipectomy.

- **Complications of brachioplasty: 40%**[16]
  - Seroma: 24%
  - Dehiscence: 9%
  - Infection: 3%
  - Hematoma: 4%

### Face and Neck[12]

- Skin redundancy exceeds that of the superficial musculoaponeurotic system (SMAS) laxity after massive weight loss.
- Appearance of premature aging develops.
- The aged facial appearance may be more displeasing to younger patients than redundant skin elsewhere, which can be hidden with clothing.
- **Surgical goals**
  - Redrape the skin over the face and neck to restore a normal-appearing jawline and neck.
  - Harmonize facial appearance with the contouring of the rest of the body.
- Modify SMAS rhytidectomy for massive-weight-loss patients.[8]
  - Correction of facial skin redundancy requires **more skin undermining** to produce a smooth contour relative to a typical rhytidectomy.
  - Less elevation of SMAS is required, because laxity at this tissue level is not the structural problem; normal SMAS plication is performed.
  - Platysmaplasty should be performed if platysmal banding is present.
  - Perform suction-assisted or direct lipectomy of remaining fat deposits in jowls and submental triangle.
  - The skin incision can enter the temporal hairline above the helical root if the planned vector of facial elevation is posterior and superior.
  - Carry the incision around the earlobe and onto the conchal bowl posteriorly.
    - The vector of elevation on the neck can be mostly superior, which prevents an incision across the occipital hairline.
    - Use a traditional postauricular incision with occipital hairline extension if the neck has severe skin laxity.

## COMPLICATIONS[1,5-8]

### Hematomas: 1%-5%

- Typically occur in the immediate postoperative period
- Require operative drainage and exploration
- Might have increased risk with low-molecular-weight heparin

### Seromas: 13%-37%

- A higher incidence is seen in patients with BMI >35 kg/m$^2$, primarily in the lower back after belt lipectomy/lower body lift.
- Maintain drains until output is <30 ml over 24 hours.
- Drain seromas early, before capsule formation.
- Aspiration can be performed in the office; may need serial aspiration.
- Large seromas can be drained by percutaneous closed-suction drains.
- Inject cavity with doxycycline to sclerose walls, if necessary.

### Lymphoceles

- Seen primarily in the inguinal region after aggressive resection into femoral triangle
- Serial aspirations
- Percutaneous drainage with placement of closed-suction drain
- Doxycycline injection
- Requires operative exploration and ligation of leaking lymphatic channels if nonoperative management fails

## Deep Venous Thrombosis and Pulmonary Embolism

- Risk is at least 1% and increases with increasing BMI.
- Truncal lipectomies create higher risk; increased intraabdominal pressure leads to decreased venous return from lower extremities.
- **Prophylaxis**
  - Administration of low-molecular-weight heparin 6 hours after surgery; this can be continued for 7 days.
  - Epidural analgesia decreases incidence in orthopedic literature; the efficacy is unknown in body contouring.
  - Place sequential compression devices before inducing general anesthesia, and maintain them postoperatively.
  - Patients should start ambulating with assistance the day of surgery.
  - Patients should perform incentive spirometry.

## Wound Complications

- **Dehiscence: 22%-30%**
  - Most occur within first few days of surgery as a result of excess tension.
- **Skin necrosis: 6%-10%**
- **Wound infection/cellulitis: 1%-7%**
- **Factors that increase incidence of wound complications:**
  - Tobacco use
    - Patients should wait at least 1 month after cessation of smoking before having surgery.
  - Diabetes
  - Active systemic steroid use
  - BMI >40 kg/m$^2$

## Key Points

- ✓ Roux-en-Y gastric bypass is the most common reproducible and effective bariatric operation performed today.[4]
- ✓ Start body contouring surgery when the patient's weight has stabilized for at least 6 months.
- ✓ The best aesthetic outcomes with lowest perioperative risks occur in patients who are near their IBW or who have a BMI of 25-30 kg/m$^2$ after bariatric surgery.
- ✓ Define goals and plan the staged procedures with each patient.
- ✓ Lower body lifts should be performed in conjunction with or before thigh lifts.
- ✓ The abdomen generally demonstrates the greatest deformity, and most tissue ptosis is along the lateral axillary lines.
- ✓ Assess nutritional deficiencies before initiating body contouring surgery.
- ✓ Treat the trunk, lateral thigh, and buttocks as a single aesthetic unit.
- ✓ Circumferential belt lipectomy/lower body lift resects excess truncal tissue and elevates the buttocks and lateral thighs.
- ✓ Perform liposuction on the lateral thighs during a belt lipectomy to release the zones of adherence and allow more effective elevation of the lateral thigh.

- ✓ Massive-weight-loss patients may require breast reduction or mastopexy, depending on the amount of breast volume lost.
- ✓ Patients develop a prematurely aging face as a result of skin redundancy rather than SMAS laxity.
- ✓ Liposuction techniques can be used as an adjunct during or after excisional operations for additional refinement of contour.

## References

1. Aly AS. Body Contouring After Massive Weight Loss. St Louis: Quality Medical Publishing, 2006.
2. Hamad GG. The state of the art in bariatric surgery for weight loss in the morbidly obese patient. Clin Plast Surg 31:591-600, 2004.
3. A review of bariatric surgery procedures. Plast Reconstr Surg 117(1 Suppl):S8-S13, 2006.
4. Gilbert EW, Wolfe BM. Bariatric surgery for the management of obesity: state of the field. Plast Reconstr Surg 130:948-954, 2012.
5. Rubin JP, Nguyen V, Schwentker A. Perioperative management of the post-gastric-bypass patient presenting for body contouring surgery. Clin Plast Surg 31:601-610, 2004.
6. Aly AS, Cram AE, Heddens C. Truncal body contouring surgery in the massive weight loss patient. Clin Plast Surg 31:611-624, 2004.
7. Taylor J, Shermak M. Body contouring following massive weight loss. Obesity Surg 14:1080-1085, 2004.
8. Michaels J, Coon D, Rubin JP. Complications in postbariatric body contouring: postoperative management and treatment. Plast Reconstr Surg 127:1693-1700, 2011.
9. Michaels J, Coon D, Rubin JP. Complications in postbariatric body contouring: strategies for assessment and prevention. Plast Reconstr Surg 127:1353-1357, 2011.
10. Fernando da Costa L, Landecker A, Marinho Manta A. Optimizing body contour in massive weight loss patients: the modified vertical abdominoplasty. Plast Reconstr Surg 114:1917-1923, 2004.
11. Strauch B, Rohde C, Patel MK, et al. Back contouring in weight loss patients. Plast Reconstr Surg 120:1692-1696, 2007.
12. Losken A. Breast reshaping following massive weight loss: principles and techniques. Plast Reconstr Surg 126:1075-1085, 2010.
13. Song AY, Jean RD, Hurwitz DJ, et al. A classification of contour deformities after bariatric weight loss: the Pittsburgh Rating Scale. Plast Reconstr Surg 116:1535-1544, 2005.
14. Nahai F, ed. The Art of Aesthetic Surgery: Principles & Techniques, 2nd ed. St Louis: Quality Medical Publishing, 2011.
15. Strauch B, Greenspun D, Levine J, et al. A technique of brachioplasty. Plast Reconstr Surg 113:1044-1048, 2004.
16. Gusenoff JA, Coon D, Rubin JP. Brachioplasty and concomitant procedures after massive weight loss: a statistical analysis from a prospective registry. Plast Reconstr Surg 122:595-603, 2008.

# Credits

### *Chapter 1*

Table 1-3 Adapted from Sidle DM, Haena K. Keloids: prevention and management. Facial Plast Surg Clin North Am 19:505-515, 2011; and Chike-Obi CJ, Cole PD, Brissett AE. Keloids: pathogenesis, clinical features, and management. Semin Plast Surg 23:178-184, 2009.

### *Chapter 2*

Fig. 2-1 Adapted from Erba P, Ogawa R, Vyas R, et al. The reconstructive matrix: a new paradigm in reconstructive plastic surgery. Plast Reconstr Surg 126:492-498, 2010.

### *Chapter 3*

Fig. 3-4 Adapted from Levenson SM, Geever EF, Crowley LV, et al. The healing of rat skin wounds. Ann Surg 161:293-308, 1965.

### *Chapter 4*

Fig. 4-1 From Zenn MR, Jones G, eds. Reconstructive Surgery: Anatomy, Technique, and Clinical Applications. St Louis: Quality Medical Publishing, 2012.

Fig. 4-6 Adapted from Inoue G, Suzuki K. Arterialized venous flap for treating multiple skin defects of the hand. Plast Recontr Surg 91:299-302; discussion 303-306, 1993.

Fig. 4-7 Adapted from Mathes SJ, Nahai F. Classification of the vascular anatomy of muscles: experimental and clinical correlation. Plast Reconstr Surg 67:177, 1981.

Fig. 4-8 Adapted from Hallock GG. Simplified nomenclature for compound flaps. Plast Reconstr Surg 105:1465, 2000.

Fig. 4-15 Adapted from Keser A, Sensoz O, Mengi AS. Double opposing semicircular flap: a modification of opposing Z-plasty for closing circular defects. Plast Reconstr Surg 102:1001, 1998.

Fig. 4-17, *A* and *C* From Zenn MR, Jones G, eds. Reconstructive Surgery: Anatomy, Technique, and Clinical Applications. St Louis: Quality Medical Publishing, 2012.

Fig. 4-17, *B* Adapted from Daniel RK, Kerrigan CL. Principles and physiology of skin flap surgery. In McCarthy JG, ed. Plastic Surgery, vol 1. Philadelphia: WB Saunders, 1990.

Table 4-6 From Rohrich RJ, Zbar PI. A simplified algorithm for the use of Z-plasty. Plast Reconstr Surg 103:1513, 1999.

Table 4-8 From Zenn MR, Jones G. Reconstructive Surgery: Anatomy, Technique, and Clinical Applications. St Louis: Quality Medical Publishing, 2012.

Table 4-9 Adams JF, Lassen LF. Leech therapy for venous congestion following myocutaneous pectoralis flap reconstruction. ORL Head Neck Nurs 13:12, 1995.

### *Chapter 5*

Fig. 5-1, *B* Courtesy of GG Hallock, MD.

Fig. 5-5 Adapted from Saint-Cyr M, Wong C, Schaverien M, et al. The perforasome theory: vascular anatomy and clinical implications. Plast Reconstr Surg 124:1529-1544, 2009.

Fig. 5-6 From Blondeel PN, Morris SF, Hallock GG, Neligan PC, eds. Perforator Flaps: Anatomy, Technique & Clinical Applications, 2nd ed. St Louis: Quality Medical Publishing, 2013.

Fig. 5-7, *A* and *B* Adapted from Zenn MR, Jones G, eds. Reconstructive Surgery: Anatomy, Technique, and Clinical Applications. St Louis: Quality Medical Publishing, 2012.

Table 5-1 Adapted from Weinzweig J. Plastic Surgery Secrets Plus. Philadelphia: Elsevier, 2010.

### *Chapter 6*

Fig. 6-1 Adapted from Siegert R, Weerda H, Hoffmann S, et al. Clinical and experimental evaluation of intermittent intraoperative short-term expansion. Plast Reconstr Surg 92:248-254, 1993.

### *Chapter 8*

Fig. 8-7, *A-D, F, G* Adapted from Alghoul MS, Gordon CR, Yetman R, et al. From simple interrupted to complex spiral: a systematic review of various suture techniques for microvascular anastomosis. Microsurgery 31:72-80, 2011.

Fig. 8-7, *E* Adapted from Turan T, Ozcelik D, Kuran I, et al. Eversion with four sutures: an easy, fast, and reliable technique for microvascular anastomosis. Plast Reconstr Surg 107:463-470, 2001.

### *Chapter 9*

Table 9-2 Adapted from Moyer HR, Losken A. The science behind tissue biologics. Plastic Surgery Pulse News 3(4), 2011; and Cheng A, Saint-Cyr M. Comparison of different ADM materials in breast surgery. Clin Plastic Surg 39:167-175, 2012.

Table 9-3 From Parikh SN. Bone graft substitutes: past, present, future. J Postgrad Med 48:142-148, 2002.

### *Chapter 10*

Fig. 10-1 From DeFranzo AJ Jr, Argenta LC. Management of wounds with vacuum-assisted closure. In Pu LLQ, Levine, JP, Wei FC, eds. Reconstructive Surgery of the Lower Extremity. St Louis: Quality Medical Publishing, 2013.

### *Chapter 11*

Fig. 11-1 Adapted from Kenkel J, Farkas JP, Hoopman JE. Five parameters you must understand to master control of your laser/light based devices. Aesthet Surg J 2013 (in press).

Table 11-2 From Nahai F, ed. The Art of Aesthetic Surgery: Principles & Techniques, 2nd ed. St Louis: Quality Medical Publishing, 2011.

Table 11-3 From Nahai F, ed. The Art of Aesthetic Surgery: Principles & Techniques, 2nd ed. St Louis: Quality Medical Publishing, 2011.

Table 11-4 From Nahai F, ed. The Art of Aesthetic Surgery: Principles & Techniques, 2nd ed. St Louis: Quality Medical Publishing, 2011.

### *Chapter 15*

Table 15-1 From Fitzpatrick TB. The validity and practicality of sun-reactive skin types I through VI. Arch Dermatol 124:869, 1988.

Table 15-2 Adapted from Miller S, Alam M, Anderson J, et al. NCCN Guidelines: Clinical Practice Guidelines in Oncology: Basal Cell and Squamous Cell Skin Cancers Version 2.2012. Available at *nccn.org*.

Table 15-3 Adapted from Coit D, Andtbacka R, Anker C, et al. NCCN Guidelines: Clinical Practice Guidelines in Oncology: Melanoma Version 2.2013. Available at *nccn.org*.

Table 15-4 Adapted from Coit D, Andtbacka R, Anker C, et al. NCCN Guidelines: Clinical Practice Guidelines in Oncology: Melanoma Version 2.2013. Available at *nccn.org*.

Fig. 15-1 Adapted from Jacobs GH, Rippey JJ, Altini M. Predication of aggressive behavior in basal cell carcinoma. Cancer 49:533, 1982.

Fig. 15-2 Adapted from McGovern VJ, Mihm MC Jr, Bailly C, et al. The classification of malignant melanoma and its histologic reporting. Cancer 32:1446, 1973.

### *Chapter 16*

Table 16-2 Data from Herndon DN, ed. Total Burn Care, 3rd ed. London: WB Saunders, 2007; and Kaga RJ, Peck MD, Ahrenholz DH, Hickerson WL, Holmes JH, Korentager RA, Kraatz JJ, Kotoski GM. Surgical management of the burn wound and use of skin substitutes. American Burn Association White Paper. Chicago: American Burn Association, 2009.

### *Chapter 17*

Table 17-2 From Mulliken JB. Classification of vascular birthmarks. In Mulliken JB, Young AE. Vascular Birthmarks: Hemangiomas and Malformations. Philadelphia: WB Saunders, 1988.

### *Chapter 20*

Fig. 20-1 Adapted from Janis JE, Ghavami A, Lemmon JA, Leedy JE, Guyuron B. The anatomy of the corrugator supercilii muscle: Part II. Supraorbital nerve branching patterns. Plast Reconstr Surg 121:233-240, 2008.

Fig. 20-2 Adapted from Janis JE, Ghavami A, Lemmon JA, Leedy JE, Guyuron B. Anatomy of the corrugator supercilii muscle: Part I. Corrugator topography. Plast Reconstr Surg 120:1647-1653, 2007.

Fig. 20-3 Adapted from Fallucco M, Janis JE, Hagan RR. The anatomical morphology of the supraorbital notch: clinical relevance to the surgical treatment of migraine headaches. Plast Reconstr Surg 130:1227-1233, 2012.

Fig. 20-5 Adapted from Janis JE, Hatef DA, Thakar H, et al. The zygomaticotemporal branch of the trigeminal nerve: Part II. Anatomical variations. Plast Reconstr Surg 126:435-442, 2010.

Fig. 20-6 Adapted from Janis JE, Hatef DA, Ducic I, et al. The anatomy of the greater occipital nerve: Part II. Compression point topography. Plast Reconstr Surg 126:1563-1572, 2010.

Fig. 20-8 From Kung TA, Guyuron B, Cederna PS. Migraine surgery: a plastic surgery solution for refractory migraine headache. Plast Reconstr Surg 127:181-189, 2011.

Fig. 20-9 From Guyuron B, Becker D. Surgical management of migraine headaches. In Guyuron B, Eriksson E, Persing JA, eds. Plastic Surgery: Indications and Practice. Philadelphia: Elsevier, 2009.

Table 20-1 Adapted from Liu MT, Armijo BS, Guyuron B. A comparison of outcome of surgical treatment of migraine headaches using a constellation of symptoms versus botulinum toxin type A to identify the trigger sites. Plast Reconst Surg 129:413-419, 2012.

### Chapter 21

Table 21-1 From Hansen M, Mulliken JB. Frontal plagiocephaly: diagnosis and treatment. Clin Plast Surg 21:543-553, 1994.

Fig. 21-1 Adapted from Carson BS, Dufresne CR. Craniosynotosis and neurocranial asymmetry. In Dufresne CR, Carson BS, Zineich SJ, eds. Complex Craniofacial Problems. New York: Churchill Livingstone, 1992.

Fig. 21-2 Adapted from Cohen MM Jr, MacLean RE. Anatomic, genetic, nosologic, diagnostic, and psychosocial considerations. In Cohen MM Jr, MacLean RE, eds. Craniosynostosis Diagnosis, Evaluation, and Management, 2nd ed. New York: Oxford University Press, 2000.

Fig. 21-3 From Derderian C, Seaward J. Syndromic craniosynostosis. Semin Plast Surg 26:64-75, 2012.

Fig. 21-4 From Derderian C, Seaward J. Syndromic craniosynostosis. Semin Plast Surg 26:64-75, 2012.

Fig. 21-6 From Derderian CA, Barlett SP. Open cranial vault remodeling: the evolving role of distraction osteogenesis. J Craniofac Surg 23:229-234, 2012.

Fig. 21-7 Adapted from Selber J, Reid RR, Gershman B, et al. Evolution of operative techniques for the treatment of single-suture metopic synostosis. Ann Plast Surg 59:6-13, 2007.

### Chapter 22

Fig. 22-1 From Bentz ML, Bauer BS, Zuker RM. Principles & Practice of Pediatric Plastic Surgery. St Louis: Quality Medical Publishing, 2008.

Fig. 22-2 Adapted from Tessier P. Anatomical classification of facial, cranio-facial, and laterofacial clefts. J Maxillofac Surg 4:69-92, 1976.

Fig. 22-3 From Bentz ML, Bauer BS, Zuker RM. Principles & Practice of Pediatric Plastic Surgery. St Louis: Quality Medical Publishing, 2008.

Fig. 22-4 From Bentz ML, Bauer BS, Zuker RM. Principles & Practice of Pediatric Plastic Surgery. St Louis: Quality Medical Publishing, 2008.

Fig. 22-5 From Bentz ML, Bauer BS, Zuker RM. Principles & Practice of Pediatric Plastic Surgery. St Louis: Quality Medical Publishing, 2008.

Fig. 22-6 From Bentz ML, Bauer BS, Zuker RM. Principles & Practice of Pediatric Plastic Surgery. St Louis: Quality Medical Publishing, 2008.

Fig. 22-7 Courtesy of Craniofacial Clinic, UT Southwestern, Dallas, Texas.

Fig. 22-8 Courtesy of Craniofacial Clinic, UT Southwestern, Dallas, Texas.

### Chapter 23

Fig. 23-1 Adapted from Yu JC, Fearon J, Havlik RJ, et al. Distraction osteogenesis of the craniofacial skeleton. Plast Reconstr Surg 114:1e-20e, 2004.

Table 23-1 From Mofid MM, Manson PN, Robertson BC, et al. Craniofacial distraction osteogenesis: a review of 3278 cases. Plast Reconstr Surg 108:1103-1114; discussion 1115-1117, 2001.

### Chapter 24

Table 24-3 Data from Millard DR. Closure of bilateral cleft lip and elongation of columella by two operations in infancy. Plast Reconstr Surg 47: 324-331, 1971; and Broadbent TR, Woolf RM. Bilateral cleft lip repairs: review of 160 cases, and description of present management. Plast Reconstr Surg 50:36-41, 1972.

Fig. 24-2 Adapted from Spira M, Hardy SB, Gerow FJ. Correction of nasal deformities accompanying unilateral cleft lip. Cleft Palate J 7:112, 1970.

Fig. 24-3 Adapted from Byrd HS. Unilateral cleft lip. In Aston SJ, Beasley RW, Thorne CHM, eds. Grabb and Smith's Plastic Surgery, 5th ed. Philadelphia: Lippincott-Raven, 1997.

Fig. 24-4 Adapted from Tajima S, Maruyama M. Reverse-U incision for secondary repair of cleft lip nose. Plast Reconstr Surg 60:256-261, 1977.

Fig. 24-5 Adapted from McComb H. Primary correction of unilateral cleft lip nasal deformity: a 10-year review. Plast Reconstr Surg 75:791-797, 1985.

Fig. 24-6 From Mulliken JB. Bilateral cleft lip. Clin Plastic Surg 31:209, 2004.

### Chapter 25

Fig. 25-2 Adapted from Ross RB, Johnston MC. Cleft Lip and Palate. Baltimore: Williams & Wilkins, 1972.

Fig. 25-3 Adapted from Smith AW, Khoo AK, Jackson IT. A modification of the Kernahan Y classification in cleft lip and palate deformities. Plast Reconstr Surg 6:1842-1847, 1998.

Fig. 25-4 Adapted from Furlow L. Cleft palate repair by double opposing Z-plasty. Plast Reconstr Surg 78:724-738, 1986.

Fig. 25-5 Adapted from Randall P, LaRossa D. Cleft palate. In McCarthy JG, ed. Plastic Surgery. Philadelphia: WB Saunders, 1990.

Fig. 25-6 Adapted from Randall P, LaRossa D. Cleft palate. In McCarthy JG, ed. Plastic Surgery. Philadelphia: WB Saunders, 1990.

Fig. 25-7 Adapted from Afifi GY, Kaidi AA, Hardesty RA. Cleft palate repair. In Evans GRD, ed. Operative Plastic Surgery. New York: McGraw-Hill, 2000.

Fig. 25-8 Adapted from Nguyen PN, Sullivan PK. Issues and controversies in the management of cleft palate. Clin Plast Surg 20:671-682, 1993.

### Chapter 26

Fig. 26-1 Adapted from Mathes SJ. Plastic Surgery, 2nd ed. Pediatric Plastic Surgery, vol 4. Philadelphia: Saunders-Elsevier, 2006.

Fig. 26-2 From Bentz ML, Bauer BS, Zuker RM. Principles & Practice of Pediatric Plastic Surgery. St Louis: Quality Medical Publishing, 2007.

Fig. 26-3 From Bentz ML, Bauer BS, Zuker RM. Principles & Practice of Pediatric Plastic Surgery. St Louis: Quality Medical Publishing, 2007.

Fig. 26-4 From Bentz ML, Bauer BS, Zuker RM. Principles & Practice of Pediatric Plastic Surgery. St Louis: Quality Medical Publishing, 2007.

### Chapter 27

Fig. 27-1 Adapted from Beahm EK, Walton RL. Auricular reconstruction for microtia. Part I: Anatomy, embryology and clinical evaluation. Plast Reconstr Surg 109:2473-2782, 2002.

Fig. 27-2, *A* Adapted from Brent B. Technical advances in ear reconstruction with autogenous rib cartilage grafts: personal experience with 1200 cases. Plast Reconstr Surg 104:319, 1999.

### Chapter 28

Fig. 28-2 Adapted from Aston SJ, Beasley RW, Thorne CHM, et al. Grabb and Smith's Plastic Surgery, 5th ed. Philadelphia: Lippincott-Raven, 1997.

Fig. 28-3 Adapted from Aston SJ, Beasley RW, Thorne CHM, et al. Grabb and Smith's Plastic Surgery, 5th ed. Philadelphia: Lippincott-Raven, 1997.

Fig. 28-5 Adapted from Aston SJ, Beasley RW, Thorne CHM, et al. Grabb and Smith's Plastic Surgery, 5th ed. Philadelphia: Lippincott-Raven, 1997.

Fig. 28-6 Adapted from Aston SJ, Beasley RW, Thorne CHM, et al. Grabb and Smith's Plastic Surgery, 5th ed. Philadelphia: Lippincott-Raven, 1997.

Box 28-1 Adapted from Janis JE, Rohrich RJ, Gutowski KA. Otoplasty. Plast Reconstr Surg 115:60e-72e, 2005; and Ha RY, Trovato MJ. Plastic surgery of the ear. SRPS 11(R3):1-46, 2011.

### Chapter 29

Table 29-1 Data from Centers for Disease Control and Prevention (CDC). Deferral of routine booster doses of tetanus and diphtheria toxoids for adolescents and adults. MMWR Morb Mortal Wkly Rep 50:418-427, 2001; and Update on adult immunization. Recommendations of the Immunization Practices Advisory Committee (ACIP). MMWR Recomm Rep 40:1-94, 1991.

Fig. 29-1 From Seckel BR. Facial Danger Zones: Avoiding Nerve Injury in Facial Plastic Surgery, 2nd ed. St Louis: Quality Medical Publishing, 2010.

Fig. 29-2 From Marcus JR. Essentials of Craniomaxillofacial Trauma. St Louis: Quality Medical Publishing, 2012.

Fig. 29-3 From Marcus JR. Essentials of Craniomaxillofacial Trauma. St Louis: Quality Medical Publishing, 2012.

### Chapter 30

Fig. 30-1 From Nahai F, Saltz R, eds. Endoscopic Plastic Surgery, 2nd ed. St Louis: Quality Medical Publishing, 2008.

Fig. 30-2 From Rohrich RJ, Hollier LH. Management of frontal sinus fractures: changing concepts. Clin Plast Surg 19:219, 1992.

Fig. 30-3 From Rohrich RJ, Hollier LH. Management of frontal sinus fractures: changing concepts. Clin Plast Surg 19:219, 1992.

Fig. 30-4 Adapted from Markowitz BL, Manson PN, Sargent L, et al. Management of the medial canthal tendon in nasoethmoid orbital fractures: the importance of the central fragment in classification and treatment. Plast Reconstr Surg 87:843-853, 1991.

Fig. 30-5 From Rohrich RJ, Adams WP. Nasal fracture management: minimizing secondary deformities. Plast Reconstr Surg 106:266, 2000.

Fig. 30-8 Adapted from Waterhouse N, Lyne J, Urdang M, et al. An investigation into the mechanism of orbital blowout fractures. Br J Plast Surg 52:607-612, 1999.

Fig. 30-9, *A* Adapted from AO North America. Review of surgical approaches to the cranial skeleton, 2010. Available at *www.aona.org.*

Fig. 30-10 From Ellis E III, Kittidumkerng W. Analysis of treatment for isolated zygomaticomaxillary complex fractures. J Oral Maxillofac Surg 54:386-400, 1996.

Table 30-1 Adapted from Follmar KE, DeBruijn M, Baccarani A, et al. Concomitant injuries in patients with panfacial fractures. J Trauma 63:831-835, 2007.

### Chapter 31

Fig. 31-1 Adapted from Aston SJ, Beasley RW, Thorne CHM, eds. Grabb and Smith's Plastic Surgery, 5th ed. Philadelphia: Lippincott-Raven, 1997.

Fig. 31-3 Adapted from Kelamis JA, Rodriguez ED. Mandible fractures. In Marcus JR, Erdmann D, Rodriguez ED, eds. Essentials of Craniomaxillofacial Trauma. St Louis: Quality Medical Publishing, 2012.

### Chapter 32

Fig. 32-1 From Marcus JR, Erdmann D, Rodriguez ED, eds. Essentials of Craniomaxillofacial Trauma. St Louis: Quality Medical Publishing, 2012.

Fig. 32-2 From Marcus JR, Erdmann D, Rodriguez ED, eds. Essentials of Craniomaxillofacial Trauma. St Louis: Quality Medical Publishing, 2012.

Fig. 32-3 From Marcus JR, Erdmann D, Rodriguez ED, eds. Essentials of Craniomaxillofacial Trauma. St Louis: Quality Medical Publishing, 2012.

Fig. 32-4 From Marcus JR, Erdmann D, Rodriguez ED, eds. Essentials of Craniomaxillofacial Trauma. St Louis: Quality Medical Publishing, 2012.

Fig. 32-5 From Jackson IT. Local Flaps in Head and Neck Reconstruction. St Louis: Quality Medical Publishing, 2007.

Fig. 32-8 From Evans G. Operative Plastic Surgery. New York: McGraw-Hill, 2000.

Table 32-2 Adapted from Ferraro JW, ed. Fundamentals of Maxillofacial Surgery. New York: Springer-Verlag, 1997.

Table 32-3 Adapted from Ferraro JW, ed. Fundamentals of Maxillofacial Surgery. New York: Springer-Verlag, 1997.

### Chapter 34

Fig. 34-6 Adapted from Arnold PG, Rangarathnam CS. Multiple-flap scalp reconstruction: Orticochea revisited. Plast Reconstr Surg 69:607, 1982.

Fig. 34-8 Adapted from Lee S, Rafii AA, Sykes J. Advances in scalp reconstruction. Curr Opin Otolaryngol Head Neck Surg 14:249-253, 2006.

### Chapter 35

Fig. 35-4 McCord CD Jr, Codner MA. Eyelid & Periorbital Surgery. St Louis: Quality Medical Publishing, 2008.

Fig. 35-5 Adapted from DiFrancesco LM, Codner MA, McCord CD Jr. Upper eyelid reconstruction. Plast Reconstr Surg 114:98e-107e, 2004.

Fig. 35-6 Adapted from DiFrancesco LM, Codner MA, McCord CD Jr. Upper eyelid reconstruction. Plast Reconstr Surg 114:98e-107e, 2004.

Fig. 35-7 Adapted from DiFrancesco LM, Codner MA, McCord CD Jr. Upper eyelid reconstruction. Plast Reconstr Surg 114:98e-107e, 2004.

Fig. 35-8 From McCord CD Jr, Codner MA. Eyelid & Periorbital Surgery. St Louis: Quality Medical Publishing, 2008.

Fig. 35-9 Adapted from DiFrancesco LM, Codner MA, McCord CD Jr. Upper eyelid reconstruction. Plast Reconstr Surg 114:98e-107e, 2004.

Fig. 35-10 Adapted from DiFrancesco LM, Codner MA, McCord CD Jr. Upper eyelid reconstruction. Plast Reconstr Surg 114:98e-107e, 2004.

Fig. 35-11 Adapted from Levine MI, Leone CR. Bipedicled musculocutaneous flap repair of cicatricial ectropion. Ophthal Plast Reconstr Surg 6:119, 1990.

Fig. 35-13 From McCord CD Jr, Codner MA. Eyelid & Periorbital Surgery. St Louis: Quality Medical Publishing, 2008.

Fig. 35-14 From McCord CD Jr, Codner MA. Eyelid & Periorbital Surgery. St Louis: Quality Medical Publishing, 2008.

Table 35-1 From Codner MA, McCord CD Jr, Mejia JD, et al. Upper and lower lid reconstruction. Plast Reconstr Surg 126:231e, 2010.

***Chapter 36***

Table 36-1 From Gonzalez-Ulloa M. Restoration of the face covering by means of selected skin in regional aesthetic units. Br J Plast Surg 9:212, 1956.

Fig. 36-1 Adapted from Funter JP, Landecker A, Cochran CS. Nomenclature for frequently used grafts in rhinoplasty. Presented at the Twenty-second Annual Dallas Rhinoplasty Symposium, Dallas, March 2005.

Fig. 36-3 Adapted from Burget GC, Menick FJ. Aesthetic Reconstruction of the Nose. St Louis: Mosby–Year Book, 1994.

Fig. 36-4 From Muzaffar AR, English JM. Nasal reconstruction. Sel Read Plast Surg 9:9, 2000.

Fig. 36-5 Adapted from Burget GC, Menick FJ. Nasal support and lining: the marriage of beauty and blood supply. Plast Reconstr Surg 84:189, 1989.

Fig. 36-6 Adapted from Burget GC, Menick FJ. Nasal support and lining: the marriage of beauty and blood supply. Plast Reconstr Surg 84:189, 1989.

Fig. 36-7 Adapted from Menick F. Nasal Reconstruction: Art and Practice. New York: Elsevier, 2008.

Fig. 36-8 From Muzaffar AB, English JM. Nasal reconstruction. Sel Read Plast Surg 9:5, 2000.

Fig. 36-9 Adapted from Gunter JP, Landecker A, Cochran CS. Nomenclature for frequently used grafts in rhinoplasty. Presented at the Twenty-second Annual Dallas Rhinoplasty Symposium, Dallas, March 2005.

Fig. 36-10 From Nahai F, ed. The Art of Aesthetic Surgery: Principles & Techniques, 2nd ed. St Louis: Quality Medical Publishing, 2011.

Fig. 36-11 Adapted from Gunter JP, Landecker A, Cochran CS. Nomenclature for frequently used grafts in rhinoplasty. Presented at the Twenty-second Annual Dallas Rhinoplasty Symposium, Dallas, March 2005.

Fig. 36-12 From Nahai F, ed. The Art of Aesthetic Surgery: Principles & Techniques, 2nd ed. St Louis: Quality Medical Publishing, 2011.

Fig. 36-13 Adapted from Becker GD, Adams LA, Levin BC. Nonsurgical repair of perinasal skin defects. Plast Reconstr Surg 88:768, 1991.

Fig. 36-14 From Muzaffar AB, English JM. Nasal reconstruction. Sel Read Plast Surg 9:13, 2000.

Fig. 36-15 Jackson IT. Local Flaps in Head and Neck Reconstruction. St Louis: Quality Medical Publishing, 2007.

Fig. 36-16 Jackson IT. Local Flaps in Head and Neck Reconstruction. St Louis: Quality Medical Publishing, 2007.

Fig. 36-17 From Zenn MR, Jones G, eds. Reconstructive Surgery: Anatomy, Technique, and Clinical Applications, 2012.

Fig. 36-18 Adapted from Rohrich RJ, Barton FE, Hollier L. Nasal reconstruction. In Aston SJ, Beasley RW, Thorne CHM, eds. Grabb and Smith's Plastic Surgery, 5th ed. Philadelphia: Lippincott-Raven, 1997.

Fig. 36-19 From Muzaffar AB, English JM. Nasal reconstruction. Sel Read Plast Surg 9:24, 2000.

Fig. 36-21 Adapted from Rohrich RJ, Griffin JR, Adams WP Jr. Rhinophyma: review and update. Plast Reconstr Surg 110:860-869, 2002.

***Chapter 37***

Fig. 37-1 Adapted from Zide BM. Deformities of the lips and cheeks. In McCarthy JR, ed. Plastic Surgery. Philadelphia: WB Saunders, 1990.

Fig. 37-2 Adapted from Zide BM. Deformities of the lips and cheeks. In McCarthy JR, ed. Plastic Surgery. Philadelphia: WB Saunders, 1990.

Fig. 37-4 From Jackson IT. Local Flaps in Head and Neck Reconstruction. St Louis: Quality Medical Publishing, 2007.

***Chapter 38***

Fig. 38-2 Adapted from Beahm EK, Walton RL. Auricular reconstruction for microtia. Part I: Anatomy, embryology and clinical evaluation. Plast Reconstr Surg 109:2473-2482, 2002.

Fig. 38-3 Adapted from Antia NH, Buch VI. Chondrocutaneous advancement flap for the marginal defect of the ear. Plast Reconstr Surg 39:472, 1967.

Fig. 38-4 From Aguilar EA. Traumatic total or partial ear loss. In Evans GR, ed. Operative Plastic Surgery. New York: McGraw-Hill, 2000.

Fig. 38-5 From Tanzer RC. Deformities of the auricle. In Converse JM, ed. Reconstructive Plastic Surgery, 2nd ed. Philadelphia: WB Saunders, 1977.

Fig. 38-6 From Aguilar EA. Traumatic total or partial ear loss. In Evans GR, ed. Operative Plastic Surgery. New York: McGraw-Hill, 2000.

Fig. 38-7 Adapted from Orticochea M. Reconstruction of partial losses of the auricle. Plast Reconstr Surg 46:403, 1970.

Fig. 38-9 From Aguilar EA. Traumatic total or partial ear loss. In Evans GR, ed. Operative Plastic Surgery. New York: McGraw-Hill, 2000.

### *Chapter 39*

Table 39-1 From Gonzalez-Ulloa M. Restoration of the face covering by means of selected skin in regional aesthetic units. Br J Plast Surg 9:212-221, 1956.

Figs. 39-4, 39- 6, 39-7 Adapted from Behmand RA, Rees R. Reconstructive lip surgery. In Achauer BM, Eriksson E, Guyuron B, et al, eds. Plastic Surgery: Indications, Operations, and Outcomes. Philadelphia: Saunders-Elsevier, 2000.

Figs. 39-8, 39-9, 39-11 From Behmand RA, Rees R. Reconstructive lip surgery. In Achauer BM, Eriksson E, Guyuron B, et al, eds. Plastic Surgery: Indications, Operations, and Outcomes. Philadelphia: Saunders-Elsevier, 2000.

Fig. 39-10 Zenn MR, Jones G, eds. Reconstructive Surgery: Anatomy, Technique, and Clinical Applications. St Louis: Quality Medical Publishing, 2012.

Fig. 39-12 From Jackson IT. Local Flaps in Head and Neck Reconstruction. St Louis: Quality Medical Publishing, 2007.

Fig. 39-13 From Zenn MR, Jones G, eds. Reconstructive Surgery: Anatomy, Technique, and Clinical Applications. St Louis: Quality Medical Publishing, 2012.

Fig. 39-15 From Zenn MR, Jones G, eds. Reconstructive Surgery: Anatomy, Technique, and Clinical Applications. St Louis: Quality Medical Publishing, 2012.

### *Chapter 40*

Table 40-1 From Hidalgo DA, Rekow A. Review of 60 consecutive fibula free mandible reconstructions. Plast Reconstr Surg 96:585-596, 1995.

Fig. 40-1 From Zenn MR, Jones G, eds. Reconstructive Surgery: Anatomy, Technique, and Clinical Applications. St Louis: Quality Medical Publishing, 2012.

Fig. 40-2 From Zenn MR, Jones G, eds. Reconstructive Surgery: Anatomy, Technique, and Clinical Applications. St Louis: Quality Medical Publishing, 2012.

Fig. 40-3 From Zenn MR, Jones G, eds. Reconstructive Surgery: Anatomy, Technique, and Clinical Applications. St Louis: Quality Medical Publishing, 2012.

### *Chapter 41*

Fig. 41-1 Adapted from American Joint Committee on Cancer (AJCC), Chicago, Illinois. AJCC Cancer Staging Manual, 6th ed. New York: Springer-Verlag, 2002.

### *Chapter 42*

Fig. 42-1 Adapted from Alford BR, Jerger JF, Coats AC, et al. Neurophysiology of facial nerve testing. Arch Otolaryngol 97:214, 1973.

Fig. 42-2 Adapted from Davis RA, Anson BJ, Budinger JM, et al. Surgical anatomy of the facial nerve and parotid gland based upon a study of 350 cerviofacial halves. Surg Gynecol Obstet 102:385, 1956.

Fig. 42-3 From Seckel BR. Facial Danger Zones: Avoiding Nerve Injury in Facial Plastic Surgery, 2nd ed. St Louis: Quality Medical Publishing, 2010.

Fig. 42-6 From Bergeron CM, Moe KS. The evaluation and treatment of upper eyelid paralysis. Facial Plastic Surg 24:220-230, 2008.

Fig. 42-7 Adapted from Baker DC, Conley J. Facial nerve grafting: a thirty-year retrospective review. Clin Plast Surg 6:343, 1979.

Table 42-1 From May M, Schaitkin BM. The Facial Nerve, 2nd ed. New York: Thieme Medical, 2000.

Table 42-2 From May M, Hardin WB. Facial palsy: interpretation of neurologic findings. Larynoscope 88:1352, 1978.

Table 42-3 From House JW, Brackmann DE. Facial nerve grading system. Otolaryngol Head Neck Surg 93:146-147, 1985, reprinted by Permission of SAGE Publications, Inc.

Table 42-4 Adapted from Anderson RG. Facial nerve disorders and surgery. Sel Read Plast Surg 9:20, 2001.

### Chapter 43

Table 43-1 From Gordon CR, Siemionow M, Coffman K, et al. The Cleveland Clinic FACES Score: a preliminary assessment tool for identifying the optimal face transplant candidate. J Craniofac Surg 20:1969-1974, 2009.

Fig. 43-1, *A-C* Adapted from Siemionow M, Ozturk C. An update on facial transplantation cases performed between 2005 and 2010. Plast Reconstr Surg 128:707e-720e, 2011.

### Chapter 44

Fig. 44-1, *B* From Hall-Findlay EJ. Aesthetic Breast Surgery: Concepts & Techniques. St Louis: Quality Medical Publishing, 2011.

Fig. 44-4 From Jones G, ed. Bostwick's Plastic and Reconstructive Breast Surgery, 3rd ed. St Louis: Quality Medical Publishing, 2010.

Fig. 44-5 From Hall-Findlay EJ. Aesthetic Breast Surgery: Concepts & Techniques. St Louis: Quality Medical Publishing, 2011.

Fig. 44-6 From Jones G, ed. Bostwick's Plastic and Reconstructive Breast Surgery, 3rd ed. St Louis: Quality Medical Publishing, 2010.

### Chapter 45

Fig. 45-2 Adapted from Tebbetts JB. Dual plane breast augmentation: optimizing implant-soft-tissue relationships in a wide range of breast types. Plast Reconstr Surg 107:1255-1272, 2001.

Fig. 45-3 Adapted from Collis N, Coleman D, Foo IT, et al. Ten-year review of a prospective randomized controlled trial of textured versus smooth subglandular silicone gel breast implants. Plast Reconstr Surg 106:786-791, 2000.

Table 45-1 From Adams WP Jr, Mallucci P. Breast augmentation. Plast Reconstr Surg 130:598e-612e, 2012.

Table 45-2 From Hidalgo DA. Breast augmentation: choosing the optimal incision, implant, and pocket plane. Plast Reconstr Surg 105:2202-2206, 2000.

### Chapter 46

Fig. 46-1 Adapted from Kirwan L. Augmentation of the ptotic breast: simultaneous periareolar mastopexy/breast augmentation. Aesthet Surg J 19:34-39, 1999.

Fig. 46-2 Adapted from Benelli L. A new periareolar mammaplasty: the round block technique. Aesthet Plast Surg 14:99, 1990; and Grotting JC, Chen SM. Control and precision in mastopexy. In Nahai F, ed. The Art of Aesthetic Surgery: Principles & Techniques, 2nd ed. St Louis: Quality Medical Publishing, 2011.

Fig. 46-3 Adapted from Lassus C. A 30-year experience with vertical mammaplasty. Plast Reconstr Surg 97:373-380, 1996.

Figs. 46-4 and 46-5 Adapted from Rohrich RJ, Thornton JF, Jakubietz RG, et al. The limited scar mastopexy: current concepts and approaches to correct breast ptosis. Plast Reconstr Surg 114:1622-1630, 2004.

Fig. 46-6 From Rubin JP, Toy J. Mastopexy and breast reduction in massive-weight-loss patients. In Nahai F, ed. The Art of Aesthetic Surgery: Principles & Techniques, 2nd ed. St Louis: Quality Medical Publishing, 2011.

Figs. 46-7, 46-8, 46-9 From Rubin JP, Toy J. Mastopexy and breast reduction in massive-weight-loss patients. In Nahai F, ed. The Art of Aesthetic Surgery: Principles & Techniques, 2nd ed. St Louis: Quality Medical Publishing, 2011.

Table 46-1 From Rohrich RJ, Beran SJ, Restifo RJ, et al. Aesthetic management of the breast following explanation: evaluation and mastopexy options. Plast Reconstr Surg 101:827-837, 1998.

### Chapter 47

Fig. 47-1 Adapted from Kirwan L. Augmentation of the ptotic breast: simultaneous periareolar mastopexy/breast augmentation. Aesthet Surg J 19:34-39, 1999.

Fig. 47-2 From Hall-Findlay EJ. Aesthetic Breast Surgery: Concepts & Techniques. St Louis: Quality Medical Publishing, 2011.

Fig. 47-3 Adapted from Lee MR, Unger JG, Adams WP. The tissue triad: a process approach to augmentation mastopexy. Plast Reconstr Surg (in press).

Fig. 47-4 From Lee MR, Unger JG, Adams WP. The tissue triad: a process approach to augmentation mastopexy. Plast Reconstr Surg (in press).

Table 47-1 Adapted from Stevens WG, Freeman ME, Stoker DA, et al. One-stage mastopexy with breast augmentation: a review of 321 patients. Plast Reconstr Surg 120:1674-1679, 2007; and Calobrace MB, Herdt DR, Cothron KJ. Simultaneous augmentation/mastopexy: a retrospective 5-year review of 332 consecutive cases. Plast Reconstr Surg 131:145-156, 2013.

Table 47-2 From Lee MR, Unger JG, Adams WP. The tissue triad: a process approach to augmentation mastopexy. Plast Reconstr Surg (in press).

### Chapter 48

Fig. 48-1, *B* From Hall-Findlay EJ. Aesthetic Breast Surgery: Concepts & Techniques. St Louis: Quality Medical Publishing, 2011.

Fig. 48-3 From Hall-Findlay EJ. Aesthetic Breast Surgery: Concepts & Techniques. St Louis: Quality Medical Publishing, 2011.

Fig. 48-4 Adapted from Penn J. Breast reduction. Br J Plast Surg 7:357, 1955.

Fig. 48-9 From Nahai F, ed. The Art of Aesthetic Surgery: Principles & Techniques, 2nd ed. St Louis: Quality Medical Publishing, 2011.

Fig. 48-10 From Nahai F, ed. The Art of Aesthetic Surgery: Principles & Techniques, 2nd ed. St Louis: Quality Medical Publishing, 2011.

Fig. 48-14 From Nahai F, ed. The Art of Aesthetic Surgery: Principles & Techniques, 2nd ed. St Louis: Quality Medical Publishing, 2011.

Fig. 48-15 From Jones G, ed. Bostwick's Plastic and Reconstructive Breast Surgery, 3rd ed. St Louis: Quality Medical Publishing, 2010.

Fig. 48-16 From Jones G, ed. Bostwick's Plastic and Reconstructive Breast Surgery, 3rd ed. St Louis: Quality Medical Publishing, 2010.

Fig. 48-17 From Rohrich RJ, Thornton JF, Sorokin ES. Recurrent mammary hyperplasia: current concepts. Plast Reconstr Surg 111:387-393, 2003.

### Chapter 49

Table 49-1 From Deepinder F, Braunsein GD. Gynecomastia: incidence, causes and treatment. Expert Rev Endocrinol Metab 6:723-730, 2011.

Table 49-2 From Deepinder F, Braunsein GD. Gynecomastia: incidence, causes and treatment. Expert Rev Endocrinol Metab 6:723-730, 2011.

### Chapter 50

Fig. 50-1 Adapted from Zenn MR, Jones G, eds. Reconstructive Surgery: Anatomy, Technique, and Clinical Applications. St Louis: Quality Medical Publishing, 2012.

Fig. 50-2 Adapted from Zenn MR, Jones G, eds. Reconstructive Surgery: Anatomy, Technique, and Clinical Applications. St Louis: Quality Medical Publishing, 2012.

Table 50-1 From Berger K, Bostwick J III, Jones G. A Woman's Decision: Breast Care, Treatment, & Reconstruction, 4th ed. St Louis: Quality Medical Publishing, 2011.

### Chapter 51

Fig. 51-1 From Losken A, Hamdi M. Partial Breast Reconstruction: Techniques in Oncoplastic Surgery. St Louis: Quality Medical Publishing, 2009.

Fig. 51-2 From Losken A, Hamdi M. Partial Breast Reconstruction: Techniques in Oncoplastic Surgery. St Louis: Quality Medical Publishing, 2009.

Fig. 51-3 Adapted from Spear SL, Little JW, Bogue DP. Nipple areola reconstruction. In Spear SL, Willey SW, Robb GL, et al, eds. Surgery of the Breast: Principles and Art, 2nd ed. Philadelphia: Lippincott Williams & Wilkins, 2006.

Fig. 51-4 From Jones G. Bostwick's Plastic and Reconstructive Breast Surgery, 3rd ed. St Louis: Quality Medical Publishing, 2010.

Fig. 51-5 From Bostwick J III. Nipple-areolar reconstruction. In Bostwick J III, ed. Plastic and Reconstructive Breast Surgery, 2nd ed. St Louis: Quality Medical Publishing, 2000.

Fig. 51-6 From Jones G. Bostwick's Plastic and Reconstructive Breast Surgery, 3rd ed. St Louis: Quality Medical Publishing, 2010.

Fig. 51-7 Adapted from Hartrampf CR, Culbertson JH. A dermal-fat flap for nipple reconstruction. Plast Reconstr Surg 73:982, 1984.

Fig. 51-8 Adapted from Spear SL, Little JW, Bogue DP. Nipple areola reconstruction. In Spear SL, Willey SW, Robb GL, et al, eds. Surgery of the Breast: Principles and Art, 2nd ed. Philadelphia: Lippincott Williams & Wilkins, 2006.

Fig. 51-9 Adapted from Spear SL, Little JW, Bogue DP. Nipple areola reconstruction. In Spear SL, Willey SW, Robb GL, et al, eds. Surgery of the Breast: Principles and Art, 2nd ed. Philadelphia: Lippincott Williams & Wilkins, 2006.

51-10 Adapted from Spear SL, Little JW, Bogue DP. Nipple areola reconstruction. In Spear SL, Willey SW, Robb GL, et al, eds. Surgery of the Breast: Principles and Art, 2nd ed. Philadelphia: Lippincott Williams & Wilkins, 2006.

Fig. 51-11 Adapted from Spear SL, Little JW, Bogue DP. Nipple areola reconstruction. In Spear SL, Willey SW, Robb GL, et al, eds. Surgery of the Breast: Principles and Art, 2nd ed. Philadelphia: Lippincott Williams & Wilkins, 2006.

Fig. 51-12 From Jones G. Bostwick's Plastic and Reconstructive Breast Surgery, 3rd ed. St Louis: Quality Medical Publishing, 2010.

### Chapter 52

Fig. 52-2 Adapted from Moore KL. Clinically Oriented Anatomy, 3rd ed. Baltimore: Williams & Wilkins, 1992.

Fig. 52-3 Adapted from Synthes Brochure: Titanium Sternal Plating System.

Table 52-1 From Starzynski TE, Snyderman RK, Beattie BJ. Problems of major chest wall reconstruction. Plast Reconstr Surg 44:525, 1969.

### Chapter 53

Fig. 53-2 Adapted from Ramirez OM, Ruas E, Dellon AL. Components separation method for closure of abdominal-wall defects: an anatomic and clinical study. Plast Reconstr Surg 86:519, 1990; and Shestak KC, Edington HJ, Johnson RR. The separation of anatomic components, technique for the reconstruction of massive midline abdominal wall defects: anatomy, surgical technique, applications, and limitations revisited. Plast Reconstr Surg 105:731, 2000.

### Chapter 54

Fig. 54-1 Adapted from Cordeiro PG, Pusic AL, Disa JJ. A classification system and reconstructive algorithm for acquired vaginal defects. Plast Reconstr Surg 110:1058-1065, 2002.

Fig. 54-2 From Marsh J, Perlyn C. Decision Making in Plastic Surgery. St Louis: Quality Medical Publishing, 2010.

Fig. 54-3 From Horton CE, Devine CJ. Hypospadia. In Converse JM, ed. Reconstructive Plastic Surgery. Principles and Procedures in Correction Reconstruction and Transplantation, vol 7, 2nd ed. Philadelphia: WB Saunders, 1977.

### Chapter 55

Fig. 55-1 Adapted from Lindan O, Greenway RM, Piazza JM. Pressure distribution on the surface of the human body. I. Evaluation in lying and sitting positions using a bed of springs and nails. Arch Phys Med Rehabil 46:378, 1965.

Fig. 55-2 Adapted from National Pressure Ulcer Advisory Panel (NPUAP). Pressure ulcer stages/categories 2007. Available at *http://www.npuap.org/resources/educational-and-clinical-resources/*.

Fig. 55-3 From Ladin DA. Understanding dressings. Clin Plast Surg 25:433, 1998.

### Chapter 56

Fig. 56-1 Adapted from Byrd HS, Spicer TE, Cierny G III. Management of open tibial fractures. Plast Reconstr Surg 76:729, 1985.

Fig. 56-4 From Pu LLQ, Levine JP, Wei F, eds. Reconstructive Surgery of the Lower Extremity. St Louis: Quality Medical Publishing, 2013.

Fig. 56-5 Adapted from Nakajima H, Fujino T, Adachi S. A new concept of vascular supply to the skin and classification of skin flaps according to their vascularization. Ann Plast Surg 16:1-19, 1986.

Fig. 56-6 Adapted from Teo TC. The propeller flap concept. Clin Plast Surg 37:615-626, 2010.

Table 56-1 Data from Gustilo RB, Anderson JT. Prevention of infection in the treatment of one thousand and twenty-five open fractures of long bones. J Bone Joint Surg Am 58:453, 1976; and Gustilo RB, Mendoza RM, Williams DN. Problems in the management of type III (severe) open fractures: a new classification of type III open fractures. J Trauma 24:742, 1984.

Table 56-2 From Byrd HS, Spicer TE, Cierny G III. Management of open tibial fractures. Plast Reconstr Surg 76:719-730, 1985.

Table 56-3 From Byrd HS, Spicer TE, Cierny G III. Management of open tibial fractures. Plast Reconstr Surg 76:719-730, 1985.

***Chapter 57***

Fig. 57-1 Illustration by Vileikyte L. From Boulton AJM. The diabetic foot: from art to science. The 18th Camillo Golgi lecture. Diabetologia 47:1343-1353, 2004.

Fig. 57-2 Adapted from Zenn MR, Jones G, eds. Reconstructive Surgery: Anatomy, Technique, and Clinical Applications. St Louis: Quality Medical Publishing, 2012.

Table 57-1 Adapted from Armstrong DG, Lavery LA, Harkless LB. Validation of a diabetic wound classification system: the contribution of depth, infection and ischemia to risk of amputation. Diabetes Care 21:855-859, 1998.

Table 57-2 Adapted from Lipsky BA, Berendt AR, Cornia PB, et al. IDSA guidelines: 2012 Infectious Diseases Society of America. Clinical Practice Guideline for the Diagnosis and Treatment of Diabetic Foot Infections. Clin Infect Dis 54:132-173, 2012.

***Chapter 58***

Fig. 58-2 Adapted from The University of Texas M.D. Anderson Cancer Center as printed in Suami H, Chang DW. Overview of surgical treatments for breast cancer-related lymphedema. Plast Reconstr Surg 126:1853-1863, 2010.

Fig. 58-3 Adapted from The University of Texas M.D. Anderson Cancer Center as printed in Suami H, Chang DW. Overview of surgical treatments for breast cancer-related lymphedema. Plast Reconstr Surg 126:1853-1863, 2010.

***Chapter 59***

Fig. 59-1 Adapted from Doyle JR, Botte MJ, eds. Surgical Anatomy of the Upper Extremity. Philadelphia: Lippincott Williams & Wilkins, 2003.

Fig. 59-2 Adapted from Bentz ML, Bauer BS, Zuker RM. Principles & Practice of Pediatric Plastic Surgery. St Louis: Quality Medical Publishing, 2008.

Fig. 59-4 Adapted from Lluch AL. Repair of the extensor tendon system. In Aston SJ, Beasley RW, Thorne CHM, eds. Grabb and Smith's Plastic Surgery, 5th ed. Philadelphia: Lippincott-Raven, 1997.

Fig. 59-5 Adapted from Zidel P. Tendon healing and flexor tendon surgery. In Aston SJ, Beasley RW, Thorne CHM, eds. Grabb and Smith's Plastic Surgery, 5th ed. Philadelphia: Lippincott-Raven, 1997.

Fig. 59-6 Adapted from Zidel P. Tendon healing and flexor tendon surgery. In Aston SJ, Beasley RW, Thorne CHM, eds. Grabb and Smith's Plastic Surgery, 5th ed. Philadelphia: Lippincott-Raven, 1997.

Fig. 59-8 Adapted from Beasley RW, ed. Beasley's Surgery of the Hand. New York: Thieme, 2003.

***Chapter 60***

Figs. 60-1 through 60-25 Adapted from American Society for Surgery of the Hand. The Hand: Examination and Diagnosis, 3rd ed. Philadelphia: Churchill Livingstone, 1990.

***Chapter 61***

Fig. 61-2 From Carter P, Ezaki M. Disorders of the upper extremity. In Herring JA, Tachdjian MO, eds. Tachdjian's Pediatric Orthopedics: From the Texas Scottish Rite Hospital for Children, vol 1, 3rd ed. Philadelphia: WB Saunders, 2001.

Fig. 61-6 From Carter P, Ezaki M. Disorders of the upper extremity. In Herring JA, Tachdjian MO, eds. Tachdjian's Pediatric Orthopedics: From the Texas Scottish Rite Hospital for Children, vol 1, 3rd ed. Philadelphia: WB Saunders, 2001.

***Chapter 62***

Fig. 62-2 Adapted from Wolfe SW. Fractures of the carpus: scaphoid fractures. In Berger RA, Weiss A-PC, eds. Hand Surgery. Philadelphia: Lippincott Williams & Wilkins, 2004.

Fig. 62-3 Adapted from Wolfe SW. Fractures of the carpus: scaphoid fractures. In Berger RA, Weiss A-PC, eds. Hand Surgery. Philadelphia: Lippincott Williams & Wilkins, 2004.

Fig. 62-4 From Shah MA, Viegas SF. Fractures of the carpal bones excluding the scaphoid. J Am Soc Surg Hand 2:129-139, 2002.

***Chapter 63***

Fig. 63-1 Adapted from Wolfe SW, Garcia-Elias M, Kitay A. Carpal instability nondissociative. J Am Acad Orthop Surg 20:575-585, 2012.

Fig. 63-2 Adapted from Wolfe SW, Garcia-Elias M, Kitay A. Carpal instability nondissociative. J Am Acad Orthop Surg 20:575-585, 2012.

Fig. 63-3 Adapted from Butterfield WL, Joshi A, Lichtman D. Lunotriquetral injuries. J Am Soc Surg Hand 2:195-203, 2002.

Fig. 63-4 Adapted from Walsh JJ, Berger RA, Cooney WP. Current status of scapholunate interosseous ligament injuries. J Am Acad Orthop Surg 10:32-42, 2002.

Fig. 63-6 Adapted from Muzaffar AR, Hand. V. Fractures and dislocations. The wrist: congenital anomalies. Sel Read Plast Surg 9:36, 2003.

Fig. 63-8 Adapted from Butterfield WL, Joshi A, Lichtman D. Lunotriquetral injuries. J Am Soc Surg Hand 2:195-203, 2002.

Fig. 63-9 Adapted from Mayfield JK, Johnson RP, Kilcoyne RK. Carpal dislocation: pathomechanics and progressive periulnar instability. J Hand Surg Am 5:226-241, 1980.

Fig. 63-13 From Walsh JJ, Berger RA, Cooney WP. Current status of scapholunate interosseous ligament injuries. J Am Acad Orthop Surg 10:32-42, 2002.

Fig. 63-15 Adapted from Walsh JJ, Berger RA, Cooney WP. Current status of scapholunate interosseous ligament injuries. J Am Acad Orthop Surg 10:32-42, 2002.

Fig. 63-18 From Rosenwasser M, Miyasajsa K, Strauch R. The RASL procedure: reduction and association of the scaphoid and lunate using the Herbert screw. Tech Hand U Extrem Surg 1:263-272, 1997.

Fig. 63-19 Adapted from Butterfield WL, Joshi A, Lichtman D. Lunotriquetral injuries. J Am Soc Surg Hand 2:195-203, 2002.

Fig. 63-20 From Taljanovic MS, Goldberg MR, Sheppard JE, et al. US of the intrinsic and extrinsic wrist ligaments and triangular fibrocartilage complex—normal anatomy and imaging technique. Radiographics 31:79-80, 2011.

Fig. 63-21 Adapted from Taljanovic MS, Goldberg MR, Sheppard JE, et al. US of the intrinsic and extrinsic wrist ligaments and triangular fibrocartilage complex—normal anatomy and imaging technique. Radiographics 31:79-80, 2011.

Fig. 63-23 From Yaghoubian R, Goebel F, Musgrave DS, et al. Diagnosis and management of acute fracture-dislocation of the carpus. Orthop Clin North Am 32:295-305, 2001.

Table 63-1 From Larsen CF, Amadio PC, Gilula LA, et al. Analysis of carpal instability: I. Description of the scheme. J Hand Surg 20:757-764, 1995.

Table 63-2 From Geissler WB, Freeland AE. Arthroscopically assisted reduction of intraarticular distal radial fractures. Clin Orthop Rel Res 327:125-134, 1996.

Table 63-3 From Walsh JJ, Berger RA, Cooney WP. Current status of scapholunate interosseous ligament injuries. J Am Acad Orthop Surg 10:32-42, 2002.

Table 63-4 From Wolf JM, Dukas A, Pensak M. Advances in wrist arthroscopy. J Am Acad Orthop Surg 20:725-734, 2012.

Table 63-5 From Adams CH. Green's Operative Hand Surgery Textbook. St Louis: Mosby-Elsevier, 2011.

### Chapter 64

Fig. 64-1 Adapted from Smith DW, Brou KE, Henry MH. Early active rehabilitation for operatively stabilized distal radius fractures. J Hand Ther 17:43-49, 2004.

Fig. 64-2 Adapted from Spinner EB. Kaplan's Functional and Surgical Anatomy of the Hand, 3rd ed. Philadelphia: Lippincott Williams & Wilkins, 1984.

Fig. 64-3 Adapted from Berger RA, Weiss APC. Hand Surgery. Philadelphia: Lippincott Williams & Wilkins, 2004.

Fig. 64-4 Adapted from Wolfe S, Hotchkiss RN, Pederson W, Kozin S. Green's Operative Hand Surgery, 6th ed. Philadelphia: Saunders-Elsevier, 2010.

Fig. 64-6 From Trumble TE, Budoff JE. Hand Surgery Update IV. Chicago: American Society for the Surgery of the Hand, 2007.

### Chapter 65

Fig. 65-1 Adapted from Zenn MR, Jones G, eds. Reconstructive Surgery: Anatomy, Technique, and Clinical Applications. St Louis: Quality Medical Publishing, 2012.

Fig. 65-2 Adapted from American Society for Surgery of the Hand. Available at *http://www.assh.org/Public/HandAnatomy/Pages/default.aspx*.

Fig. 65-3 Adapted from PediatricEducation.org. Available at *http://www.pediatriceducation.org/2005/10/03/*.

Fig. 65-4 Adapted from Day CS, Stern PJ. Fractures of the metacarpals and phalanges. In Green DP, Hotchkiss RN, Pederson WC, eds. Green's Operative Hand Surgery, 6th ed. Philadelphia: Elsevier, 2011.

Fig. 65-5 Adapted from Hamilton SW, Aboud H. Finite element analysis, mechanical assessment and material comparison of two volar slab constructs. Injury 40:397-399, 2009.

Fig. 65-6 Adapted from Day CS, Stern PJ. Fractures of the metacarpals and phalanges. In Green DP, Hotchkiss RN, Pederson WC, eds. Green's Operative Hand Surgery, 6th ed. Philadelphia: Elsevier, 2011.

Fig. 65-7 From Hand Innovations. The first percutaneous locked flexible intramedullary nail system for hand fractures. Photo courtesy of Biomet Trauma. Reprinted with the permission of Biomet, Inc, Warsaw, IN.

Fig. 65-8 Adapted from Day CS, Stern PJ. Fractures of the metacarpals and phalanges. In Green DP, Hotchkiss RN, Pederson WC, eds. Green's Operative Hand Surgery, 6th ed. Philadelphia: Elsevier, 2011.

Fig. 65-9 Adapted from Day CS, Stern PJ. Fractures of the metacarpals and phalanges. In Green DP, Hotchkiss RN, Pederson WC, eds. Green's Operative Hand Surgery, 6th ed. Philadelphia: Elsevier, 2011.

Fig. 65-10 Adapted from Day CS, Stern PJ. Fractures of the metacarpals and phalanges. In Green DP, Hotchkiss RN, Pederson WC, eds. Green's Operative Hand Surgery, 6th ed. Philadelphia: Elsevier, 2011.

Fig. 65-12, *A* Adapted from Ruland RT, Hogan CJ, Cannon DL, et al. Use of dynamic distraction external fixation for unstable fracture-dislocations of the proximal interphalangeal joint. J Hand Surg Am 33:19-25, 2008.

Fig. 65-12, *B-C* From Ruland RT, Hogan CJ, Cannon DL, et al. Use of dynamic distraction external fixation for unstable fracture-dislocations of the proximal interphalangeal joint. J Hand Surg Am 33:19-25, Copyright 2008, with permission from Elsevier.

Fig. 65-13 Adapted from Kang GC, Yam A, Phoon ES, et al. The hook plate technique for fixation of phalangeal avulsion fractures. J Bone Joint Surg Am 94:e72, 2012.

Box 65-1 From Stern PJ. Fractures of the metacarpals and phalanges. In Green DP, Hotchkiss RN, Pederson WC, eds. Green's Operative Hand Surgery, 4th ed. Philadelphia: Churchill Livingstone, 1999.

### *Chapter 66*

Fig. 66-1 Adapted from Eaton RG, Littler JW. Joint injuries and their sequelae. Clin Plast Surg 3:85-98, 1976.

Fig. 66-3 From Calfee RP, Kiefhaber TR, Sommerkamp TG, et al. Hemi-hamate arthroplasty provides functional reconstruction of acute and chronic proximal interphalangeal fracture-dislocations. J Hand Surg 34:1232-1241, 2009.

### *Chapter 67*

Fig. 67-4 Adapted from Fassier PR. Fingertip injuries: evaluation and treatment. J Am Acad Orthop Surg 4:84-92, 1996.

Fig. 67-5 From Chao JD, Huang JM, Wiedrich TA. Local hand flaps. J Am Soc Surg Hand 1:28, 2002.

Fig. 67-6 Adapted from Rohrich RJ, Antrobus SD. Volar advancement flaps. In Blair WF, ed. Techniques in Hand Surgery. Baltimore: Williams & Wilkins, 1996.

Fig. 67-7 From Chao JD, Huang JM, Wiedrich TA. Local hand flaps. J Am Soc Surg Hand 1:28, 2002.

Fig. 67-9 Adapted from Green DP, Hotchkiss RN, Pederson WC, eds. Green's Operative Hand Surgery, 4th ed. Philadelphia: Churchill Livingstone, 1999.

Fig. 67-10 Adapted from Green DP, Hotchkiss RN, Pederson WC, eds. Green's Operative Hand Surgery, 4th ed. Philadelphia: Churchill Livingstone, 1999.

### *Chapter 68*

Fig. 68-2 From Hung VS, Bodavula VK, Dubin NH. Digital anaesthesia: comparison of the efficacy and pain associated with three digital nerve block techniques. J Hand Surg Br 30:581-584, 2005.

Fig. 68-3 From Jellinek NJ. Nail surgery: practical tips and treatment options. Dermatol Ther 20:68-74, 2007.

Fig. 68-5 Adapted from Strick MJ, Bremner-Smith AT, Tonkin MA. Antenna procedure for the correction of hook nail deformity. J Hand Surg Br 29B:3-7, 2004.

### *Chapter 69*

Fig. 69-1 From Idler RS. Anatomy and biomechanics of the digital flexor tendons. Hand Clin 1:4, 1985.

69-2, *A* From Idler RS. Anatomy and biomechanics of the digital flexor tendons. Hand Clin 1:4, 1985.

Fig. 69-2, *B* Adapted from Idler RS. Anatomy and biomechanics of the digital flexor tendons. Hand Clin 1:4, 1985.

Fig. 69-3 Adapted from Kleinert HE, Lubahn JD. Current state of flexor tendon surgery. Ann Chir Main 3:10, 1984.

Fig. 69-4 Adapted from Strickland JW. Flexor tendon repair. Hand Clin 1:56, 1985.

Fig. 69-6 From Seiler JG. Flexor tendon repair. J Am Soc Surg Hand 1:177, Copyright 2001, with permission from Elsevier.

### Chapter 70

Fig. 70-3 Adapted from Green DP, Hotchkiss RN, Pederson WC, et al, eds. Green's Operative Hand Surgery, 5th ed. Philadelphia: Churchill Livingstone, 2005.

Fig. 70-4 From Coon MS, Green SM. Boutonniere deformity. Hand Clin 11:387-402, Copyright 1995, with permission from Elsevier.

Fig. 70-6 Adapted from Green DP, Hotchkiss RN, Pederson WC, et al, eds. Green's Operative Hand Surgery, 5th ed. Philadelphia: Churchill Livingstone, 2005.

Fig. 70-7 Adapted from Lister G. Rheumatoid arthritis, its variants, and osteoarthritis. In Smith P, ed. Lister's The Hand, 4th ed. London: Churchill Livingstone, 2002.

### Chapter 71

Table 71-2 From Lieber RL, Jacobson MD, Fazeli BM, et al. Architecture of selected muscles of the arm and forearm: anatomy and implications for tendon transfer. J Hand Surg Am 17:787-798, Copyright 1992, with permission from Elsevier.

Table 71-3 Sammer DM, Chung KC. Tendon transfers: Part I. Principles of transfer and transfers for radial nerve palsy. Plast Reconstr Surg 123:169e-177e, 2009.

### Chapter 73

Fig. 73-1 Adapted from Sebastin SJ, Chung KC. A systematic review of the outcomes of replantation of distal digital amputation. Plast Reconstr Surg 128:723-737, 2011.

Fig. 73-2 Adapted from Sebastin SJ, Chung KC. A systematic review of the outcomes of replantation of distal digital amputation. Plast Reconstr Surg 128:723-737, 2011.

Fig. 73-3 Adapted from Callico CG. Replantation and revascularization of the upper extremity. In May JW Jr, Littler JW, eds. McCarthy's Plastic Surgery, vol 7. The Hand. Philadelphia: WB Saunders, 1990.

Fig. 73-4 From Callico CG. Replantation and revascularization of the upper extremity. In May JW Jr, Littler JW, eds. McCarthy's Plastic Surgery, vol 7. The Hand. Philadelphia: WB Saunders, 1990.

### Chapter 74

Fig. 74-1 Adapted from Gordon CR, Siemionow M. Requirements for the development of a hand transplantation program. Ann Plast Surg 63:262-273, 2009.

Fig. 74-2 From Azari KK, Imbriglia JE, Goitz RJ, et al. Technical aspects of the recipient operation in hand transplantation. J Reconstr Microsurg 28:27-34, 2012 (reprinted by permission of Thieme Medical).

### Chapter 75

Fig. 75-5 From Canale ST. Campbell's Operative Orthopedics, vol 4, 10th ed. St Louis: Mosby-Elsevier, 2003.

### Chapter 76

Fig. 76-1 From Zenn MR, Jones G, eds. Reconstructive Surgery: Anatomy, Technique, and Clinical Applications. St Louis: Quality Medical Publishing, 2012.

### Chapter 77

Fig. 77-1 Adapted from Aston SJ, Beasley RQ, Thorne CHM, eds. Grabb and Smith's Plastic Surgery, 5th ed. Philadelphia: Lippincott-Raven, 1997.

Fig. 77-2 Adapted from Aston SJ, Beasley RQ, Thorne CHM, eds. Grabb and Smith's Plastic Surgery, 5th ed. Philadelphia: Lippincott-Raven, 1997.

Fig. 77-3 From Velmahos GC, Toutouzas KG. Vascular trauma and compartment syndromes. Surg Clin North Am 82:125, Copyright 2002, with permission from Elsevier.

Fig. 77-4 From Velmahos GC, Toutouzas KG. Vascular trauma and compartment syndromes. Surg Clin North Am 82:125, Copyright 2002, with permission from Elsevier.

Fig. 77-5 From Velmahos GC, Toutouzas KG. Vascular trauma and compartment syndromes. Surg Clin North Am 82:125, Copyright 2002, with permission from Elsevier.

Fig. 77-6 From Velmahos GC, Toutouzas KG. Vascular trauma and compartment syndromes. Surg Clin North Am 82:125, Copyright 2002, with permission from Elsevier.

Fig. 77-7 From Velmahos GC, Toutouzas KG. Vascular trauma and compartment syndromes. Surg Clin North Am 82:125, Copyright 2002, with permission from Elsevier.

Table 77-1 Kavouni A, Ion L. Bilateral well-leg compartment syndrome after supine position surgery. Ann Plast Surg 44:462e-463e, 2000.

Fig. 77-8 From Velmahos GC, Toutouzas KG. Vascular trauma and compartment syndromes. Surg Clin North Am 82:125, Copyright 2002, with permission from Elsevier.

### Chapter 78

Fig. 78-4 Adapted from Lanz U. Anatomical variations of the median nerve in the carpal tunnel. J Hand Surg 2:44, 1977.

### Chapter 79

Fig. 79-1 Illustration by Michael Yeh.

Fig. 79-2 Illustration by Michael Yeh.

Table 79-1 Adapted from Waters PM. Pediatric brachial plexus palsy. In Wolfe S, Hotchkiss RN, Pederson W, Kozin S, eds. Green's Operative Hand Surgery, 6th ed. Philadelphia: Elsevier, 2011.

Table 79-2 Adapted from Spinner R, Shin AY, Hebert-Blouin M, et al. Traumatic brachial plexus injury. In Wolfe S, Hotchkiss RN, Pederson W, Kozin S, eds. Green's Operative Hand Surgery, 6th ed. Philadelphia: Elsevier, 2011; and Terzis JK, Papakonstantinou KC. The surgical treatment of brachial plexus injuries in adults. Plast Reconstr Surg 106:1097-1122, 2000.

Table 79-3 Adapted from Mackinnon SE, Dellon AL. Surgery of the Peripheral Nerve. New York: Thieme Medical, 1988.

Table 79-4 © 2012 American Academy of Orthopaedic Surgeons. From the Journal of the American Academy of Orthopaedic Surgeons, 20:506-517, with permission.

Table 79-5 © 2012 American Academy of Orthopaedic Surgeons. From the Journal of the American Academy of Orthopaedic Surgeons, 20:506-517, with permission.

Table 79-6 © 2012 American Academy of Orthopaedic Surgeons. From the Journal of the American Academy of Orthopaedic Surgeons, 20:506-517, with permission.

### Chapter 80

Fig. 80-1 From Brandt KE, Mackinnon SE. Microsurgical repair of peripheral nerves and nerve grafts. In Aston JS, Beasley RW, Thorne CHM, eds. Grabb and Smith's Plastic Surgery, 5th ed. Philadelphia: Lippincott-Raven, 1997.

Fig. 80-2 From Brushart T. Nerve repair and grafting. In Green DP, Hotchkiss RN, Pederson WC, eds. Green's Operative Hand Surgery, vol 2, 4th ed. Philadelphia: Churchill Livingstone, 1998.

Table 80-1 From Gutowski KA. Hand. II: Peripheral nerve and tendon transfers. Sel Read Plast Surg 9:1-19, 2003.

### Chapter 81

Fig. 81-1 Adapted from Green DP, Hotchkiss RN, Pederson WC, eds. Green's Operative Hand Surgery, 5th ed. Philadelphia: Churchill Livingstone, 2005.

Fig. 81-2 Adapted from Stevanovic MV, Sharpe F, Wolfe SW, eds. Green's Operative Hand Surgery, 6th ed. Philadelphia: Elsevier, 2011.

Fig. 81-3 Adapted from Stevanovic MV, Sharpe F, Wolfe SW, eds. Green's Operative Hand Surgery, 6th ed. Philadelphia: Elsevier, 2011.

Fig. 81-4 Adapted from Netter FH. Atlas of Human Anatomy. New York: Novartis, 1997.

Fig. 81-5 Adapted from Green DP, Hotchkiss RN, Pederson WC, et al, eds. Green's Operative Hand Surgery, 5th ed. Philadelphia: Churchill Livingstone, 2005.

Fig. 81-6 Adapted from Stevanovic MV, Sharpe F, Wolfe SW. Green's Operative Hand Surgery, 6th ed. Philadelphia: Elsevier, 2011.

Fig. 81-7 Adapted from Costerton J. Biofilm theory can guide treatment for device-related orthopaedic infections. Clin Orthop Rel Res 437:7-11, 2005.

### Chapter 84

Fig. 84-1 Courtesy of Denton Watumull, MD.

Fig. 84-2 Adapted from Smith P, ed. Lister's The Hand, 4th ed. London: Churchill Livingstone, 2002.

Fig. 84-4 From Flatt AE. Care of the Arthritic Hand, 5th ed. St Louis: Quality Medical Publishing, 1995.

### Chapter 85

Table 85-1 Data from Smith P, ed. Lister's The Hand, 4th ed. London: Churchill Livingstone, 2002.

Fig. 85-1 From Lister G. Rheumatoid arthritis, its variants, and osteoarthritis. In Smith P, ed. Lister's The Hand, 4th ed. London: Churchill Livingstone, 2002.

### Chapter 86

Fig. 86-1 From Connell D, Koulouris G, Thorn D, et al. Contrast-enhanced MR angiography of the hand. Radiographics 22:583-599, 2002.

Fig. 86-2 From Huang J, Zager E. Thoracic outlet syndrome. Neurosurgery 55:897-903, 2004.

Fig. 86-3 From Al-Qattan M, Al-Namla A, Al-Thunayan A, et al. Magnetic resonance imaging in the diagnosis of glomus tumours of the hand. J Hand Surg Br 30:535-540, 2005.

Fig. 86-4 From Drape J. Imaging of tumors of the nail unit. Clin Pod Med Surg 21:493-511, Copyright 2004, with permission from Elsevier.

Table 86-1 Data from Lee BB, Do YS, Yakes W, et al. Management of arteriovenous malformations: a multidisciplinary approach. J Vasc Surg 39:590-600, 2004; Menzoian JO, Doyle JE, LoGerfo FW, et al. Evaluation and management of vascular injuries of the extremities. Arch Surg 118:93-95, 1983; and Newmeyer W. Vascular disorders. In Green DP, ed. Operative Hand Surgery, 3rd ed. Philadelphia: Churchill Livingstone, 1993.

Table 86-2 Data from Perry MO, Thal ER, Shires GT. Management of arterial injuries. Ann Surg 173:403-408, 1971; Gelberman RH, Blasingame JP, Fronek A, et al. Forearm arterial injuries. J Hand Surg Am 4:401-408, 1979; Leclercq DC, Carlier AJ, Khuc T, et al. Improvement in the results in sixty-four ulnar nerve sections associated with arterial repair. J Hand Surg Am 10:997-999, 1985; and Katz SG, Kohl RD. Direct revascularization for the treatment of forearm and hand ischemia. Am J Surg 165:312-316, 1993.

Table 86-3 Adapted from Chang MW. Updated classification of hemangiomas and other vascular anomalies. Lymphat Res Biol 1:259-265, 2003; and the International Society for the Study of Vascular Anomalies, Brussels, Belgium. Available at *www.http://www.issva.org/.*

Table 86-4 Data from Lee BB, Do YS, Yakes W, et al. Management of arteriovenous malformations: a multidisciplinary approach. J Vasc Surg 39:590-600, 2004; and Newmeyer W. Vascular disorders. In Green DP, ed. Operative Hand Surgery, 3rd ed. Philadelphia: Churchill Livingstone, 1993.

Table 86-5 From Sofocleous CT, Rosen RJ, Raskin K, et al. Congenital vascular malformations in the hand and forearm. J Endovasc Ther (© International Society of Endovascular Specialists) 8:484-494, 2001.

Box 86-1 From Wigley FM, Flavahan NA. Raynaud's phenomenon. Rheum Dis Clin North Am 22:765-781, Copyright 1996, with permission from Elsevier.

### Chapter 87

Box 87-1 Adapted from Janis JE, Rohrich RJ, Gutowski KA. Otoplasty. Plast Reconstr Surg 115:60e-72e, 2005; and Ha RY, Trovato MJ. Plastic surgery of the ear. SRPS 11(R3):1-46, 2011.

Fig. 87-1 Adapted from Bashour M. History and current concepts in the analysis of facial attractiveness. Plast Reconstr Surg 118:741-756, 2006.

Fig. 87-2 through 87-12 Adapted from Gunter JP, Rohrich RJ, Adams WP Jr. Dallas Rhinoplasty: Nasal Surgery by the Masters. St Louis: Quality Medical Publishing, 2002.

Fig. 87-13 McCord CD Jr, Codner MA. Eyelid & Periorbital Surgery. St Louis: Quality Medical Publishing, 2008.

Fig. 87-14 through 87-28 Adapted from Gunter JP, Rohrich RJ, Adams WP Jr. Dallas Rhinoplasty: Nasal Surgery by the Masters. St Louis: Quality Medical Publishing, 2002.

Box 87-1 Adapted from Janis JE, Rohrich RJ, Gutowski KA. Otoplasty. Plast Reconstr Surg 115:60e-72e, 2005; and Ha RY, Trovato MJ. Plastic surgery of the ear. SRPS 11(R3):1-46, 2011.

### Chapter 88

Fig. 88-2 Adapted from Carruthers J, Fagien S, Matarasso SL; Botox Consensus Group. Consensus recommendations on the use of botulinum toxin type a in facial aesthetics. Plast Reconstr Surg 114 (Suppl 6):S1-S22, 2004.

Fig. 88-3 Adapted from Carruthers J, Fagien S, Matarasso SL; Botox Consensus Group. Consensus recommendations on the use of botulinum toxin type a in facial aesthetics. Plast Reconstr Surg 114(Suppl 6):S1-S22, 2004.

Fig. 88-4 Adapted from Carruthers J, Fagien S, Matarasso SL; Botox Consensus Group. Consensus recommendations on the use of botulinum toxin type a in facial aesthetics. Plast Reconstr Surg 114(Suppl 6):S1-S22, 2004.

Fig. 88-5 Adapted from Carruthers J, Fagien S, Matarasso SL; Botox Consensus Group. Consensus recommendations on the use of botulinum toxin type a in facial aesthetics. Plast Reconstr Surg 114(Suppl 6):S1-S22, 2004.

Table 88-1 Adapted from Glogau RG. Chemical peeling and aging skin. J Geriatr Dermatol 2:30-35, 1994.

Table 88-2 Adapted from Fitzpatrick RE, Goldman MP, Satur NM, et al. Pulsed carbon dioxide laser resurfacing of photo-aged facial skin. Arch Dermatol 132:395-402, 1996.

Table 88-4 Data from Moy LS, Murad H, Moy RL. Glycolic acid peels for the treatment of wrinkles and photoaging. J Dermatol Surg Oncol 19:243-246, 1993.

Table 88-5 From Hetter GP. An examination of the phenol-croton oil peel. Part IV. Face peel results with different concentrations of phenol and croton oil. Plast Reconstr Surg 105:1061-1083, 2000.

Box 88-1 From Baumann L, Blyumin M, Saghari S. Dermal fillers. In Baumann L. Cosmetic Dermatology: Principals and Practice, 2nd ed. New York: McGraw-Hill, 2009.

### Chapter 89

Fig. 89-1 From Khouri RK, Del Vecchio DA. Breast reconstruction and augmentation with Brava external expansion and fat grafting. In Coleman SR, Mazzola RF, eds. Fat Injection: From Filling to Rejuvenation, vol II. St Louis: Quality Medical Publishing, 2009.

Fig. 89-3 From Coleman SR. Structural Fat Grafting, vol I. St Louis: Quality Medical Publishing, 2004.

Fig. 89-6, *A* From Coleman SR. Overview of structural fat grafting. In Coleman SR, Mazzola RF, eds. Fat Injection: From Filling to Rejuvenation, vol II. St Louis: Quality Medical Publishing, 2009.

Fig. 89-6, *B* From Coleman SR. Structural Fat Grafting, vol I. St Louis: Quality Medical Publishing, 2004.

### Chapter 90

Fig. 90-3 From Norwood OT, Shiell RC. Hair Transplant Surgery, 2nd ed. Springfield, IL: Charles C Thomas, 1984.

Fig. 90-4 From Ludwig E. Classification of the types of androgenic alopecia (common baldness) arising in the female sex. Br J Dermatol 97:247, 1977.

Fig. 90-7 Adapted from Vogel JE, Jimenez F, Cole J, Keene SA, Harris JA, Barrera A, Rose PT. Hair Restoration Surgery: The State of the Art. Aesthet Surg J 33:128-151, 2013.

### Chapter 91

Fig. 91-1 From Nahai F, Saltz R, eds. Endoscopic Plastic Surgery, 2nd ed. St Louis: Quality Medical Publishing, 2008.

Fig. 91-2 From Nahai F, ed. The Art of Aesthetic Surgery: Principles & Techniques, 2nd ed. St Louis: Quality Medical Publishing, 2011.

Fig. 91-3 From McCord CD Jr, Codner MA. Eyelid & Periorbital Surgery. St Louis: Quality Medical Publishing, 2008.

Fig. 91-4 From Nahai F, ed. The Art of Aesthetic Surgery: Principles & Techniques, 2nd ed. St Louis: Quality Medical Publishing, 2011.

Fig. 91-5 From Nahai F, ed. The Art of Aesthetic Surgery: Principles & Techniques, 2nd ed. St Louis: Quality Medical Publishing, 2011.

Fig. 91-6 From McCord CD Jr, Codner MA. Eyelid & Periorbital Surgery. St Louis: Quality Medical Publishing, 2008.

Table 91-1 From Nahai F, ed. The Art of Aesthetic Surgery: Principles & Techniques, 2nd ed. St Louis: Quality Medical Publishing, 2011.

### Chapter 92

Fig. 92-2 From Nahai F, ed. The Art of Aesthetic Surgery: Principles & Techniques, 2nd ed. St Louis: Quality Medical Publishing, 2011.

Fig. 92-6 From McCord CD Jr, Codner MA. Eyelid & Periorbital Surgery. St Louis: Quality Medical Publishing, 2008.

Fig. 92-8 From Barton F. Facial Rejuvenation. St Louis: Quality Medical Publishing, 2008.

Fig. 92-9 Adapted from Loeb R. Fat pad sliding and fat grafting for leveling lid depressions. Clin Plast Surg 8:774, 1981.

Fig. 92-11 Adapted from Hamra ST. The role of the septal reset in creating a youthful eyelid-cheek complex in facial rejuvenation. Plast Reconstr Surg 113:2124-2141, 2004.

Fig. 92-12 From McCord CD Jr, Codner MA. Eyelid & Periorbital Surgery. St Louis: Quality Medical Publishing, 2008.

Fig. 92-13 From McCord CD Jr, Codner MA. Eyelid & Periorbital Surgery. St Louis: Quality Medical Publishing, 2008.

### Chapter 93

Fig. 93-1 From McCord CD Jr, Codner MA. Eyelid & Periorbital Surgery. St Louis: Quality Medical Publishing, 2008.

Fig. 93-2 From McCord CD Jr, Codner MA. Eyelid & Periorbital Surgery. St Louis: Quality Medical Publishing, 2008.

Fig. 93-3 From Bentz ML, Bauer BS, Zuker RM. Principles and Practice of Pediatric Plastic Surgery. St Louis: Quality Medical Publishing, 2008.

Fig. 93-5 From Marsh J, Perlyn C. Decision Making in Plastic Surgery. St Louis: Quality Medical Publishing, 2010.

Fig. 93-6 From McCord CD Jr, Codner MA. Eyelid & Periorbital Surgery. St Louis: Quality Medical Publishing, 2008.

Fig. 93-7 From Bentz ML, Bauer BS, Zuker RM. Principles & Practice of Pediatric Plastic Surgery. St Louis: Quality Medical Publishing, 2008.

Table 93-3 From Liu MT, Totonchi A, Katira K, Daggett J, Guyuron B. Outcomes of mild to moderate upper eyelid ptosis correction using Müller's muscle-conjunctival resection. Plast Reconstr Surg 130(5 Suppl 1):46-47, 2012.

### Chapter 94

Fig. 94-3 Adapted from Rohrich RJ, Pessa JE. The fat compartments of the face: anatomy and clinical implications for cosmetic surgery. Plast Reconstr Surg 119:2219-2227, 2007.

Fig. 94-4, *A* Adapted from Moss JC, Mendelson BC, Taylor GI. Surgical anatomy of the ligamentous attachments in the temple and periorbital regions. Plast Reconstr Surg 105:1475-1490, 2000.

Fig. 94-7 Adapted from Barton FE Jr. Aesthetic surgery of the face and neck. Aesthet Surg J 29:449-463, 2009.

Fig. 94-8 Adapted from Barton FE Jr. Aesthetic surgery of the face and neck. Aesthet Surg J 29:449-463, 2009.

Fig. 94-10 Adapted from Seckel BR. Facial Danger Zones: Avoiding Nerve Injury in Facial Plastic Surgery, 2nd ed. St Louis: Quality Medical Publishing, 2010.

Fig. 94-14 From Tonnard PL, Verpaele AM. The MACS-Lift Short-Scar Rhytidectomy. St Louis: Quality Medical Publishing, 2004.

Fig. 94-15 Adapted from Barton FE Jr. Aesthetic surgery of the face and neck. Aesthet Surg J 29:449-463, 2009.

Table 94-1 From Seckel, BR. Facial Danger Zones: Avoiding Nerve Injury in Facial Plastic Surgery, 2nd ed. St Louis: Quality Medical Publishing, 2010.

### Chapter 95

Fig. 95-4 Adapted from Netter FH. Atlas of Human Anatomy. Summit, NJ: CIBA-GEIGY, 1989.

Fig. 95-8 Adapted from Rohrich RJ, Rios JL, Smith PD, et al. Neck rejuvenation revisited. Plast Reconstr Surg 118:1251-1263, 2006.

### Chapter 96

Fig. 96-21 From Gunter JP, Rohrich RJ, Adams WP Jr, eds. Dallas Rhinoplasty: Nasal Surgery by the Masters, 2nd ed. St Louis: Quality Medical Publishing, 2007.

Fig. 96-38 From Rohrich RJ, Gunter JP, Deuber MA, Adams WP Jr. The deviated nose: optimizing results using a simplified classification and algorithmic approach. Plast Reconstr Surg 110:1509-1523, 2002.

### Chapter 97

Fig. 97-1 Adapted from Cohen SR. Genioplasty. In Achauer BH, Eriksson E, Guyuron B, et al, eds. Plastic Surgery: Indications, Operations, and Outcomes, vol 5. St Louis: Mosby-Elsevier, 2000.

Fig. 97-5 From Gunter JP, Rohrich RJ, Adams WP Jr, eds. Dallas Rhinoplasty: Nasal Surgery by the Masters, 2nd ed. St Louis: Quality Medical Publishing, 2007.

Fig. 97-6 Adapted from Cohen SR. Genioplasty. In Achauer BH, Eriksson E, Guyuron B, et al, eds. Plastic Surgery: Indications, Operations, and Outcomes, vol 5. St Louis: Mosby-Elsevier, 2000.

### Chapter 98

Fig. 98-1 Adapted from Markman B, Barton FE Jr. Anatomy of the subcutaneous tissue of the trunk and lower extremity. Plast Reconstr Surg 80:248, 1987.

Table 98-1 From Rohrich RJ, Beran SJ, Fodor PB. The role of subcutaneous infiltration in suction-assisted lipoplasty: a review. Plast Reconstr Surg 99:514, 1997.

Table 98-2 From Rohrich RJ, Beran SJ, Fodor PB. The role of subcutaneous infiltration in suction-assisted lipoplasty: a review. Plast Reconstr Surg 99:514, 1997.

Box 98-1 Rohrich RJ. Discussion of Grazer FM, de Jong RH. Fatal outcomes from liposuction: census survey of cosmetic surgeons. Plast Reconstr Surg 105:447, 2000.

### Chapter 99

Table 99-1 From Appelt EA, Janis JE, Rohich RJ. An algorithmic approach to upper arm contouring. Plast Reconstr Surg 118:237-246, 2006.

Fig. 99-7 From Appelt EA, Janis JE, Rohich RJ. An algorithmic approach to upper arm contouring. Plast Reconstr Surg 118:237-246, 2006.

Fig. 99-11 From Aly A. Body Contouring After Massive Weight Loss. St Louis, Quality Medical Publishing, 2006.

Fig. 99-9 From Nahai F, ed. The Art of Aesthetic Surgery: Principles & Techniques, 2nd ed. St Louis: Quality Medical Publishing, 2011.

Fig. 99-10 From Nahai F, ed. The Art of Aesthetic Surgery: Principles & Techniques, 2nd ed. St Louis: Quality Medical Publishing, 2011.

### Chapter 100

Fig. 100-2 Adapted from Huger WE Jr. The anatomic rationale for abdominal lipectomy. Am Surg 45:612-617, 1979.

Fig. 100-7 Adapted from Pollock H, Pollock T. Progressive tension sutures: a technique to reduce local complications in abdominoplasty. Plast Reconstr Surg 105:2583-2586; discussion 2587-2588, 2000.

Fig. 100-8 Adapted from Heller JB. Outcome analysis of combined lipoabdominoplasty versus conventional abdominoplasty. Plastic Reconstr Surg 121:1821-1829, 2008.

### Chapter 102

Table 102-2 From Song AY, Jean RD, Hurwitz D, et al. A classification of contour deformities after bariatric weight loss: the Pittsburgh Rating Scale. Plast Reconstr Surg 116:1535-1544, 2005.

Table 102-4 From Losken A. Breast reshaping following massive weight loss: principles and techniques. Plast Reconstr Surg 126:1075-1085, 2010.

Fig. 102-1 Adapted from Gilbert E, Wolfe B. Bariatric surgery for the management of obesity: state of the field. Plast Reconstr Surg 130:948-954, 2012.

Fig. 102-3 Adapted from Fernando da Costa L, Landecker A, Marinho Manta A. Optimizing body contour in massive weight loss patients: the modified vertical abdominoplasty. Plast Reconstr Surg 114:1917-1923, 2004.

Fig. 102-5 From Aly A. Body Contouring After Massive Weight Loss. St Louis: Quality Medical Publishing, 2006.

Fig. 102-6 From Nahai F, ed. The Art of Aesthetic Surgery: Principles & Techniques, 2nd ed. St Louis: Quality Medical Publishing, 2011.

Fig. 102-7 From Aly A. Body Contouring After Massive Weight Loss. St Louis: Quality Medical Publishing, 2006.

Fig. 102-8 From Aly A. Body Contouring After Massive Weight Loss. St Louis: Quality Medical Publishing, 2006.

# Index

## C

Kos

Costancostantini , Rosa

Amlin

Flexeril 5mg.